HANDBOOK OF OBESITY TREATMENT

Handbook of Obesity Treatment

SECOND EDITION

edited by
Thomas A. Wadden
George A. Bray

THE GUILFORD PRESS
New York   London

Copyright © 2018 The Guilford Press
A Division of Guilford Publications, Inc.
370 Seventh Avenue, Suite 1200, New York, NY 10001
www.guilford.com

All rights reserved

No part of this book may be reproduced, translated, stored in a retrieval system, or transmitted, in any form or by any means, electronic, mechanical, photocopying, microfilming, recording, or otherwise, without written permission from the publisher.

Printed in the United States of America

This book is printed on acid-free paper.

Last digit is print number: 9 8 7 6 5 4 3 2 1

The authors have checked with sources believed to be reliable in their efforts to provide information that is complete and generally in accord with the standards of practice that are accepted at the time of publication. However, in view of the possibility of human error or changes in behavioral, mental health, or medical sciences, neither the authors, nor the editors and publisher, nor any other party who has been involved in the preparation or publication of this work warrants that the information contained herein is in every respect accurate or complete, and they are not responsible for any errors or omissions or the results obtained from the use of such information. Readers are encouraged to confirm the information contained in this book with other sources.

Library of Congress Cataloging-in-Publication Data
Names: Wadden, Thomas A. | Bray, George A.
Title: Handbook of obesity treatment / edited by Thomas A. Wadden, George A. Bray.
Other titles: Obesity.
Description: Second edition. | New York : The Guilford Press, [2018] | Revision of: Obesity. 2nd ed. 1993. | Includes bibliographical references and index.
Identifiers: LCCN 2018027803 | ISBN 9781462535569 (hardback)
Subjects: LCSH: Obesity. | BISAC: PSYCHOLOGY / Psychopathology / Eating Disorders. | MEDICAL / Psychiatry / General. | PSYCHOLOGY / Psychotherapy / General. | MEDICAL / Nutrition.
Classification: LCC RC628 .O32 2018 | DDC 616.3/98—dc23
LC record available at *https://lccn.loc.gov/2018027803*

*In memory of
Albert J. "Mickey" Stunkard, MD,
and George L. Blackburn, MD, PhD*

*And to Jan and Mitzi,
with deepest love, affection, and admiration*

About the Editors

Thomas A. Wadden, PhD, is the Albert J. Stunkard Professor of Psychology in Psychiatry at the Perelman School of Medicine, University of Pennsylvania. He also is Visiting Professor of Psychology at Haverford College. Dr. Wadden's more than 500 scientific publications have focused on the treatment of obesity by methods including diet, physical activity, behavior therapy, medication, and surgery. He also has investigated the health and psychosocial consequences of obesity and its associated eating disorders. Dr. Wadden is past president of the Obesity Society and has served on numerous panels for the National Institutes of Health. He is the recipient of multiple honors, including the TOPS Research Achievement Award from the Obesity Society, mentoring awards from the Perelman School of Medicine and the Obesity Society, and the Distinguished Alumni Award from the Department of Psychology at The University of North Carolina at Chapel Hill.

George A. Bray, MD, is Boyd Professor Emeritus at the Pennington Biomedical Research Center, Louisiana State University; Professor of Medicine Emeritus at the Louisiana State University Medical Center; and Visiting Scientist at the Children's Hospital of Oakland Research Institute. With over 2,000 scientific publications, Dr. Bray has conducted influential research on the causes of obesity, dietary approaches to the prevention of hypertension and diabetes, and dietary approaches to weight loss. He is a Master in the American College of Physicians, the American College of Endocrinology, and the American Board of Obesity Medicine. Other honors include the Lifetime Achievement Award from the North American Association for the Study of Obesity, induction into the Johns Hopkins Society of Scholars, and the Presidential Medal from the Obesity Society.

Contributors

Naji Alamuddin, MD, Department of Medicine, Perelman School of Medicine, University of Pennsylvania, Philadelphia, Pennsylvania

Kelly C. Allison, PhD, Center for Weight and Eating Disorders, Department of Psychiatry, Perelman School of Medicine, University of Pennsylvania, Philadelphia, Pennsylvania

Ali Aminian, MD, Department of General Surgery, Cleveland Clinic Foundation, and Learner College of Medicine, Case Western Reserve University, Cleveland, Ohio

Aviva H. Ariel-Donges, MA, Department of Clinical and Health Psychology, College of Public Health and Health Professions, University of Florida, Gainesville, Florida

Louis J. Aronne, MD, Comprehensive Weight Control Center, Division of Endocrinology, Diabetes, and Metabolism, Weill Cornell Medical College, Cornell University, New York, New York

Arne Astrup, MD, PhD, Department of Nutrition, Exercise and Sports, Faculty of Science, University of Copenhagen, Copenhagen, Denmark

Zayna M. Bakizada, BA, Center for Weight and Eating Disorders, Department of Psychiatry, Perelman School of Medicine, University of Pennsylvania, Philadelphia, Pennsylvania

Katherine N. Balantekin, PhD, RD, Department of Exercise and Nutrition Sciences, University at Buffalo, The State University of New York, Buffalo, New York

Andrew J. Beamish, MBBCh, MSc, MD, Department of Gastrosurgical Research, Institute of Clinical Sciences, Gothenburg University, Gothenburg, Sweden; and Department of Research, The Royal College of Surgeons of England, London, United Kingdom

Robert I. Berkowitz, MD, Department of Child and Adolescent Psychiatry and Behavioral Science, Children's Hospital of Philadelphia; and Center for Weight and Eating Disorders, Department of Psychiatry, Perelman School of Medicine, University of Pennsylvania, Philadelphia, Pennsylvania

Claude Bouchard, PhD, Pennington Biomedical Research Institute, Louisiana State University, Baton Rouge, Louisiana

George A. Bray, MD, Pennington Biomedical Research Institute, Louisiana State University, Baton Rouge, Louisiana

Kelly D. Brownell, PhD, Sanford School of Public Policy, Duke University, Durham, North Carolina

Johannes Brug, PhD, Faculty of Social and Behavioural Sciences, University of Amsterdam, Amsterdam, The Netherlands

Meghan L. Butryn, PhD, Department of Psychology, College of Arts and Sciences, Drexel University, Philadelphia, Pennsylvania

Ariana M. Chao, PhD, CRNP, Center for Weight and Eating Disorders, Department of Psychiatry, Perelman School of Medicine, University of Pennsylvania; and University of Pennsylvania School of Nursing, Philadelphia, Pennsylvania

Jeanne M. Clark, MD, MPH, Division of General Internal Medicine, Johns Hopkins University School of Medicine, Baltimore, Maryland

Graham A. Colditz, DrPH, MD, MPH, Division of Public Health Sciences, Washington University School of Medicine in St. Louis, St. Louis, Missouri

Hank Dart, MS, Siteman Cancer Center, Washington University School of Medicine in St. Louis, St. Louis, Missouri

David F. Dinges, PhD, Division of Sleep and Chronobiology, Department of Psychiatry, Perelman School of Medicine, University of Pennsylvania, Philadelphia, Pennsylvania

Morgan Downey, JD, *The Downey Obesity Report,* Washington, DC

Kristoffel R. Dumon, MD, Department of Surgery, Perelman School of Medicine, University of Pennsylvania, Philadelphia, Pennsylvania

Leonard H. Epstein, PhD, Division of Behavioral Medicine, University at Buffalo, The State University of New York, Buffalo, New York

I. Sadaf Farooqi, MD, Department of Clinical Biochemistry, Cambridge Institute for Medical Research, University of Cambridge, Cambridge, United Kingdom

Marcela Rodriguez Flores, MD, Instituto Nacional de Ciencias Médicas y Nutrición Salvador Zubirán, Mexico City, Mexico

Evan M. Forman, PhD, Eating and Lifestyle Science (WELL) Center and Department of Psychology, College of Arts and Sciences, Drexel University, Philadelphia, Pennsylvania

Gary D. Foster, PhD, Weight Watchers International, New York, New York; Center for Weight and Eating Disorders, Department of Psychiatry, Perelman School of Medicine, University of Pennsylvania; and Center for Obesity Research and Education, College of Public Health, Temple University, Philadelphia, Pennsylvania

Stephanie Gomez-Rubalcava, BS, Kinesiology Department, College of Science and Mathematics, California Polytechnic State University, San Luis Obispo, California

Edward W. Gregg, PhD, Epidemiology and Statistics Branch, Division of Diabetes Translation, Centers for Disease Control and Prevention, Atlanta, Georgia

Carlos M. Grilo, PhD, Program for Obesity, Weight and Eating Research (POWER), Department of Psychiatry, Yale School of Medicine, Yale University, New Haven, Connecticut

Kimberly A. Gudzune, MD, MPH, Division of General Internal Medicine, Johns Hopkins University School of Medicine, Baltimore, Maryland

Casey H. Halpern, MD, Department of Neurosurgery, Stanford University Medical Center, Stanford, California

Matthew R. Hayes, PhD, Translational Neuroscience Program and Center for Weight and Eating Disorders, Department of Psychiatry, Perelman School of Medicine, University of Pennsylvania, Philadelphia, Pennsylvania

Thomas H. Inge, MD, PhD, Department of Pediatric Surgery, Cincinnati Children's Hospital Medical Center, University of Cincinnati College of Medicine, Cincinnati, Ohio

John M. Jakicic, PhD, Physical Activity and Weight Management Research Center, Department of Health and Physical Activity, School of Education, University of Pittsburgh, Pittsburgh, Pennsylvania

Carol A. Johnson, MA, Largely Positive, Inc., Ashtabula, Ohio

Scott Kahan, MD, MPH, Department of Health Policy and Management, Johns Hopkins Bloomberg School of Public Health, Baltimore, Maryland

Peter T. Katzmarzyk, PhD, Pennington Biomedical Research Institute, Louisiana State University, Baton Rouge, Louisiana

Sara J. Kovacs, MS, Physical Activity and Weight Management Research Center, Department of Health and Physical Activity, School of Education, University of Pittsburgh, Pittsburgh, Pennsylvania

Tanja V. E. Kral, PhD, University of Pennsylvania School of Nursing and Center for Weight and Eating Disorders, Department of Psychiatry, Perelman School of Medicine, University of Pennsylvania, Philadelphia, Pennsylvania

Rebecca A. Krukowski, PhD, Department of Preventive Medicine, University of Tennessee Health Sciences Center, Memphis, Tennessee

Shiriki K. Kumanyika, PhD, MPH, Department of Community Health and Prevention, Dornsife School of Public Health, Drexel University, Philadelphia, Pennsylvania

Rekha B. Kumar, MD, Comprehensive Weight Control Center, Division of Endocrinology, Diabetes, and Metabolism, Weill Cornell Medical College, Cornell University, New York, New York

Robert F. Kushner, MD, Center for Lifestyle Medicine, Feinberg School of Medicine, Northwestern University, Chicago, Illinois

Theodore K. Kyle, RPh, MBA, ConscienHealth.org, Pittsburgh, Pennsylvania

Jeroen Lakerveld, PhD, Department of Epidemiology and Biostatistics, VU University Medical Center, Amsterdam, The Netherlands

Chelsea A. Larsen, MPH, Technology Center for Healthful Lifestyles, Arnold School of Public Health, University of South Carolina, Columbia, South Carolina

Hannah G. Lawman, PhD, Philadelphia Department of Public Health, Philadelphia, Pennsylvania

Rudolph L. Leibel, MD, Division of Molecular Genetics and the Naomi Berrie Diabetes Center, College of Physicians and Surgeons, Columbia University, New York, New York

Joreintje Dingena Mackenbach, MSc, Department of Epidemiology and Biostatistics, VU University Medical Center, Amsterdam, The Netherlands

Kara L. Marlatt, PhD, MPH, Pennington Biomedical Research Institute, Louisiana State University, Baton Rouge, Louisiana

Corby K. Martin, PhD, Pennington Biomedical Research Institute, Louisiana State University, Baton Rouge, Louisiana

Courtney McCuen-Wurst, PsyD, LCSW, Center for Weight and Eating Disorders, Department of Psychiatry, Perelman School of Medicine, University of Pennsylvania, Philadelphia, Pennsylvania

Candice A. Myers, PhD, Pennington Biomedical Research Institute, Louisiana State University, Baton Rouge, Louisiana

Brooke T. Nezami, PhD, Department of Health Behavior, Gillings School of Global Public Health, University of North Carolina at Chapel Hill, Chapel Hill, North Carolina

Zubaidah Nor Hanipah, MD, Bariatric and Metabolic Institute, Cleveland Clinic Foundation, Cleveland, Ohio; and Department of Surgery, Faculty of Medicine and Health Sciences, University Putra Malaysia, Selangor, Malaysia

Mitesh S. Patel, MD, MBA, MS, Leonard Davis Institute Center for Health Incentives and Behavioral Economics, Department of Medicine, Perelman School of Medicine, University of Pennsylvania; Department of Health Care Management, Wharton School of Business, University of Pennsylvania; Penn Medicine Center for Health Care Innovation, University of Pennsylvania; and Crescenz Veterans Affairs Medical Center, Philadelphia, Pennsylvania

Rebecca L. Pearl, PhD, Center for Weight and Eating Disorders, Department of Psychiatry, Perelman School of Medicine, University of Pennsylvania, Philadelphia, Pennsylvania

Michael G. Perri, PhD, College of Public Health and Health Professions, University of Florida, Gainesville, Florida

Suzanne Phelan, PhD, Kinesiology Department, College of Science and Mathematics, California Polytechnic State University, San Luis Obispo, California

Heather M. Polonsky, BS, Center for Obesity Research and Education, College of Public Health, Temple University, Philadelphia, Pennsylvania

Rebecca M. Puhl, PhD, UConn Rudd Center for Food Policy and Obesity, Hartford, Connecticut; and Department of Human Development and Family Studies, University of Connecticut, Storrs, Connecticut

Eric Ravussin, PhD, Nutrition Obesity Research Center, Pennington Biomedical Research Institute, Louisiana State University, Baton Rouge, Louisiana

W. Jack Rejeski, PhD, Translational Science Center, Wake Forest University, Winston-Salem, North Carolina

Contributors

Renee J. Rogers, PhD, Physical Activity and Weight Management Research Center, Department of Health and Physical Activity, School of Education, University of Pittsburgh, Pittsburgh, Pennsylvania

Barbara J. Rolls, PhD, Department of Nutritional Sciences, The Pennsylvania State University, State College, Pennsylvania

Michael Rosenbaum, MD, Department of Pediatrics, Division of Molecular Genetics, Columbia University Medical Center, New York, New York

Robert Ross, PhD, School of Kinesiology and Health Studies, Queen's University, Kingston, Ontario, Canada

Donna H. Ryan, MD, Pennington Biomedical Research Institute, Louisiana State University, Baton Rouge, Louisiana

David B. Sarwer, PhD, Center for Obesity Research and Education, College of Public Health, Temple University, Philadelphia, Pennsylvania

Philip R. Schauer, MD, Bariatric and Metabolic Institute, Cleveland Clinic Foundation, and Learner College of Medicine, Case Western Reserve University, Cleveland, Ohio

Leah M. Schumacher, BS, Department of Psychology, College of Arts and Sciences, Drexel University, Philadelphia, Pennsylvania

Marlene B. Schwartz, PhD, UConn Rudd Center for Food Policy and Obesity, Hartford, Connecticut; and Department of Human Development and Family Studies, University of Connecticut, Storrs, Connecticut

Sally A. Sherman, PhD, Physical Activity and Weight Management Research Center, Department of Health and Physical Activity, School of Education, University of Pittsburgh, Pittsburgh, Pennsylvania

Jacqueline M. Soegaard Ballester, MD, Department of Surgery, Perelman School of Medicine, University of Pennsylvania, Philadelphia, Pennsylvania

Andrea M. Spaeth, PhD, Center for Obesity Research and Education, Temple University, Philadelphia, Pennsylvania

Kaitlin Stabbert, BS, Kinesiology Department, College of Science and Mathematics, California Polytechnic State University, San Luis Obispo, California

Deborah F. Tate, PhD, Departments of Health Behavior and Nutrition, Gillings School of Global Public Health, University of North Carolina at Chapel Hill, Chapel Hill, North Carolina

Colleen M. Tewksbury, MPH, RD, LDN, Department of Surgery, University of Pennsylvania Health System, Philadelphia, Pennsylvania

Jena Shaw Tronieri, PhD, Center for Weight and Eating Disorders, Department of Psychiatry, Perelman School of Medicine, University of Pennsylvania, Philadelphia, Pennsylvania

Adam G. Tsai, MD, MSc, Center for Human Nutrition, Division of General Internal Medicine, University of Colorado Denver, Denver, Colorado

Carmina G. Valle, PhD, Department of Health Behavior, Gillings School of Global Public Health, University of North Carolina at Chapel Hill, Chapel Hill, North Carolina

Kevin G. M. Volpp, MD, PhD, Leonard Davis Institute Center for Health Incentives and Behavioral Economics, Departments of Medicine and Medical Ethics and Health Policy, Perelman School of Medicine, University of Pennsylvania; Department of Health Care Management, Wharton School of Business, University of Pennsylvania; Penn Medicine Center for Health Care Innovation, University of Pennsylvania; and Crescenz Veterans Affairs Medical Center, Philadelphia, Pennsylvania

Steven Z. Wadden, AB, Center for Weight and Eating Disorders, Department of Psychiatry, Perelman School of Medicine, University of Pennsylvania, Philadelphia, Pennsylvania

Thomas A. Wadden, PhD, Center for Weight and Eating Disorders, Department of Psychiatry, Perelman School of Medicine, University of Pennsylvania, Philadelphia, Pennsylvania; and Department of Psychology, Haverford College, Haverford, Pennsylvania

Delia S. West, PhD, Technology Center for Healthful Lifestyles, Arnold School of Public Health, University of South Carolina, Columbia, South Carolina

Denise E. Wilfley, PhD, Department of Psychiatry, Washington University School of Medicine in St. Louis, St. Louis, Missouri

Noel N. Williams, MD, Department of Surgery, Perelman School of Medicine, University of Pennsylvania, Philadelphia, Pennsylvania

Donald A. Williamson, PhD, Pennington Biomedical Research Institute, Louisiana State University, Baton Rouge, Louisiana

Alexis C. Wojtanowski, BA, Weight Watchers International, New York, New York

Preface

The first edition of *Handbook of Obesity Treatment* appeared in 2002, 4 years after the publication of the *Clinical Guidelines on the Identification, Evaluation, and Treatment of Overweight and Obesity in the Adults: The Evidence Report*, produced by the National Heart, Lung, and Blood Institute (1998). The second edition now appears 4 years after publication of the revised guidelines, which were issued by a joint committee of the American Heart Association/American College of Cardiology/The Obesity Society (Jensen et al., 2014).

Sixteen years thus separate the publication of the first and second National Heart, Lung, and Blood Institute-supported guidelines, as they do the first and second editions of this handbook. This period has been marked by a dramatic increase in the sheer volume of research on obesity and on its health complications and management, as well as by a welcome change in the manner in which obesity is viewed by both health professionals and the public. In 2013, the American Medical Association classified obesity as a disease, challenging the longstanding view that this condition is instead a lifestyle choice, attributable to poor eating and activity habits, purportedly rooted in a lack of willpower. Continued advances over the past two decades in our understanding of the genetically based regulation of body weight, as well as of the pernicious consequences of a toxic food environment, have revealed the simplistic and stigmatizing nature of explanations that blame individuals for their obesity and suffering.

Further progress has come with the increasing recognition that obesity is a disease. In 2012, the U.S. Preventive Services Task Force recommended that primary care practitioners screen all adults for obesity and offer intensive behavioral intervention to affected individuals. At the same time, the Centers for Medicare and Medicaid Services approved the coverage of this therapy for beneficiaries treated in primary care settings, a move that likely will increase reimbursement by other insurers. Growing numbers of physicians should be prepared (with other health practitioners) to provide comprehensive care for persons with obesity as a result of the emerging field of obesity medicine, which provides board certification in this area of practice. Advocacy efforts, supported by The Obesity Society, the Obesity Action Coalition, and the American Society for Metabolic and Bariatric Surgery also are improving patients' access to weight reduction therapies, while also beginning to address the prejudice and discrimination to which persons with obesity are subjected in other aspects of their lives, beyond health care.

Plan of the Book

The first edition of this *Handbook* contained 27 chapters presented in six parts. This second edition includes 42 chapters, presented in seven parts, an increase that reflects the marked increase in research and practice in this area. Although the title of this volume continues to emphasize the treatment of obesity, the 42 chapters provide a comprehensive overview of the epidemiology, multifactorial etiology, and health consequences of this disease, in addition to the focus on obesity management. We hope that all seven parts of the volume will be of interest to readers; however, researchers likely will be drawn particularly to the first three parts, and practitioners especially to the latter four.

The parts are as follows:

• *Part I. Prevalence, Consequences, and Etiology of Obesity*. This part includes four chapters from the first edition that address (1) the epidemiology and health consequences of obesity, (2) the regulation of body weight, (3) energy metabolism and obesity, and (4) genetic influences. A new, fifth chapter examines exciting findings on the role of the microbiome in obesity.

• *Part II. Behavioral, Environmental, and Psychosocial Contributors to Obesity*. This newly added part of the volume contains six chapters that provide a full examination of behavioral factors associated with obesity. These include a consideration of (1) food intake and eating behavior, (2) physical activity, (3) sleep, (4) environmental and economic influences, (5) psychosocial factors, and (6) eating disorders and addiction. The first four chapters are new to this edition.

• *Part III. Health Consequences of Weight Reduction*. The three chapters that comprise this part of the book examine the effects of intentional weight loss on (1) all-cause morbidity and mortality, (2) psychological and cognitive function, and (3) physical function and quality of life. Findings from the Look AHEAD (Action for Health in Diabetes) trial, which has examined the long-term (i.e., 18 years) health benefits of intentional weight loss in patients with type 2 diabetes and overweight/obesity, are reviewed at length.

• *Part IV. Assessment of Patients with Obesity*. The two chapters in this part provide guidance and practical advice on conducting a medical evaluation of patients with obesity, as well as a behavioral–psychosocial assessment. The former evaluation is usually performed by a physician, nurse practitioner, or physician assistant, and the latter assessment by a mental health professional who may be meeting with individuals who seek bariatric surgery or suffer from a mood or eating disorder associated with their obesity.

• *Part V. Treatment of Obesity in Adults*. This part of the volume, presented in seven chapters, provides a comprehensive examination of the management of obesity using the three most common approaches recommended by expert panels: (1) diet, physical activity, and behavior therapy, collectively referred to as *intensive lifestyle intervention* or *behavioral weight control*; (2) pharmacotherapy, prescribed as an adjunct to lifestyle intervention; and (3) bariatric surgery. Since the publication of the first edition of the *Handbook* in 2002, four new medications have been approved for chronic weight management by the Food and Drug Administration, and sleeve gastrectomy, which was only introduced in 2007, has emerged as the most widely used form of bariatric surgery. The chapters describe these and other developments, including the head-to-head "diet contests" of the past 16 years.

• *Part VI. Additional Approaches to and Resources for the Treatment of Obesity*. Part VI contains 13 chapters, seven of which are new to this volume and present important developments that include the emerging field of obesity medicine and the current coverage of obesity treatments by insurers and employers. Practitioners will be particularly interested in chapters that describe the effectiveness of lifestyle interventions that are delivered remotely (e.g., via Internet, text, smartphone) or in community or commercial settings. Efforts to improve weight loss with traditional lifestyle intervention through the incorporation of weight loss devices (e.g., gastric balloons), as well as principles from behavioral economics, acceptance and commitment therapy, and motivational interviewing, also are examined.

- *Part VII. Childhood Obesity and Obesity Prevention.* The six chapters that comprise this final part of the volume address the pressing problem of childhood obesity and its prevention and treatment. The three new chapters that have been added address (1) the effectiveness of school-based interventions in preventing overweight/obesity, (2) the anticipated approval of weight loss medications for youth, and (3) the increasing use of bariatric surgery in adolescents with severe obesity. The volume's closing chapter describes progress in the primary prevention of obesity through the use of public policy and legislative approaches, including the taxation of sugar-sweetened beverages.

Acknowledgments

We are fortunate to have received contributions for this volume from an outstanding group of investigators who are the world's experts in their areas of research and practice. We count many of them among our closest friends and colleagues; all have our deepest thanks and appreciation. We also give thanks to our departed and much revered colleague, Albert J. "Mickey" Stunkard, who was coeditor of the first edition of the *Handbook* and who inspired hundreds of investigators, young and old, over the course of his 60-year career in obesity research. He was a dear friend, mentor, and colleague to us both, as was George L. Blackburn, another giant in the field of obesity, whose recent passing so many of us still mourn.

We thank Jim Nageotte, Senior Editor at The Guilford Press, for his invaluable counsel on all aspects of the book, from framing the big picture to addressing the smallest details. We particularly appreciate his support in expanding the size of the second edition to present the many important developments in the field in recent years. We also acknowledge Jane Keislar, Senior Assistant Editor at Guilford, for her careful review of all aspects of the manuscript and her gracious reminders of items that needed to be addressed to reach publication. Jeannie Tang, Senior Production Editor at Guilford, played a similarly important role as the book proceeded to its last stages of production. In addition, we thank Seymour Weingarten, Editor-in-Chief, for making this book possible (as he did Tom Wadden's first book in 1992).

This book also would not have been completed without the outstanding editorial assistance generously provided by Zayna Bakizada and Steven Wadden at the University of Pennsylvania's Center for Weight and Eating Disorders. Both read all chapters; reformatted many drafts to adhere to Guilford's publication style; and tracked down missing references, figures, and permission requests—all the while maintaining exceptionally good humor. Both also shared their excellent research and writing skills in serving as coauthors of a chapter. Olivia Walsh and Callie Fisher, both from the Center for Weight and Eating Disorders, also provided critical last-stage editorial assistance for which we are grateful. We also thank Landy Anderton, Mary Lloyd Craddock, Gary Gordon, Michael James, David Joseph, John H. Kennedy, Maurice Lemon, Judy Mozersky, Anne Peck, Saideep Raj, Avery Rimer, Michael Van Ness, Rick Weissbourd, and Douglas Whittaker for their support and inspiration in completing this volume.

Our research on obesity has been funded for many years by the National Institutes of Health, to which we both are grateful. In particular, we acknowledge the National Institute of Diabetes and Digestive and Kidney Diseases for supporting the Diabetes Prevention Program and the Look AHEAD study, which have facilitated such a rich and productive collaboration among investigators at academic medical centers across the nation, and indirectly fostered our collaboration on the second edition of this book. We also pay tribute to our alma mater, Brown University, which we both attended as undergraduates, more than 20 years apart, and left inspired to pursue careers in science. Little did we know that our paths would cross again in our efforts to treat obesity and diabetes.

And finally, we thank our wives (whom we both met at Brown) for their love, support, and understanding. They ultimately have contributed to this volume, as they have to all significant events in our lives.

References

Jensen, M. D., Ryan, D. H., Apovian, C. M., Ard, J. D., Comuzzie, A. G., Donato, K. A., et al. (2014). 2013 AHA/ACC/TOS guidelines for the management of overweight and obesity in adults: A report of the American College of Cardiology/American Heart Association Task Force on Practice Guidelines and The Obesity Society. *Circulation, 129*(25, Suppl. 2), S102–S138.

National Heart, Lung, and Blood Institute. (1998). *Clinical guidelines on the identification, evaluation, and treatment of overweight and obesity in adults: The evidence report* (NIH Publication No. 98-4083). Bethesda, MD: Author.

Contents

PART I. Prevalence, Consequences, and Etiology of Obesity

1. Epidemiology and Health and Economic Consequences of Obesity ... 3
   Graham A. Colditz and Hank Dart

2. Gut-to-Brain Mechanisms of Body Weight Regulation ... 24
   Matthew R. Hayes

3. Energy Expenditure and Obesity ... 38
   Kara L. Marlatt and Eric Ravussin

4. Genetics of Obesity ... 64
   I. Sadaf Farooqi

5. Human Energy Homeostasis and the Gut Microbiome ... 75
   Michael Rosenbaum and Rudolph L. Leibel

PART II. Behavioral, Environmental, and Psychosocial Contributors to Obesity

6. The Role of Portion Size, Energy Density, and Variety in Obesity and Weight Management ... 93
   Barbara J. Rolls

7. Physical Activity and the Development of Obesity ... 105
   Claude Bouchard, Peter T. Katzmarzyk, and Robert Ross

8. Sleep and Obesity ... 123
   Andrea M. Spaeth and David F. Dinges

9. Social, Economic, and Physical Environmental Contributors to Obesity among Adults ... 137
   Joreintje Dingena Mackenbach, Jeroen Lakerveld, and Johannes Brug

10. Psychosocial Contributors to and Consequences of Obesity 149
    Rebecca M. Puhl and Rebecca L. Pearl

11. Obesity, Eating Disorders, and Addiction 169
    Courtney McCuen-Wurst and Kelly C. Allison

PART III. Health Consequences of Weight Reduction

12. The Impact of Intentional Weight Loss on Major Morbidity and Mortality 185
    Edward W. Gregg and Marcela Rodriguez Flores

13. Weight Loss and Changes in Psychosocial Status and Cognitive Function 208
    Candice A. Myers and Corby K. Martin

14. Effects of Lifestyle Interventions on Health-Related Quality of Life and Physical Functioning 223
    W. Jack Rejeski and Donald A. Williamson

PART IV. Assessment of Patients with Obesity

15. Medical Evaluation of Patients with Obesity 243
    Rekha B. Kumar and Louis J. Aronne

16. Behavioral Assessment of Patients with Obesity 253
    Jena Shaw Tronieri and Thomas A. Wadden

PART V. Treatment of Obesity in Adults

17. An Overview of the Treatment of Obesity in Adults 283
    Thomas A. Wadden, Zayna M. Bakizada, Steven Z. Wadden, and Naji Alamuddin

18. Dietary Treatment of Overweight and Obesity 309
    Arne Astrup

19. Physical Activity and Weight Management 322
    John M. Jakicic, Renee J. Rogers, Sally A. Sherman, and Sara J. Kovacs

20. Behavioral Treatment of Obesity 336
    Stephanie Gomez-Rubalcava, Kaitlin Stabbert, and Suzanne Phelan

21. The Role of Medications in Weight Management 349
    George A. Bray and Donna H. Ryan

22. Surgical Treatment of Obesity 367
    Zubaidah Nor Hanipah, Ali Aminian, and Philip R. Schauer

23. Maintenance of Weight Lost in Behavioral Treatment of Obesity 393
    Michael G. Perri and Aviva H. Ariel-Donges

PART VI. Additional Approaches to and Resources for the Treatment of Obesity

24. The Emerging Field of Obesity Medicine   413
Robert F. Kushner and Scott Kahan

25. Coverage of Obesity Treatment: Costs and Benefits   425
Morgan Downey and Theodore K. Kyle

26. Obesity Treatment Perspectives in U.S. Racial/Ethnic Minority Populations   437
Shiriki K. Kumanyika

27. Treatment of Obesity in Primary Care   453
Adam G. Tsai and Thomas A. Wadden

28. Remotely Delivered Interventions for Obesity   466
Deborah F. Tate, Brooke T. Nezami, and Carmina G. Valle

29. Commercial Weight Loss Programs   480
Kimberly A. Gudzune and Jeanne M. Clark

30. Treatment of Obesity in Community Settings   492
Delia S. West, Rebecca A. Krukowski, and Chelsea A. Larsen

31. Alternative Behavioral Weight Loss Approaches: Acceptance and Commitment Therapy and Motivational Interviewing   508
Meghan L. Butryn, Leah M. Schumacher, and Evan M. Forman

32. Behavioral Economics and Weight Management   522
Mitesh S. Patel and Kevin G. M. Volpp

33. Nonsurgical Interventional Modalities for the Treatment of Obesity   531
Jacqueline M. Soegaard Ballester, Casey H. Halpern, Noel N. Williams, and Kristoffel R. Dumon

34. Treatment of Eating Disorders in Persons with Obesity   552
Carlos M. Grilo

35. Obesity and Body Image Dissatisfaction   565
David B. Sarwer, Colleen M. Tewksbury, and Heather M. Polonsky

36. Obesity, Weight Management, and Self-Esteem   576
Carol A. Johnson

PART VII. Childhood Obesity and Obesity Prevention

37. The Development of Childhood Obesity   593
Tanja V. E. Kral and Robert I. Berkowitz

38. Prevention of Obesity in Youth: Findings from Controlled Trials   605
Hannah G. Lawman, Alexis C. Wojtanowski, and Gary D. Foster

39. Behavioral Treatment of Obesity in Youth   622
Katherine N. Balantekin, Denise E. Wilfley, and Leonard H. Epstein

40. Pharmacological Treatment of Pediatric Obesity　　　636
    Robert I. Berkowitz and Ariana M. Chao

41. Bariatric Surgery in Adolescents with Severe Obesity　　　644
    Andrew J. Beamish and Thomas H. Inge

42. Using Public Policy to Address Obesity: Past, Present, and Future　　　659
    Marlene B. Schwartz and Kelly D. Brownell

    Author Index　　　671

    Subject Index　　　699

Purchasers of this book can access the Weight and Lifestyle Inventory (WALI) at *www.guilford.com/wadden2-materials* for personal use or use with patients.

PART I
Prevalence, Consequences, and Etiology of Obesity

CHAPTER 1

Epidemiology and Health and Economic Consequences of Obesity

Graham A. Colditz
Hank Dart

The obesity epidemic has gone largely unchecked for more than three decades (Finucane et al., 2011; Malik, Willett, & Hu, 2013). Its impact on rates of chronic disease, quality of life, and health economics is felt strongly the world over, in high- and low-income countries alike. Data from the National Health and Nutrition Examination Survey show that in 2013–2014, 37.8% of adults in the United States were obese, with an additional 32.6% classified as overweight (National Center for Health Statistics, 2016). The prevalence of obesity in adult women has surpassed 40% (Flegal, Kruszon-Moran, Carroll, Fryar, & Ogden, 2016), with rates varying significantly by ethnic population. Whereas 38.2% of non-Hispanic white women are obese, the obesity rate in Hispanic women is 46.9%. In non-Hispanic black women, it is 57.2% (Flegal et al., 2016). Globally in 2014, 13% of adults were obese—more than twice the prevalence in 1980 (World Health Organization, 2016).

The categories "overweight" and "obesity" are used to describe levels of excess body fat that can influence the risk of disease and other measures of health. Body mass index (BMI) is the formula most commonly used to determine weight status, with a BMI of 25–29.9 kg/m^2 generally defined as overweight and a BMI of ≥ 30 kg/m^2 defined as obesity. In 2013, high BMI accounted for over 4 million deaths globally (GBD 2013 Risk Factor Collaborators et al., 2015). Overweight and obesity are established risk factors for numerous serious conditions, including cardiovascular disease (CVD), hypertension, cancer, asthma, osteoarthritis, and infertility. Additionally, weight status impacts, among other outcomes, health-related quality of life, disability-adjusted life years, employment status, and lifelong earnings. When all effects are combined, obesity results in major national and worldwide health and economic burdens. In the United States, the direct and indirect economic impact of obesity is estimated to be over $215 billion each year (Hammond & Levine, 2010). Globally, the direct medical costs for obesity alone account for an estimated 0.7% to 2.7% of a nation's spending on health care (Withrow & Alter, 2011).

Definitions, Prevalence, and Age-Related Changes

Definitions of Overweight and Obesity

BMI, a formula that combines weight and height, is commonly used in epidemiological studies assessing the relationship between weight and disease. In addition, the public health recommendations for body weight are based on BMI, which is computed as weight (in kilograms) divided by height (in meters) squared. The advantage of using BMI instead of weight in pounds or kilograms is that it accounts for height—an essential piece of information when one is evaluating weight. For example, a woman who weighs 150 pounds (68 kg) is overweight if she is 5 feet 4 inches (163 cm) tall, but a healthy weight if she is 5 feet 8 inches (173 cm).

BMI correlates with adiposity (Hu, 2008). However, because BMI is an indirect method of assessment, it can overestimate or underestimate adiposity in certain individuals or groups, such as well-trained athletes or the elderly (Willett, 2013). The Centers for Disease Control and Prevention classify underweight as a BMI of < 18.5 kg/m^2; normal weight as 18.5–24.9 kg/m^2; overweight as 25–29.9 kg/m^2; and obese as ≥ 30 kg/m^2. The obese category is further stratified as class 1 (30–34.9 kg/m^2), class 2 (35–39.9 kg/m^2), and class 3 (≥ 40 kg/m^2). The World Health Organization (2016) uses the same general BMI categories but classifies BMI ≥ 25 kg/m^2 as overweight, with a BMI of 25–29.9 kg/m^2 classified as pre-obese. For this chapter, overweight is defined as a BMI of 25–29.9 kg/m^2, and obesity is defined as a BMI ≥ 30 kg/m^2. As can be seen in Figure 1.1, a woman, who at 5 feet, 4 inches (163 cm) tall and 150 pounds (68 kg) is considered overweight, would be considered obese if she weighed 180 pounds (82 kg).

These BMI cutpoints are used worldwide in epidemiological research and health recommendations, although there can be variance across ethnicities in the specific links between BMI and certain conditions. For example, compared to whites, Asians have been found to have a higher risk of cardiometabolic effects for a given BMI level (Haldar, Chia, & Henry, 2015). Although research must continue to document such relationships so that they can be translated into practice, BMI remains an efficient and useful measure for tracking global health.

Prevalence of Obesity

In the period of 2011–2014, 73% of adult men in the United States and 66.2% of adult women were either overweight or obese (National Center for Health Statistics, 2016). Currently, 40.4% of adult women and 35% of adult men are obese, with the prevalence of class 3 obesity at 9.9% and 5.5%, respectively (Flegal et al., 2016). Since 2005, the rates of obesity and class 3 obesity in U.S. women have increased significantly, whereas the rates in U.S. men they have remained relatively stable.

The prevalence of obesity can vary greatly by gender, race/ethnicity, and socioeconomic status. In 2011–2014 in the United States, the rate of obesity was 56.5% in black women and 37.9% in black men; 45.6% in Hispanic women and 39.1% in Hispanic men; 35.3% in white women and 34% in white men; and 11.9% in Asian women and 11.3% in Asian men (National Center for Health Statistics, 2016). Among adults with incomes under the U.S. federal poverty level, 39.2% are obese. Among those with incomes 400% or greater than the poverty level, the rate is 29.7% (National Center for Health Statistics, 2016). Approximately 17% of U.S. children and youth ages 2–19 years are obese (Ogden et al., 2016). Although the rates of obesity in younger children have been declining or leveling off, they continue to rise in adolescents ages 12–19 years old. Overweight or obese youth are more likely than normal-weight youth to become overweight or obese adults (Singh, Mulder, Twisk, van Mechelen, & Chinapaw, 2008).

Globally in 2014, 1.9 billion adults and 41 million young children were either overweight or obese, and excess weight now leads to more deaths than underweight (World Health Organization, 2016). Since 1975, there have been sharp increases in obesity and severe obesity (BMI ≥ 35 kg/m^2) in many regions of the globe (N.C.D. Risk Factor Collaboration, 2016).

Body Mass Index Table

BMI	19	20	21	22	23	24	25	26	27	28	29	30	31	32	33	34	35	36	37	38	39	40	41	42	43	44	45	46	47	48	49	50	51	52	53	54
	Normal						Overweight					Obese									Extreme Obesity															
Height (inches)																	Body Weight (pounds)																			
58	91	96	100	105	110	115	119	124	129	134	138	143	148	153	158	162	167	172	177	181	186	191	196	201	205	210	215	220	224	229	234	239	244	248	253	258
59	94	99	104	109	114	119	124	128	133	138	143	148	153	158	163	168	173	178	183	188	193	198	203	208	212	217	222	227	232	237	242	247	252	257	262	267
60	97	102	107	112	118	123	128	133	138	143	148	153	158	163	168	174	179	184	189	194	199	204	209	215	220	225	230	235	240	245	250	255	261	266	271	276
61	100	106	111	116	122	127	132	137	143	148	153	158	164	169	174	180	185	190	195	201	206	211	217	222	227	232	238	243	248	254	259	264	269	275	280	285
62	104	109	115	120	126	131	136	142	147	153	158	164	169	175	180	186	191	196	202	207	213	218	224	229	235	240	246	251	256	262	267	273	278	284	289	295
63	107	113	118	124	130	135	141	146	152	158	163	169	175	180	186	191	197	203	208	214	220	225	231	237	242	248	254	259	265	270	278	282	287	293	299	304
64	110	116	122	128	134	140	145	151	157	163	169	174	180	186	192	197	204	209	215	221	227	232	238	244	250	256	262	267	273	279	285	291	296	302	308	314
65	114	120	126	132	138	144	150	156	162	168	174	180	186	192	198	204	210	216	222	228	234	240	246	252	258	264	270	276	282	288	294	300	306	312	318	324
66	118	124	130	136	142	148	155	161	167	173	179	186	192	198	204	210	216	223	229	235	241	247	253	260	266	272	278	284	291	297	303	309	315	322	328	334
67	121	127	134	140	146	153	159	166	172	178	185	191	198	204	211	217	223	230	236	242	249	255	261	268	274	280	287	293	299	306	312	319	325	331	338	344
68	125	131	138	144	151	158	164	171	177	184	190	197	203	210	216	223	230	236	243	249	256	262	269	276	282	289	295	302	308	315	322	328	335	341	348	354
69	128	135	142	149	155	162	169	176	182	189	196	203	209	216	223	230	236	243	250	257	263	270	277	284	291	297	304	311	318	324	331	338	345	351	358	365
70	132	139	146	153	160	167	174	181	188	195	202	209	216	222	229	236	243	250	257	264	271	278	285	292	299	306	313	320	327	334	341	348	355	362	369	376
71	136	143	150	157	165	172	179	186	193	200	208	215	222	229	236	243	250	257	265	272	279	286	293	301	308	315	322	329	338	343	351	358	365	372	379	386
72	140	147	154	162	169	177	184	191	199	206	213	221	228	235	242	250	258	265	272	279	287	294	302	309	316	324	331	338	346	353	361	368	375	383	390	397
73	144	151	159	166	174	182	189	197	204	212	219	227	235	242	250	257	265	272	280	288	295	302	310	318	325	333	340	348	355	363	371	378	386	393	401	408
74	148	155	163	171	179	186	194	202	210	218	225	233	241	249	256	264	272	280	287	295	303	311	319	326	334	342	350	358	365	373	381	389	396	404	412	420
75	152	160	168	176	184	192	200	208	216	224	232	240	248	256	264	272	279	287	295	303	311	319	327	335	343	351	359	367	375	383	391	399	407	415	423	431
76	156	164	172	180	189	197	205	213	221	230	238	246	254	263	271	279	287	295	304	312	320	328	336	344	353	361	369	377	385	394	402	410	418	426	435	443

FIGURE 1.1. BMI (body mass index) chart. Data from the National Heart, Lung, and Blood Institute.

Body Weight and Age

Body weight and body composition are a function of genetics, health status, basal metabolic factors, dietary intake, physical activity, race, and hormonal factors (Heymsfield & Wadden, 2017). The onset (i.e., childhood, adolescence, or adulthood) and duration of obesity, as well as weight change, may have an important impact on health. Changes over time in basal metabolic rate, hormones, dietary intake, and physical activity result in changes in body weight and composition.

Although BMI does an adequate job of classifying young and middle-age people in terms of body weight, it is less accurate among elderly individuals. Older age is frequently accompanied by a decline in lean body mass and changes in the distribution of body fat. Therefore, when body weight and risk of disease are being assessed among elderly persons, both BMI and waist circumference should be used.

Consequences of Overweight and Obesity

Mortality

It is now well established that there is a J-shaped relationship between BMI and premature mortality (Aune et al., 2016; Flegal, Kit, Orpana, & Graubard, 2013; Manson et al., 1995; Prospective Studies Collaborative et al., 2009). Both excess weight and underweight can increase risk of death. Some debate remains, however, about the specific shape of this curve and the BMI range that marks the nadir of risk (Aune et al., 2016; Berrington de Gonzalez et al., 2010; Flegal et al., 2013; Prospective Studies Collaborative et al., 2009). Because existing or latent illness can lead to weight loss, it is essential that studies of weight and mortality adequately control for such factors and their correlates. Most large, well-designed studies and pooled analyses that have done so have found that overweight (BMI 25–29.9 kg/m^2) and obesity (BMI ≥ 30 kg/m^2) increase the risk of premature mortality, with the optimal level of BMI within the normal range of 18.5–24.9 kg/m^2.

A meta-analysis of 230 cohort studies by Aune et al. (2016) found that among healthy individuals who had never smoked, the lowest risk of mortality was at BMI 22–23 kg/m^2. When the analyses were restricted to those with the longest duration of follow-up—and therefore the lowest level of possible confounding by preclinical weight loss—the lowest risk was BMI between 20 and 22 kg/m^2. Among healthy never-smokers, the relative risk (RR) for premature mortality was 1.24 (95% confidence interval [CI] = 1.14–1.36) in those with BMI 30 kg/m^2, 1.66 (95% CI = 1.43–1.94) in those with BMI 35 kg/m^2, and 2.37 (95% CI = 1.91–2.95) in those with BMI 40 kg/m^2. Every 5 kg/m^2 increase in BMI in healthy never-smokers increased risk by 21% (95% CI = 1.18–1.25). Pooled analyses from the National Cancer Institute Cohort Consortium and the Prospective Studies Collaborative have reported similar findings (Berrington de Gonzalez et al., 2010; Prospective Studies Collaborative et al., 2009) (see Figure 1.2).

Looking at survival, the Prospective Studies Collaborative et al. (2009) estimated that overweight reduced median survival time by 1–2 years, class 1 obesity by 2–4 years, and class 3 obesity by 8–10 years—an amount of time, the authors note, on par with cigarette smoking. Early-life BMI also appears to play an important role in determining risk of adult chronic disease and premature mortality. In a study of 227,000 adolescents with 8 million person-years of follow-up, researchers found that adolescents with a BMI in the 85th percentile or higher had an RR of death of 1.4 (95% CI = 1.3–1.6) compared to those with a BMI in the 25th–74th percentile (Bjorge, Engeland, Tverdal, & Smith, 2008). Although mortality is a clearly defined outcome, the results of mortality analyses can be difficult to interpret. Except for diseases that are almost always fatal regardless of treatment, mortality is a function of incidence of disease, stage of illness at diagnosis, and the effectiveness of treatment. Many forms of CVD are treatable by either pharmacotherapy or intervention (i.e., angioplasty or surgery). Thus the relationship between excess weight and death from CVD does not necessarily translate to the same relationship with the development of CVD.

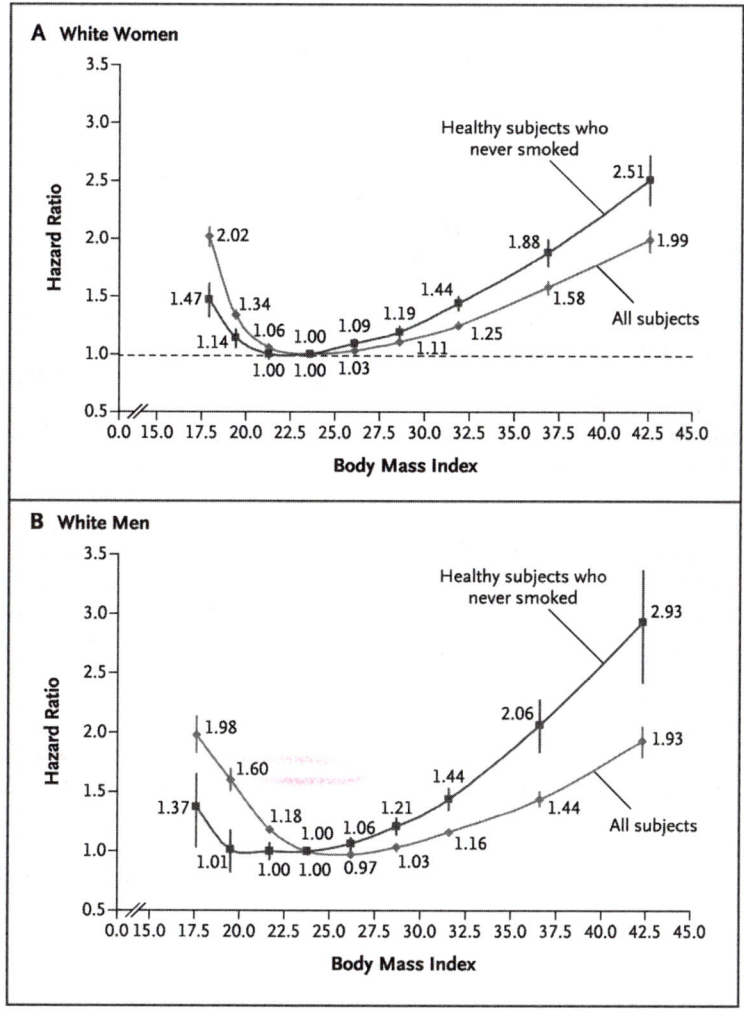

FIGURE 1.2. Risk of death with BMI. From Berrington de Gonzalez, Hartge, Cerhan, Flint, Hannan, MacInnis, et al. (2010). Body-mass index and mortality among 1.46 million white adults. *New England Journal of Medicine, 363*(23), 2211–2219. Copyright © 2010 the Massachusetts Medical Society. Reprinted by permission.

Morbidity

Coronary Heart Disease

Heart disease is the leading cause of death in the United States, accounting for 23.5% of all deaths (Xu, Murphy, Kochanek, & Bastian, 2016). Results from large cohort studies convincingly show a linear relationship between adult BMI and risk of incident coronary heart disease. Combining two large prospective cohort studies—the Nurses' Health Study and the Health Professionals Follow-Up Study—Flint et al. (2010) found that, compared to BMI 18.5–22.9 kg/m², obesity had an RR of coronary heart disease (CHD) of 2.13 (95% CI = 1.82–2.48) in men and 2.48 (95% CI = 2.20–2.80) in women. Risk of CHD was also significantly increased for overweight, beginning at the lower end of the range (BMI 25–26.9 kg/m²) for both men and women, with a suggestion of increased risk at the upper end of the normal range (BMI 23–24.9 kg/m²). The authors estimated the population attributable risk fraction for increased BMI compared to BMI 18.5–22.9 kg/m² to be 38.7% in men and 43.5% in women.

The Million Women Study, a U.K. population-based cohort study with over 1 million female participants, estimated CHD risk with BMI from ages 55 to 74 years. Researchers found a largely linear increase in cumulative incidence of CHD between BMI 20 and 34 kg/m², with a near doubling of cumulative incidence comparing highest BMI to lowest (see Figure 1.3; Canoy et al., 2013).

A meta-analysis by Guh et al. (2009) found that overweight and obesity determined by BMI or waist circumference (WC) increased risk of coronary artery disease (CAD) in both men and women. In men, the RR of CAD from obesity based on WC (≥ 102 cm) was 1.81 (95% CI = 1.45–2.5), and the RR based on BMI was 1.72 (95% CI = 1.51–1.96). Risks with obesity were higher in women, with an RR based on WC (≥ 88 cm) of 2.69 (95% CI = 2.05–3.53) and an RR based on BMI of 3.10 (95% CI = 2.81–3.43).

Excessive weight earlier in life is also predictive of CHD mortality. Must and colleagues followed 508 adolescents who participated in the Harvard Growth Study of 1922 to 1935 (Must, Jacques, Dallal, Bajema, & Dietz, 1992). The adolescents who were overweight were twice as likely as their lean peers to die from CHD during adulthood (relative risk [RR] = 2.3, 95% CI = 1.4–4.1). In Bjorge and colleagues' prospective study of 230,000 adolescents, early-life BMI in the 85th percentile nearly tripled the risk of dying of CHD later in life (RR = 2.9; 95% CI = 2.3–3.6) (Bjorge et al., 2008). Obesity influences a number of important risk factors for CHD. Increasing BMI is correlated with type 2 diabetes, hypertension, increased triglyceride levels, and unfavorable serum cholesterol levels (Zalesin, Franklin, Miller, Peterson, & McCullough, 2008). Excess weight may also raise CHD risk through other mechanisms, such as promoting inflammatory responses, thrombosis, and obstructive sleep apnea (Flint et al., 2010; Zalesin et al., 2008).

Ischemic Stroke

Cerebrovascular disease is the fifth leading cause of death in the United States, accounting for 5% of all deaths (Xu et al., 2016). Overweight and obesity are important risk factors for ischemic but likely not hemorrhagic stroke. In a meta-analysis by Guh et al. (2009), the relative risk of stroke for BMI ≥ 30 kg/m² was 1.51 (95% CI = 1.33–1.72) for men and 1.49 (95% CI = 1.27–1.74) for women. Overweight was linked to an increased risk in men but not women. Strazzullo et al. (2010) performed a meta-analysis of 25 prospective studies with over 2 million participants. They found that, for men and women combined, the relative risk for ischemic stroke with overweight was 1.22 (95% CI = 1.05–1.41) and the relative risk with obesity was 1.64 (95% CI = 1.36–1.99). Results for hemorrhagic stroke were null.

Hypertension

Approximately 30% of adult Americans have high blood pressure (hypertension), around half of which is properly controlled (Nwankwo, Yoon, Burt, & Gu, 2013). Hypertension increases the risk of both CHD and stroke, and the combination of obesity and hypertension is associated with an in-

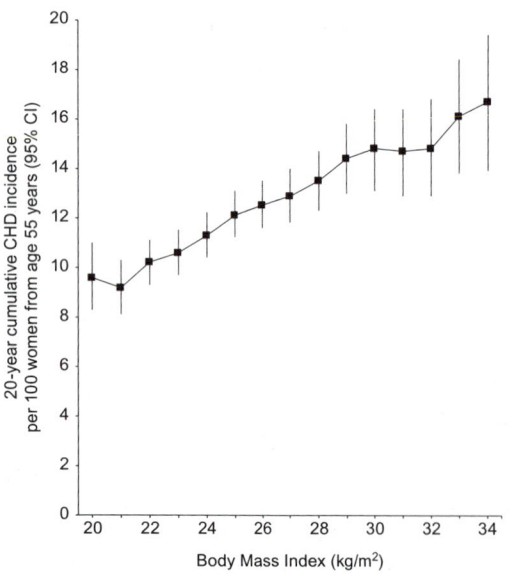

FIGURE 1.3. Cumulative incidence of heart disease in women from age 55 years in relation to BMI. From Canoy et al. (2013).

creased risk of cardiac failure due to thickening of the ventricular wall and increased heart volume (Alpert & Hashimi, 1993). Both body weight (Ascherio et al., 1992; Folsom, Prineas, Kaye, & Soler, 1989; Guh et al., 2009; Huang et al., 1998; Shihab et al., 2012; Witteman et al., 1989) and weight gain (Field et al., 1999; Huang et al., 1998; Shihab et al., 2012; Yong, Kuller, Rutan, & Bunker, 1993) increase the risk of hypertension. Even beginning at BMI well within the normal range, blood pressure rises steadily with body weight. Huang et al. (1998) studied 82,000 women over 923,544 person-years of follow-up and observed a relative risk of 6.31 (95% CI = 5.80–6.87) for BMI ≥ 31 kg/m² compared to BMI < 20 kg/m². Risk increased, however, with BMI as low as 20–20.9 kg/m², and every 1-unit increase in BMI was linked with a 12% higher risk of hypertension. BMI at age 18 years also had a significant impact on risk, with a BMI over 25 kg/m² more than doubling the risk of hypertension in later adulthood (RR = 2.28; 95% CI = 2.12–2.45), and every 1-unit increase in BMI increasing the risk of later adult hypertension by 8%. Adult weight gain had a significant impact as well, with every 1 kg gained since age 18 years increasing the risk of hypertension by approximately 5%.

Findings similar to those of Huang et al. (1998) were reported in the Johns Hopkins Precursor Study, which followed 1,100 men for a median of 46 years and observed a significant impact of early adult weight on hypertension risk (Shihab et al., 2012). Young-adult men who were overweight at study outset had a 50% increase in risk of hypertension (RR = 1.58; 95% CI = 1.28–1.96) compared to normal-weight men. This relative risk jumped to 4.17 (95% CI = 2.34–7.42) for young adult men who were obese. Weight gain was also associated with increased risk. Men who had been a normal weight in young adulthood but later became overweight or obese by age 45 years had a relative risk of hypertension of 1.57 (95% CI = 1.20–2.07).

In the all-male Physicians' Health Study, Gelber, Gaziano, Manson, Buring, and Sesso (2007) followed over 13,000 men for a median of 14.5 years and observed significant increases in the risk of hypertension beginning with BMI 22.4–23.6 kg/m² compared to BMI < 22.4 kg/m². Finally, the meta-analysis by Guh et al. (2009) observed relative risks of hypertension in men of 1.28 (95% CI = 1.10–1.50) for BMI 25–29.9 kg/m² and 1.84 (95% CI = 1.51–2.24) for BMI ≥ 30 kg/m². Observed risks in women were 1.65 (95% CI = 1.24–2.19) for BMI 25–29.9 kg/m² and 2.42 (95% CI = 1.59–3.67) for BMI ≥ 30 kg/m² (Guh et al., 2009). There are several mechanisms through which obesity causes hypertension. Hyperinsulinemia, which is common among overweight and obese individuals, can cause activation of the sympathetic nervous system as well as sodium retention, both of which increase the risk of developing hypertension (Mikhail, Golub, & Tuck, 1999).

Diabetes

The incidence of type 2 diabetes has risen steadily over the last decades, in step with the rise in overweight and obesity. Diabetes is a prevalent and serious disease, affecting approximately 29 million people in the United States, 8 million of whom are undiagnosed (Centers for Disease Control and Prevention, 2014). Individuals with diabetes are at substantially elevated risk for blindness, kidney disease, heart disease, stroke, and premature mortality. Diabetes is the seventh leading cause of death in the United States (Xu et al., 2016). Excess weight increases the risk of type 2 diabetes through mechanisms such as chronic inflammation, insulin resistance, and β-cell stress (DeFronzo et al., 2015; Mahler & Adler, 1999).

Not only are overweight and obese men and women at substantially increased risk for developing type 2 diabetes (Chan, Rimm, Colditz, Stampfer, & Willett, 1994; Guh et al., 2009), but adults at the upper end of the normal range (BMI of 20–24.9 kg/m²) are also at risk because of the strong linear relation between BMI and risk (Carey et al., 1997). In the meta-analysis by Guh et al. (2009), the relative risk for type 2 diabetes for overweight was 2.40 (95% CI = 2.12–2.72) in men and 3.92 (95% CI = 3.10–4.97) in women, with risk increasing for obesity to 6.74 (95% CI = 5.55–8.19) in men and 12.41 (95% CI = 9.03–17.06) in women. Carey et al. (1997), in an analysis of Nurses' Health Study data, observed a significant trend (p

for trend = < .0001) in increasing risk with BMI beginning as low as BMI 21–22.9 kg/m² (see Figure 1.4).

In addition, even after adjustment for weight, weight gain has been observed to be strongly associated with the risk of developing diabetes (Colditz, Willett, Rotnitzky, & Manson, 1995). Colditz et al. (1995) observed that among 114,281 female nurses 30–55 years of age, even a modest weight gain (5–7.9 kg) since age 18 years was associated with a 90% increase in risk of diabetes (RR = 1.9; 95% CI = 1.5–2.3). Similar results were observed in a parallel study among men (Chan et al., 1994). A study of male alumni of Harvard University and the University of Pennsylvania observed that in those with initially low BMIs (BMI < 21 kg/m²) early in adulthood, an increase in BMI of 1.5 units over a decade nearly doubled the risk of diabetes, compared to those with little or no change in BMI (RR = 1.93; 95% CI = 1.26–2.94; Oguma, Sesso, Paffenbarger, & Lee, 2005). Risk increased in a dose–response relationship with BMI (p for trend = < .0001), with a relative risk of 7.68 (95% CI = 4.72–12.50) for a greater than 3-unit increase in BMI over a decade.

Independent of weight, location of adiposity has an important role in the development of type 2 diabetes. Carey et al. (1997) observed that women with a large WC (36.2 inches [91.9 cm]) were more than five times as likely as their peers with small waists (26.2 inches [66.5cm]) to develop type 2 diabetes, regardless of their overall adiposity (measured by body mass index [BMI]). Moreover, among 15,432 women, Hartz and colleagues found that the prevalence of diabetes within each weight stratum (nonobese, moderately obese, and severely obese) increased with waist-to-hip ratio (WHR; Hartz, Rupley, Kalkhoff, & Rimm, 1983). Among the nonobese women, the risk increased in a gradual, linear fashion. Among the severely obese women, the risk increased sharply from approximately 6% for those with a WHR under 0.72 to 16.5% among women with a WHR over 0.81. Similar associations have been seen in men. In an analysis of 27,270 men in the Health Professionals Follow-Up Study, both abdominal adiposity

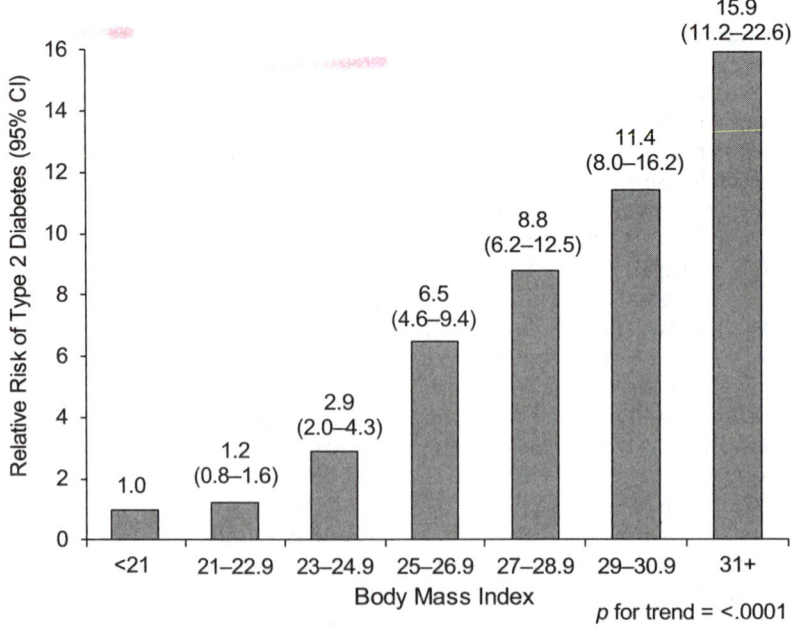

FIGURE 1.4. Relative risk of type 2 diabetes in women in relation to BMI. Data from Carey et al. (1997).

and overall obesity were observed to have independent and important effects on the risk of type 2 diabetes (Wang, Rimm, Stampfer, Willett, & Hu, 2005). Compared to WCs between 73.7 and 86.4 cm, BMI-adjusted multivariate relative risks were 1.7 (95% CI 1.1–2.5) for 87.0–91.4 cm, 2.0 (95% CI 1.3–3.0) for 92.1–95.9 cm, 3.0 (95% CI 2.0–4.5) for 96.5–101.0 cm, and 4.5 (95% CI 3.0–6.7) for 101.6–157.5 cm. Compared to BMI 14.2–22.8 kg/m², the WC-adjusted multivariate relative risk was 2.7 (95% CI 1.9–3.7) for BMI 27.2–54.2 kg/m².

In addition, solid evidence now shows that early-life weight can have an important impact on later-adult risk of type 2 diabetes. A pooled analysis by Juonala et al. (2011) of data from four long-running cohort studies observed an overall relative risk of type 2 diabetes of 2.4 (95% CI = 1.6–3.6) for participants who were overweight or obese in childhood. In participants who were overweight or obese as children and then obese as adults, the observed relative risk was 5.4 (95% CI = 3.4–8.5).

Cancers

Excessive weight is associated with the development of at least 13 different types of cancer, including breast, colon and rectum, endometrial, esophageal (adenocarcinoma), gallbladder, gastric, kidney (renal cell), liver, multiple myeloma, ovary, pancreas, and thyroid (Lauby-Secretan et al., 2016; Renehan, Tyson, Egger, Heller, & Zwahlen, 2008; see Table 1.1). The specific mechanisms through which obesity increases cancer risk are not clear (Renehan, Zwahlen, & Egger, 2015). However, there are multiple possible mechanisms. The impact of body weight on sex hormone levels is thought to play a primary role, especially for cancers such as breast and ovary. Other mechanisms thought to be involved in carcinogenesis include the influence of weight on cellular inflammation as well as insulin resistance. Newer theories explore the importance of local effects of fat tissue that may promote tumor development (Renehan et al., 2015). Overweight in youth and young adulthood has also been observed to increase the risk of many cancers linked to adult weight (Genkinger et al., 2015; Teras et al., 2014).

Breast Cancer

Breast cancer is the most common cancer in U.S. women and is the leading killer of women in midlife. There is consistent evidence that excess weight and weight gain increase the risk of postmenopausal breast cancer. Renehan et al. (2008), in a meta-analysis of 221 datasets from prospective cohort studies, found a relative risk of postmenopausal breast cancer of 1.12 (95% CI = 1.08–1.16) for every 5 kg/m² increase in BMI. The Nurses' Health Study analysis, which followed women for up to 46 years, found that women who had gained 25 kg since age 18 years had a relative risk of postmenopausal breast cancer of 1.45 (95% CI = 1.27–1.66), which increased to 1.98 (95% CI = 1.55–2.53) in those who had never taken postmenopausal hormones. Adipose tissue is the primary source of estrogen among postmenopausal women who do not use postmenopausal hormones. Therefore, it is not surprising that the weight-related increases in risk are often higher in women who do not use postmenopausal hormones.

Whereas weight gain across the years increases postmenopausal risk of breast cancer, in premenopausal women, excess weight has consistently been linked to a lower risk of the disease (Renehan et al., 2008). However, growing evidence suggests that short-term weight gain could increase breast cancer risk in the premenopausal years. A study by Rosner et al. (2015) that followed 77,000 women for 26 years found that a weight gain of 15 or more pounds (≥ 6.8 kg) over a 4-year period increased risk of premenopausal breast cancer by nearly 40% (RR 1.38; 95% CI = 1.13–1.69). This risk was higher in receptor-negative (ER–/PR–) disease (RR 2.06; 95% CI = 1.21–3.51)—a type of disease that is more common in premenopausal women.

Colon Cancer

Colon cancer is the third most common cancer in U.S. men and women, and the third most common cause of cancer death. Consistent evidence points to a dose–response relationship between BMI, as well as WC, and increased risk of the disease—with risk generally higher in men than women.

TABLE 1.1. Strength of the Evidence for a Cancer-Preventive Effect of the Absence of Excess Body Fatness, According to Cancer Site or Type

Cancer site or type	Strength of the evidence in humans[a]	RR of the highest BMI category evaluated versus normal BMI (95% CI)[b]
Esophagus: adenocarcinoma	Sufficient	4.8 (3.0–7.7)
Gastric cardia	Sufficient	1.8 (1.3–2.5)
Colon and rectum	Sufficient	1.3 (1.3–1.4)
Liver	Sufficient	1.8 (1.6–2.1)
Gallbladder	Sufficient	1.3 (1.2–1.4)
Pancreas	Sufficient	1.5 (1.2–1.8)
Breast: postmenopausal	Sufficient	1.1 (1.1–1.2)[c]
Corpus uteri	Sufficient	7.1 (6.3–8.1)
Ovary	Sufficient	1.1 (1.1–1.2)
Kidney: renal-cell	Sufficient	1.8 (1.7–1.9)
Meningioma	Sufficient	1.5 (1.3–1.8)
Thyroid	Sufficient	1.1 (1.0–1.1)[c]
Multiple myeloma	Sufficient	1.5 (1.2–2.0)
Male breast cancer	Limited	NA
Fatal prostate cancer	Limited	NA
Diffuse large B-cell lymphoma	Limited	NA
Esophagus: squamous-cell carcinoma	Inadequate	NA
Gastric noncardia	Inadequate	NA
Extrahepatic bilary tract	Inadequate	NA
Lung	Inadequate	NA
Skin: cutaneous melanoma	Inadequate	NA
Testis	Inadequate	NA
Urinary bladder	Inadequate	NA
Brain or spinal cord: glioma	Inadequate	NA

Note. Reprinted from Lauby-Secretan, Scoccianti, Loomis, Grosse, Bianchini, Straif, et al. (2016). Body fatness and cancer—Viewpoint of the IARC working group. *New England Journal of Medicine, 375*(8), 794–798. Copyright © 2016 the Massachusetts Medical Society. Reprinted by permission. BMI, body mass index; CI, confidence interval; NA, not applicable; RR, relative risk.

[a]Sufficient evidence indicates that the International Agency for Research on Cancer Handbook Working Group considers that a preventive relationship has been established between the intervention (in this case, the absence of excess body fatness) and the risk of cancer in humans; that is, a preventive association has been observed in studies in which chance, bias, or confounding could not be ruled out with confidence. Inadequate evidence indicates that the available studies are not of sufficient quality, consistency, or statistical power to permit a conclusion regarding the presence or absence of a cancer-preventive effect of the intervention or that no data on the prevention of cancer by this intervention in humans are available. Additional information on the criteria for classification of the evidence is available at *http://handbooks.iarc.fr/docs/Handbook16_Working-Procedures.PrimaryPrevention.pdf*.

[b]For cancer sites with sufficient evidence, the RR reported in the most recent or comprehensive meta-analysis or pooled analysis is presented. The evaluation in the previous column is based on the entire body of data available at the time of the meeting (April 5–12, 2016) and reviewed by the working group and not solely on the RR presented in this column. Normal BMI is defined as 18.5–24.9.

[c]Shown is the RR per 5 BMI units.

A meta-analysis of 30 prospective studies by Larsson and Wolk (2007) found that for every 5-unit increase in BMI, the risk of colon cancer increased by 30% (RR = 1.30; 95% CI = 1.25–1.35) in men and 12% (RR = 1.12; 95% CI = 1.07–1.18) in women. The findings were similar across genders for every 10 cm increase in WC. A pooled analysis by Matsuo et al. (2012) that combined data from eight large prospective cohort studies also observed a significant trend in colorectal cancer risk with increasing BMI (males, p for trend = < .001; females, p for trend = .032). For each 1-unit increase in BMI the adjusted hazard ratio was 1.03 (95% CI = 1.02–1.04) in men and 1.02 (95% CI = 1.00–1.03) in women.

Endometrial Cancer

Endometrial cancer is the most common reproductive cancer in the United States, with approximately 60,000 women diagnosed with the disease each year. Excess weight is a key risk factor for endometrial cancer. In a meta-analysis of 30 prospective studies, Aune, Navarro Rosenblatt, et al. (2015) found an overall relative risk of 1.54 (95% CI = 1.47–1.61) for every 5-unit increase in BMI and a relative risk of 1.27 (95% CI = 1.17–1.39) for every 10 cm increase in WC (Figure 1.5). In looking at specific types of endometrial cancer, weight was a particularly strong risk factor for type 1 endometrial cancer, which is most common and consists largely of endometrioid adenocarcinomas. From a pooled analysis of 10 cohort studies and 14 case–control studies, Setiawan et al. (2013) found a relative risk for type 1 endometrial cancer with overweight of 1.45 (95% CI = 1.37 to 1.53); with class 1 obesity of 2.52 (95% CI = 2.35 to 2.69); with class 2 obesity of 4.45 (95% CI = 4.05 to 4.89); and with class 3 obesity of 7.14 (95% CI = 6.33 to 8.06)—all compared to normal-weight women.

Esophageal Adenocarcinoma

There is strong evidence showing that the risk of esophageal adenocarcinoma increases with excess weight. In a pooled analysis of 10 case–control studies and two cohort studies by Hoyo et al. (2012), the odds ratio for esophageal adenocarcinoma, compared to normal-weight individuals, was 1.54 (95% CI = 1.26–1.88) for BMI of 25–29.9 kg/m^2, 2.39 (95% CI = 1.86–3.06) for BMI of 30–34.9 kg/m^2, 2.79 (95% CI = 1.89–4.12) for BMI of 35–39.9 kg/m^2, and 4.76 (95% CI = 2.96–7.66) for BMI of 40 kg/m^2 or higher.

Other Cancers

Based on results from pooled and meta-analyses, the relative risks for cancers of the gastric cardia, liver, gall bladder, pancreas, and kidney generally fall between 1.2 and 1.5 for BMI of 25–29.9 kg/m^2 and 1.5–1.8 for BMI ≥ 30 kg/m^2 (Lauby-Secretan et al., 2016).

Gallstones

Gallstones are a fairly common and often quite painful condition, and they are most common among overweight adults. Gallstones are believed to form when bile contains excess cholesterol or bilirubin or not enough bile salts, or when the gallbladder does not empty properly. Stones can range in size, and many of them are asymptomatic; however, if the stones lodge in any of the ducts that carry bile from the liver, problems can arise. The trapped bile in the ducts can lead to inflammation in the gallbladder, the ducts themselves, or the liver. If prolonged, the blockages can have severe consequences affecting the gallbladder, liver, or pancreas. Gallstones that are symptomatic can be very painful.

Although gallstones do form in lean adults, the relationship among weight, weight change, and gallstone formation is very strong, with the risk in women generally higher than that in men. Aune, Norat, and Vatten (2015) assessed the links between BMI, WC, and the risk of gallbladder disease, a grouping that included gallstones, gallstones with cholecystitis, and cholecystectomy. The authors found that the risk of gallbladder disease increased substantially with BMI, even within the normal range. Overall, relative risk for gallbladder disease was 1.63 (95% CI = 1.49–1.78) for each 5-unit increase in BMI, with the risk higher in women (RR = 1.73; 95% CI = 1.57–1.91) than in men (RR = 1.46; 95% CI = 1.29–

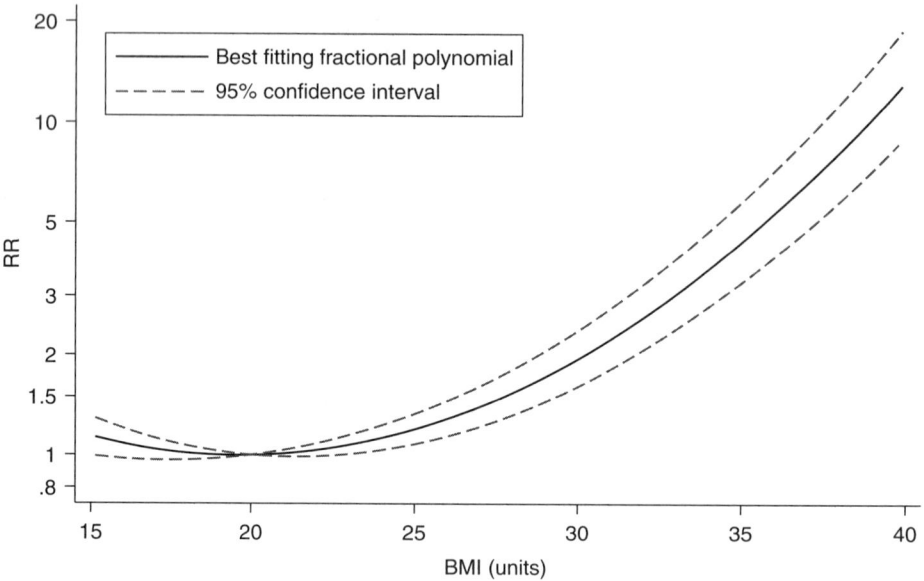

FIGURE 1.5. Relative risk of endometrial cancer with BMI. Reprinted from Aune, Navarro Rosenblatt, Chan, Vingeliene, Abar, Vieira, et al. (2015). Anthropometric factors and endometrial cancer risk: A systematic review and dose–response meta-analysis of prospective studies. *Annals of Oncology, 26*(8), 1635–1648. Copyright © 2015 Oxford University Press. Reprinted by permission.

1.65). In men and women combined, there was a relative risk of 1.46 (95% CI = 1.24–1.72) with each 10 cm increase in WC. Excess weight is linked to increased secretion of cholesterol into the bile, which is one possible mechanism through which weight may influence the risk of developing gallstones (Aune, Norat, et al., 2015).

Osteoarthritis

In 2008–2011, over 31 million adults in the United States had osteoarthritis, a disease that causes the breakdown of cartilage in joints (Centers for Disease Control and Prevention, 2016a). The hips, knees, and spine are the most common sites of osteoarthritis. As a result of the degeneration of the cartilage, bones that were previously cushioned by cartilage rub together and cause considerable pain. Approximately 16% of adults with a BMI < 25 kg/m² report a diagnosis of arthritis. This proportion rises to close to 50% for those with a BMI ≥ 25 kg/m² (Centers for Disease Control & Prevention, 2013).

The meta-analysis by Guh et al. (2009) of comorbidities related to excess weight reported significant links between BMI and osteoarthritis risk. The relative risks associated with overweight were 2.76 (95% CI = 2.05–3.70) in men and 1.80 (95% CI = 1.75–1.85) in women, and with obesity were 4.20 (95% CI = 2.76–6.41) in men and 1.96 (95% CI = 1.88–2.04) in women. Excessive weight causes additional strain on the joints and can lead to their degradation.

Benign Prostatic Hyperplasia and Lower Urinary Tract Symptoms

Benign prostatic hyperplasia (BPH) and the lower urinary tract symptoms (LUTS) that can result from it are extremely common among men (Wang et al., 2012). BPH is marked by nonmalignant enlargement of the prostate gland, with LUTS including symptoms such as urgency to urinate, weak urine flow, and incontinence. Approximately half of men over 40 years old have BPH, with around a third to a half of those men experiencing significant LUTS (Roehrborn, 2011).

As age increases, so too does the prevalence of each.

Excess weight and central adiposity have been found to increase both BPH and LUTS (Wang et al., 2012). In a meta-analysis of 19 cohort and case–control studies, Wang et al. (2012) found an overall positive link between BMI and the combination of BPH and LUTS (odds ratio [OR] = 1.27; 95% CI = 1.05–1.53); however, no relationship was observed when the analysis was limited to cohort studies (OR = 1.00; 95% CI = 0.77–1.31). In a cross-sectional analysis of the Baltimore Longitudinal Study, the odds ratio for BPH in men with BMI ≥ 35 kg/m^2 was 3.52 (95% CI = 1.45–8.56; Parsons et al., 2006). Among 25,892 men in the Health Professionals Follow-Up Study, men with a large WC (≥ 109 cm vs. < 89 cm) were more than twice as likely (OR = 2.4; 95% CI = 1.4–4.0) to develop BPH and have a prostatectomy (Giovannucci et al., 1994). Among other possible mechanisms, centrally located adiposity may increase the risk of developing BPH by increasing the estrogen-to-androgen ratio and sympathetic nervous activity (De Nunzio, Aronson, Freedland, Giovannucci, & Parsons, 2012).

Nonalcoholic Fatty Liver Disease

Nonalcoholic fatty liver disease (NAFLD) is an increasingly common liver disorder marked by increased liver fat content (steotosis) in those who abstain from alcohol or drink at moderate or lower levels, and it encompasses a broad range of conditions. The majority of those with NAFLD have simple steotosis, but in some cases, it can progress to nonalcoholic steatohepatitis (NASH), cryptogenic cirrhosis, and possibly liver cancer (Than & Newsome, 2015). In the general U.S. population between the years 2005 and 2008, the estimated prevalence of NAFLD and NASH was 11% and 1%, respectively (Younossi et al., 2011). This is a near doubling in prevalence since 1988–1994.

Obesity is an important risk factor for both NAFLD and NASH, so it is not surprising to see a steady increase in rates of these disorders with the rising rates of overweight and obesity. Very high rates of NAFLD and NASH have been found in bariatric surgery patients (Clark, 2006). A meta-analysis of 21 prospective and retrospective cohort studies observed a relative risk of 3.5 (95% CI 2.48–5.03) for NAFLD comparing obese to normal-weight individuals, with every 1-unit increase in BMI increasing the risk of NAFLD by 20% (RR = 1.20; 95% CI 1.14–1.26) (Li et al., 2016). A meta-analysis by Pang et al. (2015) observed a strong relationship between central adiposity and NAFLD independent of BMI. The relative risk of NAFLD with obesity measured by WC and WHR was 2.34 (95% CI 1.83–3.0) and 4.06 (95% CI 1.53–10.79), respectively, compared to nonobese levels. Obesity-associated insulin resistance, inflammation, and dyslipidemia are key contributors to the development of NAFLD (Li et al., 2016; Than & Newsome, 2015).

Other Health Outcomes

Asthma

In 2014, the prevalence of asthma in the United States was 7.4% in adults and 8.6% of youth under 18 years old. Asthma leads to approximately 1.8 million emergency room visits and 10.5 million doctor's office visits annually (Centers for Disease Control and Prevention, 2016b). Though evidence is still developing, meta-analyses suggest links between both childhood BMI, adult BMI, and risk of asthma (Egan, Ettinger, & Bracken, 2013; Guh et al., 2009).

Infertility

Infertility affects approximately 12% of women 15–44 years of age in the United States, and good evidence links weight with fertility (Brewer & Balen, 2010). In an investigation of the Nurses' Health Study II, both BMI under 20 kg/m^2 and above 24 kg/m^2 were observed to increase the risk of ovulatory infertility (Rich-Edwards et al., 2002), with the authors estimating that a quarter (95% CI = 20–31%) of ovulatory infertility in the United States may be linked to overweight and obesity.

Disability-Adjusted Life Years

Excess weight is a major contributor to disability-adjusted life years (DALYs). DALYs is a measure of the burden of a disease or risk factor that takes into account years of life lost, as well as years of life living with disability. A systematic analysis by the Global Burden of Disease (GBD) study 2013 estimated that, globally, high BMI was among the top risk factors contributing to DALYs, accounting for 134 million DALYs (95% uncertainty interval = 112 million–156 million) in 2013 (GBD 2013 Risk Factor Collaborators et al., 2015).

Health-Related Quality of Life

Overweight and obesity have an important impact on many aspects of quality of life. Ul-Haq, Mackay, Fenwick, and Pell (2013a) conducted a meta-analysis of eight studies assessing the link between BMI and health-related quality of life (HQoL), measured using the Medical Outcome Study 36-Item Short-Form Health Survey (SF-36), and observed decreasing physical health scores with increasing BMI. For mental health, significantly lower scores were linked only to class 3 obesity, with significantly higher mental health scores seen in the overweight category. In youth, obesity and overweight have also been linked to lower physical and psychosocial quality of life (Ul-Haq, Mackay, Fenwick, & Pell, 2013b).

Outside of body weight alone, weight gain has been found to affect HQOL as well. Pan et al. (2014) followed over 100,000 participants in the Nurses' Health Study and Nurses' Health Study II, and found in a multivariate analysis that a gain of 15 or more pounds (≥ 6.8 kg) over a 4-year period negatively impacted physical domains, including bodily pain, general health, physical functioning, and vitality.

Discrimination and Lifestyle Outcomes

Despite the high prevalence of overweight and obesity in the United States, there are considerable social consequences of being overweight in a Westernized society that values thinness and fitness. Overweight and obese individuals perceive or experience stigma and discrimination across multiple domains, from work to health care to mass media (Table 1.2; Puhl & Heuer, 2009). An analysis within the Coronary Artery Risk Development in Young Adults (CARDIA) study found that combined class 2 and 3 obesity was linked to significantly higher risk of perceived weight discrimination in multiple groups (Dutton et al., 2014). Overweight individuals are also less likely than their leaner peers to be promoted at work (Wadden & Stunkard, 1985), and obese individuals, particularly women, are more likely to experience discrimination in job hiring (Bartels & Nordstrom, 2013; Flint et al., 2016). Sonne-Holm and Sorensen (1986) observed that among 3,267 men in Copenhagen at each level of education attainment, the attained level of social class was significantly lower for obese men. Gortmaker, Must, Perrin, Sobol, and Dietz (1993) followed a sample of 16- to 24-year-old people over 8 years and observed that women and men who were overweight were approximately 20% and 11%, respectively, less likely to marry than persons of average weight.

Economic Costs of Obesity

Society bears the burden of overweight and obesity—from premature mortality, higher incidence of chronic conditions, lower HQOL, increased DALYs, and a range of other factors. One metric that can help quantify the overall burden of overweight and obesity on the medical system and society at large is to assess their economic costs.

Economic costs related to excess weight can be split into direct and indirect costs. The direct costs of illness include the costs of diagnosis and treatment related to any disease (i.e., hospital stays, nursing homes, medications, physician visits). Indirect costs include the value of lost productivity, including wages lost by people unable to work because of disease and wages forgone due to premature mortality. It is important to not lose sight of the fact that although the aggregated economic burden of overweight and obesity is a very important metric, these numbers reflect, in part, significant personal costs and burdens experienced by overweight individuals (Dor, Ferguson, Langwith, & Tan, 2010). In the United States, the direct cost of overweight and obesity has been estimated to range from approximately 9% to up to 20% of annual health care expendi-

TABLE 1.2. Evidence on Weight Bias

Summary of key findings in existing weight bias research	Strength of evidence		
	Limited	Moderate	Strong
Employment settings			
Obese employees perceive weight-based disparities in employment			X
Obese employees experience a wage penalty (controlling for sociodemographic variables)			X
Obese applicants face weight bias in job evaluations and hiring decisions			X
Obese employees face disadvantaged employment outcomes due to weight bias		X	
Health care settings			
Health care professionals endorse stereotypes and negative attitudes about obese patients			X
Weight bias negatively affects providers' weight management practices	X		
Obese patients perceive biased treatment in health care		X	
Weight bias negatively impacts health care utilization	X		
Educational settings			
Weight bias contributes to educational disparities for obese students	X		
Educators endorse negative weight-based stereotypes and antifat attitudes	X		
Other students perceive weight bias from educators	X		
Interpersonal relationships			
Weight bias negatively impacts romantic relationship for obese adults	X		
Obese individuals perceive weight bias from family members and friends		X	
Family/friends report stereotypes and negative attitudes about obese persons	X		
Media			
Overweight/obese characters are stigmatized in television and film			X
Overweight/obese characters are stereotyped in children's media (TV, DVDs, cartoons)		X	
Weight bias exists in news media		X	
Media and television exposure is positively related to stigmatization of obese persons	X		
Psychological and physical health consequences			
Weight bias increases vulnerability to depression, low self-esteem, and poor body image		X	
Weight bias contributes to maladaptive eating behaviors among obese individuals			X
Weight bias contributes to less participation/avoidance of physical activity	X		
Weight bias negatively impacts cardiovascular health outcomes	X		
Stigma-reduction strategies			
Effective intervention strategies have been identified to reduce weight bias	X		

Note. Reprinted from Puhl and Heuer (2009). The stigma of obesity: A review and update. *Obesity (Silver Spring), 17*(5), 941–964. Copyright © 2009 Wiley. Reprinted by permission.

tures (Cawley & Meyerhoefer, 2012; Finkelstein, Trogdon, Cohen, & Dietz, 2009). In other developed countries, directs costs as a percent of health care spending generally range between 2 and 5% (Lehnert, Sonntag, Konnopka, Riedel-Heller, & Konig, 2013). Using projected obesity rates for 2030—and the impact that they may have on rates of chronic disease—Wang, McPherson, Marsh, Gortmaker, and Brown (2011) estimated that direct, obesity-related medical spending in the United States may increase by $48–$66 billon per year (Figure 1.6).

Assessing indirect costs further defines the full economic burden of overweight and obesity and takes into account factors such as lost wages, absenteeism, disability, and loss of productivity. An analysis by Finkelstein, DiBonaventura, Burgess, and Hale (2010) assessed the economic impact in the workplace of both absenteeism and presenteeism (i.e., working while sick), a metric intended to capture losses in work productivity. Using data from the 2006 Medical Expenditure Panel Survey (MEPS) and 2008 U.S. National Health and Wellness Survey (NHWS), the authors estimated that obesity-related costs from absenteeism and presenteeism were over $40 billion among full-time workers. Adding direct medical costs, the total impact rose to $73.1 billion. Adopting data from Finklestein et al. (2010), Wang et al. (2011) estimated that by 2030, in the United States, excess weight may lead to the loss of 1.7–3 million productive person-years in working U.S. adults. The total cost of such a loss could be up to $390–$580 billon. All told, the direct and indirect economic impact of obesity in the United States has been estimated to be over $215 billion each year (Hammond & Levine, 2010). CHD is the major weight-related contributor to indirect costs, with other key contributors being type 2 diabetes

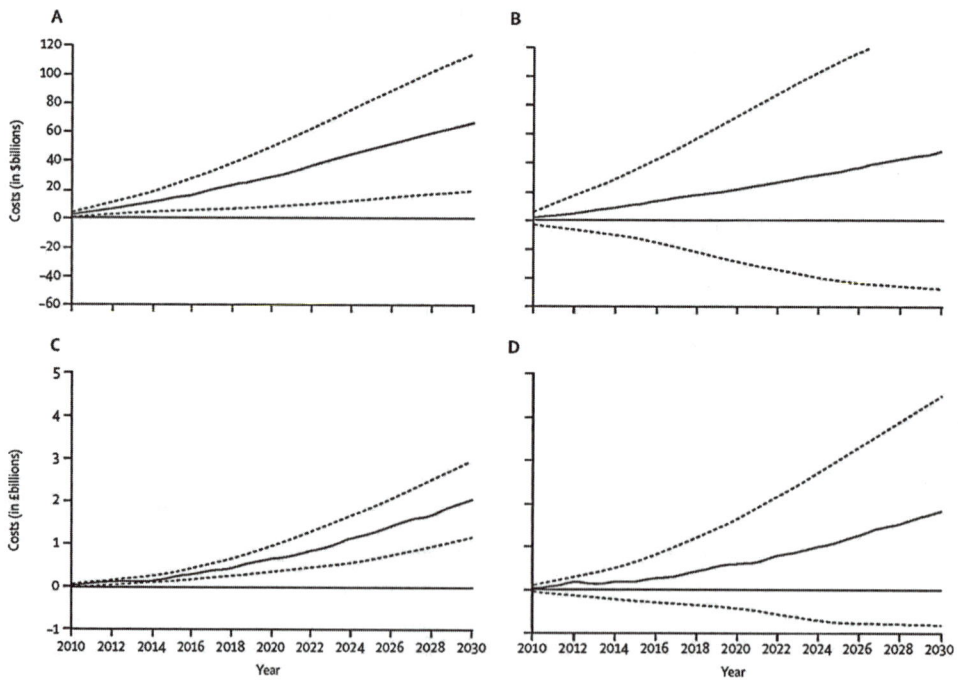

FIGURE 1.6. Projected health care related to obesity: United States and United Kingdom, 2010–2030. (A) United States, historic trend; (B) United States, recent trend; (C) United Kingdom, historic trend; (D) United Kingdom, recent trend. Dashed lines indicate 95% CI. Costs are $ for United States and £ for United Kingdom. Reprinted from Wang, McPherson, Marsh, Gortmaker, & Brown, M. (2011). Health and economic burden of the projected obesity trends in the USA and the UK. *Lancet*, *378*(9793), 815–825. Copyright © 2011, with permission from Elsevier.

and osteoarthritis; combined, they have a major impact on premature mortality, workdays lost, and restricted-activity days. The health care costs that have been estimated to date are likely underestimates of the true direct and indirect costs, since they do not take into account the full spectrum of negative outcomes caused by or associated with overweight or obesity. Moreover, rates of obesity continue to rise in many groups. It is possible that increased rates of health insurance coverage in the United States through the Affordable Care Act and the expansion of Medicaid in most states could help mitigate or stabilize costs associated with overweight and obesity. However, data are not yet available to adequately address that question, and the health insurance environment is currently in flux.

Conclusion

Overweight and obesity are major burdens on societies and individuals the world over. In the United States, rates of obesity continue to increase in many populations, with few signs of substantial slowing. Globally, in 2013, high BMI accounted for over four million deaths (GBD 2013 Risk Factor Collaborators et al., 2015). Among other serious outcomes, excess weight is a key contributor to premature mortality, heart disease, stroke, type 2 diabetes, hypertension, and osteoarthritis, as well as lower quality of life and increased DALYs. Obesity is also associated with social stigma, discrimination, absenteeism, lost wages, and lower work productivity. All told, overweight and obesity are responsible for a substantial proportion of medical spending in the United States and other Westernized countries. Indirect costs related to weight-related issues such as quality of life, disability, and employment further add to the economic burden. Trends suggest that these costs are likely to continue to increase.

However, overweight and obesity are modifiable risk factors, and evidence shows that weight loss leads to lower risk of many weight-related diseases (Rueda-Clausen, Ogunleye, & Sharma, 2015). Even small shifts downward in population BMI can have an enormous effect on societal burden (Wang et al., 2011). As with the fight against tobacco, making progress against the obesity epidemic will require multipronged, multilayered approaches—such as improved food and activity offerings in schools and workplaces, taxes on unhealthy foods, subsidies for healthy foods, widespread communication campaigns, and infrastructure that allows individuals to easily and safely fit activity into their days. The social, financial, and structural environment that surrounds individuals is key to making and sustaining healthy behaviors. Garnering the resources and political will to make and sustain such efforts will be key to effectively addressing the burden of overweight and obesity.

References

Alpert, M. A., & Hashimi, M. W. (1993). Obesity and the heart. *American Journal of the Medical Sciences, 306*(2), 117–123.

Ascherio, A., Rimm, E. B., Giovannucci, E. L., Colditz, G. A., Rosner, B., Willett, W. C., et al. (1992). A prospective study of nutritional factors and hypertension among U.S. men. *Circulation, 86*(5), 1475–1484.

Aune, D., Navarro Rosenblatt, D. A., Chan, D. S., Vingeliene, S., Abar, L., Vieira, A. R., et al. (2015). Anthropometric factors and endometrial cancer risk: A systematic review and dose–response meta-analysis of prospective studies. *Annals of Oncology, 26*(8), 1635–1648.

Aune, D., Norat, T., & Vatten, L. J. (2015). Body mass index, abdominal fatness and the risk of gallbladder disease. *European Journal of Epidemiology, 30*(9), 1009–1019.

Aune, D., Sen, A., Prasad, M., Norat, T., Janszky, I., Tonstad, S., et al. (2016). BMI and all cause mortality: Systematic review and non-linear dose–response meta-analysis of 230 cohort studies with 3.74 million deaths among 30.3 million participants. *BMJ, 353*, i2156.

Bartels, L. K., & Nordstrom, C. R. (2013). Too big to hire: Factors impacting weight discrimination. *Management Research Review, 36*(9), 868–881.

Berrington de Gonzalez, A., Hartge, P., Cerhan, J. R., Flint, A. J., Hannan, L., MacInnis, R. J., et al. (2010). Body-mass index and mortality among 1.46 million white adults. *New England Journal of Medicine, 363*(23), 2211–2219.

Bjorge, T., Engeland, A., Tverdal, A., & Smith, G. D. (2008). Body mass index in adolescence in relation to cause-specific mortality: A follow-up of 230,000 Norwegian adolescents. *American Journal of Epidemiology, 168*(1), 30–37.

Brewer, C. J., & Balen, A. H. (2010). The adverse effects of obesity on conception and implantation. *Reproduction, 140*(3), 347–364.

Canoy, D., Cairns, B. J., Balkwill, A., Wright, F. L., Green, J., Reeves, G., et al. (2013). Body mass index and incident coronary heart disease in women: A population-based prospective study. *BMC Medicine, 11,* 87.

Carey, V. J., Walters, E. E., Colditz, G. A., Solomon, C. G., Willett, W. C., Rosner, B. A., et al. (1997). Body fat distribution and risk of non-insulin-dependent diabetes mellitus in women: The Nurses' Health Study. *American Journal of Epidemiology, 145*(7), 614–619.

Cawley, J., & Meyerhoefer, C. (2012). The medical care costs of obesity: An instrumental variables approach. *Journal of Health Economics, 31*(1), 219–230.

Centers for Disease Control and Prevention. (2013). Prevalence of doctor-diagnosed arthritis and arthritis-attributable activity limitation—United States, 2010–2012. *Morbidity and Mortality Weekly Report, 62*(44), 869–873.

Centers for Disease Control and Prevention. (2014). *National Diabetes Statistics Report: Estimates of diabetes and its burden in the United States, 2014.* Atlanta, GA: Author.

Centers for Disease Control and Prevention. (2016a). Arthritis-related statistics. Retrieved August 3, 2016, from *www.cdc.gov/arthritis/data_statistics/arthritis-related-stats.htm*.

Centers for Disease Control and Prevention. (2016b). Most recent asthma data. Retrieved August 3, 2016, from *www.cdc.gov/asthma/most_recent_data.htm*.

Chan, J. M., Rimm, E. B., Colditz, G. A., Stampfer, M. J., & Willett, W. C. (1994). Obesity, fat distribution, and weight gain as risk factors for clinical diabetes in men. *Diabetes Care, 17*(9), 961–969.

Clark, J. M. (2006). The epidemiology of nonalcoholic fatty liver disease in adults. *Journal of Clinical Gastroenterology, 40*(Suppl. 1), S5–10.

Colditz, G. A., Willett, W. C., Rotnitzky, A., & Manson, J. E. (1995). Weight gain as a risk factor for clinical diabetes in women. *Annals of Internal Medicine, 122*(7), 481–486.

De Nunzio, C., Aronson, W., Freedland, S. J., Giovannucci, E., & Parsons, J. K. (2012). The correlation between metabolic syndrome and prostatic diseases. *European Urology, 61*(3), 560–570.

DeFronzo, R. A., Ferrannini, E., Groop, L., Henry, R. R., Herman, W. H., Holst, J. J., et al. (2015). Type 2 diabetes mellitus. *Nature Reviews Disease Primers, 32,* 657–664.

Dor, A., Ferguson, C., Langwith, C., & Tan, E. (2010). *A heavy burden: The individual costs of being overweight and obese in the United States.* Washington, DC: George Washington University School of Public Health and Health Services.

Dutton, G. R., Lewis, T. T., Durant, N., Halanych, J., Kiefe, C. I., Sidney, S., et al. (2014). Perceived weight discrimination in the CARDIA study: Differences by race, sex, and weight status. *Obesity (Silver Spring), 22*(2), 530–536.

Egan, K. B., Ettinger, A. S., & Bracken, M. B. (2013). Childhood body mass index and subsequent physician-diagnosed asthma: A systematic review and meta-analysis of prospective cohort studies. *BMC Pediatrics, 13,* 121.

Field, A. E., Byers, T., Hunter, D. J., Laird, N. M., Manson, J. E., Williamson, D. F., et al. (1999). Weight cycling, weight gain, and risk of hypertension in women. *American Journal of Epidemiology, 150*(6), 573–579.

Finkelstein, E. A., DiBonaventura, M., Burgess, S. M., & Hale, B. C. (2010). The costs of obesity in the workplace. *Journal of Occupational and Environmental Medicine, 52*(10), 971–976.

Finkelstein, E. A., Trogdon, J. G., Cohen, J. W., & Dietz, W. (2009). Annual medical spending attributable to obesity: Payer- and service-specific estimates. *Health Affairs, 28*(5), w822–w831.

Finucane, M. M., Stevens, G. A., Cowan, M. J., Danaei, G., Lin, J. K., Paciorek, C. J., et al. (2011). National, regional, and global trends in body-mass index since 1980: Systematic analysis of health examination surveys and epidemiological studies with 960 country-years and 9.1 million participants. *Lancet, 377*(9765), 557–567.

Flegal, K. M., Kit, B. K., Orpana, H., & Graubard, B. I. (2013). Association of all-cause mortality with overweight and obesity using standard body mass index categories: A systematic review and meta-analysis. *Journal of the American Medical Association, 309*(1), 71–82.

Flegal, K. M., Kruszon-Moran, D., Carroll, M. D., Fryar, C. D., & Ogden, C. L. (2016). Trends in obesity among adults in the United States, 2005 to 2014. *Journal of the American Medical Association, 315*(21), 2284–2291.

Flint, A. J., Hu, F. B., Glynn, R. J., Caspard, H., Manson, J. E., Willett, W. C., et al. (2010). Excess weight and the risk of incident coronary heart disease among men and women. *Obesity (Silver Spring), 18*(2), 377–383.

Flint, S. W., Cadek, M., Codreanu, S. C., Ivic, V., Zomer, C., & Gomoiu, A. (2016). Obesity discrimination in the recruitment process: "You're not hired!" *Frontiers in Psychology, 7,* 647.

Folsom, A. R., Prineas, R. J., Kaye, S. A., & Soler, J. T. (1989). Body fat distribution and self-reported prevalence of hypertension, heart attack, and other heart disease in older women. *International Journal of Epidemiology, 18*(2), 361–367.

GBD 2013 Risk Factor Collaborators, Forouzanfar, M. H., Alexander, L., Anderson, H. R., Bachman, V. F., Biryukov, S., et al. (2015). Global, regional, and national comparative risk assessment of 79 behavioural, environmental and occupational, and metabolic risks or clusters of risks in 188 countries, 1990–2013: A systematic analysis for the Global Burden of Disease Study 2013. *Lancet, 386*(10010), 2287–2323.

Gelber, R. P., Gaziano, J. M., Manson, J. E., Buring, J. E., & Sesso, H. D. (2007). A prospective study of body mass index and the risk of developing hypertension in men. *American Journal of Hypertension, 20*(4), 370–377.

Genkinger, J. M., Kitahara, C. M., Bernstein, L., Berrington de Gonzalez, A., Brotzman, M., Elena, J. W., et al. (2015). Central adiposity, obesity during early adulthood, and pancreatic cancer mortality in a pooled analysis of cohort studies. *Annals of Oncology, 26*(11), 2257–2266.

Giovannucci, E., Rimm, E. B., Chute, C. G., Kawachi, I., Colditz, G. A., Stampfer, M. J., et al. (1994). Obesity and benign prostatic hyperplasia. *American Journal of Epidemiology, 140*(6, Suppl.), 989–1002.

Gortmaker, S. L., Must, A., Perrin, J. M., Sobol, A. M., & Dietz, W. H. (1993). Social and economic consequences of overweight in adolescence and young adulthood. *New England Journal of Medicine, 329*(14), 1008–1012.

Guh, D. P., Zhang, W., Bansback, N., Amarsi, Z., Birmingham, C. L., & Anis, A. H. (2009). The incidence of co-morbidities related to obesity and overweight: A systematic review and meta-analysis. *BMC Public Health, 9*, 88.

Haldar, S., Chia, S. C., & Henry, C. J. (2015). Body composition in Asians and Caucasians: Comparative analyses and influences on cardiometabolic outcomes. *Advances in Food and Nutrition Research, 75*, 97–154.

Hammond, R. A., & Levine, R. (2010). The economic impact of obesity in the United States. *Diabetes, Metabolic Syndrome and Obesity, 3*, 285–295.

Hartz, A. J., Rupley, D. C., Jr., Kalkhoff, R. D., & Rimm, A. A. (1983). Relationship of obesity to diabetes: Influence of obesity level and body fat distribution. *Preventive Medicine, 12*(2), 351–357.

Heymsfield, S. B., & Wadden, T. A. (2017). Mechanisms, pathophysiology, and management of obesity. *New England Journal of Medicine, 376*(3), 254–266.

Hoyo, C., Cook, M. B., Kamangar, F., Freedman, N. D., Whiteman, D. C., Bernstein, L., et al. (2012). Body mass index in relation to oesophageal and oesophagogastric junction adenocarcinomas: A pooled analysis from the International BEACON Consortium. *International Journal of Epidemiology, 41*(6), 1706–1718.

Hu, F. B. (2008). Measurements of adiposity and body composition. In F. B. Hu (Ed.), *Obesity epidemiology* (pp. 55–83). Oxford, UK: Oxford University Press.

Huang, Z., Willett, W. C., Manson, J. E., Rosner, B., Stampfer, M. J., Speizer, F. E., et al. (1998). Body weight, weight change, and risk for hypertension in women. *Annals of Internal Medicine, 128*(2), 81–88.

Juonala, M., Magnussen, C. G., Berenson, G. S., Venn, A., Burns, T. L., Sabin, M. A., et al. (2011). Childhood adiposity, adult adiposity, and cardiovascular risk factors. *New England Journal of Medicine, 365*(20), 1876–1885.

Larsson, S. C., & Wolk, A. (2007). Obesity and colon and rectal cancer risk: A meta-analysis of prospective studies. *American Journal of Clinical Nutrition, 86*(3), 556–565.

Lauby-Secretan, B., Scoccianti, C., Loomis, D., Grosse, Y., Bianchini, F., Straif, K., et al. (2016). Body fatness and cancer—Viewpoint of the IARC working group. *New England Journal of Medicine, 375*(8), 794–798.

Lehnert, T., Sonntag, D., Konnopka, A., Riedel-Heller, S., & Konig, H. H. (2013). Economic costs of overweight and obesity. *Best Practice and Research: Clinical Endocrinology and Metabolism, 27*(2), 105–115.

Li, L., Liu, D. W., Yan, H. Y., Wang, Z. Y., Zhao, S. H., & Wang, B. (2016). Obesity is an independent risk factor for non-alcoholic fatty liver disease: Evidence from a meta-analysis of 21 cohort studies. *Obesity Reviews, 17*(6), 510–519.

Mahler, R. J., & Adler, M. L. (1999). Clinical review 102: Type 2 diabetes mellitus: Update on diagnosis, pathophysiology, and treatment. *Journal of Clinical Endocrinology and Metabolism, 84*(4), 1165–1171.

Malik, V. S., Willett, W. C., & Hu, F. B. (2013). Global obesity: Trends, risk factors and policy implications. *Nature Reviews: Endocrinology, 9*(1), 13–27.

Manson, J. E., Willett, W. C., Stampfer, M. J., Colditz, G. A., Hunter, D. J., Hankinson, S. E., et al. (1995). Body weight and mortality among women. *New England Journal of Medicine, 333*(11), 677–685.

Matsuo, K., Mizoue, T., Tanaka, K., Tsuji, I., Sugawara, Y., Sasazuki, S., et al. (2012). Association between body mass index and the colorectal cancer risk in Japan: Pooled analysis of population-based cohort studies in Japan. *Annals of Oncology, 23*(2), 479–490.

Mikhail, N., Golub, M. S., & Tuck, M. L. (1999). Obesity and hypertension. *Progress in Cardiovascular Diseases, 42*(1), 39–58.

Must, A., Jacques, P. F., Dallal, G. E., Bajema, C. J., & Dietz, W. H. (1992). Long-term morbidity and mortality of overweight adolescents: A follow-up of the Harvard Growth Study of 1922 to 1935. *New England Journal of Medicine, 327*(19), 1350–1355.

National Center for Health Statistics. (2016). *Health, United States, 2015: With special feature on racial and ethnic health disparities*. Hyattsville, MD: Author.

N.C.D. Risk Factor Collaboration. (2016). Trends in adult body-mass index in 200 countries from 1975 to 2014: A pooled analysis of 1698 population-based measurement studies with 19.2 million participants. *Lancet, 387*(10026), 1377–1396.

Nwankwo, T., Yoon, S. S., Burt, V., & Gu, Q. (2013). Hypertension among adults in the United States: National Health and Nutrition Examination Survey, 2011–2012. *NCHS Data Brief* (133), 1–8.

Ogden, C. L., Carroll, M. D., Lawman, H. G., Fryar, C. D., Kruszon-Moran, D., Kit, B. K., et al. (2016). Trends in obesity prevalence among children and adolescents in the United States, 1988–1994 through 2013–2014. *Journal of the American Medical Association, 315*(21), 2292–2299.

Oguma, Y., Sesso, H. D., Paffenbarger, R. S., Jr., & Lee, I. M. (2005). Weight change and risk of developing Type 2 diabetes. *Obesity Research, 13*(5), 945–951.

Pan, A., Kawachi, I., Luo, N., Manson, J. E., Willett, W. C., Hu, F. B., et al. (2014). Changes in body weight and health-related quality of life: 2 cohorts of US women. *American Journal of Epidemiology, 180*(3), 254–262.

Pang, Q., Zhang, J. Y., Song, S. D., Qu, K., Xu, X. S., Liu, S. S., et al. (2015). Central obesity and nonalcoholic fatty liver disease risk after adjusting for body mass index. *World Journal of Gastroenterology, 21*(5), 1650–1662.

Parsons, J. K., Carter, H. B., Partin, A. W., Windham, B. G., Metter, E. J., Ferrucci, L., et al. (2006). Metabolic factors associated with benign prostatic hyperplasia. *Journal of Clinical Endocrinology and Metabolism, 91*(7), 2562–2568.

Prospective Studies Collaborative, Whitlock, G., Lewington, S., Sherliker, P., Clarke, R., Emberson, J., et al. (2009). Body-mass index and cause-specific mortality in 900,000 adults: Collaborative analyses of 57 prospective studies. *Lancet, 373*(9669), 1083–1096.

Puhl, R. M., & Heuer, C. A. (2009). The stigma of obesity: A review and update. *Obesity (Silver Spring), 17*(5), 941–964.

Renehan, A. G., Tyson, M., Egger, M., Heller, R. F., & Zwahlen, M. (2008). Body-mass index and incidence of cancer: A systematic review and meta-analysis of prospective observational studies. *Lancet, 371*(9612), 569–578.

Renehan, A. G., Zwahlen, M., & Egger, M. (2015). Adiposity and cancer risk: New mechanistic insights from epidemiology. *Nature Reviews Cancer, 15*(8), 484–498.

Rich-Edwards, J. W., Spiegelman, D., Garland, M., Hertzmark, E., Hunter, D. J., Colditz, G. A., et al. (2002). Physical activity, body mass index, and ovulatory disorder infertility. *Epidemiology, 13*(2), 184–190.

Roehrborn, C. G. (2011). Male lower urinary tract symptoms (LUTS) and benign prostatic hyperplasia (BPH). *Medical Clinics of North America, 95*(1), 87–100.

Rosner, B., Eliassen, A. H., Toriola, A. T., Hankinson, S. E., Willett, W. C., Natarajan, L., et al. (2015). Short-term weight gain and breast cancer risk by hormone receptor classification among pre- and postmenopausal women. *Breast Cancer Research and Treatment, 150*(3), 643–653.

Rueda-Clausen, C. F., Ogunleye, A. A., & Sharma, A. M. (2015). Health benefits of long-term weight-loss maintenance. *Annual Review of Nutrition, 35*, 475–516.

Setiawan, V. W., Yang, H. P., Pike, M. C., McCann, S. E., Yu, H., Xiang, Y. B., et al. (2013). Type I and II endometrial cancers: Have they different risk factors? *Journal of Clinical Oncology, 31*(20), 2607–2618.

Shihab, H. M., Meoni, L. A., Chu, A. Y., Wang, N. Y., Ford, D. E., Liang, K. Y., et al. (2012). Body mass index and risk of incident hypertension over the life course: The Johns Hopkins Precursors Study. *Circulation, 126*(25), 2983–2989.

Singh, A. S., Mulder, C., Twisk, J. W., van Mechelen, W., & Chinapaw, M. J. (2008). Tracking of childhood overweight into adulthood: A systematic review of the literature. *Obesity Reviews, 9*(5), 474–488.

Sonne-Holm, S., & Sorensen, T. I. (1986). Prospective study of attainment of social class of severely obese subjects in relation to parental social class, intelligence, and education. *British Medical Journal (Clinical Research Ed.), 292*(6520), 586–589.

Strazzullo, P., D'Elia, L., Cairella, G., Garbagnati, F., Cappuccio, F. P., & Scalfi, L. (2010). Excess body weight and incidence of stroke: Meta-analysis of prospective studies with 2 million participants. *Stroke, 41*(5), e418–e426.

Teras, L. R., Kitahara, C. M., Birmann, B. M., Hartge, P. A., Wang, S. S., Robien, K., et al. (2014). Body size and multiple myeloma mortality: A pooled analysis of 20 prospective studies. *British Journal of Haematology, 166*(5), 667–676.

Than, N. N., & Newsome, P. N. (2015). A concise review of non-alcoholic fatty liver disease. *Atherosclerosis, 239*(1), 192–202.

Ul-Haq, Z., Mackay, D. F., Fenwick, E., & Pell, J. P. (2013a). Meta-analysis of the association between body mass index and health-related quality of life among adults, assessed by the SF-36. *Obesity (Silver Spring), 21*(3), E322–E327.

Ul-Haq, Z., Mackay, D. F., Fenwick, E., & Pell, J. P. (2013b). Meta-analysis of the association between body mass index and health-related quality of life among children and adolescents, assessed using the Pediatric Quality Of Life Inventory index. *Journal of Pediatrics, 162*(2), 280–286.

Wadden, T. A., & Stunkard, A. J. (1985). Social and psychological consequences of obesity. *Annals of Internal Medicine, 103*(6, Pt. 2), 1062–1067.

Wang, S., Mao, Q., Lin, Y., Wu, J., Wang, X., Zheng, X., et al. (2012). Body mass index and risk of BPH: A meta-analysis. *Prostate Cancer and Prostatic Diseases, 15*(3), 265–272.

Wang, Y. C., McPherson, K., Marsh, T., Gortmaker, S. L., & Brown, M. (2011). Health and economic burden of the projected obesity trends in the USA and the UK. *Lancet, 378*(9793), 815–825.

Wang, Y., Rimm, E. B., Stampfer, M. J., Willett, W. C., & Hu, F. B. (2005). Comparison of abdominal adiposity and overall obesity in predicting risk of type 2 diabetes among men. *American Journal of Clinical Nutrition, 81*(3), 555–563.

Willett, W. (2013). *Nutritional epidemiology* (3rd ed.). Oxford, UK: Oxford University Press.

Withrow, D., & Alter, D. A. (2011). The economic burden of obesity worldwide: A systematic review of the direct costs of obesity. *Obesity Reviews, 12*(2), 131–141.

Witteman, J. C., Willett, W. C., Stampfer, M. J., Colditz, G. A., Sacks, F. M., Speizer, F. E., et al. (1989). A prospective study of nutritional factors and hypertension among US women. *Circulation, 80*(5), 1320–1327.

World Health Organization. (2016). Obesity and overweight: Fact sheet. Retrieved July 18, 2016, from *www.who.int/mediacentre/factsheets/fs311/en*.

Xu, J., Murphy, S. L., Kochanek, K. D., & Bastian, B. A. (2016). Deaths: Final data for 2013. *National Vital Statistics Reports, 64*(2), 1–119.

Yong, L. C., Kuller, L. H., Rutan, G., & Bunker, C. (1993). Longitudinal study of blood pressure: Changes and determinants from adolescence to middle age: The Dormont High School follow-up study, 1957–1963 to 1989–1990. *American Journal of Epidemiology, 138*(11), 973–983.

Younossi, Z. M., Stepanova, M., Afendy, M., Fang, Y., Younossi, Y., Mir, H., et al. (2011). Changes in the prevalence of the most common causes of chronic liver diseases in the United States from 1988 to 2008. *Clinical Gastroenterology and Hepatology, 9*(6), 524–530.

Zalesin, K. C., Franklin, B. A., Miller, W. M., Peterson, E. D., & McCullough, P. A. (2008). Impact of obesity on cardiovascular disease. *Endocrinology and Metabolism Clinics of North America, 37*(3), 663–684, ix.

CHAPTER 2

Gut-to-Brain Mechanisms of Body Weight Regulation

Matthew R. Hayes

Although energy balance is ultimately regulated by the central nervous system (CNS), the organs of the alimentary canal and supporting organs of the peritoneal cavity supply numerous neuroendocrine signals that are necessary for the physiological and behavioral processes that affect energy balance. This chapter provides a brief overview of "gut hormones" and their contribution to energy balance regulation. Here, gastrointestinal (GI)- and pancreatic-derived peptides that have been extensively studied both in the context of normal physiology and in the pathophysiological state of obesity are discussed. Accordingly, the hormonal systems reviewed here are likely those systems that represent the greatest opportunity for future pharmacological targets to treat obesity. It is also worth noting that some of the gut peptides discussed in this chapter are also synthesized centrally within the brain and are more accurately referred to as *neuropeptides*. Thus, an important consideration for all of the peptides described is a discussion about the mechanisms (behavioral, endocrine, and autonomic) and neuroanatomical sites-of-action within the brain and periphery.

Gut peptides regulate feeding behavior by negatively or positively influencing food intake during a meal and/or between meals (influencing the intermeal interval and the frequency of meal taking; Grill & Hayes, 2012; Moran, 2006; Ritter, 2004). This process involves a constant stream of gut-to-brain communication through humoral mechanisms as well as neuronal signaling predominately via the vagus nerve and, to a smaller extent, splanchnic pathways. Once a meal has begun and food enters the oral cavity, cranial nerves VII, IX, and X relay various properties of the ingesta (e.g., taste and texture) to the brainstem, which promotes further feeding if the food is perceived as palatable (Norgren, 1983). As food is swallowed and enters the GI tract, information about the volume of the food is sensed through the mechanical distension of the stomach and subsequently relayed to the nucleus tractus solitarius (NTS) by the vagus nerve. These gastric inhibitory signals begin to counteract the positive meal-promoting signals from the oral cavity. The various chemical and nutritive properties of the food stimulate the release of gut peptides and neurotransmitters from the GI tract and supporting organs of the alimentary canal (e.g., pancreas). This process enhances communication to the brain via humoral (i.e., endocrine) and neuronal pathways about the ongoing status of the meal. These within-meal food-intake-inhibitory signals are collectively referred to as *satiation signals* (Ritter, 2004). The accumulation of these satiation signals is perpetually sensed by the brain and eventually leads to *satiety*, or meal termination. Satiety then persists from the end of one meal to the start of the next meal.

Given the redundant number of gut peptides, neuropeptides, and neurotransmitter systems that exist in the body to inhibit food intake and promote satiety, it seems initially paradoxical that obesity rates continue to rise worldwide. One interpretation of this phenomenon is that humans lack true homeostatic equilibrium when it comes to energy balance. Many theories have been proposed, discussed, heavily reviewed, and cited on this topic (McAllister et al., 2009; Thomas et al., 2012). A growing evolutionary theory states that our energy balance neuroendocrine systems have developed not to maintain leanness or normal energy equilibrium, but rather to defend adiposity and the surplus of energy storage (Rosenbaum, Kissileff, Mayer, Hirsch, & Leibel, 2010). From this perspective, it is worth noting that the brain initiates autonomic, behavioral, and endocrine responses not just in response to the accumulation of a given neuropeptide signal and receptor activation, but also in response to the *reduction* of a given signal.

GI Satiation Signals

The abundant vagal afferent innervation and proximal location of the stomach within the GI tract provide an early monitoring system for the status of meal ingestion. Specifically, the food-intake-inhibitory signals produced by the stomach arise from the mechanical distension of the stomach (rather than the chemical/nutritive properties of the ingested food; Mathis, Moran, & Schwartz, 1998; Phillips & Powley, 1996; Powley & Phillips, 2004). Unlike the satiation signals that arise from the intestine, the intake-inhibitory signals arising from the stomach are not mediated by gut peptides. Rather, a portion of the dendritic vagal sensory endings innervating the stomach is specialized to be responsive to stretch and/or tension. These sensory endings are referred to as *intraganglionic laminar endings* and *intramuscular arrays* (see Ritter, 2004, for review). The vagal dendritic detection of tension and stretch within the gastric wall results in neuronal transmission from vagal axon projections to NTS neurons in the caudal brainstem (see Grill & Hayes, 2012, for review). In addition, as the gastric wall is distended, the neurotransmitter serotonin (5-HT) is secreted from gastric enterochromaffin (EC) cells and is thought to provide the principal stomach-derived intake-inhibitory signal. This 5-HT-mediated hypophagic response engaged by gastric distension occurs principally through the activation of ionotropic 5-HT type-3 receptors (5-HT3_R) expressed on the dendritic terminals of vagal afferents innervating the stomach (Glatzle et al., 2002; Hayes, Moore, Shah, & Covasa, 2004; Mazda, Yamamoto, Fujimura, & Fujimiya, 2004). Where appropriate, gastric distension and GI-derived satiation signaling interactions with gut peptides that control energy balance are discussed further in this chapter.

Cholecystokinin

The neuropeptide cholecystokinin (CCK), released peripherally from intestinal "I" cells in response to ingestion of nutrients, is arguably one of the most well-studied satiation signals (see Moran, 2006, and Ritter, 2004, for review). Indeed, over four decades ago, Gibbs, Young, and Smith (1973) first reported that exogenous, systemic administration of CCK produced a dose-dependent decrease in meal size. This initial finding was the first to demonstrate that a GI-derived peptide could negatively influence food intake, providing the seminal discovery for future scientific fields investigating the gut-to-brain communication involved in the control of energy balance.

Systemic CCK acts via CCK-1 receptors (historically referred to as CCK-A receptors) that are densely distributed in the periphery on the afferent terminals of the vagus nerve and in select regions of the CNS. Importantly, though, the primary site-of-action for either endogenous or exogenous systemic CCK is not the CNS, but rather the vagal afferents (Smith, Jerome, & Norgren, 1985). Support for the physiological requirement of endogenous CCK-1 receptor signaling in controlling meal size, as well as energy balance more broadly, comes from the findings that blockade of CCK-1 receptors, using selective antagonists, results in a short-term increase in food intake. Other supporting data show that rats with genetic deletion of the CCK-1 receptor are chronically hyperphagic and obese (see Moran, 2006, and Ritter, 2004, for review).

The suppression of food intake by CCK administration is enhanced when combined with other GI-derived satiation signals. For example, data from Schwartz and Moran show that CCK and gastric distension combine in a dose- and volume-dependent fashion to increase firing rate and total spike number of electrophysiological recordings made on single vagal afferent fibers (Schwartz, McHugh, & Moran, 1993; Schwartz & Moran, 1996). This vagal integration is further postulated to mediate the enhanced behavioral suppression of food intake when CCK and gastric distension are combined (Moran, Ladenheim, & Schwartz, 2001; Ritter, 2004; Schwartz & Moran, 1996). Interestingly, these two GI-derived satiation signals also mechanistically interact within a meal to suppress the ongoing meal. Specifically, CCK-1 receptor activation reduces gastric emptying and thereby enhances gastric distension as the animal/human continues to feed (Moran & McHugh, 1982). Further, this interaction between CCK and gastric distension involves participation of other GI-derived satiating signals, such as 5-HT, which is released in response to gastric distension (Mazda et al., 2004) and interacts with CCK to reduce food intake. Indeed, blockade of $5-HT3_R$ attenuates the suppression of food intake by CCK (Daughters et al., 2001; Hayes et al., 2004).

In addition to the traditional role of CCK as a within-meal satiation signal, CCK interacts with hormonal systems such as insulin and leptin, which serve as a readout of long-term energy stores (see Begg & Woods, 2012, and Grill & Hayes, 2012, for review). Looking at leptin as the example of this interaction, leptin potentiates the anorectic effects of CCK and other GI-derived satiation signals (see Grill & Hayes, 2012, for review). This leptin–CCK interaction is not confined to one nucleus within the brain, but rather involves distributed sites of action throughout the body that include vagal afferents (Peters, Karpiel, Ritter, & Simasko, 2004; Peters, Ritter, & Simasko, 2006), the NTS (Hayes et al., 2010), the parabrachial nucleus (Flak et al., 2014), and hypothalamic nuclei (Barrachina, Martinez, Wang, Wei, & Tache, 1997; Emond, Schwartz, Ladenheim, & Moran, 1999).

Despite extensive examination of the CCK system, there are a number of hurdles blocking the development of safe and efficacious pharmacological tools targeting CCK as a means to facilitate weight loss in obese humans. One major obstacle is the pronounced tachyphylaxis that develops with repetitive CCK administrations (Crawley & Beinfeld, 1983). Perhaps most important for CCK-1 receptor agonists is the need for analogs that remain efficacious without producing pancreatitis, a well-known response to chronic CCK-like treatments in mammals (Lampel & Kern, 1977; Makovec et al., 1986). To this end, at least one compound, GI181771X (GlaxoSmithKline), appears to have little effect on pancreatic endpoints in overweight/obese humans (Myer, Romach, & Elangbam, 2014). Unfortunately, chronic treatment with this therapeutic did not reduce food intake and body weight in overweight and obese humans (Jordan et al., 2008), possibly for the aforementioned tachyphylaxis and reduced responsiveness that occurs with continuous CCK-1 receptor activation.

Glucagon–Like Peptide-1

Multiple biological processes are regulated by the glucagon-like peptide-1 (GLP-1) system, including insulin secretion; blood glucose regulation; suppression of gastric emptying; cardiovascular and thermogenic effects; modulation of reward- and goal-directed behaviors; and, importantly, a physiological role in food intake and energy balance (see Hayes, Mietlicki-Baase, Kanoski, & De Jonghe, 2014, and Holst, 2007, for review). Within the periphery, GLP-1 is principally secreted by enteroendocrine "L" cells of the distal small intestine and large intestine in response to the ingestion of food. GLP-1 is rapidly degraded by the enzyme dipeptidyl peptidase-4 (DPP-IV) to inactive metabolites, and therefore has a short circulating half-life of less than 10 minutes

(Holst, 2007), rendering native GLP-1 inappropriate for the treatment of obesity. GLP-1 acts on the GLP-1 receptor (GLP-1R), a G protein-coupled receptor, which has a varied tissue distribution in mammals (brain, pancreas, intestine, heart, etc.; see Holst, 2007, for review). Under normal physiological circumstances, intestinally derived GLP-1 activates GLP-1R, expressed on the dendritic terminals of the vagal afferents innervating the GI tract in a paracrine-like mode of action (see Hayes et al., 2014, for review). However, the relevant GLP-1R populations mediating the suppression of food intake through GLP-1R pharmacological agonists (e.g., liraglutide, exendin-4) or inhibitors of DPP-IV (e.g., sitagliptin) are more diverse. For example, when the long-lasting GLP-1R agonist liraglutide or exendin-4 is administered systemically, each can sufficiently penetrate the blood–brain barrier and gain access to the brain in amounts sufficient to drive physiological and behavioral responses. Indeed, activation of GLP-1R expressed in the CNS will recapitulate many of the same behavioral and physiological responses that are observed following peripheral GLP-1R ligand administration (see Hayes et al., 2014, for review). This makes it difficult to disentangle the effects originating in the periphery from those effects mediated by direct CNS activation. Therefore, one of the current challenges in the obesity field is to characterize the energy balance responses mediated by individual GLP-1R-expressing nuclei and the physiological mechanisms mediating these responses.

Whereas research pursuant to the exploration of GLP-1-mediated effects in a multitude of CNS nuclei is certainly warranted, of particular interest is research aimed at identifying GLP-1 modulation of food reward processes. Given that the excessive food intake that contributes to human obesity is not driven by metabolic need alone, a number of laboratories have made major advances in our understanding of the role that GLP-1 signaling in the nuclei of the mesolimbic reward system has on control of energy balance (Alhadeff, Rupprecht, & Hayes, 2012; Dickson et al., 2012; Dossat, Lilly, Kay, & Williams, 2011). Perhaps most attractive from the perspective of obesity treatment is the finding that some of these mesolimbic nuclei (e.g., ventral tegmental area [VTA]) are directly activated by systemic administration of GLP-1R agonists to suppress food intake and body weight (Mietlicki-Baase, Ortinski, et al., 2013). Recently, the GLP-1R agonist liraglutide (Saxenda) was approved for the treatment of obesity (Mordes, Liu, & Xu, 2015). We now need further basic science investigations to identify adjunct behavioral and pharmacological therapies that can be combined with GLP-1R ligands to enhance the suppression of food intake and body weight by these pharmacotherapies.

Gastric Inhibitory Polypeptide

Gastric inhibitory polypeptide (GIP) stimulates glucose-dependent insulin secretion, insulin transcription/translation, as well as betacell growth and preservation of betacell survival under normal physiological conditions (see Sadry & Drucker, 2013, for review). However, there is limited evidence supporting consistent effects of GIP on energy balance produced by GIP treatment alone. Further, much of the beneficial glycemic effect of GIP signaling is impaired in states of chronic hyperglycemia (Jones, Owens, Vora, Luzio, & Hayes, 1989). The latter fact has greatly precluded any significant pharmacological advancement for the GIP system as a primary treatment strategy for type 2 diabetes mellitus (T2DM). There is also a multitude of conflicting reports showing opposing metabolic effects arising from activation or inhibition of GIP receptors. For example, GIP administration in hyperglycemic patients with T2DM promotes glucagon secretion and worsens glucose tolerance (Chia et al., 2009), an effect contrary to GIP-mediated effects in euglycemic nondiabetic conditions. In mouse models, genetic deletion of the GIP receptor improves glucose tolerance and insulin sensitivity (see Sadry & Drucker, 2013, for review). Thus, although emerging combination therapies involving GIP signaling are being pursued as a potential treatment strategy for metabolic diseases (Sadry & Drucker, 2013), the cautious view at this moment indicates that further extensive preclinical and clinical trials for GIP-based pharmacotherapy are needed before considering any GIP-based compound as a viable treatment option for T2DM and/or obesity.

Peptide YY

Peptide YY (PYY) is co-released with GLP-1 from the L cells of the small and large intestines after the ingestion of food (Lundberg et al., 1982). PYY is initially secreted in a longer form (PYY[1–36]) that has no effect on food intake (Sloth, Davidsen, Holst, Flint, & Astrup, 2007), but like GLP-1, PYY is rapidly cleaved by DPP-IV) to form PYY(3–36) (Medeiros & Turner, 1994). Although first identified in the early 1980s (Tatemoto, 1982), the effects of PYY(3–36) on energy balance remained controversial for many years (Batterham & Bloom, 2003; Batterham et al., 2002; Boggiano et al., 2005; Tschop et al., 2004), due in part to the fact that the two endogenous circulating isoforms of PYY (PYY[1–36] and PYY[3–36]) bind to Y1, Y2, and Y5 receptors with different affinities (Blomqvist & Herzog, 1997; Silva, Cavadas, & Grouzmann, 2002). Importantly, PYY(1–36) binds to all of these receptors, whereas PYY(3–36) is thought to have the highest affinity for the Y2 receptor (Keire, Bowers, Solomon, & Reeve, 2002). Further contributing to the controversy is the bidirectional effect on feeding seen with peripheral versus central delivery. Specifically, peripheral administration of PYY(3–36) suppresses feeding and body weight in humans and in animal models (Batterham & Bloom, 2003), whereas central (lateral, third, and fourth intracerebroventricular [ICV]) administration of either PYY(1–36) or PYY(3–36) robustly *stimulates* food intake (Clark, Sahu, Kalra, Balasubramaniam, & Kalra, 1987). Thus, although there is growing research attention to the PYY system as a potential future target for obesity treatment, it is clear that an abundance of work is needed to discern the physiological effects mediated by Y-receptor signaling.

From the perspective of creating pharmacotherapies to treat obesity, it is worth noting that chronic systemic administration of PYY(3–36) reduces food intake (Reidelberger, Haver, Chelikani, & Buescher, 2008). This peptide can cross the blood–brain barrier (Nonaka, Shioda, Niehoff, & Banks, 2003) and is thought to act primarily within the CNS to exert its hypophagic effects. Like ghrelin (discussed later), particular attention has been paid to the actions of PYY on the neuropeptide Y (NPY) system (Ballantyne, 2006). Indeed, PYY(3–36) is thought to exert its anorectic effects, in part, via agonism of the Y2 receptor, and specifically the Y2 receptors expressed on arcuate nucleus of the hypothalamus (ARC) NPY/agouti-related peptide (AgRP) neurons (Teubner & Bartness, 2013). However, further research is needed to determine if all of the CNS action results in a decrease or increase in food intake, if there is a hope that PYY-based pharmacotherapies could be used to treat human obesity.

Ghrelin: The Sole GI "Hunger Hormone"

The conscious decision made by humans and animals to procure food and initiate ingestion of a meal is made after neural assimilation of a multitude of internal and external stimuli. Meal initiation occurs in response to internal hunger signals that communicate energy need, as well as to external environmental cues and appetite signals that include entrainment and the social, memory, cognitive, and sensory aspects of feeding behavior. With regard to the subjective feeling of hunger, it is important to note that hunger is generated by an accumulation of central and peripheral orexigenic signals that promote feeding, as well as the reduction of GI-derived satiation signals once the previous meal has been digested and absorbed. To date, ghrelin represents the sole gut peptide that is classified as a hunger (orexigenic) hormone.

Upon its original discovery, ghrelin was recognized for its ability to promote growth hormone secretion (Kojima et al., 1999). The role of this peptide as a hunger hormone was identified shortly after its discovery (Tschop, Smiley, & Heiman, 2000). Ghrelin is produced primarily in the X/A-like cells of the stomach (Date et al., 2000), although some reports suggest that ghrelin is also synthesized centrally (Cowley et al., 2003). Within the circulation, ghrelin exists in two major forms: des-acyl ghrelin and acylated ghrelin (Hosoda, Kojima, Matsuo, & Kangawa, 2000). Acylation is accomplished by the actions of the enzyme ghrelin-O-acyltransferase (GOAT; Yang, Brown, Liang, Grishin, & Goldstein, 2008). Circulating levels of acylated ghrelin are lower than des-acyl ghrelin (Hosoda et al., 2000); however, the orexigenic effects of ghrelin are attributed predominantly to its acylated form. Toshinai et al. (2006) have reported a hyperphagic effect of des-acyl ghrelin, but more recent studies show a reduction in food intake and body weight with des-acyl ghrelin administration (Heppner et al., 2014). In fact, there is a growing consensus that des-acyl ghrelin may act as an endogenous competitive antagonist for the hyperphagic effects of acylated ghrelin (Delhanty, Neggers, & van der Lely, 2012). Given the controversy and limited number of reports on des-acyl ghrelin's actions on food intake, for the duration of this section, *ghrelin* refers to the acylated form of the peptide.

One of the most remarkable and unique features of ghrelin with regard to GI-derived hormones is that circulating levels of ghrelin increase with fasting (Tschop et al., 2001). Individuals who take meals on a regular schedule from day to day will eventually exhibit an entrainment of ghrelin levels to their mealtimes (Cummings et al., 2001). This temporal link between peak ghrelin levels and the onset of feeding has led to the notion that ghrelin may serve as a meal initiation signal (Cummings et al., 2001). Once food is ingested, circulating ghrelin declines (Tschop et al., 2001). Interestingly, the postprandial suppression of ghrelin is related to the macronutrient content of the meal, with ghrelin being more effective at reducing carbohydrates than intake of fats or proteins (Overduin, Frayo, Grill, Kaplan, & Cummings, 2005).

The ghrelin receptor, or growth hormone secretagogue receptor (GHS-R), is widely distributed throughout the body, including the brain (Asakawa et al., 2003; Shuto et al., 2002). Given that ghrelin crosses the blood–brain barrier (Banks, Burney, & Robinson, 2008), circulating ghrelin can potentially activate both central and peripheral receptor populations. Indeed, most of the research on ghrelin's hyperphagic effects has focused on its actions within the brain. Some of the initial research on the neuronal mechanisms mediating ghrelin's orexigenic effects examined the ability of ghrelin to regulate feeding via effects in the ARC nucleus of the hypothalamus (Cowley et al., 2003). Specifically, ghrelin activating the GHS-R expressed on NPY/AgRP neurons in the ARC (Willesen, Kristensen, & Romer, 1999) increases expression of NPY and AgRP, neuropeptides with orexigenic effects (Kamegai et al., 2001). At the same time, ghrelin is thought to activate GHS-R expressed on adjacent ARC NPY/AgRP neurons to stimulate the release of gamma-aminobutyric acid (GABA) onto proopiomelanocortin (POMC) neurons within the ARC (Cowley et al., 2003), reducing the activity of this hypophagia-producing neuronal population. These complementary effects of increasing NPY/AgRP activity, while concomitantly suppressing POMC activity, contribute to the overall stimulation of feeding by ghrelin.

Beyond the hypothalamus, ghrelin has been well documented to activate a number of other nuclei within the brain to promote positive energy balance. These include hindbrain sites such as the dorsal vagal complex (Faulconbridge, Cummings, Kaplan, & Grill, 2003), as well as a number of forebrain nuclei, including the paraventricular nucleus of the hypothalamus (Currie, Mirza, Fuld, Park, & Vasselli, 2005), the lateral hypothalamus (Olszewski et al., 2003), the hippocampus (Kanoski, Fortin, Ricks, & Grill, 2013), and the amygdala (Alvarez-Crespo et al., 2012). Several recent studies have focused on the ability of ghrelin to modulate activity of the mesolimbic dopamine pathway, including the VTA, and to increase food intake and the motivation to obtain palatable food (Egecioglu et al., 2010). Collectively, these studies suggest that ghrelin may have interesting effects on reward and motivational processes involved in feeding.

Though it may seem paradoxical, obese individuals typically have lower plasma levels of ghrelin than do lean individuals. This is observed in fasting levels of ghrelin. Additionally, the postprandial suppression of ghrelin is not as large in obese individuals as in lean individuals (Tschop et al., 2001). Weight loss results in an increase in plasma ghrelin (Cummings et al., 2002), which may contribute to the increased hunger experienced during and after dieting-induced weight loss. Because ghrelin stimulates hunger and increases feeding, a number of laboratories have attempted to reduce the bioactivity of ghrelin in an attempt to promote weight loss. In animal models, reduction of ghrelin levels has been accomplished through the use of anti-ghrelin immunoglobulins (Teubner & Bartness, 2013). Unfortunately, the bioavailability of these compounds, as well as multiple undesired side effects, have limited the translation of this type of pharmacological approach for humans.

Pancreatic Beta-Cell-Derived Hormones

Meal taking presents a challenge to many aspects of metabolic homeostasis, including glycemia. Maintenance of blood glucose levels is largely regulated by pancreatic-derived hormones glucagon and insulin, released from pancreatic alpha and beta cells, respectively. As nutrients enter the GI tract during meal taking, it is critical that adequate and rapid communication occur between the GI tract, brain, and pancreas to facilitate glycemic control. Interestingly, some of the hormonal signals produced by the pancreas also have potent effects on feeding and body weight.

Insulin

In addition to insulin's ability to regulate glucose levels, insulin receptor signaling also affects food intake, although the reliability of insulin-mediated energy balance effects are sometimes questioned (see Begg & Woods, 2012, and Woods & Langhans, 2012, for review). Although insulin obviously promotes the lowering of plasma blood glucose—an effect that, in itself, may affect subsequent food intake—the energy balance effects of insulin receptor signaling are thought to be independent from its effects on glycemia (Woods, Stein, McKay, & Porte, 1984). Thus, whereas some of the energy balance effects of insulin may be mediated by peripheral organs such as the liver (see Begg & Woods, 2012, for review), the majority of the intake-suppressive effects of peripheral insulin are thought to be centrally mediated (Woods, Seeley, Baskin, & Schwartz, 2003), following CNS penetrance via facilitated transport (Baura et al., 1993).

Within the CNS, insulin receptor signaling reduces food intake and body weight in baboons, rats, sheep, mice, and possibly humans (Brown, Clegg, Benoit, & Woods, 2006). Many studies have examined the ability of insulin to regulate feeding via actions in the hypothalamus, particularly in the ARC. Insulin receptors are tyrosine kinase receptors that are expressed on NPY-containing, as well as on POMC-expressing, ARC neurons. To this end, ICV administration of insulin reduces NPY expression in the ARC (Schwartz et al., 1991), as well as in the paraventricular nucleus (Schwartz et al., 1992), possibly via recruitment of GABAergic circuits. Insulin also increases POMC expression (Kim, Grace, Welsh, Billington, & Levin, 1999), consistent with an overall reduction in food intake.

Activation of the insulin receptor results in rapid phosphorylation of insulin receptor substrates (IRS). In particular, IRS-2 appears to be important for the control of energy balance by insulin, in that whole-body (Burks et al., 2000) or hypothalamic knockdown (Kubota et al., 2004) of IRS-2 promotes obesity in murine models. A number of intracellular pathways downstream of IRS have been documented as required signaling events to mediate the suppression of food intake by activation of insulin receptors. Principal among these is the . . . phosphatidylinositol-3-kinases (PI3K) signaling pathway (Niswender et al., 2003). Pharmacological inhibition of PI3K attenuates the ability of centrally delivered insulin to suppress food intake (Niswender et al., 2003), indicating the requirement of PI3K activation to facilitate the anorectic effects of insulin. Engagement of the PI3K pathway is also important for insulin-mediated control of energy balance in extrahypothalamic sites such as the amygdala (Castro et al., 2013).

In the context of obesity, insulin is often referred to as a lipostatic signal (Benoit, Clegg, Seeley, & Woods, 2004), in that circulating concentrations of insulin reflect levels of adiposity (Ahren, 1999). This concept fails, to some extent. Despite an accumulating magnitude of insulin signaling as adiposity increases, insulin resistance develops, and the obese individual does not subsequently reduce energy intake and increase energy expenditure to reduce adiposity levels. Thus, despite their higher plasma insulin, obese individuals are resistant to the intake- and body-weight-suppressive effects of the peptide (see Begg & Woods, 2012, for review). These effects are not entirely due to an insufficient penetration of insulin into the CNS (Kaiyala, Prigeon, Kahn, Woods, & Schwartz, 2000), as direct, central administration of insulin is less effective at reducing food intake in obese animals maintained on a high-fat diet.

Amylin (Islet Amyloid Polypeptide)

The peptide hormone amylin is co-secreted with insulin at a 1-to-100 ratio from pancreatic beta cells after food is consumed (Ogawa, Harris, McCorkle, Unger, & Luskey, 1990). As one might expect, given its association with insulin release, amylin has complementary effects to insulin on glycemic control (Schmitz, Brock, & Rungby, 2004), mainly mediated through delayed gastric emptying (Clementi et al., 1996), inhibition of glucagon release (Fehmann et al., 1990), and potent anorectic effects (Lutz, 2010). Specifically, amylin is well documented as a satiation signal, given its robust ability to reduce food intake via suppression of meal size (Lutz, 2010).

Because surgical vagotomy does not block amylin-induced hypophagia (Lutz, Del Prete, & Scharrer, 1995), the effects of the peptide on feeding are thought to be mediated by direct activation of amylin receptors in the brain (Lutz, 2005). Amylin receptors are fairly unique, in that they contain one of two splice variants of the calcitonin receptor (CTa/CTb; a G-protein-coupled receptor) that heterodimerizes with one of the receptor activity modifying proteins (RAMP1, RAMP2 or RAMP3; Hay, Christopoulos, Christopoulos, & Sexton, 2004). Despite the widespread expression of amylin receptors throughout the central neuraxis, investigations of CNS nuclei and neuronal mechanisms mediating the anorectic effects of amylin have, until recently, focused on classic homeostatic circuitry (Hilton, Chai, & Sexton, 1995; Sexton, Paxinos, Kenney, Wookey, & Beaumont, 1994). The majority of reports describing the hypophagic effect of amylin have focused on its ability to regulate food intake via actions at the area postrema (AP) of the hindbrain, because lesions of this nucleus attenuate the hypophagic effects of systemic amylin administration (Lutz, Mollet, Rushing, Riediger, & Scharrer, 2001; Lutz et al., 1998). Importantly, though, amylin binding is distributed throughout the brain (Paxinos et al., 2004; Sexton et al., 1994), and amylin can cross the blood–brain barrier (Banks & Kastin, 1998; Banks, Kastin, Maness, Huang, & Jaspan, 1995). These data suggest that amylin's access to the CNS is not limited to circumventricular structures such as the AP. Indeed, recent research has shown that amylin can act directly in the VTA to control food intake (Mietlicki-Baase et al., 2015; Mietlicki-Baase, Rupprecht, et al., 2013). VTA amylin receptor activation appears to have especially potent suppressive effects on palatable food intake, as well as on the motivation to obtain a palatable food (Mietlicki-Baase et al., 2015; Mietlicki-Baase, Rupprecht, et al., 2013). This is an interesting finding given the role of the VTA and the mesolimbic system in regulating the intake of palatable and rewarding ingesta. Additionally, a few studies have investigated the actions of amylin in the ventromedial nucleus of the hypothalamus (VMH). Results indicate that amylin may enhance the intake-suppressive effects of the adipose-derived hormone leptin through actions in the VMH (Le Foll et al., 2014; Turek et al., 2010).

A unique feature of amylin receptor activation as a potential treatment for obesity is that it remains effective in its ability to suppress food intake and body weight in obese rodents and humans (Boyle, Rossier, & Lutz, 2011). Studies using the amylin agonist pramlintide, which is FDA approved for the treatment of diabetes (Singh-Franco, Robles, & Gazze, 2007), show that pramlintide treatment in obese humans reduces body weight and enhances control over feeding behavior (Chapman et al., 2005; Ravussin et al., 2009; Roth et al., 2008). This ability of amylin to exert its effects in obese individuals contrasts with other hormonal signals, such as those of leptin and insulin, where sensitivity to suppressing food intake is reduced in the obese state (Munzberg, Flier, & Bjorbaek, 2004). Thus, the absence of amylin resistance in obesity has intensified interest in amylin-based pharmaceuticals as potential future treatments for obesity (Mietlicki-Baase & Hayes, 2014).

Adipose-Derived Hormones

Leptin

Research examining the adipose-tissue-derived hormone leptin has transformed our understanding of the function of white adipose tissue from one of a simple energy storage depot to the view that adipose tissue is an active endocrine organ. We now appreciate that the greater the fat mass of an individual, the larger the available circulating levels of leptin. Given that leptin, acting on its receptors (LepRb, a.k.a. ObRb) in the brain, is known to suppress food intake and energy expenditure, it seems somewhat paradoxical that obesity, a chronic state of elevated adipose mass, is able to occur. Under normal physiological conditions in a lean human or animal, both the total amount of adiposity and the fluctuation in adiposity levels are minimal. Under these conditions, slight variations in circulating leptin levels, which communicate energy storage within the adipose tissue, are sensed by the brain. Appropriate CNS signaling pathways are engaged to either increase or decrease food intake and energy expenditure to normalize energy balance. Unfortunately, however, in the case of obesity, leptin levels are chronically elevated and the brain fails to correctly perceive and respond to the overaccumulation of the leptin signal. Such a response is known as *leptin resistance*.

Under conditions in which the body is challenged by a constant oversupply of nutrients, the normal functioning of the physiological mechanisms maintaining energy balance is disrupted. A state of chronic nutrient excess (caused by over consumption of calorically dense foods) leads eventually to a blunting of signaling in the insulin and leptin pathways, a concept referred to as *resistance*. As described previously, under normal conditions, elevated leptin levels act centrally to decrease feeding and prevent obesity. Under conditions of excess (i.e., obesity), even though large amounts of leptin circulate in the blood, there are disruptions in the receptor and intracellular signaling responses for these hormones. In short, the oversaturation of the hormone at the transporter into the CNS, as well as at the LepRb themselves, decreases the receptor response to the hormone such that leptin fails to appropriately suppress food intake and increase energy expenditure. Thus, weight gain continues, further exacerbating the obesity phenotype. A vicious cycle develops, in which the person who is already consuming too many calories now has less sensitivity to the normal neurochemical signals that should be leading to meal termination. Over time, this resistance to leptin signaling further predisposes the individual toward T2DM and obesity.

Conclusions and Future Directions for Obesity Treatment

Although this chapter considers the individual contributions of several gut-derived and pancreatic hormonal signals to energy balance control, it is crucial to reiterate that these signals do not act in isolation in mammals. Ingestion of food affects many neural and hormonal processes, including those described here, as well as numerous other peripheral and central systems, each of which contributes to the overall control of food intake and body weight. The redundancy of some of these signals is important for preserving and maintaining energy storage, but has also presented a major challenge to the development of pharmacological strategies for the treatment of obesity.

Historically, attempts to treat obesity by targeting a single neuroendocrine system have failed to produce meaningful and long-lasting suppression of body weight, and some have been plagued by serious side effects (Gadde, 2014; James et al., 2010). New monotherapeutic strategies continue to be developed and tested as potential anti-obesity drugs. However, the notion that combination approaches will be more effective for producing sustained reductions in body weight has become increasingly accepted by the scientific community (Phelan & Wadden, 2002). Such approaches include using pharmacotherapy in conjunction with behavioral intervention (Vetter, Faulconbridge, Webb, & Wadden, 2010) and/or pharmacologically targeting more than one neurotransmitter/neuropeptide system (Bray, 2014; Rodgers, Tschop, & Wilding, 2012). It is clear that further development of effective, noninvasive pharmacological strategies for obesity treatment is urgently required.

Acknowlegments

This work was supported in part by National Institutes of Health Grant Nos. DK096139 and DK105155.

References

Ahren, B. (1999). Plasma leptin and insulin in C57Bl/6J mice on a high-fat diet: Relation to subsequent changes in body weight. *Acta Physiologica Scandinavica*, 165(2), 233–240.

Alhadeff, A. L., Rupprecht, L. E., & Hayes, M. R. (2012). GLP-1 neurons in the nucleus of the solitary tract project directly to the ventral tegmental area and nucleus accumbens to control for food intake. *Endocrinology*, 153(2), 647–658.

Alvarez-Crespo, M., Skibicka, K. P., Farkas, I., Molnar, C. S., Egecioglu, E., Hrabovszky, E., et al. (2012). The amygdala as a neurobiological target for ghrelin in rats: Neuroanatomical, electrophysiological and behavioral evidence. *PLOS ONE*, 7(10), e46321.

Asakawa, A., Inui, A., Kaga, T., Katsuura, G., Fujimiya, M., Fujino, M. A., et al. (2003). Antagonism of ghrelin receptor reduces food intake and body weight gain in mice. *Gut*, 52(7), 947–952.

Ballantyne, G. H. (2006). Peptide YY(1–36) and peptide YY(3–36): Part I. Distribution, release and actions. *Obesity Surgery*, 16(5), 651–658.

Banks, W. A., Burney, B. O., & Robinson, S. M. (2008). Effects of triglycerides, obesity, and starvation on ghrelin transport across the blood–brain barrier. *Peptides*, 29(11), 2061–2065.

Banks, W. A., & Kastin, A. J. (1998). Differential permeability of the blood–brain barrier to two pancreatic peptides: Insulin and amylin. *Peptides*, 19(5), 883–889.

Banks, W. A., Kastin, A. J., Maness, L. M., Huang, W., & Jaspan, J. B. (1995). Permeability of the blood–brain barrier to amylin. *Life Sciences*, 57(22), 1993–2001.

Barrachina, M. D., Martinez, V., Wang, L., Wei, J. Y., & Tache, Y. (1997). Synergistic interaction between leptin and cholecystokinin to reduce short-term food intake in lean mice. *Proceedings of the National Academy of Sciences of the USA*, 94(19), 10455–10460.

Batterham, R. L., & Bloom, S. R. (2003). The gut hormone peptide YY regulates appetite. *Annals of the New York Academy of Sciences*, 994, 162–168.

Batterham, R. L., Cowley, M. A., Small, C. J., Herzog, H., Cohen, M. A., Dakin, C. L., et al. (2002). Gut hormone PYY(3–36) physiologically inhibits food intake. *Nature*, 418(6898), 650–654.

Baura, G. D., Foster, D. M., Porte, D., Jr., Kahn, S. E., Bergman, R. N., Cobelli, C., et al. (1993). Saturable transport of insulin from plasma into the central nervous system of dogs in vivo. A mechanism for regulated insulin delivery to the brain. *Journal of Clinical Investigation*, 92(4), 1824–1830.

Begg, D. P., & Woods, S. C. (2012). The central insulin system and energy balance. In H.-G. Joost (Ed.), *Handbook of Experimental Pharmacology*, 209, 111–129.

Benoit, S. C., Clegg, D. J., Seeley, R. J., & Woods, S. C. (2004). Insulin and leptin as adiposity signals. *Recent Progress in Hormone Research*, 59, 267–285.

Blomqvist, A. G., & Herzog, H. (1997). Y-receptor subtypes—how many more? *Trends in Neurosciences*, 20(7), 294–298.

Boggiano, M. M., Chandler, P. C., Oswald, K. D., Rodgers, R. J., Blundell, J. E., Ishii, Y., et al. (2005). PYY3-36 as an anti-obesity drug target. *Obesity Reviews: An Official Journal of the International Association for the Study of Obesity*, 6(4), 307–322.

Boyle, C. N., Rossier, M. M., & Lutz, T. A. (2011). Influence of high-fat feeding, diet-induced obesity, and hyperamylinemia on the sensitivity to acute amylin. *Physiology and Behavior*, 104(1), 20–28.

Bray, G. A. (2014). Medical treatment of obesity: The past, the present and the future. *Best Practice and Research: Clinical Gastroenterology*, 28(4), 665–684.

Brown, L. M., Clegg, D. J., Benoit, S. C., & Woods, S. C. (2006). Intraventricular insulin and leptin reduce food intake and body weight in C57BL/6J mice. *Physiology and Behavior*, 89(5), 687–691.

Burks, D. J., Font de Mora, J., Schubert, M., Withers, D. J., Myers, M. G., Towery, H. H., et al. (2000). IRS-2 pathways integrate female reproduction and energy homeostasis. *Nature*, 407(6802), 377–382.

Castro, G. C., Areias, M. F., Weissmann, L., Quaresma, P. G., Katashima, C. K., Saad, M. J., et al. (2013). Diet-induced obesity induces endoplasmic reticulum stress and insulin resistance in the amygdala of rats. *FEBS Open Bio*, 3, 443–449.

Chapman, I., Parker, B., Doran, S., Feinle-Bisset, C., Wishart, J., Strobel, S., et al. (2005). Effect of pramlintide on satiety and food intake in obese subjects and subjects with type 2 diabetes. *Diabetologia*, 48(5), 838–848.

Chia, C. W., Carlson, O. D., Kim, W., Shin, Y. K., Charles, C. P., Kim, H. S., et al. (2009). Exogenous glucose-dependent insulinotropic polypeptide worsens post prandial hyperglycemia in type 2 diabetes. *Diabetes*, 58(6), 1342–1349.

Clark, J. T., Sahu, A., Kalra, P. S., Balasubramaniam, A., & Kalra, S. P. (1987). Neuropeptide Y (NPY)-induced feeding behavior in female rats: Comparison with human NPY ([Met17]NPY), NPY analog ([norLeu4]NPY) and peptide YY. *Regulatory Peptides*, 17(1), 31–39.

Clementi, G., Caruso, A., Cutuli, V. M., de Bernardis, E., Prato, A., & Amico-Roxas, M. (1996). Amylin given by central or peripheral routes decreases gastric emptying and intestinal transit in the rat. *Experientia*, 52(7), 677–679.

Cowley, M. A., Smith, R. G., Diano, S., Tschop, M., Pronchuk, N., Grove, K. L., et al. (2003). The distribution and mechanism of action of ghrelin in the CNS demonstrates a novel hypothalamic circuit regulating energy homeostasis. *Neuron*, 37(4), 649–661.

Crawley, J. N., & Beinfeld, M. C. (1983). Rapid development of tolerance to the behavioural actions of cholecystokinin. *Nature, 302*(5910), 703–706.

Cummings, D. E., Purnell, J. Q., Frayo, R. S., Schmidova, K., Wisse, B. E., & Weigle, D. S. (2001). A preprandial rise in plasma ghrelin levels suggests a role in meal initiation in humans. *Diabetes, 50*(8), 1714–1719.

Cummings, D. E., Weigle, D. S., Frayo, R. S., Breen, P. A., Ma, M. K., Dellinger, E. P., et al. (2002). Plasma ghrelin levels after diet-induced weight loss or gastric bypass surgery. *New England Journal of Medicine, 346*(21), 1623–1630.

Currie, P. J., Mirza, A., Fuld, R., Park, D., & Vasselli, J. R. (2005). Ghrelin is an orexigenic and metabolic signaling peptide in the arcuate and paraventricular nuclei. *American Journal of Physiology: Regulatory, Integrative, and Comparative Physiology, 289*(2), R353–R358.

Date, Y., Kojima, M., Hosoda, H., Sawaguchi, A., Mondal, M. S., Suganuma, T., et al. (2000). Ghrelin, a novel growth hormone-releasing acylated peptide, is synthesized in a distinct endocrine cell type in the gastrointestinal tracts of rats and humans. *Endocrinology, 141*(11), 4255–4261.

Daughters, R. S., Hofbauer, R. D., Grossman, A. W., Marshall, A. M., Brown, E. M., Hartman, B. K., et al. (2001). Ondansetron attenuates CCK induced satiety and c-fos labeling in the dorsal medulla. *Peptides, 22*(8), 1331–1338.

Delhanty, P. J., Neggers, S. J., & van der Lely, A. J. (2012). Mechanisms in endocrinology: Ghrelin—the differences between acyl- and des-acyl ghrelin. *European Journal of Endocrinology/European Federation of Endocrine Societies, 167*(5), 601–608.

Dickson, S. L., Shirazi, R. H., Hansson, C., Bergquist, F., Nissbrandt, H., & Skibicka, K. P. (2012). The glucagon-like peptide 1 (GLP-1) analogue, exendin-4, decreases the rewarding value of food: A new role for mesolimbic GLP-1 receptors. *Journal of Neuroscience, 32*(14).

Dossat, A. M., Lilly, N., Kay, K., & Williams, D. L. (2011). Glucagon-like peptide 1 receptors in nucleus accumbens affect food intake. *Journal of Neuroscience, 31*(41), 14453–14457.

Egecioglu, E., Jerlhag, E., Salome, N., Skibicka, K. P., Haage, D., Bohlooly, Y. M., et al. (2010). Ghrelin increases intake of rewarding food in rodents. *Addiction Biology, 15*(3), 304–311.

Emond, M., Schwartz, G. J., Ladenheim, E. E., & Moran, T. H. (1999). Central leptin modulates behavioral and neural responsivity to CCK. *American Journal of Physiology, 276*(5, Pt. 2), R1545–R1549.

Faulconbridge, L. F., Cummings, D. E., Kaplan, J. M., & Grill, H. J. (2003). Hyperphagic effects of brainstem ghrelin administration. *Diabetes, 52*(9), 2260–2265.

Fehmann, H. C., Weber, V., Goke, R., Goke, B., Eissele, R., & Arnold, R. (1990). Islet amyloid polypeptide (IAPP; amylin) influences the endocrine but not the exocrine rat pancreas. *Biochemical and Biophysical Research Communications, 167*(3), 1102–1108.

Flak, J. N., Patterson, C. M., Garfield, A. S., D'Agostino, G., Goforth, P. B., Sutton, A. K., et al. (2014). Leptin-inhibited PBN neurons enhance responses to hypoglycemia in negative energy balance. *Nature Neuroscience, 17*(12), 1744–1750.

Gadde, K. M. (2014). Current pharmacotherapy for obesity: Extrapolation of clinical trials data to practice. *Expert Opinion on Pharmacotherapy, 15*(6), 809–822.

Gibbs, J., Young, R. C., & Smith, G. P. (1973). Cholecystokinin decreases food intake in rats. *Journal of Comparative and Physiological Psychology, 84*(3), 488–495.

Glatzle, J., Sternini, C., Robin, C., Zittel, T. T., Wong, H., Reeve, J. R., Jr., et al. (2002). Expression of 5-HT3 receptors in the rat gastrointestinal tract. *Gastroenterology, 123*(1), 217–226.

Grill, H. J., & Hayes, M. R. (2012). Hindbrain neurons as an essential hub in the neuroanatomically distributed control of energy balance. *Cell Metabolism, 16*(3), 296–309.

Hay, D. L., Christopoulos, G., Christopoulos, A., & Sexton, P. M. (2004). Amylin receptors: Molecular composition and pharmacology. *Biochemical Society Transactions, 32*(Pt. 5), 865–867.

Hayes, M. R., Mietlicki-Baase, E. G., Kanoski, S. E., & De Jonghe, B. C. (2014). Incretins and amylin: Neuroendocrine communication between the gut, pancreas, and brain in control of food intake and blood glucose. *Annual Review of Nutrition, 34*, 237–260.

Hayes, M. R., Moore, R. L., Shah, S. M., & Covasa, M. (2004). 5-HT3 receptors participate in CCK-induced suppression of food intake by delaying gastric emptying. *American Journal of Physiology: Regulatory, Integrative and Comparative Physiology, 287*(4), R817–R823.

Hayes, M. R., Skibicka, K. P., Leichner, T. M., Guarnieri, D. J., DiLeone, R. J., Bence, K. K., et al. (2010). Endogenous leptin signaling in the caudal nucleus tractus solitarius and area postrema is required for energy balance regulation. *Cellular Metabolism, 11*(1), 77–83.

Heppner, K. M., Piechowski, C. L., Muller, A., Ottaway, N., Sisley, S., Smiley, D. L., et al. (2014). Both acyl and des-acyl ghrelin regulate adiposity and glucose metabolism via central nervous system ghrelin receptors. *Diabetes, 63*(1), 122–131.

Hilton, J. M., Chai, S. Y., & Sexton, P. M. (1995). In vitro autoradiographic localization of the calcitonin receptor isoforms, C1a and C1b, in rat brain. *Neuroscience, 69*(4), 1223–1237.

Holst, J. J. (2007). The physiology of glucagon-like peptide 1. *Physiological Reviews, 87*(4), 1409–1439.

Hosoda, H., Kojima, M., Matsuo, H., & Kangawa, K. (2000). Ghrelin and des-acyl ghrelin: Two major forms of rat ghrelin peptide in gastrointestinal tissue. *Biochemical and Biophysical Research Communications, 279*(3), 909–913.

James, W. P., Caterson, I. D., Coutinho, W., Finer, N., Van Gaal, L. F., Maggioni, A. P., et al. (2010). Effect of sibutramine on cardiovascular outcomes in overweight and obese subjects. *New England Journal of Medicine, 363*(10), 905–917.

Jones, I. R., Owens, D. R., Vora, J., Luzio, S. D., & Hayes, T. M. (1989). A supplementary infusion of glucose-dependent insulinotropic polypeptide (GIP) with a meal does not significantly improve the beta cell response or glucose tolerance in type 2 diabetes mellitus. *Diabetes Research and Clinical Practice, 7*(4), 263–269.

Jordan, J., Greenway, F. L., Leiter, L. A., Li, Z., Jacobson, P., Murphy, K., et al. (2008). Stimulation of cholecystokinin-A receptors with GI181771X does not cause weight loss in overweight or obese patients. *Clinical Pharmacology and Therapeutics, 83*(2), 281–287.

Kaiyala, K. J., Prigeon, R. L., Kahn, S. E., Woods, S. C., & Schwartz, M. W. (2000). Obesity induced by a high-fat diet is associated with reduced brain insulin transport in dogs. *Diabetes, 49*(9), 1525–1533.

Kamegai, J., Tamura, H., Shimizu, T., Ishii, S., Sugihara, H., & Wakabayashi, I. (2001). Chronic central infusion of ghrelin increases hypothalamic neuropeptide Y and agouti-related protein mRNA levels and body weight in rats. *Diabetes, 50*(11), 2438–2443.

Kanoski, S. E., Fortin, S. M., Ricks, K. M., & Grill, H. J. (2013). Ghrelin signaling in the ventral hippocampus stimulates learned and motivational aspects of feeding via PI3K-Akt signaling. *Biological Psychiatry, 73*(9), 915–923.

Keire, D. A., Bowers, C. W., Solomon, T. E., & Reeve, J. R., Jr. (2002). Structure and receptor binding of PYY analogs. *Peptides, 23*(2), 305–321.

Kim, E. M., Grace, M. S., Welch, C. C., Billington, C. J., & Levine, A. S. (1999). STZ-induced diabetes decreases and insulin normalizes POMC mRNA in arcuate nucleus and pituitary in rats. *American Journal of Physiology, 276*(5, Pt. 2), R1320–R1326.

Kojima, M., Hosoda, H., Date, Y., Nakazato, M., Matsuo, H., & Kangawa, K. (1999). Ghrelin is a growth-hormone-releasing acylated peptide from stomach. *Nature, 402*(6762), 656–660.

Kubota, N., Terauchi, Y., Tobe, K., Yano, W., Suzuki, R., Ueki, K., et al. (2004). Insulin receptor substrate 2 plays a crucial role in beta cells and the hypothalamus. *Journal of Clinical Investigation, 114*(7), 917–927.

Lampel, M., & Kern, H. F. (1977). Acute interstitial pancreatitis in the rat induced by excessive doses of a pancreatic secretagogue. *Virchows Archive A: Pathological Anatomy and Histology, 373*(2), 97–117.

Le Foll, C., Johnson, M. D., Dunn-Meynell, A., Boyle, C. N., Lutz, T. A., & Levin, B. E. (2014). Amylin-induced central IL-6 production enhances ventromedial hypothalamic leptin signaling. *Diabetes, 64*(5), 1621–1631.

Lundberg, J. M., Tatemoto, K., Terenius, L., Hellstrom, P. M., Mutt, V., Hokfelt, T., et al. (1982). Localization of peptide YY (PYY) in gastrointestinal endocrine cells and effects on intestinal blood flow and motility. *Proceedings of the National Academy of Sciences of the United States of America, 79*(14), 4471–4475.

Lutz, T. A. (2005). Pancreatic amylin as a centrally acting satiating hormone. *Current Drug Targets, 6*(2), 181–189.

Lutz, T. A. (2010). Roles of amylin in satiation, adiposity and brain development. *Forum of Nutrition, 63*, 64–74.

Lutz, T. A., Del Prete, E., & Scharrer, E. (1995). Subdiaphragmatic vagotomy does not influence the anorectic effect of amylin. *Peptides, 16*(3), 457–462.

Lutz, T. A., Mollet, A., Rushing, P. A., Riediger, T., & Scharrer, E. (2001). The anorectic effect of a chronic peripheral infusion of amylin is abolished in area postrema/nucleus of the solitary tract (AP/NTS) lesioned rats. *International Journal of Obesity and Related Metabolic Disorders, 25*(7), 1005–1011.

Lutz, T. A., Senn, M., Althaus, J., Del Prete, E., Ehrensperger, F., & Scharrer, E. (1998). Lesion of the area postrema/nucleus of the solitary tract (AP/NTS) attenuates the anorectic effects of amylin and calcitonin gene-related peptide (CGRP) in rats. *Peptides, 19*(2), 309–317.

Makovec, F., Bani, M., Cereda, R., Chiste, R., Revel, L., Rovati, L. C., et al. (1986). Protective effect of CR 1409 (cholecystokinin antagonist) on experimental pancreatitis in rats and mice. *Peptides, 7*(6), 1159–1164.

Mathis, C., Moran, T. H., & Schwartz, G. J. (1998). Load-sensitive rat gastric vagal afferents encode volume but not gastric nutrients. *American Journal of Physiology, 274*(2, Pt. 2), R280–R286.

Mazda, T., Yamamoto, H., Fujimura, M., & Fujimiya, M. (2004). Gastric distension-induced release of 5-HT stimulates c-fos expression in specific brain nuclei via 5-HT3 receptors in conscious rats. *American Journal of Physiology: Gastrointestinal Liver Physiology, 287*(1), G228–G235.

McAllister, E. J., Dhurandhar, N. V., Keith, S. W., Aronne, L. J., Barger, J., Baskin, M., et al. (2009). Ten putative contributors to the obesity epidemic. *Critical Reviews in Food Science and Nutrition, 49*(10), 868–913.

Medeiros, M. D., & Turner, A. J. (1994). Processing and metabolism of peptide-YY: Pivotal roles of dipeptidylpeptidase-IV, aminopeptidase-P, and endopeptidase-24.11. *Endocrinology, 134*(5), 2088–2094.

Mietlicki-Baase, E. G., & Hayes, M. R. (2014). Amylin activates distributed CNS nuclei to control energy balance. *Physiology and Behavior, 136*, 39–46.

Mietlicki-Baase, E. G., Ortinski, P. I., Rupprecht, L. E., Olivos, D. R., Alhadeff, A. L., Pierce, R. C., et al. (2013). The food intake-suppressive effects of glucagon-like peptide-1 receptor signaling in the ventral tegmental area are mediated by AMPA/kainate receptors. *American Journal of Physiology: Endocrinology and Metabolism, 305*(11), E1367–E1374.

Mietlicki-Baase, E. G., Reiner, D. J., Cone, J. J., Olivos, D. R., McGrath, L. E., Zimmer, D. J., et al. (2015). Amylin modulates the mesolimbic dopamine system to control energy balance. *Neuropsychopharmacology, 40*(2), 372–385.

Mietlicki-Baase, E. G., Rupprecht, L. E., Olivos, D. R., Zimmer, D. J., Alter, M. D., Pierce, R. C., et al. (2013). Amylin receptor signaling in the ventral tegmental area is physiologically relevant for the control of food intake. *Neuropsychopharmacology, 38*(9), 1685–1697.

Moran, T. H. (2006). Gut peptide signaling in the controls of food intake. *Obesity, 14*(Suppl. 5), 250S–253S.

Moran, T. H., Ladenheim, E. E., & Schwartz, G. J. (2001). Within-meal gut feedback signaling. *International Journal of Obesity and Related Metabolic Disorders, 25*(Suppl. 5), S39–S41.

Moran, T. H., & McHugh, P. R. (1982). Cholecystokinin suppresses food intake by inhibiting gastric emptying. *American Journal of Physiology, 242*(5), R491–R497.

Mordes, J. P., Liu, C., & Xu, S. (2015). Medications for weight loss. *Current Opinion in Endocrinology, Diabetes, and Obesity, 22*(2), 91–97.

Munzberg, H., Flier, J. S., & Bjorbaek, C. (2004). Region-specific leptin resistance within the hypothalamus of diet-induced obese mice. *Endocrinology, 145*(11), 4880–4889.

Myer, J. R., Romach, E. H., & Elangbam, C. S. (2014). Species- and dose-specific pancreatic responses and progression in single- and repeat-dose studies with GI181771X: A novel cholecystokinin 1 receptor agonist in mice, rats, and monkeys. *Toxicologic Pathology, 42*(1), 260–274.

Niswender, K. D., Morrison, C. D., Clegg, D. J., Olson, R., Baskin, D. G., Myers, M. G., Jr., et al. (2003). Insulin activation of phosphatidylinositol 3-kinase in the hypothalamic arcuate nucleus: A key mediator of insulin-induced anorexia. *Diabetes, 52*(2), 227–231.

Nonaka, N., Shioda, S., Niehoff, M. L., & Banks, W. A. (2003). Characterization of blood–brain barrier permeability to PYY3-36 in the mouse. *Journal of Pharmacology and Experimental Therapeutics, 306*(3), 948–953.

Norgren, R. (1983). The gustatory system in mammals. *American Journal of Otolaryngology, 4*(4), 234–237.

Ogawa, A., Harris, V., McCorkle, S. K., Unger, R. H., & Luskey, K. L. (1990). Amylin secretion from the rat pancreas and its selective loss after streptozotocin treatment. *Journal of Clinical Investigation, 85*(3), 973–976.

Olszewski, P. K., Li, D., Grace, M. K., Billington, C. J., Kotz, C. M., & Levine, A. S. (2003). Neural basis of orexigenic effects of ghrelin acting within lateral hypothalamus. *Peptides, 24*(4), 597–602.

Overduin, J., Frayo, R. S., Grill, H. J., Kaplan, J. M., & Cummings, D. E. (2005). Role of the duodenum and macronutrient type in ghrelin regulation. *Endocrinology, 146*(2), 845–850.

Paxinos, G., Chai, S. Y., Christopoulos, G., Huang, X. F., Toga, A. W., Wang, H. Q., et al. (2004). In vitro autoradiographic localization of calcitonin and amylin binding sites in monkey brain. *Journal of Chemical Neuroanatomy, 27*(4), 217–236.

Peters, J. H., Karpiel, A. B., Ritter, R. C., & Simasko, S. M. (2004). Cooperative activation of cultured vagal afferent neurons by leptin and cholecystokinin. *Endocrinology, 145*(8), 3652–3657.

Peters, J. H., Ritter, R. C., & Simasko, S. M. (2006). Leptin and CCK selectively activate vagal afferent neurons innervating the stomach and duodenum. *American Journal of Physiology: Regulatory, Integrative and Comparative Physiology, 290*(6), R1544–R1549.

Phelan, S., & Wadden, T. A. (2002). Combining behavioral and pharmacological treatments for obesity. *Obesity Research, 10*(6), 560–574.

Phillips, R. J., & Powley, T. L. (1996). Gastric volume rather than nutrient content inhibits food intake. *American Journal of Physiology, 271*(3, Pt. 2), R766–R769.

Powley, T. L., & Phillips, R. J. (2004). Gastric satiation is volumetric, intestinal satiation is nutritive. *Physiology and Behavior, 82*(1), 69–74.

Ravussin, E., Smith, S. R., Mitchell, J. A., Shringarpure, R., Shan, K., Maier, H., et al. (2009). Enhanced weight loss with pramlintide/metreleptin: An integrated neurohormonal approach to obesity pharmacotherapy. *Obesity, 17*(9), 1736–1743.

Reidelberger, R. D., Haver, A. C., Chelikani, P. K., & Buescher, J. L. (2008). Effects of different intermittent peptide YY (3–36) dosing strategies on food intake, body weight, and adiposity in diet-induced obese rats. *American Journal of Physiology: Regulatory, Integrative and Comparative Physiology, 295*(2), R449–R458.

Ritter, R. C. (2004). Gastrointestinal mechanisms of satiation for food. *Physiology and Behavior, 81*(2), 249–273.

Rodgers, R. J., Tschop, M. H., & Wilding, J. P. (2012). Anti-obesity drugs: Past, present and future. *Disease Models and Mechanisms, 5*(5), 621–626.

Rosenbaum, M., Kissileff, H. R., Mayer, L. E., Hirsch, J., & Leibel, R. L. (2010). Energy intake in weight-reduced humans. *Brain Research, 1350*, 95–102.

Roth, J. D., Roland, B. L., Cole, R. L., Trevaskis, J. L., Weyer, C., Koda, J. E., et al. (2008). Leptin responsiveness restored by amylin agonism in diet-induced obesity: Evidence from nonclinical and clinical studies. *Proceedings of the National Academy of Sciences of the USA, 105*(20), 7257–7262.

Sadry, S. A., & Drucker, D. J. (2013). Emerging combinatorial hormone therapies for the treatment of obesity and T2DM. *Nature Reviews: Endocrinology, 9*(7), 425–433.

Schmitz, O., Brock, B., & Rungby, J. (2004). Amylin agonists: A novel approach in the treatment of diabetes. *Diabetes, 53*(Suppl. 3), S233–S238.

Schwartz, G. J., McHugh, P. R., & Moran, T. H. (1993). Gastric loads and cholecystokinin synergistically stimulate rat gastric vagal afferents. *American Journal of Physiology, 265*(4, Pt. 2), R872–R876.

Schwartz, G. J., & Moran, T. H. (1996). Sub-diaphragmatic vagal afferent integration of meal-related gastrointestinal signals. *Neuroscience and Biobehavioral Reviews, 20*(1), 47–56.

Schwartz, M. W., Marks, J. L., Sipols, A. J., Baskin, D. G., Woods, S. C., Kahn, S. E., et al. (1991). Central insulin administration reduces neuropeptide Y mRNA expression in the arcuate nucleus of food-deprived lean (Fa/Fa) but not obese (fa/fa) Zucker rats. *Endocrinology, 128*(5), 2645–2647.

Schwartz, M. W., Sipols, A. J., Marks, J. L., Sanacora,

G., White, J. D., Scheurink, A., et al. (1992). Inhibition of hypothalamic neuropeptide Y gene expression by insulin. *Endocrinology, 130*(6), 3608–3616.

Sexton, P. M., Paxinos, G., Kenney, M. A., Wookey, P. J., & Beaumont, K. (1994). In vitro autoradiographic localization of amylin binding sites in rat brain. *Neuroscience, 62*(2), 553–567.

Shuto, Y., Shibasaki, T., Otagiri, A., Kuriyama, H., Ohata, H., Tamura, H., et al. (2002). Hypothalamic growth hormone secretagogue receptor regulates growth hormone secretion, feeding, and adiposity. *Journal of Clinical Investigation, 109*(11), 1429–1436.

Silva, A. P., Cavadas, C., & Grouzmann, E. (2002). Neuropeptide Y and its receptors as potential therapeutic drug targets. *Clinica Chimica Acta, 326*(1–2), 3–25.

Singh-Franco, D., Robles, G., & Gazze, D. (2007). Pramlintide acetate injection for the treatment of type 1 and type 2 diabetes mellitus. *Clinical Therapeutics, 29*(4), 535–562.

Sloth, B., Davidsen, L., Holst, J. J., Flint, A., & Astrup, A. (2007). Effect of subcutaneous injections of PYY1–36 and PYY3–36 on appetite, ad libitum energy intake, and plasma free fatty acid concentration in obese males. *American Journal of Physiology: Endocrinology and Metabolism, 293*(2), E604–E609.

Smith, G. P., Jerome, C., & Norgren, R. (1985). Afferent axons in abdominal vagus mediate satiety effect of cholecystokinin in rats. *American Journal of Physiology, 249*(5, Pt. 2), R638–R641.

Tatemoto, K. (1982). Isolation and characterization of peptide YY (PYY), a candidate gut hormone that inhibits pancreatic exocrine secretion. *Proceedings of the National Academy of Sciences of the USA, 79*(8), 2514–2518.

Teubner, B. J., & Bartness, T. J. (2013). Anti-ghrelin Spiegelmer inhibits exogenous ghrelin-induced increases in food intake, hoarding, and neural activation, but not food deprivation-induced increases. *American Journal of Physiology: Regulatory, Integrative and Comparative Physiology, 305*(4), R323–R333.

Thomas, D. M., Bouchard, C., Church, T., Slentz, C., Kraus, W. E., Redman, L. M., et al. (2012). Why do individuals not lose more weight from an exercise intervention at a defined dose?: An energy balance analysis. *Obesity Reviews, 13*(10), 835–847.

Toshinai, K., Yamaguchi, H., Sun, Y., Smith, R. G., Yamanaka, A., Sakurai, T., et al. (2006). Des-acyl ghrelin induces food intake by a mechanism independent of the growth hormone secretagogue receptor. *Endocrinology, 147*(5), 2306–2314.

Tschop, M., Castaneda, T. R., Joost, H. G., Thone-Reineke, C., Ortmann, S., Klaus, S., et al. (2004). Physiology: Does gut hormone PYY3–36 decrease food intake in rodents? *Nature, 430*(6996), 165.

Tschop, M., Smiley, D. L., & Heiman, M. L. (2000). Ghrelin induces adiposity in rodents. *Nature, 407*(6806), 908–913.

Tschop, M., Wawarta, R., Riepl, R. L., Friedrich, S., Bidlingmaier, M., Landgraf, R., et al. (2001). Postprandial decrease of circulating human ghrelin levels. *Journal of Endocrinological Investigation, 24*(6), RC19–RC21.

Turek, V. F., Trevaskis, J. L., Levin, B. E., Dunn-Meynell, A. A., Irani, B., Gu, G., et al. (2010). Mechanisms of amylin/leptin synergy in rodent models. *Endocrinology, 151*(1), 143–152.

Vetter, M. L., Faulconbridge, L. F., Webb, V. L., & Wadden, T. A. (2010). Behavioral and pharmacologic therapies for obesity. *Nature Reviews: Endocrinology, 6*(10), 578–588.

Willesen, M. G., Kristensen, P., & Romer, J. (1999). Co-localization of growth hormone secretagogue receptor and NPY mRNA in the arcuate nucleus of the rat. *Neuroendocrinology, 70*(5), 306–316.

Woods, S. C., & Langhans, W. (2012). Inconsistencies in the assessment of food intake. *American Journal of Physiology: Endocrinology and Metabolism, 303*(12), E1408–E1418.

Woods, S. C., Seeley, R. J., Baskin, D. G., & Schwartz, M. W. (2003). Insulin and the blood–brain barrier. *Current Pharmaceutical Design, 9*(10), 795–800.

Woods, S. C., Stein, L. J., McKay, L. D., & Porte, D., Jr. (1984). Suppression of food intake by intravenous nutrients and insulin in the baboon. *American Journal of Physiology, 247*(2, Pt. 2), R393–R401.

Yang, J., Brown, M. S., Liang, G., Grishin, N. V., & Goldstein, J. L. (2008). Identification of the acyltransferase that octanoylates ghrelin, an appetite-stimulating peptide hormone. *Cell, 132*(3), 387–396.

CHAPTER 3

Energy Expenditure and Obesity

Kara L. Marlatt
Eric Ravussin

Throughout history, humans and animals have evolved to exhibit complex mechanisms that regulate energy homeostasis, or the energy intake and energy expenditure required to maintain body weight. However, what was once an evolutionary asset has become a liability in the current "pathoenvironment" or "obesogenic" environment (Ravussin, 1995). The "thrifty genotype" was thought to enable individuals to efficiently collect and process food to deposit fat during periods of food abundance, so that periods of food shortage were offset (feast and famine) (Neel, 1962). These once historically advantageous genes have now become a detriment in the modern obesogenic world where famine never occurs. Recently, the "thrifty genotype" hypothesis has been challenged by Speakman (2007), who offers an alternative explanation to the theory of obesity susceptibility, called the *predation release* hypothesis. Speakman argues that around 2 million years ago, predation was removed as a significant factor by the development of social behaviors, weapons, and fire. The absence of predation led to a change in the population distribution of body fatness due to random mutations and genetic drift. According to Speakman, such random drift, rather than directed selection, explains why some individuals are able to remain thin while living in an obesogenic environment.

Regardless of the origin of the genetic predisposition to obesity, obesity has reached epidemic proportions, with rates more than doubling over the last 40 years in both industrialized countries and in urbanized populations around the world. This epidemic is the result of a normal physiology (genetic variability) in a pathoenvironment (Figure 3.1). The Centers for Disease Control and Prevention reported that 35.0% of men and 40.4% of women in the United States were obese in 2013–2014. Importantly, the prevalence of obesity has more than doubled in children and quadrupled in adolescents in the past 30 years (National Center for Health Statistics Report, 2012), with approximately 18% of children and 21% of teenagers reported as obese and more than one-third of children and adolescents reported as overweight or obese (National Center for Health Statistics Report, 2012). As a result, the World Health Organization has identified obesity as one of the major emerging chronic diseases.

Obesity results from a chronic imbalance between energy intake and energy expenditure, where energy intake exceeds energy expenditure over an extended period of time. In order to understand and better treat indi-

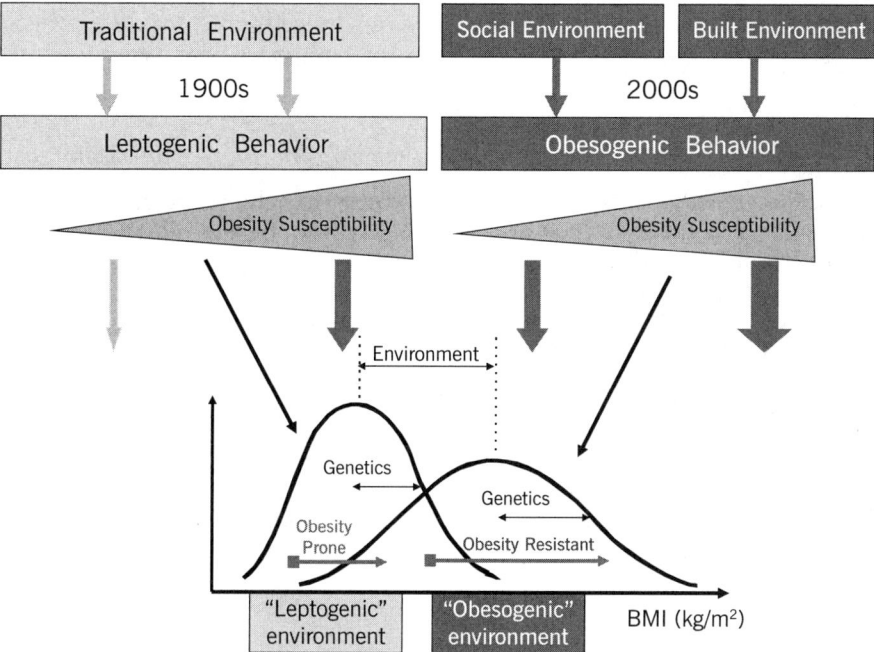

FIGURE 3.1. The potential effect of genes and environment on adiposity assessed by body mass index (BMI). Some of the concepts described in this figure were originally proposed by Bouchard (2007). Our environment has evolved over the past century from a "traditional" environment to a new "westernized" environment. The left part of the figure presents the "traditional" environment in which food was rather scarce and energy expenditure was high, mostly related to occupational physical activity. Such an environment leads to "leptogenic" behaviors in which the variability of BMI will be dependent on individuals' genetic propensity to weight gain. On the right part of the figure, the modern "social" and "built" environment, characterized by plenty of cheap high-calorie density food and little need for physical activity, leads to "obesogenic" behaviors. Similarly, the variability in BMI will also depend on the genetic propensity to weight gain of individuals. Compared with the "leptogenic" environment, the distribution of BMI will have a higher mean and higher standard deviation. Such a paradigm can be applied to populations with similar genetic backgrounds living in drastically different environments like the Pima Indians in Arizona and in Mexico.

viduals who currently suffer from obesity or any complications associated with chronic energy balance, we need to understand the metabolic factors underlying the interindividual variability of energy metabolism. We know that weight gain is characterized by a combination of increased energy (food) intake and/or reduced energy expenditure. We also know that a variety of metabolic characteristics, such as a low metabolic rate or low rates of fat oxidation, can exacerbate the susceptibility to weight gain in humans beyond just imbalances between energy intake and energy expenditure. Although dietary intake assessment can be assessed in free-living conditions, this measure is not accurate and is usually imprecise. Conversely, dietary intake assessment in a laboratory setting is also not ideal because it does not mimic normal habitual daily intake. Research scientists, therefore, have concentrated on the contributions of energy expenditure to understand overall energy balance. This chapter reviews the concepts of energy balance, substrate utilization, and balance; methods by which energy expenditure can be measured in humans; and the components of daily energy expenditure, their inherent interindividual variability, and their contribution to weight gain in adults. Finally, recent advances in our understanding of some of the molecular mechanisms underlying the regulation of energy expenditure are discussed.

Energy Balance Equations

The balance between energy intake (dietary calories consumed) and energy expenditure (calories burned) determines energy stores (and body weight) (Figure 3.2). Since living organisms must obey the first law of thermodynamics, energy balance equations are used to predict changes in body weight when energy intake or expenditure is changed. The classic equation of energy balance, which states that energy stored by the body is equal to energy intake minus energy expenditure, has provided new insight and confusion in the understanding of energy balance in humans. Indeed, much of the confusion comes from inappropriate energy calculations using the static equation of energy balance.

Equations during Weight Maintenance

In order to achieve weight maintenance (stability), both of the following equations must be true:

Energy intake = Energy expenditure   (3.1)

Macronutrient intake   (3.2)
(protein, carbohydrate, fat) =
Macronutrient oxidation
(protein, carbohydrate, fat)

These equations are quite accurate under conditions of weight maintenance, as only

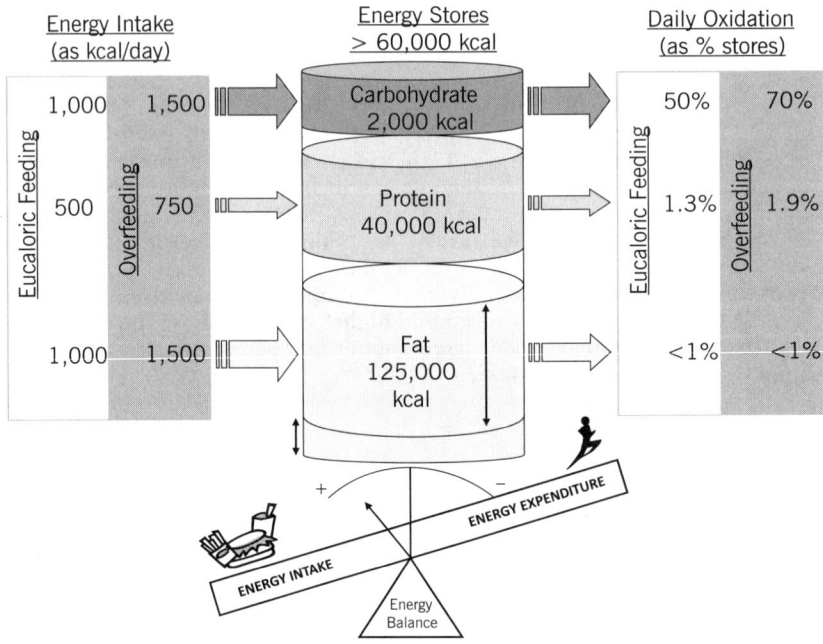

FIGURE 3.2. The daily energy and nutrient balance of a 70-kg man (20% body fat) in relationship to macronutrient energy stores, intake, and oxidation. Each macronutrient intake and oxidation on a 2,500 kcal/day standard American diet (i.e., 40% fat, 40% carbohydrate, and 20% protein) is shown on the left as absolute intake in kilocalories and on the right as a percentage of its respective nutrient body store. Because carbohydrate, protein, and alcohol intakes and oxidation rates are tightly regulated on a daily basis, any inherent differences between energy intake and energy expenditure predominantly impact body fat stores. During overfeeding, the oxidation of carbohydrate and protein is increased to compensate for the increased intake at the expense of fat intake, yet the increase in oxidation is not equally coupled with intake. Thus, if sustained fat kilocalories are stored, fat stores will expand and body weight will increase.

limited changes in body composition are possible without changing body weight. These simple weight maintenance equations have been most useful in uncovering problems with reported energy intake.

Most dietary intake studies show either no correlation or a negative correlation between energy intake and body weight (Heymsfield et al., 1995). This finding is in marked contrast to the findings in studies of energy expenditure, which show a positive relationship between the two. In addition to their greater fat mass, obese individuals have a greater fat-free mass (FFM), which is the main determinant of both basal (resting) metabolic rate (BMR) and 24-hour metabolic rate as measured in a respiratory chamber (Ravussin, Lillioja, Anderson, Christin, & Bogardus, 1986). Studies involving free-living individuals have simultaneously measured energy expenditure via the doubly labeled water technique and energy intake via continuous recording of diet diaries (Mertz et al., 1991). Under these careful conditions of food intake assessment, obese individuals reported only 50–67% of their total energy intake; by contrast, lean individuals reported 80–100%. This gap between the food that people who are obese perceive themselves to eat and what they actually eat has been termed the *eye–mouth gap*. It represents a major challenge for psychologists interested in obesity and food intake behaviors.

Static Energy Balance Equation

During energy imbalance, the most common equation used by scientists in the calculation of energy balance is

Change in energy stores = (3.3)
Energy intake − Energy expenditure

However, Alpert (1990) elegantly demonstrated that this equation is inadequate for calculating the energy needs of living organisms, because it does not take into account the increasing energy expenditure with increasing weight or the reverse during weight loss (Jequier & Schutz, 1983; Ravussin et al., 1986). Thus, a small initial increase in energy intake sustained over a number of years cannot lead to a large weight gain, as is often claimed. Therefore, a more dynamic equation is necessary to capture time-dependent factors related to weight gain.

Dynamic Energy Balance Equation

Indeed, the most valid equation to use is dynamic and states that

Rate of change of energy stores = (3.4)
Rate of energy intake −
Rate of energy expenditure

The use of *rates* in this equation introduces time dependency, thereby allowing the effect of changing energy stores (especially FFM and weight) on energy expenditure to enter into the calculation (Alpert, 1990). This explains why a small initial positive energy balance (e.g., from an increased energy intake or a decrease in physical activity) will not lead to large weight increases over a number of years. After a period of positive energy balance, the energy stores (fat mass and FFM) will increase and cause an increase in energy expenditure, which will balance the increased energy intake. The individual will then, once again, be in energy balance, but with a higher energy intake, higher energy expenditure, and higher energy stores. Weight gain can therefore be viewed not only as the consequence of an initial positive energy balance but also as the mechanism by which energy balance is eventually restored. Importantly, the "3,500 kilocalories (kcal) per pound" rule, a static weight loss concept that states that cutting food intake by 3,500 kcal results in 1 pound of weight loss, has recently been challenged (Thomas et al., 2013). Indeed, the 3,500 kcal per pound concept ignores dynamic physiological adaptations that occur as a result of altered body weight (Leibel, Rosenbaum, & Hirsch, 1995); specifically, both resting metabolic rate (RMR) and the energy cost of physical activity decrease in response to weight loss, thus resisting further weight loss. A more accurate assessment of the amount and time course of predicted weight change is very valuable (Hall et al., 2011; Thomas et al., 2013). Furthermore, a more dynamic model has postulated that every permanent change of energy intake of 100 kilojoules (kJ) per day will lead to an eventual weight change of about 1 kg (equivalently, 10 kcal/day per pound of weight change), and that it will take about 1 year to achieve half of the total weight change and 3 years to achieve 95% of the total weight change (Hall et al., 2011).

How is intake balanced against expenditure, and how might a chronic mismatch between the two occur? A fruitful approach to these questions has been to dissect the energy balance equation into its various macronutrients.

Substrate Balance

If the origins of a positive energy balance lie in the chronic imbalance of energy intake and expenditure, an appropriate question is: "What conditions allow a long-lasting imbalance between intake and expenditure?" An examination of each nutrient balance equation to determine whether a chronic imbalance between nutrient intake and oxidation exists is only valid if each macronutrient has a separate balance equation, implying separate regulation (Figure 3.2). In practical terms, is each macronutrient either oxidized or stored in its own compartment (separate regulation), or does it get converted into another compartment for storage? This question applies particularly to the issue of whether dietary carbohydrate is stored as fat (de novo lipogenesis). In contrast to animals, de novo lipogenesis is very limited in humans and occurs only when large excesses of carbohydrate are ingested (Acheson, Schutz, Bessard, Flatt, & Jequier, 1987; Acheson et al., 1988). Because de novo lipogenesis is quite negligible in humans under physiological conditions, it seems reasonable to consider each nutrient balance equation as a separate entity.

Protein Balance

Protein intake usually accounts for about 15% of daily consumed calories, and the protein stores in the body represent approximately one-third of the total calories in a man weighing 70 kg. The daily protein intake amounts to a little over 1% of the total protein stores (Bray, 1991; Snyder et al., 1975) (Figure 3.2). The protein stores increase in size in response to such growth stimuli as growth hormone, androgens, physical training, and weight gain, but have been thought to *not* increase simply from increased dietary protein. Protein stores are thus thought to be tightly controlled; protein balance is achieved on a day-to-day basis (Abbott et al., 1988). Nonetheless, a recent study did demonstrate that 8 weeks of protein overfeeding (25%) resulted in increased body protein (lean body mass) of 3.18 kg (Bray et al., 2012). Although protein imbalance cannot be implicated with certainty as a direct cause of obesity, protein intake may affect the fat balance equation (Snyder et al., 1975).

Carbohydrate Balance

Carbohydrate is usually the main source of dietary calories, yet the body stores of glycogen are very limited: 500–1,000 g on average (Acheson et al., 1988). Daily intake of carbohydrate corresponds to about 50–100% of the carbohydrate stores, compared to about 1% for protein or fat (Schutz, Flatt, & Jequier, 1989) (Figure 3.2); therefore, over a period of hours and days, the carbohydrate stores fluctuate markedly compared to those of protein and fat. However, as with protein stores, carbohydrate stores are tightly controlled (Rising, Keys, Ravussin, & Bogardus, 1992). Whether this control is based on humoral and/or nervous signals exchanged between the muscle and liver and the brain remains to be established. Dietary carbohydrate stimulates both glycogen storage and glucose oxidation and suppresses fat oxidation (Flatt, Ravussin, Acheson, & Jequier, 1985). That which is not stored as glycogen is oxidized (not converted to fat), and carbohydrate balance is achieved (Abbott et al., 1988; Flatt et al., 1985). Therefore, as with the other nonfat nutrients, a chronic imbalance between carbohydrate intake and oxidation cannot be the basis of weight gain. Storage capacity is limited and controlled; conversion to fat is an option that occurs only under extreme conditions in humans.

Fat Balance

In marked contrast to the other nutrients, body fat stores are large, and fat intake has very little influence on fat oxidation (Flatt et al., 1985; Schutz et al., 1989). As with protein, the daily fat intake represents less than 1% of the total energy stored as fat, but the fat stores contain about six times the energy of the protein stores (Bray, 1991) (Figure 3.2). These fat stores are the energy buffer for the body, and the slope of the relationship between energy balance and fat balance is almost 1 in conditions of day-to-day small positive or negative energy balances (Abbott et al., 1988). A deficit of 200 kcal of energy over 24 hours means that 200 kcal must come from fat stores, whereas an excess of 200 kcal of energy means that 200 kcal are deposited in fat stores. Even in conditions of spontaneous overfeeding, the entire excess fat intake is stored as body fat (Rising, Alger, et al., 1992). Ingestion of a mixed meal is followed by an increase in carbohydrate oxidation and a decrease in fat oxidation, and the addition of extra fat does not alter the mix of nutrient oxidation (Flatt et al., 1985; Schutz et al., 1989). What does promote fat oxidation, if it is not dietary fat intake? The amount of total body fat exerts a small but significant effect on fat oxidation. Therefore, progressive increase in body fat levels may represent a mechanism for the attenuation of the rate of fat storage and, thus, weight gain (Zurlo, Larson, et al., 1990). Energy balance is the driving force for fat oxidation (Abbott et al., 1988; Zurlo, Lillioja, et al., 1990); when it is negative (i.e., energy expenditure exceeding intake), fat oxidation increases. Indeed, a recent study of obese adults showed that selectively reducing dietary fat compared to carbohydrate for 6 days in an isocaloric setting resulted in significant increases in fat oxidation following carbohydrate restriction, where fat oxidation by fat restriction was unchanged yet resulted in significantly greater body fat loss than carbohydrate restriction (Hall et al., 2015).

In summary, when one considers energy balance in humans under physiological conditions, fat is the only nutrient that maintains a chronic imbalance between intake and oxidation, thus directly contributing to the increase in adipose mass. The other nutrients will indirectly influence adiposity by their contribution to overall energy balance, and thus to fat balance, as emphasized by Frayn (1995). The use of the fat balance equation instead of the energy balance equation offers a new framework for understanding the pathogenesis of obesity.

Alcohol Balance

There is an inconsistent relationship between reported alcohol intake and body mass index, with many studies showing a negative relationship (Sayon-Orea, Martinez-Gonzalez, & Bes-Rastrollo, 2011). However, it has been shown that in healthy individuals, the fate of ingested alcohol is oxidation and not storage (as fat). Thus, perfect alcohol balance is achieved (Shelmet et al., 1988) in a matter of hours. In the same manner as dietary carbohydrate and protein, alcohol diverts dietary fat away from oxidation and toward storage and inhibits lipolysis. Therefore, alcohol contributes to overall energy balance by indirectly impacting fat balance.

Methods of Measuring Energy Expenditure

Several methods have been developed to measure daily energy expenditure in humans. The most accurate methods involve continuous measurement of heat output (direct calorimetry) or gas exchange (indirect calorimetry) in individuals confined to small metabolic chambers. Confined individuals, however, are unable to pursue habitual activities, and hence several field methods have been developed to measure energy expenditure in free-living conditions. These include doubly labeled water, self-reports, and portable monitors.

Direct Calorimetry

Heat, water, and carbon dioxide are the ultimate fate of all the body's metabolic processes, and energy expenditure, therefore, can be measured directly as total heat loss. First described in the late 1800s by Zuntz and Hagerman, direct calorimetry involves placing an individual in a small, insulated chamber in which all the heat released in the form of dry heat (radiation and convection heat losses, ~80%) or evaporative heat (from the evaporation of water from the skin and lungs, ~20%) is measured. This method has been applied to various animal and human studies, but has become largely obsolete because these studies are expensive to conduct and require individuals to be confined in a very small room.

Indirect Calorimetry

The term *indirect calorimetry* arises from the premise that heat released from the metabolic processes in the body can be indirectly measured from oxygen consumption. Under normal physiological conditions, neither oxygen nor carbon dioxide is stored within the body; therefore, an indirect method of assessing energy expenditure is to measure oxygen consumption, carbon dioxide production, and nitrogen excretion. Indirect calorimetry has proved useful for the study of energy expenditure and/or substrate oxidation in normal and diseased states and can be measured using open-circuit or closed-circuit systems.

Importantly, open-circuit indirect calorimetry provides a relatively simple way to measure oxygen consumption at rest and during exercise. It is typically performed using a mouthpiece, mask, or canopy taking measurements of oxygen and carbon dioxide percentages in the inspired and expired air. During the last three decades, the indirect calorimetry method has been applied to respiratory (or metabolic) chambers. These are rooms large enough (12,000–40,000 liters) for an individual to live comfortably for up to several days. The measurements from the chamber are accurate and are now used extensively to assess the determinants of daily sedentary energy expenditure in humans. Respiratory chambers enable us to measure the different components of energy expenditure, including the sleeping metabolic rate, the energy cost of arousal, the thermic effect of food (TEF), and the energy cost of spontaneous physical activity (SPA) (Figure 3.3). The only disadvantage is the confinement of the subjects in a relatively small room, which reduces energy expenditure from physical activity. With an average coefficient of variation (CV) of 1–3% (Donahoo, Levine, & Melanson, 2004), respiratory chambers are used as the gold standard to validate newer methods of measuring energy expenditure, such as doubly labeled water

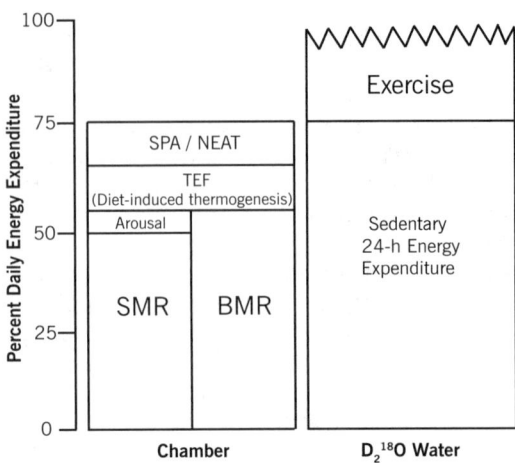

FIGURE 3.3. Total daily energy expenditure is comprised of three major physiological compartments: (1) *basal metabolic rate* (BMR) (60–70%) includes the energy cost required to maintain the integrated systems of the body and homeostatic temperature at rest, and can be divided into sleeping metabolic rate (SMR) and the energy cost of arousal; (2) *thermic effect of food* (TEF) (10%) is the increase in energy cost associated with the digestion, absorption, and storage of food; and (3) *activity thermogenesis* (20–30%) is the energy expended during volitional (structured exercise) and nonvolitional activities. The latter is termed spontaneous physical activity (SPA) or nonexercise activity thermogenesis (NEAT). This includes the energy cost of sitting, maintaining posture, fidgeting, shopping, etc. Total daily energy expenditure and its components can be measured in free-living conditions using the doubly labeled water ($D_2^{18}O$ Water) method. The left panel indicates the measurement of daily energy expenditure for 24 hours in an indirect room calorimeter and the right panel depicts the total daily energy expenditure measured over 7–10 days using the doubly labeled water method in free-living conditions.

(Ravussin, Harper, Rising, & Bogardus, 1991; Schoeller et al., 1986).

Doubly Labeled Water

Developed by Lifson, the doubly labeled water (DLW) method is a form of "indirect" calorimetry (Lifson, 1966). It is based on the differential elimination of two nonradioactive isotopes, deuterium (^2H) and

^{18}oxygen (^{18}O), from body water following a single oral dose of the two isotopes. Oxygen tagged with the ^{18}O tracer will equilibrate not only in body water but also in circulating bicarbonate and expired carbon dioxide. Over time, the ^{18}O tracer in body water will decrease as CO_2 is expired and water is lost in respiration, perspiration, and urine. The hydrogen molecule tagged with the ^{2}H tracer will distribute only in the circulating water and bicarbonate, and over time will decrease as water is lost. The elimination rates of the two isotopes from the body are measured by isotope ratio mass spectroscopy in blood, saliva, or most commonly urine. The difference between the elimination rates (^{18}O − ^{2}H) of the two isotopes therefore provides a measure of carbon dioxide production from which total daily energy expenditure (TDEE) can be calculated from classical indirect calorimetry equations (Schoeller et al., 1986). The major advantage of the DLW method is that it provides an integrated measure of total carbon dioxide production over periods of 1–2 weeks, yet requires only periodic sampling of blood, saliva, or most commonly, urine, for measurements of ^{2}H and ^{18}O enrichments. Importantly, the DLW method allows individuals to be studied in the free-living state without being influenced or limited in their activity by wearing cumbersome monitors. The DLW technique has been validated repeatedly with excellent accuracy (1–3%) and precision (3–8%) against the gold standard indirect calorimetry (Ravussin et al., 1991; Schoeller et al., 1986).

In conjunction with other determinations of resting energy expenditure using indirect calorimetry, DLW is the best and most accurate way of assessing the energy cost of physical activity in humans. The major drawbacks of the method are the high costs of the ^{18}O isotope for large clinical trials, the mass spectrometer necessary to determine the isotopic enrichments of ^{2}H and ^{18}O, and the inability to quantify substrate oxidation.

Questionnaires and Activity Logs

An individual's habitual and occupational physical activity can also be captured with the use of activity diaries, questionnaires, interviews, or time and motion studies, with the energy cost of the activities estimated from energy expenditure tables. This method is called the *factorial method*. The energy cost of each activity is then estimated from energy-equivalent tables and multiplied by the time spent in any given activity. This method, therefore, is extremely time-consuming for individuals and investigators. Substantial variability with the technique has been reported, which is due to poor and inaccurate recall by individuals, as well as to the availability of numerous energy coefficients that can be applied to determine the energy cost of the activities.

Portable Devices with the Future of Smart Devices

Pedometers and accelerometers are devices worn by an individual to quantify movement. Pedometers assess displacement of the body with a single stride, and the output represents steps taken or steps/day. Because they are relatively cheap, pedometers are commonly used by individuals, researchers, and practitioners to monitor physical activity. Accelerometers, on the other hand, are devices that detect body displacement in terms of acceleration. Accelerometers can assess movements via piezoelectric sensors in a single plane, usually vertical (uniaxial accelerometer), or within three planes, anterior–posterior, medio–lateral, and vertical (triaxial accelerometer). Accelerometers are worn on the wrist or more commonly on the hip or waist. They capture the duration and intensity of activities and can provide data storage for a number of days, which can be downloaded directly to a computer (Westerterp & Plasqui, 2004). The triaxial devices tend to provide the best precision and correlation with activity energy expenditure measured by indirect calorimetry and doubly labelled water (Bonomi, Goris, Yin, & Westerterp, 2009). With the inability of the free-living assessments of energy expenditure to differentiate between the type, intensity, and duration of activities, several laboratories have begun to incorporate the use of multiple accelerometers on various body parts (Foerster & Fahrenberg, 2000; Levine et al., 2005). These studies have proven that multiple accelerometers can quantify varying activities and posture allocations.

Components of Energy Expenditure and Their Relevance to Human Obesity

TDEE varies substantially in humans (Black, Coward, Cole, & Prentice, 1996), such that two adults of the same size could have an EE that varies by 1,500 kcal/day. The largest determinants of TDEE are weight (specifically FFM and fat mass), height, age, and sex (Black et al., 1996). Whereas both height and weight are positively associated with higher TDEE, older age is negatively associated with TDEE in adults. Across all ages, TDEE is approximately 11% higher in males, after adjustments for body size (Black et al., 1996). With the increasing prevalence of obesity, understanding the inherent interindividual variation in TDEE is important. The variability in daily energy requirements is related to the variability in the energy expended in its three major components: (1) BMR, (2) TEF (or diet-induced thermogenesis), and (3) the energy cost of physical activity (or *activity thermogenesis,* including both exercise and nonexercise components) (Figure 3.3).

Further contributing to an individual's overall metabolic rate are the specific individual metabolic rates of major organs and tissues. Indeed, differences in organ and tissue mass contribute to differences in resting energy expenditure between underweight, overweight, and obese individuals (Bosy-Westphal et al., 2014). Studies also have reported distinct trends for reduced specific organ and tissue metabolic rates and, thus, lower resting energy expenditures at identical organ masses. This has been observed in both obese versus lean individuals and older versus younger individuals, an effect that can be explained by either lower cellularity or lower specific metabolic rates of the respective organs and tissues (Wang et al., 2010, 2012).

Basal Metabolic Rate

The BMR is the energy expended by an individual who is resting, yet awake and fasted, in comfortable ambient conditions. Under standard conditions, BMR is measured using the ventilated hood technique while the participant is awake and resting in a thermo-neutral environment (i.e., temperatures between 28° and 33° C) following an 8- to 12-hour fast and at least 12 hours of abstinence from exercise, smoking, and caffeine. BMR accounts for approximately 60–70% of daily energy expenditure in sedentary adults (Ravussin et al., 1986) and is therefore the largest component of TDEE. There is a close relationship between BMR and body size, and this association has led to the development of widely used equations to predict BMR from height and weight, based on the classical Harris and Benedict equation proposed in 1919 (Harris & Benedict, 1919), the Schofield equation in 1985 (Schofield, 1985), and many others (e.g., Cunningham, 1991; Mifflin et al., 1990). Up to three-quarters of the variance in BMR is determined by FFM (Bogardus et al., 1986; Tataranni & Ravussin, 1995) and to a lesser extent by fat mass, sex, and age. Together, these four components explain 80–85% of the interindividual variance in BMR (Bogardus et al., 1986; Tataranni & Ravussin, 1995). Interestingly, 11% of the remaining variance can be further explained by family membership; therefore, we know that genetic factors also influence the variability in BMR (Bogardus et al., 1986). It is important to mention that FFM is not metabolically uniform, since it is composed of different tissue and organs, and thus will have tissue or organ-specific metabolic rates contributing to further variability in measured BMR (Elia, 1992; Muller et al., 2011).

Interestingly, BMR adjusted for differences in FFM, fat mass, and age is related to the variability in body temperature (Rising, Keys, et al., 1992). Such results indicate that body temperature could be a marker for a high or low relative metabolic rate. Some of the variability in BMR has also been shown to be related to variability in muscle sympathetic nerve activity (Spraul et al., 1993). Resting skeletal muscle metabolism also seems to be a significant determinant of whole-body metabolism (Zurlo, Larson, Bogardus, & Ravussin, 1990), and studies suggest that uncoupling protein 3 (UCP3) expression (Schrauwen, Xia, Bogardus, Pratley, & Ravussin, 1999) and uncoupling protein 2 (UCP2) polymorphisms (Kovacs et al., 2005) appear to underlie some of this variability.

Thermic Effect of Food

TEF is the increase in energy expenditure associated with the chewing, digestion, absorption, and storage of food in response to a single meal. By contrast, diet-induced thermogenesis (DIT) is the increase in energy expenditure not accounted for by the increase in body weight after days or weeks of overfeeding. TEF and DIT are often confused in the literature. The TEF is the smallest component of daily energy expenditure, accounting for approximately 5–15% of TDEE (Donahoo et al., 2004; Tataranni, Larson, Snitker, & Ravussin, 1995). The TEF is, however, the most difficult and least reproducible component of energy expenditure to measure, and therefore its role in the etiology of obesity is controversial. In contrast to BMR with a CV of 3–8%, the CV of TEF measured with indirect calorimetry is typically around 20% (Tataranni et al., 1995). The measurement of TEF is performed in response to a test meal, either continuously or intermittently for 3–6 hours, under similar conditions as BMR. A comprehensive review of 49 studies comparing TEF in lean versus obese individuals reported that obesity was associated with an impaired TEF and was related to the degree of insulin resistance (de Jonge & Bray, 1997). However, Granata and Brandon (2002) identified substantial shortcomings in the methods used to calculate TEF, questioning the role of low TEF in the development of obesity.

The measurement of TEF is influenced by a myriad of factors, including meal size and delivery, nutrient composition (protein exerts higher TEF), palatability of the meal, and meal frequency, as well as an individual's genetic background, age, physical activity, and sensitivity to insulin (de Jonge & Bray, 1997; Granata & Brandon, 2002). Importantly, prospective studies have not identified a relationship between TEF and weight change (Tataranni et al., 1995). Furthermore, TEF recently has been shown to increase significantly with higher dietary protein intake, yet no differences in metabolic adaptation across levels of dietary protein were observed (Sutton, Bray, Burton, Smith, & Redman, 2016). It is safe to say that a decrease in TEF amounts to only a small number of calories and, therefore, is very unlikely to explain significant degrees of obesity.

In distinction to the TEF (energy expenditure increase in response to a single meal), DIT is the cumulative response to prolonged overfeeding. In classical studies conducted more than 3 decades ago, Rothwell and Stock (1979) reported that overfeeding resulted in less weight gain than anticipated. The fact that the predicted weight gain was observed when animals were given propranolol suggested that the activation of the sympathetic system was the mediator of the DIT, in concert with an increase in brown adipose tissue (BAT) mass. Over the past few years, it has been debated whether BAT can be stimulated in humans to induce a larger DIT and can therefore be involved in the resistance to weight gain in some individuals. However, our recent data in humans seem to indicate that unlike cold-induced thermogenesis (CIT), DIT is probably not mediated by BAT in humans (Peterson et al., 2016). Additionally, we recently found that BAT did not mediate metabolic adaptation following 8 weeks of overfeeding in men, and BAT activity did not correlate with metabolic adaptation or with body weight (Peterson et al., 2017).

Activity Thermogenesis

Activity thermogenesis, defined as body movement produced by skeletal muscle, is the most variable component of TDEE. It comprises two distinct types of energy expenditure: (1) the energy expended during exercise or structured physical activity (normally planned activities); and (2) the energy expended in all other nonexercise activities (normally unplanned activities). The latter activity, originally described as SPA (Ravussin et al., 1986) and subsequently called nonexercise activity thermogenesis (NEAT; Levine, Eberhardt, & Jensen, 1999), includes activities such as the energy cost of sitting, standing, maintaining posture, talking, fidgeting, and performing leisure activities such as playing guitar, shopping, etc.

Activity thermogenesis can account for a significant number of calories in very active people. However, sedentary adult individuals exhibit a range of physical activity, which represents only 20–30% of total energy expenditure. Therefore, the hypothesis that reduced physical activity is the cause of the worldwide obesity epidemic is an obvious and attractive one. Nonetheless, the amount of structured physical activity has remained relatively stable over the years, thereby leaving occupational physical activity to have even greater potential to impact energy balance. Indeed, physical activity energy expenditure, as examined in one European study, demonstrated no significant decline over a similar time period of increased obesity, supporting the argument that reduced energy expenditure due to lower physical activity expenditure is unlikely to have fueled the obesity epidemic (Westerterp & Speakman, 2008).

Indeed, for the vast majority of people living in developed countries, exercise-related activity thermogenesis is becoming negligible (with the exception of devoted exercisers). Therefore, for most people NEAT is the predominant component of activity thermogenesis. Furthermore, NEAT is the most variable component of TDEE, varying by 200 kcal/day (Levine, 2007) and may, therefore, be a determinant of body weight control.

Some of the most carefully controlled studies examining the role of NEAT in weight gain have been performed by Levine and colleagues, who found that resistance to the development of obesity may be related to the ability of individuals to increase NEAT (Levine et al., 1999; Levine, 2007). In response to overfeeding (1,000 kcal/day), participants who were able to increase NEAT gained the least fat mass, whereas changes in BMR and TEF did not predict changes in fat gain (Levine et al., 1999). In a follow-up study, Levine et al. (2005) attempted to identify whether there was a defect in NEAT in obese individuals. Using an integrated system of microsensors in undergarments to assess body posture and movements for 10 days, they found that obese individuals remained seated 2.5 hours longer than lean individuals, equivalent to an energy surplus of approximately 350 kcal/day. Next, they examined whether weight loss in the obese participants and weight gain in the lean would reverse this usual pattern of posture allocation. Similar to previous studies (e.g., Zurlo et al., 1992), they showed that both the lean and obese groups maintained their original posture allocation, suggesting that some of the interindividual variation in NEAT is probably explained by genetic factors (Levine et al., 2005). Taken together, these studies suggest that NEAT in our daily environment may be significant but is unlikely to be a real target for managing weight control.

Normalizing Energy Expenditure Data in Humans According to Body Size

Regardless of the technique used to measure daily energy expenditure, adjustment for metabolic body size is essential for valid interpretation of the data. Traditionally, investigators have used the ratio method and simply divided energy expenditure by the amount of metabolic mass (body weight, FFM of surface area), which leads to erroneous results (Goran, 2005; Ravussin & Bogardus, 1989) because this method fails to take into account the non-zero intercept in the relationship between energy expenditure and metabolic mass. As a consequence, the adjusted metabolic rate is artificially increased as the FFM decreases. An alternative and more valid approach is a regression-based approach that derives prediction equations from simple available measures (FFM, fat mass [FM], sex, and age) to determine size-adjusted energy expenditure (Goran, 2005; Ravussin & Bogardus, 1989). As one would expect, the method chosen for normalization of metabolic size is particularly crucial when assessing the effects of an intervention (weight loss, drug intervention, etc.) on energy expenditure.

Metabolic Risk Factors for Body Weight Gain

Cross-sectional studies that compare lean and obese individuals have not added as much as longitudinal studies to our understanding of the physiological mechanisms predisposing individuals to weight gain (Ravussin & Swinburn, 1996). An understanding of the etiology of human obesity demands longitudinal studies to reveal predictors or risk factors. Several studies have prospectively examined these predictors in the Pima Indian population in Arizona, a population in which obesity is extremely prevalent (Knowler et al., 1991) and, therefore, weight gain is common in young adults. Indeed, the Pimas are one of the most obese populations in the world, with the highest reported prevalence of type 2 diabetes (Knowler et al., 1991). As such, they provided opportunities to examine predictors of weight gain. In these individuals at least six metabolic parameters have been found to be associated with (and probably predictive of) weight gain. In particular, low metabolic rate, low activity thermogenesis, low sympathetic nervous system (SNS) activity, and low fat oxidation are related to energy expenditure and relevant to understanding the etiology of obesity.

Low Metabolic Rate

Obesity is associated with a high absolute metabolic rate, both in resting conditions and over 24 hours (Ravussin et al., 1986). Whether a low energy metabolism is involved or not in the propensity to gain weight is, however, still controversial (Flatt, 2007). One of the reasons for this controversy may be related to the way that energy expenditure is compared in people of different body sizes. It is obvious that BMR is higher in obese individuals in absolute terms, but when adjusted for differences in body size (i.e., BMR divided by body weight, surface area, FFM, or even adjusted for body size by multiple regression analysis), the results are not always clear. Indeed, there is wide variability in the association between metabolic rate and body size, such that two individuals with the same FFM and FM can still differ in metabolic rate by up to 500 kcal/day (Ravussin, 1993).

In 126 adult nondiabetic Pima Indians, body composition and metabolic rate (measured with a ventilated hood) were assessed at baseline and follow-up 4 years later, on average (Ravussin et al., 1988). Using an arbitrary definition of weight gain of 10 kg, subjects were divided retrospectively into gainers and non-gainers. Despite the gainers and non-gainers having similar body composition at baseline, the gainers had metabolic rates that were 100 kcal/day lower than the non-gainers, suggesting that a low "relative" metabolic rate predicts weight gain. This possibility was further supported by tertile analysis in the whole group, demonstrating that the risk of weight gain at follow-up was approximately seven times greater in subjects with the lowest metabolic rate compared to those with the highest metabolic rate (Ravussin et al., 1988). In another group of 95 Pima Indians in whom 24-hour energy expenditure was measured in a metabolic chamber, 24-hour energy expenditure adjusted for body size, age, and sex correlated negatively with the change in body weight and rate of change in body weight 2 years later (Ravussin et al., 1988), a relationship that was not found in all other populations (Katzmarzyk, Perusse, Tremblay, & Bouchard, 2000).

Taken together, the results demonstrate that low rates of energy expenditure (adjusted for body size, age, and sex) are significant predictors of weight gain, at least in a population prone to obesity. Most interestingly, in response to weight gain, the mean adjusted metabolic rate of individuals who gained weight became similar to the mean adjusted metabolic rate of individuals who remained weight-stable. This finding implies that weight gain may be a compensatory mechanism that results in an increased rate of energy expenditure, engaging a mechanism of resistance to further weight gain. This *metabolic adaptation*, defined as a greater than predicted increase in energy expenditure beyond changes in FM and FFM, is highly variable between individuals and occurs in both lean and obese individuals. Similarly, a reduction in energy expenditure in response to weight loss can counteract further weight loss or even predispose to weight regain (Johanssen et al., 2012). Specifically, individuals who participated in a nationally televised weight loss competition (*The Biggest Loser*), which consisted of an intensive exercise program in combination with calorie restriction, exhibited dramatic slowing of resting metabolism out of proportion with weight loss (i.e., metabolic adaptation), despite relative preservation of FFM (Johanssen et al., 2012). Surprisingly, such metabolic adaptation persisted 6 years after the initial weight loss (~500 kcal/day lower than expected) (Fothergill et al., 2016). Indeed, metabolic adaptation is thought to counter weight loss and contribute to weight regain and energy restabilization (Rosenbaum & Leibel, 2010).

Importantly, a low metabolic rate explains a relatively low percentage of the variance in weight gain, and therefore other factors such as excessive energy intake and reduced activity levels are likely culprits (Tataranni et al., 2003). The recent report that greater decreases in energy expenditure during caloric restriction predicted less weight loss in subsequent weight reduction attempts confirms the presence of "thrifty" and "spendthrift" phenotypes in obese humans and their role in weight control (Reinhardt et al., 2015). Interestingly, one study found that energy expenditure responses to both fasting and overfeeding conditions within individuals are correlated, and that it is not so much a response to calorie restriction but, rather, the response to protein restriction that defines the thrifty phenotype (Schlögl et al., 2015). Another study (Bray et al., 2012) demonstrated the critical role of protein and how metabolism responds to an imposed (and presumably restricted) calorie load. Specifically, with respect to increases in body fat, calories were found to be more important than protein when consuming excess amounts of energy (Bray et al., 2012).

Low Activity Thermogenesis

The energy cost of exercise and NEAT accounts for 10–20% of TDEE. The most variable component of activity thermogenesis is NEAT, also known as SPA (Zurlo et al., 1992). Using whole-room calorimetry, longitudinal studies in the Pima Indians demonstrated that SPA, defined as the percentage of time that subjects were active in the chamber, accounted for a significant portion of 24-hour energy expenditure in males and females (Zurlo et al., 1992). Fifty-seven percent of the variance in SPA was related to family membership (i.e., probably to genetic background). Furthermore, SPA correlated inversely with the rate of weight change assessed 3 years later in males but not in females (Zurlo et al., 1992). The confined environment of a respiratory chamber does not reflect physical activity levels in free-living conditions. However, physical activity measured in a respiratory chamber correlated with habitual physical activity level assessed by doubly labeled water in 50 nondiabetic Pima Indians (Snitker, Tataranni, & Ravussin, 2001). Several longitudinal studies have clearly demonstrated the association between reduced NEAT/SPA and weight gain (Levine et al., 2005; Snitker et al., 2001). Whether a similar association exists for habitual or structured physical activity is not clear (Wareham, van Sluijs, & Ekelund, 2005; Westerterp & Speakman, 2008). A study of 92 nondiabetic Pima Indians showed that physical activity level (assessed by doubly labeled water) was not associated with changes in body weight 4 years later (Tataranni et al., 2003).

Low SNS Activity

Reduced SNS plays a causative role in several models of obesity in rodent models (Bray, York, & Fisler, 1989). In humans, SNS activity can be directly measured in the muscle by microneurographic recordings (Spraul et al., 1993). Studies indicate that muscle sympathetic nervous activity (MSNA) correlates well with indirect measures of SNS activity (plasma norepinephrine turnover) and is independently related to TDEE and to each of the major components of energy expenditure: that is, RMR (Spraul et al., 1993), TEF (Schwartz, Jaeger, & Veith, 1988), and SPA (Christin, O'Connell, Bogardus, Danforth, & Ravussin, 1993). SNS activity is also negatively correlated with the 24-hour respiratory quotient (Snitker, Tataranni, & Ravussin, 1998).

Cross-sectional studies indicate that the obesity-prone Pima Indians have lower rates of TDEE preceding weight gain (Ravussin et al., 1988) as well as reduced SNS (Spraul et al., 1993). Together, these two factors may represent potential mechanisms predisposing Pima Indians to body weight gain. Indeed, baseline SNS activity (24-hour urinary epinephrine excretion rates) was negatively associated with weight gain at a 3-year follow-up (Tataranni, Young, Bogardus, & Ravussin, 1997). Importantly, beta-blocker treatment is often associated with a 0.5–3.5 kg increase in body weight after 6–12 months of treatment compared with other antihypertensive agents (Sharma, Pischon, Hardt, Kunz, & Luft, 2001). Further indications of the possible role of SNS activity in the regulation of energy balance in humans come from a study showing that low SNS activity was associated with a poor weight loss outcome in obese individuals treated with a dietary restriction intervention (Spraul et al., 1993).

Low Fat Oxidation

The choice of nutrient substrate (carbohydrate vs. fat) used for oxidation may be an important factor in the etiology of obesity. The respiratory quotient ($RQ = VCO_2/VO_2$) reflects the ratio of carbohydrate to fat oxidation and can vary between ~0.7 after an overnight fast when fat is the primary substrate, up to values close to 1.0 after a high-carbohydrate meal when glucose is the principal energy substrate (Flatt et al., 1985). Apart from the obvious impact of diet composition, RQ is also influenced by recent energy balance (i.e., negative balance causing more fat oxidation), sex (i.e., females tend to have reduced fat oxidation), adiposity (i.e., higher fat mass leads to higher fat oxidation), and family membership, suggesting a genetic component to RQ (Zurlo, Lillioja, et al., 1990).

Low fat oxidation has been suggested to be a factor in the development of obesity. In 111 Pima Indians, 24-hour RQ (measured in a metabolic chamber) was correlated with subsequent changes in body weight and FM at follow-up 3 years later. In fact, individuals in the top 90th percentile for RQ—that is, "low fat oxidizers"—had a 2.5 times greater risk of gaining 5 kg or more of body weight compared to individuals in the bottom 10th percentile of RQ—that is, "high fat oxidizers" (Zurlo, Lillioja, et al., 1990). This effect was independent of a relatively low or high 24-hour metabolic rate. In support of these observations, others have demonstrated that postobese volunteers have high RQs—that is, low rates of fat oxidation (Larson, Ferraro, Robertson, & Ravussin, 1995)—and those who are able to maintain weight loss have lower RQs compared to those experiencing weight relapse (Froidevaux, Schutz, Christin, & Jequier, 1993). Furthermore, a dietary shift to a high-fat, low-carbohydrate diet with a failure to compensate for the positive fat balance with increased energy expenditure or decreased food intake has been previously evaluated (Smith, de Jonge, Zachwieja, Roy, et al., 2000). Interestingly, concurrent physical activity has also been shown to increase fat oxidation during the shift to a high-fat diet (Smith, de Jonge, Zachwieja, Nguyen, et al., 2000).

Low Plasma Concentration of Leptin

Leptin, the product of the *OB* gene, is a hormone produced by the adipose tissue that inhibits food intake and increases energy expenditure (Caro, Sinha, Kaloczynski, Zhang, & Considine, 1997). To investigate whether individuals prone to weight gain are hypoleptinemic, we measured fasting plasma leptin concentrations in two groups of weight-matched, nondiabetic Pima Indians and followed their weight change for approximately 3 years. Nineteen individuals subsequently gained weight (average weight gain 23 kg), and 17 maintained their weight within 0.5 kg. After adjustment for initial percent body fat, mean plasma leptin concentration was lower in those who gained weight than in those whose weight was stable (Ravussin et al., 1997). Despite the leptin resistance apparent in obesity (Caro et al., 1997), these data indicate that relatively low plasma leptin concentrations may play a role in the development of obesity in some Pima Indians. Interestingly, declines in circulating leptin contributed to the degree of metabolic adaptation and therefore may be a trigger toward weight regain (Knuth et al., 2014).

In summary, cross-sectional studies have not been informative about the determinants of weight gain, since low metabolic rate, low activity energy expenditure, low SNS activity, low fat oxidation, and low plasma leptin concentration are all predictive of weight gain, whereas people with obesity have high metabolic rate, high energy expenditure for activity, high SNS activity, high fat oxidation, and high plasma leptin concentration.

An alternative and important hypothesis about the mechanisms of weight gain has been postulated as being directly related to the carbohydrate–insulin model (Ludwig & Friedman, 2014), which postulates that diet composition matters. The prevailing hypothesis suggests that environmental influences, such as poor dietary habits and sedentary lifestyle, alongside genetic predisposition, result in fat storage and ultimately can lead to obesity. By contrast, the recently proposed carbohydrate–insulin model of obesity posits that genetic and lifestyle factors alongside diet quality, especially habitual consumption of a high-carbohydrate diet with abundant simple sugars, sequesters fat within adipose tissue due to hyperinsulinemia and thereby results in adaptive suppression of energy expenditure and increased hunger and appetite. Both hypotheses are important to consider, and future studies will yield more fruitful conclusions about this debate.

In an initial study by Ebbeling and colleagues (2012), participants achieved a 10–15% weight loss during a run-in diet, followed by the presentation, in random order, of isocaloric diets that were low-fat, low-glycemic-index, or very-low-carbohydrate in macronutrient composition. Each diet was consumed for 4 weeks. Among the study's overweight and obese young adults, compared with pre-weight-loss energy expenditure, the isocaloric diets resulted in decreases in resting energy expenditure (REE) and total energy expenditure (TEE) that were greatest with the low-fat diet, intermediate with the low-glycemic-index diet, and least with the very-low-carbohydrate diet. Conversely, a recent study by Hall et al. (2016) found that an isocaloric ketogenic diet was not accompanied by increased body fat loss but was associated with a relatively small increase in energy expenditure (57 ± 13 kcal/day) that was near the limits of detection using state-of-the-art technology. Indeed, Hall et al. (2016) suggested that the data did not support the increased energy expenditure of ~300–600 kcal/day reported in the prior studies (Ebbeling et al., 2012). Further investigation is needed to fully elucidate the conclusions of these studies.

Metabolic Adaptation

Studies in adult Pima Indians have allowed us to identify metabolic risk factors of body weight gain such as a relatively low metabolic rate, low SPA, and a high RQ. We have also observed that upon gaining weight, the original abnormal state becomes normalized. Because the change in metabolic risk factors is greater than the cross-sectional data would predict, this may be a mechanism to counteract further weight gain.

Changes in metabolic factors that are not explained by changes in body weight and composition are the hallmark of metabolic adaptation. The concept of metabolic adaptation was introduced in 1950 by the pioneering work of Ancel Keys, who defined the drop in energy expenditure observed in healthy men in response to semi-starvation as a useful adjustment to changed circumstances (Keys, Brozek, Henschel, Mickelsen, & Taylor, 1950). A definition of adaptation was proposed in the 1985 FAO/WHO/UNU report as "a process by which a new or different steady state is reached in response to a change or difference in the intake of food and nutrients" (United Nations University, 2018). Results from most overfeeding studies indicate that short-term experimental weight gain is accompanied by an overcompensatory increase in energy expenditure (Tremblay, Despres, Theriault, Fournier, & Bouchard, 1992). A study by Levine et al. (1999) found that most of the overcompensatory response may be due to an increase in NEAT. A recent study suggests that metabolic adaption may be a function of the amount of protein that is consumed in the overfeeding (Bray et al., 2015). Similarly, most underfeeding studies reveal that in the short term, intentional weight loss leads to a decrease in energy expenditure beyond predicted values (Johanssen et al., 2012). Therefore, there is substantial evidence that metabolic adaptation occurs in response to large perturbations in body weight over a relatively short period of time, but it is unknown whether similar adaptive mechanisms also operate in response to long-term weight changes in free-living conditions.

We examined longitudinal changes in energy expenditure and RQ associated with spontaneous long-term weight change in Pima Indians (Weyer et al., 2000). Results indicated that metabolic adaptation does occur in response to spontaneous long-term weight change, but the magnitude of the adaptive changes is small, and the interindividual variability is large. Based on these and other data, we have developed a theoretical model to explain how metabolic propensity to obesity (or resistance to weight loss) might thus depend not only on initial rates of energy expenditure and fat oxidation, but also on how these measures change in response to weight change (Reinhardt et al., 2015).

Molecular Mechanisms of Energy Expenditure Variability and Avenues for Treatment

Leptin

Leptin is a hormone, secreted predominantly by adipocytes, which binds primarily to receptors in the hypothalamus (and in the entire central nervous system) as a "lipostat," and which plays a key role in regulating long-term energy homeostasis and the body's energy stores. Zhang, Proenca, Maffei, Barone, Leopold, et al. (1994) described the genetic mutation that caused massive obesity in *ob/ob* mice. Mice homozygous for the *ob* mutation completely lack the presence of circulating leptin, and these animals develop severe, early-onset obesity, with many associated metabolic and hormonal abnormalities, including hyperphagia, defective thermogenesis, infertility, and type 2 diabetes. Subsequent experiments demonstrated that these metabolic and physiological abnormalities were rapidly corrected by leptin administration, which caused significant reductions in food intake and increased energy expenditure, resulting in weight loss after only a few days of leptin administration (Pelleymounter et al., 1995). These findings led to optimism that leptin therapy might be important for treating human obesity. The human gene encoding leptin has been screened in a large number of obese individuals, and a growing number of families have been shown to have mutations resulting in complete leptin deficiency (Farooqi & O'Rahilly, 2014). Indeed, humans with the *ob* mutation lack circulating levels of leptin and therefore develop severe, early-onset obesity with associated metabolic and behavioral consequences, including hyperphagia, defective thermogenesis, and type 2 diabetes. Leptin replacement therapy using daily subcutaneous injections has been shown to completely reverse these symptoms in patients with congenital leptin deficiency, as well as lipodystrophy, largely through the dramatic weight loss that occurs in these patients (Martos et al., 2006). Treatment of three known leptin-deficient adults (with a functional recessive mutation in the leptin gene), using recombinant human leptin for 3 months, resulted in drastic changes in energy metabolism with normalization of energy expenditure and large increases in fat oxidation (Galgani et al., 2010).

These early findings in leptin-deficient patients suggested that administering leptin to obese patients would be a stand-alone solution for the treatment of obesity. Unfortunately, this theory was short-lived. In 1999, a randomized controlled trial of daily subcutaneous recombinant leptin injection was performed in 54 lean and 73 obese subjects. In the initial phase of the study lasting 4 weeks, lean and obese subjects lost similar amounts of weight with leptin (Heymsfield et al., 1999). Obese subjects were studied for a further 20 weeks. Of the 47 patients who completed the study, the eight receiving the highest dose of leptin lost 7.1 kg, whereas the placebo lost 1.3 kg. However, this weight change varied widely among patients, from a loss of about 15 kg to a gain of 5 kg in the group treated with the highest dose. Moreover, these doses induced skin irritation and swelling at the injection site in 62% of patients and headache in half the patients. The use of leptin therapy as a panacea for obesity was a failure. However, leptin replacement therapy may be more pertinent for patients during weight loss maintenance. In calorie-restricted animals and humans, exogenous leptin administration has been shown to reverse the metabolic adaptation induced by caloric restriction and restore energy expenditure, catecholamine and thyroid hormone levels, and skeletal muscle efficiency back to baseline values (Rosenbaum, Murphy, Heymsfield, Matthews, & Leibel, 2002; Rosenbaum et al., 2005). Some of our recent studies (Johanssen et al., 2012; Knuth et al., 2014) showed drastic metabolic adaptations (i.e., drop in BMR beyond what was expected on the basis of the losses in fat-free and fat masses) in response to massive weight losses with bariatric surgery (201 ± 182 kcal/day) or by intensive behavioral changes in the *The Biggest Losers* contestants (504 ± 171 kcal/day). Interestingly, the metabolic adaptation was strongly related to the decrease in plasma leptin concentration. As previously mentioned, metabolic adaptation is thought to counter weight loss and contribute to weight regain and energy restabilization (Muller & Bosy-Westphal, 2013; Rosenbaum et al., 2010), yet Fothergill et al. (2016) found that metabolic adaptation following weight loss in *The Biggest Loser* was not associated with weight regain.

Beta-3-Adrenergic Receptors

Beta-3-adrenergic receptor (beta-3-AR) agonists are very effective thermogenic and anti-obesity and insulin-sensitizing agents in rodents, with the main sites of action in skeletal muscle (Astrup, Bulow, Madsen, & Christensen, 1985) as well as white (Foster & Frydman, 1978) and brown (Schiffelers, Brouwer, Saris, & van Baak, 1998) adipocytes. Mice lacking beta-3-ARs have a modest increase in body fat, indicating that beta-3-ARs play a role in regulating energy balance. Acute treatment of normal animals with beta-3-selective agonists leads to increased serum free fatty acid (FFA) and insulin levels, increased whole-body energy expenditure, and decreased food intake. When these agonists were administered to beta-3-AR-/- mice, each of these effects was completely absent, indicating that these responses are mediated exclusively by beta-3-ARs (Susulic et al., 1995). Testing in humans with the first generation of beta-3-AR agonists (BRL 26830A and CL 316243) revealed promising anti-diabetic and anti-obesity effects on energy metabolism (Weyer, Tataranni, Snitker, Danforth, & Ravussin, 1998). However, some of these compounds shared substantial selectivity with the beta-1- and beta-2-AR subtypes, inducing some undesired effects. The second generation of beta-3-ARs had improved selectivity but poor oral availability or pharmokinetics. Given these problems, we are not aware of any beta-3-ARs that have progressed beyond Phase II clinical trials. However, given the recent findings that BAT is present in adult humans (Cypess et al., 2009; van Marken Lichtenbelt et al., 2009; Virtanen et al., 2009), the potential of beta-3-AR agonists for increasing the amount and activity of BAT is an active area of exploration.

Uncoupling Proteins and Activation of BAT and Beiging

Discovered in 1978, uncoupling protein 1 (or UCP1) is only expressed in BAT and plays an important role in thermogenesis in rodents. The uncoupling proteins (UCPs) gene, and especially *UCP1*, encodes for mitochondrial protein carriers, which uncouples respiration from adenosine triphosphate (ATP) production, thereby stimulating heat production. Therefore, activation of such proteins may decrease metabolic efficiency and thus help in weight control. *UCP1* was generally believed not to play a major role in energy balance, as adults were thought to have very little BAT stores. However, recent studies using positron emission tomography (PET) with 2-deoxy-2-[fluorine-18]-fluorodeoxyglucose integrated with computed tomography (CT) (^{18}F-FDG PET/CT) revealed the presence of BAT in adult humans, with a prevalence estimated to be between 2 and 100% (closer to 100%).

The two other mitochondrial UCPs that were discovered later, UCP2 (widely distributed in a variety of tissues) and UCP3 (abundantly expressed in skeletal muscle), did not turn out to be targets for obesity management (Clapham et al., 2000; Schrauwen, Xia, Bogardus, et al., 1999). Specifically, phenotypes of mice in which UCP3 genes have been inactivated do not indicate that these homologues have a function in regulating either body temperature or body weight (Arsenijevic et al., 2000; Zhang et al., 2001). In one study in which UCP3 was overexpressed in skeletal muscle of transgenic mice, the mice showed a resistance to diet-induced obesity and an improvement in insulin sensitivity (Clapham et al., 2000). Since the amount of UCP3 in the muscle of the transgenic mice was at a level that had been shown previously, by the same group of investigators, to be toxic to the mitochondria of mammalian cells, it is possible that the mitochondria of the transgenic mice were leaky due to toxicity from the high levels of UCP3 (Stuart, Harper, Brindle, Jekabsons, & Brand, 2001). Consequently, the effects of the UCP3 transgene expression were not indicative of a normal physiological function. A recent study in which UCP3 was induced in human muscle by a high-fat diet, and then the rate of recovery of energy stores (i.e., creatine phosphate) was determined, failed to find an effect, suggesting that UCP3 in humans does not uncouple muscle mitochondria (Hesselink et al., 2003). It is interesting to note that a genetic variation at UCP2–UCP3 is associated with low metabolic rate in Pima Indians (Walder et al., 1998). However, whether UCPs play a significant role in human obesity remains to be established.

Currently, there is intense investigation into mechanisms for stimulating existing BAT or to induce BAT (or beiging) in white adipose tissue (WAT) as a means of promoting thermogenesis and energy expenditure (Tam, Lecoultre, & Ravussin, 2012). Both BAT and WAT make up the adipose organ. WAT is the primary site of energy storage and of release of hormones and cytokines that modulate whole-body metabolism and insulin resistance (Ronti, Lupattelli, & Mannarino, 2006; Rosen & Spiegelman, 2006). On the other hand, BAT is important for both basal and inducible energy expenditure in the form of thermogenesis, mediated by the expression of the tissue-specific UCP1 and the abundance of mitochondria (contributing to a brown appearance). BAT affects whole-body metabolism and may alter insulin sensitivity (Yang, Enerbäck, & Smith, 2003) and modify susceptibility to weight gain. Whereas an abundance of BAT was originally thought to exist only in newborns and hibernating animals, within the last decade BAT has been (re)discovered in the anterior neck and thorax region of adult humans undergoing PET and CT scanning (Cypess et al., 2009; Enerbäck, 2010; van Marken Lichtenbelt et al., 2009; Virtanen et al., 2009).

Besides the results reported by Cypress et al. (2009), two other independent publications reported in a comprehensive manner the presence of BAT in adult humans (van Marken Lichtenbelt et al., 2009; Virtanen et al., 2009). Virtanen and colleagues (2009) used ^{18}F-FDG in combination with PET/CT technologies to examine five subjects during cold exposure (2 hours at 17–19° C; one of the subject's feet was placed intermittently in ice water 5–9° C for 5 minutes) and warm conditions. In response to cold, a 15-fold increase in FDG uptake in the supraclavicular area was observed. WAT and BAT biopsies were taken from three of the volunteers to measure the expression of informative genes for cellular origin. Increased expression of UCP1, deiodinase iodothyronine type II (DIO2), peroxisome proliferator-activated receptor gamma (PPARγ) coactivator 1 alpha (or PGC1α), protein domain containing 16 (PRDM16), beta-3-AR, and cytochrome c were observed in BAT versus WAT from surrounding areas. Van Marken Lichtenbelt et al. (2009) used a similar approach in a larger group of subjects (10 lean, 14 overweight/obese) and found increased FDG uptake, potentially attributable to BAT activity, in the neck, supraclavicular region, chest, and abdomen. Importantly, the activity of BAT was approximately fourfold higher in the lean group than in the overweight/obese group. These same investigators reported a positive association between BMR and BAT activity at thermoneutrality or during cold exposure, whereas an inverse association between BAT amount/activity and BMI was found. Similarly, an inverse association between cold-stimulated FDG uptake and BMI was reported by Saito et al. (2009) in healthy volunteers ages 23–65 years. The latter study also pointed out a seasonal variation, with increased cold-activated FDG uptake during winter versus summer. Importantly, the amount of BAT is inversely correlated with BMI, especially in older people, suggesting a potential role of BAT in adult human metabolism as it relates to energy-efficient heat production (Cypess et al., 2009). This (re)discovery of BAT and its known role in the regulation of adaptive thermogenesis has opened an interest in activating BAT and enhancing energy expenditure in order to control body weight and prevent metabolic disorders (Ravussin & Kozak, 2009). However, although BAT has been proposed to mediate both CIT and DIT, a recent study found that cold acclimation resulted in increased CIT but not DIT (via TEF150%), suggesting that CIT and DIT are mediated by distinct regulatory mechanisms.

More recent discussion has lent itself to examining the potential "beiging" (or "browning") of white fat cells to reduce adverse effects of WAT and potentially improve metabolic health (Bartelt & Heeren, 2014). The idea of using beige adipocytes and browning of WAT therapeutically has gained a lot of attention, because the actual amount of BAT found in adults is typically quite low and correlates inversely with BMI and age. Beige adipocytes are generated by both de novo recruitment from progenitor cells and transdifferentiation from white adipocytes—independent processes that might coexist. Although cellular energy sensing and sympathetic tone are driving forces that regulate the transcriptional networks controlling browning, cold exposure and other metabolic challenges elicit complex hormonal responses that facilitate communication between tissues and prepare the body for adaptive thermogenesis. Whereas BAT, and potentially beige cells, are critical regulators of metabolic health in mice, it remains unclear whether the induction of browning will be a promising avenue for treatment in humans.

Diacylglycerol Transferase and Acetyl CoA Carboxylase2

Triglyceride synthesis occurs through the acyl CoA:diacylglycerol transferases (DGATs), enzymes that catalyze the final and only committed reaction in the glycerol phosphate pathway. DGAT enzymes are highly expressed in tissues associated with triglyceride synthesis. In humans, an abundant expression of DGAT enzymes has been observed in adipose tissue and liver. Mice deficient in the diacylglycerol acyltransferase 1 enzyme ($DGAT1^{-/-}$) are leaner than wild-type mice and have smaller adipocytes (Smith, Cases, et al., 2000; Chen et al., 2002), are resistant to high-fat-induced obesity, and are protected from hepatic steatosis (Smith et al., 2000). These effects are likely due in part to increased energy expenditure. Moreover, $DGAT^{-/-}$ mice have increased SPA (Chen & Farese, 2005), increased expression of UCP1 (Chen et al., 2002), and increased leptin sensitivity (Chen et al., 2002). Conversely, overexpression of DGAT1 in adipose tissue results in impaired insulin sensitivity and hepatic steatosis (Chen, Liu, Zhang, Ginsberg, & Yu, 2005). These findings suggest that pharmacological inhibition of DGAT may be a potential therapeutic target for obesity in humans. Preclinical studies indicate that DGAT inhibitors (e.g., T863) inhibit lipid absorption, cause weight loss, improve insulin resistance, and alleviate hepatic steatosis in mice fed a high-fat diet (Cao et al., 2011). Due to the profound effects of DGAT deficiency on energy metabolism, studies are underway to identify suitable natural and synthetic compounds that can specifically inhibit its action.

Acetyl CoA carboxylase (ACC), which exists in at least two isoforms in humans, is responsible for synthesizing malonyl coenzyme A, a potent inhibitor of fatty acid oxidation. ACC1 is expressed mainly in lipogenic tissues such as the liver and adipose tissue, and ACC2 is expressed in the heart and skeletal muscle. Although mice lacking ACC1 die young, mice lacking ACC2 ($ACC2^{-/-}$) have increased fat oxidation and therefore decreased weight and fat stores compared to wild-type mice (Abu-Elheiga, Oh, Kordari, & Wakil, 2003). Furthermore, when fed a high-fat/high-carbohydrate diet, $ACC2^{-/-}$ mice are resistant to obesity and the development of diabetes (Abu-Elheiga et al., 2003). This preclinical evidence suggests that ACC inhibitors may serve as therapeutic targets for obesity, and clinical trials are ongoing. To date, more than 600 genetic markers and chromosomal regions have been associated or linked with human obesity phenotypes. In humans, both isoforms have central roles in fatty acid biosynthesis and oxidation (Tong, 2005). A recent genomewide association study (GWAS) suggests that 97 BMI-associated loci, 56 of which are novel, highlight genetic relevance to BMI alone (Locke et al., 2015). Future studies will, no doubt, report that additional genetic loci have proven to impact energy metabolism.

Targeting Energy Expenditure for Weight Loss Maintenance

Lifetime body weight change is evident and not confined to certain individuals. Although the degree of weight gain is individual, no one is immune to the decreases in energy expenditure associated with the aging process. One potential modality for weight loss treatment is the use of a tiered approach to both weight loss and weight loss maintenance. Targeting energy expenditure for therapeutic purposes may not be efficacious for producing the initial weight loss but may be an effective strategy for weight loss maintenance. Although lifetime weight change is inevitable, with degrees of weight gain variable across individuals, it has been suggested that interventions combining lifestyle improvements with appetite-suppressant drug therapy would elicit an initial decrement in body weight that may only be successfully maintained through methods that increase energy expenditure (Figure 3.4). Furthermore, the usage of targeted fat oxidation drug therapies alongside methods to target increases in energy expenditure may be a critical component to sustaining weight loss when metabolic adaptation is attempting to counteract the degree of weight loss via decreases in daily energy expenditure.

Conclusions

The global obesity epidemic has stimulated intense interest in the genetic and molecular basis of body weight regulation. Changes in the components of energy expenditure, comprised of BMR, TEF, and physical activity thermogenesis have important roles in modulating energy balance. However, what ultimately determines "metabolic efficiency" is extremely complex. All components of energy expenditure are likely influenced by interactions between our individual genes and the environment, affecting many physiological and biochemical processes. Recent progress in gene targeting and other technologies has pushed mouse models to the forefront of this effort. Whether these preclinical findings will translate into therapeutic utility for human obesity is not yet known. There is no doubt that the field of energy expenditure has developed tremendously over the years and that understanding the homeostatic balance between energy intake and energy expenditure will continue to be an active research endeavor. Indeed, different

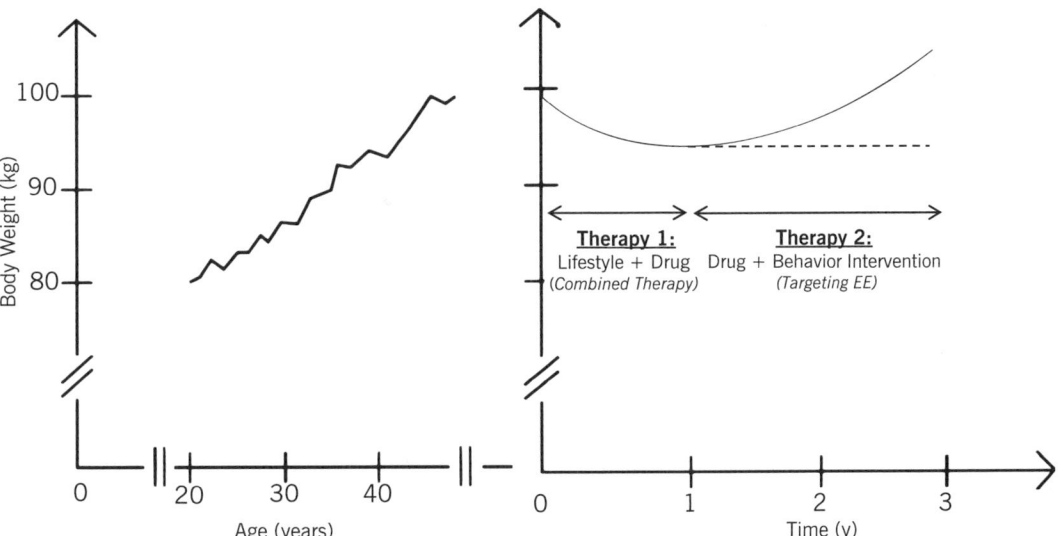

FIGURE 3.4. Body weight tends to increase steadily as we age (as depicted in the left panel). If we intervene (right panel) with lifestyle modifications (e.g., dieting via caloric restriction, exercise) and/or a drug therapy, we can expect to see a weight loss plateau around 6–12 months after lifestyle and/or drug therapy intervention. Given the tendency toward weight regain (due to metabolic adaptation often observed with weight loss), it might be fruitful to intervene with drug therapies and/or behavioral interventions targeting energy expenditure.

tiered therapeutic approaches to weight loss therapy are available and may contribute to improvements in weight loss success, and increasing the mass and activity of brown adipocytes (beige and brown) may help in the maintenance of weight loss as well. Furthermore, personalized treatment for weight loss and weight loss maintenance should also be at the forefront of research priorities.

References

Abbott, W. G. H., Howard, B. V., Christin, L., Freymond, S., Lillioja, L. V., Boyce, T. E., et al. (1988). Short-term energy balance: Relationship with protein, carbohydrate, and fat balances. *American Journal of Physiology, 255*(3, Pt. 1), E332–E337.

Abu-Elheiga, L., Oh, W., Kordari, P., & Wakil, S. J. (2003). Acetyl-CoA carboxylase 2 mutant mice are protected against obesity and diabetes induced by high-fat/high-carbohydrate diets. *Proceedings of the National Academy of Sciences of the United States of America, 100*(18), 10207–10212.

Acheson, K. J., Schutz, Y., Bessard, T., Anantharaman, K., Flatt, J. P., & Jequier, E. (1988). Glycogen storage capacity and de novo lipogenesis during massive carbohydrate overfeeding in man. *American Journal of Clinical Nutrition, 48*(2), 240–247.

Acheson, K. J., Schutz, Y., Bessard, T., Flatt, J. P., & Jequier, E. (1987). Carbohydrate metabolism and de novo lipogenesis in human obesity. *American Journal of Clinical Nutrition, 45*(1), 78–85.

Alpert, S. (1990). Growth, thermogenesis, and hyperphagia. *American Journal of Clinical Nutrition, 52*(5), 784–792.

Arsenijevic, D., Onuma, H., Pecqueur, C., Raimbault, S., Manning, B. S., Miroux, B., et al. (2000). Disruption of the uncoupling protein-2 gene in mice reveals a role in immunity and reactive oxygen species production. *Nature Genetics, 26*(4), 435–439.

Astrup, A., Bulow, J., Madsen, J., & Christensen, N. J. (1985). Contribution of BAT and skeletal muscle to thermogenesis induced by ephedrine in man. *American Journal of Physiology, 248*(5, Pt. 1), E507–E515.

Bartelt, A., & Heeren, J. (2014). Adipose tissue browning and metabolic health. *Nature Reviews Endocrinology, 10*(1), 24–36.

Black, A. E., Coward, W. A., Cole, T. J., & Prentice, A. M. (1996). Human energy expenditure in affluent societies: An analysis of 574 doubly-labeled water measurements. *European Journal of Clinical Nutrition, 50*(2), 72–92.

Bogardus, C., Lillioja, S., Ravussin, E., Abbott, W., Zawadzki, J. K., Young, A., et al. (1986). Familial dependence of the resting metabolic rate. *New England Journal of Medicine, 315*(2), 96–100.

Bonomi, A. G., Goris, A. H., Yin, B., & Westerterp, K. R. (2009). Detection of type, duration, and intensity of physical activity using an accelerometer. *Medicine and Science in Sports and Exercise, 41*(9), 1770–1777.

Bosy-Westphal, A., Reinecke, U., Schorke, T., Illner, K., Kutzner, D., Heller, M., et al. (2014). Effect of organ and tissue masses on resting energy expenditure in underweight, normal weight and obese adults. *International Journal of Obesity and Related Metabolic Disorders, 28*(1), 72–79.

Bray, G. A. (1991). Treatment for obesity: A nutrient balance/nutrient partition approach. *Nutrition Reviews, 49*(2), 33–45.

Bray, G. A., Redman, L. R., de Jonge, L., Covington, J., Rood, J., Brock, C., et al. (2015). Effect of protein overfeeding on energy expenditure measured in a metabolic chamber. *American Journal of Clinical Nutrition, 101*, 496–505.

Bray, G. A., Smith, S. R., de Jonge, L., Xie, H., Rood, J., Martin, C. K., et al. (2012). Effect of dietary protein content on weight gain, energy expenditure, and body composition during overeating: A randomized controlled trial. *Journal of the American Medical Association, 307*(1), 47–55.

Bray, G. A., York, D. A., & Fisler, J. S. (1989). Experimental obesity: A homeostatic failure due to defective nutrient stimulation of the sympathetic nervous system. *Vitamins and Hormones, 45*, 1–125.

Cao, J., Zhou, Y., Peng, H., Huang, X., Stahler, S., Suri, V., et al. (2011). Targeting acyl-CoA:diacylglycerol acyltransferase 1 (DGAT1) with small molecule inhibitors for the treatment of metabolic diseases. *Journal of Biological Chemistry, 286*(48), 41838–41851.

Caro, J. F., Sinha, M. K., Kolaczynski, J. W., Zhang, P. L., & Considine, R. V. (1997). Leptin: The tale of an obesity gene. *Diabetes, 45*(11), 1455–1462.

Chen, H. C., & Farese, R. V., Jr. (2005). Inhibition of triglyceride synthesis as a treatment strategy for obesity: Lessons from DGAT1-deficient mice. *Arteriosclerosis, Thrombosis, and Vascular Biology, 25*(3), 482–486.

Chen, H. C., Smith, S. J., Ladha, Z., Jensen, D. R., Ferreira, L. D., Pulawa, L. K., et al. (2002). Increased insulin and leptin sensitivity in mice lacking acyl CoA:diacylglycerol acyltransferase 1. *Journal of Clinical Investigation, 109*(8), 1049–1055.

Chen, N., Liu, L., Zhang, Y., Ginsberg, H. N., & Yu, Y. H. (2005). Whole-body insulin resistance in the absence of obesity in FVB mice with overexpression of Dgat1 in adipose tissue. *Diabetes, 54*(12), 3379–3386.

Christin, L., O'Connell, M., Bogardus, C., Danforth, E., Jr., & Ravussin, E. (1993). Norepinephrine turnover and energy expenditure in Pima Indian and white men. *Metabolism, 42*(6), 723–729.

Clapham, J. C., Arch, J. R., Chapman, H., Haynes, A., Lister, C., Moore, G. B., et al. (2000). Mice overexpressing human uncoupling protein-3 in skeletal muscle are hyperphagic and lean. *Nature, 406*(6794), 415–418.

Cunningham, J. J. (1991). Body composition as a determinant of energy expenditure: A synthetic review and a proposed general prediction equation. *American Journal of Clinical Nutrition, 54*(6), 963–969.

Cypess, A. M., Lehman, S., Williams, G., Tal, I., Rodman, D., Goldfine, A. B., et al. (2009). Identification and importance of brown adipose tissue in adult humans. *New England Journal of Medicine, 360*(15), 1509–1517.

de Jonge, L., & Bray, G. A. (1997). The thermic effect of food and obesity: A critical review. *Obesity Research, 5*(6), 622–631.

Donahoo, W. T., Levine, J. A., & Melanson, E. L. (2004). Variability in energy expenditure and its components. *Current Opinion in Clinical Nutrition and Metabolic Care, 7*(6), 599–605.

Ebbeling, C. B., Swain, J. F., Feldman, H. A., Wong, W. W., Hachey, D. L., Garcia-Lago, E., et al. (2012). Effects of dietary composition on energy expenditure during weight-loss maintenance. *Journal of the American Medical Association, 307*(24), 2627–2634.

Elia, M. (1992). Organ and tissue contribution to metabolic rate. In J. M. Kinney & H. N. Tucker (Eds.), *Energy metabolism: Tissue determinants and cellular corollaries* (pp. 61–77). New York: Raven Press.

Enerback, S. (2010). Human brown adipose tissue. *Cell Metabolism, 11*(4), 248–252.

Farooqi, I. S., & O'Rahilly, S. (2014). 20 years of leptin: Human disorders of leptin action. *Journal of Endocrinology, 223*(1), T63–T70.

Flatt, J. P. (2007). Differences in basal energy expenditure and obesity. *Obesity (Silver Spring), 15*(11), 2546–2548.

Flatt, J. P., Ravussin, E., Acheson, K. J., & Jequier, E. (1985). Effects of dietary fat on postprandial substrate oxidation and on carbohydrate and fat balance. *Journal of Clinical Investigation, 76*(3), 1019–1024.

Foerster, F., & Fahrenberg, J. (2000). Motion pattern and posture: Correctly assessed by calibrated accelerometers. *Behavioral Research Methods, Instruments, and Computers, 32*(3), 450–457.

Foster, D. O., & Frydman, M. L. (1978). Brown adipose tissue: The dominant site of nonshivering thermogenesis in the rat. *Experientia Supplementum, 32*, 147–151.

Fothergill, E., Guo, J., Howard, L., Kerns, J. C., Knuth, N. D., Brychta, R., et al. (2016). Persistent metabolic adaptation 6 years after "The Biggest Loser" competition. *Obesity (Silver Spring), 24*(8), 1612–1619.

Frayn, K. N. (1995). Physiological regulation of macronutrient balance. *International Journal of Obesity, 19*(5, Suppl.), S4–S10.

Froidevaux, F., Schutz, Y., Christin, L., & Jequier, E. (1993). Energy expenditure in obese women before and during weight loss, after refeeding, and in the weight-relapse period. *American Journal of Clinical Nutrition, 57*(1), 35–42.

Galgani, J. E., Greenway, F. L., Caglayan, S., Wong, M. L., Licinio, J., & Ravussin, E. (2010). Leptin replacement prevents weight loss-induced metabolic adaptation in congenital leptin-deficient patients. *Journal of Clinical Endocrinology and Metabolism, 95*(2), 851–855.

Goran, M. I. (2005). Estimating energy requirements: Regression based prediction equations or multiples of resting metabolic rate. *Public Health Nutrition, 8*(7A), 1184–1186.

Granata, G. P., & Brandon, L. J. (2002). The thermic effect of food and obesity: Discrepant results and methodological variations. *Nutrition Reviews, 60*(8), 223–233.

Hall, K. D., Bemis, T., Brychta, R., Chen, K. Y., Courville, A., Crayner, E. J., et al. (2015). Calorie for calorie, dietary fat restriction results in more body fat loss than carbohydrate restriction in people with obesity. *Cell Metabolism, 22*(3), 427–436.

Hall, K. D., Chen, K. Y., Guo, J., Lam, Y. Y., Leibel, R. L., Mayer, L. E. S., et al. (2016). Energy expenditure and body composition changes after an isocaloric ketogenic diet in overweight and obese men. *American Journal of Clinical Nutrition, 104*(2), 324–333.

Hall, K. D., Sacks, G., Chandramohan, D., Chow, C. C., Wang, Y. C., Gortmaker, S. L., et al. (2011). Quantifying the effect of energy imbalance on body weight change. *Lancet, 378*(9793), 826–837.

Harris, J. A., & Benedict, F. G. (1919). *A biometric study of basal metabolism in man.* Washington, DC: Carnegie Institution of Washington.

Hesselink, M. K., Greenhaff, P. L., Constantin-Teodosiu, D., Hultman, E., Saris, W. H., Nieuwlaat, R., et al. (2003). Increased uncoupling protein 3 content does not affect mitochondrial function in human skeletal muscle in vivo. *Journal of Clinical Investigation, 111*(4), 479–486.

Heymsfield, S. B., Darby, P. C., Muhlheim, L. S., Gallagher, D., Wolper, C., & Allison, D. B. (1995). The calorie: Myth, measurement, and reality. *American Journal of Clinical Nutrition, 62*(5, Suppl.), 1034S–1041S.

Heymsfield, S. B., Greenberg, A. S., Fujioka, K., Dixon, R. M., Kushner, R., Hunt, T., et al. (1999). Recombinant leptin for weight loss in obese and lean adults: A randomized, controlled, dose-escalation trial. *Journal of the American Medical Association, 282*(16), 1568–1575.

Jequier, E., & Schutz, Y. (1983). Long-term measurements of energy expenditure in humans using a respiration chamber. *American Journal of Clinical Nutrition, 38*(6), 989–998.

Johanssen, D. L., Knuth, N. D., Huizenga, R., Rood, J. C., Ravussin, E., & Hall, K. D. (2012). Metabolic slowing with massive weight loss despite preservation of fat-free mass. *Journal of Clinical Endocrinology and Metabolism, 97*(7), 2489–2496.

Katzmarzyk, P. T., Perusse, L., Tremblay, A., & Bouchard, C. (2000). No association between resting metabolic rate or respiratory exchange ratio and subsequent changes in body mass and fatness: 5½ year follow-up of the Quebec family study. *European Journal of Clinical Nutrition, 54*(8), 610–614.

Keys, A., Brozek, J., Henschel, A., Mickelsen, O., & Taylor, H. L. (1950). *The biology of human starvation.* Minneapolis: University of Minnesota Press.

Knowler, W. C., Pettitt, D. J., Saad, M. F., Charles, M. A., Nelson, R. G., Howard, B. V., et al. (1991). Obesity in the Pima Indians: Its magnitude and relationship with diabetes. *American Journal of Clinical Nutrition, 53*(6, Suppl.), 1543S–1551S.

Knuth, N. D., Johannsen, D. L., Tamboli, R. A., Marks-Shulman, P. A., Huizenga, R., Chen, K. Y., et al. (2014). Metabolic adaptation following massive weight loss is related to the degree of energy imbalance and changes in circulating leptin. *Obesity, 22*(12), 2563–2569.

Kovacs, P., Ma, L., Hanson, R. L., Franks, P., Stumvoll, M., Bogardus, C., et al. (2005). Genetic variation in UCP2 (uncoupling protein-2) is associated with energy metabolism in Pima Indians. *Diabetologia, 48*(11), 2292–2295.

Larson, D. E., Ferraro, R. T., Robertson, D. S., & Ravussin, E. (1995). Energy metabolism in weight-stable postobese individuals. *American Journal of Clinical Nutrition, 62*(4), 735–739.

Leibel, R. L., Rosenbaum, M., & Hirsch, J. (1995). Changes in energy expenditure resulting from altered body weight. *New England Journal of Medicine, 332*(10), 621–628.

Levine, J. A. (2007). Nonexercise activity thermogenesis: Liberating the life-force. *Journal of Internal Medicine, 262*(3), 273–287.

Levine, J. A., Eberhardt, N. L., & Jensen, M. D. (1999). Role of nonexercise activity thermogenesis in resistance to fat gain in humans. *Science, 283*(5399), 212–214.

Levine, J. A., Lanningham-Foster, L. M., McCrady, S. K., Krizan, A. C., Olson, L. R., Kane, P. H., et al. (2005). Interindividual variation in posture allocation: Possible role in human obesity. *Science, 307*(5709), 584–586.

Lifson, N. (1966). Theory of use of the turnover rates of body water for measuring energy and material balance. *Journal of Theoretical Biology, 12*(1), 46–74.

Locke, A. E., Kahali, B., Berndt, S. I., Justice, A. E., Pers, T. H., Day, F. R., et al. (2015). Genetic studies of body mass index yield new insights for obesity biology. *Nature, 518*(7538), 197–206.

Ludwig, D. S., & Friedman, M. I. (2014). Increasing adiposity: Consequence or cause of overeating? *Journal of the American Medical Association, 311*(21), 2167–2168.

Martos, R., Valle, M., Morales, R., Canete, R., Gavilan, M. I., & Sanchez-Margalet, V. (2006). Hyperhomocysteinemia correlates with insulin resistance and low-grade systemic inflammation in obese prepubertal children. *Metabolism: Clinical and Experimental, 55*(1), 72–77.

Mertz, W., Tsui, J. C., Judd, J. T., Reiser, S., Hallfrisch, J., Morris, E. R., et al. (1991). What are people really eating?: The relation between energy derived from estimated diet records and intake determined to maintain body weight. *American Journal of Clinical Nutrition, 54*(2), 291–295.

Mifflin, M. D., St. Jeor, S. T., Hill, L. A., Scott, B. J., Daugherty, S. A., & Koh, Y. O. (1990). A new predictive equation for resting energy expenditure in healthy individuals. *American Journal of Clinical Nutrition, 51*(2), 241–247.

Muller, M. J., & Bosy-Westphal, A. (2013). Adaptive thermogenesis with weight loss in humans. *Obesity, 21*(2), 218–228.

Muller, M. J., Langemann, D., Gehrke, I., Later, W., Heller, M., Gluer, C. C., et al. (2011). Effect of constitution on mass of individual organs and their association with metabolic rate in humans: A detailed view on allometric scaling. *PLOS ONE, 6*(7), E22732.

National Center for Health Statistics. (2012). *Health, United States, 2011: With special features on socioeconomic status and health.* Hyattsville, MD: U.S. Department of Health and Human Services.

Neel, J. V. (1962). Diabetes mellitus: A "thrifty" genotype rendered detrimental by "progress"? *American Journal of Human Genetics, 14*(4), 353–362.

Pelleymounter, M. A., Cullen, M. J., Baker, M. B., Hecht, R., Winters, D., Boone, T., et al. (1995). Effects of the obese gene product on body weight regulation in ob/ob mice. *Science, 269*(5233), 540–543.

Peterson, C. M., Lecoultre, V., Frost, E. A., Simmons, J., Redman, L. M., & Ravussin, E. (2016). The thermogenic responses to overfeeding and cold are differentially regulated. *Obesity (Silver Spring), 24*(1), 96–101.

Peterson, C. M., Orooji, M., Johnson, D. N., Naraghi-Pour, M., & Ravussin, E. (2017). Brown adipose tissue does not mediate metabolic adaptation to overfeeding in men. *Obesity (Silver Spring), 25*(3), 502–505.

Ravussin, E. (1993). Energy metabolism in obesity: Studies in the Pima Indians. *Diabetes Care, 16*(1), 232–238.

Ravussin, E. (1995). Obesity in Britain: Rising trend may be due to "pathoenvironment" [letter]. *British Medical Journal, 311*(7019), 1569.

Ravussin, E., & Bogardus, C. (1989). Relationship of genetics, age, and physical fitness to daily energy expenditure and fuel utilization. *American Journal of Clinical Nutrition, 49*(5, Suppl.), 968–975.

Ravussin, E., Harper, I. T., Rising, R., & Bogardus, C. (1991). Energy expenditure by doubly labeled water: Validation in lean and obese subjects. *American Journal of Physiology, 261*(3, Pt. 1), E402–E409.

Ravussin, E., & Kozak, L. P. (2009). Have we entered the brown adipose tissue renaissance? *Obesity Reviews, 10*(3), 265–268.

Ravussin, E., Lillioja, S., Anderson, T. E., Christin, L., & Bogardus, C. (1986). Determinants of 24-hour energy expenditure in man: Methods and results using a respiratory chamber. *Journal of Clinical Investigation, 78*(6), 1568–1578.

Ravussin, E., Lillioja, S., Knowler, W. C., Christin, L., Freymond, D., Abbott, W. G., et al. (1988). Reduced rate of energy expenditure as a risk factor for body-weight gain. *New England Journal of Medicine, 318*(8), 467–672.

Ravussin, E., Pratley, R. E., Maffei, M., Wang, H., Friedman, J. M., Bennett, P. H., et al. (1997). Relatively low plasma leptin concentrations precede weight gain in Pima Indians. *Nature Medicine, 3*(2), 238–240.

Ravussin, E., & Swinburn, B. A. (1996). Energy expenditure and obesity. *Diabetes Reviews, 4*, 403–422.

Reinhardt, M., Thearle, M. S., Ibrahim, M., Hohenadel, M. G., Bogardus, C., Krakoff, J., et al. (2015). A human thrifty phenotype associated with less weight loss during caloric restriction. *Diabetes, 64*(8), 2859–2867.

Rising, R., Alger, S., Boyce, V., Seagle, H., Ferraro, R., Fontvieille, A. M., et al. (1992). Food intake measured by an automated food-selection system: Relationship to energy expenditure. *American Journal of Clinical Nutrition, 55*(2), 343–349.

Rising, R., Keys, A., Ravussin, E., & Bogardus, C. (1992). Concomitant interindividual variation in body temperature and metabolic rate. *American Journal of Physiology, 263*(4, Pt. 1), E730–E734.

Ronti, T., Lupattelli, G., & Mannarino, E. (2006). The endocrine function of adipose tissue: An update. *Clinical Endocrinology (Oxford), 64*(4), 355–365.

Rosen, E. D., & Spiegelman, B. M. (2006). Adipocytes as regulators of energy balance and glucose homeostasis. *Nature, 444*(7121), 847–853.

Rosenbaum, M., Goldsmith, R., Bloomfield, D., Magnano, A., Weimer, J., Heymsfield, S., et al. (2005). Low-dose leptin reverses skeletal muscle, autonomic, and neuroendocrine adaptations to maintenance of reduced weight. *Journal of Clinical Investigation, 115*(12), 3579–3586.

Rosenbaum, M., & Leibel, R. L. (2010). Adaptive thermogenesis in humans. *International Journal of Obesity (London), 34*(1), S47–S55.

Rosenbaum, M., Murphy, E. M., Heymsfield, S. B., Matthews, D. E., & Leibel, R. L. (2002). Low dose leptin administration reverses effects of sustained weight-reduction on energy expenditure and circulating concentrations of thyroid hormones. *Journal of Clinical Endocrinology and Metabolism, 87*(5), 2391–2394.

Rothwell, N. J., & Stock, M. J. (1979). A role for brown adipose tissue in diet-induced thermogenesis. *Nature, 281*(5726), 31–35.

Saito, M., Okamatsu-Ogura, Y., Matsushita, M., Watanabe, K., Yoneshiro, T., Nio-Kobayashi, J., et al. (2009). High incidence of metabolically active brown adipose tissue in healthy adult humans: Effects of cold exposure and adiposity. *Diabetes, 58*(7), 1526–1531.

Sayon-Orea, C., Martinez-Gonzalez, M. A., & Bes-Rastrollo, M. (2011). Alcohol consumption and body weight: A systematic review. *Nutrition Reviews, 69*(8), 419–431.

Schiffelers, S. L., Brouwer, E. M., Saris, W. H., & van Baak, M. A. (1998). Inhibition of lipolysis reduces beta1-adrenoceptor-mediated thermogenesis in man. *Metabolism, 47*(12), 1462–1467.

Schlögl, M., Piaggi, P., Pannacciulli, N., Bonfiglio, S. M., Krakoff, J., & Thearle, M. S. (2015). Energy expenditure responses to fasting and overfeeding identify phenotypes associated with weight change. *Diabetes, 64*(11), 3680–3689.

Schoeller, D. A., Ravussin, E., Schutz, Y., Acheson, K. J., Baertschi, P., & Jequier, E. (1986). Energy expenditure by doubly labeled water: Validation in humans and proposed calculation. *American Journal of Physiology, 250*(5, Pt. 2), R823–R830.

Schofield, W. N. (1985). Predicting basal metabolic rate: New standards and review of previous work. *Human Nutrition: Clinical Nutrition, 39*(1, Suppl.), 5–41.

Schrauwen, P., Xia, J., Bogardus, C., Pratley, R. E., & Ravussin, E. (1999). Skeletal muscle uncoupling protein 3 expression is a determinant of energy expenditure in Pima Indians. *Diabetes, 48*(1), 146–149.

Schutz, Y., Flatt, J. P., & Jequier, E. (1989). Failure of dietary fat intake to promote fat oxidation: A factor favoring the development of obesity. *American Journal of Clinical Nutrition, 50*(2), 307–314.

Schwartz, R. S., Jaeger, L. F., & Veith, R. C. (1988). Effect of clonidine on the thermic effect of feeding in humans. *American Journal of Physiology, 254*(1, Pt. 2), R90–R94.

Sharma, A. M., Pischon, T., Hardt, S., Kunz, I., & Luft, F. C. (2001). Hypothesis: β-adrenergic receptor blockers and weight gain: A systematic analysis. *Hypertension, 37*(2), 250–254.

Shelmet, J. J., Reichard, G. A., Skutches, C. L., Hoeldtke, R. D., Owen, O. E., & Boden, G. (1988). Ethanol causes acute inhibition of carbohydrate, fat, and protein oxidation and insulin resistance. *Journal of Clinical Investigation, 81*(4), 1137–1145.

Smith, S. J., Cases, S., Jensen, D. R., Chen, H. C., Sande, E., Tow, B., et al. (2000). Obesity resistance and multiple mechanisms of triglyceride synthesis in mice lacking Dgat. *Nature Genetics, 25*(1), 87–90.

Smith, S. R., de Jonge, L., Zachwieja, J. J., Roy, H., Nguyen, T., Rood, J. C., et al. (2000). Fat and carbohydrate balances during adaptation to a high-fat diet. *American Journal of Clinical Nutrition, 71*(2), 450–457.

Smith, S. R., de Jonge, L., Zachwieja, J. J., Nguyen, T., Rood, J. C., & Bray, G. A. (2000). Concurrent physical activity increases fat oxidation during the shift to a high fat diet. *American Journal of Clinical Nutrition, 72*(1), 131–138.

Snitker, S., Tataranni, P. A., & Ravussin, E. (1998). Respiratory quotient is inversely associated with muscle sympathetic nerve activity. *Journal of Clinical Endocrinology and Metabolism, 83*(11), 3977–3979.

Snitker, S., Tataranni, P. A., & Ravussin, E. (2001). Spontaneous physical activity in a respiratory chamber is correlated to habitual physical activity. *International Journal of Obesity and Related Metabolic Disorders, 25*(10), 1481–1486.

Snyder, W. S., Cook, M. J., Nasset, E. S., Karhausen, L. R., Howells, G. P., & Tipton, I. H. (1975). *Report of the task group on reference man* (International Commission on Radiological Protection, No. 23). New York: Pergamon Press.

Speakman, J. R. (2007). A nonadaptive scenario explaining the genetic predisposition to obesity: The "predation release" hypothesis. *Cell Metabolism, 6*(1), 5–12.

Spraul, M., Ravussin, E., Fontvieille, A. M., Rising, R., Larson, D. E., & Anderson, E. A. (1993). Reduced sympathetic nervous activity: A potential mechanism predisposing to body weight gain. *Journal of Clinical Investigation, 92*(4), 1730–1735.

Stuart, J. A., Harper, J. A., Brindle, K. M., Jekabsons, M. B., & Brand, M. D. (2001). Physiological levels of mammalian uncoupling protein 2 do not uncouple yeast mitochondria. *Journal of Biological Chemistry, 276*, 18633–18639.

Susulic, V. S., Frederich, R. C., Lawitts, J., Tozzo, E., Kahn, B. B., Harper, E. E., et al. (1995). Targeted disruption of the beta 3-adrenergic receptor gene. *Journal of Biological Chemistry, 270*(49), 29483–29492.

Sutton, E. F., Bray, G. A., Burton, J. H., Smith, S. R., & Redman, L. M. (2016). No evidence for metabolic adaptation in thermic effect of food by dietary protein. *Obesity (Silver Spring), 24*(8), 1639–1642.

Tam, C. S., Lecoultre, V., & Ravussin, E. (2012). Brown adipose tissue: Mechanisms and potential therapeutic targets. *Circulation, 125*(22), 2782–2791.

Tataranni, P. A., Harper, I. T., Snitker, S., Del, P. A., Vozarova, B., Bunt, J., et al. (2003). Body weight gain in free-living Pima Indians: Effect of energy intake vs expenditure. *International Journal of Obesity and Related Metabolic Disorders, 27*(12), 1578–1583.

Tataranni, P. A., Larson, D. E., Snitker, S., & Ravussin, E. (1995). Thermic effect of food in humans: Methods and results from use of a respiratory chamber. *American Journal of Clinical Nutrition, 61*(5), 1013–1019.

Tataranni, P. A., & Ravussin, E. (1995). Variability in metabolic rate: Biological sites of regulation. *International Journal of Obesity and Related Metabolic Disorders, 19*(4, Suppl.), S102–S106.

Tataranni, P. A., Young, J. B., Bogardus, C., & Ravussin, E. (1997). A low sympathoadrenal activity is associated with body weight gain and development of central adiposity in Pima Indian men. *Obesity Research, 5*(4), 341–347.

Thomas, D. M., Martin, C. K., Lettieri, S., Bredlau, C., Kaiser, K., Church, T., et al. (2013). Can a weight loss of one pound a week be achieved with a 3500-kcal deficit?: Commentary on a commonly accepted rule. *International Journal of Obesity (London), 37*(12), 1611–1613.

Tong, L. (2005). Acetyl-coenzyme A carboxylase: Crucial metabolic enzyme and attractive target for drug discovery. *Cellular and Molecular Life Sciences, 62*(16), 1784–1803.

Tremblay, A., Despres, J. P., Theriault, G., Fournier, G., & Bouchard, C. (1992). Overfeeding and energy expenditure in humans. *American Journal of Clinical Nutrition, 56*(5), 857–862.

United Nations University. (2018). Adaptation and energy requirements. Retrieved February 28. 2018 from http://archive.unu.edu/unupress/food2/UID01E/UID01E07.HTM.

van Marken Lichtenbelt, W. D., Vanhommerig, J. W., Smulders, N. M., Drossaerts, J. M., Kemerink, G. J., Bouvy, N. D., et al. (2009). Cold-activated brown adipose tissue in healthy men. *New England Journal of Medicine, 360*(15), 1500–1508.

Virtanen, K. A., Lidell, M. E., Orava, J., Heglind, M., Westergren, R., Niemi, T., et al. (2009). Functional brown adipose tissue in healthy adults. *New England Journal of Medicine, 360*(15), 1518–1525.

Walder, K., Norman, R. A., Hanson, R. L., Schrauwen, P., Neverova, M., Jenkinson, C. P., et al. (1998). Association between uncoupling protein polymorphisms (UCP2-UCP3) and energy metabolism/obesity in Pima Indians. *Human Molecular Genetics, 7*(9), 1431–1435.

Wang, Z., Ying, Z., Bosy-Westphal, A., Zhang, J., Heller, M., Later, W., et al. (2012). Evaluation of specific metabolic rates of major organs and tissues: Comparison between nonobese and obese women. *Obesity (Silver Spring), 20*(1), 95–100.

Wang, Z., Ying, Z., Bosy-Westphal, A., Zhang, J., Schautz, B., Later, W., et al. (2010). Specific metabolic rates of major organs and tissues across adulthood: Evaluation by mechanistic model of resting energy expenditure. *American Journal of Clinical Nutrition, 92*(6), 1369–1377.

Wareham, N. J., van Sluijs, E. M., & Ekelund, U. (2005). Physical activity and obesity prevention: A review of the current evidence. *Proceedings of the Nutrition Society, 64*(2), 229–247.

Westerterp, K. R., & Plasqui, G. (2004). Physical activity and human energy expenditure. *Current Opinion in Clinical Nutrition and Metabolic Care, 7*(6), 607–613.

Westerterp, K. R., & Speakman, J. R. (2008). Physical activity energy expenditure has not declined since the 1980s and matches energy expenditures of wild mammals. *International Journal of Obesity (London), 32*(8), 1256–1263.

Weyer, C., Pratley, R. E., Salbe, A., Bogardus, C., Ravussin, E., & Tataranni, P. A. (2000). Energy expenditure, fat oxidation, and body weight regulation: A study of metabolic adaptation to long term weight change. *Journal of Clinical Endocrinology and Metabolism, 85*(3), 1087–1094.

Weyer, C., Tataranni, P. A., Snitker, S., Danforth, E., Jr., & Ravussin, E. (1998). Increase in insulin action and fat oxidation after treatment with CL 316,243, a highly selective beta3-adrenoceptor agonist in humans. *Diabetes, 47*(10), 1555–1561.

Yang, X., Enerbäck, S., & Smith, U. (2003). Reduced expression of FOXC2 and brown adipogenic genes in human subjects with insulin resistance. *Obesity Research, 11*(10), 1182–1191.

Zhang, C. Y., Baffy, G., Perret, P., Krauss, S., Peroni, O., Grujic, D., et al. (2001). Uncoupling protein-2 negatively regulates insulin secretion and is a major link between obesity, beta cell dysfunction, and type 2 diabetes. *Cell, 105*(6), 745–755.

Zhang, Y., Proenca, R., Maffei, M., Barone, M., Leopold, L., & Friedman, J. M. (1994). Positional cloning of the mouse obese gene and its human homologue. *Nature, 372*, 425–432.

Zurlo, F., Ferraro, R. T., Fontvielle, A. M., Rising, R.,

Bogardus, C., & Ravussin, E. (1992). Spontaneous physical activity and obesity: Cross-sectional and longitudinal studies in Pima Indians. *American Journal of Physiology, 263*(2, Pt. 1), E296–E300.

Zurlo, F., Larson, K., Bogardus, C., & Ravussin, E. (1990). Skeletal muscle metabolism is a major determinant of resting energy expenditure. *Journal of Clinical Investigation, 86*(5), 1423–1427.

Zurlo, F., Lillioja, S., Esposito-Del Puente, A., Nyomba, B. L., Baz, I., Saad, M. F., et al. (1990). Low ratio of fat to carbohydrate oxidation as a predictor of weight gain: Study of 24-h RQ. *American Journal of Physiology, 259*(5, Pt. 1), E650–E657.

CHAPTER 4

Genetics of Obesity

I. Sadaf Farooqi

Major contributors to the rising prevalence of obesity are factors that promote an increase in energy intake (an abundance of inexpensive, easily available, energy-rich, highly palatable foods) and factors that contribute to a decrease in energy expenditure. Such factors affecting energy expenditure include sedentary lifestyles (television watching, driving to work), reduced physical activity at work (office work rather than manual work), and reduced physical activity in leisure time. However, within this obesogenic environment, there is considerable variation in body weight and fat mass among individuals (Friedman, 2003). Some people are much more likely to gain weight, whereas others tend to stay lean. This variability is influenced by complex interactions between environmental factors and biological (genetic, developmental, and behavioral) factors that influence where an individual falls on the body mass index (BMI) distribution (Bray, 2015). As the mean BMI has increased in many populations, the proportion of people at the upper end of the distribution—children and adults with severe obesity—has also increased (Garnett, Baur, Jones, & Hardy, 2016; Skinner & Skelton, 2014). There is also evidence to demonstrate that the response to dietary restriction and physical activity is highly variable, as are the responses to weight loss medications and bariatric surgery (Bray, 2015; Hatoum et al., 2011; King et al., 2007). Understanding the mechanisms that underpin the variability in BMI and in the response to interventions may inform strategies to prevent and treat obesity and related disorders.

Genetic Contributors to Obesity: The Evidence

The biological factors that influence interindividual variability in body weight are, to a large extent, inherited (Friedman, 2000; Maes, Neale, & Eaves, 1997; Perusse et al., 1988). Evidence for the genetic contribution to body weight comes from twin studies that have informed estimates of heritability—defined as the proportion of total phenotypic variance attributable to genetic variation in a specified environment. Multiple twin studies have suggested that the heritability of body BMI is between 0.71 and 0.86 (Silventoinen, Magnusson, Tynelius, Kaprio, & Rasmussen, 2008). Recent studies in over 5,000 U.K. twins, ages 8–11 years, growing up during a time of dramatic rises in obesity, support the substantial heritability of BMI (~77%). In this study by Wardle and colleagues, there was a very modest effect of the shared environment (which can inflate heritability estimates); the remaining environmental variance was largely unshared (Wardle, Carnell, Haworth, & Plomin, 2008). Similar heritability estimates were found when studying identical twins who were reared together and apart (Allison et al., 1996) and in large studies of adopted children whose body weights tended to be more similar to those of their biological parents than to their adopted parents (Sorensen, Price, Stunkard, & Schulsinger, 1989). Family-based studies generally report somewhat lower heritability estimates.

It is likely that genetic factors influence how much weight people gain and how much they lose in response to changes in the amount of food consumed and the amount of exercise undertaken. Carefully controlled experimental studies of identical twins, conducted under direct supervision, have shown that the amount of weight gained in response to a fixed number of excess calories and the amount of weight lost after a fixed amount of physical activity is very similar between twins, but varies across different sets of twins (Bouchard et al., 1990, 1996; Poehlman et al., 1986). These studies demonstrate that the variability in body weight and in the physiological response to energy intake and energy expenditure is very strongly influenced by genetic factors (Elder et al., 2012; Fabsitz, Sholinsky, & Carmelli, 1994; Perusse, Tremblay, Leblanc, & Bouchard, 1989).

Common Genetic Variants in the Population

Genomewide association studies (GWASs) have led to the identification of common genetic variants (i.e., those present in at least 5% of people) that contribute to obesity or increased BMI. By comparing very large numbers of people on whom BMI data are available, more than 100 genetic loci associated with BMI and body fat distribution (often measured by waist-to-hip ratio) have been identified (Dina et al., 2007; Frayling et al., 2007; Loos et al., 2008). Many of these findings have been replicated in different ethnic groups (Locke et al., 2015). GWAS-associated loci are often identified by the name of the nearest gene, although it is important to note that this may not be the gene in which variation contributes to variation in BMI. Some obesity-associated GWAS loci encompass genes previously shown to play a role in energy balance in animals and in people with severe obesity (e.g., *LEPR, SH2B1, MC4R, BDNF*; Wheeler et al., 2013). Other loci contain genes that seem to be plausible biological candidates (Locke et al., 2015). A large proportion of obesity/BMI loci contain genes that are expressed in the brain (Locke et al., 2015). In well-powered studies that have been performed for the more frequently occurring variants, obesity-associated variants seem to be associated with increased energy intake rather than with decreased energy expenditure, although energy expenditure measurements have only been performed in a few cohorts (Cecil, Tavendale, Watt, Hetherington, & Palmer, 2008; Timpson et al., 2008; Wardle, Carnell, Haworth, Farooqi, et al., 2008). This contrasts with loci associated with body fat distribution, which are enriched for genes expressed in adipose tissue and overlap with loci for insulin resistance, which has a shared pathogenesis (Shungin et al., 2015).

Cumulatively, the common variants identified in obesity/BMI GWAS are characterized by modest effect sizes, and the proportion of the variance in BMI explained by GWAS-identified loci remains relatively modest (< 5%). At the most, single variants predict that a person's weight may increase by a few kilograms over several years. Given the large number of common genetic variants identified, one way of estimating their cumulative burden is to use genetic risk scores (GRS), which aggregate information from multiple GWASs to summarize risk-associated variation across the genome (Belsky & Israel, 2014; Loos, 2012). Some studies have shown that people with a high GRS consume more food based on dietary records and have a higher BMI (Qi et al., 2014); some have shown that higher GRS is associated with reduced levels of physical activity (Ahmad et al., 2013; Zhu et al., 2014). However, the effects of these associations remain modest. Therefore, genotyping healthy individuals to identify those who carry a high burden of "obesogenic alleles" is not currently warranted, nor, at this time, would such genetic information usefully guide interventions in people with common forms of obesity

Genetic Discoveries in Severe Obesity

Genetic studies focussed on children with severe childhood-onset obesity have led to the identification of multiple genes in which rare, highly penetrant variants cause obesity (Jackson et al., 1997; Krude et al., 1998; Montague et al., 1997; Ramachandrappa et al., 2013; Yeo et al., 1998). Whereas individually these disorders are rare, cumulatively, at least 10% of children with severe obesity have rare chromosomal abnormalities and/or highly penetrant genetic mutations that drive their obesity (Bochukova et al., 2010). This figure is likely to increase with wider accessibility to genetic testing in clinical practice and as new genes are identified from exome and genome sequencing in large research programs.

Some genetic obesity syndromes are associated with learning difficulties and developmental delay (e.g., Prader–Willi syndrome) and major clinical problems, which means that children come to medical attention at a young age. However, over the last 15 years there has been increasing recognition of a large and growing group of genetic disorders in which *severe obesity itself* is the presenting feature (Farooqi et al., 2003, 2007). Children who suffer from these disorders are often identified as a result of early and marked weight gain, but the lack of other clinical features often means that a genetic diagnosis is not considered and may only be offered when the children reach secondary care.

The diagnosis of a genetic obesity syndrome can provide information that has diagnostic value for the family through genetic counselling. There is particular value in a genetic diagnosis for severe obesity, which, unlike other clinical disorders, is often not recognized as a medical condition by some health care professionals, educators, and employers. The making of a genetic diagnosis can help children and their families deal with the social stigma that comes with severe obesity. In some instances where the persistence of severe obesity despite medical advice has been considered a reason to invoke parental neglect, making a genetic diagnosis has prevented children from being taken into care.

A genetic diagnosis can inform management (many such patients are relatively refractory to weight loss through changes in diet and exercise) and can inform clinical decision making regarding the use of bariatric surgery (feasible in some; high risk in others). Importantly, some genetic obesity syndromes are treatable (Farooqi et al., 1999, 2002). There are a number of drugs in Phase Ib and Phase II clinical trials targeted specifically at patients with genetic obesity syndromes (*www.rhythmtx.com*).

Genetic Obesity Syndromes without Developmental Delay

To date, many of the genetic disorders that are characterised by severe obesity alone affect the leptin–melanocortin pathway (van der Klaauw & Farooqi, 2015), which, from an evolutionary perspective, is critical to defend against starvation and ensure sufficient energy stores for survival (Ahima et al., 1996; Schwartz et al., 2003).

Leptin, a hormone made by adipose tissue, circulates in the bloodstream as a signal reflecting energy stores (Ahima et al., 1996; Maffei et al., 1995). Leptin signals pass through the long isoform of the leptin receptor to stimulate the expression of proopiomelanocortin (POMC) in the arcuate nucleus of the hypothalamus. POMC is extensively modified post-translationally to generate the melanocortin peptides (adrenocorticotropic hormone [ACTH] and alpha-, beta-, gamma-melanocyte-stimulating hormone [MSH]). These peptides activate melanocortin receptors in the skin (melanocortin-1 receptor [MC1R]), to modulate pigmentation, in the adrenal gland (melanocortin-2 receptor [MC2R]) to regulate glucocorticoid synthesis, and in the brain (melanocortin-3 receptor and melanocortin-4 receptor [MC3R and MC4R]) to reduce energy intake and increase energy expenditure. In parallel, leptin inhibits pathways that stimulate food intake (orexigenic), effects that are mediated by neurons expressing the melanocortin antagonist agouti-related protein (AgRP) and neuropeptide Y (NPY).

These two sets of primary leptin-responsive neurons project to second-order neurons expressing the MC4R in the paraventricular nucleus of the hypothalamus and other brain regions. Together, these neurons constitute a critical circuit that regulates energy homeostasis (Schwartz, Woods, Porte, Seeley, & Baskin, 2000).

Leptin and Leptin Receptor Deficiency

Approximately 1% of patients with severe childhood-onset obesity from consanguineous families may have mutations in the gene encoding leptin; 2–3% may have mutations affecting the leptin receptor. Serum leptin is a useful test in patients with severe early-onset obesity, as an undetectable serum leptin is highly suggestive of a diagnosis of congenital leptin deficiency. Very rare leptin mutations that result in a bioactive form of leptin have been reported (Wabitsch et al., 2015). Serum leptin concentrations are appropriate for the degree of obesity in leptin-receptor deficient patients, and as such, an elevated serum leptin concentration is not necessarily a predictor of leptin receptor deficiency (Farooqi et al., 2007). However, a subset of patients harbor *LEPR* mutations, which result in abnormal cleavage of the extracellular domain of LEPR (which can then act as a leptin-binding protein) and are associated with markedly elevated leptin levels (Clement et al., 1998; Lahlou et al., 2000).

The clinical phenotypes associated with congenital leptin and leptin receptor deficiencies are similar. Leptin- and leptin-receptor-deficient infants are born of normal birth weight but exhibit rapid weight gain in the first few months of life, resulting in severe obesity (Farooqi et al., 2002). These infants are characterized by intense hyperphagia, with food-seeking behavior and aggressive behavior when food is denied. Although measurable changes in resting metabolic rate or total energy expenditure have not been demonstrated, abnormalities of sympathetic nerve function in leptin-deficient adults suggest that autonomic dysfunction may contribute to the observed obesity phenotype. Leptin and leptin receptor deficiency are associated with hypothalamic hypothyroidism; normal pubertal development does not occur in adolescents with leptin or leptin receptor deficiency, with biochemical evidence of hypogonadotropic hypogonadism. However, there is some evidence for the delayed but spontaneous onset of menses in some leptin- and leptin-receptor-deficient females. Leptin- and leptin-receptor-deficient children have normal linear growth in childhood and normal insulin-like growth factor-1 (IGF-1) levels. However, the final height of adults is reduced due to the absence of a pubertal growth spurt. Children with leptin deficiency have impaired T cell number and function, consistent with high rates of childhood infection and a high reported rate of childhood mortality from infection (Farooqi et al., 2002).

Although leptin deficiency appears to be rare, it is entirely treatable with daily subcutaneous injections of recombinant human leptin (Farooqi et al., 2002), which are currently available to patients on a named patient basis in a small number of centers around the world. The major effect of leptin treatment is on food intake, with normalization of hyperphagia and enhanced satiety (Farooqi et al., 1999, 2002). Leptin also has permissive effects on the development of puberty and, if given in early childhood, permits appropriate linear growth (Farooqi et al., 2002).

Disorders of POMC Synthesis and Processing

Children who are homozygous or compound heterozygous for mutations in the POMC gene present in neonatal life with adrenal crisis due to ACTH deficiency (POMC is a precursor of ACTH in the pituitary) and require long-term corticosteroid replacement (Krude et al., 2003). Such children have pale skin, and white infants often have red hair due to the lack of MSH function at MC1Rs in the skin. Although red hair may be an important diagnostic clue in patients of white origin, its absence in patients originating from other ethnic groups should not result in this diagnostic consideration being excluded. Children from different ethnic backgrounds may have a less obvious phenotype, such as dark hair with red roots (Farooqi et al., 2006). POMC deficiency results in hyperphagia and early-onset obesity due to loss of melanocortin signaling at the

MC4R. The clinical features are comparable to those reported in patients with mutations in the receptor for POMC derived ligands, MC4R. Selective melanocortin receptor agonists are in clinical trials and appear to be effective therapies for such patients (Kuhnen et al., 2016).

Proprotein convertases (PCs) are a family of serine endoproteases that cleave inactive propeptides into biologically active peptides (Seidah, 2011). Proprotein convertase subtilisin/kexin type 1 and 2 (PCSK1 and PCSK2) are expressed in neuroendocrine tissues where they cleave prohormones, including POMC, pro-thyrotrophin-releasing hormone (TRH), proinsulin, proglucagon, and pro-gonadotrophin-releasing hormone (GnRH) to release biologically active peptides. Compound heterozygous or homozygous mutations in the PCSK1 gene, which encodes PC1/3, cause small-bowel enteropathy. Patients may present in neonatal life/early infancy with persistent diarrhea requiring parenteral feeding. Other important clinical features include hypoglycemia and complex neuroendocrine effects (including diabetes insipidus) due to a failure to process a number of prohormones. Hyperphagia and severe obesity tend to become apparent by 2–3 years of age (Jackson et al., 1997, 2003).

MC4R Deficiency

MC4R deficiency is the most common genetic form of obesity. Assessment of the sequence of the MC4R is increasingly seen as a necessary part of the clinical evaluation of the severely obese child. The prevalence of pathogenic *MC4R* mutations has varied from 0.5 to 2.5% of people, with a BMI >30 kg/m^2 in U.K. and European populations to 5% in patients with severe childhood obesity (Farooqi et al., 2003; Stutzmann et al., 2008). Given the large number of potential influences on body weight, it is perhaps not surprising that both genetic and environmental modifiers will have important effects on the severity of obesity associated with *MC4R* mutations in some pedigrees. Most patients have heterozygous mutations; codominance, with modulation of expressivity and penetrance of the phenotype, is the most appropriate descriptor for the mode of inheritance. Homozygous mutations in *MC4R* have been identified in children from consanguineous families (Farooqi et al., 2003).

The clinical features of MC4R deficiency include hyperphagia in early childhood and accelerated linear growth, which may be a consequence of disproportionate early hyperinsulinemia and effects on pulsatile growth hormone (GH) secretion, which is retained in contrast to common forms of obesity (Martinelli et al., 2011). Reduced sympathetic nervous system activity in MC4R-deficient patients is likely to explain the lower prevalence of hypertension and lower systolic and diastolic blood pressures seen in adults (Greenfield et al., 2009). Central leptin–melanocortin signaling appears to play an important role in the regulation of blood pressure and its coupling to changes in weight (Simonds et al., 2014).

Several studies have now shown that adolescents and adults with heterozygous MC4R mutations do respond to Roux-en-Y gastric bypass surgery (Hatoum et al., 2012). Additionally, as most patients are heterozygotes with one functional allele intact, it is possible that small molecule MC4R agonists or pharmacological chaperones that improve receptor trafficking to the cell surface might be appropriate treatments for this disorder. More recently, a potent melanocortin receptor agonist, RM-493, has been administered as part of a Phase Ib proof-of-concept clinical trial in obese patients. This trial included one cohort of patients with heterozygous loss of function mutations in *MC4R*, who showed promising weight loss after 4 weeks. If this compound moves forward, it may be one of the first examples of a personalized medicine approach for treating obesity in people with a genetically characterized subtype of obesity.

Src Homology 2B Adapter Protein 1 Deficiency

Severe obesity without developmental delay is associated with a significantly increased burden of rare, typically singleton copy number variants (deletions/duplications; Wheeler et al., 2013). Deletion of a 220-kb segment of 16p11.2 is associated with highly penetrant familial severe early-onset obesity and severe insulin resistance (Bochukova et al., 2010). This deletion includes a small number of genes, one of which is Src homology 2B adapter protein 1 (*SH2B1*), known to be involved in leptin and insulin signaling. These patients gain weight in the first years of life, with hyperphagia and fasting plasma insulin levels that are disproportionately elevated compared to age- and obesity-matched controls. Several mutations in the *SH2B1* gene have also been reported in association with early-onset obesity, severe insulin resistance, and behavioral abnormalities, including aggression (Doche et al., 2012).

Genetic Obesity Syndromes with Developmental Delay

Prader–Willi Syndrome

The prevalence of Prader–Willi syndrome (PWS) is approximately 1 in 25,000 live births. Key clinical features include hypotonia and failure to thrive in infancy, mental retardation, short stature, hyperphagic obesity, and hypogonadotropic hypogonadism (Goldstone, 2004). Children with PWS have reduced lean body mass, increased fat mass, and abnormalities that resemble those seen in GH deficiency. GH treatment decreases body fat and increases linear growth, muscle mass, fat oxidation, and energy expenditure in these individuals (Carrel & Allen, 2001). Plasma levels of the stomach-derived hormone ghrelin are markedly elevated in children and adults with PWS, compared to obese controls and patients with other genetic obesity syndromes. The significance of this finding and its possible role in the pathogenesis of hyperphagia in these patients is unknown.

PWS is caused by the deletion of a critical segment on the paternally inherited copy of chromosome 15q11.2-q12, or loss of the entire paternal chromosome 15 with the presence of two maternal copies (uniparental maternal disomy). Most chromosomal abnormalities in PWS occur sporadically. Deletions account for 70–80% of cases; the majority are interstitial deletions, many of which can be visualized by karyotype analysis. There are distinct differences in DNA methylation of the parental alleles. DNA methylation can be used as a reliable postnatal diagnostic tool in PWS. Small deletions encompassing only the HBII-85 family of snoRNAs have been reported in association with the cardinal features of PWS, including obesity (de Smith et al., 2009; Sahoo et al., 2008), suggesting that these noncoding RNAs and the genes that they regulate may be important in the etiology of PWS.

Albright Hereditary Osteodystrophy

Mutations in *GNAS1* that decrease the expression or function of the G alpha s protein result in Albright hereditary osteodystrophy (AHO), which is an autosomal-dominant disorder. Maternal transmission of *GNAS1* mutations leads to classical AHO (characterized by short stature, obesity, skeletal defects, and impaired olfaction) plus resistance to several hormones (e.g., parathyroid hormone) that activate Gs in their target tissues (pseudohypoparathyroidism type IA), whereas paternal transmission leads only to AHO (pseudopseudohypoparathyroidism). Studies in both mice and humans demonstrate that *GNAS1* is imprinted in a tissue-specific manner, being expressed primarily from the maternal allele in some tissues and bi-allelically in other tissues; thus, multi-hormone resistance occurs only when Gs (alpha) mutations are inherited maternally (Weinstein, Chen, & Liu, 2002). Some patients with *GNAS1* mutations may present with obesity without the classical features; the reasons for this phenotypic variation are not as yet known.

Bardet–Biedl Syndrome

Bardet–Biedl syndrome (BBS) is a rare (prevalence < 1/100,000) autosomal-recessive disease characterized by obesity, learning disability, dysmorphic extremities (syndactyly, brachydactyly, or polydactyly), retinal dystrophy or pigmentary retinopathy, hypogonadism, and structural abnormalities of the kidney or functional renal impairment. BBS is a genetically heterogeneous disorder that is now known to map to at least 16 loci, with mutations in more than one locus sometimes required for complete expression of the phenotype. Many BBS genes appear to affect proteins localized to the basal body, a key element of the monocilium thought to be important for intercellular sensing in mammalian cells, including neurons (Ansley et al., 2003). Other disorders of ciliary function (e.g., Alström syndrome [retinal dystrophy, severe insulin resistance, deafness]) and Carpenter syndrome are also associated with obesity. The link between ciliary function and obesity remains unclear, although studies in mice have suggested that ciliary dysfunction can affect leptin signaling and activity of POMC neurons (Seo et al., 2009).

Brain-Derived Neurotrophic Factor Disruption

A small number of children with severe hyperphagia and obesity, impaired short-term memory, hyperactivity, and learning disability who have mutations or chromosomal deletions that disrupt brain-derived neurotrophic factor (BDNF) or its tyrosine kinase receptor tropomycin-related kinase B (TrkB) have been reported (Yeo et al., 2004; Gray et al., 2006). Yanovski and colleagues showed that in patients with Wilms tumor, aniridia, genitourinary anomalies, mental retardation/intellectual disability (WAGR) syndrome, a subset of deletions on chromosome 11p.12 that encompasses the BDNF locus were associated with early-onset obesity (Han et al., 2008). Given the severe developmental phenotype of these patients, it is not surprising that mutations seem to arise de novo, and as such, they should be considered when both parents are of normal weight and IQ.

SIM1 Deficiency

Single-minded 1 (*SIM1*) is a basic helix–loop–helix transcription factor involved in the development and function of the paraventricular nucleus of the hypothalamus. Chromosomal deletions affecting *SIM1* (Faivre et al., 2002; Holder, Butte, & Zinn, 2000) (often de novo) and dominantly inherited heterozygous loss of function mutations in *SIM1* have been reported (Bonnefond et al., 2013; Ramachandrappa et al., 2013). SIM1-deficient patients are hyperphagic with evidence of autonomic dysfunction (characterized by low systolic blood pressures) as seen in MC4R deficiency, which suggests that some aspects of the clinical phenotype can be explained by altered melanocortin signaling. However, many *SIM1* mutation carriers have speech and language delays and exhibit neurobehavioral abnormalities, including autistic-type behaviors. These features are not recognized features of MC4R deficiency but show some overlap with the behavioral phenotypes seen in PWS. As the hyperphagia of *SIM1* haplo-insufficient mice is partly ameliorated by the central administration of oxytocin (Kublaoui, Gemelli, Tolson, Wang, & Zinn, 2008), a neurotransmitter involved in the modulation of emotion and social interaction, impaired oxytocinergic signaling is one possible mechanism implicated in the obesity and behavioral phenotype seen in SIM1 deficiency.

KSR2 Deficiency

A number of large family-based population studies have addressed the contribution of genetic versus environmental factors to energy expenditure, including physical activity (Perusse et al., 1989). For example, exercise participation within families is entirely accounted for by shared family environment. However, basal metabolic rate (BMR), which is the major determinant of energy expenditure (70%), is highly heritable (Bouchard & Tremblay, 1990). Whereas most of the genes that promote severe obesity do so by affecting appetite, the recent finding that obese people harboring genetic variants in *KSR2* (kinase suppressor of ras2) have reduced BMR demonstrates that genetic variation in energy expenditure can contribute to weight gain in some individuals (Pearce et al., 2013).

Summary

Cumulatively, work in the genetics of obesity has shown that the variability in BMI in the population has a large genetic component. The finding of multiple common variants in GWASs currently has limited utility in predicting weight-related problems and the potential impact of interventions. Many of the GWAS signals identified to date map to noncoding regions of the genome that may potentially be involved in gene regulation (rather than by directly disrupting particular genes). Further experimental work is needed to understand the mechanisms that underlie these associations.

Exome sequencing of cohorts of obese, normal-weight, and lean people are well underway and are likely to lead to the identification of additional rare variants in new genes. The functions of these genes need to be explored in cells, model organisms, and humans. Establishing the functional relevance of rare variants (which outnumber common variants in the human genome) has diagnostic value, can inform drug development, and provides opportunities for the development of precision/stratified medicine. Adding genetic evidence to support the role of a drug target in disease can increase the chances of success in drug development (Nelson et al., 2016), in turn reducing the timeline from target discovery to clinical trials and the cost burden of failed clinical trials due to ineffective drugs that lack efficacy.

References

Ahima, R. S., Prabakaran, D., Mantzoros, C., Qu, D., Lowell, B., Maratos-Flier, E., et al. (1996). Role of leptin in the neuroendocrine response to fasting. *Nature, 382*(6588), 250–252.

Ahmad, S., Rukh, G., Varga, T. V., Ali, A., Kurbasic, A., Shungin, D., et al. (2013). Gene × physical activity interactions in obesity: Combined analysis of 111,421 individuals of European ancestry. *PLOS Genetics, 9*(7), e1003607.

Allison, D. B., Kaprio, J., Korkeila, M., Koskenvuo, M., Neale, M. C., & Hayakawa, K. (1996). The heritability of body mass index among an international sample of monozygotic twins reared apart. *International Journal of Obesity and Related Metabolic Disorders, 20*(6), 501–506.

Ansley, S. J., Badano, J. L., Blacque, O. E., Hill, J., Hoskins, B. E., Leitch, C. C., et al. (2003). Basal body dysfunction is a likely cause of pleiotropic Bardet–Biedl syndrome. *Nature, 425*(6958), 628–633.

Belsky, D. W., & Israel, S. (2014). Integrating genetics and social science: Genetic risk scores. *Biodemography and Social Biology, 60*(2), 137–155.

Bochukova, E. G., Huang, N., Keogh, J., Henning, E., Purmann, C., Blaszczyk, K., et al. (2010). Large, rare chromosomal deletions associated with severe early-onset obesity. *Nature, 463*(7281), 666–670.

Bonnefond, A., Raimondo, A., Stutzmann, F., Ghoussaini, M., Ramachandrappa, S., Bersten, D. C., et al. (2013). Loss-of-function mutations in SIM1 contribute to obesity and Prader–Willi-like features. *Journal of Clinical Investigation, 123*(7), 3037–3041.

Bouchard, C., & Tremblay, A. (1990). Genetic effects in human energy expenditure components. *International Journal of Obesity, 14*(Suppl. 1), 49–55.

Bouchard, C., Tremblay, A., Despres, J. P., Nadeau, A., Lupien, P. J., Moorjani, S., et al. (1996). Overfeeding in identical twins: 5-year postoverfeeding results. *Metabolism, 45*(8), 1042–1050.

Bouchard, C., Tremblay, A., Despres, J. P., Nadeau, A., Lupien, P. J., Theriault, G., et al. (1990). The response to long-term overfeeding in identical twins. *New England Journal of Medicine, 322*(21), 1477–1482.

Bray, G. A. (2015). From farm to fat cell: Why aren't we all fat? *Metabolism, 64*(3), 349–353.

Carrel, A. L., & Allen, D. B. (2001). Prader–Willi syndrome: How does growth hormone affect body composition and physical function? *Journal of Pediatric Endocrinology and Metabolism, 14*(6, Suppl.), 1445–1451.

Cecil, J. E., Tavendale, R., Watt, P., Hetherington, M. M., & Palmer, C. N. (2008). An obesity-associated FTO gene variant and increased energy intake in children. *New England Journal of Medicine, 359*(24), 2558–2566.

Clement, K., Vaisse, C., Lahlou, N., Cabrol, S., Pelloux, V., Cassuto, D., et al. (1998). A mutation in the human leptin receptor gene causes obesity and pituitary dysfunction. *Nature, 392*(6674), 398–401.

de Smith, A. J., Purmann, C., Walters, R. G., Ellis, R. J., Holder, S. E., Van Haelst, M. M., et al. (2009). A deletion of the HBII-85 class of small nucleolar RNAs (snoRNAs) is associated with hyperphagia, obesity and hypogonadism. *Human Molecular Genetics, 18*(17), 3257–3265.

Dina, C., Meyre, D., Gallina, S., Durand, E., Korner, A., Jacobson, P., et al. (2007). Variation in FTO contributes to childhood obesity and severe adult obesity. *Nature Genetics, 39*(6), 724–726.

Doche, M. E., Bochukova, E. G., Su, H. W., Pearce, L. R., Keogh, J. M., Henning, E., et al. (2012). Human SH2B1 mutations are associated with maladaptive behaviors and obesity. *Journal of Clinical Investigation, 122*(12), 4732–4736.

Elder, S. J., Neale, M. C., Fuss, P. J., Lichtenstein, A. H., Greenberg, A. S., McCrory, M. A., et al. (2012). Genetic and environmental influences on eating behavior: A study of twin pairs reared apart or reared together. *Open Nutrition Journal, 6*, 59–70.

Fabsitz, R. R., Sholinsky, P., & Carmelli, D. (1994). Genetic influences on adult weight gain and maximum body mass index in male twins. *American Journal of Epidemiology, 140*(8), 711–720.

Faivre, L., Cormier-Daire, V., Lapierre, J. M., Colleaux, L., Jacquemont, S., Genevieve, D., et al. (2002). Deletion of the SIM1 gene (6q16.2) in a patient with a Prader–Willi-like phenotype. *Journal of Medical Genetics, 39*(8), 594–596.

Farooqi, I. S., Drop, S., Clements, A., Keogh, J. M., Biernacka, J., Lowenbein, S., et al. (2006). Heterozygosity for a POMC-null mutation and increased obesity risk in humans. *Diabetes, 55*(9), 2549–2553.

Farooqi, I. S., Jebb, S. A., Langmack, G., Lawrence, E., Cheetham, C. H., Prentice, A. M., et al. (1999). Effects of recombinant leptin therapy in a child with congenital leptin deficiency. *New England Journal of Medicine, 341*(12), 879–884.

Farooqi, I. S., Keogh, J. M., Yeo, G. S., Lank, E. J., Cheetham, T., & O'Rahilly, S. (2003). Clinical spectrum of obesity and mutations in the melanocortin 4 receptor gene. *New England Journal of Medicine, 348*(12), 1085–1095.

Farooqi, I. S., Matarese, G., Lord, G. M., Keogh, J. M., Lawrence, E., Agwu, C., et al. (2002). Beneficial effects of leptin on obesity, T cell hyporesponsiveness, and neuroendocrine/metabolic dysfunction of human congenital leptin deficiency. *Journal of Clinical Investigation, 110*(8), 1093–1103.

Farooqi, I. S., Wangensteen, T., Collins, S., Kimber, W., Matarese, G., Keogh, J. M., et al. (2007). Clinical and molecular genetic spectrum of congenital deficiency of the leptin receptor. *New England Journal of Medicine, 356*(3), 237–247.

Frayling, T. M., Timpson, N. J., Weedon, M. N., Zeggini, E., Freathy, R. M., Lindgren, C. M., et al. (2007). A common variant in the FTO gene is associated with body mass index and predisposes to childhood and adult obesity. *Science, 316*(5826), 889–894.

Friedman, J. M. (2000). Obesity in the new millennium. *Nature, 404*(6778), 632–634.

Friedman, J. M. (2003). A war on obesity, not the obese. *Science, 299*(5608), 856–858.

Garnett, S. P., Baur, L. A., Jones, A. M., & Hardy, L. L. (2016). Trends in the prevalence of morbid and severe obesity in Australian children aged 7–15 years, 1985–2012. *PLOS ONE, 11*(5), e0154879.

Goldstone, A. P. (2004). Prader–Willi syndrome: Advances in genetics, pathophysiology and treatment. *Trends in Endocrinology and Metabolism, 15*(1), 12–20.

Gray, J., Yeo, G. S., Cox, J. J., Morton, J., Adlam, A. L., Keogh, J. M., et al. (2006). Hyperphagia, severe obesity, impaired cognitive function, and hyperactivity associated with functional loss of one copy of the brain-derived neurotrophic factor (BDNF) gene. *Diabetes, 55*(12), 3366–3371.

Greenfield, J. R., Miller, J. W., Keogh, J. M., Henning, E., Satterwhite, J. H., Cameron, G. S., et al. (2009). Modulation of blood pressure by central melanocortinergic pathways. *New England Journal of Medicine, 360*(1), 44–52.

Han, J. C., Liu, Q. R., Jones, M., Levinn, R. L., Menzie, C. M., Jefferson-George, K. S., et al. (2008). Brain-derived neurotrophic factor and obesity in the WAGR syndrome. *New England Journal of Medicine, 359*(9), 918–927.

Hatoum, I. J., Greenawalt, D. M., Cotsapas, C., Reitman, M. L., Daly, M. J., & Kaplan, L. M. (2011). Heritability of the weight loss response to gastric bypass surgery. *Journal of Clinical Endocrinology and Metabolism, 96*(10), E1630–E1633.

Hatoum, I. J., Stylopoulos, N., Vanhoose, A. M., Boyd, K. L., Yin, D. P., Ellacott, K. L., et al. (2012). Melanocortin-4 receptor signaling is required for weight loss after gastric bypass surgery. *Journal of Clinical Endocrinology and Metabolism, 97*(6), E1023–E1031.

Holder, J. L., Jr., Butte, N. F., & Zinn, A. R. (2000). Profound obesity associated with a balanced translocation that disrupts the SIM1 gene. *Human Molecular Genetics, 9*(1), 101–108.

Jackson, R. S., Creemers, J. W., Farooqi, I. S., Raffin-Sanson, M. L., Varro, A., Dockray, G. J. et al. (2003). Small-intestinal dysfunction accompanies the complex endocrinopathy of human proprotein convertase 1 deficiency. *Journal of Clinical Investigation, 112*(10), 1550–1560.

Jackson, R. S., Creemers, J. W., Ohagi, S., Raffin-Sanson, M. L., Sanders, L., Montague, C. T. et al. (1997). Obesity and impaired prohormone processing associated with mutations in the human prohormone convertase 1 gene. *Nature Genetics, 16*(3), 303–306.

King, N. A., Caudwell, P., Hopkins, M., Byrne, N. M., Colley, R., Hills, A. P., et al. (2007). Metabolic and behavioral compensatory responses to exercise interventions: Barriers to weight loss. *Obesity (Silver Spring), 15*(6), 1373–1383.

Krude, H., Biebermann, H., Luck, W., Horn, R., Brabant, G., & Gruters, A. (1998). Severe early-onset obesity, adrenal insufficiency and red hair pigmentation caused by POMC mutations in humans. *Nature Genetics, 19*(2), 155–157.

Krude, H., Biebermann, H., Schnabel, D., Tansek, M. Z., Theunissen, P., Mullis, P. E., et al. (2003). Obesity due to proopiomelanocortin deficiency: Three new cases and treatment trials with thyroid hormone and ACTH4-10. *Journal of Clinical Endocrinology and Metabolism, 88*(10), 4633–4640.

Kublaoui, B. M., Gemelli, T., Tolson, K. P., Wang, Y., & Zinn, A. R. (2008). Oxytocin deficiency mediates hyperphagic obesity of Sim1 haploinsufficient mice. *Molecular Endocrinology, 22*(7), 1723–1734.

Kuhnen, P., Clement, K., Wiegand, S., Blankenstein, O., Gottesdiener, K., Martini, L. L., et al. (2016). Proopiomelanocortin deficiency treated with a melanocortin-4 receptor agonist. *New England Journal of Medicine, 375*(3), 240–246.

Lahlou, N., Clement, K., Carel, J. C., Vaisse, C., Lotton, C., Le Bihan, Y., et al. (2000). Soluble leptin receptor in serum of subjects with complete resistance to leptin: Relation to fat mass. *Diabetes, 49*(8), 1347–1352.

Locke, A. E., Kahali, B., Berndt, S. I., Justice, A. E., Pers, T. H., Day, F. R., et al. (2015). Genetic studies of body mass index yield new insights for obesity biology. *Nature, 518*(7538), 197–206.

Loos, R. J. (2012). Genetic determinants of common obesity and their value in prediction. *Best Practice and Research: Clinical Endocrinology and Metabolism, 26*(2), 211–226.

Loos, R. J., Lindgren, C. M., Li, S., Wheeler, E., Zhao, J. H., Prokopenko, I., et al. (2008). Common variants near MC4R are associated with fat mass, weight and risk of obesity. *Nature Genetics, 40*(6), 768–775.

Maes, H. H., Neale, M. C., & Eaves, L. J. (1997).

Genetic and environmental factors in relative body weight and human adiposity. *Behavior Genetics, 27*(4), 325–351.

Maffei, M., Halaas, J., Ravussin, E., Pratley, R. E., Lee, G. H., Zhang, Y., et al. (1995). Leptin levels in human and rodent: Measurement of plasma leptin and ob RNA in obese and weight-reduced subjects. *Nature Medicine, 1*(11), 1155–1161.

Martinelli, C. E., Keogh, J. M., Greenfield, J. R., Henning, E., van der Klaauw, A. A., Blackwood, A., et al. (2011). Obesity due to melanocortin 4 receptor (MC4R) deficiency is associated with increased linear growth and final height, fasting hyperinsulinemia, and incompletely suppressed growth hormone secretion. *Journal of Clinical Endocrinology and Metabolism, 96*(1), E181–E188.

Montague, C. T., Farooqi, I. S., Whitehead, J. P., Soos, M. A., Rau, H., Wareham, N. J., et al. (1997). Congenital leptin deficiency is associated with severe early-onset obesity in humans. *Nature, 387*(6636), 903–908.

Nelson, M. R., Johnson, T., Warren, L., Hughes, A. R., Chissoe, S. L., Xu, C. F., et al. (2016). The genetics of drug efficacy: Opportunities and challenges. *Nature Reviews Genetics, 17*(4), 197–206.

Pearce, L. R., Atanassova, N., Banton, M. C., Bottomley, B., van der Klaauw, A. A., Revelli, J. P., et al. (2013). KSR2 mutations are associated with obesity, insulin resistance, and impaired cellular fuel oxidation. *Cell, 155*(4), 765–777.

Perusse, L., Tremblay, A., Leblanc, C., & Bouchard, C. (1989). Genetic and environmental influences on level of habitual physical activity and exercise participation. *American Journal of Epidemiology, 129*(5), 1012–1022.

Perusse, L., Tremblay, A., Leblanc, C., Cloninger, C. R., Reich, T., Rice, J., et al. (1988). Familial resemblance in energy intake: Contribution of genetic and environmental factors. *American Journal of Clinical Nutrition, 47*(4), 629–635.

Poehlman, E. T., Tremblay, A., Despres, J. P., Fontaine, E., Perusse, L., Theriault, G., et al. (1986). Genotype-controlled changes in body composition and fat morphology following overfeeding in twins. *American Journal of Clinical Nutrition, 43*(5), 723–731.

Qi, Q., Kilpelainen, T. O., Downer, M. K., Tanaka, T., Smith, C. E., Sluijs, I., et al. (2014). FTO genetic variants, dietary intake and body mass index: Insights from 177,330 individuals. *Human Molecular Genetics, 23*(25), 6961–6972.

Ramachandrappa, S., Raimondo, A., Cali, A. M., Keogh, J. M., Henning, E., Saeed, S., et al. (2013). Rare variants in single-minded 1 (SIM1) are associated with severe obesity. *Journal of Clinical Investigation, 123*(7), 3042–3050.

Sahoo, T., del Gaudio, D., German, J. R., Shinawi, M., Peters, S. U., Person, R. E., et al. (2008). Prader–Willi phenotype caused by paternal deficiency for the HBII-85 C/D box small nucleolar RNA cluster. *Nature Genetics, 40*(6), 719–721.

Schwartz, M. W., Woods, S. C., Porte, D., Jr., Seeley, R. J., & Baskin, D. G. (2000). Central nervous system control of food intake. *Nature, 404*(6778), 661–671.

Schwartz, M. W., Woods, S. C., Seeley, R. J., Barsh, G. S., Baskin, D. G., & Leibel, R. L. (2003). Is the energy homeostasis system inherently biased toward weight gain? *Diabetes, 52*(2), 232–238.

Seidah, N. G. (2011). The proprotein convertases, 20 years later. *Methods in Molecular Biology, 768*, 23–57.

Seo, S., Guo, D. F., Bugge, K., Morgan, D. A., Rahmouni, K., & Sheffield, V. C. (2009). Requirement of Bardet–Biedl syndrome proteins for leptin receptor signaling. *Human Molecular Genetics, 18*(7), 1323–1331.

Shungin, D., Winkler, T. W., Croteau-Chonka, D. C., Ferreira, T., Locke, A. E., Magi, R., et al. (2015). New genetic loci link adipose and insulin biology to body fat distribution. *Nature, 518*(7538), 187–196.

Silventoinen, K., Magnusson, P. K., Tynelius, P., Kaprio, J., & Rasmussen, F. (2008). Heritability of body size and muscle strength in young adulthood: A study of one million Swedish men. *Genetic Epidemiology, 32*(4), 341–349.

Simonds, S. E., Pryor, J. T., Ravussin, E., Greenway, F. L., Dileone, R., Allen, A. M., et al. (2014). Leptin mediates the increase in blood pressure associated with obesity. *Cell, 159*(6), 1404–1416.

Skinner, A. C., & Skelton, J. A. (2014). Prevalence and trends in obesity and severe obesity among children in the United States, 1999–2012. *JAMA Pediatrics, 168*(6), 561–566.

Sorensen, T. I., Price, R. A., Stunkard, A. J., & Schulsinger, F. (1989). Genetics of obesity in adult adoptees and their biological siblings. *British Medical Journal, 298*(6666), 87–90.

Stutzmann, F., Tan, K., Vatin, V., Dina, C., Jouret, B., Tichet, J., et al. (2008). Prevalence of melanocortin-4 receptor deficiency in Europeans and their age-dependent penetrance in multigenerational pedigrees. *Diabetes, 57*(9), 2511–2518.

Timpson, N. J., Emmett, P. M., Frayling, T. M., Rogers, I., Hattersley, A. T., McCarthy, M. I., et al. (2008). The fat mass- and obesity-associated locus and dietary intake in children. *American Journal of Clinical Nutrition, 88*(4), 971–978.

van der Klaauw, A. A., & Farooqi, I. S. (2015). The hunger genes: Pathways to obesity. *Cell, 161*(1), 119–132.

Wabitsch, M., Funcke, J. B., Lennerz, B., Kuhnle-Krahl, U., Lahr, G., Debatin, K. M., et al. (2015). Biologically inactive leptin and early-onset extreme obesity. *New England Journal of Medicine, 372*(1), 48–54.

Wardle, J., Carnell, S., Haworth, C. M., Farooqi, I. S., O'Rahilly, S., & Plomin, R. (2008). Obesity associated genetic variation in FTO is associated with diminished satiety. *Journal of Clinical Endocrinology and Metabolism, 93*(9), 3640–3643.

Wardle, J., Carnell, S., Haworth, C. M., & Plomin, R. (2008). Evidence for a strong genetic influence on childhood adiposity despite the force of the obesogenic environment. *American Journal of Clinical Nutrition, 87*(2), 398–404.

Weinstein, L. S., Chen, M., & Liu, J. (2002). Gs(alpha) mutations and imprinting defects in human disease. *Annals of the New York Academy of Sciences, 968*, 173–197.

Wheeler, E., Huang, N., Bochukova, E. G., Keogh, J. M., Lindsay, S., Garg, S., et al. (2013). Genome-wide SNP and CNV analysis identifies common and low-frequency variants associated with severe early-onset obesity. *Nature Genetics, 45*(5), 513–517.

Yeo, G. S., Connie Hung, C. C., Rochford, J., Keogh, J., Gray, J., Sivaramakrishnan, S., et al. (2004). A de novo mutation affecting human TrkB associated with severe obesity and developmental delay. *Nature Neuroscience, 7*(11), 1187–1189.

Yeo, G. S., Farooqi, I. S., Aminian, S., Halsall, D. J., Stanhope, R. G., & O'Rahilly, S. (1998). A frameshift mutation in MC4R associated with dominantly inherited human obesity. *Nature Genetics, 20*(2), 111–112.

Zhu, J., Loos, R. J., Lu, L., Zong, G., Gan, W., Ye, X., et al. (2014). Associations of genetic risk score with obesity and related traits and the modifying effect of physical activity in a Chinese Han population. *PLOS ONE, 9*(3), e91442.

CHAPTER 5

Human Energy Homeostasis and the Gut Microbiome

Michael Rosenbaum
Rudolph L. Leibel

The ecological community of commensal, symbiotic, and pathogenic microorganisms that live throughout and on our bodies is collectively referred to as the *microbiota*. The human gut microbiota consists of up to 100 trillion microbes that exist in a largely symbiotic relationship with their human hosts. In the aggregate, these microbes include at least 150 times the number of genes present in the entire human genome (Hamady & Knight, 2009; Ursell et al., 2014). These genes are collectively referred to as the *microbiome*. Interplay between the gut microbiota and human health has been posited for over a century (Metchnikoff & Mitchell, 1908). However, due largely to the inability to characterize the intestinal bacterial population, much of which remains uncultureable, evidence that these microbes may participate in energy intake and expenditure did not emerge until this millennium (Backhed et al., 2004). Recently developed techniques to directly sequence the microbiome have enabled characterization of the microbiota in ways that were not previously possible (Goodman et al., 2011) and opened up exciting new avenues for studying the role of these microbes in the development and treatment of obesity.

The gut microbiome varies substantially in size and composition, both cross-sectionally between individuals and longitudinally within individuals. For example, the microbiome is affected by age, diet, medication, weight, and overall metabolic state of the host. In turn, various subpopulations of the gut microbiota are capable of affecting the production of molecules that may influence energy balance and substrate metabolism (Tehrani, Nezami, Gewirtz, & Srinivasan, 2012; Tagliabue & Eli, 2013). Based predominantly on rodent studies, the microbiota thus constitutes a responsive enteroendocrine organ that may participate in the pathogenesis of human obesity and diabetes, and, for this reason, could provide therapeutic targets. This chapter reviews what has been done and what may be done to determine how translatable rodent microbiota-related data are to humans, as well as the implications for use of human gut microbiota as an index of risk for obesity and as a target for the treatment and prevention of obesity.

The Microbiota

Although phylum-level and even family-level groupings of microbes are very broad and can conceal potentially important variation at finer levels (including at the strain level), some general trends emerge. The major gut microbial phyla, expressed as the percentage of the total population, are *Bacteroidetes* (~20–25%), *Firmicutes* (~60–65%), *Proteobacteria* (~5–10%), and *Actinobacteria* (~3%). Together, these phyla constitute over 97% of the gut microbe population (see Table 5.1). The taxonomic variability (reflecting both the number of operational taxonomic units [OTUs] and the diversity within those OTUs) is much greater than the functional variability (the variability in categories of gene [COG] functions relevant to energy homeostasis performed by these OTUs) as measured by a variety of methods. This finding suggests that multiple microbiotal configurations may lead to essentially the same functional result, making it more complicated to assess whether taxonomic changes are of clinical significance (Turnbaugh et al., 2009; Human Microbiome Project Consortium, 2012).

Studies in Rodents

Effects of Weight and Diet Composition on the Microbiota in Rodents

As discussed above, the two most abundant phyla in the gut are *Bacteroidetes* and *Firmicutes*. In genetically obese Lep^{ob} mice, the relative proportion of *Bacteroidetes* is decreased and the relative proportion of *Firmicutes* is increased across all subgroups within these phyla (Clarke et al., 2012). However, the taxonomic variability is not different from that of lean mice. These data suggest that in the genetically obese mouse, obesity per se alters microbial ecology (relative proportion of different phyla) without affecting diversity. In contrast, dietary manipulations affect both microbial ecology and diversity (greater diversity on diets high in polysaccharides, plus the same changes in microbial ecology seen with weight loss or weight gain in mice on a high-fat Western diet; Turnbaugh, Backhed, Fulton, & Gordon, 2008). When fed a high-fat diet, both wild-type and obesity-resistant RELM-β knockout (KO) mice still show significant decreases in *Bacteroidetes* independent of their substantially different rates of fat accretion (less weight gain in the KO mice; Hildebrandt et al., 2009). Changes in the microbiome due to weight reduction are also affected by diet composition. Weight-reduced, diet-induced obese (DIO) mice eating a high-fat diet have a more diverse microbiome after weight reduction than control mice at the same weight on chow or than weight-reduced control mice eating a chow diet (Ravussin et al., 2012). As discussed below, there is much greater variability in results comparing humans who are obese with humans who have never been obese (Walters, Xu, & Knight, 2014).

Effects of Changes in the Microbiota on Energy Homeostasis in Rodents

The importance of the gut microbiota in rodent energy homeostasis is emphasized by the consequences of its absence and repletion in studies of germ-free mice, especially those that were colonized with a defined microbial community (*gnotobiotic mice*). The lack of microbiota in germ-free mice results in food-processing inefficiency (impaired harvesting of energy from the diet). Inoculation of germ-free mice with "conventional" (mice on standard chow diet, not overfed or underfed) microbes results in weight gain to similar levels of fatness as the donor mice, despite an approximate 30% increase in energy expenditure and 30% decline in energy intake (Backhed et al., 2004)—that is, a reversal of the food-processing inefficiency.

Changes in energy homeostasis and weight in gnotobiotic mice are dependent upon the status of the donor. Germ-free mice inoculated with microbes from leptin-deficient (Lep^{ob}) mice containing higher absolute and relative proportions of *Firmicutes* gain about twice as much fat mass as gnotobiotic mice given inoculations from wild-type mice, despite no significant differences in absolute energy intake. The increase in fat mass without changes in caloric intake reflect an approximate 15% decrease in the number of unabsorbed calories remaining in the distal intestines of the mice inoculated with the Lep^{ob} microbiota—that is, an increase in energy harvest efficiency (Turnbaugh et al., 2006). This donor effect is also seen following inoculation of germ-free mice with the microbiota from monozygotic (MZ) and dizygotic (DZ) human twin pairs discordant for obesity. Despite no donor-related differences in daily chow consumption, gnotobiotic animals with microbes from the obese twin (designated as Ob mice) experienced an approximately 10-fold greater increase in percentage of body fat than gnotobiotic animals with microbes from the lean twin (designated as Ln mice).

Surprisingly, instead of any regression toward a "mean microbiome" and level of fatness, co-housing of Ob and Ln mice (designated as Ob–Ln pairs, and individual mice in each pair designated as Ob^{ch} and Ln^{ch} depending on whether animals were inoculated initially with an obese or lean twin microbiota, respectively) resulted in the Ob^{ch} mice acquiring the microbiome of Ln^{ch} animals and only a 2–3% gain in fat mass in the Ob^{ch} mice (vs. ~11% in Ob–Ob pairs). In contrast, there was no change in the somatotype or microbiome of the Ln^{ch} mice. The degree of adoption of the Ln^{ch} microbiome in roommate Ob^{ch} mice was even greater if the mice were fed a low-saturated-fat, high-fruit and -vegetable diet, rather than a high-saturated-fat, low-fruit and -vegetable diet, which is considered reflective of the Western diet. On the non-Western low-saturated fat, high-fruit and -vegetable diet, Ob-Ob cage mates gained significantly more fat mass (~6%) and weight (~8%) than all other mice (Ln–Ln, Ln^{ch}, and Ob^{ch}), for whom body composition changes were insignificant over a 10-day period. However, on the Western high-saturated-fat, low-fruit and -vegetable diet, the greater weight gain (~8% in Ln–Ln and Ln^{ch} mice and ~14% in Ob–Ob and Ob^{ch} mice) and fat gain (~2–3% in Ln–Ln and Ln^{ch} mice and ~9% in Ob–Ob and Ob^{ch} mice) in Ob^{ch} mice was not affected by co-housing with Ln^{ch} mice (Ridaura, et al., 2013). In other words, the dietary composition not only affected the microbiome of both lean and obese mice, but also affected the "susceptibility" of obese mice to acquiring the microbiome and somatotype of their lean cage mates. The effects of microbiome inoculation on somatotype in mice are not limited to obese verses lean donors. Studies of germ-free mice inoculated with microbiota from obesity-prone (OP, higher *Firmicutes:Bacteroidetes* ratio) versus obesity-resistant (OR) rats show that there is greater weight gain in the OP-treated group, but only in the setting of a high-fat diet (Duca et al., 2014); that is, the microbiota effect of OP donors is dependent on diet composition.

It has been observed that probiotics, defined as live microorganisms that confer a health benefit on the host when administered in adequate amounts (Bindels, Delzenne, Cani, & Walter, 2015)—such as certain species of *Lactobacillus*—reduce weight and body fat in DIO mice without changing energy intake (Lee et al., 2006). This finding is in contrast to the transfer of intestinal flora from lean mice to germ-free mice, which results in weight (fat) gain despite *decreased* energy intake and *increased* energy expenditure (Backhed et al., 2004).

The mouse microbiome is somewhat strain-dependent (Kovacs et al., 2011), but these host genotype effects are outweighed by the environment. Ericsson et al. (2015) compared mouse strain and vendor effects on the microbiomes of six strains of female mice (3.5 weeks to 24 weeks of age, some strains duplicated) purchased from three different commercial resources. All mice were housed at a single site and fed standard chow diets consisting of approximately 20% of kilocalories (kcal) as protein, 60% as carbohydrate, and 20% as fat. Within populations of *Bacteroidetes, Firmicutes,* and *Proteobacteria,* twice as many significant effects of vendor source (within inbred strains) were noted than differences among strains. There was a greater effect for the vendor than for the specific strain of mouse on the density of the most common microbiota. The significant initial effects of vendor, and to a lesser degree, of strain, did not seem to increase or decrease significantly as the mice aged (between 3.5 and 24 weeks of age), suggesting the importance of early gut colonization and inbred strain × vendor interactions. On the other hand, Parks et al. (2013) reported significant heritability of weight gain and gut microbial composition and plasticity (potential for change) in response to a high-fat, high-sugar diet. However, neither the baseline "enterotype" nor the degree of plasticity (amount of change in response to diet) was independently predictive of weight gain in mice. In humans, the predominance of the environment in determining the composition of the gut microbiome is also evident (Wu et al., 2011).

TABLE 5.1. Overview of the Composition of the Human Microbiome

Phylum	% of microbiome	Genus or species	Relevant function	Sources	References
			Major phyla (> 1% of most individuals)		
Firmicutes	~60–65%	*Clostridium* *Eubacterium* *Faecalibacterium* *Lactobacilli* *Roseburia* *Ruminococcus*	Some species ferment fiber into butyrate; other functions range from symbionts to pathogens; butyrate production		Backhed et al. (2004); Eckburg et al. (2005); Ley, Peterson, & Gordon (2006); Turnbaugh et al. (2009); Human Microbiome Project Consortium (2012); Yatsunenko et al. (2012)
Bacteroidetes	~20–25%	*Alistipes* *Bacteroides* *Parabacteroides* *Prophyromonas* *Prevotella*	Polysaccharide degradation; some species ferment fiber into butyrate	Increase in protein-rich, high-meat diets; increase in grain-rich, high-fiber diets	Xu et al. (2003); Backhed et al. (2004); Eckburg et al. (2005); Ley, Peterson, & Gordon (2006); Xu et al. (2007); Turnbaugh et al. (2009); Wu et al. (2011); Human Microbiome Project Consortium (2012); Walters, Xu, & Knight (2014)
Proteobacteria	~5–10%	*E. coli*			Backhed et al. (2004); Eckburg et al. (2005); Ley, Peterson, et al. (2006); Turnbaugh et al. (2009); Human Microbiome Project Consortium (2012)
Actinobacteria	~3%	*Bifidobacterium* *Colinsella*	Vitamin biosynthesis, especially folic acid	Common probiotic	Backhed et al. (2004); Eckburg et al. (2005); Ley, Peterson, et al. (2006); Turnbaugh et al. (2009); Human Microbiome Project Consortium (2012)

			Minor phyla (< 1% of most individuals)		
Archaea	< 1%	*Methanobrevibacter* *Methanosphera*	Both convert hydrogen gas to methane (methanogens)		Gaci, Borrel, Tottey, O'Toole, & Brugere (2014); Remely et al. (2015)
Deferribacteres	< 1%		Reduce iron	Increased in gastrointerestinal bleeding	Xu et al. (2003, 2007); Wu et al. (2011); Walters et al. (2014)
Fusobacteria	< 1%	*Fusobacterium nucleatum*	Pro-inflammatory colonic tumorigenic factor	Increased in high-meat diets	Strauss, White, Ambrose, McDonald, & Allen-Vercoe (2008); Wu et al. (2011); Castellarin et al. (2012)
Melainabacteria	< 1%		Synthesize vitamins B and K; ferment carbohydrate into ethanol, lactate, and formate	Increased in high-plant diets; present in groundwater	Wu et al., 2011; Yatsunenko et al. (2012); Soo et al. (2014)
Spirochaetes	< 1%	Predominantly *Treponema*		More common in rural communities and in high-fiber diets	Wu et al. (2011); Schnorr et al. (2014)
Verrucomicrobia	< 1%	*Akkermansia muciniphila*	Degrade mucin, diminish inflammation, and increase gut butyrate and mucus layer thickness		Everard et al. (2013)

Studies in Humans

Effects of the Intrauterine Environment and Mode of Delivery

The establishment of the gut microbial population in a neonate is a complex process involving interactions among the maternal and fetal genotypes and the intrauterine (e.g., gestation length), perinatal (delivery type), and postnatal (diet, antibiotics) environments (Guaraldi & Salvatori, 2012). Recent data have challenged the view that the intrauterine environment is normally sterile, and that therefore fetal/neonatal microbial colonization begins at birth. There is apparent in utero colonization of the infant gut, which is influenced by such factors as maternal history or allergies/atopy and antibiotic therapy, with possible implications for infant health (Koleva, Kim, Scott, & Kozysrskyi, 2015). Maternal exposures to antibiotics in the second and third trimesters of pregnancy (or early infancy) are associated with decreased bacterial diversity of the neonate's stool, reduced abundance of lactobacilli and bifidobacteria in the infant gut, and an increased risk of childhood obesity (Ajslev, Andeersen, Gamborg, Sorensen, & Jess, 2011; Mueller et al., 2013; Murphy et al., 2014). The mechanisms for this increase are not clear, but animal studies have suggested that low-dose penicillin administered early in life increases susceptibility to high-fat-diet (HFD)-induced obesity, and that this susceptibility can be transferred to gnotobiotic animals (Cox et al., 2014).

The vaginally delivered neonate is initially colonized postnatally with the vaginal and distal gut bacteria of the mother, whereas babies delivered by Cesarean section (C-section) are initially colonized predominantly with the skin bacteria from the mother (Huurre et al., 2008; Mueller, Bakacs, Cornbellick, Grigoryan, & Dominguez-Bello, 2014). Premature infants and those delivered by C-section initially develop a less diverse microbiome, characterized by an increased predominance of *Proteobacteria* and *Firmicutes* versus *Bacteroidetes* species, compared, respectively, to term infants and those delivered vaginally (Barrett et al., 2013, Chernikova et al., 2016).

Regardless of gestational age at delivery, babies delivered by C-section have a less diverse microbiome that contains absolutely and relatively smaller populations of *Bacteroides* and *Bifidobacteria* species (Costello, Stagaman, Dethlefsen, Bohannan, & Reiman, 2012) that persist for months to years (Guaraldi & Salvatori, 2012). The observations that decreased *Bacteroidetes* populations are present in both obese adults and children born by C-section (Ravussin et al., 2012) suggest that the infant microbiome may contribute to the subsequent increased risk of obesity of approximately 40% in children (Mueller et al., 2013) and young adults (Blustein et al., 2013; Mesquita et al., 2013) delivered by C-section.

Effects of the Extrauterine Environment

In so-called *ecological models,* childhood adiposity is influenced by home and school environments, parental eating behaviors, and food availability (both within and outside of the home), in addition to the adiposity of parents (Larson, Wall, Story, & Neumark-Sztainer, 2013). Although there are genetic influences on the human microbiome (based on studies of the variance in the microbiome between MZ and DZ twin and within-twin pairs raised together vs. apart), particularly in the first 3 years of life, these effects are small compared to those associated with the extrauterine environment (Turnbaugh et al., 2009; Yatsunenko et al., 2012; Goodrich et al., 2014). The UniFrac distance, a measure of the phylogenetic distance between sets of taxa, is only about 2–4% higher within DZ (shared environment and 50% genotype) versus MZ (shared environment and 100% genotype) twin pairs. In contrast, it is about 10–15% higher within pairs of unrelated children. In a study of 54 twin pairs (23 DZ and 31 MZ), Turnbaugh et al. (2009) found no significant zygosity effect on the UniFrac distance, as did Yatsunenko et al. (2012). The small differences based on zygosity and large differences based on being reared in different homes suggest that the environment contributes more than do shared genes to the gut microbe composition (Turnbaugh et al., 2009).

The relative contributions of genes and environment may be taxa-dependent. In a study of 416 (171 MZ, 245 DZ) twin pairs in the TwinsUK population, there was a significantly higher correlation within MZ twin pairs for certain taxa, in particular, for the family *Christensenellaceae*. The abundance of the *Christensenellaceae* species was negatively associated with fatness in humans and reduced weight gain when transplanted into gnotobiotic mice (Goodrich et al., 2014), indicating that colonization by physiologically important microbes may still be heritable at narrower taxonomic levels.

Studies using multivariate analyses to compare industrialized societies such as the United States or Europe with nonindustrialized societies, such as the Hadza hunter-gatherers (Schnorr et al., 2014) or groups in Papua New Guinea (Martinez et al., 2015), indicate that industrialization is associated with a lower diversity of fecal bacteria within individuals (α-diversity) and greater diversity between individuals (β-diversity). Regardless of environmental effects on the microbiome due to climate, geography, industrialization, diet, etc., the diversity of the microbiome within a community increases with age (Yatsunenko et al., 2012).

Adult Human Gut Microbiota and Energy Homeostasis

Several mechanisms have been postulated by which the microbiome might affect energy balance. These mechanisms are inadequately studied in humans.

It is important to consider the possible interactions between the human microbiota and adiposity within the framework of what is known about human energy homeostasis. Within a stable environment, individual energy stores remain relatively constant over extended periods of time, suggesting that energy intake and output are coupled (co-vary) in a manner that "defends" a relatively constant level of energy stores (Du et al., 2009; Forouhi et al., 2009). Specifically, weight loss (negative energy balance) and the maintenance of a reduced body weight (energy balance at reduced weight) invoke similar but not identical declines in energy expenditure (exceeding those predicted by concurrent changes in body weight and composition) and intake. The disproportionate decline in energy expenditure predominantly reflects increased chemomechanical contractile efficiency of skeletal muscle. The increased energy intake reflects increased food reward (hunger) and decreased food restraint (delayed satiation and decreased perception of how much has been eaten), which do not abate over time (Ravussin, Burnand, Schutz, & Jéquier, 1985; Weyer et al., 2000; Leibel & Rosenbaum, 2010; Myers, Leibel, Seeley, & Schwartz, 2010). These effects are largely mediated by the declines in circulating concentrations of the adipocyte-derived hormone leptin, acting directly on "feeding centers" in the brain, and via the autonomic nervous (ANS) and neuroendocrine systems. The increase in parasympathetic nervous system (PNS) tone following weight loss is associated with a slowing of heart rate and decline in resting energy expenditure (Leibel & Rosenbaum 2010). The decrease in sympathetic nervous system (SNS) tone following weight loss modulates feeding behavior via effects on various gut peptides and transmission of nutrient-derived signals to the brainstem (Bellocchio et al., 2013), and directly decreases heart rate and secretion of thyroid hormone (Aronne, Mackintosh, Rosenbaum, Leibel, & Hirsch, 1995; Lang, Rayos, Chomsky, Wood, & Wilson, 1997). Thyroid hormone increases energy expenditure by increasing heart rate, blood pressure, and muscle ATP consumption (largely by stimulating production of muscle ATPase and favoring expression of the less mechanically efficient myosin heavy chain II [MHCII] isoform) (Jakubiec-Puka, Ciechomska, Mackiewicz, Langford, & Chomontowska, 1999; Baldwin et al., 2011). The increase in PNS tone and the declines in SNS tone and circulating concentrations of leptin and bioactive thyroid hormones during and following weight loss effectively conspire to favor the regain of lost weight (McGuire, Wing, Klem, & Hill, 1999; DelParigi et al., 2004; Wing & Phelan, 2005; Rosenbaum, Hirsch, Gallagher, & Leibel, 2008; Phelan et al., 2011; Sumithran et al., 2011).

Before extrapolating from studies of body weight and the mouse microbiome to humans, it should be noted that murine and sapien energy homeostatic systems differ in a number of key areas. There are obvious differences in natural diet composition (greater carbohydrate and less fat in murine diet) and biorhythms relevant to energy intake and expenditure (nocturnal vs. diurnal). Perhaps most striking are the interspecies differences in thermogenesis by brown (BAT) and beige (Brite) adipose tissue, which accounts for over 50% of adaptive thermogenesis in rodents versus < 5% in adult humans (Cannon & Nedergaard, 2004; Vosselman, van Marken Lichtenbelt, & Schrauwen, 2013). In mice, both the quantity and activity of BAT are affected by diet composition and the gut microbiota (Mestdagh et al., 2012; Okubo, Takemura, Yoshida, & Sonoyama, 2013), which will clearly have a much more substantial effect on energy expenditure in rodents than it would in humans. As discussed later, there are many hypotheses regarding the mechanisms by which the human gut microbiota might affect these phenotypes. However, these hypotheses are largely based on animal studies or indirect measurements of the effects of experimental alterations of gut flora on other molecules known to affect energy output and intake, without direct measures of these variables.

Effects of Weight and Diet Composition on the Gut Microbiome in Humans

The human intestinal microbial population is sensitive to adiposity (obese vs. lean), weight loss history (formerly obese vs. never obese), diet composition, and energy balance (dynamic weight loss vs. static weight maintenance). In most (Turnbaugh et al., 2006, 2009) but not all (Walters et al., 2014) studies, the proportion of *Bacteroidetes* species relative to *Firmicutes* species is decreased in subjects who are obese (similar to rodents) and is increased compared to never-obese humans in formerly-obese subjects following dietary weight loss (Cotillard et al., 2013). In subjects studied before, during, and after weight loss while ingesting the same liquid formula diet of identical macronutrient composition (Faith et al., 2013), the relative proportion of *Bacteroidetes* species and microbial diversity were increased following weight loss, even though dietary macronutrient content remained identical and the subjects were weight stable. In other studies of subjects during weight loss, this effect was augmented by ingestion of a low carbohydrate versus a low-fat weight reduction diet (Ley, Turnbaugh, Klein, & Gordon, 2006).

In humans undergoing dynamic weight gain or loss, the slope of the line relating degree of overfeeding and underfeeding to changes in the relative abundance of *Bacteroidetes* and *Firmicutes* is almost identical—making it unclear whether these changes in the microbiome reflect nutrient balance or nutrient stores (Jumpertz et al., 2011). In theory, the positive association of the relative abundance of *Firmicutes* and negative association of the relative abundance of *Bacteroidetes* with changes in body weight could be direct effects of the degree and duration of negative or positive energy balance, or of changes in energy stores as fat mass. Studies of changes in the microbiome induced by liposuction—that is, reducing fat stores without inducing a negative energy balance—might address this issue more directly.

Effects of Changes in the Gut Microbiota on Energy Homeostasis in Humans

There are few studies examining the effects of intentional manipulation of the human gut microbiota on body weight. However, manipulation of body weight and diet have been associated with changes in the microbiome and energy homeostasis. Kocelak et al. (2013) examined resting energy expenditure (REE), body composition, and the gut microbial populations in 50 obese and 30 lean subjects who were healthy and weight-stable. The investigators reported that the obese subjects had a significantly greater total microbial count without significant differences in the ratio of *Bacteroidetes* to *Firmicutes*. However, in multiple regression analyses, including fat mass, none of these correlations between the microbiota and cardiorespiratory fitness remained significant. It should also be noted that other studies reported a significantly lower and less diverse microbial count in obese versus lean subjects (Turnbaugh et al., 2006, 2009). In a study of cardiorespiratory fitness (defined as VO_2max), there was a significant correlation (adjusted $R^2 = 0.20$, $p < .001$) and taxonomic diversity in multivariate analyses of 39 healthy adults (Estaki et al., 2016), with shifts in the microbiome that predicted metagenomic functions aligning positively with genes related to bacterial chemotaxis, motility, and fatty acid biosynthesis. The correlation was confirmed by gut short-chain fatty acid (butyrate) content.

The observation that administration of conventional mouse microbiota to germ-free mice results in decreased energy intake suggests a role of the microbiome in appetite regulation, possibly including the efficiency of energy harvest from food (Backhed et al., 2004; Harstra, Bouter, Backhed, & Nieuwdorp, 2011). Though there is no direct evidence linking the microbiome to energy intake, the microbiota metabolizes fiber and complex carbohydrates into short-chain fatty acids (SCFAs), particularly acetate, butyrate, and propionate. These SCFAs are capable of crossing the blood–brain barrier and can interact with hypothalamic feeding circuitry (Frost et al., 2014). Specifically, increasing acetate production by feeding mice a high fermentable carbohydrate diet has an anorexigenic effect. Intraperitoneal administration of acetate is similarly anorexigenic and also increases central synthesis and release of glutamate, gamma-aminobutyric acid (GABA), and proopiomelanocortin (POMC), and decreases expression of the orexigenic agouti-related peptide (AgRP; Frost et al., 2014).

Prebiotics, defined as selectively fermented nondigestible food ingredients or substances specifically supporting the growth and/or activity of health-promoting bacteria that colonize the gastrointestinal tract (Bindels et al., 2015), are useful tools for modulating the human gut microflora (Macfarlane, Macfarlane, & Cummings, 2006). For example, small amounts of dietary inulin-type fructo-oligosaccharides given to humans stimulate growth of health-promoting *Bifidobacterium, Lactobacillus, Roseburia,* and *Faecalibacterium* species (Macfarlane et al., 2006). In a double-blind placebo-controlled study of 16 adults, Cani et al. (2009) administered an inulin-like prebiotic fiber versus a similar tasting placebo (dextrin-maltose). They found that prebiotic administration was associated with a significant decrease in hunger and postprandial glucose excursions, significantly greater satiation after a meal, as well as increases in plasma glucagon-like peptide 1 (GLP-1) and peptide YY (PYY), both of which are gut-derived peptides known to promote satiation and glucose homeostasis (Moran & Dailey, 2011).

Overview of Possible Mechanisms
Energy Harvest

Inoculation of gnotobiotic mice with conventional mouse gut biota provokes weight gain (increased energy stores) despite decreased energy intake and increased energy expenditure (Backhed et al., 2004; Ley, Turnbaugh, et al., 2006; Turnbaugh et al., 2006). The most logical explanation for weight gain in the setting of decreased energy intake and increased expenditure is that the addition of microbiota to a formerly germ-free mouse results in increased efficiency of nutrient absorption (a.k.a. *energy harvest,* the extraction of calories from ingested dietary substances). In studies of colonization of gnotobiotic mice with the caecal microbiota from *ob/ob* mice, Turnbaugh et al. (2006) reported that inoculation increased energy harvesting, including increased absorption of monosaccharides from the gut. In turn, this greater absorption led to increased hepatic lipogenesis and stimulation of both hepatic lipoprotein lipase (LPL) and hepTIC sterol regulatory element-binding proteins (SREBPs). An unanswered question regarding the germ-free mouse is what mechanisms allow it to maintain a lower level of energy stores in the germ-free state than the level that it will "defend" once inoculated with a microbiome. The identification of these factors might increase the utility of dietary manipulations, medications, surgeries, etc., that decrease energy harvest in humans (O'Donovan, Feinte-Bisset, Wishart, & Horowitz, 2003; Little et al., 2006).

As discussed above, increased efficiency of energy harvest has been reported to be associated with increased *Firmicutes* and decreased *Bacteroidetes* species in gnotobiotic mice (Turnbaugh et al., 2006). Similar studies examining energy harvest after manipulating the gut microbial population have not, to our knowledge, been done with humans. Jumpertz et al. (2011) examined the effects of underfeeding (2,400 kcal/day) and overfeeding (3,400 kcal/day) on the human microbiota of 12 lean and 9 obese individuals. They reported that the differences between caloric intake and weight maintenance calories were positively correlated with the relative abundance of *Firmicutes* species and were negatively correlated with the relative abundance of *Bacteroidetes* species in lean and obese humans. These differences suggest that microbiota are responsive to energy balance (i.e., to the degree of overfeeding or underfeeding) as well as to adiposity. An approximate 20% increase in abundance of *Firmicutes* and corresponding decrease in *Bacteroidetes* (which is what would occur during weight gain) was associated with a 150 kcal/day (approximately 5% of ingested calories) increase in energy harvest (measured by bomb calorimetry to determine the number of calories remaining in the stool; Jumpertz et al., 2011). Therefore, it is conceivable that inoculation of obese humans with a "leaner microbiome" *might* promote weight loss by decreasing energy harvest, as has been observed in mice.

The mechanisms by which the microbiome might affect energy harvest remain hypothetical. Nutrient absorption is clearly influenced by the length of exposure to the gut mucosa. Kashyap et al. (2013) reported that colonization of germ-free mice with human or rodent (mouse or rat) bacteria was associated with a decrease in gastrointestinal (GI) transit time, and that shortening or increasing GI transit time resulted, respectively, in increased abundance of *Bacteroidaceae* and *Porphyromonadaceae*. This type of study is clearly replicable in humans, but to our knowledge a replication has not yet been attempted.

Leptin Signaling

Introduction of conventional gut bacteria in gnotobiotic mice increases fatness but does not appear to affect the secretion of the anorexigenic hormone leptin. Neither does this manipulation increase expression of hypothalamic POMC and cocaine-amphetamine-related transcript (CART) nor decrease expression of the orexigenic peptides agouti-related peptide (AgRP) and neuropeptide Y (NPY; Schele et al., 2013; Everard & Cani, 2014). However, the colonization of germ-free mice with conventional microbiota significantly blunts both the weight loss and the decline in *AgRP* and *NPY* expression following leptin administration (Schele et al., 2013; Everard & Cani, 2014). Prebiotic manipulation of the microbiota in leptin-deficient mice to decrease *Firmicutes* and increase *Bacteroidetes* phyla resulted in increased leptin sensitivity (Everard et al., 2011), suggesting that the gut microbiota may affect CNS leptin signaling. Germ-free mice have significantly increased brainstem expression of proglucagon (GCG), which is the precursor for the incretin and anti-obesity molecule, glucagon-like peptide-1 (GLP-1). Reductions are also seen in the anorexigenic brain-derived neurotrophic factor (BDNF) and leptin-resistance-associated suppressor of cytokine signaling-3 in both the brainstem and hypothalamus, compared to conventionally raised mice. Microbe-induced suppression of any or all of these molecules might promote weight gain.

Inflammation

Increased circulating concentrations of inflammatory cytokines induced by an HFD has been proposed as a mechanism by which an HFD induces obesity and opposes weight loss in the setting of a high-fat versus a chow diet (McNay & Speakman, 2013; de Git & Adan, 2015). This may be due to increased colonic and ileal expression of lipolysacchardie (LPS, which can also be released from intestinal microbes), NF-kappaB, and TNFα (Belkaid & Hand, 2014; Khan, Gerasimidis, Edwards, & Shaikh, 2016). Cani et al. (2008) suggested that production of endotoxin by gut microbiota as well as ileal and colonic cells (Tehrani et al., 2012) results in a metabolic endotoxemia that acts centrally at the hypothalamus to promote hyperphagia and also increases permeability to nutrients. This metabolic endotoxemia, and resultant fat gain, are exacerbated by a high-fat diet and ameliorated by antibiotic treatment.

Short-Chain Fatty Acids

SCFAs, predominantly butyrate, acetate, and propionate, are the products of microbial (predominantly *Firmicutes* and *Bacteroidetes* as well as the minor phyla *Melainabacteria* [Hester et al., 2015]) fermentation of dietary fiber (germ-free mice produce almost no SCFAs [Maslowski et al., 2009]). SCFAs are bioactive molecules and are relevant to energy homeostasis beyond serving as an energy source for the colonic epithelia (butyrate), hepatocytes (propionate), and other peripheral tissues (e.g., acetate; Lin et al., 2012).

SCFAs engage two orphan G-protein-coupled receptors (GPCRs). GPR41 (also known as free fatty acid receptor 3 or FFAR3) is expressed in the gut, the peripheral nervous system (promotes growth and activation of the SNS), liver (promotes hepatic lipogenesis), and adipose tissue (promotes leptin release primarily via activation of the $G_{i/o}$ protein). GPR43 (FFAR2) primarily activates $G_{i/o}$ and G_q proteins in adipose tissue and the gut, where it enhances the density of PYY cells and release of PYY (Brooks et al., 2016). SCFA-induced activation of intestinal GPR43 decreases release of inflammatory cytokines (Maslowski et al., 2009), an effect that could indirectly increase hypothalamic sensitivity to leptin (McNay & Speakman, 2013; de Git & Adan, 2015). GPR 41 is equally activated by propionate and butyrate, whereas GPR43 is more responsive to propionate and acetate than to butyrate (Inoue, Tsujimoto, & Kimura, 2014; Kimura, Inoue, Hirano, & Tsujimoto, 2014). Butyrate inhibits histone deacetylases (HDACs), thereby inducing histone hypermethylation with subsequent changes in transcription of genes affecting pathways involved in fatty acid oxidation, epithelial integrity, and apoptosis (Waldecker, Kautenburger, Daumann, Busch, & Schrenk, 2008; Vanhoutvin et al., 2009; Matsuki et al., 2013).

Similarly, there are distinct effects of each of these SCFAs on various gut peptides (incretins and hormones) and energy homeostasis. For example, oral administration of butyrate significantly increases circulating concentrations of gastric inhibitory polypeptide (GIP), GLP-1, PYY, insulin, and amylin. This increase could have a net effect of slowing digestion and nutrient intestinal transit time, promoting satiety, and increasing plasma insulin. Propionate administration causes a more modest but still significant increase in circulating GIP, insulin, and amylin. Acetate administration has no effect on any of these hormones, but does increase leptin release by fat cells. Butyric acid and propionate increase G-protein-mediated secretion of PYY and GLP-1 in the gut, rates of isoproterenol-stimulated lipolysis, rates of basal and insulin-stimulated de novo lipogenesis in fat cells, and insulin-stimulated glucose uptake (Inoue et al., 2014; Kimura et al., 2014).

In mice, butyrate and acetate have been reported to protect against diet-induced obesity without hypophagia, and propionate has been reported to reduce food intake and increase locomotor activity (Lin et al., 2012). Collectively, these data suggest that acetate, since it has little effect on activity or energy intake, exerts its actions primarily via effects on basal thermogenesis (as evidenced by increased oxygen consumption in rats given oral acetate [Yamashita et al., 2009]), whereas butyrate and propionate have more direct effects on feeding behavior and physical activity.

Conclusions

Research, predominantly in rodents, indicates that the microbiome affects energy intake, expenditure, and nutrient harvest in ways that suggest that specific alterations of the gut microbiota might constitute a potential therapeutic intervention to prevent obesity and/or to promote and sustain weight loss in humans. Based on rodent studies, the effects of the microbiome on energy homeostasis are unique in that inoculation of mice with the microbiota from lean donors not only results in weight loss, but apparently does so without inducing the metabolic and behavioral opposition that would normally favor weight regain.

Further studies are clearly necessary, using manipulations involving prebiotics, probiotics, and diet composition, before any recommendations can be made regarding microbial therapeutics for human obesity. Specifically, studies of obesity and the human microbiome thus far have been mainly epidemiological and have failed to distinguish whether alterations of the microbiota are a cause or consequence of changes in fat mass.

Manipulation of the gut microbiome by transplantation, diet, or prebiotics in humans with varying somatotypes (obese, formerly obese, and never obese) and genetic predispositions could be used to isolate the possible role(s) of the microbiota in the regulation of energy homeostasis. Efforts should be made to identify those individuals for whom the gut microbiome is most likely to be salient in the regulation of energy homeostasis—much like the vendor- and strain-specific studies in rodents. Data from larger-scale studies could identify specific behavioral, microbiotic, and metabolic phenotypes that might be predictive of response to different types of behavioral, pharmacological, pro-/prebiotic, or surgical therapies. Of particular interest would be the consequences of bariatric surgical procedures on the gut microbiome and the correlation of any changes in flora with the effects of surgery on body weight and glucose homeostasis.

Finally, it should be recognized that the effects of the intestinal microbial populations extend to other systems, including glucose and lipid homeostasis, blood pressure, inflammation, and other adiposity-related comorbidities (Le Chatelier et al., 2013).

Acknowledgments

Our work cited in this manuscript has been supported by the National Institutes of Health (Nos. DK30292, DK078669, DK70977, DK64774, HG4872, DK P30 26687, and UL1TR000040).

References

Ajslev, T. A., Andeersen, C. S., Gamborg, M., Sorensen, T. I., & Jess, T. (2011). Childhood overweight after establishment of the gut microbiota: The role of delivery mode, pre-pregnancy weight and early administration of antibiotics. *International Journal of Obesity, 35*(4), 522–529.

Aronne, L. J., Mackintosh, R., Rosenbaum, M., Leibel, R. L., & Hirsch, J. (1995). Autonomic nervous system activity in weight gain and weight loss. *American Journal of Physiology, 269*(1, Pt. 2), R222–R225.

Backhed, F., Ding, H., Wang, T., Hopper, L. V., Koh, G. Y., Nagy, A., et al. (2004). The gut microbiota as an environmental factor that regulates fat storage. *Proceedings of the National Academy of Sciences of the United States of America, 101*(44), 15718–15723.

Baldwin, K. M., Joanisse, D. R., Haddad, F., Goldsmith, R. L., Gallagher, D., Pavlovich, K. H., et al. (2011). Effects of weight loss and leptin on skeletal muscle in human subjects. *American Journal of Physiology: Regulatory, Integrative, and Comparative Physiology, 301*(5), R1259–R1266.

Barrett, E., Kerr, C., Murphy, K., O'Sullivan, O., Ryan, C. A., Dempsey, E. M., et al. (2013). The individual-specific and diverse nature of the preterm infant microbiota. *Archives of Disease in Childhood: Fetal and Neonatal Edition, 98*(4), F334–F340.

Belkaid, Y., & Hand, T. W. (2014). Role of the microbiota in immunity and inflammation. *Cell, 157*(1), 121–141.

Bellocchio, L., Soria-Gomez, E., Quarta, C., Methna-Laurent, M., Cardinal, P., Binder, E., et al. (2013). Activation of the sympathetic nervous system mediates hypophagic and anxiety-like effects of CB1 receptor blockade. *Proceedings of the National Academy of Sciences of the United States of America, 110*(12), 4786–4791.

Bindels, L. B., Delzenne, N. M., Cani, P. D., & Walter, J. (2015). Towards a more comprehensive concept for prebiotics. *Nature Reviews Gastroenterology and Hepatology, 12*(5), 303–310.

Blustein, J., Attina, T., Liu, M., Ryan, A. M., Cox, L. M., Blaser, M. J., et al. (2013). Association of caesarean delivery with child adiposity from age 6 weeks to 15 years. *International Journal of Obesity, 37*(7), 900–906.

Brooks, L., Viardot, A., Tsakmaki, A., Stolarczyk, E., Howard, J. K., Cani, P. D., Everard, A., et al. (2016). Fermentable carbohydrate stimulates FFAR2-dependent colonic PYY cell expansion to increase satiety. *Molecular Metabolism, 6*, 48–60.

Cani, P. D., Bibiloni, R., Knauf, C., Waget, A., Neyrinck, A. M., Delzenne, N. M., et al. (2008). Changes in gut microbiota control metabolic endotoxemia-induced inflammation in high-fat induced obesity and diabetes in mice. *Diabetes, 57*(6), 1470–1481.

Cani, P. D., Lecourt, E., Dewulf, E. M., Sohet, F. M., Pachikian, B. D., Naslain, D., et al. (2009). Gut microbiota fermentation of prebiotics increases satietogenic and incretin gut peptide production with consequences for appetite sensation and glucose response after a meal. *American Journal of Clinical Nutrition, 90*(5), 1236–1243.

Cannon, B., & Nedergaard, J. (2004). Brown adipose tissue: Function and physiological significance. *Physiological Reviews, 84*(1), 277–359.

Castellarin, M., Warren, R. L., Freeman, J. D., Dreolini, L., Krzywinski, M., Strauss, J., et al. (2012). *Fusobacterium nucleatum* infection is prevalent in human colorectal carcinoma. *Genome Research, 22*(2), 299–306.

Chernikova, D. A., Koestler, D. C., Hoen, A. G., Housman, M. L., Hibberd, P. L., Moore, J. H., et al. (2016). Fetal exposures and perinatal infoluences on the stool microbiota of premature infants. *Journal* of Maternal-Fetal and Neonatal Medicine, 29(1), 99–105.

Clarke, S. F., Murphy, E. F., Nilaweera, K., Ross, P. R., Shanahan, F., O'Toole, P. W., et al. (2012). The gut microbiota and its relationship to diet and obesity. Gut Microbes, 3(3), 186–202.

Costello, E. K., Stagaman, K., Dethlefsen, L., Bohannan, B. J., & Reiman, D. (2012). The application of ecological theory toward an understanding of the human microbiome. Science, 336(6086), 1256–1262.

Cotillard, A., Kennedy, S. P., Kong, L. C., Prifti, E., Pons, N., Le Chatelier, E., et al. (2013). Dietary intervention impact on gut microbial gene richness. Nature, 500(7464), 585–588.

Cox, L. M., Yamanishi, S., Sohn, J., Alekseyenko, A. V., Leung, J. M., Cho, I., et al. (2014). Altering the intestinal microbiota during a critical development window has lasting metabolic consequences. Cell, 158(4), 705–721.

de Git, K. C., & Adan, R. A. (2015). Leptin resistance in diet-induced obesity: The role of hypothalamic inflammation. Obesity Review, 16(3), 207–224.

DelParigi, A., Chen, K., Salbe, A. D., Hill, J. O., Wing, R. R., Reiman, E. M., et al. (2004). Persistence of abnormal neural response to a meal in postobese individuals. International Journal of Obesity, 28(3), 370–407.

Du, H., van der A, D. L., Ginder, V., Jebb, S. A., Forouhi, N. G., Wareham, N. J., et al. (2009). Dietary energy density in relation to subsequent changes of weight and waist circumference in European men and women. PLOS ONE, 4(4), e5339.

Duca, F. A., Sakar, Y., Lepage, P., Devime, F., Langelier, B., Dore, J., et al. (2014). Replication of obesity and associated signaling pathways through transfer of microbiota from obese-prone rats. Diabetes, 63(5), 1624–1636.

Eckburg, P. B., Bik, E. M., Bernstein, C. N., Purdom, E., Dethlefsen, L., Sargent, M., et al. (2005). Diveristy of the human intestinal microbial flora. Science, 308(5728), 1635–1638.

Ericsson, A. C., Davis, J. W., Spollen, W., Bivens, N., Givan, S., Hagan, C. E., et al. (2015). Effects of vendor and genetic background on the composition of the fetal microbiota of inbred mice. PLOS ONE, 10(2), e0116704.

Estaki, M., Pither, J., Baumeister, P., Little, J. P., Gill, S. K., Ghost, S., et al. (2016). Cardiorespiratory fitness as a predictor of intestinal microbial diversity and distinct metagenomic functions. Microbiome, 4(1), 42–55.

Everard, A., Belzer, C., Geurts, L., Ouwekerk, J. P., Druart, C., Bindels, L. B., et al. (2013). Cross-talk between Akkermansia muciniphila and intestinal epithelium controls diet-induced obesity. Proceedings of the National Academy of Sciences of the United States of America, 110(22), 9066–9071.

Everard, A., & Cani, P. D. (2014). Gut microbiota and GLP-1. Reviews in Endocrine and Metabolic Disorders, 15(3), 189–196.

Everard, A., Lazarevic, V., Derrien, M., Girard, M., Muccioli, G. G., Neyrinck, A. M., et al. (2011). Responses of gut microbiota and glucose and lipid metabolism to prebiotics in genetic obese and diet-induced leptin-resistant mice. Diabetes, 60(11), 2775–2786.

Faith, J. J., Guruge, J. L., Charbonneau, M., Subramanian, S., Seedorf, H., Goodman, A. L., et al. (2013). The long-term stability of the human gut microbiota. Science, 341(6141), 1237439.

Forouhi, N. G., Sharp, S. J., Du, H., van der A, D. L., Halkjaer, J., Schultze, M. B., et al. (2009). Dietary fat intake and subsequent weight change in adults: Results from the European prospective investigation in cancer and nutrition cohorts. American Journal of Clinical Nutrition, 90(6), 1632–1641.

Frost, G., Sleeth, M. L., Sahuri-Arisoylu, M., Lizarbe, B., Cerdan, S., Brody, L., et al. (2014). The short-chain fatty acid acetate reduces appetite via a central homeostatic mechanism. Nature Communications, 5, 3611.

Gaci, N., Borrel, G., Tottey, W., O'Toole, P. W., & Brugere, J. F. (2014). Archaea and the human gut: New beginning of an old story. World Journal of Gastroenterology, 20(43), 16062–16078.

Goodman, A. L., Kallstrom, G., Faith, J. J., Reyes, A., Moore, A., Dantas, G., et al. (2011). Extensive personal human gut microbiota culture collections characterized and manipulated in gnotobiotic mice. Proceedings of the National Academy of Sciences of the United States of America, 108(15), 6252–6257.

Goodrich, J. K., Waters, J. L., Poole, A. C., Sutter, J. L., Koren, O., Blekhman, R., et al. (2014). Human genetics shape the gut microbiome. Cell, 159(4), 789–799.

Guaraldi, F., & Salvatori, G. (2012). Effect of breast and formula feeding on gut microbiota shaping in newborns. Frontiers in Cellular Infection Microbiology, 2, 94.

Hamady, M., & Knight, R. (2009). Microbial community profiling for human microbiome projects: Tools, techniques, and challenges. Genome Research, 19(7), 1141–1152.

Harstra, A. V., Bouter, K. E., Backhed, F., & Nieuwdorp, M. (2011). Insights into the role of the microbiome in obesity and type 2 diabetes. Diabetes Care, 38(1), 1159–1165.

Hester, C. M., Jala, V. R., Langille, M. G. I., Umar, S., Greiner, K. A., & Haribabu, B. (2015). Fecal microbes, short chain fatty acids, and colorectal cancer across racial/ethnic groups. World Journal of Gastroenterology, 21(9), 2759–2769.

Hildebrandt, M. A., Hoffman, C., Sherrill-Mix, S. A., Keilbaugh, S. A., Hamady, M., Chen, Y. Y., et al. (2009). High-fat diet determines the composition of the murine gut microbiome independently of obesity. Gastroenterology, 137(5), 1716–1724.

Human Microbiome Project Consortium. (2012). Structure, function and diveristy of the health human microbiome. Nature, 486(7402), 207–214.

Huurre, A., Kalliomake, M., Rautava, S., Rinne, M.,

Salminen, S., & Isolauri, E. (2008). Mode of delivery: Effects on gut microbiota and humoral immunity. *Neonatology, 93*(4), 236–240.

Inoue, D., Tsujimoto, G., & Kimura, I. (2014). Regulation of energy homeostasis by GPR41. *Frontiers in Endocrinology, 5*, 81.

Jakubiec-Puka, A., Ciechomska, I., Mackiewicz, U., Langford, J., & Chomontowska, H. (1999). Effect of thyroid hormone on the myosin heavy chain isoforms in slow and fast muscles of the rat. *Acta Biochimica Polonica, 46*(3), 823–835.

Jumpertz, R., Le, D. S., Turnbaugh, P. J., Trinidad, C., Bogardus, C., Gordon, J. I., et al. (2011). Energy-balance studies reveal assocations between gut microbes, caloric load, and nutrient absorption in humans. *American Journal of Clinical Nutrition, 94*(1), 58–65.

Kashyap, P. C., Marcobal, A., Ursell, L. K., Larauche, M., Duboc, H., Earle, K. A., et al. (2013). Complex interactions among diet, gastrointestinal transit, and gut microbiota in humanized mice. *Gastroenterology, 144*(5), 967–977.

Khan, M. J., Gerasimidis, K., Edwards, C. A., & Shaikh, M. G. (2016). Role of gut microbiota in the aetiology of obesity: Proposed mechanisms and review of the literature. *Journal of Obesity, 2016*, 7353642.

Kimura, I., Inoue, D., Hirano, K., & Tsujimoto, G. (2014). The SCFA receptor GPR43 and energy metabolism. *Frontiers in Endocrinology, 5*, 85.

Kocelak, P., Zak-Golab, A., Zahorska-Markiewicz, B., Aptekorz, M. Zientara, M., Martirosian, G., et al. (2013). Resting energy expenditure and gut microbiota in obese and normal weight subjects. *European Review for Medical and Pharacological Sciences, 17*(20), 2816–2821.

Koleva, P. T., Kim, J. S., Scott, J. A., & Kozyrskyi, A. L. (2015). Microbial programming of health and disease starts during fetal life. *Birth Defect Research Part C: Embryo Today, 105*(4), 265–277.

Kovacs, A., Ben-Jacob, N., Tayem, H., Halperin, E., Iraqi, F. A., & Gophna, U. (2011). Genotype is a stronger determinant than sex of the mouse gut microbiota. *Microbial Ecology, 61*(2), 423–428.

Lang, C. C., Rayos, G. H., Chomsky, D. B., Wood, A. J. J., & Wilson, J. R. (1997). Effect of sympathoinhibition on exercise performance in patients with heart failure. *Circulation, 96*, 238–245.

Larson, N. I., Wall, M. M., Story, M. T., & Neumark-Sztainer, D. R. (2013). Home/family, peer, school, and neighborhood correlates of obesity in adolescents. *Obesity, 21*(9), 1858–1869.

Le Chatelier, E., Nielsen, T., Qin, J., Prifti, E., Hildebrand, F., Falony, G., et al. (2013). Richness of human gut microbiome correlates with metabolic markers. *Nature, 500*(7464), 541–546.

Lee, H. Y., Park, J. H., Seok, S. H., Baej, M. W., Kim, D. J., Lee, K. E., et al. (2006). Human originated bacteria, Lactobacillus rhamnosus PL60, produce conjugated linoleic acid and show anti-obesity effects in diet-induced obese mice. *Biochimica et Biophysica Acta, 1761*(7), 736–744.

Leibel, R. L., & Rosenbaum, M. (2010). Metabolic response to weight perturbation. In K. Clement, B. M. Spiegelman, & Y. Christen (Eds.), *Novel insights into adipose cell functions, research and perspectives in endocrine interactions* (pp. 121–133). Heidelberg, Germany: Springer-Verlag.

Ley, R. E., Peterson, D. A., & Gordon, J. I. (2006). Ecological and evolutionary forces shaping microbial diversity in the human intestines. *Cell, 124*(4), 837–848.

Ley, R. E., Turnbaugh, P. J., Klein, S., & Gordon, J. I. (2006). Microbial ecology: Human gut microbes associated with obesity. *Nature, 444*, 1022–1023.

Lin, H. V., Frassetto, A., Kowelik, E. J., Jr., Nawrocki, A. R., Lu, M. M., Kosinski, J. R., et al. (2012). Butyrate and propionate protect against diet-induced obesity and regulate gut hormones via free fatty acid receptor-3 independent mechanisms. *PLOS ONE, 7*(4), e35240.

Little, T. J., Doran, S., Meyer, J. H., Smout, A. J., O'Donovan, D. G., Wu, K. L., et al. (2006). The release of GLP-1 and ghrelin, but not GIP and CCK, by glucose is dependent upon the length of small intestine exposed. *American Journal of Phyiology: Endocrinology and Metabolism, 291*(3), E647–E655.

Macfarlane, S., Macfarlane, G. T., & Cummings, J. H. (2006). Review article: Prebiotics in the gastrointestinal tract. *Alimentary Pharmacology and Therapeutics, 24*(5), 701–714.

Martinez, I., Stegen, J. C., Maldonado-Gomez, M. X., Eren, A. M., Siba, P. M., Greenhill, A. R., et al. (2015). The gut microbiota of rural Papua New Guineans: Composition, diversity patterns, and ecological processes. *Cell Reports, 11*(4), 527–538.

Maslowski, K. M., Vieira, A. T., Ng, A., Kranch, J., Sierro, F., Yu, D., et al. (2009). Regulation of inflammatory responses by gut microbiota and chemoattractant receptor GPR43. *Nature, 461*(7268), 1282–1286.

Matsuki, T., Pedron, T., Regnault, B., Mulet, C., Hara, T., & Samsonetti, P. J. (2013). Epithelial cell proliferation arrest induced by lactate and acetate from Lactobacillus casei and Bifidobacterium breve. *PLOS ONE, 8*(4), e63053.

McGuire, M. T., Wing, R. R., Klem, M. L., & Hill, J. O. (1999). Behavioral strategies of individuals who have maintained long-term weight losses. *Obesity Research, 7*(4), 334–341.

McNay, D. E. G., & Speakman, J. R. (2013). High fat diet causes rebound weight gain. *Molecular Metabolism, 2*(2), 103–109.

Mesquita, D. N., Barbieri, M. A., Goldani, H. A., Cardoso, V. C., Goldani, M. Z., Kac, G., et al. (2013). Cesarean section is associated with increased peripheral and central adiposity in young adulthood: Cohort study. *PLOS ONE, 8*(6), e66827.

Mestdagh, R., Dumas, M. E., Rezzi, S., Kochar, S., Holmes, E., Claus, S. P., et al. (2012). Gut microbiota modulate the metaboism of brown adipose tissue in mice. *Journal of Proteome Research, 11*(12), 620–630.

Metchnikoff, E., & Mitchell, P. C. (1908). *The prolongation of life: Optimistic studies. New York: G. P. Putnam's Sons.

Moran, T. H., & Dailey, M. J. (2011). Intestinal feedback signaling and satiety. *Physiological Behavior, 105*(1), 77–82.

Mueller, N. T., Bakacs, E., Combellick, J., Grigoryan, Z., & Dominguez-Bello, M. G. (2014). The infant microbiome development: Mom matters. *Trends in Molecular Medicine, 21*(2), 109–117.

Mueller, N. T., Whyatt, R., Hoepner, L., Oberfield, S., Dominguez-Bello, M. G., Widen, E. M., et al. (2013). Prenatal exposure to antibiotics, cesarean section and risk of childhood obesity. *International Journal of Obesity, 39*(4), 665–670.

Murphy, R., Stewart, A. W., Braithwaite, I., Beasley, R., Hancox, R. J., Mitchell, E. A., et al. (2014). Antibiotic treatment during infancy and increased body mass index in body: An international cross-sectional study. *International Journal of Obesity, 38*(8), 1115–1119.

Myers, M. G., Jr., Leibel, R. L., Seeley, R. J., & Schwartz, M. W. (2010). Obesity and leptin resistance: Distinguishing cause from effect. *Trends in Endocrinology and Metabolism, 21*(11), 643–651.

O'Donovan, D., Feinle-Bisset, C., Wishart, J., & Horowitz, M. (2003). Lipase inhibition attenuates the acute inhibitory effects of oral fat on food intake in healthy subjects. *British Journal of Nutrition, 90*(5), 849–852.

Okubo, T., Takemura, N., Yoshida, A., & Sonoyama, K. (2013). KK/Ta mice administered *Lactobacillus plantarum* strain no. 14 have lower adiposity and higher insulin sensitivity. *Bioscience of Microbiota, Food and Health, 32*(3), 93–100.

Parks, B. W., Nam, E., Org, E., Kostem, E., Norheim, F., Hui, S. T., et al. (2013). Genetic control of obesity and gut microbiota composition in response to high-fat, high-sucrose diet in mice. *Cell Metabolism, 17*(1), 141–152.

Phelan, S., Hassenstab, J., McCaffery, J. M., Sweet, L., Raynor, H. A., Cohen, R. A., et al. (2011). Cognitive interference from food cues in weight loss maintainers, normal weight, and obese individuals. *Obesity, 19*(1), 69–73.

Ravussin, E., Burnand, B., Schutz, Y., & Jequier, E. (1985). Energy expenditure before and during energy restriction in obese patients. *American Journal of Clinical Nutrition, 41*(4), 753–759.

Ravussin, Y., Koren, O., Spor, A., LeDuc, C., Gutman, R., Stombagh, J., et al. (2012). Response of gut microbiota to diet compositon and weight loss in lean and obese mice. *Obesity, 20*(4), 738–747.

Remely, M., Tesar, I., Hippe, B., Gnauer, S., Rust, P., & Haslberger, A. G. (2015). Gut microbiota composition correlates with changes in body fat content due to weight loss. *Beneficial Microbes, 6*(4), 431–439.

Ridaura, V. K., Faith, J. J., Rey, F. E., Cheng, J., Duncan, A. E., Kau, A. L., et al. (2013). Gut microbiota from twins discordant for obesity modulates metabolism in mice. *Science, 341*(6150), 1241214.

Rosenbaum, M., Hirsch, J., Gallagher, D. A., & Leibel, R. L. (2008). Long-term persistence of adaptive thermogenesis in subjects who have maintained a reduced body weight. *American Journal of Clinical Nutrition, 88*(4), 906–912.

Schele, E., Grahnemo, L., Anestein, F., Hallen, A., Backhed, F., & Jansson, J. O. (2013). The gut microbiota reduces leptin sensitivity and the expression of the obesity-suppressing neuropeptides proglucagon (GCG) and brain-derived neurotrophic factor (BDNF) in the central nervous system. *Endocrinology, 154*(10), 3643–3651.

Schnorr, S. L., Candela, M., Rampelli, S., Centanni, M., Consolandi, C., Basaglia, G., et al. (2014). Gut microbiome of the Hadza hunter-gatherers. *Nature Communications, 5*, 3654.

Soo, R. M., Skennerton, C. T., Sekiguchi, Y., Imelfort, M., Paech, S. J., Dennis, P. G., et al. (2014). An expanded genomic respresentation of the phylum cyanobacteria. *Genome Biology and Evolution, 6*(5), 1031–1045.

Strauss, J., White, A., Ambrose, C., McDonald, J., & Allen-Vercoe, E. (2008). Phenotypic and genomic analyses of clinical *Fusobacterium nucleatum* and *Fusobacterium periodonticum* isolates from the human gut. *Anaerobe, 14*(6), 301–309.

Sumithran, P., Prendergast, L. A., Delbridge, E., Purcell, K., Shulkes, A., Kriketos, A., et al. (2011). Long-term persistence of hormonal adaptations to weight loss. *New England Journal of Medicine, 365*(17), 1597–1604.

Tagliabue, A., & Elli, M. (2013). The role of gut microbiota in human obesity: Recent findings and future perspectives. *Nutrition, Metabolism, and Cardiovascular Diseases, 23*(3), 160–168.

Tehrani, A. B., Nezami, B. G., Gewirtz, A., & Srinivasan, S. (2012). Obesity and its associated diseases: A role for microbiota? *Neurogastroenterology and Motility, 24*(4), 305–311.

Turnbaugh, P. J., Backhed, F., Fulton, L., & Gordon, J. I. (2008). Marked alterations in the distal gut micorbiome linked to diet-induced obesity. *Cell Host and Microbe, 3*(4), 213–223.

Turnbaugh, P. J., Hamady, M., Yatsunenko, T., Cantarel, B. L., Duncan, A., Ley, R. E., et al. (2009). A core gut microbiome in obese and lean twins. *Nature, 457*(7228), 480–484.

Turnbaugh, P. J., Ley, R. E., Mahowald, M. A., Magrini, V., Mardis, E. R., & Gordon, J. I. (2006). An obesity-associated gut microbiome with increased capacity for energy harvest. *Nature, 444*, 1027–1031.

Ursell, L. K., Haiser, H. J., Van Treuren, W., Garg, N., Reddivari, L., Vanamala, J., et al. (2014). The intestinal metabolone: An intersection between microbiota and host. *Gastroenterology, 146*(6), 1470–1476.

Vanhoutvin, S. A., Troost, F. J., Hamer, H. M., Lindsey, P. J., Koek, G. H., Jonkers, D. M., et al. (2009). Butyrate-induced transcriptional changes in human colonic mucosa. *PLOS ONE, 4*(8), e6759.

Vosselman, M. J., van Marken Lichtenbelt, W. D., & Schrauwen, P. (2013). Energy dissipation in brown adipose tissue: From mice to men. *Molecular and Cellular Endocrinology, 379*(1–2), 43–50.

Waldecker, M., Kautenburger, T., Daumann, H., Busch, C., & Schrenk, D. (2008). Inhibition of histone-deacetylase activity by short-chain fatty acids and some polyphenol metabolites formed in the colon. *Journal of Nutritional Biochemistry, 19*(9), 587–593.

Walters, W. A., Xu, Z., & Knight, R. (2014). Meta-analyses of human gut microbes associated with obesity and IBD. *FEBS Letters, 588*(22), 4223–4233.

Weyer, C., Walford, R. L., Harper, I. T., Milner, M., MacCallum, T., Tataranni, P. A., et al. (2000). Energy metabolism after 2 y of energy restriction: The biosphere 2 experiment. *American Journal of Clinical Nutrition, 72*(4), 946–953.

Wing, R. R., & Phelan, S. (2005). Long-term weight maintenance. *American Journal of Clinical Nutrition, 82*(1, Suppl.), 222S–225S.

Wu, G. D., Chen, J., Hoffmann, C., Bittinger, K., Chen, Y. Y., Keilbaugh, S. A., et al. (2011). Linking long-term dietary patterns with gut microbial enterotypes. *Science, 334*(6052), 105–108.

Xu, J., Bjursell, M. K., Himrod, J., Dent, S., Carmichael, L. K., Chiang, H. C., et al. (2003). A genomic view of the human–Bacteroides thetaiotaomicron symbiosis. *Science, 299*(5615), 2074–2076.

Xu, J., Mahowald, M. A., Ley, R. E., Lozupone, C. A., Hamady, M., Martens, E. C., et al. (2007). Evolution of symbiotic bacteria in the distal human intestine. *PLOS Biology, 5*(7), e156.

Yamashita, H., Maruta, H., Jozuka, M., Kimura, R., Iwabuchi, H., Yamato, M., et al. (2009). Effects of acetate on lipid metabolism in muscles and adipose tissues of type 2 diabetic Otsuka Long-Evans Tokushima Fatty (OLETF) rats. *Bioscience, Biotechnology, and Biochemistry, 73*(3), 570–576.

Yatsunenko, T., Rey, F. E., Manary, M. J., Trehan, I., Dominguez-Bello, M. G., Contreras, M., et al. (2012). Human gut micorbiome viewed across age and geography. *Nature, 486*(7402), 222–227.

PART II

Behavioral, Environmental, and Psychosocial Contributors to Obesity

CHAPTER 6

The Role of Portion Size, Energy Density, and Variety in Obesity and Weight Management

Barbara J. Rolls

Recent research has revealed multiple properties of food that have effects on eating behavior and the overconsumption of energy that could lead to the development of obesity. This chapter reviews some of the most robust of these dietary influences and discusses implications of the findings for obesity treatment. Emphasis is placed on the importance of adopting sustainable dietary patterns that support optimal health while controlling hunger and enhancing satiety. Consideration is given to the challenges of translating current evidence into practical and sustainable dietary interventions to curb unwanted weight gain and regain.

The focus on properties of food that drive intake is not meant to diminish the critical role that physical activity plays in energy balance and optimal health, but is based on the premise that it is easier to overeat than to burn off excess calories. Dietary influences on consumption are numerous and complex, and include food amount, composition, form, cost, palatability, variety, and availability, as well as the combined impact of these factors. The next sections consider recent studies aimed at characterizing some of these food properties and how they can be utilized to help manage intake, control hunger, and increase satiety.

Portion Size

Experimental Evidence That Portion Size Affects Energy Intake

Portion size has received considerable attention in relation to the recent surge in rates of obesity (Dobbs et al., 2014; Kral & Rolls, 2011; Rolls, 2014). Portion sizes of many foods and beverages have increased in restaurants, supermarkets, and homes in parallel with the rise in the prevalence of obesity (Young & Nestle, 2002). In establishing a link between portion size and body weight, a crucial step has been to demonstrate that portion size affects energy intake. Controlled studies show that when adults and children are offered bigger portions, they consume more. The influence of portion size is seen for all types of foods, including those with indistinct shapes such as pasta (Rolls, Morris, & Roe, 2002), for which it is difficult to judge the size, as well as for foods with clearly defined shapes or units, such as sandwiches (Rolls, Roe, Meengs, & Wall, 2004) and packaged snacks (Rolls, Roe, Kral, Meengs, & Wall, 2004). Studies in natural eating environments such as restaurants confirm that food portions influence energy intake. For example, when the portion size of a pasta entrée served in a campus cafeteria was increased by 50%, customers rated the standard and larger portions as equally appropriate, and most ate all of the bigger portion (Diliberti, Bordi, Conklin, Roe, & Rolls, 2004).

Although intake of all types of food can be influenced by portion size, this effect is strongest for the foods that are best liked. It is obvious that food palatability is a major determinant of both food choice and intake; a recent study showed that when a number of oversized foods were offered, it was the relative liking among those foods that influenced the extent of overeating of a particular food. In a meal with multiple items, large portions had the greatest effect on foods ranked highest in palatability (Roe, Kling, & Rolls, 2016). The effect of portion size becomes particularly relevant for weight management if it persists over multiple eating occasions. Studies have questioned whether, after a bout of overeating in response to large portions, people compensate by eating less later, and whether when large portions are continuously available, the effect is sustained over time. In several studies, the effect has been shown to persist from meal to meal (Rolls, Roe, & Meengs, 2007). When men and women were provided with all of their foods and beverages during two 11-day periods, the effect of a 50% increase in portion size did not diminish significantly over time and led to a mean cumulative increase in intake of 4,636 kilocalories (kcal). Thus, the availability of large portions of palatable, energy-dense foods can override biological signals for satiety and promote a sustained accumulation of excess energy.

An even longer intervention conducted in a work site cafeteria over 6 months offered participants a free box lunch of 400, 800, or 1,600 kcal every weekday and compared body weight change to a no-lunch provision condition. The 1,600-kcal group gained around a kilogram more than the other lunch box groups, but not more than a control group that ate their usual lunch (French et al., 2014). The lack of a systematic relationship between lunch portion and weight change has been used to challenge the notion that large portions are related to obesity (Herman, Polivy, Vartanian, & Pliner, 2016). But another interpretation is that the provision of the smaller portion-controlled meals moderated the exposure to the usual obesogenic lunch environment experienced by the control group. As explained later, evidence suggests that portion-controlled foods can be an effective tool for weight loss.

Strategies to Counter the Portion-Size Effect

A number of instructional materials related to portion size are available from health organizations and can be found online. Individuals receiving dietary counseling are often taught to use measuring tools (scales, cups and spoons, and photographs). An evaluation of such portion-size estimation aides found that household measures such as cups easiest to use and most likely to be used again (Faulkner et al., 2016), whereas another study showed that use of most portion-control strategies was not sustained over time (Spence et al., 2015). One portion-control tool showing promise for weight management is a plate that clearly defines the proportions of foods that should comprise one's diet. Several studies have shown that using this type of portion-control plate for 6 months was associated with significant weight loss (Huber et al., 2015; Kesman, Ebbert, Harris, & Schroeder, 2011; Pedersen, Kang, & Kline, 2007). It is not clear, however, whether using such tools leads to better understanding of appropriate portions or to persistent changes in food selection, or whether such tools or education about appropriate portions will promote maintenance of weight loss.

The portion-control strategy best supported by clinical evidence is the provision of liquid meal replacements or portion-controlled snacks or frozen meals (Heymsfield, 2010; Raynor & Champagne, 2016). Preportioned foods are a component of several commercial weight loss programs, and it is likely that their provision contributes to improved weight loss and weight loss maintenance (Foster et al., 2013). Portion-controlled foods, whether as liquid shakes, meal bars, or prepared servings of conventional foods, are beneficial and can induce significantly greater weight loss than advice to consume a self-selected diet with similar energy content (Heymsfield, 2010; Rolls, 2014). It is not clear whether improved weight loss is related to portion control or to reduced exposure to large portions of other foods and the structure that food provision gives to the eating environment (Wing, 1997).

Although a number of strategies have been proposed to counter the effects of portion size, there are only limited data from randomized clinical trials indicating which are likely to be both effective and sustainable (Rolls, 2014). A recent study compared the efficacy of three different strategies for weight management in the year-long randomized Portion Control Strategies Trial (Rolls, Roe, James, & Sanchez, 2017). Women with overweight or obesity received one of three equally intensive behavioral treatments: the *standard advice group* followed guidelines to eat less of all foods while making healthy choices; the *portion selection group* chose foods based on energy density and received tools such as food scales; and the *preportioned foods group* structured meals around preportioned foods and received vouchers to encourage their use. During the first 3 months the preportioned foods group lost weight at a greater rate than the other groups, supporting the findings of another recent trial (Rock et al., 2016), but this early success did not persist. After a year, weight loss did not differ among groups, with an average loss of 4.5 kg. In all groups, reported use of target strategies indicated adherence for the first several months, but use of the strategies declined and converged over time. Although all three groups lost weight and kept most of it off over 1 year, maintaining behavior changes to manage portion size remains a challenge. This conclusion is supported by another large randomized controlled trial that found that teaching portion-control strategies helped with weight loss at the 3-month follow-up but that effects on weight were not observed at 6 and 12 months (Poelman et al., 2015).

It is likely that no one portion-control strategy will be effective for everyone, and further research is needed to develop tailored treatments suited for different individuals. Techniques for maintaining adherence to interventions that incorporate portion-control strategies into sustainable lifestyle changes are likely to improve long-term outcomes. Strategies to use the robust effect of portion size to promote consumption of healthy food options is considered later, as well as possible changes in the eating environment that make it easier to avoid the overconsumption associated with large portions of energy-dense foods.

Energy Density

Evidence That Energy Density Affects Energy Intake

Foods low in nutrients but high in energy density (kcal/g or calories per gram), such as chips, crackers, candy, and cake, are pervasive and dominate the choices available in a variety of settings. Shifting people to healthier choices is difficult, not only because energy-dense foods are palatable and often preferred, but also because foods lower in energy density are frequently less available, less convenient, and more expensive. This is particularly problematic because the energy density of foods and beverages has a robust and significant effect on energy intake. Numerous studies show that people tend to eat a consistent weight or volume of food over a day, and if calories are densely packed into each bite, energy intake increases (Perez-Escamilla et al., 2012; Rolls, Roe, & Meengs, 2010). Until recently, it was presumed that the fat in foods, which has more than twice as many calories per gram (9 kcal/g) as carbohydrates or protein (4 kcal/g), was the main determinant of energy density. However, of the components of foods, water (0 kcal/g) has the greatest influence, since it adds substantial weight without adding energy and is the largest component on average of commonly consumed foods.

For the same amount of energy, a larger, more satiating portion can be consumed when the energy density is low. For example, a 100 kcal snack of grape tomatoes (0.2 kcal/g) would provide around 20 times more food by weight than 100 kcal of potato chips (4.0 kcal/g). Figure 6.1 shows how the range of energy densities found in typical diets influences the amount of food that can be consumed in a day at four different levels of daily energy intake. A growing body of evidence indicates that lowering the energy density of the diet by increasing the water content through the incorporation of foods such as vegetables or fruit, or by decreasing

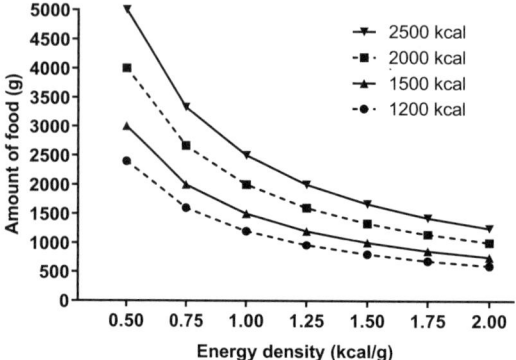

FIGURE 6.1. For a given level of daily energy intake, as the energy density of the diet is decreased, a greater weight of food can be eaten.

the proportion of unhealthy fats or carbohydrates, not only allows consumption of a satisfying amount of food but also reduces energy intake and improves diet quality (Perez-Escamilla et al., 2012; Rolls et al., 2010).

Energy Density and Body Weight

Both laboratory and clinical trial data indicate that reducing dietary energy density can be an effective approach for weight management. For example, in a year-long trial, women with obesity who were counseled to increase intake of vegetables and fruits and reduce fat intake had a larger reduction in dietary energy density and greater weight loss than those who were advised only to reduce fat intake (Ello Martin, Roe, Ledikwe, Beach, & Rolls, 2007). In the multicenter PREMIER trial that included three different lifestyle interventions, dietary changes that led to a lower-energy-dense diet were correlated with greater weight loss after 6 months, though as with all weight loss treatments, there was considerable individual variability in response (Ledikwe et al., 2007; Figure 6.2). In addition to weight loss, reductions in energy density were associated with improved diet quality, indicating that this is a healthy strategy for weight management (Ledikwe et al., 2006). Furthermore, participants who decreased dietary energy density reported eating a significantly greater weight of food. Increasing the amount of food consumed while decreasing energy intake could contribute to the long-term acceptability of a low-energy-dense eating pattern because it could help to control hunger. In support of this possibility, additional clinical trials have reported that lowering dietary energy density helped patients maintain their weight loss. Greene et al. (2006) examined energy density values 2 years after participation in a weight loss program that encouraged consumption of low-energy-dense foods. They found that individuals who maintained their weight loss reported eating a lower-energy-dense diet than those who regained 5% or more of their body weight. In another trial, instruction on reducing dietary energy density led to sustained weight loss 36 months after the start of the intervention (Lowe, Butryn, Thomas, & Coletta, 2014).

Longitudinal studies of free-living individuals support data from clinical trials. In a 6-year study, young women who reported a diet higher in energy density gained two and a half times as much weight as those reporting a diet lower in energy density (Savage, Marini, & Birch, 2008). Furthermore, increases in dietary energy density were associated with greater weight gain over 8 years

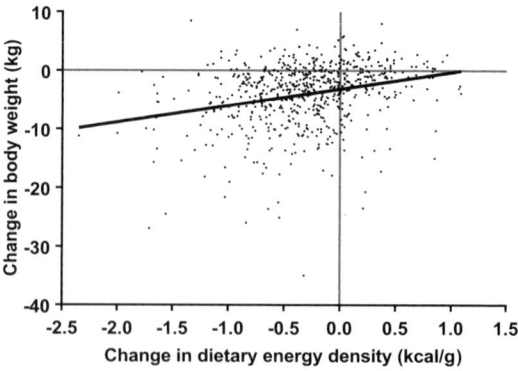

FIGURE 6.2. The relationship between dietary energy density and weight change after 6 months in the multicenter PREMIER trial that tested three weight loss strategies ($n = 658$). When results from participants in all three groups were combined, weight loss was significantly correlated with a decrease in food energy density. From Ledikwe et al. (2007). Reprinted by permission.

in a prospective study of 50,000 middle-age women (Bes-Rastrollo et al., 2008). Several systematic reviews (Perez-Escamilla et al., 2012; Rouhani, Haghighatdoost, Surkan, & Azadbakht, 2016) and a meta-analysis (Stelmach-Mardas et al., 2016) confirmed that lower-energy-dense diets were associated with lower body weight.

Additionally, an analysis of data from a nationally representative sample of U.S. adults found that reported energy intake was lowest for people eating a low-energy-dense diet, even though they reported consuming the greatest amount of food in grams (Ledikwe et al., 2006). This further indicates that a reduction in calories does not necessarily need to be accomplished by eating less food. A diet plan that severely restricts the amount of food a person consumes would likely lead to feelings of hunger and have unfavorable influences on the satisfaction with the diet and long-term compliance. However, laboratory data, clinical trials, and observational data indicate that with a low-energy-dense diet, people can manage their energy intake without the need to eat less than they habitually consume.

Practical Strategies to Manage the Effects of Energy Density on Intake

An advantage to advocating a reduction in dietary energy density is that this approach is flexible and can be modified to fit with many types of healthy diets and personal preferences. It does not rely on restriction of food groups; instead, it emphasizes consuming larger portions of low-energy-dense foods and controlling portions of higher-energy-dense foods. Using energy density as a guide to food choices not only enhances satiety but also directs consumers to foods that health professional encourage: vegetables, fruit, whole grains, legumes, soups, and lean protein sources. A number of well-controlled studies have investigated different methods for reducing energy density, such as decreasing fat, increasing vegetables and fruits, adding water, and using fat or sugar substitutes (Bray et al., 2002; Rolls, 2009, 2010). Although the sensory and biological effects of these methods differ, they are all associated with decreased energy intake (Williams, Roe, & Rolls, 2013). This research shows that individuals can use a variety of methods to reduce energy density, all of which can effectively decrease energy intake. Furthermore, a combination of methods can be used in order to modify foods for a more personalized and flexible dietary approach. Research suggests several specific strategies that can help individuals reduce the overall energy density of their diet.

Fill Up at the Start of a Meal

The standard method for determining the satiety value of a food is to ask study participants to consume a preload or first course of a fixed amount of food and then measure its effect on intake at the rest of the meal. Studies indicate that having a first course that was low in energy density (e.g., soup, salad, or fruit) reduced energy intake during the entire meal, compared with having a first course higher in energy density or compared to having no first course at all (Flood-Obbagy & Rolls, 2009; Flood & Rolls, 2007; Rolls, Roe, & Meengs, 2004). This strategy is most effective if the first course is a large portion of a very-low-energy-dense food that is less than 100 calories total. It is important to note that if the foods served at the rest of the meal are palatable and energy dense, people are still at risk of eating excess calories (Williams, Roe, & Rolls, 2014). Nevertheless, this strategy could have utility for weight management when incorporated into comprehensive behavioral programs. A small study found that consuming a low-energy-dense first course of salad and yogurt prior to the main course at both lunch and dinner reduced body weight over 3 months, compared to consuming these foods with the main course (Azadbakht, Haghighatdoost, Karimi, & Esmaillzadeh, 2013).

Substitute Lower-Energy-Dense Foods for Those Higher in Energy Density

• Palatability and preferences play critical roles in food selection and intake; thus, modifying a person's usual diet has the greatest likelihood of being sustained. Since people tend to eat a consistent weight of food over a day, the goal is to help them find ways to substitute lower-energy-dense foods for those higher in energy density without sacrificing acceptability. One of the most effective strategies is to incorporate more water-rich foods. For example, increasing consumption of broth-based soups can increase satiety (Flood & Rolls, 2007), and if overall dietary energy density is reduced, can facilitate weight loss (Rolls, Roe, Beach, & Kris-Etherton, 2005). Simply drinking more water as a beverage along with a meal has not been found to be as effective in enhancing satiety as incorporating water into foods (Casazza et al., 2015; Rolls et al., 1999).

Substituting vegetables and fruits for more energy dense meal components can also be beneficial, not only because it lowers energy density, but also because it improves diet quality. Much recent research has focused on strategies to encourage consumption of vegetables. They can be incorporated into meals in a variety of ways; for example, they can be served whole, chopped, shredded, or puréed, depending on whether they are provided as a side dish or incorporated into a main dish (Bell, Castellanos, Pelkman, Thorwart, & Rolls, 1998; Rolls, Roe, & Meengs, 2006). Covertly incorporating puréed vegetables has been shown to be particularly effective in increasing vegetable intake and lowering daily energy intake, even in people who dislike vegetables (Blatt, Roe, & Rolls, 2011).

A number of short-term studies indicate that reductions in energy density related to the incorporation of vegetables have a significant impact on energy intake over several days. However, simply advising people to eat more vegetables has not been found to reduce body weight unless dietary energy density is reduced (Casazza et al., 2015). The available data indicate that weight management messages about increasing vegetable and fruit intake should be accompanied by specific strategies to reduce energy intake, such as filling up on them first and incorporating them into recipes. These messages must emphasize that it is important to *substitute* vegetables and fruits for more energy dense foods with the goal of reducing the overall energy density of the diet.

Tools are available to help people shift the proportions of foods that compose meals or snacks so that lower-energy-dense options displace those higher in energy density. For example, a variety of plates can be found online that illustrate the message in Dietary Guidelines MyPlate, published by the U.S. Department of Agriculture (2016), which encourages consumers to fill half their plate with vegetables and fruits. In support of the effectiveness of this advice, a study found that increasing the portion size of a low-energy-dense vegetable served at a meal significantly increased vegetable intake (Rolls et al., 2010). An increased serving of vegetables to replace other more energy-dense meal components also reduced overall energy intake. Although plates that encourage increased proportions of healthy meal components have some efficacy for weight management (Huber et al., 2015; Kesman et al., 2011; Pedersen et al., 2007), this strategy may be effective only if those components are palatable enough to displace higher-calorie options (Roe et al., 2016). Another cautionary note is that simply reducing the size of dishware, a strategy often suggested to counter the portion-size effect (Hollands et al., 2015), has not been consistently shown to influence intake (Robinson et al., 2014; Rolls, Roe, Halverson, & Meengs, 2007). Indeed, one study found that with smaller plates, people cut down on the proportion of vegetables rather than high-energy-dense items when serving themselves from a buffet (Libotte, Siegrist, & Bucher, 2014).

Data indicate that reducing dietary energy density can facilitate weight management, and resources are available that teach proper implementation of this approach (Centers for Disease Control and Prevention, Division of Nutrition, Physical Activity, and Obesity, 2008; Rolls, 2012). However, more studies are needed to understand how to increase preferences for healthy, low-energy-density foods and to facilitate the maintenance of low-energy-dense eating habits. If people were to adopt these habits, they would be able to eat satisfying amounts of foods, appropriate for meeting both energy and nutrient needs. However, long-term compliance with any diet that requires deliberate and sustained changes in established eating habits is difficult. A key question addressed later is how the food environment can be modified to help people lower the energy density of their diets and eat appropriate amounts.

Dietary Variety

Evidence That Dietary Variety Affects Energy Intake

For omnivores such as humans, variety in the diet is key for obtaining nutritional balance. However, the availability of a wide variety of palatable, high-calorie foods makes selection of nutritious, lower-energy-dense options difficult and can drive up energy intake. Laboratory-based studies show that people eat more during a meal consisting of a variety of foods than during a meal with a single food (Rolls et al., 1981). Even similar foods presented in a variety of flavors or forms can enhance intake. Offering sandwiches with different flavors of fillings or pasta with different shapes increased energy intake compared to when the participants were offered a single flavor or a single shape. The variety of available foods and beverages is one of the most consistent influences on energy intake and affects people regardless of weight status (Johnson & Wardle, 2014). This holds true for individuals of all ages, though the effect declines over the lifespan, as do most variety-seeking behaviors (Rolls & McDermott, 1991).

The influence of variety on energy intake is related to changes in the palatability of a food as it is consumed. Although palatability is a primary determinant of food choice and intake, the palatability of a particular food is not constant; it declines as that food is consumed. This decrease in the palatability of a food as it is eaten, relative to other foods, is called sensory-specific satiety (Rolls, 1986). Sensory-specific satiety leads to cessation of consumption of the food being eaten and promotes consumption of other foods, especially those with very different sensory properties.

When a variety of foods and beverages are available, sensory-specific satiety helps to ensure that a balance of nutrients is consumed; however, increased variety can lead to persistent excess energy intake and promote obesity. In a laboratory-based study, access to a greater variety of foods and beverages with different sensory properties led to a sustained increase in energy intake over 7 days (Stubbs, Johnstone, Mazlan, Mbaiwa, & Ferris, 2001). Observational data support a relationship between food variety and body weight, but this relationship depends upon the types of foods that participants report they have consumed. Roberts and colleagues found that a dietary pattern consisting of a variety of foods with a high-energy content was associated with higher body mass index values among a representative sample of older U.S. adults (Roberts, Hajduk, Howarth, Russell, & McCrory, 2005). In another study examining food consumption patterns, there was a direct correlation between intake of relatively high-energy-dense foods and adiposity (McCrory et al., 1999). Body fatness was positively correlated with the variety of sweets, snacks, condiments, entrées, and carbohydrates consumed by study participants. Conversely, consuming a greater variety of lower-energy-dense foods such as vegetables was associated with having less body fat.

Variety and Weight Management

The role of dietary variety in weight management is not well understood, despite the role that restriction of variety plays in many regimes (Johnson & Wardle, 2014; McCrory, Burke, & Roberts, 2012). Several investigators have conducted secondary analyses of the association between weight loss and food variety in diets consumed by participants in behavioral weight loss trials. In an 18-month clinical trial, greater weight loss was associated with increases in the variety of vegetables consumed and with decreases in the variety of high-fat foods and sweets (Raynor, Jeffery, Tate, & Wing, 2004). A similar association of greater healthful dietary variety with changes in body weight and adiposity over 2 years was found in the multicenter POUNDS Lost trial (Vadiveloo, Sacks, Champagne, Bray, & Mattei, 2016). Despite the clear association of dietary variety to the overconsumption of energy, the extrapolation of this understanding to clinical practice remains a challenge. In an 18-month randomized clinical trial aimed at evaluating the effect of limiting the variety of energy-dense foods, reduced intake of the targeted foods was found, but weight loss was not increased (Raynor & Osterholt, 2012). The authors concluded that they may have needed to limit the variety of more foods than they targeted.

In a thoughtful review, Johnson and Wardle (2014) suggest several approaches to countering the variety effect. One approach could be to help people structure their personal environment to reduce their exposure to varied energy-dense foods. Another approach could be to teach people to be aware of the effects of variety and provide skills to manage intake when many choices are available. Although there are few data to support these suggestions, several studies indicate that the greater availability of a variety of fruits or vegetables can increase intake of such foods (Meengs, Roe, & Rolls, 2012; Raynor & Osterholt, 2012). Thus, rather than restricting variety, which is difficult to maintain for omnivores, perhaps people should be urged to stock their environments with an appealing variety of nutritious, low-energy-dense options that will help them to resist tempting, high-calorie foods (Rolls, 2012).

A key issue with all strategies that aim to limit energy intake by changing properties of foods and diets that could influence intake is obtaining a balance between what is effective and what is sustainable. Reductions in portion size, energy density, and dietary variety are all associated with lower intake and can facilitate weight loss. However, in the current obesogenic environment characterized by large portions of a variety of palatable, energy-dense foods, the maintenance of long-term energy balance remains a challenge (MacLean et al., 2015).

Managing the Obesogenic Food Environment

A dominant question among researchers, clinicians, and policymakers is how to counter the environmental facilitation of overconsumption. A range of strategies has been proposed, including education and nutritional information such as menu labeling, restriction of sugar-sweetened beverages, increased promotion and availability of low-energy-dense foods such as vegetables and fruits, more opportunities to choose smaller portions of energy-dense foods, and pricing or tax incentives to encourage selection of appropriate portions of nutrient-dense, low-energy-dense foods. A summary of some interventions that have been proposed to modify the food environment is provided in Figure 6.3 (Kral & Rolls, 2011; Marteau, Hollands, Shemilt, & Jebb, 2015; Riis, Fisher, & Rowe, 2016; Steenhuis & Vermeer, 2009). Although the long-term effectiveness of such interventions is not known, policymakers have begun to implement some that could provide immediate benefit to consumers. Consideration of the numerous proposed strategies is beyond the scope of this review, but several related to portion control and food choice that have immediate potential to be incorporated into weight-management programs are introduced.

Among the food properties of concern, portion size has often been targeted for intervention. The dietary guidelines published in 2010 by the U.S. Department of Agriculture and the U.S. Department of Health and Human Services encouraged the public to "enjoy your food, but eat less" and to "avoid oversized portions." Although the 2015 dietary guidelines abandoned this portion-control strategy in favor of a recommendation to adopt a healthy eating pattern with appropriate calorie levels, the use of MyPlate guidance remains, and similar advice about appropriate proportions of meal components is utilized in other countries (U.S. Department of Health and Human Services & U.S. Department of Agriculture, 2015). As mentioned previously, this type of tool can be used easily in weight loss treatments to help patients make appropriate decisions about what and how much to eat. This approach can be particularly helpful since many such decisions are often made before eating starts; for example, when shopping and ordering, as well as when determining how much to serve at a meal (Brunstrom, 2014).

Several other recent policies have the potential to help consumers make better choices. One of these—labeling the energy content on menus—could assist customers not only in making comparisons of similar offerings, but also could encourage restaurants to provide lower-calorie options (Bleich, Wolfson, Jarlenski, & Block, 2015). To determine effectiveness, a recent review and meta-analysis found that menu labeling did help to reduce energy ordered and consumed (Bleich et al., 2015; Littlewood, Lourenco,

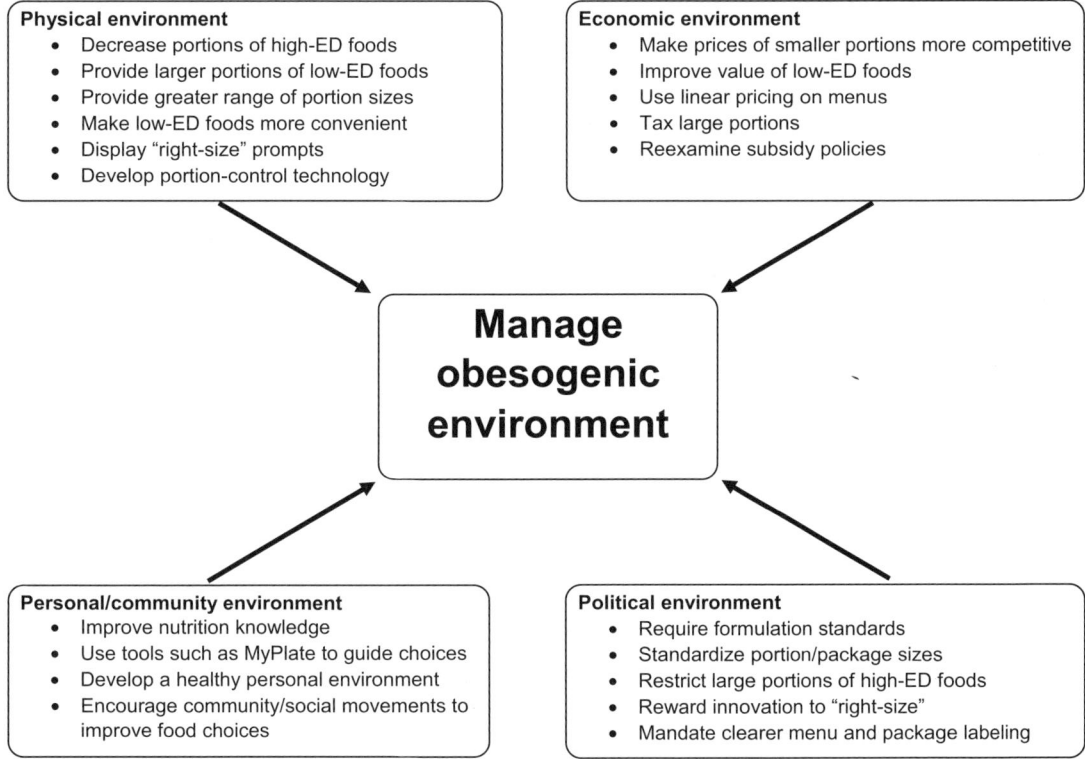

FIGURE 6.3. Schematic of some of the numerous interventions that provide opportunities to moderate the current obesogenic eating environment. ED, energy density.

Iversen, & Hansen, 2016); however, another review questioned the effectiveness for individuals in lower socioeconomic positions (Sarink et al., 2016), perhaps because they do not use the labels or do not understand them (Schindler, Kiszko, Abrams, Islam, & Elbel, 2013). Consumer use of nutritional labels, not only on menus but also on foods, is driven primarily by consumer belief in the importance of a healthy diet and motivation (Kerr, McCann, & Livingstone, 2015). As policymakers and food providers work to make labels clearer and more salient, it will be important to include education about their use in weight management programs.

Concluding Remarks

Increases in portion size, energy density, and variety can promote overconsumption leading to excess body weight. Even minor changes in these food properties could help moderate energy consumption and produce a more healthful eating environment. In addition to such changes, it is important for consumers to recognize the influence of various environmental factors on their food choices and intake. Ultimately, consumers must understand and accept the value to their overall health of eating a nutritious and balanced diet. Weight management programs should encourage the consumption of a variety of foods that are low in energy density, such as vegetables and fruits, while promoting more moderate portions of nutrient-poor foods that are high in energy density. Educational messages that encompass interrelationships between the various nutritional and environmental factors that can influence food intake and body weight are more likely to be effective than messages focusing on a single property of food or aspect of the obesogenic environment.

Acknowledgments

This work was supported by the National Institute of Diabetes and Digestive and Kidney Diseases (Grant Nos. R01-DK059853 and R01-DK082580).

References

Azadbakht, L., Haghighatdoost, F., Karimi, G., & Esmaillzadeh, A. (2013). Effect of consuming salad and yogurt as preload on body weight management and cardiovascular risk factors: A randomized clinical trial. *International Journal of Food Sciences and Nutrition, 64*(4), 392–399.

Bell, E. A., Castellanos, V. H., Pelkman, C. L., Thorwart, M. L., & Rolls, B. J. (1998). Energy density of foods affects energy intake in normal-weight women. *American Journal of Clinical Nutrition, 67*(3), 412–420.

Bes-Rastrollo, M., van Dam, R. M., Martinez-Gonzalez, M. A., Li, T. Y., Sampson, L. L., & Hu, F. B. (2008). Prospective study of dietary energy density and weight gain in women. *American Journal of Clinical Nutrition, 88*(3), 769–777.

Blatt, A. D., Roe, L. S., & Rolls, B. J. (2011). Hidden vegetables: An effective strategy to reduce energy intake and increase vegetable intake in adults. *American Journal of Clinical Nutrition, 93*(4), 756–763.

Bleich, S. N., Wolfson, J. A., Jarlenski, M. P., & Block, J. P. (2015). Restaurants with calories displayed on menus had lower calorie counts compared to restaurants without such labels. *Health Affairs, 34*(11), 1877–1884.

Bray, G. A., Lovejoy, J. C., Most-Windhauser, M., Smith, S. R., Volaufova, J., Denkins, Y., et al. (2002). A 9-mo randomized clinical trial comparing fat-substituted and fat-reduced diets in healthy obese men: The Ole Study. *American Journal of Clinical Nutrition, 76*(5), 928–934.

Brunstrom, J. M. (2014). Mind over platter: Pre-meal planning and the control of meal size in humans. *International Journal of Obesity, 38*(Suppl. 1), S9–S12.

Casazza, K., Brown, A., Astrup, A., Bertz, F., Baum, C., Bohan Brown, M., et al. (2015). Weighing the evidence of common beliefs in obesity research. *Critical Reviews in Food Science and Nutrition, 55*(14), 2014–2053.

Centers for Disease Control and Prevention, Division of Nutrition, Physical Activity, and Obesity. (2008). *Research to Practice Series, No. 5: Low-energy-dense foods and weight management: Cutting calories while controlling hunger*. Atlanta, GA: Author.

Diliberti, N., Bordi, P., Conklin, M. T., Roe, L. S., & Rolls, B. J. (2004). Increased portion size leads to increased energy intake in a restaurant meal. *Obesity Research, 12*(3), 562–568.

Dobbs, R., Sawers, C., Thompson, F., Manyika, J., Woetzel, J., Child, P., et al. (2014). *Overcoming obesity: An initial economic analysis*. New York: McKinsey Global Institute.

Ello Martin, J. A., Roe, L. S., Ledikwe, J. H., Beach, A. M., & Rolls, B. J. (2007). Dietary energy density in the treatment of obesity: A year-long trial comparing 2 weight-loss diets. *American Journal of Clinical Nutrition, 85*(6), 1465–1477.

Faulkner, G. P., Livingstone, M. B., Pourshahidi, L. K., Spence, M., Dean, M., O'Brien, S., et al. (2016). An evaluation of portion size estimation aids: Precision, ease of use and likelihood of future use. *Public Health Nutrition, 19*(13), 2377–2387.

Flood, J. E., & Rolls, B. J. (2007). Soup preloads in a variety of forms reduce meal energy intake. *Appetite, 49*(3), 626–634.

Flood-Obbagy, J. E., & Rolls, B. J. (2009). The effect of fruit in different forms on energy intake and satiety at a meal. *Appetite, 52*(2), 416–422.

Foster, G. D., Wadden, T. A., Lagrotte, C. A., Vander Veur, S. S., Hesson, L. A., Homko, C. J., et al. (2013). A randomized comparison of a commercially available portion-controlled weight-loss intervention with a diabetes self-management education program. *Nutrition and Diabetes, 3*, e63.

French, S. A., Mitchell, N. R., Wolfson, J., Harnack, L. J., Jeffery, R. W., Gerlach, A. F., et al. (2014). Portion size effects on weight gain in a free living setting. *Obesity, 22*(6), 1400–1405.

Greene, L. F., Malpede, C. Z., Henson, C. S., Hubbert, K. A., Heimburger, D. C., & Ard, J. D. (2006). Weight maintenance 2 years after participation in a weight loss program promoting low-energy density foods. *Obesity, 14*(10), 1795–1801.

Herman, C. P., Polivy, J., Vartanian, L. R., & Pliner, P. (2016). Are large portions responsible for the obesity epidemic? *Physiology and Behavior, 156*, 177–181.

Heymsfield, S. B. (2010). Meal replacements and energy balance. *Physiology and Behavior, 100*(1), 90–94.

Hollands, G. J., Shemilt, I., Marteau, T. M., Jebb, S. A., Lewis, H. B., Wei, Y., et al. (2015). Portion, package or tableware size for changing selection and consumption of food, alcohol and tobacco. *Cochrane Database of Systematic Reviews*, (9), 1–387.

Huber, J. M., Shapiro, J. S., Wieland, M. L., Croghan, I. T., Vickers Douglas, K. S., Schroeder, D. R., et al. (2015). Telecoaching plus a portion control plate for weight care management: A randomized trial. *Trials, 16*, 323.

Johnson, F., & Wardle, J. (2014). Variety, palatability, and obesity. *Advances in Nutrition, 5*(6), 851–859.

Kerr, M. A., McCann, M. T., & Livingstone, M. B. (2015). Food and the consumer: Could labelling be the answer? *Proceedings of the Nutrition Society, 74*(2), 158–163.

Kesman, R. L., Ebbert, J. O., Harris, K. I., & Schroeder, D. R. (2011). Portion control for the treatment of obesity in the primary care setting. *BMC Research Notes, 4*, 346.

Kral, T. V. E., & Rolls, B. J. (2011). Portion size and the obesity epidemic. In J. Cawley (Ed.), *The Oxford handbook of the social science of obesity: The causes and correlates of diet, physical activity and obesity* (pp. 367–384). Oxford, UK: Oxford University Press.

Ledikwe, J. H., Blanck, H. M., Khan, L. K., Serdula, M. K., Seymour, J. D., Tohill, B. C., et al. (2006). Low-energy-density diets are associated with high diet quality in adults in the United States. *Journal of the American Dietetic Association, 106*(8), 1172–1180.

Ledikwe, J. H., Rolls, B. J., Smiciklas-Wright, H., Mitchell, D. C., Ard, J. D., Champagne, C., et al. (2007). Reductions in dietary energy density are associated with weight loss in overweight and obese participants in the PREMIER trial. *American Journal of Clinical Nutrition, 85*(5), 1212–1221.

Libotte, E., Siegrist, M., & Bucher, T. (2014). The influence of plate size on meal composition: Literature review and experiment. *Appetite, 82,* 91–96.

Littlewood, J. A., Lourenco, S., Iversen, C. L., & Hansen, G. L. (2016). Menu labelling is effective in reducing energy ordered and consumed: A systematic review and meta-analysis of recent studies. *Public Health Nutrition, 19*(12), 2106–2121.

Lowe, M. R., Butryn, M. L., Thomas, J. G., & Coletta, M. (2014). Meal replacements, reduced energy density eating, and weight loss maintenance in primary care patients: A randomized controlled trial. *Obesity, 22*(1), 94–100.

MacLean, P. S., Wing, R. R., Davidson, T., Epstein, L., Goodpaster, B., Hall, K. D., et al. (2015). NIH working group report: Innovative research to improve maintenance of weight loss. *Obesity, 23*(1), 7–15.

Marteau, T. M., Hollands, G. J., Shemilt, I., & Jebb, S. A. (2015). Downsizing: Policy options to reduce portion sizes to help tackle obesity. *BMJ, 351,* h5863.

McCrory, M. A., Burke, A., & Roberts, S. B. (2012). Dietary (sensory) variety and energy balance. *Physiology and Behavior, 107*(4), 576–583.

McCrory, M. A., Fuss, P. J., McCallum, J. E., Yao, M., Vinken, A. G., Hays, N. P., et al. (1999). Dietary variety within food groups: Association with energy intake and body fatness in men and woman. *American Journal of Clinical Nutrition, 69*(3), 440–447.

Meengs, J. S., Roe, L. S., & Rolls, B. J. (2012). Vegetable variety: An effective strategy to increase vegetable intake in adults. *Journal of the Academy of Nutrition and Dietetics, 112*(8), 1211–1215.

Pedersen, S. D., Kang, J., & Kline, G. A. (2007). Portion control plate for weight loss in obese patients with type 2 diabetes mellitus: A controlled clinical trial. *Archives of Internal Medicine, 167*(12), 1277–1283.

Perez-Escamilla, R., Obbagy, J. E., Altman, J. M., Essery, E. V., McGrane, M. M., Wong, Y. P., et al. (2012). Dietary energy density and body weight in adults and children: A systematic review. *Journal of the Academy of Nutrition and Dietetics, 112*(5), 671–684.

Poelman, M. P., de Vet, E., Velema, E., de Boer, M. R., Seidell, J. C., & Steenhuis, I. H. (2015). PortionControl@HOME: Results of a randomized controlled trial evaluating the effect of a multi-component portion size intervention on portion control behavior and body mass index. *Annals of Behavioral Medicine, 49*(1), 18–28.

Raynor, H. A., & Champagne, C. M. (2016). Position of the Academy of Nutrition and Dietetics: Interventions for the treatment of overweight and obesity in adults. *Journal of the Academy of Nutrition and Dietetics, 116*(1), 129–147.

Raynor, H. A., Jeffery, R. W., Tate, D. F., & Wing, R. R. (2004). Relationship between changes in food group variety, dietary intake, and weight during obesity treatment. *International Journal of Obesity, 28*(6), 813–820.

Raynor, H. A., & Osterholt, K. M. (2012). Greater variety of fruit served in a four-course snack increases fruit consumption. *Appetite, 59*(3), 662–667.

Riis, J., Fisher, J. O., & Rowe, S. (2016). How food marketers can sell smaller portions: Consumer insights and product innovation. *Appetite, 103,* 423–424.

Roberts, S. B., Hajduk, C. L., Howarth, N. C., Russell, R., & McCrory, M. A. (2005). Dietary variety predicts low body mass index and inadequate macronutrient and micronutrient intakes in community-dwelling older adults. *Journals of Gerontology. Series A, Biological Sciences and Medical Sciences, 60*(5), 613–621.

Robinson, E., Nolan, S., Tudur-Smith, C., Boyland, E. J., Harrold, J. A., Hardman, C. A., et al. (2014). Will smaller plates lead to smaller waists?: A systematic review and meta-analysis of the effect that experimental manipulation of dishware size has on energy consumption. *Obesity Reviews, 15*(10), 812–821.

Rock, C. L., Flatt, S. W., Pakiz, B., Barkai, H. S., Heath, D. D., & Krumhar, K. C. (2016). Randomized clinical trial of portion-controlled prepackaged foods to promote weight loss. *Obesity, 24*(6), 1230–1237.

Roe, L. S., Kling, S. M., & Rolls, B. J. (2016). What is eaten when all of the foods at a meal are served in large portions? *Appetite, 99,* 1–9.

Rolls, B. J. (1986). Sensory-specific satiety. *Nutrition Reviews, 44*(3), 93–101.

Rolls, B. J. (2009). The relationship between dietary energy density and energy intake. *Physiology and Behavior, 97*(5), 609–615.

Rolls, B. J. (2010). Plenary Lecture 1: Dietary strategies for the prevention and treatment of obesity. *Proceedings of the Nutrition Society, 69*(1), 70–79.

Rolls, B. J. (2012). *The ultimate volumetrics diet.* New York: Morrow.

Rolls, B. J. (2014). What is the role of portion control in weight management? *International Journal of Obesity, 38*(Suppl. 1), S1–S8.

Rolls, B. J., Bell, E. A., Castellanos, V. H., Chow, M., Pelkman, C. L., & Thorwart, M. L. (1999). Energy density but not fat content of foods affected energy intake in lean and obese women. *American Journal of Clinical Nutrition, 69*(5), 863–871.

Rolls, B. J., & McDermott, T. M. (1991). Effects of age on sensory-specific satiety. *American Journal of Clinical Nutrition, 54*(6), 988–996.

Rolls, B. J., Morris, E. L., & Roe, L. S. (2002). Portion size of food affects energy intake in normal-weight and overweight men and women. *American Journal of Clinical Nutrition, 76*(6), 1207–1213.

Rolls, B. J., Roe, L. S., Beach, A. M., & Kris-Etherton, P. M. (2005). Provision of foods differing in energy density affects long-term weight loss. *Obesity Research, 13*(6), 1052–1060.

Rolls, B. J., Roe, L. S., Halverson, K. H., & Meengs, J. S. (2007). Using a smaller plate did not reduce energy intake at meals. *Appetite, 49*(3), 652–660.

Rolls, B. J., Roe, L. S., James, B. L., & Sanchez, C. E. (2017). Does the incorporation of portion-control strategies in a behavioral program improve weight loss in a 1-year randomized controlled trial? *International Journal of Obesity, 41*(3), 434–442.

Rolls, B. J., Roe, L. S., Kral, T. V., Meengs, J. S., & Wall, D. E. (2004). Increasing the portion size of a packaged snack increases energy intake in men and women. *Appetite, 42*(1), 63–69.

Rolls, B. J., Roe, L. S., Meengs, J. S., & Wall, D. E. (2004). Increasing the portion size of a sandwich increases energy intake. *Journal of the American Dietetic Association, 104*(3), 367–372.

Rolls, B. J., Roe, L. S., & Meengs, J. S. (2004). Salad and satiety: Energy density and portion size of a first course salad affect energy intake at lunch. *Journal of the American Dietetic Association, 104*(10), 1570–1576.

Rolls, B. J., Roe, L. S., & Meengs, J. S. (2006). Reductions in portion size and energy density of foods are additive and lead to sustained decreases in energy intake. *American Journal of Clinical Nutrition, 83*(1), 11–17.

Rolls, B. J., Roe, L. S., & Meengs, J. S. (2007). The effect of large portion sizes on energy intake is sustained for 11 days. *Obesity, 15*(6), 1535–1543.

Rolls, B. J., Roe, L. S., & Meengs, J. S. (2010). Portion size can be used strategically to increase vegetable consumption in adults. *American Journal of Clinical Nutrition, 91*(4), 913–922.

Rolls, B. J., Rowe, E. A., Rolls, E. T., Kingston, B., Megson, A., & Gunary, R. (1981). Variety in a meal enhances food intake in man. *Physiology and Behavior, 26*(2), 215–221.

Rouhani, M. H., Haghighatdoost, F., Surkan, P. J., & Azadbakht, L. (2016). Associations between dietary energy density and obesity: A systematic review and meta-analysis of observational studies. *Nutrition, 32*(10), 1037–1047.

Sarink, D., Peeters, A., Freak-Poli, R., Beauchamp, A., Woods, J., Ball, K., et al. (2016). The impact of menu energy labelling across socioeconomic groups: A systematic review. *Appetite, 99*, 59–75.

Savage, J. S., Marini, M., & Birch, L. L. (2008). Dietary energy density predicts women's weight change over 6 y. *American Journal of Clinical Nutrition, 88*(3), 677–684.

Schindler, J., Kiszko, K., Abrams, C., Islam, N., & Elbel, B. (2013). Environmental and individual factors affecting menu labeling utilization: A qualitative research study. *Journal of the Academy of Nutrition and Dietetics, 113*(5), 667–672.

Spence, M., Lahteenmaki, L., Stefan, V., Livingstone, M. B., Gibney, E. R., & Dean, M. (2015). Quantifying consumer portion control practices: A cross-sectional study. *Appetite, 92*, 240–246.

Steenhuis, I. H., & Vermeer, W. M. (2009). Portion size: Review and framework for interventions. *International Journal of Behavior Nutrition and Physical Activity, 6*, 58.

Stelmach-Mardas, M., Rodacki, T., Dobrowolska-Iwanek, J., Brzozowska, A., Walkowiak, J., Wojtanowska-Krosniak, A., et al. (2016). Link between food energy density and body weight changes in obese adults. *Nutrients, 8*(4), 229.

Stubbs, R. J., Johnstone, A. M., Mazlan, N., Mbaiwa, S. E., & Ferris, S. (2001). Effect of altering the variety of sensorially distinct foods, of the same macronutrient content, on food intake and body weight in men. *European Journal of Clinical Nutrition, 55*(1), 19–28.

U.S. Department of Agriculture. (2016). *ChooseMyPlate.gov Home Page*. Retrieved August 23, 2016, from *www.choosemyplate.gov*.

U.S. Department of Agriculture & U.S. Department of Health and Human Services. (2010). *Dietary guidelines for Americans, 2010* (7th ed.). Washington, DC: U.S. Government Printing Office. Retrieved August 23, 2016, from *www.cnpp.usda.gov/sites/default/files/dietary_guidelines_for_americans/PolicyDoc.pdf*.

U.S. Department of Health and Human Services and U.S. Department of Agriculture. (2015). *2015–2020 dietary guidelines for Americans* (8th ed.). Retrieved August 23, 2016, from *http://health.gov/dietaryguidelines/2015/guidelines*.

Vadiveloo, M., Sacks, F. M., Champagne, C. M., Bray, G. A., & Mattei, J. (2016). Greater healthful dietary variety is associated with greater 2-year changes in weight and adiposity in the Preventing Overweight Using Novel Dietary Strategies (POUNDS Lost) Trial. *Journal of Nutrition, 146*(8), 1552–1559.

Williams, R. A., Roe, L. S., & Rolls, B. J. (2013). Comparison of three methods to reduce energy density: Effects on daily energy intake. *Appetite, 66*, 75–83.

Williams, R. A., Roe, L. S., & Rolls, B. J. (2014). Assessment of satiety depends on the energy density and portion size of the test meal. *Obesity, 22*(2), 318–324.

Wing, R. R. (1997). Food provision in dietary intervention studies. *American Journal of Clinical Nutrition, 66*(2), 421–422.

Young, L. R., & Nestle, M. (2002). The contribution of expanding portion sizes to the U.S. obesity epidemic. *American Journal of Public Health, 92*(2), 246–249.

CHAPTER 7

Physical Activity and the Development of Obesity

Claude Bouchard
Peter T. Katzmarzyk
Robert Ross

Physical activity as a behavior is central to the global health problem of obesity and its associated morbidities. In the present chapter, we focus on the metabolic demands of physical activity and the contributions of regular physical activity to the prevention and etiology of weight gain and obesity. This review emphasizes adult weight gain and regain, all types of activities, metabolic responses to physical activity, and the regulation of energy balance. The role of physical activity level in the treatment of obesity and its effects on the metabolic profile of obese individuals is not addressed.

A central issue is whether physical activity energy expenditure associated with occupational work, leisure-time activities, spontaneous activities, and fidgeting makes a significant contribution to energy balance or attenuates weight gain when energy intake exceeds total energy expenditure. Even though commonsense reasoning suggests that the response to the above queries is a resounding "yes," and is a truism in a sense, strong and irrefutable evidence in support of this reasoning has been difficult to obtain. Moreover, the science reported to date has emphasized group-level differences and mean effect sizes, and it is now critical to evaluate to what extent group-level evidence tracks at the individual level.

Until an "obesity vaccine" is found, and it is a long shot (Ruttimann, 2012), or until we learn how to tweak the biology of some aspects of the regulation of energy balance (e.g., enticing some white fat cells to become more thermogenic), we are left with a limited number of options in the endeavor to prevent unhealthy weight gain. Hence, the current obesity research literature reveals a persistent interest in energy expenditure from physical activity as a means to maintain a healthy body weight.

Physical Activity Metrics and Energetics

There is still a lot of debate about the specific events in our evolutionary history that have led to current body mass, body proportion and composition, and the systems regulating energy balance. However, there is general agreement that a better understanding of the evolutionary biology of body weight would provide insights on biological and behavioral mechanisms. On this topic, the science is still in a state of flux, with widely divergent positions. Some have proposed that a sedentary lifestyle devoid of periodic bouts of physical activity betrays our evolutionary history and biology (Mattson, 2012). In contrast, others have gone as far as to proclaim that "it is time to bust the myth of physical inactivity and obesity," as if sustained physical inactivity had nothing to do with the variability of body weight (Malhotra, Noakes, & Phinney, 2015).

It is obvious to a biologist that the human body is "built" to be able to perform physical activity of multiple types with variable intensities and durations. Along with many others, we believe that our capacity for sustained physical activity, and perhaps our high muscular and physiological fitness, evolved under evolutionary pressures that rewarded those who were sufficiently gifted to survive until the age of reproduction. It is also likely that enhanced coordination and motor skill development were also selected for during the process (Malina & Little, 2008). In this context, it would be surprising if there had been no selective pressure on the capacity to store energy during periods of affluence and to mobilize energy stores in times of need. However, these systems are extremely complex, and their evolutionary roots have not yet been fully elucidated, despite decades of intensive research.

Classification of Physical Activity Intensities

One important issue is normative: What are the intensity and duration levels of activity that can be executed by adults of both genders in relation to the level of stress that these levels impose on the organism? We begin to address this question with a table displaying the intensity of physical activity expressed as the number of METs (metabolic equivalent; multiples of the resting energy expenditure measured in the sitting position), defined in ml O_2/kg weight/minute, with 1 MET being equal to 3.5 ml O_2/kg/minute (Table 7.1). Expressing the intensity values in METs has the advantage of standardizing the values for differences in body weight and essen-

TABLE 7.1. Classification of Physical Activity Intensities for Four Levels of Maximal Aerobic Power

Categories	Rest	Light	Moderate	Hard	Very hard to maximal
% HR max[a]	Variable	30–50	51–75	76–90	91–100
Perceived exertion[b]	0	1–3	4–6	7–8	9–10
Breathing[c]	Normal	Slight increase	Greater increase	More out of breath	Completely out of breath
Body temperature[c]	Normal	Start to feel warm	Warmer	Quite warm	Very hot; perspiring heavily
VO_2 max = 15 METs[d]	1	4–7.4	7.5–11.2	11.3–13.5	13.6–15
VO_2 max = 10 METs[d]	1	3–4.9	5.0–7.4	7.5–8.9	9–10
VO_2 max = 5 METs[d]	1	1.5–2.5	2.6–3.7	3.8–4.5	4.6–5

Note. HR max, maximal heart rate; VO_2 max, maximal oxygen consumption.
[a]Percentage of maximal heart rate reached in a progressive test to exhaustion.
[b]Perceived exertion as assessed on a 10-point scale.
[c]From Warburton (2010).
[d]Estimated from previous classification schemes (Bouchard & Shephard, 1994; Howley, 2001; Warburton, 2010).

tially eliminates the need for gender-specific values when scaled to maximal aerobic capacity. The table recognizes four levels of intensity ranging from "light" to "very hard to maximal." It also provides indications on the energy costs of these intensity categories (expressed in METs) for three levels of cardiorespiratory fitness. These three levels of fitness are typical of the average values observed in adults of increasing age: 15 METs for active young-adult males; 10 METs for healthy adults 40–60 years; and 5 METs for males around 80 years. The average MET values in women are about 2 METs lower than the average male, except in the older age category, where both genders have comparable values.

Intensity is the most challenging dimension of any physical activity program to define. It is greatly influenced by multiple factors, including the cardiorespiratory fitness level and exercise tolerance of the participant, level of habituation with the activity and history of recent exposures, age of the participant, overall cardiometabolic health, etc. In the case of weight gain and obesity prevention, there may be an advantage in focusing on an intensity range that would allow for longer duration of physical activity sessions and a higher frequency of exposures to maximize energy expenditure. These intensity conditions are typically found in the class of moderate intensity as defined in Table 7.1. However, this does not mean that activities performed at lower or higher intensities do not contribute to the prevention of weight gain. Quite the contrary! If substantial levels of physical-activity-related daily energy expenditure can be accumulated through activities executed at light or hard intensities, one can expect to experience weight control benefits. Actually, there may be additional weight control benefits from engaging in activities in the hard and very-hard intensity range. For instance, these activities generate higher sympathetic nervous system activity, require flexibility in the metabolic fuel mix oxidized to meet the energy demands, cause a higher muscle glycogen mobilization, and result in a larger and more prolonged excess postexercise oxygen consumption (EPOC). However, it has been challenging to obtain convincing evidence for these benefits in free-living individuals.

Measuring Physical Activity Level Outside of the Laboratory

Quantifying the energy expenditure of a physical activity program outside of the laboratory represents a challenge, but it can be done. Reasonable estimates of energy expenditure can be obtained by taking into account the nature of the particular activity, its intensity, the duration of each session, and the frequency of these sessions. Of these factors, the intensity of activity is the most difficult one to quantify in free-living persons. One practical solution is to rely on existing tables of the average or median MET values of commonly practiced activities. The most comprehensive of these resources is that produced by Barbara Ainsworth and colleagues (Ainsworth et al., 2011a). The most recent version of the *Compendium of Physical Activities* (the MET values) is available and updated periodically at *https://sites.google.com/site/compendiumofphysicalactivities/compendia* (Ainsworth et al., 2011b). Fine-tuning of the estimated value of an activity can be attempted using some of the indicators of intensity as defined in Table 7.1, such as perceived exertion, breathing, and body temperature indicators. The overarching goal is to come up with a global estimate of MET-minutes per week of physical activity so that progressive increases in the dose of physical activity can be programmed in an orderly manner.

Historically, physical activity has been measured using questionnaires, the vast majority of which rely on self-report of physical activity to determine the frequency, duration, intensity, and type of physical activity (Epstein, Miller, Stitt, & Morris, 1976). The principal concern with the use of questionnaires to assess physical activity is related to the accuracy of recall and reporting bias, which is well documented. Self-report questionnaires were shown to be accurate when describing high-intensity physical activity but not low-to-moderate intensity physical activity (Ainsworth, Richardson, Jacobs, Leon, & Sternfeld, 1999), a finding confirmed by others (Strath, Bassett, & Swartz, 2004). Of further concern is the inability to reconcile self-reports with direct measures of physical activity such as the accelerometry. Several reports suggest that the subjective error inherent in self-reported physical activity is not systematic but random, and thus the direction of the error in self-reported assessment of physical activity is unclear (Welk et al., 2014).

The recent development of wearable monitors that provide measures of physical activity in free-living settings represents a major advancement in the field. Wearable monitors provide more accurate assessments of physical activity in comparison to self-reported physical activity behaviors obtained from questionnaires (Westerterp, 2009). However, the availability of numerous monitors that vary in complexity, placement, and output presents a challenge to the practitioner, because at present there is no single gold-standard wearable monitor (Freedson, Bowles, Troiano, & Haskell, 2012). Monitor selection varies greatly and depends on a number of factors, including the specific component of physical activity of interest, the target population of interest, cost, and the required precision (Table 7.2). For a more detailed consideration of the strengths and weaknesses of available wearable devices, the reader is encouraged to review Ainsworth, Cahalin, Buman, and Ross (2015).

Depending on the physical activity that is pursued, step counting may provide a useful approach to the quantification of the amount of activity performed (Tudor-Locke et al., 2012). Step counting works particularly well with walking and jogging programs. The number of steps per session, together with information on the number of sessions per week, can provide valuable information on the volume of activity and allow for a systematic increment in the dose of energy expended over time. However, for the derivation of the energy expenditure of such programs, it would still be important to start with the estimated MET values from the *Compendium*. The number of steps executed over a known period of time would offer an additional means to fine-tune the

TABLE 7.2. Overview of Qualitative and Quantitative Components of Physical Activity and Related Metrics and Recommended Wearable Monitor Use in Free-Living Settings

Component	Common outputs (*units*)	Self-report tool recommendations	Wearable monitor		
			Type	Placement	Cost
Quantitative Components					
Total PA	Energy expenditure (kcal)	Diary; quantitative history	HRM, MSS	Upper and lower body	+++
Duration, frequency, intensity, and domain	Sedentary (minute); light (minute), moderate (minute); and vigorous (minute)	Short-term recall; quantitative history	Accelerometer, HRM	Hip, wrist	++
Qualitative Components					
General PA level	Meeting guidelines vs. no; active vs. inactive	Global; PA log	Accelerometer	Hip	++
Postural allocation	Sitting (% time); sit-to-stand transitions (no./hour)	Short-term recall	Inclinometer, accelerometer	Thigh	++
Walking	Steps (no./day); cadence (steps/minute); distance (m)	n/a	Pedometer	Ankle, hip, wrist	+
Activity type	Jogging (minute); running (minute); cycling (minute)	Short-term recall; quantitative history	Accelerometer, MSS	Unknown	++

Note. PA, physical activity; MSS, multisensor system; HRM, heart rate monitor; +, relatively inexpensive; ++, moderately expensive; +++, relatively expensive. From Ainsworth, Cahalin, Buman, & Ross (2015). The current state of physical activity assessment tools. *Progress in Cardiovascular Diseases, 57*(4), 387–395. Copyright © 2015 Elsevier. Reprinted by permission.

definition of the intensity of the activity. Other approaches with potential application at the individual level are also available (see Westerterp, 2013).

Physical Activity Guidelines and Prevention of Weight Gain

What is a reasonable level of activity-related energy expenditure that could be of value in prevention of weight gain? Common sense suggests that the higher the energy expenditure resulting from a physically active lifestyle, the greater the benefit in preventing weight gain. For adults, the Physical Activity Guidelines for Americans recommend 150–300 minutes of activity at moderate intensity per week (U.S. Department of Health and Human Services, 2008). This translates into 500–1,000 MET minutes/week of physical activity. What does this mean for body weight regulation? One approach is to use the guidelines' recommendation to estimate the number of calories potentially expended.

If we assume that an adult woman weighing 70 kg is walking 50 minutes/day, five times a week, at an intensity of 4 METs, we have a total of 1,000 MET minutes/week. To derive the caloric expenditure of this level of physical activity, we can use the following:

4 METs × 3.5 × 70 kg/200 =
4.9 kilocalories (kcal)/minute

where 3.5 and 200 are both constants. Then we have

4.9 kcal × 250 minutes =
1,225 kcals/week of energy expenditure

To obtain the net energy expenditure associated with this physical activity program, we need to subtract the amount of energy that would have been expended at rest. In this case, the resting expenditure for a woman of her weight would be about 225 kcal over the 250 minutes. Thus, the net energy expenditure of her physical activity regimen would be about 1,000 kcal/week. This level of expenditure would be lower for a lighter-weight person or higher for a heavier person. Age, gender, or ethnicity would have little effect on this estimate. If the same person was engaging in physical activity only at the low end of the guidelines—that is, for 150 minutes/week at the same intensity—her program net energy expenditure would be about 600 kcal/week. *What is the potential impact of this level of physical activity on the mobilization of fat stores and on carbohydrate and lipid balance?*

When someone engages in physical activity in a relative steady state, information on the proportion of lipids and carbohydrates oxidized to meet the energy demands of the activity can be derived from the measurement of the respiratory exchange ratio (RER). The RER is the ratio of carbon dioxide expired (VCO_2) to oxygen consumed (VO_2) under steady-state conditions, assuming that there is no contribution from proteins to the metabolic fuel being oxidized (VCO_2/VO_2) or correcting for nitrogen catabolism when appropriate. Based on chemical studies, we know that when a gram of lipid is fully oxidized, the RER is 0.70, whereas it reaches 1.0 when a gram of carbohydrate is fully oxidized. RER values across the 0.70–1.0 range are listed in Table 7.3 along with the % lipids and carbohydrates that contribute to the metabolic fuel oxidized for various classes of RER. The lower the RER, the higher the proportion of lipids in the metabolic fuel mix oxidized. In contrast, a high RER reflects a high proportion of metabolized carbohydrates.

RER measurements performed when engaging in steady-state physical activity can give useful information about the contributions of carbohydrates and lipids to the energy demands of the workload. Such experiments have been performed across a whole range of physical activity intensities; the main findings are graphed in Figure 7.1. The two curves represent the contribution of each metabolic fuel to the energy requirements of exercise in the range from 20 to 100% of maximal working capacity. As intensity increases, the proportion of lipids oxidized in the metabolic fuel mix decreases. Conversely, the proportion of carbohydrates oxidized increases, until almost all of the energy needs are met by carbohydrates at maximal intensity. Of particular interest for the topic of the present chapter is the intensity zone ranging from about 40 to 75% of maximal working capacity. Lipid oxidation contributes about 50% of the energy needs

TABLE 7.3. Percentage of Carbohydrates and Lipids Oxidized to Meet the Energy Needs, Assuming no Contribution from Proteins, Based on the Respiratory Exchange Ratio

RER	% lipid	% carbohydrate	kcal/L of O_2	Grams of lipids/L of O_2
0.70	100	0	4.69	0.50
0.75	83	17	4.74	0.43
0.80	67	33	4.80	0.35
0.85	50	50	4.86	0.26
0.90	33	67	4.92	0.18
0.95	17	83	4.98	0.09
1.00	0	100	5.05	0.00

Note. RER, respiratory exchange ratio; O_2, oxygen.

in the lower intensity end of this exercise range, decreasing to 25% in the higher intensity end of the energy needs. This finding suggests that engaging regularly in physical activity pursuits in this intensity range could play an important role in maintaining lipid balance or inducing a negative lipid balance. However, higher-intensity exercise programs resulting in high levels of energy expenditure can also lead to negative lipid balance. Recall that 1 g of fat is the energy equivalent of 9 kcal.

At light intensity, after fasting for several hours, the energy needs of activity are primarily met by the oxidation of fatty acids. Interestingly, the proportion and the amount of lipids oxidized increase with the duration of exercise, particularly when the intensity is in the range of about 40–75% of maximal working capacity. This is schematically illustrated in Figure 7.2. In this case, a moderately active person is exercising at about 65% of maximal for a period of 2 hours. In the first 30 minutes, muscle glycogen and blood glucose contribute about 50% of the energy needs, and the remainder comes from oxidation of plasma free fatty acids (FFA) and muscle triglycerides. Over time, plasma FFA provides a growing proportion of the energy needs of the exercising individual—that is, up to about 40% at 2 hours. This increase in plasma FFA oxidation is supported by FFA releases from adipose tissue depots. Oxidation of glucose after muscle uptake from circulating blood glucose is also on the rise over time, and the contribution of muscle glycogen decreases progressively over the 2-hour period. With regular expo-

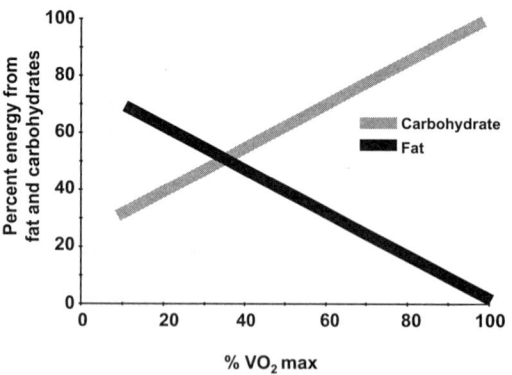

FIGURE 7.1. Changes in the predominant source of metabolic fuel with increases in the intensity of activity being pursued. With increasing intensity, carbohydrate sources contribute more of the energy needs.

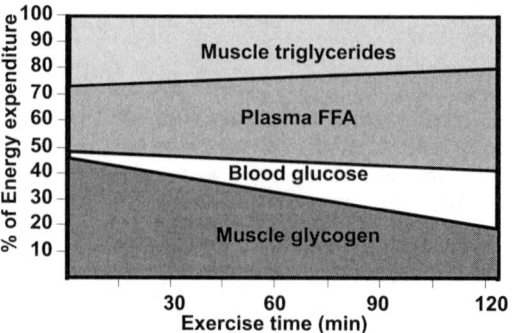

FIGURE 7.2. Changes in the sources of metabolic fuel over a 2-hour period of physical activity at moderate intensity, defined as about 50–75% of maximal aerobic capacity.

sure to exercise, the contribution of lipids to the metabolic fuel mix increases even more. This increase is a reflection of an improving metabolic flexibility that is progressively acquired by most individuals when they are physically active. The interested reader will find a more detailed treatment of these bioenergetics issues elsewhere (Brooks, 2012; Coyle, 1995; Kenney, Wilmore, & Costill, 2015; McArdle, Katch, & Katch, 2016; Powers & Howley, 2015).

Among the lessons learned from the preceding comments on bioenergetics that are particularly relevant to maintaining a healthy body weight, a fundamental lesson is that moderate to large amounts of calories can be expended by regular physical activity, provided the activity is in an appropriate intensity range and for long duration. The higher the volume of physical activity, the higher the energy expenditure. One other important lesson is that an exercising person mobilizes and oxidizes many grams of fat to meet the energy needs of the physical work being performed. Since the maintenance of a normal body weight requires the prevention of excessive fat storage, engaging in physical activity for a sufficiently long duration offers a strong behavioral approach to preventing positive fat balance, which is the cornerstone of adipose tissue mass expansion. Moreover, regular exposure to physical activity improves metabolic flexibility, which is an important health benefit, in and of itself, but also favors a stable and healthy body weight.

Sedentary Time and Risk of Weight Gain and Obesity

Although this chapter focuses on the role of physical activity in regulating body weight, there is emerging interest in the health effects associated with sedentary behavior, including the risk of obesity. Sedentary behavior has been defined as "any waking behavior characterized by an energy expenditure ≤1.5 METs while in a sitting or reclining posture" (Sedentary Behaviour Research Network, 2012, p. 540). In recent years, there has been a move to consider sedentary behavior as a distinct behavioral paradigm, one that may be somewhat independent of physical activity per se (Owen, Healy, Matthews, & Dunstan, 2010). For example, one could easily envision a situation where someone is meeting the recommendations for moderate-to-vigorous physical activity, yet is still excessively sedentary for the remainder of the day.

Recent technological advances such as the development of accelerometers and inclinometers have allowed for the quantitative measurement of time spent in sedentary behavior. Although these measurement techniques are beginning to be applied more widely in large-scale epidemiological studies, most of the research on the health effects of sedentary behavior has been conducted using questionnaires that ask about time spent in specific sedentary behaviors such as TV viewing (Grontved & Hu, 2011) or time spent sitting (Katzmarzyk, Church, Craig, & Bouchard, 2009). Cross-sectional studies have shown that obese individuals sit for a longer duration on a daily basis compared to lean individuals (Harrington, Barreira, Staiano, & Katzmarzyk, 2014; Levine et al., 2005). For example, results from the U.S. National Health and Nutrition Examination Survey (NHANES) indicated that obese women sat for a significantly greater amount of time compared to overweight and normal-weight women (Harrington et al., 2014). However, there were no significant differences in sitting time between body mass index (BMI) categories in men.

There is suggestive but conflicting evidence based on longitudinal studies as to whether or not sedentary behavior is positively related to weight gain and obesity in adults (Proper, Singh, van Mechelen, & Chinapaw, 2011; Thorp, Owen, Neuhaus, & Dunstan, 2011). Given the lack of high-quality studies and the inconsistent measures of sedentary behavior used in the literature (i.e., TV viewing vs. sitting vs. total sedentary time), it is difficult to derive summary estimates of risk based on meta-analyses. However, prospective results from the Nurses' Health Study demonstrate a dose–response association between baseline levels of TV viewing and the subsequent development of obesity over 6 years of follow-up among 30- to 55-year-old women who were not obese at baseline (Figure 7.3; Hu, Li, Colditz, Willett, & Manson, 2003).

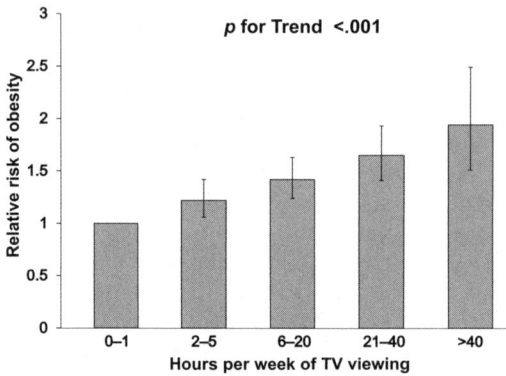

FIGURE 7.3. Relative risk of developing obesity over 6 years, according to television viewing at baseline, among 50,277 women ages 30–55 from the Nurses' Health Study. Relative risk ratios are adjusted for age, smoking, alcohol use, hormone use, physical activity, total fat, cereal fiber, glycemic load, and total calories. Error bars represent 95% confidence intervals. Drawn from data in Table 2 of Hu et al. (2003).

Leisure Time Physical Activity and Risk of Weight Gain and Obesity

Based on a literature review of available longitudinal studies, Di Pietro (1999) concluded that physical activity was effective at attenuating weight gain among adults, even more so than it was at inducing weight loss. Subsequently, Di Pietro and colleagues explored the association between changes in physical activity and the trajectory of weight change over 5 years in 2,501 healthy middle-age men in the Aerobics Center Longitudinal Study (Di Pietro, Dziura, & Blair, 2004). The results showed that men who maintained their initial level of physical activity over time experienced weight gain over the 5-year period, whereas men who increased their physical activity levels from baseline to follow-up (either from low to moderate or from low to high) experienced attenuation of weight gain or even some weight loss (Di Pietro, 1999). These results demonstrate that physical activity is important in maintaining body weight over time.

A common limitation in studies of physical activity and obesity has been the inability to precisely measure physical activity levels. A recent study attempted to overcome this limitation by carefully monitoring moderate-to-vigorous physical activity (MVPA) levels with a wearable monitor (multisensor armband) and measuring changes in adiposity over time using dual-energy X-ray absorptiometry (DXA; Shook et al., 2015). Among 421 adults, MVPA measured at baseline was a significant predictor of changes in fat mass over 1 year, such that those in the lowest quintile of baseline MVPA gained significantly more fat mass (1.7 kg) than the other groups (Shook et al., 2015; see Figure 7.4). These results suggest that very low physical activity levels are predictive of weight gain among adults.

Support for this notion comes from many studies that show that a high level of physical activity is associated with low weight gain over time, whereas comparatively low levels of physical activity are associated with higher weight gain over time (Hankinson et al., 2010). Using data from the Coronary Artery Risk Development in Young Adults (CARDIA) prospective study, Hankinson et al. (2010) observed that relative to lower activity levels, sustaining higher levels of activity over 20 years was associated with less weight gain among men and women transitioning from young adulthood to middle age. Men and women who sustained higher levels of physical activity gained 2.6 and 6.1 fewer kg over the 20 years, respectively, compared to the low-activity referent group. Higher physical activity levels in this study approximated 60 minutes/day in men and about 35 minutes/day in women.

The amount of physical activity required to prevent weight gain remains a topic of debate (Erlichman, Kerbey, & James, 2002; Saris et al., 2003). Results from other observational cohort studies suggest that 30 minutes of daily activity is not sufficient to prevent weight gain in women (Lee, Djousse, Sesso, Wang, & Buring, 2010) and that at least 60 minutes of daily activity is required to prevent weight gain in men (Di Pietro et al., 2004). Discrepancies may be partially explained by differences in the manner in which levels of physical activity are derived from self-report and/or issues related to the accurate measurement of energy intake. Nevertheless, taken together, these observations confirm the notion that increasing levels of physical activity may offset a corre-

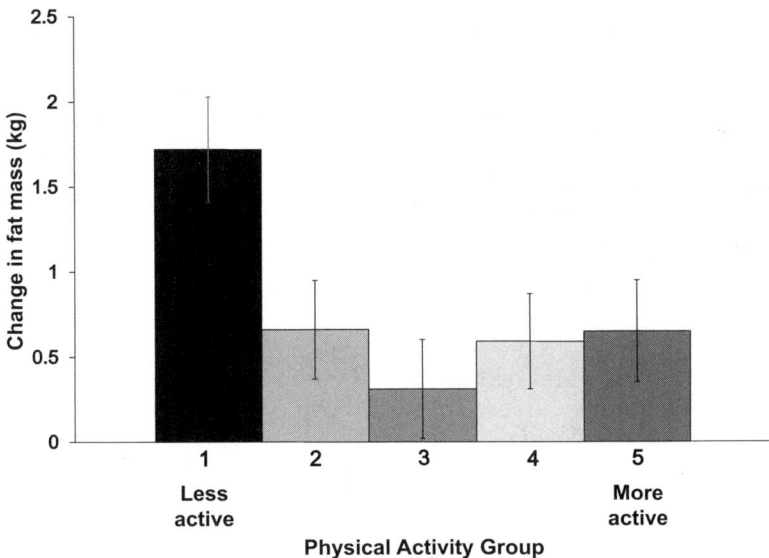

FIGURE 7.4. Change in fat mass from baseline to 1 year of follow-up across quintiles of baseline physical activity in 421 adults, adjusted for change in moderate-to-vigorous physical activity and baseline fat mass. Error bars represent standard errors. Redrawn from Shook, Hand, Drenowatz, Hebert, Paluch, Blundell, et al. (2015). Low levels of physical activity are associated with dysregulation of energy intake and fat mass gain over 1 year. *American Journal of Clinical Nutrition, 102*(6), 1332–1338.

sponding increase in energy intake resulting in the prevention of weight gain.

Based on the available scientific evidence, the American College of Sports Medicine recommends between 150 and 250 minutes of physical activity per week for the prevention of weight gain in adults (Donnelly et al., 2009), which translates into a higher physical activity amount than reported in the Physical Activity Guidelines (U.S. Department of Health and Human Services, 2008).

High Levels of Exercise and Obesity Prevention

The notion that high levels of physical activity are required to maintain energy balance and hence prevent weight gain was first proposed by Jean Mayer in the 1950s (Mayer et al., 1954; Mayer, Roy, & Mitra, 1956). In a series of studies in both animals and humans, Mayer and colleagues observed that the matching of energy intake with energy expenditure was very poor when levels of physical activity were either very low (weight gain), or very high (slight weight loss). At high levels of daily physical activity, Mayer observed that the increase in energy intake often prevented weight gain but, in some, was insufficient to prevent weight loss (Mayer et al., 1954, 1956). These observations were controversial at the time and remain in need of clear experimental validation today.

Studies in which participants perform extremely high amounts of exercise have confirmed that energy intake may not be able to match the energy expenditure associated with higher levels of physical activity (Rosenkilde et al., 2015). Rosenkilde et al. (2015) studied a small group of older men to investigate whether extreme increases in daily energy expenditure during prolonged cycling are sufficiently matched by an increase in energy intake. Over 14 days, six older men (61 ± 3 years) covered a distance of 2,706 km from Copenhagen, Denmark to Nordkapp, Norway. During the 14 days, the increase in energy expenditure measured by doubly labeled water reached 83% above baseline or 30.1 ± 1.5 megajoules (MJ)/day. This is an extraordinary increase in energy expenditure similar to that observed in much younger male professional cyclists during the Tour de France (Saris, van Erp-Baart, Brouns, Westerterp, & ten Hoor, 1989). The principal finding in this study was that increases in energy intake were insufficient to maintain body weight, suggesting that, despite the increase in their motivation to eat, energy balance was not maintained and weight loss was observed. These observations confirm the hypothesis first described by Mayer and colleagues (1956) that beyond a certain threshold level of physical activity, increases in energy intake are no longer coupled with energy expenditure. Although the mechanisms that would explain this phenomenon remain to be elucidated, the importance of increasing physical activity as a means of preventing weight gain is established.

Energy Expenditure of Occupational Work and Risk of Obesity

The technological revolution has changed the energy demands associated with most occupations, in addition to changing the types of occupations that predominate in the Western world. Church et al. (2011) explored the role that temporal changes in occupational energy expenditure may have played in the observed increases in obesity in the United States. By combining data from the U.S. Bureau of Labor Statistics with NHANES, the authors concluded that the energy expenditure associated with occupational work has declined by over 100 calories/day over the last 50 years, and that this decrease accounts for a significant portion of the observed increases in body weights in the U.S. population (Church et al., 2011). The decline in energy expenditure associated with work in the United States is largely the result of a significant reduction in "goods-producing" and "agricultural" jobs and a significant increase in "service" jobs over the last five decades. Another study conducted in several countries around the world (Brazil, China, India, United Kingdom, and United States) has also demonstrated significant reductions in occupational energy expenditure over recent decades (Ng & Popkin, 2012). Given the important role of physical activity at maintaining energy balance, the significant decline in occupational physical activity is undoubtedly an important factor in explaining the global trends in weight gain and obesity.

Some studies have specifically addressed the association between occupational activity and sedentary behavior with obesity. For example, an analysis of data from the NHANES demonstrated that people who were working in occupations classified as "high activity" had lower odds of being abdominally obese (high waist circumference) compared to people in occupations classified as "low activity" (Steeves, Bassett, Thompson, & Fitzhugh, 2012). Further, in those people with little or no nonoccupational physical activity, the odds of being abdominally obese were about 50% lower if they had a highly active occupation (Steeves et al., 2012). In another study of working adults in Denmark, an increase in occupational sitting over 5 years was associated with a significant increase in BMI among women, but not in men (Eriksen, Rosthoj, Burr, & Holtermann, 2015).

The results from systematic reviews have indicated that workplace interventions that include dietary and physical activity components are effective at reducing obesity (Gudzune, Hutfless, Maruthur, Wilson, & Segal, 2013; Verweij, Coffeng, van Mechelen, & Proper, 2011). Further, interventions that focus on increasing physical activity alone in the workplace have been shown to be effective at reducing body weight and BMI (Verweij et al., 2011). However, there have been very few workplace interventions that specifically target increases in physical activity. This area is a priority for future research.

Modes of Transportation and Risk of Obesity

The use of "active" means of transportation (walking, cycling, etc.) has been shown to be associated with a higher level of daily physical activity compared to "passive" means of transportation (e.g., riding in a car; Rissel, Curac, Greenaway, & Bauman, 2012). The results of an international study conducted among 153,996 adults from 17 low-, middle-, and high-income countries demonstrated that car ownership was associated with significantly higher (14%) odds of obesity compared to not owning a car (Lear et al., 2014). Although these results could be interpreted as an association between socioeconomic status (SES) and obesity (i.e., owning a car is related to higher SES), car ownership might also result in lower physical activity levels, given the reliance on passive rather than active transportation.

Indeed, systematic reviews of the existing literature have provided some evidence that active transportation may be associated with a lower risk of obesity (Wanner, Gotschi, Martin-Diener, Kahlmeier, & Martin, 2012; Xu, Wen, & Rissel, 2013). In one review, 40 of 69 studies reported a significant negative association between active transportation and body weight (Xu et al., 2013). In a second review, 25 of 30 studies reported negative associations between active transportation and body weight or reduced odds of obesity (Wanner et al., 2012). However, most of the studies contributing data to these reviews were cross-sectional, which limits inferences about causal associations. Nevertheless, these results are further supported by a recent analysis of data from 156,666 adult participants in the UK Biobank project that demonstrated a strong negative association between active commuting and both BMI and percentage of body fat (Flint & Cummins, 2016). Compared to car-only commuters, mixed public transport and active commuters had significantly lower BMI and percentage of body fat, as did both walking and cycling commuters (Flint & Cummins, 2016). Although these results represent suggestive cross-sectional associations between active transportation and body weight, there is a need for future research that addresses these associations using longitudinal and intervention study designs.

Effects of Exercise on EPOC

The increased oxygen uptake required to meet the energy needs during exercise does not return to resting levels immediately postexercise and may remain elevated for extended periods. The term *excess postexercise oxygen consumption* was introduced as a means of capturing both the rapid and prolonged components of the observed increase in oxygen uptake after exercising (Brooks, Hittelman, Faulkner, & Beyer, 1971). A detailed description of the EPOC components and their associated mechanisms is beyond the scope of this chapter. The reader is referred to the reviews of Borsheim and Bahr (2003) and Gaesser and Brooks (1984) for details.

Acute exercise is generally associated with increases in EPOC, which are greatest immediately following the exercise session (rapid or short-term EPOC), with rapid declines within 2 hours of termination. Prolonged or long-term elevations in EPOC, albeit slight, may persist for 48 hours or more postexercise (Hunter, Byrne, Gower, Sirikul, & Hills, 2006; Speakman & Selman, 2003). Here we consider whether exercise may influence the magnitude and duration of EPOC, whether exercise intensity and duration (amount) have separate effects, and whether the magnitude of EPOC may be of value for preventing weight gain.

Two prior reviews have carefully considered current knowledge with respect to the separate influence of exercise intensity and duration on EPOC (Borsheim & Bahr, 2003; LaForgia, Withers, & Gore, 2006). Consistent with the conclusions of these reviews is the notion that duration and intensity of exercise act synergistically to influence EPOC; however, it appears that at exercise intensities above 50% of VO_2 max, exercise intensity is more important (Borsheim & Bahr, 2003). This observation is illustrated by the work of Gore and Withers (1990). Their study included nine experimental treatments ($N = 9$ trained men), each with different combinations of exercise durations (i.e., 20, 50, and 80 minutes) and intensities (30%, 50%, and 70% VO_2 max). The authors observed a strong interaction between exercise duration and exercise intensity. With the exception of exercise performed at 30% VO_2 max, the magnitude of the EPOC was elevated as exercise duration increased, whereas exercise intensity was held constant. Although the magnitude of the EPOC also increased with increasing exercise intensity, whereas duration was held constant, compared to exercise duration (7%), exercise intensity contributed far more to the increase in EPOC (~45%). In response to 80 minutes of exercise, the EPOC ranged from a low value of 1.0 L, equivalent to 5.2 kcal at 30% VO_2 max, to a high value of 14.6 L, equivalent to 73 kcal at 70% VO_2

max. EPOC was determined over 8 hours postexercise.

Although the vast majority of studies report that a synergistic relation exists between exercise intensity, duration, and EPOC, it is apparent that with increasing exercise duration, total energy expenditure is increased, thus confounding this interpretation. Whether exercise intensity is positively associated with EPOC when exercise amount (caloric expenditure in kilocalories) is held constant remains unclear. Four studies in which the investigators held exercise amount constant while varying intensity have been reported (Frey, Byrnes, & Mazzeo, 1993; Phelain, Reinke, Harris, & Melby, 1997; Sedlock, 1991; Sedlock, Fissinger, & Melby, 1989). Sedlock et al. (1989) was one of the first studies to consider the separate effects of exercise intensity and amount of exercise on EPOC. Highly trained men exercised at (1) high (~75%) and low (~50%) intensity with caloric expenditure held constant (~300 kcal) and (2) equal exercise intensity with varying duration. The primary observation was that exercise intensity affected both the magnitude and the duration of the EPOC. Holding exercise amount constant revealed a longer EPOC duration for the high-intensity group (33.3 minutes) compared to the low-intensity group (19.8 minutes) and a greater caloric expenditure during EPOC.

This finding is consistent with Frey et al. (1993), who examined trained and untrained women who exercised at high (~80%) and low (~65%) intensity with exercise amount held constant (~300 kcal/session). The authors also observed that EPOC at high intensity was greater than EPOC at low intensity, despite a shorter duration for the high-intensity exercise. Phelain et al. (1997) observed similar results with trained women exercising at high (~75%) and low (~50%) intensity with constant caloric expenditure (~500 kcal). In contrast to these findings, Sedlock (1991) found no effect of exercise intensity and duration on EPOC magnitude. This study was also performed with trained women who exercised at high (~60%) and low (~40%) intensity, with caloric expenditure held constant (~200 kcal). The fact that exercise intensity did not affect the EPOC magnitude might have been due to a lower exercise amount (200 kcal) as opposed to the other studies (300 kcal and above). In general, however, these findings support the notion that exercise intensity contributes substantially to the observed EPOC.

Whether the EPOC is of value in preventing gains in body fat depends on whether the individual sustains exercise over the long term. Although EPOC appears to be modest in response to a single exercise session, the potential energy expenditure increase associated with EPOC may be substantial if exercise is sustained long term. Based on their comprehensive review, Borsheim and Bahr (2003) reported that for a single session of moderate-intensity (less than 1 hour at ~50% VO_2 max) exercise, EPOC will approximate 12–24 kcal, equivalent to ~2,800 kcal a year, which translates to a loss of 311g fat (assuming exercise is performed 3 days/week). In response to vigorous exercise (at least 1 hour at a minimum of 70% VO_2 max), EPOC will approximate 170 kcal/session or approximately 26,000 kcal/year, which translates to a loss of 3.0 kg fat. Clearly, 1 hour of exercise performed at about 70% of VO_2 max may be difficult to sustain for many, if not most, overweight or obese persons. Although from a physiological perspective, the EPOC consequent to sustained high-intensity exercise may be helpful for prevention of weight gain, the sustainability of this exercise behavior pattern would represent a challenge for most adults.

Physical Activity and Regulation of Energy Balance

One question raised from time to time in the popular press and the scientific literature is whether physical activity influences the level at which energy balance is regulated. Another way to pose the question is to ask whether there is coupling between the energy expended for physical activity on a daily basis and the energy intake on the same day. Despite decades of research, we still do not have a complete understanding of the process, and currently there is no consensus on what exactly the data signify. A number of models have been put forward over the years in attempts to recapitulate data from various sources and their implications for the regulation of energy balance and body weight.

An overview of four of these models—the set point model, the settling point model, the general intake model, and the dual intervention point model—was given in a summary a few years ago (Speakman et al., 2011). The interested reader can refer to this publication for a detailed discussion.

Common sense suggests that there is poor coupling between energy expenditure from physical activity and dietary caloric intake at the low end of the activity continuum. This idea is supported by the high-population prevalence of overweight and obesity in sedentary people in many countries of the developed world. There is also support for this notion in observational prospective studies that utilize careful monitoring of activity and caloric intake (Shook et al., 2015). For some reasons yet to be uncovered, the regulation of caloric intake at very low levels of energy expenditure is a challenge for a large fraction of adults. It is also suggested that the coupling between energy expenditure and caloric intake is not very tight at slightly higher levels of physical activity energy expenditure in the range of 100–150 kcal/day. However, coupling seems to be better for this group than for completely sedentary individuals.

With increasing amounts of physical activity energy expenditure, the coupling with caloric intake gets better and becomes tight at high levels of activity. Interestingly, the same coupling is true with cold exposure. Those who expend large amounts of calories, such as endurance athletes in training or people whose occupation requires large-calorie expenditures, are typically of normal body weight with low levels of adiposity. Excess weight and obesity would clearly be a major handicap for long-distance runners, cyclists, and other endurance athletes. These athletes have no choice but to consume large amounts of calories just to maintain body weight. In other words, when people expend 200 kcal/day, or more, on purposeful activity-related energy expenditure, there is a pretty tight coupling between energy intake and energy expenditure. This coupling is even more precise at high levels of caloric output. For instance, many types of athletes in training or in their competitive season consume around 5,000 kcal/day, and still they have to be careful about maintaining a healthy body weight because they tend to lose weight unintentionally. There are even more extreme examples, such as the 6,000–9,000 kcal of energy expenditure per day for 21 days of the professional cyclists who compete in the Tour de France. Interestingly, as we discussed in a previous section, when older men who were recreationally active increased their rate of energy expenditure to 6,000 kcal/day for 14 days, this change resulted in a negative energy balance (about 1,000 kcal/day). This loss was due to their inability to increase caloric intake sufficiently to match energy expenditure (Rosenkilde et al., 2015).

In spite of all the limitations in the body of knowledge, there is some justification for the belief that physical activity is a powerful regulator of energy balance. Potential mechanisms for a role of physical activity in the regulation of energy balance when the activity-related energy expenditure ranges from very low to very high include, at a minimum, the following paths.

At low levels of activity, which is also typically low intensity, the muscular demands are met mainly by the recruitment of slow motor units and muscle fibers. With increasing exercise intensity and amount, the recruitment of fast motor units and muscle fibers is increased. The fast contracting motor fibers rely more on a carbohydrate-derived substrate to sustain muscle contractions than slow contracting fibers. The progressive shift in metabolic fuel takes place in the presence of more sympathetic nervous system activation, growing levels of norepinephrine and other hormones, and increased secretions of myokines by the active muscles and adipokines by adipose tissue depots. The EPOC recovery period following a high-intensity activity bout is also more substantial.

In the first phase, O_2 debt recovery accounts for the elevated metabolic rate post-activity (replenishing muscle and blood O_2 stores, lactate removal, regeneration of adenosine triphosphate [ATP] and C-reactive protein levels, etc.). In the second extended phase of EPOC, continuing recovery of circulatory and pulmonary functions, normalization of body temperature, progressive shift of metabolic fuel from carbohydrate to lipid oxidation, replenishment of glycogen levels, elevated synthesis and breakdown of proteins, and undoubtedly other mechanisms participate in the prolonged, elevated energy expenditure above resting metabolic rate (Borsheim, 2010). These descriptions suggest that metabolic flexibility is needed at high amounts of physical activity executed at moderate and high intensities, and that multiple biological signals arising under these conditions may favor coupling between the energy expenditure of activity and caloric intake.

There are undoubtedly other mechanisms at play, as suggested by a study of pairs of monozygotic twins, in which one member was a sustained runner and the other was not (Williams, 2012). The difference between the active twin and the less active co-twin was more than 2 BMI units. These observations suggest the presence of a genotype-by-physical-activity interaction, which translates into a better regulation of energy intake and an attenuation of the genetic risk of excess weight. The apparent uncoupling of energy intake and energy expenditure at the low end of the physical activity level is not fully understood. A sedentary state requires less metabolic flexibility and is undoubtedly characterized by much lower trafficking levels of activity-induced myokines and adipokines. It is also a state in which fast twitch muscle fibers are not solicited to a large and sustained extent. Moreover, there is no need to recover from the metabolic demands of a physical activity period, and therefore EPOC is nonexistent.

Physical Activity, Appetite, and Satiety

Are there any effects of acute and chronic exposure to physical activity on appetite and satiety? The topic is of considerable importance, as the popular press seems to believe that being physically active makes you eat more. Let's begin with a few definitions. *Appetite* is defined as the desire to eat food due to hunger. *Satiation* occurs while eating and brings the consumption of food to an end. Finally, *satiety* is the state of being satiated; it is characterized by the feeling of being full after eating food. Appetite and satiety are complex states regulated by hormonal secretions from the stomach, gut, pancreas, and hypothalamus as well as vagal afferent from the stomach, gastrointestinal tract, and other organs signaling to hypothalamic neurons. There is a strong neural basis to the regulation of appetite and satiety, and the brain is likely to be the site of some of the genetic predisposition favoring the adoption of obesogenic behavior (Farooqi, 2014). However, even though there is some evidence for a genetic component to these behavioral traits (Melhorn et al., 2016), identifying the specific genes and variants driving individual differences in appetite and satiety has proven to be very difficult (van Vliet-Ostaptchouk, Hofker, van der Schouw, Wijmenga, & Onland-Moret, 2009).

The neurobiology of appetite and satiety (and of energy balance regulation) with exposure to physical activity across ranges of intensity, duration, and frequency of exposures has the potential to shed light on critical aspects of this highly complex topic (Dishman et al., 2006). Importantly, a sustained physically active lifestyle has the potential to alter brain functions in a direction favoring better adaptation (Mattson, 2012). Unfortunately, the full power of the modern neuroscience technologies has not been applied to address these issues as of yet. However, a number of generalizations can be made based on existing observational and experimental studies. There is a large body of evidence supporting a beneficial role of physical activity on appetite regulation (Martins, Morgan, & Truby, 2008). Engaging in physical activity increases hunger and food intake, but the latter increase is commensurate with the activity-induced energy expenditure. This is generally observed for activities extending from light to moderate to vigorous to hard intensities, although there are individual differences.

A different trend is observed when the intensity of physical activity is maximal or near maximal. In brief, activities in these intensity ranges are typically followed by periods of appetite suppression. Blundell and colleagues have referred to this as "post exercise anorexia," and it is typically observed after an acute exposure to a high-intensity exercise bout (King et al., 2009; Martins, Kulseng, King, Holst, & Blundell, 2010). This appetite suppressive effect can be seen at times in the fasted state but is more consistently observed in a postprandial state. In comparing two doses of physical activity at moderate intensity, only the highest dose (60 min/day) was associated with an increase in fasting and meal-related ratings of fullness and satiety (Rosenkilde et al., 2013). Another dimension of the relationship between being physically active and the regulation of appetite or satiety was evidenced in a study demonstrating that active individuals had a greater ability to compensate for high-energy preloads through reductions in energy intake in comparison with inactive controls (Beaulieu, Hopkins, Blundell, & Finlayson, 2016).

This is an area of considerable importance for the maintenance of a healthy body weight. More research is needed to clarify the mechanisms behind the improvement in short-term appetite control observed with exercise and the long-term implications of these mechanisms (Martins et al., 2008). The regulation of appetite and satiety is influenced by multiple factors, including hormonal and cytokine status, metabolic factors, physiological and psychological states, the intensity and duration of the physical activity exposure, and undoubtedly other factors as well. The response of appetite and satiety indicators to physical activity exposures is highly variable, and it may be difficult to ever achieve generalization and prediction (Blundell, Gibbons, Caudwell, Finlayson, & Hopkins, 2015).

Summary

Physical activity energy expenditure is highly variable among adults. We take strong objection with the notion that physical inactivity has nothing to do with variation in body weight and the obesity epidemic. The time spent in a sedentary state is predictive of weight gain over the years. The shift in the occupational activity profile over several decades is associated with the increase in the prevalence of overweight and obesity. Even though physical activities performed at low to moderate intensities can result in substantial energy expenditure, activities at high intensities carry not only weight control benefits but multiple metabolic advantages as well. Among others, these metabolic advantages include entrainment of metabolic flexibility and an elevated EPOC lasting for hours.

Measuring and monitoring physical activity energy expenditures outside of the laboratory can be challenging, but there are practical ways to obtain reasonable estimates. Adherence to the current Physical Activity Guidelines can result in true weight gain prevention benefits. However, it is becoming widely recognized that higher volumes of regular physical activity have the potential to achieve even better weight gain prevention results. Globally, energy intake is well matched to physical activity level across the continuum of intensity and volume, with the exception of sedentary condition and high-intensity, very-high-volume conditions resulting in very large activity-related energy expenditure. Potential mechanisms for a role of physical activity in the regulation of caloric intake and energy balance have been proposed. We conclude that there is strong evidence from multiple lines of research that being physically active on a regular basis offers some protection against weight gain over the years.

Acknowledgments

Claude Bouchard is partially funded by the John W. Barton Sr. Chair in Genetics and Nutrition and by a Centers of Biomedical Excellence grant from the National Institutes of Health (No. NIH 8 P20 GM103528). Peter T. Katzmarzyk is partially funded by the Marie Edana Corcoran Endowed Chair in Pediatric Obesity and Diabetes. We would like to express our gratitude to Melanie Peterson for her valuable assistance with the preparation of the manuscript.

References

Ainsworth, B. E., Cahalin, L., Buman, M., & Ross, R. (2015). The current state of physical activity assessment tools. *Progress in Cardiovascular Diseases, 57*(4), 387–395.

Ainsworth, B. E., Haskell, W. L., Herrmann, S. D., Meckes, N., Bassett, D. R., Jr., Tudor-Locke, C., et al. (2011a). 2011 Compendium of physical activities: A second update of codes and MET values. *Medicine and Science in Sports and Exercise, 43*(8), 1575–1581.

Ainsworth, B. E., Haskell, W. L., Herrmann, S. D., Meckes, N., Bassett, D. R., Jr., Tudor-Locke, C., et al. (2011b). Compendium of physical activities tracking guide. Retrieved from *https://sites.google.com/site/compendiumofphysicalactivities*.

Ainsworth, B. E., Richardson, M. T., Jacobs, D. R.,

Jr., Leon, A. S., & Sternfeld, B. (1999). Accuracy of recall of occupational physical activity by questionnaire. *Journal of Clinical Epidemiology, 52*(3), 219–227.

Beaulieu, K., Hopkins, M., Blundell, J., & Finlayson, G. (2016). Does habitual physical activity increase the sensitivity of the appetite control system?: A systematic review. *Sports Medicine, 46*(12), 1897–1919.

Blundell, J. E., Gibbons, C., Caudwell, P., Finlayson, G., & Hopkins, M. (2015). Appetite control and energy balance: Impact of exercise. *Obesity Review, 16*(1, Suppl.), 67–76.

Borsheim, E. (2010). Post-exercise energy expenditure or EPOC. In C. Bouchard & P. T. Katzmarzyk (Eds.), *Physical activity and obesity* (2nd ed., pp. 174–177). Champaign, IL: Human Kinetics.

Borsheim, E., & Bahr, R. (2003). Effect of exercise intensity, duration and mode on post-exercise oxygen consumption. *Sports Medicine, 33*(14), 1037–1060.

Bouchard, C., & Shephard, R. J. (1994). Physical activity, fitness, and health: The model and key concepts. In C. Bouchard, R. J. Shephard, & T. Stephens (Eds.), *Physical activity, fitness, and health: International proceedings and consensus statement* (pp. 77–88). Champaign, IL: Human Kinetics.

Brooks, G. A. (2012). Bioenergetics of exercising humans. *Comprehensive Physiology, 2*(1), 537–562.

Brooks, G. A., Hittelman, K. J., Faulkner, J. A., & Beyer, R. E. (1971). Tissue temperatures and whole-animal oxygen consumption after exercise. *American Journal of Physiology, 221*(2), 427–431.

Church, T. S., Thomas, D. M., Tudor-Locke, C., Katzmarzyk, P. T., Earnest, C. P., Rodarte, R. Q., et al. (2011). Trends over 5 decades in U.S. occupation-related physical activity and their associations with obesity. *PLOS ONE, 6*(5), e19657.

Coyle, E. F. (1995). Substrate utilization during exercise in active people. *American Journal of Clinical Nutrition, 61*(4, Suppl.), 968S–979S.

Di Pietro, L. (1999). Physical activity in the prevention of obesity: Current evidence and research issues. *Medicine and Science in Sports and Exercise, 31*(11, Suppl.), S542–S546.

Di Pietro, L., Dziura, J., & Blair, S. N. (2004). Estimated change in physical activity level (PAL) and prediction of 5-year weight change in men: The Aerobics Center Longitudinal Study. *International Journal of Obesity and Related Metabolic Disorders, 28*(12), 1541–1547.

Dishman, R. K., Berthoud, H. R., Booth, F. W., Cotman, C. W., Edgerton, V. R., Fleshner, M. R., et al. (2006). Neurobiology of exercise. *Obesity (Silver Spring), 14*(3), 345–356.

Donnelly, J. E., Blair, S. N., Jakicic, J. M., Manore, M. M., Rankin, J. W., & Smith, B. K. (2009). American College of Sports Medicine position stand: Appropriate physical activity intervention strategies for weight loss and prevention of weight regain for adults. *Medicine and Scients in Sports and Exercise, 41*(2), 459–471.

Epstein, L., Miller, G. J., Stitt, F. W., & Morris, J. N. (1976). Vigorous exercise in leisure time, coronary risk-factors, and resting electrocardiogram in middle-aged male civil servants. *British Heart Journal, 38*(4), 403–409.

Eriksen, D., Rosthoj, S., Burr, H., & Holtermann, A. (2015). Sedentary work: Associations between five-year changes in occupational sitting time and body mass index. *Preventive Medicine, 73*, 1–5.

Erlichman, J., Kerbey, A. L., & James, W. P. (2002). Physical activity and its impact on health outcomes: Paper 2. Prevention of unhealthy weight gain and obesity by physical activity—an analysis of the evidence. *Obesity Review, 3*(4), 273–287.

Farooqi, I. S. (2014). Defining the neural basis of appetite and obesity: From genes to behaviour. *Clinical Medicine (London), 14*(3), 286–289.

Flint, E., & Cummins, S. (2016). Active commuting and obesity in mid-life: Cross-sectional, observational evidence from UK Biobank. *Lancet Diabetes and Endocrinology, 4*(5), 420–435.

Freedson, P., Bowles, H. R., Troiano, R., & Haskell, W. (2012). Assessment of physical activity using wearable monitors: Recommendations for monitor calibration and use in the field. *Medicine and Science in Sports and Exercise, 44*(1, Suppl. 1), S1–S4.

Frey, G. C., Byrnes, W. C., & Mazzeo, R. S. (1993). Factors influencing excess postexercise oxygen consumption in trained and untrained women. *Metabolism, 42*(7), 822–828.

Gaesser, G. A., & Brooks, G. A. (1984). Metabolic bases of excess post-exercise oxygen consumption: A review. *Medicine and Science in Sports and Exercise, 16*(1), 29–43.

Gore, C. J., & Withers, R. T. (1990). The effect of exercise intensity and duration on the oxygen deficit and excess post-exercise oxygen consumption. *European Journal of Applied Physiology and Occupational Physiology, 60*(3), 169–174.

Grontved, A., & Hu, F. B. (2011). Television viewing and risk of type 2 diabetes, cardiovascular disease, and all-cause mortality: A meta-analysis. *Journal of the American Medical Association, 305*(23), 2448–2455.

Gudzune, K., Hutfless, S., Maruthur, N., Wilson, R., & Segal, J. (2013). Strategies to prevent weight gain in workplace and college settings: A systematic review. *Preventive Medicine, 57*(4), 268–277.

Hankinson, A. L., Daviglus, M. L., Bouchard, C., Carnethon, M., Lewis, C. E., Schreiner, P. J., et al. (2010). Maintaining a high physical activity level over 20 years and weight gain. *Journal of the American Medical Association, 304*(23), 2603–2610.

Harrington, D. M., Barreira, T. V., Staiano, A. E., & Katzmarzyk, P. T. (2014). The descriptive epidemiology of sitting among US adults, NHANES 2009/2010. *Journal of Science and Medicine in Sport, 17*(4), 371–375.

Howley, E. T. (2001). Type of activity: Resistance, aerobic and leisure versus occupational physical activity. *Medicine and Science in Sports and Exercise, 33*(6, Suppl.), S364–S369; discussion S419–S420.

Hu, F. B., Li, T. Y., Colditz, G. A., Willett, W. C., & Manson, J. E. (2003). Television watching and other sedentary behaviors in relation to risk of obesity and type 2 diabetes mellitus in women. *Journal of the American Medical Association, 289*(14), 1785–1791.

Hunter, G. R., Byrne, N. M., Gower, B. A., Sirikul, B., & Hills, A. P. (2006). Increased resting energy expenditure after 40 minutes of aerobic but not resistance exercise. *Obesity (Silver Spring), 14*(11), 2018–2025.

Katzmarzyk, P. T., Church, T. S., Craig, C. L., & Bouchard, C. (2009). Sitting time and mortality from all causes, cardiovascular disease, and cancer. *Medicine and Science in Sports and Exercise, 41*(5), 998–1005.

Kenney, W. L., Wilmore, J. H., & Costill, D. L. (2015). *Physiology of sport and exercise* (6th ed.). Champaign, IL: Human Kinetics.

King, N. A., Caudwell, P. P., Hopkins, M., Stubbs, J. R., Naslund, E., & Blundell, J. E. (2009). Dual-process action of exercise on appetite control: Increase in orexigenic drive but improvement in meal-induced satiety. *American Journal of Clinical Nutrition, 90*(4), 921–927.

LaForgia, J., Withers, R. T., & Gore, C. J. (2006). Effects of exercise intensity and duration on the excess post-exercise oxygen consumption. *Journal of Sports Sciences, 24*(12), 1247–1264.

Lear, S. A., Teo, K., Gasevic, D., Zhang, X., Poirier, P. P., Rangarajan, S., et al. (2014). The association between ownership of common household devices and obesity and diabetes in high, middle and low income countries. *Canadian Medical Association Journal, 186*(4), 258–266.

Lee, I. M., Djousse, L., Sesso, H. D., Wang, L., & Buring, J. E. (2010). Physical activity and weight gain prevention. *Journal of the American Medical Association, 303*(12), 1173–1179.

Levine, J. A., Lanningham-Foster, L. M., McCrady, S. K., Krizan, A. C., Olson, L. R., Kane, P. H., et al. (2005). Interindividual variation in posture allocation: Possible role in human obesity. *Science, 307*(5709), 584–586.

Malhotra, A., Noakes, T., & Phinney, S. (2015). It is time to bust the myth of physical inactivity and obesity: You cannot outrun a bad diet. *British Journal of Sports Medicine, 49*(15), 967–968.

Malina, R. M., & Little, B. B. (2008). Physical activity: The present in the context of the past. *American Journal of Human Biology, 20*(4), 373–391.

Martins, C., Kulseng, B., King, N. A., Holst, J. J., & Blundell, J. E. (2010). The effects of exercise-induced weight loss on appetite-related peptides and motivation to eat. *Journal of Clinical Endocrinology and Metabolism, 95*(4), 1609–1616.

Martins, C., Morgan, L., & Truby, H. (2008). A review of the effects of exercise on appetite regulation: An obesity perspective. *International Journal of Obesity (London), 32*(9), 1337–1347.

Mattson, M. P. (2012). Evolutionary aspects of human exercise: Born to run purposefully. *Ageing Research Reviews, 11*(3), 347–352.

Mayer, J., Marshall, N. B., Vitale, J. J., Christensen, J. H., Mashayekhi, M. B., & Stare, F. J. (1954). Exercise, food intake and body weight in normal rats and genetically obese adult mice. *American Journal of Physiology, 177*(3), 544–548.

Mayer, J., Roy, P., & Mitra, K. P. (1956). Relation between caloric intake, body weight, and physical work: Studies in an industrial male population in West Bengal. *American Journal of Clinical Nutrition, 4*(2), 169–175.

McArdle, W. D., Katch, F. I., & Katch, V. L. (2016). *Essentials of exercise physiology* (5th ed.). Philadelphia: Wolters Kluwer.

Melhorn, S. J., Mehta, S., Kratz, M., Tyagi, V., Webb, M. F., Noonan, C. J., et al. (2016). Brain regulation of appetite in twins. *American Journal of Clinical Nutrition, 103*(2), 314–322.

Ng, S. W., & Popkin, B. M. (2012). Time use and physical activity: A shift away from movement across the globe. *Obesity Review, 13*(8), 659–680.

Owen, N., Healy, G. N., Matthews, C. E., & Dunstan, D. (2010). Too much sitting: The population science of sedentary behavior. *Exercise and Sport Sciences Review, 38*(3), 105–13.

Phelain, J. F., Reinke, E., Harris, M. A., & Melby, C. L. (1997). Postexercise energy expenditure and substrate oxidation in young women resulting from exercise bouts of different intensity. *Journal of the American College of Nutrition, 16*(2), 140–146.

Powers, S. K., & Howley, E. T. (2015). *Exercise physiology: Theory and application to fitness and performance* (9th ed.). New York: McGraw-Hill Education.

Proper, K. I., Singh, A. S., van Mechelen, W., & Chinapaw, M. J. (2011). Sedentary behaviors and health outcomes among adults: A systematic review of prospective studies. *American Journal of Preventive Medicine, 40*(2), 174–182.

Rissel, C., Curac, N., Greenaway, M., & Bauman, A. (2012). Physical activity associated with public transport use: A review and modelling of potential benefits. *International Journal of Environmental Research and Public Health, 9*(7), 2454–2478.

Rosenkilde, M., Morville, T., Andersen, P. R., Kjaer, K., Rasmusen, H., Holst, J. J., et al. (2015). Inability to match energy intake with energy expenditure at sustained near-maximal rates of energy expenditure in older men during a 14-d cycling expedition. *American Journal of Clinical Nutrition, 102*(6), 1398–1405.

Rosenkilde, M., Reichkendler, M. H., Auerbach, P., Torang, S., Gram, A. S., Ploug, T., et al. (2013). Appetite regulation in overweight, sedentary men after different amounts of endurance exercise: A randomized controlled trial. *Journal of Applied Physiology, 115*(11), 1599–1609.

Ruttimann, J. (2012). Obesity vaccines: A long shot? *Endocrine News*, pp. 20–23.

Saris, W. H., Blair, S. N., van Baak, M. A., Eaton, S. B., Davies, P. S., Di Pietro, L., et al. (2003). How much physical activity is enough to prevent unhealthy weight gain?: Outcome of the IASO 1st Stock Conference and consensus statement. *Obesity Review, 4*(2), 101–114.

Saris, W. H., van Erp-Baart, M. A., Brouns, F., Westerterp, K. R., & ten Hoor, F. (1989). Study on food intake and energy expenditure during extreme sustained exercise: The Tour de France. *International Journal of Sports Medicine, 10*(Suppl. 1), S26–S31.

Sedentary Behaviour Research Network. (2012). Letter to the editor: Standardized use of the terms "sedentary" and "sedentary behaviours." *Applied Physiology, Nutrition, and Metabolism, 37*(3), 540–542.

Sedlock, D. A. (1991). Effect of exercise intensity on postexercise energy expenditure in women. *British Journal of Sports Medicine, 25*(1), 38–40.

Sedlock, D. A., Fissinger, J. A., & Melby, C. L. (1989). Effect of exercise intensity and duration on postexercise energy expenditure. *Medicine and Science in Sports and Exercise, 21*(6), 662–666.

Shook, R. P., Hand, G. A., Drenowatz, C., Hebert, J. R., Paluch, A. E., Blundell, J. E., et al. (2015). Low levels of physical activity are associated with dysregulation of energy intake and fat mass gain over 1 year. *American Journal of Clinical Nutrition, 102*(6), 1332–1338.

Speakman, J. R., Levitsky, D. A., Allison, D. B., Bray, M. S., de Castro, J. M., Clegg, D. J., et al. (2011). Set points, settling points and some alternative models: Theoretical options to understand how genes and environments combine to regulate body adiposity. *Disease Models and Mechanisms, 4*(6), 733–745.

Speakman, J. R., & Selman, C. (2003). Physical activity and resting metabolic rate. *Proceedings of the Nutrition Society, 62*(3), 621–634.

Steeves, J. A., Bassett, D. R., Jr., Thompson, D. L., & Fitzhugh, E. C. (2012). Relationships of occupational and non-occupational physical activity to abdominal obesity. *International Journal of Obesity, 36*(1), 100–106.

Strath, S. J., Bassett, D. R., Jr., & Swartz, A. M. (2004). Comparison of the College Alumnus Questionnaire Physical Activity Index with objective monitoring. *Annals of Epidemiology, 14*(6), 409–415.

Thorp, A. A., Owen, N., Neuhaus, M., & Dunstan, D. W. (2011). Sedentary behaviors and subsequent health outcomes in adults: A systematic review of longitudinal studies, 1996–2011. *American Journal of Preventive Medicine, 41*(2), 207–215.

Tudor-Locke, C., Martin, C. K., Brashear, M. M., Rood, J. C., Katzmarzyk, P. T., & Johnson, W. D. (2012). Predicting doubly labeled water energy expenditure from ambulatory activity. *Applied Physiology, Nutrition, and Metabolism, 37*(6), 1091–1100.

U.S. Department of Health and Human Services. (2008). 2008 Physical Activity Guidelines for Americans. Retrieved from *http://health.gov/paguidelines/guidelines*.

van Vliet-Ostaptchouk, J. V., Hofker, M. H., van der Schouw, Y. T., Wijmenga, C., & Onland-Moret, N. C. (2009). Genetic variation in the hypothalamic pathways and its role on obesity. *Obesity Review, 10*(6), 593–609.

Verweij, L. M., Coffeng, J., van Mechelen, W., & Proper, K. I. (2011). Meta-analyses of workplace physical activity and dietary behaviour interventions on weight outcomes. *Obesity Review, 12*(6), 406–429.

Wanner, M., Gotschi, T., Martin-Diener, E., Kahlmeier, S., & Martin, B. W. (2012). Active transport, physical activity, and body weight in adults: A systematic review. *American Journal of Preventive Medicine, 42*(5), 493–502.

Warburton, D. (2010). The physical activity and exercise continuum. In C. Bouchard & P. T. Katzmarzyk (Eds.), *Physical activity and obesity* (2nd ed., pp. 7–12). Champaign, IL: Human Kinetics.

Welk, G. J., Kim, Y., Stanfill, B., Osthus, D. A., Calabro, M. A., Nusser, S. M., et al. (2014). Validity of 24-h physical activity recall: Physical activity measurement survey. *Medicine and Science in Sports and Exercise, 46*(10), 2014–2024.

Westerterp, K. R. (2009). Assessment of physical activity: A critical appraisal. *European Journal of Applied Physiology, 105*(6), 823–828.

Westerterp, K. R. (2013). Physical activity and physical activity induced energy expenditure in humans: Measurement, determinants, and effects. *Frontiers in Physiology, 4*, 90.

Williams, P. T. (2012). Attenuated inheritance of body weight by running in monozygotic twins. *Medicine and Science in Sports and Exercise, 44*(1), 98–103.

Xu, H., Wen, L. M., & Rissel, C. (2013). The relationships between active transport to work or school and cardiovascular health or body weight: A systematic review. *Asia Pacific Journal of Public Health, 25*(4), 298–315.

CHAPTER 8

Sleep and Obesity

Andrea M. Spaeth
David F. Dinges

Sleeping, like eating, is a biological need. It consumes approximately one-third of human life. Just as missing a day's worth of meals produces strong feelings of hunger, being deprived of a night's sleep leads to severe sleepiness. Recently, a large body of research has focused on the relationship between sleep and energy balance.

Sleep Duration

In healthy humans, the timing, intensity, and duration of sleep are primarily regulated by two processes: homeostatic regulation and circadian timing. The term *sleep homeostasis* refers to the drive for sleep that increases progressively during wakefulness and decreases progressively during sleep. The circadian process that controls sleep is described as the *24-hour oscillatory variation in the propensity for sleep*. Human sleep is naturally regulated by these two processes, with sunrise and sunset providing the photic signals necessary to entrain the sleep–wake cycle.

Sleep duration changes markedly across the lifespan with sleep need decreasing as we age. The latest recommendations for sleep by age group are shown in Table 8.1 (Hirschkowitz et al., 2015). Although the majority of people need these recommended amounts of sleep to function optimally, there are individual differences in sleep need, sleep ability, and sleep opportunity such that a variety of factors determine actual sleep duration. A large proportion (approximately one-third) of American adults self-report habitually sleeping less than the

TABLE 8.1. Recommended Sleep across the Lifespan

Age range	Recommended sleep duration/24 hours
Newborns (0–3 months)	14–17 hours
Infants (4–11 months)	12–15 hours
Toddlers (1–2 years)	11–14 hours
Preschoolers (3–5 years)	10–13 hours
School-age children (6–13 years)	9–11 hours
Teenagers (14–17 years)	8–10 hours
Young adults (18–25 years)	7–9 hours
Adults (26–64 years)	7–9 hours
Older adults (≥65 years)	7–9 hours

Note. Based on the report of an expert panel convened by the U.S.-based National Sleep Foundation and published in Hirschkowitz, Whiton, Albert, Alessi, Bruni, DonCarlos, et al. (2015). National Sleep Foundation's sleep time duration recommendations: Methodology and results summary. *Sleep Health, 1*(1), 40–43.

recommended 7 hours/night, prompting the Centers for Disease Control and Prevention (CDC) to declare insufficient sleep a public health epidemic (CDC, 2016). Insufficient sleep has also become a concern in regard to children and adolescents. When parents were asked to estimate how much sleep their child obtained at night, 31% of 6- to 11-year-olds and 71% of 12- to 14-year-olds were reported to sleep less than the recommended 9 hours/night, and 56% of 15- to 17-year-olds were reported to sleep less than the recommended 8 hours/night (National Sleep Foundation, 2014). In response to the large proportion of adolescents obtaining less than the recommended amount of sleep, the American Academy of Pediatrics issued a policy statement urging middle and high schools to modify start times to no earlier than 8:30 A.M. (American Academy of Pediatrics, 2014).

Evidence suggests that the vast majority of habitual short sleepers (those routinely sleeping less than the recommended amount for their age) do not *require* less sleep than others but rather are limiting their sleep opportunity in order to accommodate school/work, family, and social obligations. Adults who routinely sleep less than 7.5 hours/night are more likely to report unintentionally falling asleep during the day and nodding off or falling asleep while driving. They also fall asleep faster during a standardized assessment of daytime sleep tendency. In addition to compromised waking performance, several adverse health outcomes, including weight gain, have been linked with habitual short sleep duration among children, adolescents, and adults.

Short Sleep Duration and Increased Risk for Obesity

A growing body of epidemiological evidence demonstrates that habitual short sleep duration is a risk factor for obesity. In adults, cross-sectional and longitudinal studies show that adults who report sleeping ≤ 5–6 hours/day gain more weight over time (Xiao, Arem, Moore, Hollenbeck, & Matthews, 2013), have larger waist circumferences (Sperry, Scully, Gramzow, & Jorgensen, 2015), and exhibit greater incidence of obesity (Wu, Zhai, & Zhang, 2014). For example, in a study examining data for 13,742 participants ages ≥ 20 years from the National Health and Nutrition Examination Survey (2005–2010), short sleepers (≤ 6 hours/day) were 1.0 kg/m² heavier and had a 2.2 cm larger waistline than sufficient sleepers (7–9 hours/day; Ford et al., 2014). The relationship between short sleep duration and body mass index (BMI) may be stronger among young (18–29 years) and middle-age (30–64 years) adults than among older (> 65 years) adults (Grandner, Schopfer, Sands-Lincoln, Jackson, & Malhotra, 2015). In 2015, a panel representing the American Academy of Sleep Medicine and the Sleep Research Society reviewed over 1,250 scientific publications and used the Oxford grading system and a modified RAND/UCLA Appropriateness Method to seek consensus on sleep recommendations. The panel concluded that at least 7 hours sleep/day were recommended for metabolic and cardiovascular health (Watson et al., 2015).

The relationship between short sleep duration and obesity risk has also been demonstrated in pediatric populations. Short sleep duration during infancy has been identified as a risk factor for obesity at 2–3 years old (Halal et al., 2016), and cross-sectional studies have revealed an association between short sleep duration and obesity in preschoolers, school-age children, and teenagers (Jiang et al., 2009; Katzmarzyk et al., 2015; Mitchell, Rodriguez, Schmitz, & Audrain-McGovern, 2013; Wu, Gong, Zou, Li, & Zhang, 2016). A recent meta-analysis examining the longitudinal impact of sleep duration on weight status in children and adolescents found that short sleepers had twice the risk for being overweight/obese (Fatima, Doi, & Mamun, 2015). Furthermore, several studies have demonstrated that sleep duration is positively associated with diet quality and fruit/vegetable intake and negatively associated with daily caloric intake, diet energy density, sugar intake, and soda consumption in children and adolescents (Bel et al., 2013; Börnhorst et al., 2015; Fisher et al., 2014; Franckle et al., 2015; Hjorth et al., 2014; Weiss et al., 2010).

Several population studies have found a stronger association between sleep duration and BMI in men than in women (Meyer, Wall, Larson, Laska, & Neumark-Sztainer, 2012; Watanabe, Kikuchhi, Tanaka, & Takahashi, 2010). This pattern has also been observed in adolescents and in children (Araujo, Severo, & Ramos, 2012; Suglia, Kara, & Robinson, 2014; Tatone-Tokuda et al., 2012); however, it has not been observed in all studies. Race differences may also exist in the relationship between sleep duration and weight. African Americans are more likely to be short sleepers than whites (Hale & Do, 2007; Singh, Drake, Roehrs, Hudgel, & Roth, 2005), and two epidemiological studies found that the association between short sleep duration and obesity risk was stronger in African Americans than whites (Donat et al., 2013; Grandner, Chakravorty, Perlis, Oliver, & Gurubhagavatula, 2014). Future studies are needed to examine gender and race differences in the relationship between sleep duration and risk for obesity.

Experimental Sleep Restriction and Energy Balance

Energy expended during sleep is less than energy expended during wake; therefore, the increased energy requirement associated with sleep restriction would produce negative energy balance and weight loss over time if diet remained constant. To protect against this state, investigators have hypothesized that the body employs compensatory responses to increase energy intake and conserve energy when sleep is restricted. However, if more energy is consumed and conserved than needed, positive energy balance and weight gain would occur. Recent research supports this compensatory hypothesis.

Spiegel and colleagues found that men undergoing 2 nights of sleep restriction (4 hours time in bed [TIB]/night) with controlled energy intake via an intravenous glucose infusion, exhibited increased levels of ghrelin (an orexigenic hormone released from the stomach) and decreased levels of leptin (an anorexigenic hormone released from adipocytes). These neuroendocrine changes were accompanied by significant increases in self-reported ratings of hunger and appetite (Spiegel, Tasali, Penev, & Van Cauter, 2004). By contrast, laboratory studies using *ad libitum* food access have demonstrated that sleep-restricted participants exhibit increased caloric intake and either no change in ghrelin or leptin or an increase in leptin levels (Markwald et al., 2013; Nedeltcheva et al., 2009; Spaeth, Dinges, & Goel, 2013; St-Onge et al., 2011). Thus, evidence suggests that sleep loss leads to changes in appetite-regulating hormones that promote increased energy intake. Research to determine how sleep loss impacts the release of other appetite regulating hormones (e.g., glucagon-like peptide-1, peptide YY(3–36), endocannabinoids) is ongoing.

Preliminary data suggest that the additional energy required for extended wakefulness from partial sleep restriction is ~100 kcal/day (Markwald et al., 2013; Shechter, Rising, Albu, & St-Onge, 2013). Healthy, normal-to-overweight adults in our in-laboratory sleep restriction protocol (5 nights, 4 hours TIB/night) overcompensated for the moderate increase in energy cost with marked increases in energy intake (~500 kcal/day) and gained significantly more weight during the study than control participants (Figures 8.1A and 8.2; Spaeth et al., 2013). Consistent with our findings in adults, children exhibited increased energy intake and weight gain when sleep was restricted by 1.5 hours/night for 1 week compared to when sleep was prolonged by 1.5 hours/night for 1 week in a counterbalanced crossover study (Hart et al., 2013).

Similar to epidemiological findings, we observed gender and race differences in the relationship between sleep restriction and energy balance. Among sleep-restricted participants, African Americans gained more weight than European Americans and men gained more weight than women (Figure 8.1B; Spaeth et al., 2013). Men exhibited a greater increase in daily caloric intake and consumed more calories during late-night hours under sleep-restricted conditions compared to women, but African Americans and European Americans showed similar changes in caloric intake and late-night eating (Spaeth, Dinges, & Goel, 2014).

In addition to changes in daily intake, laboratory studies have also demonstrated that sleep restriction leads to more food purchases (Chapman et al., 2013), greater consumption of snacks (Nedeltcheva et al., 2009; St-Onge et al., 2011), increased portion sizes (Hogenkamp et al., 2013), increased impulsivity in response to food

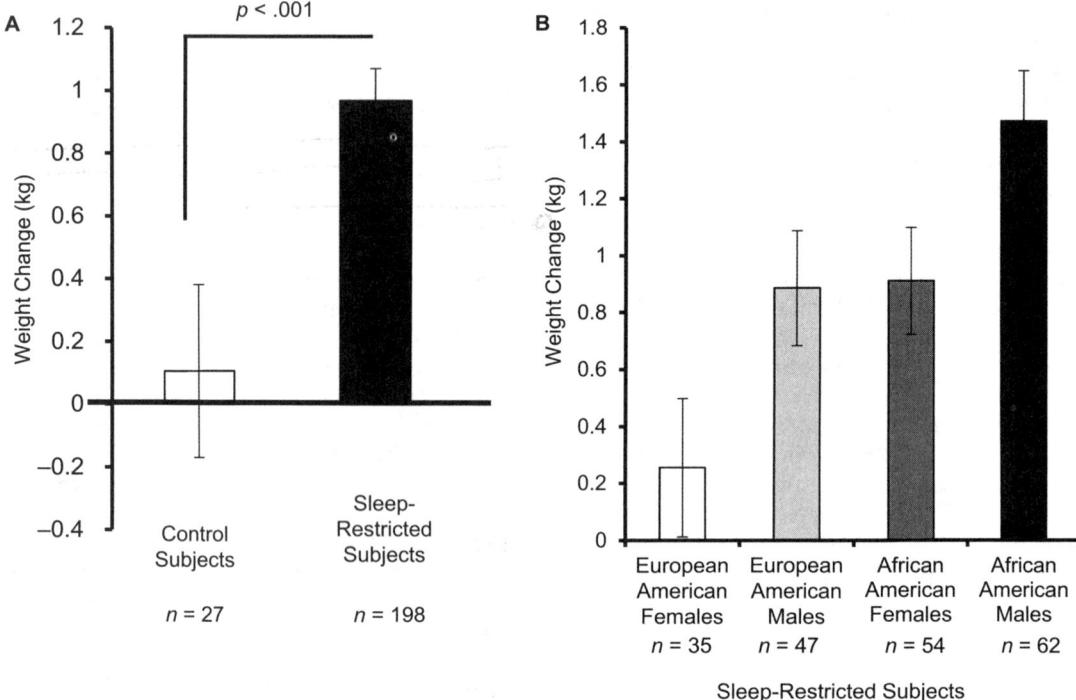

FIGURE 8.1. Effect of sleep loss on weight gain. Participants were healthy adults, ages 22–50 years, with a BMI ranging between 19 and 30. (A) Sleep-restricted participants gained significantly more weight than control participants ($d = 0.51$). (B) Among sleep-restricted participants, African Americans gained more weight than European Americans ($p = .003$, $d = 0.37$), and males gained more weight than females ($p = .004$, $d = 0.38$). Data are expressed as mean ± standard error of the mean. From Spaeth, Dinges, and Goel (2013). Reprinted by permission.

cues (Cedernaes et al., 2014), and changes in macronutrient intake. Some studies have shown that sleep restriction leads to greater consumption of carbohydrates (Nedeltcheva et al., 2009; Spiegel et al., 2004), and others have reported greater consumption of fats (St-Onge et al., 2011; Spaeth et al., 2014; Fang et al., 2015). Adolescents consumed foods with a higher glycemic index and more desserts/sweets when assigned 6.5 hours TIB/night for 5 nights than when assigned 10 hours TIB/night for 5 nights (Beebe et al., 2013). Table 8.2 illustrates changes in the consumption of various foods and drinks during an in-laboratory sleep restriction protocol (Spaeth et al., 2014). In general, sleep restriction has been associated with greater intake of unhealthy foods. Neuroimaging studies have shown that sleep loss alters activity in limbic, reward, and salience network regions (see Fang et al., 2015, for a review of the literature). These changes are associated with altered feeding behaviors and responses to food cues.

Recent research has highlighted the critical contribution of meal timing to weight regulation (Garaulet et al., 2013; Jakubowicz, Barnea, Wainstein, & Froy, 2013), with evening intake associated with adverse outcomes. During our sleep restriction protocol, we observed a shift in the timing of caloric intake. When bedtime was delayed from 2200 hours to 0400 hours, participants consumed ~500 additional calories during the late-night period (2200 hours–0359 hours), ~100 fewer calories the following morning (0800 hours–1459 hours), and a similar number of calories from 1500 hours to 2159 hours (Spaeth et al., 2013, 2014). Thus, during baseline, participants consumed the majority of calories in morning/early afternoon hours, whereas during sleep restriction, participants consumed the majority of calories in early-evening/late-night hours (Figure 8.3A). We also observed an increase in the proportion of calories from fat consumed during late-night hours (Figure 8.3B; Spaeth et al., 2013). Late-night fat consumption has been positively associated with daily caloric intake, BMI, and weight gain (Baron, Reid, Horn, & Zee, 2013; Spaeth, Dinges, & Goel, 2015a).

Whereas increased energy intake has been identified as a behavioral mechanism underlying the relationship between short sleep duration and weight gain, the role of energy expenditure is less clear. Some laboratory studies (but not all) have observed decreases in resting metabolic rate, diet-induced thermogenesis, and physical activity during the day following sleep loss, suggesting a metabolic adaptation to conserve energy in re-

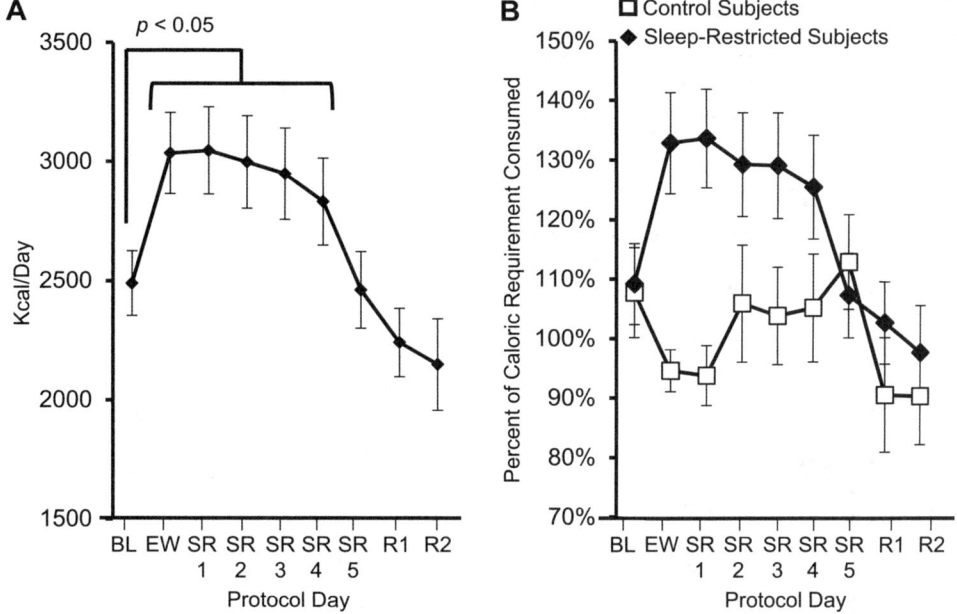

FIGURE 8.2. Caloric intake during an in-laboratory sleep restriction protocol. Participants were randomized to either a sleep restriction or control condition after 2 nights of baseline sleep. Sleep opportunity was restricted by delaying bedtime from 2200h (10:00 P.M.) until 0400h (4:00 A.M.) and maintaining wake time at 0800h (8:00 A.M.). Participants were given a 10-hour sleep opportunity (2200h–0800h [10:00 P.M.–8:00 A.M.) for 2 consecutive baseline nights. During the day following the second night of baseline sleep, participants who were randomized to the sleep restriction condition were kept awake until 0400h (4:00 A.M.) (EW). For the next five nights, these participants were given a 4-hour sleep opportunity per night (0400h–0800h [4:00 A.M.–8:00 A.M.]), and on the fifth day following sleep restriction, bedtime returned to 2200h (10:00 P.M.) in order to begin the recovery phase (12-hour sleep opportunity, 2200h–1000h [10:00 P.M.–10:00 A.M.]). Participants who were randomized to the control condition experienced no change in sleep opportunity across protocol days (bedtime: 2200h [10:00 P.M.], wake time: 0800h [8:00 A.M.]). (A) Compared to BL, sleep-restricted participants consumed more calories during days when bedtime was delayed (EW-SR4). Caloric intake did not differ between BL and SR5 (when waking hours and bedtime were equivalent). (B) Sleep-restricted participants consumed extra calories (130.0 ± 43.0% of daily caloric requirement) during days with a delayed bedtime (0400h [4:00 A.M.]) compared with control participants who did not consume extra calories (100.6 ± 11.4%) during corresponding days ($p = .003$, $d = 0.94$). Data are expressed as mean ± standard error of the mean. BL, baseline; EW, extended wakefulness; R, recovery; SR, sleep restriction. From Spaeth, Dinges, and Goel (2013). Effects of experimental sleep restriction on weight gain, caloric intake, and meal timing in healthy adults. *Sleep*, 36(7), 981–990. Reprinted by permission of Oxford University Press.

TABLE 8.2. Caloric Intake (Mean ± *SD*) by Food/Drink Category in a Diverse Sample of Healthy Normal-to-Overweight Adults (*N* = 44)

Food/drink category	Baseline days 1–2 (kcal)	Sleep restriction days 1–3 (kcal)
Meat, eggs, and fish	381.55 ± 128.92	419.77 ± 149.36
Fruit, vegetables, and salad	177.65 ± 149.61	170.66 ± 138.02
Bread, cereal, plain rice, and pasta	572.27 ± 192.71	659.51 ± 259.88[a]
Condiments	231.69 ± 139.55	276.44 ± 181.81[a]
Desserts	343.38 ± 286.83	544.34 ± 284.23[a]
Chips, pretzels, crackers, and popcorn	78.88 ± 123.72	150.91 ± 202.57[a]
Caffeine-free soda and juice	272.64 ± 160.91	346.18 ± 219.36[a]
Milk	84.16 ± 98.45	119.78 ± 152.89

Note. Modified from Spaeth, Dinges, & Goel, N. (2014). Adapted by permission.
[a]Significantly higher than baseline (repeated-measures analysis of variance; $p < .05$).

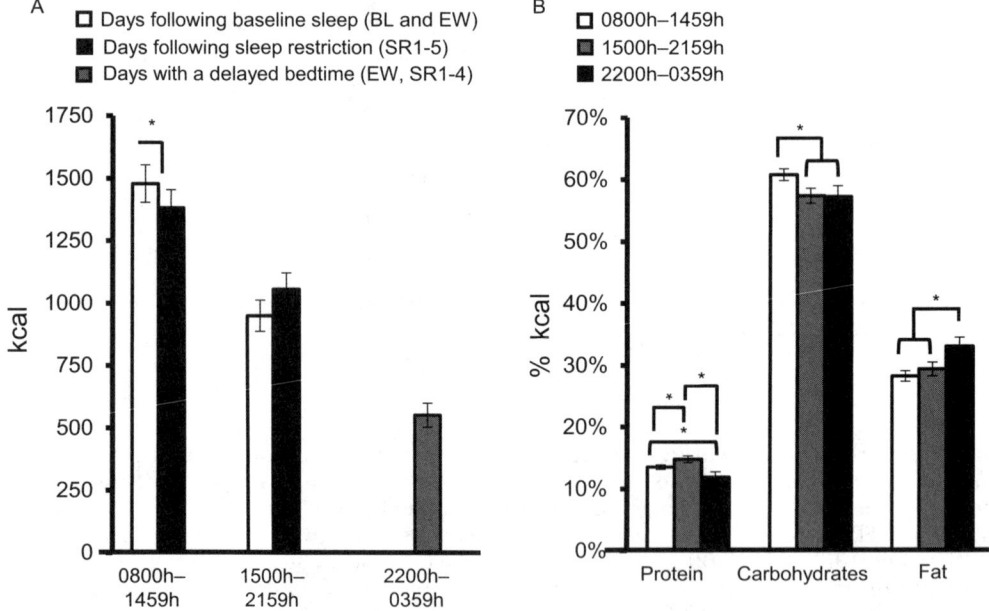

FIGURE 8.3. Effect of sleep loss on meal timing. (A) Participants consumed significantly fewer calories from 0800h (8:00 A.M.) to 1459h (2:59 P.M.) on days following sleep restriction (SR1-5) compared to days following baseline sleep (BL and EW). During days with a delayed bedtime (EW, SR1-4), participants consumed on average of 552.9 calories from 2200h (10:00 P.M.) to 0359h (3:59 A.M.). (B) The amount of calories derived from protein was significantly greater during 1500–2159h (3:00 P.M.–9:59 P.M.) and was significantly reduced during 2200h (10:00 P.M.)–0359h (3:59 A.M.) compared to the other two time intervals. Compared to the other two time intervals, the amount of calories derived from carbohydrates was significantly greater during 0800h (8:00 A.M.)–1459h (2:59 P.M.), and the amount of calories derived from fat was significantly greater during 2200h (10:00 P.M.)–0359h (3:59 A.M.). Data are expressed as mean ± standard error of the mean, *$p < .05$. BL, baseline; EW, extended wakefulness; SR, sleep restriction. From Spaeth, Dinges, and Goel (2013). Effects of experimental sleep restriction on weight gain, caloric intake, and meal timing in healthy adults. *Sleep, 36*(7), 981–990. Reprinted by permission of Oxford University Press.

sponse to the previous day's extended wakefulness (see Capers, Fobian, Kaiser, Borah, & Allison, 2015, and Spaeth, Dinges, & Goel, 2015b, for reviews of the literature). Thus, decreased energy expenditure, particularly when combined with the increased consumption of unhealthy foods caused by sleep restriction, may contribute to positive energy balance and weight gain over time.

Sleep Timing

Humans are less efficient sleepers when attempting to sleep outside of their endogenous circadian phase for sleep; therefore, limitations in the timing of sleep opportunities can lead to the accumulation of sleep debt over time. *Social jetlag* describes a misalignment between biological and social time. For example, a woman's internal biological phase for waking may be 7:00 A.M., but she must wake up at 5:00 A.M. to perform household tasks before going to work. In an attempt to recover some sleep debt, individuals with social jetlag sleep longer on weekends and exhibit marked differences in sleep duration and/or in the midpoint of sleep between work and nonwork days (Roenneberg, Allebrandt, Merrow, & Vetter, 2012). Many adults experience chronic social jetlag for the duration of their working career. These weekly changes in sleep timing resemble "traveling across several time zones to the West on Friday evenings and 'flying' back on Monday mornings" (Roenneberg et al., 2012, p. 939). Shift work represents more extreme circadian misalignment, as shift work schedules often require work to occur during the night when the circadian system is promoting sleep and require sleep to occur during the day when the circadian system is promoting wakefulness. Night-shift workers sleep 2–4 hours less per day than day-shift workers and are more likely to experience excessive sleepiness.

Although humans exhibit a diurnal circadian rhythm (active during the day, sleep during the night), there are individual differences in the optimal timing of activity and sleep. Some individuals prefer activity in the morning (larks) and exhibit an advanced (earlier) sleep period, whereas others prefer activity in the evening (owls) and exhibit a delayed (later) sleep period. Morning-type and evening-type individuals differ endogenously in the circadian phase of their biological clocks. Individual differences in preference are due to age, gender, and genetic factors. The interaction between Earth's light–dark cycle and current school/work schedules complement individuals who function best in the morning rather than in the evening. Because owls experience heightened alertness in the late evening, they often delay bedtime but still have to wake up early in the morning to accommodate school/work schedules. Thus, owls are more likely to experience social jetlag and sleep restriction during the school/work week.

Altered Sleep Timing and Increased Risk for Obesity

When quantifying social jetlag as the difference in mid-sleep time between free days and workdays, Roenneberg and colleagues observed that 69% of participants experienced at least 1 hour of social jetlag and that social jetlag significantly increased the probability of being overweight/obese (Roenneberg et al., 2012). Among those who were overweight/obese, social jetlag positively correlated with weight. Social jetlag has also been associated with cardiovascular risk factors, fat mass, and incidence of metabolic syndrome (Parsons et al., 2015; Rutters et al., 2014). Observational studies of shift workers as well as experimental studies that mimic shift work schedules have consistently demonstrated that this type of circadian misalignment leads to altered meal timing and increased risk for obesity (Banks, Dorrian, Grant, & Coates, 2015; Depner, Stothard, & Wright, 2014).

When examining the role of chronotype, there is some evidence that adolescents and adults with an evening preference are at increased risk for weight gain/obesity (Arora & Taheri, 2015; Yu et al., 2015), consume a less healthy diet (Maukonen et al., 2016), and exhibit delayed meal timing (Lucassen et al., 2013). Baron and colleagues found that late sleepers (sleep midpoint > 0530 hours) exhibited a shorter sleep duration, consumed more calories at dinner and after 2000 hours, consumed more fast food and full-calorie soda, and had a higher BMI compared to normal sleepers (sleep midpoint < 0530 hours; Baron, Reid, Kern, & Zee, 2011). In a large sample of severely obese adults undergoing bariatric surgery, evening-type individuals weighed more before surgery, lost less weight after surgery, and regained more weight at follow-up (Ruiz-Lozano et al., 2016). Given that this is a new area of research and findings are somewhat mixed, more work is needed to examine the influence of social jetlag and chronotype on obesity.

Recent research has also focused on how bedtime, independent from sleep duration, relates to weight gain and obesity. Increased variability in bedtime and going to bed later have been associated with unhealthy diet and higher BMI in children, adolescents, and adults (Asarnow, McGlinchey, & Harvey, 2015; Golley, Maher, Matricciani, & Olds, 2013; Scharf & DeBoer, 2015; Thivel et al., 2015). These associations are consistent with our experimental findings (Spaeth et al., 2013). During our sleep restriction protocol, caloric intake was increased on all days with a delayed bedtime, including the first day of the sleep restriction phase, when participants woke up after sufficient sleep but were kept awake for 20 hours and went to bed at 0400 hours (Figure 8.2A). Caloric intake was not increased on the last day of the sleep restriction phase, when participants woke up after five consecutive nights of insufficient sleep but were only kept awake for 14 hours and went to bed at 2200 hours (Figure 8.2A). This pattern suggests that bedtime and/or hours of wakefulness are better predictors of daily intake than hours of sleep during the preceding night(s). The timing and variability of bedtime should be targets for improving sleep and promoting weight maintenance, particularly for low-income families in which sleep habits are less stable and the risk for obesity is greater (Appelhans et al., 2014; Miller et al., 2014).

Sleep Disorders and Risk for Obesity

Sleep disorders such as insomnia, obstructive sleep apnea (OSA), and narcolepsy may also affect energy balance. Insomnia is diagnosed or suspected when an individual complains of having difficulty initiating or maintaining sleep, waking up earlier than desired, and experiencing impaired daytime functioning, despite having sufficient opportunities for sleep. Insomnia is highly comorbid with psychiatric disorders (e.g., anxiety and depression) and is not always associated with objectively measured short sleep duration (Vgontzas, Fernandez-Mendoza, Liao, & Bixler, 2013). There is a paucity of research examining the relationship between insomnia and obesity, and results have been mixed (Crönlein, Langguth, Busch, Rupprecht, & Wetter, 2015). However, insomnia with objectively measured short sleep duration has been associated with other markers of metabolic dysregulation (i.e., hypertension and type 2 diabetes; Vgontzas, et al., 2013). The primary treatment for insomnia involves decreasing sleep opportunity; therefore, more research is needed to understand the relationship between insomnia and weight regulation.

OSA occurs when an individual exhibits shallow breathing or ceases to breathe during sleep. Symptoms include loud snoring, gasping for air, reduced airflow during sleep, and impaired daytime functioning. The most common cause of OSA is obesity. It is estimated that 50% of children and adults with obesity have OSA, and studies have consistently demonstrated that weight loss improves OSA symptoms (Depner et al., 2014; Foster et al., 2009; Narang & Mathew, 2012). OSA is also associated with metabolic dysregulation, independent of obesity. Treatment of OSA with continuous positive airway pressure (CPAP) leads to improvements in daytime functioning and metabolic health (Chirinos et al., 2014). Given the serious adverse cognitive and health consequences of untreated OSA, it is critical for physicians to screen for and treat this condition in patients with obesity.

Narcolepsy occurs when an individual experiences excessive sleepiness with uncontrolled need for sleep or lapses into sleep during the day. It can occur with (type 1) or without (type 2) cataplexy and cerebral spinal fluid hypocretin-1 deficiency. Patients with narcolepsy exhibit a higher BMI than those without narcolepsy. This association has been observed in children, adolescents, and adults (Kotagal, Krahn, & Slocumb, 2004; Schuld, Hebebrand, Geller, &

Pollmächer, 2000). Orexin deficiency and decreased energy expenditure have been identified as mechanisms that may underlie this relationship (Chabas et al., 2007; Dahmen, Tonn, Messroghli, Ghezl-Ahmadi, & Engel, 2009). Individuals with narcolepsy are also more likely to experience persistent food cravings, to binge eat, and to have an eating disorder (Chabas et al., 2007; Dimitrova et al., 2011; Fortuyn et al., 2008). Patients who have been treated for narcolepsy continue to exhibit a higher BMI than those who have never been diagnosed with the disease (Depner et al., 2014); therefore, more research is needed to better prevent and treat obesity in narcoleptic patients.

Sleep in Individuals with Obesity

Poor sleep quality and excessive daytime sleepiness are frequent complaints among individuals with obesity (Fatima, Doi, & Mamun, 2016; Rahe, Czira, Teismann, & Berger, 2015; Resta et al., 2003). Weight loss (after diet/exercise programs or bariatric surgery) leads to improvements in sleep and daytime functioning (Fernandez-Mendoza et al., 2015; Thomson et al., 2012; Toor, Kim, & Buffington, 2012). Depression and psychological distress play an important role in the relationships between obesity, sleep, and daytime functioning (Vgontzas, Bixler, Chrousos, & Pekovic, 2008). Although few studies have objectively measured sleep in obese individuals, there is evidence that excessive adiposity relates to changes in sleep architecture.

Sleep is comprised of rapid-eye-movement (REM) sleep and non-REM sleep, with the latter comprised of stage 1, stage 2, and slow-wave sleep (SWS). SWS duration has been negatively correlated with BMI, waist circumference, ghrelin levels, intake during an *ad libitum* meal, saturated fat intake, and hunger ratings and has also been positively related with fiber intake, lean body mass, and growth hormone release (see Spaeth, Dinges, & Goel, 2017, for a review of the literature). REM sleep duration has been positively correlated with hunger ratings, body fat percentage, BMI, and overeating; however, other studies have shown that REM sleep duration is negatively correlated with waist circumference and BMI (see Spaeth et al., 2017, for a review of the literature).

In adults, those who are normal weight have exhibited higher sleep efficiency (total sleep time/TIB) than those who are overweight/obese (Bailey et al., 2014; Kahlhöfer, Karschin, Breusing, & Bosy-Westphal, 2016; Wirth et al., 2015); however, results have been more mixed in pediatric populations (Arora & Taheri, 2015; Chamorro et al., 2014; McNeil et al., 2015). More research is needed to examine differences in sleep architecture between normal, overweight, and obese individuals and to assess how changes in weight and/or body composition affect subjective and objective measures of sleep.

The Role of Sleep in Weight Loss Interventions

Recent research has highlighted the importance of sleep during weight loss interventions and assessed the efficacy of sleep extension in promoting healthy weight maintenance. Children (ages 2–5), enrolled in a randomized trial to improve household routines, exhibited increased sleep duration and decreased BMI (Haines et al., 2013). Longer sleep duration was also associated with lower BMI and caloric intake in a sample of obese preschool-age children in a weight management program (Clifford et al., 2012). Similarly, in obese adolescents, long sleep duration and better sleep quality at baseline were associated with greater weight loss during weight management programs (Sallinen et al., 2013; Valrie, Bond, Lutes, Carraway, & Collier, 2015). Among women randomized to a weight management program, better subjective sleep quality and sleeping > 7 hours/night at baseline significantly increased the likelihood of weight loss success (Thomson et al., 2012). Other studies have observed similar results in adults (Alfaris et al., 2015; Elder et al., 2012; Filiatrault, Chaput, Drapeau, & Tremblay, 2014). Future studies are needed to examine how sleep can be used to increase weight loss success.

During an in-laboratory experimental study, overweight/obese women were placed on a hypocaloric diet for 14 days with either 8.5 hours or 5.5 hours of sleep opportunity each night. During the 5.5-hour sleep condition, women lost a similar amount of weight as during the 8.5-hour condition; however, they lost less fat, reported greater hunger, and exhibited a higher respiratory quotient (RQ; Nedeltcheva, Kilkus, Imperial, Schoeller, & Penev, 2010). More work is needed to understand how sleep influences the changes in physiology that occur during weight loss and weight loss maintenance. Recently, sleep extension interventions in children and adults have been proposed for weight loss (Cizza et al., 2010; Yoong et al., 2016). Preliminary data demonstrate that sleep extension decreases desire for high-calorie foods, improves blood pressure, and is associated with increased insulin sensitivity in adults (Haack et al., 2013; Tasali, Chapotot, Wroblewski, & Schoeller, 2014; Leproult, Deliens, Gilson, & Peigneux, 2015).

Conclusion

Impaired sleep, due to lifestyle factors, chronotype, or sleep disorders, is associated with an increased risk for obesity in children, adolescents, and adults. Experimental studies demonstrate that sleep curtailment leads to increased daily caloric intake, greater consumption of unhealthy foods and drinks, and delayed meal timing. It also leads to alterations in brain activity, metabolism, and metabolic hormones that promote positive energy balance and weight gain over time. Addressing sleep issues with individuals who are obese or at risk for uncontrolled weight gain will improve daytime functioning and may increase the likelihood of weight loss success.

References

Alfaris, N., Wadden, T. A., Sarwer, D. B., Diwald, L., Volger, S., Hong P., et al. (2015). Effects of a 2-year behavioral weight loss intervention on sleep and mood in obese individuals treated in primary care practice. *Obesity, 23*(3), 558–564.

American Academy of Pediatrics. (2014). Policy statement: School start times for adolescents. *Pediatrics, 134*(3), 642–649.

Appelhans, B. M., Fitzpatrick, S. L., Li, H., Cail, V., Waring, M. E., Schneider, K. L., et al. (2014). The home environment and childhood obesity in low-income households: Indirect effects via sleep duration and screen time. *BMC Public Health, 14*, 1160.

Araujo, J., Severo, M., & Ramos, E. (2012). Sleep duration and adiposity during adolescence. *Pediatrics, 130*(5), e1146–e1154.

Arora, T., & Taheri, S. (2015). Associations among late chronotype, body mass index and dietary behaviors in young adolescents. *International Journal of Obesity, 39*(1), 39–44.

Asarnow, L. D., McGlinchey, E., & Harvey, A. G. (2015). Evidence for a possible link between bedtime and change in body mass index. *Sleep, 38*(10), 1523–1527.

Bailey, B. W., Allen, M. D., LeCheminant, J. D., Tucker, L. A., Errico, W. K., Christensen, W. F., et al. (2014). Objectively measured sleep patterns in young adult women and the relationship to adiposity. *American Journal of Health Promotion, 29*(1), 46–54.

Banks, S., Dorrian, J., Grant, C., & Coates, A. (2015). Circadian misalignment and metabolic consequences: Shiftwork and altered meal times. In R. R. Watson (Ed.), *Modulation of sleep by obesity, diabetes, age and diet* (pp. 155–164). Amsterdam, The Netherlands: Elsevier.

Baron, K. G., Reid, K. J., Horn, L. V., & Zee, P. C. (2013). Contribution of evening macro-nutrient intake to total caloric intake and body mass index. *Appetite, 60*(1), 246–251.

Baron, K. G., Reid, K. J., Kern, A. S., & Zee, P. C. (2011). Role of sleep timing in caloric intake and BMI. *Obesity, 19*(7), 1374–1381.

Beebe, D. W., Simon, S., Summer, S., Hemmer, S., Strotman, D., & Dolan, L. M. (2013). Dietary intake following experimentally restricted sleep in adolescents. *Sleep, 36*(6), 827–834.

Bel, S., Michels, N., De Vriendt, T., Patterson, E., Cuenca-García, M., Diethelm, K., et al. (2013). Association between self-reported sleep duration and dietary quality in European adolescents. *British Journal of Nutrition, 110*(5), 949–959.

Börnhorst, C., Wijnhoven, T. M., Kunešová, M., Yngve, A., Rito, A. I., Lissner, L., et al. (2015). WHO European Childhood Obesity Surveillance Initiative: Associations between sleep duration, screen time and food consumption frequencies. *BMC Public Health, 15*, 442.

Capers, P. L., Fobian, A. D., Kaiser, K. A., Borah, R., & Allison, D. B. (2015). A systematic review and meta-analysis of randomized controlled trials of the impact of sleep duration on adiposity and components of energy balance. *Obesity Reviews, 16*(9), 771–782.

Cedernaes, J., Brandell, J., Ros, O., Broman, J. E., Hogenkamp, P. S., Schiöth, H. B., et al. (2014). Increased impulsivity in response to food cues after sleep loss in healthy young men. *Obesity, 22*(8), 1786–1791.

Centers for Disease Control and Prevention. (2016). Insufficient sleep is a public health problem. Retrieved August 1, 2016, from *www.cdc.gov/features/dssleep*.

Chabas, D., Foulon, C., Gonzalez, J., Nasr, M., Lyon-Caen, O., Willer, J. C., et al. (2007). Eating disorder and metabolism in narcoleptic patients. *Sleep, 30*(10), 1267–1273.

Chamorro, R., Algarín, C., Garrido, M., Causa, L., Held, C., Lozoff, B., et al. (2014). Night time sleep macrostructure is altered in otherwise healthy 10-year-old overweight children. *International Journal of Obesity, 38*(8), 1120–1125.

Chapman, C. D., Nilsson, E. K., Nilsson, V. C., Cedernaes, J., Rångtell, F. H., Vogel, H., et al. (2013). Acute sleep deprivation increases food purchasing in men. *Obesity, 21*(12), 555–560.

Chirinos, J. A., Gurubhagavatula, I., Teff, K., Rader, D. J., Wadden, T. A., Townsend, R., et al. (2014). CPAP, weight loss, or both for obstructive sleep apnea. *New England Journal of Medicine, 370*(24), 2265–2275.

Cizza, G., Marincola, P., Mattingly, M., Williams, L., Mitler, M., Skarulis, M., et al. (2010). Treatment of obesity with extension of sleep duration: A randomized, prospective, controlled trial. *Clinical Trials, 7*(3), 274–285.

Clifford, L. M., Beebe, D. W., Simon, S. L., Kuhl, E. S., Filigno, S. S., Rausch, J. R., et al. (2012). The association between sleep duration and weight in treatment-seeking preschoolers with obesity. *Sleep Medicine, 13*(8), 1102–1105.

Crönlein, T., Langguth, B., Busch, V., Rupprecht, R., & Wetter, T. C. (2015). Severe chronic insomnia is not associated with higher body mass index. *Journal of Sleep Research, 24*(5), 514–517.

Dahmen, N., Tonn, P., Messroghli, L., Ghezel-Ahmadi, D., & Engel, A. (2009). Basal metabolic rate in narcoleptic patients. *Sleep, 32*(7), 962–964.

Depner, C. M., Stothard, E. R., & Wright, K. P. (2014). Metabolic consequences of sleep and circadian disorders. *Current Diabetes Reports, 14*(7), 507.

Dimitrova, A., Fronczek, R., Van der Ploeg, J., Scammell, T., Gautam, S., Pascual-Leone, A., et al. (2011). Reward-seeking behavior in human narcolepsy. *Journal of Clinical Sleep Medicine, 7*(3), 293–300.

Donat, M., Brown, C., Williams, N., Pandey, A., Racine, C., McFarlane, S. I., et al. (2013). Linking sleep duration and obesity among black and white US adults. *Clinical Practice, 10*(5), 661–667.

Elder, C. R., Gullion, C. M., Funk, K. L., Debar, L. L., Lindberg, N. M., & Stevens, V. J. (2012). Impact of sleep, screen time, depression and stress on weight change in the intensive weight loss phase of the LIFE study. *International Journal of Obesity, 36*(1), 86–92.

Fang, Z., Spaeth, A. M., Ma, N., Zhu, S., Hu, S., Goel, N., et al. (2015). Altered salience network connectivity predicts macronutrient intake after sleep deprivation. *Scientific Reports, 5*, 8215.

Fatima, Y., Doi, S. A., & Mamun, A. A. (2015). Longitudinal impact of sleep on overweight and obesity in children and adolescents: A systematic review and bias-adjusted meta-analysis. *Obesity Reviews, 16*(2), 137–149.

Fatima, Y., Doi, S. A., & Mamun, A. A. (2016). Sleep quality and obesity in young subjects: A meta-analysis. *Obesity Reviews, 17*(11), 1154–1166.

Fernandez-Mendoza, J., Vgontzas, A. N., Kritikou, I., Calhoun, S. L., Liao, D., & Bixler, E. O. (2015). Natural history of excessive daytime sleepiness: Role of obesity, weight loss, depression, and sleep propensity. *Sleep, 38*(3), 351–360.

Filiatrault, M. L., Chaput, J. P., Drapeau, V., & Tremblay, A. (2014). Eating behavior traits and sleep as determinants of weight loss in overweight and obese adults. *Nutrition and Diabetes, 4*, e140.

Fisher, A., McDonald, L., van Jaarsveld, C. H., Llewellyn, C., Fildes, A., Schrempft, S., et al. (2014). Sleep and energy intake in early childhood. *International Journal of Obesity, 38*(7), 926–929.

Ford, E. S., Li, C., Wheaton, A. G., Chapman, D. P., Perry, G. S., & Croft, J. B. (2014). Sleep duration and body mass index and waist circumference among U.S. adults. *Obesity, 22*(2), 598–607.

Fortuyn, H. A., Swinkels, S., Buitelaar, J., Renier, W. O., Furer, J. W., Rijnders, C. A., et al. (2008). High prevalence of eating disorders in narcolepsy with cataplexy: A case-control study. *Sleep, 31*(3), 335–341.

Foster, G. D., Borradaile, K. E., Sanders, M. H., Millman, R., Zammit, G., Newman, A. B., et al. (2009). A randomized study on the effect of weight loss on obstructive sleep apnea among obese patients with type 2 diabetes: The Sleep AHEAD study. *Archives of Internal Medicine, 169*(17), 1619–1626.

Franckle, R. L., Falbe, J., Gortmaker, S., Ganter, C., Taveras, E. M., Land, T., et al. (2015). Insufficient sleep among elementary and middle school students is linked with elevated soda consumption and other unhealthy dietary behaviors. *Preventative Medicine, 74*, 36–41.

Garaulet, M., Gomez-Abellan, P., Alburquerque-Bejar, J. J., Lee, Y. C., Ordovas, J. M., & Scheer, F. A. (2013). Timing of food intake predicts weight loss effectiveness. *International Journal of Obesity, 37*(4), 604–611.

Golley, R. K., Maher, C. A., Matricciani, L., & Olds, T. S. (2013). Sleep duration or bedtime?: Exploring the association between sleep timing behaviour, diet and BMI in children and adolescents. *International Journal of Obesity, 37*(4), 546–551.

Grandner, M. A., Chakravorty, S., Perlis, M. L., Oliver, L., & Gurubhagavatula, I. (2014). Habitual sleep duration associated with self-reported and objectively determined cardiometabolic risk factors. *Sleep Medicine, 15*(1), 42–50.

Grandner, M. A., Schopfer, E. A., Sands-Lincoln, M., Jackson, N., & Malhotra, A. (2015). Relationship between sleep duration and body mass index depends on age. *Obesity, 23*(12), 2491–2498.

Haack, M., Serrador, J., Cohen, D., Simpson, N., Meier-Ewert, H., & Mullington, J. M. (2013). Increasing sleep duration to lower beat-to-beat blood pressure: A pilot study. *Journal of Sleep Research, 22*(3), 295–304.

Haines, J., McDonald, J., O'Brien, A., Sherry, B., Bottino, C. J., Schmidt, M. E., et al. (2013). Healthy habits, happy homes: Randomized trial to improve household routines for obesity prevention among preschool-aged children. *JAMA Pediatrics, 167*(11), 1072–1079.

Halal, C. S., Matijasevich, A., Howe, L. D., Santos, I. S., Barros, F. C., & Nunes, M. L. (2016). Short sleep duration in the first years of life and obesity/overweight at age 4 years: A birth cohort study. *Journal of Pediatrics, 168*, 99–103.

Hale, L., & Do, D. P. (2007). Racial differences in self-reports of sleep duration in a population-based study. *Sleep, 30*(9), 1096–1103.

Hart, C. N., Carskadon, M. A., Considine, R. V., Fava, J. L., Lawton, J., Raynor, H. A., et al. (2013). Changes in children's sleep duration on food intake, weight, and leptin. *Pediatrics, 132*(6), e1473–e1480.

Hirschkowitz, M., Whiton, K., Albert, S. M., Alessi, C., Bruni, O., DonCarlos, L., et al. (2015). National Sleep Foundation's sleep time duration recommendations: Methodology and results summary. *Sleep Health, 1*(1), 40–43.

Hjorth, M. F., Quist, J. S., Andersen, R., Michaelsen, K. F., Tetens, I., Astrup, A., et al. (2014). Change in sleep duration and proposed dietary risk factors for obesity in Danish school children. *Pediatric Obesity, 9*(6), e156–e159.

Hogenkamp, P. S., Nilsson, E., Nilsson, V. C., Chapman, C. D., Vogel, H., Lundberg, L. S., et al. (2013). Acute sleep deprivation increases portion size and affects food choice in young men. *Psychoneuroendocrinology, 38*(9), 1668–1674.

Jakubowicz, D., Barnea, M., Wainstein, J., & Froy, O. (2013). High caloric intake at breakfast vs. dinner differentially influences weight loss of overweight and obese women. *Obesity, 21*(12), 2504–2512.

Jiang, F., Zhu, S., Yan, C., Jin, X., Bandla, H., & Shen, X. (2009). Sleep and obesity in preschool children. *Journal of Pediatrics, 154*(6), 814–818.

Kahlhöfer, J., Karschin, J., Breusing, N., & Bosy-Westphal, A. (2016). Relationship between actigraphy-assessed sleep quality and fat mass in college students. *Obesity, 24*(2), 335–341.

Katzmarzyk, P. T., Barreira, T. V., Broyles, S. T., Champagne, C. M., Chaput, J. P., Fogelholm, M., et al. (2015). Relationship between lifestyle behaviors and obesity in children ages 9–11: Results from a 12-country study. *Obesity, 23*(8), 1696–1702.

Kotagal, S., Krahn, L. E., & Slocumb, N. (2004). A putative link between childhood narcolepsy and obesity. *Sleep Medicine, 5*(2), 147–150.

Leproult, R., Deliens, G., Gilson, M., & Peigneux, P. (2015). Beneficial impact of sleep extension on fasting insulin sensitivity in adults with habitual sleep restriction. *Sleep, 38*(5), 707–715.

Lucassen, E. A., Zhao, X., Rother, K. I., Mattingly, M. S., Courville, A. B., de Jonge, L., et al. (2013). Evening chronotype is associated with changes in eating behavior, more sleep apnea, and increased stress hormones in short sleeping obese individuals. *PLOS ONE, 8*(3), e56519.

Markwald, R. R., Melanson, E. L., Smith, M. R., Higgins, J., Perreault, L., Eckel, R. H., et al. (2013). Impact of insufficient sleep on total daily energy expenditure, food intake, and weight gain. *Proceedings of the National Academy of Sciences of the United States of America, 110*(14), 5695–5700.

Maukonen, M., Kanerva, N., Partonen, T., Kronholm, E., Konttinen, H., Wennman, H., et al. (2016). The associations between chronotype, a healthy diet and obesity. *Chronobiology International, 33*(8), 972–981.

McNeil, J., Tremblay, M. S., Leduc, G., Boyer, C., Bélanger, P., Leblanc, A. G., et al. (2015). Objectively-measured sleep and its association with adiposity and physical activity in a sample of Canadian children. *Journal of Sleep Research, 24*(2), 131–139.

Meyer, K. A., Wall, M. M., Larson, N. I., Laska, M. N., & Neumark-Sztainer, D. (2012). Sleep duration and BMI in a sample of young adults. *Obesity, 20*(6), 1279–1287.

Miller, A. L., Kaciroti, N., Lebourgeois, M. K., Chen, Y. P., Sturza, J., & Lumeng, J. C. (2014). Sleep timing moderates the concurrent sleep duration–body mass index association in low-income preschool-age children. *Academy of Pediatrics, 14*(2), 207–213.

Mitchell, J. A., Rodriguez, D., Schmitz, K. H., & Audrain-McGovern, J. (2013). Sleep duration and adolescent obesity. *Pediatrics, 131*(5), e1428–e1434.

Narang, I., & Mathew, J. L. (2012). Childhood obesity and obstructive sleep apnea. *Journal of Nutrition and Metabolism, 2012*, 134202.

National Sleep Foundation. (2014). Sleep in American poll: Sleep in the modern family—summary of findings. Retrieved August 1, 2016, from *https://sleepfoundation.org/sites/default/files/2014-NSF-Sleep-in-America-poll-summary-of-findings-FINAL-Updated-3-26-14-.pdf*.

Nedeltcheva, A. V., Kilkus, J. M., Imperial, J., Kasza, K., Schoeller, D. A., & Penev, P. D. (2009). Sleep curtailment is accompanied by increased intake of calories from snacks. *American Journal of Clinical Nutrition, 89*(1), 126–133.

Nedeltcheva, A. V., Kilkus, J. M., Imperial, J., Schoeller, D. A., & Penev, P. D. (2010). Insufficient sleep undermines dietary efforts to reduce adiposity. *Annals of Internal Medicine, 153*(7), 435–441.

Parsons, M. J., Moffitt, T. E., Gregory, A. M., Goldman-Mellor, S., Nolan, P. M., Poulton, R., et al. (2015). Social jetlag, obesity and metabolic disorder: Investigation in a cohort study. *International Journal of Obesity, 39*(5), 842–848.

Rahe, C., Czira, M. E., Teismann, H., & Berger, K. (2015). Associations between poor sleep quality and different measures of obesity. *Sleep Medicine, 16*(10), 1225–1228.

Resta, O., Foschino Barbaro, M. P., Bonfitto, P., Giliberti, T., Depalo, A., Pannacciulli, N., et al. (2003). Low sleep quality and daytime sleepiness in obese patients without obstructive sleep apnoea syndrome. *Journal of Internal Medicine, 253*(5), 536–543.

Roenneberg, T., Allebrandt, K. V., Merrow, M., & Vetter, C. (2012). Social jetlag and obesity. *Current Biology, 22*(10), 939–943.

Ruiz-Lozano, T., Vidal, J., de Hollanda, A., Canteras, M., Garaulet, M., & Izquierdo-Pulido, M. (2016). Evening chronotype associates with obesity in severely obese subjects: Interaction with CLOCK 3111T/C. *International Journal of Obesity, 40*(10), 1550–1557.

Rutters, F., Lemmens, S. G., Adam, T. C., Bremmer, M. A., Elders, P. J., Nijpels, G., et al. (2014). Is social jetlag associated with an adverse endocrine, behavioral, and cardiovascular risk profile? *Journal of Biological Rhythms, 29*(5), 377–383.

Sallinen, B. J., Hassan, F., Olszewski, A., Maupin, A., Hoban, T. F., Chervin, R. D., et al. (2013). Longer weekly sleep duration predicts greater 3-month BMI reduction among obese adolescents attending a clinical multidisciplinary weight management program. *Obesity Facts, 6*(3), 239–246.

Scharf, R. J., & DeBoer, M. D. (2015). Sleep timing and longitudinal weight gain in 4- and 5-year-old children. *Pediatric Obesity, 10*(2), 141–148.

Schuld, A., Hebebrand. J., Geller, F., & Pollmächer, T. (2000). Increased body-mass index in patients with narcolepsy. *Lancet, 355*(9211), 1274–1275.

Shechter, A., Rising, R., Albu, J. B., & St-Onge, M. P. (2013). Experimental sleep curtailment causes wake-dependent increases in 24-h energy expenditure as measured by whole-room indirect calorimetry. *American Journal of Clinical Nutrition, 98*(6), 1433–1439.

Singh, M., Drake, C. L., Roehrs, T., Hudgel, D. W., & Roth, T. (2005). The association between obesity and short sleep duration: A population-based study. *Journal of Clinical Sleep Medicine, 1*(4), 357–363.

Spaeth, A. M., Dinges, D. F., & Goel, N. (2013). Effects of experimental sleep restriction on weight gain, caloric intake, and meal timing in healthy adults. *Sleep, 36*(7), 981–990.

Spaeth, A. M., Dinges, D. F., & Goel, N. (2014). Sex and race differences in caloric intake during sleep restriction in healthy adults. *American Journal of Clinical Nutrition, 100*(2), 559–566.

Spaeth, A. M., Dinges, D. F., & Goel, N. (2015a). Phenotypic vulnerability of energy balance responses to sleep loss in healthy adults. *Scientific Reports, 5*, 14920.

Spaeth, A. M., Dinges, D. F., & Goel, N. (2015b). Resting metabolic rate varies by race and by sleep duration. *Obesity, 23*(12), 2349–2356.

Spaeth, A. M., Dinges, D. F., & Goel, N. (2017). Objective measures of sleep architecture correlate with energy balance in healthy adults. *Sleep, 40*(1), 1–8.

Sperry, S. D., Scully, I. D., Gramzow, R. H., & Jorgensen, R. S. (2015). Sleep duration and waist circumference in adults: A meta-analysis. *Sleep, 38*(8), 1269–1276.

Spiegel, K., Tasali, E., Penev, P., & Van Cauter, E. (2004). Brief communication: Sleep curtailment in healthy young men is associated with decreased leptin levels, elevated ghrelin levels, and increased hunger and appetite. *Annals of Internal Medicine, 141*(11), 846–850.

St-Onge, M. P., Roberts, A. L., Chen, J., Kelleman, M., O'Keeffe, M., RoyChoudhury, A. J., et al. (2011). Short sleep duration increases energy intake but does not change energy expenditure in normal-weight individuals. *American Journal of Clinical Nutrition, 94*(2), 410–416.

Suglia, S. F., Kara, S., & Robinson, W. R. (2014). Sleep duration and obesity among adolescents transitioning to adulthood: Do results differ by sex? *Journal of Pediatrics, 165*(4), 750–754.

Tasali, E., Chapotot, F., Wroblewski, K., & Schoeller, D. (2014). The effects of extended bedtimes on sleep duration and food desire in overweight young adults: A home-based intervention. *Appetite, 80*, 220–224.

Tatone-Tokuda, F., Dubois, L., Ramsay, T., Girard, M., Touchette, E., Petit, D., et al. (2012). Sex differences in the association between sleep duration, diet and body mass index: A birth cohort study. *Journal of Sleep Research, 21*(4), 448–460.

Thivel, D., Isacco, L., Aucouturier, J., Pereira, B., Lazaar, N., Ratel, S., et al. (2015). Bedtime and sleep timing but not sleep duration are associated with eating habits in primary school children. *Journal of Developmental and Behavioral Pediatrics, 36*(3), 158–165.

Thomson, C. A., Morrow, K. L., Flatt, S. W., Wertheim, B. C., Perfect, M. M., Ravia, J. J., et al. (2012). Relationship between sleep quality and quantity and weight loss in women participating in a weight-loss intervention trial. *Obesity, 20*(7), 1419–1425.

Toor, P., Kim, K., & Buffington, C. K. (2012). Sleep quality and duration before and after bariatric surgery. *Obesity Surgery, 22*(6), 890–895.

Valrie, C. R., Bond, K., Lutes, L. D., Carraway, M., & Collier, D. N. (2015). Relationship of sleep quality, baseline weight status, and weight-loss responsiveness in obese adolescents in an immersion treatment program. *Sleep Medicine, 16*(3), 432–440.

Vgontzas, A. N., Bixler, E. O., Chrousos, G. P., & Pejovic, S. (2008). Obesity and sleep disturbances: Meaningful sub-typing of obesity. *Archives of Physiology and Biochemistry, 114*(4), 224–236.

Vgontzas, A. N., Fernandez-Mendoza, J., Liao, D., & Bixler, E. O. (2013). Insomnia with objective short sleep duration: The most biologically severe phenotype of the disorder. *Sleep Medicine Reviews, 17*(4), 241–254.

Watanabe, M., Kikuchi, H., Tanaka, K., & Takahashi, M. (2010). Association of short sleep duration with weight gain and obesity at 1-year follow-up: A large-scale prospective study. *Sleep, 33*(2), 161–167.

Watson, N. F., Badr, M. S., Belenky, G., Bliwise, D. L., Buxton, O. M., Buysse, D., et al. (2015). Joint consensus statement of the American Academy of Sleep Medicine and Sleep Research Society on the recommended amount of sleep for a healthy adult: Methodology and discussion. *Sleep, 38*(8), 1161–1183.

Weiss, A., Xu, F., Storfer-Isser, A., Thomas, A., Ievers-Landis, C. E., & Redline, S. (2010). The association of sleep duration with adolescents' fat and carbohydrate consumption. *Sleep, 33*(9), 1201–1209.

Wirth, M. D., Hébert, J. R., Hand, G. A., Youngstedt, S. D., Hurley, T. G., Shook, R. P., et al. (2015). Association between actigraphic sleep metrics and body composition. *Annals of Epidemiology, 25*(10), 773–778.

Wu, Y., Gong, Q., Zou, Z., Li, H., & Zhang, X. (2016). Short sleep duration and obesity among children: A systematic review and meta-analysis of prospective studies. *Obesity Research and Clinical Practice, 11*(2), 140–150.

Wu, Y., Zhai, L., & Zhang, D. (2014). Sleep duration and obesity among adults: A meta-analysis of prospective studies. *Sleep Medicine, 15*(12), 1456–1462.

Xiao, Q., Arem, H., Moore, S. C., Hollenbeck, A. R., & Matthews, C. E. (2013). A large prospective investigation of sleep duration, weight change, and obesity in the NIH-AARP Diet and Health Study cohort. *American Journal of Epidemiology, 178*(11), 1600–1610.

Yoong, S. L., Chai, L. K., Williams, C. M., Wiggers, J., Finch, M., & Wolfenden, L. (2016). Systematic review and meta-analysis of interventions targeting sleep and their impact on child body mass index, diet, and physical activity. *Obesity, 24*(5), 1140–1147.

Yu, J. H., Yun, C. H., Ahn, J. H., Suh, S., Cho, H. J., Lee, S. K., et al. (2015). Evening chronotype is associated with metabolic disorders and body composition in middle-aged adults. *Journal of Clinical Endocrinology and Metabolism, 100*(4), 1494–1502.

CHAPTER 9

Social, Economic, and Physical Environmental Contributors to Obesity among Adults

Joreintje Dingena Mackenbach
Jeroen Lakerveld
Johannes Brug

The direct cause of obesity is a long-term positive energy balance whereby calorie intake exceeds energy expenditure. Intake and expenditure of energy are, in turn, influenced by many underlying factors. According to socioecological theory (Dahlgren & Whitehead, 2007), there are several layers of influence that directly or indirectly affect the risk of obesity, ranging from individual factors such as genetic predisposition to social, economic, and physical environmental conditions. Genetic and biological factors are unlikely to have changed to such an extent that they can explain the current obesity epidemic, but the environment that individuals live in has changed substantially over the last few decades.

The "obesogenic environment" has been described as "the sum of influences in the surroundings, opportunities, or conditions of life that promote obesity in individuals or populations" (Swinburn, Egger, & Raza, 1999, p. 564). Simply put, the obesogenic environment encompasses the range of environmental characteristics that promote overweight and obesity and hinder an individual's ability to maintain a healthy body weight. Obesogenic environments can consist of sociocultural, economic, and physical environmental factors. For example, the lack of availability of facilities such as parks, sidewalks, and bicycle lanes may hinder physical activity, whereas social norms and the availability, accessibility, and affordability of high-energy foods may promote overeating. It has been argued that our present-day "food environment" offers easy access to affordable, palatable, energy-dense, and high-calorie foods and drinks almost anywhere at almost any time. Simultaneously, our "physical activity environment" has changed so that physical activities can easily be avoided (Schmidhauser, Eichler, & Brugger, 2009). Some behaviors (e.g., sedentary behaviors) or groups (e.g., elderly persons) may be more affected by micro-environments such as family influences, design of the home, and the indoor workplace environment (Kaushal & Rhodes, 2014). Other behaviors and groups are more strongly influenced by macro-level factors. Environments do not influence obesity in isolation. The ways in which environmental factors may influence obesogenic behaviors are conceptualized in various socioecological frameworks. For instance, Kremers et al. (2006) used their environmental research framework for weight gain prevention (EnRG) to conceptualize how environmental factors may affect obesogenic behaviors, and how these environmental influences are also likely to be mediated and moderated by individual-level factors (see Figure 9.1; Kremers et al., 2006).

One example of a mediating pathway is the presence of high-quality bicycle infrastructure, which may enhance the intention to ride a bike and, in turn, to form an actual cycling habit. Further, the influence of ample availability and accessibility of sweet foods on an individual's diet may be more pronounced in people with stronger taste preference for sweet flavors (moderating pathway). Many such mediating and moderating pathways are likely to be present, and the obesogenic environment is therefore considered to act on obesogenic behaviors and obesity in a complex system. Interactions and feedback loops influence where, when, for how long, why, how, and with whom people conduct health-related activities (McPherson, Marsh, & Brown, 2007). In this chapter, we discuss the social, economic, and physical environmental contributors to obesity in adults.

Social Contributors to Obesity

One aspect of the obesogenic environment is the sociocultural environment: the sets of beliefs, customs, practices, and behaviors within a population. Four key aspects of the social environment are discussed here: socioeconomic status, income inequality, and deprivation; social capital, social cohesion, social networks, and social support; ethnic and cultural influences; and safety and

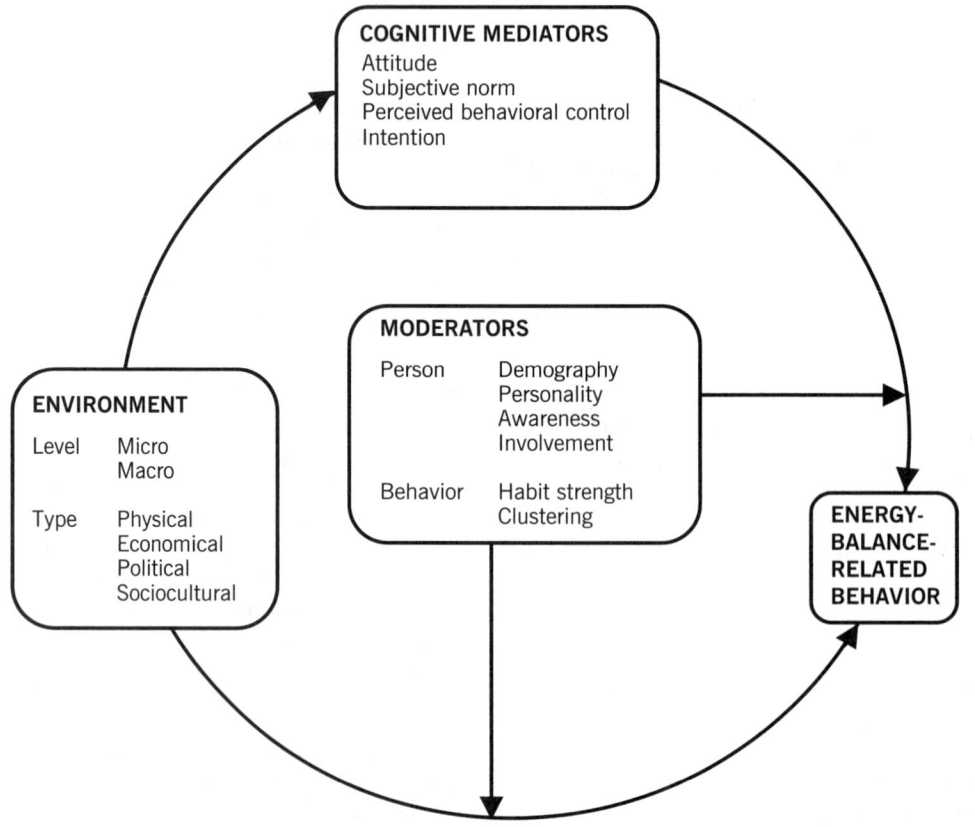

FIGURE 9.1. Environmental research framework for weight gain prevention (EnRG).

Socioeconomic Status, Income Inequality, and Deprivation

The term *socioeconomic status* (SES) describes the social standing or class of an individual or group. Often-used indicators of SES are educational attainment, occupation, employment status, and income (Galobardes, Shaw, Lawlor, Lynch, & Davey Smith, 2006). SES is strongly related to overweight and obesity (Sobal & Stunkard, 1989; Stunkard, 1996). In higher-income countries, lower SES is generally associated with higher body weight (Cohen, Rai, Rehkopf, & Abrams, 2013; Sobal & Stunkard, 1989; Stunkard, 1996), whereas in low-income countries, lower SES tends to be associated with lower body weight (Dinsa, Goryakin, Fumagalli, & Suhrcke, 2012). In higher-income countries, unhealthier lifestyles and body weights can be explained by the lack of psychosocial and material resources among individuals with lower SES; that is, lack of knowledge and social support and lack of money and means (Goldman, 2001). In lower-income countries, the association between SES and obesity follows conventional economic theories that predict that richer individuals engage in more unhealthy behaviors (Altman, 2008). The term *socioeconomic deprivation* also describes the state in which individuals (or areas) lack necessary life resources. For example, in a European setting, living in low-SES neighborhoods has been associated with consuming fewer fruits and vegetables and more sugar-sweetened beverages, as well as having a higher body mass index (BMI), compared to residents in high-SES neighborhoods (Lakerveld et al., 2015).

Income, education, and deprivation are absolute measures, but theories on the effect of *income inequality* on health suggest that not just low income, but also inequality in income, affects obesity risk. The income inequality hypothesis, as formulated by Wagstaff and Van Doorslaer (2000), states that the income gap between the rich and the poor within a country or region affects health and weight status of the poor, more so than, or in addition to, the absolute income levels. The assumed mechanism behind this influence is the fact that a perceived low position in the social hierarchy leads to social disconnection (lack of social capital) and social distress (Mackenbach, Lakerveld, van Oostveen, et al., 2016). These social impediments have been associated with risk factors for overweight and obesity, such as overeating and preferences for energy-dense foods (Oliver, Wardle, & Gibson, 2000).

Social Capital, Social Cohesion, Social Networks, and Social Support

The influence of other people, such as neighbors, family members, friends, colleagues, and other network members, is also an important correlate of obesity risk. In a landmark study, Christakis and Fowler (2007) showed that obesity seems to spread through social networks over time, mainly via siblings and friends becoming obese (Christakis & Fowler, 2007). Hammond (2010) concluded that there is increasing evidence that social influence and social network structures influence obesity, but also noted little understanding of the underlying mechanisms. Potential explanations for the role of social networks in the development of overweight and obesity include social contagion (whereby the network influences obesity-related behaviors or body weight via mirroring, aspiring, and changing), social capital (whereby sense of belonging and social support influence obesity-related behaviors and body weight), and social selection (whereby an individual's network is a function of his or her weight) (Powell et al., 2015).

A recent literature review summarized the evidence regarding several social environmental factors and their associations with weight status. The reviewers concluded that the strongest associations were found for social capital and collective efficacy, although few studies actually found significant associations (Glonti et al., 2016). Social capital and collective efficacy are two related concepts, both referring to the shared norms and values, trust, and ability to undertake collective action in a community (Sampson, Raudenbusch, & Earls, 1997). In addition, there is some preliminary evidence suggesting that enhancement of social network characteristics is associated with an improvement in weight status (Yoon & Brown, 2011), although evidence from intervention studies remains limited (Leroux, Moore, & Dubé, 2013).

Ethnicity and Culture

There are marked differences in obesity prevalence between ethnic groups. For example, in The Netherlands, all major ethnic-minority groups have a higher prevalence of overweight than the native Dutch, except for people of Moroccan descent (Cornelisse-Vermaat & Maassen van den Brink, 2007). In the United States, there are considerable differences in obesity prevalence between non-Hispanic whites, non-Hispanic blacks, and Mexican American men and women (Flegal, Carroll, Ogden, & Curtin, 2010). In New Zealand, members of Pacific ethnic groups are over 11 times more likely to be obese than European New Zealanders (Sundborn et al., 2010). There are several explanations for these differences. First, they may be due to differences in muscularity and the associated potentially inappropriate use of similar BMI cutoff points for different ethnic groups (Jih et al., 2014). Second, these ethnic differences may be mainly the result of socioeconomic differences (Ujcic-Voortman, Bos, Baan, Verhoeff, & Seidell, 2011), as ethnic minorities tend to have lower socioeconomic positions than majority populations (van Tubergen, Maas, & Flap, 2004). Third, cultural factors such as body size preferences, religious food practices, family dynamics, and gender roles may also influence dietary and physical activity behaviors (Cachelin, 2001).

In addition, evidence from the United States suggests that adults who experience more everyday racism have higher rates of obesity (Cozier et al., 2014) and that living in areas with higher levels of segregation increases risk of obesity (Kershaw, Albrecht, & Carnethon, 2013). It has been suggested that these associations are due to the sorting of racial/ethnic minorities into poor-quality neighborhoods, limiting opportunities for social and economic mobility (Acevedo-Garcia, Lochner, Osypuk, & Al, 2003). Indeed, Zenk et al. (2005) showed that racial residential segregation placed African Americans in more impoverished neighborhoods with reduced access to supermarkets.

Safety and Crime

There is increasing evidence of an association between neighborhood (un)safety and crime and adult body weight. Although some studies do not show such associations (e.g., Zhao, Kaestner, & Xu, 2014), most investigations support the hypothesis that higher levels of unsafety and crime (whether perceived or objectively observed) are associated with higher BMI and greater odds of overweight and obesity (Tamayo et al., 2016). Evidence also suggests that this association can be explained by physical activity: Inhabitants of unsafe neighborhoods are less likely to be physically active and therefore have higher body weights (Eichinger, Titze, Haditsch, Dorner, & Stronegger, 2015). Although most of this evidence originates from the United States, a recent publication from the International Physical Activity and Environment Network (IPEN) confirmed that traffic safety and safety from crime were consistently associated with BMI across 15 cities in 12 countries (De Bourdeaudhuij et al., 2015). We note, however, that it is difficult to appropriately adjust studies on safety and crime for SES. Low SES is an important risk factor for obesity, and low SES neighborhoods tend to have higher rates of crime.

Economic Contributors to Obesity

Although obesity is a topic of great economic concern (Lehnert, Sonntag, Konnopka, Riedel-Heller, & König, 2013), economic contributors have been less researched compared to other socioeconomic factors that affect weight status (Sobal & Stunkard, 1989). Economic contributors to obesity may operate at the individual level (individual purchasing power) and the macro/societal level (economic growth and prosperity).

Individual-Level Economic Factors

As described earlier in this chapter, there is a strong association between SES and obesity (Sobal & Stunkard, 1989). Income is an often-used indicator of SES (Galobardes et al., 2006) that can affect obesity via material resources such as food budgets, car and home ownership, and time use. With regard to *time use,* studies show that employed women nowadays spend significantly less time cooking, eating with their children, and playing with their children, and are more likely to purchase prepared foods (Cawley & Liu, 2012). U.S. adults consume less food at home and prepare meals from raw ingredients less frequently. It seems, however, that the reduction in time spent cooking since 1965 has leveled off, with no substantial decrease occurring after the mid-1990s (Smith, Ng, & Popkin, 2013). Although evidence suggests that time use and food patterns impact weight status (Kolodinsky & Goldstein, 2011), it is unclear whether changes in obesity prevalence can be attributed to changes in time use.

With regard to *car and home ownership,* each additional kilometer walked per day is associated with a 4.8% reduction in the likelihood of obesity. By contrast, each additional hour spent in a car per day is associated with a 6% increased risk of obesity (Frank, Andresen, & Schmid, 2004). Moreover, countries with higher levels of active transportation (i.e., transport by foot or bike) have lower obesity rates (Bassett, Pucher, Buehler, Thompson, & Crouter, 2008), and replacing car travel with more active modes of transportation could significantly improve physical activity rates (Edwards & Tsourosm, 2008). Research from the United States also suggests that area-level housing prices are strongly associated with obesity, such that women in the bottom quartile of property values were over three times as likely to be obese than women in the top quartile (Rehm, Moudon, Hurvitz, & Drewnowski, 2012).

Income may also affect the amount of money available to purchase food (*food budget*), which may affect obesity via dietary behaviors (Rao, Afshin, Singh, & Mozaffarian, 2013). Studies have shown that constraining food budgets can lower the nutritional adequacy of the diet (Drewnowski & Darmon, 2005), and that economic uncertainty may adversely affect people's food choices (Waterlander et al., 2010). Dietary costs may therefore be a barrier to the uptake and maintenance of healthy diets (Darmon, Ferguson, & Briend, 2002). Research from the United States has shown that adherence to a healthy diet (lower energy density, higher intake of vitamins, potassium, and dietary fiber) is costlier than adherence to a less healthy diet (e.g., Rao et al., 2013), and these results have been replicated in the United Kingdom (Monsivais et al., 2015). Importantly, healthy diets are also perceived to be more expensive than unhealthy diets (Monsivais et al., 2015). However, in some cases food insecurity also leads to creative strategies to make food dollars stretch—for example, using strategies such as shopping based on chain-specific discounts and in-store specials (Wiig & Smith, 2009). An intervention examining the effect of price discounts on fruit and vegetables showed higher fruit and vegetable purchases after a 50% price reduction (Waterlander, de Boer, Schuit, & Seidell, 2013), suggesting that pricing strategies may be part of an effective strategy to promote healthy diets.

In contrast to food, physical activity does not necessarily have a direct financial cost (Swinburn et al., 1999). However, there are a number of economic factors that can influence the amount of physical activity in which people engage, such as municipal budgets for the maintenance of recreational facilities and footpaths, the proportion of national budgets allowed for health promotion, traffic safety, and paid parking policies (Feeney, 1989; Swinburn et al., 1999).

Societal-Level Economic Factors

Large shifts in diet and in physical activity patterns, particularly in the last one or two decades of the 20th century, are likely to be at least partly attributable to changes in societal-level economic factors, such as economic growth and changes in food prices. *Economic growth* has a profound impact on health and weight status. For example, a study using data from postwar Japan showed that times of economic prosperity corresponded with increased consumption of tobacco, alcohol, and saturated fat (Tapia Granados, 2008). These periods also corresponded with increased rates of inactivity, work pressures, inadequate sleep, social isolation, and traffic injuries (Tapia Granados, 2008), all of which have links with chronic disease risk (Egger & Dixon, 2009). Studying the situation in reverse, there is additional support for the adverse effects of economic development. Cuba's economic decline after Russia's withdrawal in 1989 resulted in a 1,000 kcal/day average decrease in food intake. The decade that followed was characterized by a decrease in overall mortality, obesity being halved, and a reduction in cardiovascular mortality (Egger, 2011). Only cancers, which could be expected to have a longer time lag in relation to causality, had not been affected at the time of study (Egger & Dixon, 2009). These examples are related to major economic changes, showing that the affordability of high-energy foods and avoidance of physical activities have a major impact on rates of overweight and obesity. However, observations within affluent societies that the wealthiest or highest SES groups have lower obesity risk indicate that the relation between income and obesity is not linear.

National-level *food prices* are also influential and have changed during the past few decades. Economists' first law of demand implies that a decrease in the price of food will cause an increase in consumption (Finkelstein et al., 2005). As such, if the price of calorie-dense, prepackaged, and/or prepared foods (e.g., fast food) falls faster than prices for less calorie-dense foods (e.g., vegetables), individuals can be expected to shift their consumption toward these cheaper alternatives. Indeed, the relative prices of calorie-dense foods and beverages decreased from the 1980s as compared to the price of less energy-dense foods (Putnum & Allshouse, 1999; Putnum, Allshouse, & Kantor, 2002). These trends are consistent with the observed rapid increase in the consumption of products made with added sugars and fats (Cutler, Glaeser, & Shapiro, 2003; Drewnowski & Specter, 2004). Even from the year 2000 onward, there has been a growing price disparity between nutrient-dense foods and less nutritious options (Monsivais & Drewnowski, 2007; Monsivais, Mclain, & Drewnowski, 2010; Rao et al., 2013).

Given the likely contribution of economic factors to the obesity epidemic, economic instruments may also be used to help stem the rise in obesity. These may include effective health filters for agricultural policies, a caloric sweetened beverage tax, and fruit and vegetable subsidies (Faulkner et al., 2011). Several experiments have been conducted to test the effects of discounting or subsidizing healthy products and/or increasing prices of unhealthy products, showing that such financial strategies can have an impact on food-purchasing behavior and food intake (e.g., Waterlander et al., 2013). Moreover, a recent study in New Zealand suggests that health-related food taxes and subsidies could not only improve diets, but also reduce mortality from diet-related disease (Mhurchu et al., 2015).

Physical Environmental Contributors to Obesity

The physical environment influences energy intake and expenditure through the availability of food and physical activity options, including the presence and variety of food outlets, active transport options, and physical activity options at worksites (Swinburn et al., 1999). *Physical environments* include built environments and natural environments. *Built environments* refer to the places and spaces created by people (including buildings, parks, and transportation systems). *Natural environments* refer to environmental features such as beaches, mountains, and forests. The physical environment can be divided further into micro (office space, home), meso (neighborhood, worksite), and macro (state, country) environments.

Micro-Level Physical Environmental Factors

Although macro environmental factors may, by definition, affect obesity levels of entire populations, even small changes in microenvironments can, together, have a significant impact on population levels (Hill, 2009). Micro- or indoor-environmental characteristics have been studied across a range of settings, including the home, workplace, and shops. *Home environments* can influence sedentary behaviors, physical activities, and dietary behaviors via what is available in the home. For example, having more televisions and other electronic screens in the home is associated with more sedentary behavior and higher levels of obesity (Thorp et al., 2011). More long-term food storage space is also associated with obesity (Emery et al., 2015).

Workplace environments are regarded as important settings for the prevention of obesity through individual-based worksite programs (Heinen & Darling, 2009). Changes in worksite environments related to mechanization and automatization of work have led to a decrease in physical activity. As such, these changes may have contributed to the increase in obesity in the 1980s, but the shift away from manual employment largely predated this time period (Finkelstein et al., 2005). At present, worksites try to promote some physical activities among the workforce by stimulating stair use (Soler et al., 2010), decreasing occupational sedentary behavior via standing desks or "active" workstations (Neuhaus et al., 2014), and improving the healthfulness of cafeteria food (Kjøllesdal, Holmboe-Ottesen, & Wandel, 2011) and of the content of worksite vending machines (French et al., 2011). Yet it remains unclear what role present-day worksites play in promoting obesity within the larger environment (Thorndike, 2011).

The *indoor environment of shops* can influence weight status through the availability, affordability, prominence, and promotion of foods and/or restricting or (de-)marketing food types (Black et al., 2014; Glanz, Bader, & Iyer, 2012). This is because there are differences in the overall healthfulness of the foods available in different stores (Black et al., 2014). Stores in lower-income neighborhoods stock fewer healthier varieties of foods and offer much lower quality fresh produce (Andreyeva, Blumenthal, Schwartz, Long, & Brownell, 2008).

Meso-Level Physical Environmental Factors

On the meso level, neighborhood environments are often studied, as they contain physical environmental attributes that are likely to be relevant for eating and physical activity behaviors (Diez Roux, 2001). Frequently studied factors of the neighborhood environment include:

- Aesthetics—for example, indicators such as graffiti, litter, natural features, and maintenance of buildings.
- Safety—for example, safety from crime as well as traffic safety.
- Land use mix—for example, the range of land uses, including residential, commercial, and industrial, that are co-located.
- Connectivity—for example, how well areas are connected through a network of paths or roads.
- Walkability—for example, an index including indicators such as population density, residential density, land use mix, intersection density, and connectivity.
- Urban sprawl—for example, spreading of development out of a city.
- Density—for example, concentration of food outlets, recreational facilities, residences, parks, etc.

These and other factors can influence rates of obesity in residential neighborhoods (areas where people live), work neighborhoods, or even the commuter neighborhoods.

In *residential neighborhood environments,* availability and proximity of recreation facilities are generally associated with higher levels of physical activity among adults (Brownson, Baker, Housemann, Brennan, & Bacak, 2001; Mackenbach, Lakerveld, van Lenthe, et al., 2016). Findings from a cross-European study (Lakerveld et al., 2015) also showed that residents living in neighborhoods with lower speed limits and better connectivity were more likely to engage in cycling for transport (Mertens et al., 2016). These results are consistent with results from studies in other parts of the world suggesting that more destinations (e.g., shops, offices, recreational facilities, health services) and opportunities for reaching these destinations by foot or bicycle are beneficial for weight status (Mujahid et al., 2008; Oliver et al., 2015). Neighborhood food environments have also been associated with obesity. For example, higher exposure to unhealthy food outlets such as takeout restaurants has been associated with higher consumption of fast food and obesity (Burgoine, Forouhi, Griffin, Wareham, & Monsivais, 2014), whereas the presence of supermarkets has been linked to higher fruit and vegetable intake and lower prevalence of obesity (Morland, Diez Roux, & Wing, 2006). In contrast with studies conducted in the United States, findings for these associations in the United Kingdom are less consistent (Cummins & Macintyre, 2006), perhaps because affordability also has important effects on diet and obesity (Breyer & Voss-Andreae, 2013).

Because adults usually spend a large share of their time at work, there is increasing attention to the *work environment*. For example, work environments may determine what mode of transport individuals use to get to work—for example, if there are no parking spaces available in the work area, individuals are less likely to drive to work (Mackenbach, Randal, Zhao, & Howden-Chapman, 2016). Similarly, if the work neighborhood is inviting in terms of physical activity—that is, is green, safe, and pleasant to walk/cycle in—individuals are more likely to walk or cycle to work (Craig, Brownson, Cragg, & Dunn, 2002). Evidence also suggests that the food environment in the work area can affect takeout consumption and obesity (Burgoine et al., 2014). Recently, *commuting environments* have been shown to affect diets and activity levels as well (Chaix et al., 2012). If commuting environments are unpleasant or unsafe for walking or cycling, individuals may be more likely to travel by car (Panter, Griffin, & Ogilvie, 2014). In addition, individuals who commute home from work have a preference for convenient, ready-prepared meals, which may strengthen the association between exposure to takeaway restaurants and obesity (Burgoine & Monsivais, 2013).

Macro-Level Physical Environmental Factors

There is an extensive body of research on the changes in macro-environmental factors in relation to obesity (Popkin, 2005). Profound changes in global food supply and in the relative costs of foods have driven the *nutrition transition* (Popkin, 2004). The term *nutrition transition* refers to the shift in dietary consumption from traditional diets high in cereal and fiber to diets high in sugar, fat, and animal-sourced foods, coinciding with demographic and epidemiological transition. There is increased consensus that the timing and magnitude of these macro-environmental changes can explain the rapid increase in obesity over the past few decades (Popkin, 2005). In addition, environmental changes are increasingly influential in lower-income countries. Generally, these processes first affect the wealthier members of urban areas, but this is followed by a reversal of the socioeconomic gradient as obesity becomes a disease of impoverished populations (Stunkard, 1996).

Apart from a major change in the macro-food environment, changing *urbanization* rates are also affecting obesity, mainly in developing countries. This effect may be due to the increased availability of high-calorie foods from supermarket and fast-food chains, more roads for passive travel, less open public spaces, more mass-media marketing of food and beverages, and less work-related physical activity (Hawkes, 2006). For example, occupational physical activity in China has decreased due to rapid urbanization. Although light occupational activity is likely to increase with further urbanization, moderate to vigorous activity is likely to decrease (Monda, Gordon-Larsen, Stevens, & Popkin, 2007). Variation in physical environmental factors across countries may partly explain variation in physical activity and obesity. Indeed, walkability has been linked to physical activity and varies considerably across the world (Adams et al., 2014), suggesting that the design of urban environments has the potential to contribute substantially to physical activity (Sallis et al., 2016). Other macro-level factors consistently associated with obesity are urban sprawl and residential density (Mackenbach et al., 2014).

Conclusions

In conclusion, this chapter argues that the physical, social, and economic environments in which individuals live are important drivers of the obesity epidemic. Current environments often promote or facilitate excessive food intake and discourage physical activity. Maintaining a healthy body weight is too much dependent on individual motivation and ability. Social, economic, and physical environmental factors may operate at different levels (micro, meso, or macro) and interact with individual motivation and abilities in their influence on obesogenic behaviors and obesity. Researchers and policymakers should work toward creating environments that facilitate rather than hinder obesity prevention and related health behaviors.

References

Acevedo-Garcia, D., Lochner, K. A., Osypuk, T. L., & Al, E. (2003). Future direction in residential segregation and health research: A multilevel approach. *American Journal of Public Health, 93*(2), 215–221.

Adams, M. A., Frank, L. D., Schipperijn, J., Smith, G., Chapman, J., Christiansen, L. B., et al. (2014). International variation in neighborhood walkability, transit, and recreation environments using geographic information systems: The IPEN Adult study. *International Journal of Health Geographics, 13*(43), 17.

Altman, M. (2008). Behavioral economics, economic theory and public policy. Retrieved from *http://ssrn.com/abstract=1152105* or *http://dx.doi.org/10.2139/ssrn.1152105*.

Andreyeva, T., Blumenthal, D. M., Schwartz, M. B., Long, M. W., & Brownell, K. D. (2008). Availability and prices of foods across stores and neighborhoods: The case of New Haven, Connecticut. *Health Affairs, 27*(5), 1381–1388.

Bassett, D. R., Pucher, J., Buehler, R., Thompson, D. L., & Crouter, S. E. (2008). Walking, cycling, and obesity rates in Europe, North America, and Australia. *Journal of Physical Activity and Health, 5*(6), 795–814.

Black, C., Ntani, G., Inskip, H., Cooper, C., Cummins, S., Moon, G., et al. (2014). Measuring the healthfulness of food retail stores: Variations by store type and neighbourhood deprivation. *International Journal of Behavioral Nutrition and Physical Activity, 11*(1), 69.

Breyer, B., & Voss-Andreae, A. (2013). Food mirages: Geographic and economic barriers to healthful food access in Portland, Oregon. *Health and Place, 24*, 131–139.

Brownson, R. C., Baker, E. A., Housemann, R. A., Brennan, L. K., & Bacak, S. J. (2001). Environmental and policy determinants of physical activity in the United States. *American Journal of Public Health, 91*(12), 1995–2003.

Burgoine, T., Forouhi, N. G., Griffin, S. J., Wareham, N. J., & Monsivais, P. (2014). Associations between exposure to takeaway food outlets, takeaway food consumption, and body weight in Cambridgeshire, UK: Population based, cross sectional study. *British Medical Journal, 348*, 1464.

Burgoine, T., & Monsivais, P. (2013). Characterising food environment exposure at home, at work, and along commuting journeys using data on adults in the UK. *International Journal of Behavioral Nutrition and Physical Activity, 10*, 85.

Cachelin, F. M. (2001). Ethnic differences in body-size preferences: Myth or reality? *Nutrition, 17*(4), 353–354.

Cawley, J., & Liu, F. (2012). Maternal employment and childhood obesity: A search for mechanisms in time use data. *Economics and Human Biology, 10*(4), 352–364.

Chaix, B., Kestens, Y., Perchoux, C., Karusisi, N., Merlo, J., & Labadi, K. (2012). An interactive mapping tool to assess individual mobility patterns in neighbourhood studies. *American Journal of Preventive Medicine, 43*(4), 440–450.

Christakis, N. A., & Fowler, J. H. (2007). The spread of obesity in a large social network over 32 years. *New England Journal of Medicine, 357*(4), 370–379.

Cohen, A. K., Rai, M., Rehkopf, D. H., & Abrams, B. (2013). Educational attainment and obesity: A systematic review. *Obesity Reviews, 14*(12), 989–1005.

Cornelisse-Vermaat, J. R., & Maassen van den Brink, H. (2007). Ethnic differences in lifestyle and overweight in The Netherlands. *Obesity, 15*(2), 483.

Cozier, Y. C., Yu, J., Coogan, P. F., Bethea, T. N., Rosenberg, L., & Palmer, J. R. (2014). Racism, segregation, and risk of obesity in the Black Women's Health Study. *American Journal of Epidemiology, 179*(7), 875–883.

Craig, C. L., Brownson, R. C., Cragg, S. E., & Dunn, A. L. (2002). Exploring the effect of the environment on physical activity: A study examining walking to work. *American Journal of Preventive Medicine, 23*(2), 36–43.

Cummins, S., & Macintyre, S. (2006). Food environments and obesity: Neighbourhood or nation? *International Journal of Epidemiology, 35*(1), 100–104.

Cutler, D. M., Glaeser, E. L., & Shapiro, J. M. (2003). Why have Americans become more obese? *Journal of Economic Perspectives, 17*(3), 93–118.

Dahlgren, G., & Whitehead, M. (2007). *European strategies for tackling social inequities in health: Levelling up part 2*. Copenhagen, Denmark: World Health Organization.

Darmon, N., Ferguson, E. L., & Briend, A. (2002). A cost constraint alone has adverse effects on food selection and nutrient density: An analysis of human diets by linear programming. *Journal of Nutrition, 132*(12), 3764–3771.

De Bourdeaudhuij, I., Van Dyck, D., Davey Rachel, R., Reis, R. S., Schofield, G., Sarmiento, O. L., et al. (2015). International study of perceived neighbourhood environmental attributes and body mass index: IPEN Adult study in 12 countries. *International Journal of Behavioral Nutrition and Physical Activity, 12*(62), 1–10.

Diez Roux, A. V. (2001). Investigating neighborhood and area effects on health. *American Journal of Public Health, 91*(11), 1783–1789.

Dinsa, G. D., Goryakin, Y., Fumagalli, E., & Suhrcke, M. (2012). Obesity and socioeconomic status in developing countries: A systematic review. *Obesity Reviews, 13*(11), 1067–1079.

Drewnowski, A., & Darmon, N. (2005). Food choices

and diet costs: An economic analysis. *Journal of Nutrition, 135*(4), 900–904.

Drewnowski, A., & Specter, S. E. (2004). Poverty and obesity: The role of energy density and energy costs. *Journal of Clinical Nutrition, 79*(1), 6–16.

Edwards, P., & Tsourosm, A. D. (2008). *A healthy city is an active city: A physical activity planning guide.* Copenhagen, Denmark: World Health Organization.

Egger, G. (2011). Obesity, chronic disease, and economic growth: A case for "big picture" prevention. *Advances in Preventive Medicine, 2011*, 149–158.

Egger, G., & Dixon, J. (2009). Should obesity be the main game?—or do we need an environmental makeover to combat the inflammatory and chronic disease epidemics?: Viewpoint. *Obesity Reviews, 10*(2), 237–249.

Eichinger, M., Titze, S., Haditsch, B., Dorner, T. E., & Stronegger, W. J. (2015). How are physical activity behaviors and cardiovascular risk factors associated with characteristics of the built and social residential environment? *PLOS ONE, 10*(6), 1–15.

Emery, C. F., Olson, K. F., Lee, V. S., Habash, D. L., Nasar, J. L., & Bodine, A. (2015). Home environment and psychosocial predictors of obesity status among community-residing men and women. *International Journal of Obesity (London), 39*(9), 1401–1407.

Faulkner, G. E. J., Grootendorst, P., Nguyen, V., Andreyeva, T., Arbour-Nicitopoulos, K., Auld, M. C., et al. (2011). Economic instruments for obesity prevention: Results of a scoping review and modified Delphi survey. *International Journal of Behavioral Nutrition and Physical Activity, 8*(1), 109.

Feeney, B. P. (1989). A review of the impact of parking policy measures on travel demand. *Transportation Planning and Technology, 13*(4), 229–244.

Finkelstein, E. A., Ruhm, C. J., & Kosa, K. (2005). Economic causes and consequences of obesity. *Annual Review of Public Health, 26*, 239–257.

Flegal, K. M., Carroll, M. D., Ogden, C. L., & Curtin, L. R. (2010). Prevalence and trends in obesity among US adults, 1999–2008. *Journal of the American Medical Association, 303*(3), 235–241.

Frank, L. D., Andresen, M. A., & Schmid, T. L. (2004). Obesity relationships with community design, physical activity, and time spent in cars. *American Journal of Preventive Medicine, 27*(2), 87–96.

French, S. A., Hannan, P. J., Harnack, L. J., Mitchell, N. R., Toomey, T. L., & Gerlach, A. (2011). Pricing and availability intervention in vending machines at four bus garages. *Journal of Occupational and Environmental Medicine, 52*(1, Suppl.), S29.

Galobardes, B., Shaw, M., Lawlor, D. A., Lynch, J. W., & Davey Smith, G. (2006). Indicators of socioeconomic position: Part 1. *Journal of Epidemiology and Community Health, 60*(1), 7–12.

Glanz, K., Bader, M. D., & Iyer, S. (2012). Retail grocery store marketing strategies and obesity: An integrative review. *American Journal of Preventive Medicine, 42*(5), 503–512.

Glonti, K., Mackenbach, J. D., Ng, J., Lakerveld, J., Oppert, J.-M., Bardos, H., et al. (2016). Psychosocial environment: Definitions, measures and associations with weight status—a systematic review. *Obesity Reviews, 17*(1, Suppl.), 81–95.

Goldman, N. (2001). Social inequalities in health disentangling the underlying mechanisms. *Annals of the New York Academy of Sciences, 954*, 118–139.

Hammond, R. A. (2010). Social influence and obesity. *Current Opinion in Endocrinology, Diabetes and Obesity, 17*(5), 467–471.

Hawkes, C. (2006). Uneven dietary development: Linking the policies and processes of globalization with the nutrition transition, obesity and diet-related chronic diseases. *Global Health, 2*, 4.

Heinen, L., & Darling, H. (2009). Addressing obesity in the workplace: The role of employers. *Milbank Quarterly, 87*(1), 101–122.

Hill, J. O. (2009). Can a small-changes approach help address the obesity epidemic?: A report of the Joint Task Force of the American Society for Nutrition, Institute of Food Technologists, and International Food Information Council. *American Journal of Clinical Nutrition, 89*(2), 477–484.

Jih, J., Mukherjea, A., Vittinghoff, E., Nguyen, T. T., Tsoh, J. Y., Fukuoka, Y., et al. (2014). Using appropriate body mass index cut points for overweight and obesity among Asian Americans. *Preventive Medicine, 65*, 1–6.

Kaushal, N., & Rhodes, R. E. (2014). The home physical environment and its relationship with physical activity and sedentary behavior: A systematic review. *Preventive Medicine, 67*, 221–237.

Kershaw, K. N., Albrecht, S. S., & Carnethon, M. R. (2013). Racial and ethnic residential segregation, the neighborhood socioeconomic environment, and obesity among Blacks and Mexican Americans. *American Journal of Epidemiology, 177*(4), 299–309.

Kjøllesdal, M. R., Holmboe-Ottesen, G., & Wandel, M. (2011). Frequent use of staff canteens is associated with unhealthy dietary habits and obesity in a Norwegian adult population. *Public Health Nutrition, 14*(1), 133–141.

Kolodinsky, J. M., & Goldstein, A. B. (2011). Time use and food pattern influences on obesity. *Obesity (Silver Spring), 19*(12), 2327–2335.

Kremers, S. P. J., de Bruijn, G. J., Visscher, T. J. S., van Mechelen, W., de Vries, N. K., & Brug, J. (2006). Environmental influences on energy balance-related behaviors: A dual-process view. *International Journal of Behavioral Nutrition and Physical Activity, 3*, 9.

Lakerveld, J., Ben Rebah, M., Mackenbach, J. D., Charreire, H., Compernolle, S., Glonti, K., et al. (2015). Obesity-related behaviours and BMI in five urban regions across Europe: Sampling design and results from the SPOTLIGHT cross-sectional survey. *BMJ Open, 5*(10), e008505.

Lehnert, T., Sonntag, D., Konnopka, A., Riedel-Heller, S., & König, H. H. (2013). Economic costs of overweight and obesity. *Best Practice and Research Clinical Endocrinology and Metabolism, 27*(2), 105–115.

Leroux, J. S., Moore, S., & Dubé, L. (2013). Beyond the "I" in the obesity epidemic: A review of social relational and network interventions on obesity. *Journal of Obesity, 2013*, 348249.

Mackenbach, J. D., Lakerveld, J., van Lenthe, F., Teixeira, P. J., Compernolle, S., De Bourdeaudhuij, I., et al. (2016). Interactions of individual perceived barriers and neighbourhood destinations with obesity-related behaviours in Europe: The SPOTLIGHT project. *Obesity Reviews, 17*(Suppl.), 68–80.

Mackenbach, J. D., Lakerveld, J., van Oostveen, Y., Compernolle, S., De Bourdeaudhuij, I., Bárdos, H., et al. (2016). The mediating role of social capital in the association between neighbourhood income inequality and body mass index. *European Journal of Public Health, 27*(2), 218–223.

Mackenbach, J. D., Randal, E., Zhao, P., & Howden-Chapman, P. (2016). The influence of urban land-use and public transport facilities on active commuting in Wellington, New Zealand: Active transport forecasting using the WILUTE model. *Sustainability, 8*(3), 242.

Mackenbach, J. D., Rutter, H., Compernolle, S., Glonti, K., Oppert, J. M., Charreire, H., et al. (2014). Obesogenic environments: A systematic review of the association between the physical environment and adult weight status—The SPOTLIGHT project. *BMC Public Health, 14*, 233.

McNeill, L. H., Kreuter, M. W., & Subramanian, S. (2006). Social environment and physical activity: A review of concepts and evidence. *Social Science and Medicine, 63*(4), 1011–1022.

McPherson, K., Marsh, T., & Brown, M. (2007). *Foresight: Tackling obesities: Future choices—Modelling future trends in obesity and the impact on health* (Report). London, UK: Government Office for Science.

Mertens, L., Compernolle, S., Gheysen, F., Deforche, B., Brug, J., Mackenbach, J. D., et al. (2016). Perceived environmental correlates of cycling for transport among adults in five regions of Europe: The SPOTLIGHT project. *Obesity Reviews, 17*(Suppl.), 53–61.

Mhurchu, C. N., Eyles, H., Genc, M., Scarborough, P., Rayner, M., Mizdrak, A., et al. (2015). Effects of health-related food taxes and subsidies on mortality from diet-related disease in New Zealand: An econometric-epidemiologic modelling study. *PLOS ONE, 10*(7), 1–17.

Monda, K. L., Gordon-Larsen, P., Stevens, J., & Popkin, B. M. (2007). China's transition: The effect of rapid urbanization on adult occupational physical activity. *Social Science and Medicine, 64*(4), 858–870.

Monsivais, P., & Drewnowski, A. (2007). The rising cost of low-energy-density foods. *Journal of the American Dietetic Association, 107*(12), 2071–2076.

Monsivais, P., Mclain, J., & Drewnowski, A. (2010). The rising disparity in the price of healthful foods: 2004–2008. *Food Policy, 35*(6), 514–520.

Monsivais, P., Scarborough, P., Lloyd, T., Mizdrak, A., Luben, R., Mulligan, A. A., et al. (2015). Greater accordance with the Dietary Approaches to Stop Hypertension dietary pattern is associated with lower diet-related greenhouse gas production but higher dietary costs in the United Kingdom. *American Journal of Clinical Nutrition, 102*(1), 138–145.

Morland, K., Diez Roux, A. V., & Wing, S. (2006). Supermarkets, other food stores, and obesity: The atherosclerosis risk in communities study. *American Journal of Preventive Medicine, 30*(4), 333–339.

Mujahid, M. S., Diez Roux, A. V., Shen, M., Gowda, D., Sanchez, B., Shea, S., et al. (2008). Relation between neighborhood environments and obesity in the Multi-Ethnic Study of Atherosclerosis. *American Journal of Epidemiology, 167*(11), 1349–1357.

Neuhaus, M., Eakin, E. G., Straker, L., Owen, N., Dunstan, D. W., Reid, N., et al. (2014). Reducing occupational sedentary time: A systematic review and meta-analysis of evidence on activity-permissive workstations. *Obesity Reviews, 15*(10), 822–838.

Oliver, G., Wardle, J., & Gibson, E. L. (2000). Stress and food choice: A laboratory study. *Psychosomatic Medicine, 62*(6), 853–865.

Oliver, G., Witten, K., Blakely, T., Parker, K., Badland, H., Schofield, G., et al. (2015). Neighbourhood built environment associations with body size in adults: Mediating effects of activity and sedentariness in a cross-sectional study of New Zealand adults. *BMC Public Health, 15*, 956.

Panter, J., Griffin, S., & Ogilvie, D. (2014). Active commuting and perceptions of the route environment: A longitudinal analysis. *Preventive Medicine, 67*, 134–140.

Popkin, B. M. (2004). The nutrition transition: An overview of world patterns of change. *Nutrition Reviews, 62*, S140–S143.

Popkin, B. M. (2005). Using research on the obesity pandemic as a guide to a unified vision of nutrition. *Public Health Nutrition, 8*(6A), 724–729.

Powell, K., Wilcox, J., Clonan, A., Bissell, P., Preston, L., Peacock, M., et al. (2015). The role of social networks in the development of overweight and obesity among adults: A scoping review. *BMC Public Health, 15*(1), 996.

Putnum, J. J., & Allshouse, J. E. (1999). Food consumption, prices, and expenditures, 1970–97. *Statistical Bulletin No. 965*. Washington, DC: U.S. Department of Agriculture.

Putnum, J. J., Allshouse, J. E., & Kantor, L. S. (2002). U.S. per capita food supply trends: More calories, refined carbohydrates, and fats. *Food Reviews, 25*(3), 2–15.

Rao, M., Afshin, A., Singh, G., & Mozaffarian, D. (2013). Do healthier foods and diet patterns cost more than less healthy options?: A systematic review and meta-analysis. *BMJ Open, 3*(12), e004277.

Rehm, C. D., Moudon, A. V., Hurvitz, P. M., & Drewnowski, A. (2012). Residential property values are associated with obesity among women in King County, WA, USA. *Social Science and Medicine, 75*(3), 491–495.

Sallis, J. F., Cerin, E., Conway, T. L., Adams, M. A., Frank, L. D., Pratt, M., et al. (2016). Physical activity in relation to urban environments in 14 cities worldwide: A cross-sectional study. *Lancet, 387*(10034), 2207–2217.

Sampson, R. J., Raudenbush, S. W., & Earls, F. (1997).

Neighborhoods and violent crime: A multilevel study of collective efficacy. *Science, 277*(5328), 918–924.

Schmidhauser, S., Eichler, K., & Brugger, U. (2009). *Environmental determinants of overweight and obesity: Extended international literature review.* Zurich, Switzerland: Winterthur Institute of Health Economics WIG.

Smith, L. P., Ng, S. W., & Popkin, B. M. (2013). Trends in US home food preparation and consumption: Analysis of national nutrition surveys and time use studies from 1965–1966 to 2007–2008. *Nutrition Journal, 12,* 45.

Sobal, J., & Stunkard, A. J. (1989). Socioeconomic status and obesity: A review of the literature. *Psychological Bulletin, 105*(2), 260–275.

Soler, R. E., Leeks, K. D., Buchanan, L. R., Brownson, R. C., Heath, G. W., & Hopkins, D. H. (2010). Point-of-decision prompts to increase stair use: A systematic review update. *American Journal of Preventive Medicine, 38*(2), S292–S300.

Stunkard, A. J. (1996). Socioeconomic status and obesity. *Ciba Foundation Symposium, 201,* 174–193.

Sundborn, G., Metcalf, P. A., Gentles, D., Scragg, R., Dyall, L., Black, P., et al. (2010). Overweight and obesity prevalence among adult Pacific peoples and Europeans in the Diabetes Heart and Health Study (DHAHS) 2002–2003, Auckland New Zealand. *New Zealand Medical Journal, 123*(1311), 30–42.

Swinburn, B., Egger, G., & Raza, F. (1999). Dissecting obesogenic environments: The development and application of a framework for identifying and prioritizing environmental interventions for obesity. *Preventive Medicine, 29*(6, Pt. 1), 563–570.

Tamayo, A., Karter, A. J., Mujahid, M. S., Warton, E. M., Moffet, H. H., Adler, N., et al. (2016). Associations of perceived neighborhood safety and crime with cardiometabolic risk factors among a population with type 2 diabetes. *Health and Place, 39,* 116–121.

Tapia Granados, J. A. (2008). Macroeconomic fluctuations and mortality in postwar Japan. *Demography, 45*(2), 323–343.

Thorndike, A. N. (2011). Workplace interventions to reduce obesity and cardiometabolic risk. *Current Cardiovascular Risk Reports, 5*(1), 79–85.

Thorp, A. A., Owen, N., Neuhaus, M., & Dunstan, D. W. (2011). Sedentary behaviors and subsequent health outcomes in adults: A systematic review of longitudinal studies, 1996–2011. *American Journal of Preventive Medicine, 41*(2), 207–215.

Ujcic-Voortman, J. K., Bos, G., Baan, C. A., Verhoeff, A. P., & Seidell, J. C. (2011). Obesity and body fat distribution: Ethnic differences and the role of socio-economic status. *Obesity Facts, 4*(1), 53–60.

van Tubergen, F., Maas, I., & Flap, H. (2004). The economic incorporation of immigrants in 18 Western societies: Origin, destination, and community effects. *American Sociological Review, 59*(5), 704–727.

Wagstaff, A., & van Doorslaer, E. (2000). Income inequality and health: What does the literature tell us? *Annual Review of Public Health, 21,* 543–567.

Waterlander, W. E., de Boer, M. R., Schuit, A. J., & Seidell, J. C. (2013). Price discounts significantly enhance fruit and vegetable purchases when combined with nutrition education: A randomized controlled. *American Journal of Clinical Nutrition, 97*(4), 886–895.

Waterlander, W. E., de Haas, W. E., van Amstel, I., Schuit, A. J., Twisk, J. W., Visser, M., et al. (2010). Energy density, energy costs and income: How are they related? *Public Health Nutrition, 13*(10), 1599–1608.

Wiig, K., & Smith, C. (2009). The art of grocery shopping on a food stamp budget: Factors influencing the food choices of low-income women as they try to make ends meet. *Public Health Nutrition, 12*(10), 1726–1734.

Yoon, J., & Brown, T. T. (2011). Does the promotion of community social capital reduce obesity risk? *Journal of Socio-Economics, 43*(3), 296–305.

Zenk, S. N., Schulz, A. J., Israel, B. A., James, S. A., Bao, S., & Wilson, M. L. (2005). Neighborhood racial composition, neighborhood poverty, and the spatial accessibility of supermarkets in metropolitan Detroit. *American Journal of Public Health, 95*(4), 660–667.

Zhao, Z., Kaestner, R., & Xu, X. (2014). Spatial mobility and environmental effects on obesity. *Economics and Human Biology, 14*(1), 128–140.

CHAPTER 10

Psychosocial Contributors to and Consequences of Obesity

Rebecca M. Puhl
Rebecca L. Pearl

Psychosocial functioning is an imperative marker of quality of life, and has been a topic of important consideration in the context of obesity. In particular, researchers have examined psychosocial symptoms that may increase the risk for the development of obesity, as well as adverse psychosocial consequences that may result from having obesity. Prospective research is especially important for studying these relationships in order to test the direction of causal pathways linking psychosocial functioning to weight trajectories over time. This chapter summarizes recent evidence from large-scale studies of population and clinical samples to identify psychosocial factors associated with obesity, with a specific focus on the extent to which psychosocial risk factors are longitudinally associated with obesity. We review the evidence of psychosocial risk factors for weight gain and psychosocial consequences of obesity, highlighting specific subgroups that may be particularly vulnerable. In addition, we highlight societal weight stigma as an important mechanism explaining links between obesity and adverse psychological functioning, as well as the clinical implications of this evidence for practitioners working with patients who have obesity.

Psychosocial Contributors to Obesity

To what extent do adverse emotions and psychological distress contribute to obesity and weight gain? Given that some individuals with obesity experience comorbid psychological problems, longitudinal research is critical to investigate the course and predictive nature of psychological functioning on body weight. The following material summarizes recent evidence on the longitudinal associations between psychosocial factors (depression, anxiety, stress, body dissatisfaction, and binge eating) and subsequent obesity and weight gain.

Depression

The links between depression and obesity have been examined in a number of longitudinal studies. Two systematic reviews of this literature examined prospective associations between depression and the development of obesity. In Faith and colleagues' review of 25 population-based studies, 15 studies specifically assessed a "depression-to-obesity" pathway, of which eight studies (53%) demonstrated depression to be a significant predictor of obesity, body mass index (BMI), or weight gain over time (Faith et al., 2011). In general, depression was found to increase obesity risk with odds ratios (ORs) in the 2.0–3.0 range. Overall, however, this review found stronger evidence for obesity leading to depression than vice versa, suggesting that depression does not consistently or necessarily increase risk of obesity. In a second review, Luppino et al. (2010) conducted a meta-analysis of 15 longitudinal studies, nine of which examined the effect of depression on obesity over time, and showed that depression was predictive of developing obesity (OR 1.58).

The reciprocal and bidirectional link observed in these reviews underscores the complexity of the interaction between depression and obesity. In addition, the authors of these studies noted challenges in interpreting this evidence in light of the considerable methodological variability of studies included in their reviews. Differences in sample sizes, age of participants, follow-up periods, self-reported versus measured weight and height, selection of covariates, and treating weight status and/or depression as categorical or continuous variables all create difficulties in comparing studies and leave questions unanswered. Thus, additional work is warranted to clarify the strength of evidence for depression as a risk factor for obesity.

More recent evidence from longitudinal studies has demonstrated somewhat similar findings. A notable example is evidence from the Nurses' Health Study, in which 65,955 women, ages 54–79, were prospectively followed from 1996 to 2006, with assessment of body weight, depression (measured by physician-diagnosed depression and use of antidepressant medication), and covariates every 2 years (Pan, Sun, et al., 2012). After adjusting for baseline age, physical activity, comorbidities, BMI, and other covariates, depression was associated with an increased risk of obesity in women at follow-up. In addition, a prospective population-based cohort study of 3,054 adults in Switzerland found that major depressive disorder with atypical features was prospectively associated (over 5.5 years) with a higher increase in BMI, incidence of obesity, and waist circumference in both men and women (Lasserre et al., 2014). These findings remained after controlling for potential confounders, including sociodemographic and lifestyle characteristics, comorbid mental disorders, and antidepressant medication.

Proposals concerning underlying mechanisms can help explain the complex relationship between depression and obesity. Some longitudinal research has found that emotional eating acts as a mediator between depression and future weight gain, especially in women (van Strien, Konttinen, Homberg, Engels, & Winkens, 2016). Depression may also contribute to unhealthy lifestyle behaviors, such as reduced physical activity or poor eating patterns, which could induce weight gain. Other research has emphasized biological factors that may be involved: namely, that depression may lead to obesity through dysregulation of the hypothalamic–pituitary–adrenal (HPA) axis or cortisol reactivity, which may play a role in abdominal obesity (Björntorp, 2001). Although antidepressant medication can have side effects that include weight gain, most research to date has found no differences in studies of participants with depression who undergo pharmacological treatment compared to those who do not (Luppino et al., 2010). Finally, weight stigmatization could increase the risk of depression, which, as discussed later in this chapter, can have a bidirectional relationship with obesity. Thus, additional longitudinal research is warranted to establish and clarify the underlying mechanisms linking depression to the development of obesity.

Anxiety

Compared to recent evidence examining links between depression and obesity, fewer longitudinal studies have assessed anxiety as a contributor to obesity. A Norwegian prospective cohort study of 25,180 adults found that symptoms of anxiety and depression were associated with weight gain and incidence of obesity over an 11-year period (Brumpton, Langhammer, Romundstad, Chen, & Mai, 2013). Participants who endorsed any anxiety or depression had a significantly higher cumulative incidence of obesity. For men, symptoms of anxiety or depression were associated with an average increased weight of 0.81 kg after 11 years compared to men without symptoms.

Women with these symptoms averaged a 0.98-kg weight gain compared to women without anxiety or depression. Although this study used questionnaires rather than diagnostic interviews to assess anxiety and depression, the findings suggest that relatively mild emotional distress may have an effect on weight gain and obesity.

Similar findings have emerged in other recent longitudinal studies. In the Netherlands Study of Depression and Anxiety, baseline symptoms of anxiety in adults ($N = 2,126$) predicted an increase in abdominal obesity over a 2-year period, independent of potential reductions in symptom severity during the study period (van Reedt Dortland, Giltay, van Veen, Zitman, & Penninx, 2013). In a sample of 167 non-treatment-seeking adults, Manzato and colleagues observed that a lifetime history of an anxiety disorder reported at baseline predicted weight gain 1 year later (Manzato, Bolognesi, Simoni, & Cuzzolaro, 2015). Further research is still needed to clarify the predictive value of anxiety for weight gain. Earlier work has demonstrated somewhat mixed findings of the association with anxiety and future weight change, including some observed differences in outcomes for women and men (Chiriboga et al., 2008). Variability in measurement of anxiety, participant demographics, sample sizes, and follow-up periods across studies create challenges in interpreting findings. Although cross-sectional research using large, racially diverse samples has demonstrated significant associations between anxiety disorders and a greater likelihood of obesity (Bodenlos, Lemon, Schneider, August, & Pagoto, 2011), the lack of longitudinal studies in this area leaves unanswered questions about the predictive nature of anxiety for obesity and weight gain.

Psychosocial Stress

General life stress and/or experiencing stressful life events may contribute to obesity risk in women and men. In a meta-analysis of 14 longitudinal studies, Wardle and colleagues found that psychosocial stress (i.e., general life stress or work stress) was positively related to the development of adiposity (objectively measured), but effects were modest (Wardle, Chida, Gibson, Whitaker, & Steptoe, 2011). Across all analyses, 69% of studies showed no significant relationship between stress and adiposity, but among those with significant effects, more demonstrated positive (25%) than negative (6%) associations. Effects were larger in studies with longer follow-up periods, and stress seemed to play a stronger role in the onset of obesity for men than women.

More recent studies have documented fairly consistent longitudinal associations of stress and weight gain. In a national, population-based sample of Australian adults ($N = 5,118$), perceived stress and stressful life events were positively associated with weight gain (but not weight loss) over a 5-year period (Harding et al., 2014). Among those who maintained or gained weight, high levels of perceived stress at baseline predicted a 0.20–0.26 kg/m^2 greater mean change in BMI compared to those with low stress. Individuals with multiple sources of stressors were at the greatest risk of weight gain. Effects were stronger for participants who were younger, nonsmokers, and whose BMI was in the normal or overweight range. These findings are similar to those of an Australian study of 1,382 women from socioeconomically disadvantaged areas, for whom higher perceived stress was associated with an increase of 11% in the odds of being obese 3 years later (Mouchacca, Abbot, & Ball, 2013). In longitudinal studies with smaller samples of adults, work-related stress has been found to predict increased BMI (Berset, Semmer, Elfering, Jacobshagen, & Meier, 2011), and higher levels of perceived stress have been found to predict weight gain through an interaction with emotional eating (Ibrahim, Thearle, Krakoff, & Gluck, 2016).

Effects of stress on weight gain may differ across demographic characteristics and health-related variables such as baseline BMI, or physiological stress levels such as cortisol reactivity, which may lead some individuals to gain more weight than others under stressful circumstances (Harding et al., 2014). For example, findings from Wardle and colleagues' (2011) meta-analysis, which found that effects of stress on obesity were stronger for men than women, could potentially be attributable to stronger physiological responses to stress among men compared to women, including higher cortisol levels following acute exposure to stress (Wardle et al., 2011). This evidence highlights the complexity of studying the relationship between stress and weight, as well as the need for consistent measurement of stress across different populations and for increased research to identify underlying mechanisms in this relationship, such as emotional eating.

Body Dissatisfaction

Body dissatisfaction tends to increase with BMI and has been found to increase the risk of disordered eating and depressive symptoms (Calzo et al., 2012), but its association with weight outcomes has received less attention. Recent prospective research in this area has studied adolescence as an important baseline developmental period, given the salience of bodily changes and body image during this time (Alberga, Sigal, Goldfield, Prud'homme, & Kenny, 2012). A number of studies examined the predictive nature of body dissatisfaction on obesity and weight change in Project EAT (Eating and Activity in Teens and Young Adults), a 10-year longitudinal investigation of adolescents that examined factors associated with weight-related outcomes in adulthood (N = 4,746 at baseline). In Project EAT, body satisfaction was measured using a modified version of the Body Shape Satisfaction Scale (Slade, Dewey, Newton, Brodie, & Kiemle, 1990). Several recent studies with this sample found body dissatisfaction to be a risk factor for overweight in adulthood. In one study, Goldschmidt and colleagues found that for both males and females (N = 1,902), body dissatisfaction in adolescence was a shared risk factor for overweight in young adulthood (Goldschmidt, Wall, Tse-Hwei, Becker, & Neumark-Sztainer, 2016). In a second study, Quick and colleagues tracked adolescents (N = 2,134) who completed baseline surveys in 1998–1999 and follow-up surveys in 2008–2009 when they were young adults (Quick, Wall, Larson, Haines, & Neumark-Sztainer, 2013). Among both females and males, higher levels of body dissatisfaction predicted the incidence of overweight at 10-year follow-up when controlling for baseline BMI. Other factors that predicted overweight included higher levels of weight concerns, unhealthy weight control behaviors, dieting, binge eating, weight-related teasing, and parental weight-related concerns during adolescence. Finally, Loth and colleagues examined Project EAT participants who were overweight at baseline (N = 496) and found that overweight girls with the most body dissatisfaction at baseline had almost a 3-unit increase in BMI at 10-year follow-up compared to those with less body dissatisfaction. No association between body satisfaction and BMI change was observed in boys (Loth, Watts, van den Berg, & Neumark-Sztainer, 2015).

Less research has examined the predictive nature of body dissatisfaction on weight outcomes in adults or used national datasets to identify differences in body dissatisfaction across population characteristics such as sex, BMI, race/ethnicity, and age (Fiske, Fallon, Blissmer, & Redding, 2014). Still, some studies have found that as many as 72% of women and 61% of men may experience body dissatisfaction (Fiske et al., 2014), which could play a role in weight changes over time. Mintem, Gigante, and Horta (2015) examined 2004 follow-up data of 3,702 adults in the 1982 Pelotas Birth Cohort panel in Brazil. Participants with increased BMI during the study period exhibited elevated risk of body dissatisfaction, which was higher for women than for men. In contrast, a Canadian longitudinal study of 1,793 older adults (ages 67–84) found that despite higher weight dissatisfaction in women than men (and a similar prevalence of obesity in both groups), weight gain was associated with body dissatisfaction in men only (Roy, Shatenstein, Gaudreau, Morais, & Payette, 2014). Caution is warranted in interpreting these results, as measurement relied on a single item of weight satisfaction.

Thus, although body dissatisfaction has received attention as a psychosocial variable that predicts weight trajectories in the lives of young people, measurement of body dissatisfaction has varied across studies. Prospective research is needed to further investigate longitudinal links between body dissatisfaction and weight outcomes throughout middle and late adulthood and to investigate whether, like depression, there are reciprocal links between body dissatisfaction and obesity. Given established links between body dissatisfaction and disordered eating, dieting, and depressive symptoms, investigators should now focus on identifying what effect body satisfaction has on weight gain independent of other psychosocial factors.

Binge-Eating Disorder

As reviewed by McCuen-Wurst and Allison (Chapter 11, this volume) and Grilo (Chapter 34, this volume), binge-eating disorder (BED) is a common comorbid condition with obesity. Individuals with BED are more likely to have obesity, and BED becomes more prevalent with increased obesity severity. Thus, it is important to consider the predictive role of BED as a psychosocial contributor to obesity or weight gain.

Among nontreatment samples, recent longitudinal research has yielded mixed findings. Field et al. (2014) followed a national cohort of 5,527 young men from 1999 to 2010 and found no associations between BED (partial or full criteria) and the development of obesity. Manzato, Bolognesi, Simoni, and Cuzzolaro (2015) observed that baseline anxiety and poor body image, but not binge eating (assessed with the Binge Eating Scale; Gormally, Black, Daston, & Rardin, 1982), predicted weight gain 1 year later in a sample of 167 overweight adults. In contrast, a study of 16,882 youth and adolescents from 1996 to 2005 found that binge eating (but not overeating) was uniquely predictive of incident overweight and obesity at follow-up (Sonneville et al., 2013). Findings from Project EAT similarly indicated that binge eating was one of several factors that predicted the incidence of overweight in both males and females at a 10-year follow-up (Quick et al., 2013).

Research with clinical samples of adults suggests that BED may have predictive value for weight outcomes. For example, Barnes, Blomquist, and Grilo (2011) examined weight trajectories of 68 obese patients with BED in the year prior to enrollment in treatment for BED. The majority (65%) gained weight, and weight gain was associated with more frequent binge-eating episodes. Ivezaj and colleagues examined weight change trajectories among patients with overweight or obesity who either met criteria for BED ($N = 26$) or did not ($N = 71$; Ivezaj, Kalebjian, Grilo, & Barnes, 2014). Weight changes during the year prior to seeking treatment differed significantly by group: BED patients gained an average of 8.3 kg, whereas those without BED gained an average of 0.7 kg. In total, BED status and binge-eating frequency each made independent, significant contributions to predicting weight change over the course of 1 year.

Recent work in this area has increasingly focused on the impact of BED on weight outcomes, specifically in patients undergoing weight loss surgery. Wadden et al. (2011) compared 1-year changes in weight among bariatric surgery patients with and without preoperative BED. Individuals without BED lost 24% of initial weight, compared to 22% for those with BED. The lack of significant differences between these groups suggests that the preoperative presence of BED did not impair weight loss 1 year later among patients who had surgery. More recently, Meany, Conceição and Mitchell (2014) reviewed longitudinal evidence from 15 studies regarding the development of binge eating, BED, and loss of control eating on long-term weight outcomes following bariatric surgery. Fourteen of the 15 studies found prospective associations between the development of these eating disturbances and more weight regain (or less weight loss) following surgery. However, studies differed with regard to the measurement of binge eating (self-report vs. clinical interview) and weight outcomes (e.g., BMI, % weight loss, weight regain), as well as length of follow-up, indicating that more research is needed to clarify the prospective effect of BED on weight outcomes in surgical patients. Although the results in a number of studies point to a contributing role of BED in weight trajectories over time, more prospective research is needed with community, clinical, and surgery populations to determine the extent to which BED directly and independently predicts weight gain.

Summary

Recent evidence suggests that there may be some longitudinal links between weight gain and adverse emotional experiences such as depression, anxiety, stress, body dissatisfaction, and binge eating. However, findings to date are mixed. Inconsistent results may reflect methodological variability across studies, ranging from differences in sample characteristics to measurement of psychological variables and selection of covariates. To better clarify the predictive role of adverse emotions on body weight, prospective studies are needed with (1) larger populations to allow for exclusion of participants with comorbidities that might influence emotional status or body weight, (2) longer follow-up periods, (3) ethnically diverse samples, and (4) a clearer examination of the clinical significance of effect sizes. Importantly, psychosocial variables that have received more longitudinal research attention (e.g., depression) highlight the reciprocal and bidirectional nature of these associations. Compared to evidence of psychosocial contributors to obesity, there is stronger evidence that obesity leads to psychosocial consequences.

Psychosocial Consequences of Obesity

Early population studies that examined psychological functioning among individuals with obesity found minimal differences in comparison to individuals without obesity (Friedman & Brownell, 1995; Stunkard & Wadden, 1992; Wadden & Stunkard, 1985). Friedman and Brownell (1995) highlighted methodological limitations of these early studies, including small sample sizes, varying definitions of obesity, inadequate assessment of psychological status, and lack of control groups. Over the past several decades, knowledge in this area has been advanced with studies utilizing large, representative samples and longitudinal designs. Overall, findings suggest an increased risk for psychological distress and impaired quality of life among individuals with obesity. It is important to note, however, that individuals with obesity are a heterogeneous group, and the majority of individuals with obesity in the general population do *not* meet criteria for a mental health disorder. We emphasize the danger in stereotyping all individuals with obesity as struggling with emotional problems, because such an assumption can contribute to weight-based stigma. Nonetheless, we review the evidence suggesting that obesity may negatively affect mental health and quality of life, highlighting specific subgroups that may be particularly vulnerable.

Mental Health among Individuals with Obesity

Depression

Of the potential psychological consequences of obesity, depression is the most thoroughly researched (Berkowitz & Fabricatore, 2011). Two systematic reviews of cross-sectional population- and community-based studies estimated a small increased risk for depression among individuals with obesity (Atlantis & Baker, 2008; de Wit et al., 2010), with de Wit and colleagues finding an OR (based on meta-analysis) of 1.18 (see Table 10.1). When risk for depression was analyzed separately for men and women with obesity, only women were found to be at heightened risk (Atlantis & Baker, 2008; de Wit et al., 2010). In a systematic, meta-analytic review of longitudinal studies, Luppino et al. (2010) reported a pooled OR of 1.55 for the association between obesity and the development of depression. Consistent with these findings, another review of 10 prospective studies examining the impact of obesity on depression reported that ORs generally ranged from 1 to 2 for obesity-to-depression associations (Faith et al., 2011). Of note, there was considerable heterogeneity in the relationship

TABLE 10.1. Pooled Odds Ratios for Depression among Individuals with Obesity from Meta-Analyses

Publication	Overall OR (95% CI)	Women	Men
Luppino et al. (2010)	1.55 (1.22–1.98)	1.67 (1.11–2.51)	1.31 (1.13–1.15)
de Wit et al. (2010)	1.18 (1.01–1.37)	1.32 (1.23–1.40)	1.00 (0.76–1.31)

Note: Studies included in meta-analyses utilized population- or community-based samples (not clinical samples). OR, Odds ratio; CI, Confidence interval.

between obesity and depression, and gender consistently emerged as a moderator.

Subsequent longitudinal studies not included in these reviews and meta-analyses have reported mixed findings. In a recent study of 2,981 participants from the Netherlands Study of Depression and Anxiety, greater BMI and waist circumference predicted a 17% increased risk of developing major depressive disorder over a 6-year period, even when controlling for other health factors (Gibson-Smith et al., 2016). Conversely, a longitudinal study of over 10,000 adults conducted by the Canadian National Population Health Survey found that obesity was a *negative* predictor of depression among men and was not a significant predictor of depression among women over a 12-year period (Gariepy, Wang, Lesage, & Schmitz, 2010). Another study of 4,643 participants in the Coronary Artery Risk Development in Young Adults study found no relationship between initial BMI or waist circumference and subsequent depressive symptoms over a 20-year period (Needham, Epel, Adler, & Kiefe, 2010). Thus, further research is needed to clarify whether individuals with obesity in the population are, on the whole, at increased risk for developing depression.

Anxiety and Substance Use

In addition to depression, obesity may increase the risk for anxiety disorders. A systematic review of 16 population studies that assessed the relationship between obesity and anxiety disorders (2 longitudinal and 14 cross-sectional) found a moderate increased risk of anxiety disorders among individuals with obesity (Gariepy, Nitka, & Schmitz, 2010). The authors conducted a meta-analysis of 13 of the cross-sectional studies and reported a pooled OR of 1.40, with consistent results across gender. However, a subsequent prospective study conducted by Pickering et al. (2011) demonstrated no increased risk of anxiety disorders among men or women, highlighting the need for further research.

Limited research has addressed the relationship between obesity and other psychiatric disorders in the general population, but some studies suggest a *reduced* likelihood of substance use disorders among individuals with obesity (Mather, Cox, Enns, & Sareen, 2009; Scott et al., 2008; Simon et al., 2006). These effects may be particularly present among men (Pickering et al., 2011) and African Americans (Rosen-Reynosos, Alegria, Chen, Laderman, & Roberts, 2011). However, Petry, Barry, Pietrzak, and Wagner (2008) reported an *increased* lifetime prevalence of alcohol use disorders among adults with obesity. Only Pickering et al. (2011) examined this relationship prospectively, and more research is needed to delineate the potential mechanisms by which obesity may affect the likelihood of substance abuse and dependence.

Body Dissatisfaction

Although not a mental disorder in and of itself, body dissatisfaction is a well-established psychological consequence of obesity, particularly for women (Schwartz & Brownell, 2004). Friedman and Brownell (1995) conducted a meta-analysis of the relationship between obesity and body dissatisfaction and reported a large effect size ($d = 0.85$). In one study of over 1,700 U.S. women ages 40 years and older with overweight/obesity, 47.6% of women indicated that they were not satisfied with their body size (Anderson, Eyler, Galuska, Brown, & Brownson, 2002). This finding is consistent with prior work by Sarwer, Wadden, and Foster (1998), which found that women with obesity seeking weight loss ($n = 79$) reported greater body dissatisfaction than controls ($n = 43$), and 8% of women exhibited body image disturbance comparable to body dysmorphic disorder. The clinical significance of body image becomes clear when considering evidence that dissatisfaction may partially account for depression among women with obesity (Gavin, Simon, & Ludman, 2010), and weight and shape concerns may have an equivalent impact on psychosocial impairment as physical health status for both men and women (van Zutven, Mond, Latner, & Rodgers, 2015).

Risk Factors Associated with Mental Health in Individuals with Obesity

Several key demographic and clinical characteristics have been identified as potential determinants of heightened risk for psychological distress among individuals with obesity. Specifically, heightened risk of impaired mental health is associated with gender, severe obesity, seeking treatment, and BED.

Gender

Most studies to date have found no differences or conflicting findings regarding the role of demographic characteristics such as race, ethnicity, socioeconomic status (SES), and age in the relationship between obesity and mental health (Heo, Pietrobelli, Fontaine, Sirey, & Faith, 2006; Hicken et al., 2013; Preiss, Brennan, & Clarke, 2013; Rosen-Reynosos et al., 2011). However, research evidence in this area has consistently pointed to the importance of gender. As previously noted, women with obesity may be particularly vulnerable to depression. In a cross-sectional examination of 8,410 participants in the National Health and Nutrition Examination Survey (NHANES) III data, only women with obesity had increased risk for depression, with 6.7% of women with obesity meeting criteria for depression in the past month, compared to 2.9% of men (Onyike, Crum, Lee, Lyketsos, & Eaton, 2003). A 2013 systematic review of moderators in the relationship between obesity and depression found that female gender was associated with greater risk of depression in 12 of 20 cross-sectional studies (Preiss et al., 2013).

Subsequent longitudinal studies have added to the body of evidence supporting a differential and heightened risk for depression among women with obesity (Geoffroy, Li, & Power, 2014; Konttinen et al., 2014; Pan, Sun, et al., 2012; Pickering et al., 2011). Among 701 adolescents followed prospectively into adulthood in the Children in the Community Study, female (but not male) participants who had obesity in adolescence were almost four times more likely to develop a subsequent anxiety disorder or major depressive disorder across 20 years than female participants without overweight or obesity (Anderson, Cohen, Naumova, Jacques, & Must, 2007). Of note, gender differences have not consistently appeared in relation to obesity and anxiety disorders in other large-scale studies (Dalrymple, Martinez, Rosenstein, Kneeland, & Zimmerman, 2015; Mather et al., 2009). As described earlier, women are more likely to experience body dissatisfaction than men (Schwartz & Brownell, 2004).

Severe and Abdominal Obesity

Individuals with severe obesity are at heightened risk for depression (Preiss et al., 2013). In the aforementioned cross-sectional examination of the NHANES III data (Onyike et al., 2003), 6.7% of women with any level of obesity and 13% of women with class 3 obesity had depression in the preceding month (as determined by structured clinical interviews); rates among men were 2.9% and 11.5%, respectively. Analyses demonstrated that only women (and not men) with obesity had an increased prevalence of past-month depression in comparison to individuals in the normal-weight range, but *both* women and men with class 3 obesity had a heightened prevalence of past-month depression (ORs = 3.78 and 7.68, respectively). An examination of 1,857 women in the 2005–2006 NHANES sample revealed a dose-dependent relationship between BMI and depression, such that increased risk of moderate to severe depressive symptoms and major depression began at a BMI of 30 kg/m^2. Women with class 3 obesity exhibited 4.9 times the risk of depression compared to women with class 1 obesity (Ma & Xiao, 2010). The increased odds of depression among individuals with severe obesity tend to be consistent across race and gender, even when controlling for obesity-related comorbidities (Dong, Sanchez, & Price, 2004; Zhao et al., 2009).

Apart from BMI-based assessments of severe obesity, abdominal or central obesity may also be associated with increased risk for depression. In a systematic review and meta-analysis of the relationship between abdominal obesity and depression, individuals with abdominal obesity had a 38% increased risk of depression in comparison to individuals without obesity (Xu, Anderson, & Lurie-Beck, 2011). These results were consistent across age and gender, suggesting that when severe obesity is defined by waist circumference rather than BMI, its relationship with depression persists. However, a longitudinal study of 2,540 older adults not included in the review demonstrated an increased risk of depression only for men (and not women) with abdominal obesity, independent of overall obesity (Vogelzangs et al., 2010). Some studies have reported no significant associations between waist circumference and risk for depression when adjusting for BMI and medical conditions (Ma & Xiao, 2010; Zhao et al., 2011). However, one study ($N = 293$) found that individuals with central obesity who did and did not have metabolic syndrome had equivalent prevalence rates of mood and anxiety disorders (Carpiniello, Pinna, Velluzzi, & Loviselli, 2012). Another study of 1,066 individuals with type 2 diabetes reported a significant association between abdominal obesity and depressive symptoms (Labad et al., 2010). These findings suggest that the relationship between abdominal obesity and mental disorders may exist independent of obesity-related health comorbidities.

Treatment-Seeking Individuals

Several decades of research have demonstrated that individuals with obesity who seek treatment for weight loss tend to have greater psychopathology than individuals with obesity who do not seek care, suggesting that distress may be a driving motivation for individuals with obesity to seek weight reduction (Fitzgibbon, Stolley, & Kirschenbaum, 1993; Friedman & Brownell, 1995; Stunkard & Wadden, 1992). Patients seeking weight loss through bariatric surgery have particularly high rates of mental disorders. In a recent meta-analysis of 59 publications assessing the mental health of patients seeking and undergoing bariatric surgery, depression was the most common disorder (prevalence estimate = 19%), followed by BED (17%) and anxiety (12%; Dawes et al., 2016). The presence of any mood disorder was 23%, which was significantly elevated in comparison to the U.S. general population estimate of 10%. Individuals seeking bariatric surgery may exhibit elevated risk of mental disorders in comparison to other treatment-seeking individuals. Wadden et al. (2006) evaluated 149 women with class 3 obesity seeking bariatric surgery, in comparison to 90 women with class 1 or 2 obesity seeking behavioral weight control. Investigators administered the Beck Depression Inventory–II (Beck, Ward, Mendelson, Mock, & Erbaugh, 1961), Rosenberg Self-Esteem Scale (Rosenberg, 1965), and Weight and Lifestyle Inventory (Wadden & Foster, 2006). Women seeking bariatric surgery reported lower self-esteem and greater symptoms of depression than the women with less severe obesity seeking behavioral weight loss. These findings may reflect the greater severity of obesity among patients seeking bariatric surgery and/or suggest that individuals seeking more intensive forms of weight loss treatment have heightened psychological vulnerability.

BED

Eating disorders (BED, in particular) are associated with increased risk for impaired psychosocial status. In a population-based study of 2,163 twins assessed with structured clinical interviews and the 42-item Symptom Checklist (Derogatis, 1983), women who engaged in binge eating and had obesity reported worse physical health and mental health (e.g., lifetime history of depression, panic disorder, and alcohol dependence) than women with obesity who did not binge-eat (Bulik, Sullivan, & Kendler, 2002). With regard to clinical samples, a study by Rosenberger, Henderson, and Grilo (2006) assessed 174 bariatric patients via structured clinical interviews. Patients diagnosed with an eating disorder (13.8%), including BED (4.6%), were significantly more likely to have another current or lifetime psychiatric diagnosis than patients without an eating disorder (Rosenberger et al., 2006). Specifically, 66.7% of bariatric patients with an eating disorder met criteria for a lifetime comorbid diagnosis, whereas only 26.7% of patients without an eating disorder met criteria for one lifetime psychiatric diagnosis. Similar findings have been reported in other studies, in which both patients seeking bariatric surgery and community samples of individuals with obesity who meet criteria for BED exhibited greater depressive symptoms, perceived stress, eating pathology (including body dissatisfaction), negative affect, and state and trait anxiety than individuals without BED (Klatzkin, Gaffney, Cyrus, Bigus, & Brownley, 2015; Vinai et al., 2015). Evidence suggests that a BED diagnosis may be more predictive than obesity severity of poorer psychosocial quality of life (Perez & Warren, 2012), emphasizing the need to address BED symptoms when treating obesity.

Impact of Obesity on Quality of Life

In addition to specific mental disorders and symptoms, obesity negatively affects overall quality of life (QoL). Broadly defined, QoL encompasses the overall impact of disease (i.e., obesity) on functioning and well-being (Fontaine & Barofsky, 2001; Kolotkin, Meter, & Williams, 2001). A large body of research has investigated health-related quality of life (HRQoL), and more specifically, weight-related quality of life.

Health- and Weight-Related QoL

Assessed with measures such as the Medical Outcomes Study 36-Item Short-Form Health Survey (SF-36; McHorney, Ware, Lu, & Sherbourne, 1994) and the Impact of Weight on Quality of Life Lite (IWQoL; Kolotkin, Crosby, Kosloski, & Williams, 2001), health- and weight-related QoL include impairments due to perceptions of health, bodily pain, difficulty fulfilling physical or social roles, low energy, mobility, public distress, sexual dysfunction, self-esteem, and emotional problems (Fontaine & Barofsky, 2001; Kolotkin, Meter, & Williams, 2001). Two reviews published in 2001 summarized evidence from cross-sectional studies demonstrating associations between obesity and poorer physical and mental health functioning, and from longitudinal studies suggesting a link between weight gain and reductions in HRQoL (Fontaine & Barofsky, 2001; Kolotkin, Meter, & Williams, 2001). More recently, Jia and Lubetkin (2010) assessed quality-adjusted life-years (QALYs) lost due to obesity, which was defined as a measure of disease burden based on reductions in HRQoL scores in 1 year (or morbidity) and projected premature death or mortality. Results indicated that from 1993 to 2008, QALYs lost due to obesity increased by 127% among U.S. adults and were comparable to QALYs lost due to smoking. Sexual quality of life is also worse among individuals with obesity (Kolotkin et al., 2006). This relationship may be attributable, in part, to the impact of excess weight and obesity-related comorbidities (such as type 2 diabetes) on reproductive hormones and sexual dysfunction, as well as to psychosocial factors (e.g., depression and body image) that may affect sexual function and satisfaction (Sarwer, Lavery, & Spitzer, 2012).

As with specific mental health outcomes, certain subgroups of individuals with obesity may be more prone to impaired QoL. Women and African Americans with obesity seem to experience worse QoL than men and European Americans with obesity (Hassan, Joshi, Madhavan, & Amonkar, 2003; Katz, McHorney, & Atkinson, 2000; Kolotkin, Meter, & Williams, 2001), although one study found that European Americans with obesity had poorer QoL than African Americans (Kolotkin, Crosby, & Williams, 2002). Additionally, higher levels of obesity tend to be associated with poorer QoL (Kolotkin, Meter, & Williams, 2001). For example, results from a large population-based sample (N = 182,372) demonstrated that individuals with severe obesity experienced more "unhealthy" and limited activity days (due to impaired mental or physical health) than individuals in other weight categories (Hassan et al., 2003). Treatment-seeking individuals also appear to be more impaired than individuals with obesity who do not seek weight loss (Kolotkin, Crosby, & Williams, 2002).

Obesity-related physical health comorbidity—including pain, sleep apnea, metabolic syndrome, type 2 diabetes, and cardiovascular disease—is another prominent clinical risk factor for impaired QoL. In a sample of 500 patients with severe obesity, chronic pain and sleep apnea emerged as consistent predictors of reduced HRQoL (Warkentin et al., 2014). Cross-sectional data from a population-based study (N = 44,800) found that the relationship between BMI and QoL was mediated by joint pain and other obesity-related comorbidities such as diabetes and hypertension (Heo, Allison, Faith, Zhu, & Fontaine, 2003). Several cross-sectional and longitudinal studies have also documented relationships between metabolic syndrome and depression (Heiskanen et al., 2006; Kahl et al., 2015; Pan, Keum, et al., 2012), even when controlling for BMI (Skilton, Moulin, Terra, & Bonnet, 2007). Similarly, type 2 diabetes may be associated with a moderately increased risk of depression (Ali,

Stone, Peters, Davies, & Khunti, 2006) and worse HRQoL among individuals with obesity, particularly if they experience diabetes-related complications (Coffey et al., 2002; Redekop et al., 2002). Of note, some studies have not found significant associations between metabolic syndrome or type 2 diabetes and HRQoL when controlling for factors such as BMI and depression (Kolotkin, Crosby, & Williams, 2003; Tsai et al., 2008; Vetter et al., 2011). However, participants in these samples may have had particularly low levels of QoL overall (Kolotkin et al., 2003), and disease burden still emerged as a predictor of reduced HRQoL (Vetter et al., 2011).

Disability and Socioeconomic Consequences

Disability due to obesity represents another form of psychosocial impairment that impacts QoL through socioeconomic consequences. Data from the NHANES sample ($N = 9,928$) indicate that older adults with obesity are over two times more likely to report functional impairment and limitations in activities of daily living (ADLs) than individuals without obesity, and the prevalence of functional impairment among individuals with obesity increased by 5.4% between the 1988–1994 and 1999–2004 waves (Alley & Chang, 2007). Furthermore, in a sample of 12,725 older adults, hazard ratios for ADL disability over the course of 7 years were found to be heightened for individuals with classes 1, 2, or 3 obesity, with increasing risk at each class (Snih et al., 2007). Reduced mobility, functioning (including ability to work), and disability-free days due to obesity have been consistently documented in other cross-sectional and longitudinal investigations (Peeters, Bonneux, Nusselder, DeLaet, & Barendregt, 2004; Sturm, Ringel, & Andreyeva, 2004; Vincent, Vincent, & Lamb, 2010).

Disability may, in part, explain trends in reduced employment and the consequent income inequality among individuals with obesity. For example, data from a prospective national cohort study (from 1986 to 1999; $N = 4,290$) suggest that obesity leads to reduced employment and, for women, increased work limitations (Tunceli, Li, & Williams, 2006). Indeed, individuals with obesity have higher unemployment rates (even when considering educational attainment), spend fewer years employed, and, once unemployed, are less likely to regain employment (Morris, 2006; Paraponaris, Saliba, & Ventelou, 2005). Evidence of a wage penalty due to obesity exists for both men and women, and the wage gap between those with and without obesity has been increasing in recent decades (Baum & Ford, 2004). Women with obesity appear to be more affected by disability than men, with lower occupational status (i.e., less skilled work) and greater income inequality (Morris, 2006; Wardle, Waller, & Jarvis, 2002). However, health limitations do not account entirely for occupational impairment (Baum & Ford, 2004). The impact of weight-based stigma and discrimination on socioeconomic disparities and other psychosocial outcomes also must be considered.

Summary

Evidence from population-based and longitudinal studies suggests a modestly heightened risk of depression due to obesity, particularly for women. Individuals with obesity also report body dissatisfaction and impaired quality of life, including disability. More prospective research is needed to clarify the causal relationship between obesity and other mental health disorders, such as anxiety and substance use disorders. Importantly, several key risk factors consistently predict poorer psychosocial status among individuals with obesity: female gender, severe obesity, seeking treatment, and BED. In the following material we highlight a prominent mechanism in the relationship between obesity and psychosocial outcomes—weight stigmatization—and review the evidence of its impact on mental health and quality of life.

Weight Stigmatization: An Important Consideration

Individuals with obesity are vulnerable to negative societal stigma and discrimination because of their weight. In general, *weight stigma* refers to negative social devaluation of people with overweight or obesity (Tomiyama, 2014). This devaluation can lead to weight-based stereotypes (e.g., widely held beliefs that individuals with obesity tend to be lazy or lacking in discipline), prejudice (e.g., preconceived negative attitudes toward a person solely because of his or her weight), and overt discrimination (e.g., unfair treatment of people who have obesity, such as inequitable workplace practices against employees with obesity). National estimates indicate that reports of weight discrimination have increased in recent decades and that weight discrimination is among the most common forms of discrimination reported by women and men (Puhl, Andreyeva, & Brownell, 2008). Research has documented pervasive weight stigma in a range of daily life settings, including employment, educational institutions, and health care, as well as in interpersonal relationships and in the mass media (Puhl & Heuer, 2009). Thus, individuals with obesity are vulnerable to prejudice and unfair treatment in multiple life domains. These experiences of weight stigmatization may help explain why people with obesity are vulnerable to adverse psychosocial consequences. Indeed, research has increasingly highlighted societal weight stigma as an important mechanism explaining links between obesity and adverse psychological functioning (Faith et al., 2011).

Research consistently indicates that experiences of weight stigma may increase risk for adverse psychological outcomes. In a large, nationally representative study of U.S. adults with overweight or obesity (N = 22,231), perceived (self-reported) weight discrimination was significantly associated with psychiatric morbidity and comorbidity, even after adjusting for stress and BMI (Hatzenbuehler, Keyes, & Hasin, 2009). A recent review of 23 studies examining correlates of perceived weight stigma and discrimination similarly showed that these experiences are consistently associated with poor mental health—increased depression, anxiety, stress, and substance use—in both community and clinical samples of adults (Papadopoulos & Brennan, 2015). These findings support evidence from a recent meta-analysis documenting perceived weight discrimination (as with other forms of discrimination) to be negatively correlated with psychological well-being (including longitudinal evidence; Schmitt, Branscombe, Postmes, & Garcia, 2014). Furthermore, studies examining mechanisms underlying links between obesity and poor mental health have found that weight stigmatization significantly mediates associations between BMI and body dissatisfaction and between BMI and depressive symptoms (Stevens, Herbozo, Morrell, Schaefer, & Thompson, 2017). Importantly, much of the research that has examined the relationship between weight stigmatization and psychological functioning has controlled for BMI (Hatzenbuehler et al., 2009; Papadopoulos & Brennan, 2015), indicating that it is stigmatizing experiences, rather than obesity, per se, that appear to be harmful to mental health.

Beyond psychological distress, considerable research has identified adverse consequences of weight stigma for weight-related health behaviors. A systematic review of recent literature (60 studies) documented consistent evidence of health consequences associated with weight stigma, including increased food intake, binge eating, reduced physical activity, elevated physiological stress, and weight gain (Puhl & Suh, 2015). Randomized experimental studies have documented adverse effects on food consumption of exposure to weight stigma. These experiments randomly assigned women (who varied in BMI) to a manipulated exposure to weight stigma or a control condition (exposure to neutral stimuli), and showed that, immediately following exposure to stigma, women who were overweight (but not thinner women) ate significantly more calories, felt less able to control their eating, had an increased desire for food, and had an increased likelihood of binge eating compared to those in control groups (Brochu & Dovidio, 2014; Chao, Yang, & Chiou, 2012; Major, Hunger, Bunyan, & Miller, 2014; Schvey, Puhl, & Brownell, 2011). These findings suggest that individuals exposed to weight stigma may turn to food as an emotional response to these distressing experiences—a response that may help to explain why weight stigmatization has been documented as a unique predictor of binge eating beyond other established risk factors (Almeida, Savoy, & Boxer, 2011; Durso, Latner, & Hayashi, 2012). Internalization of weight stigma (i.e., the extent to which a person blames him- or herself for negative weight-based stereotypes) has also been found to make significant, independent contributions to eating disorder pathology, after controlling for depression and self-esteem, regardless of obesity or BED status (Durso, Latner, White, et al., 2012). Vartanian and Porter (2016) have provided a comprehensive review of associations between weight stigma and eating behaviors.

In addition to eating behaviors, evidence suggests that weight stigma may have negative implications for physical activity and physiological stress. Research in community and clinical samples of adults has found that experienced and internalized weight stigma negatively affects exercise motivation, willingness to participate in physical activity, and perceived competence in physical activity (Pearl, Puhl, & Dovidio, 2014; Schmalz, 2010; Vartanian & Novak, 2011). Evidence has also documented increased cortisol reactivity in response to exposure to or experiences of weight stigma, as well as greater blood pressure and oxidative stress, independent of adiposity (Dutton et al., 2014; Schvey, Puhl, & Brownell, 2014; Tomiyama et al., 2014). Perceived weight discrimination has also been identified as a stressor that increases the adverse effects of waist-to-hip ratio on glycemic control (Tsenkova, Carr, Schoeller, & Ryff, 2011). Although this area of research is still in its infancy, existing evidence suggests that perceiving oneself as a target of weight stigma or discrimination may induce physiological stress responses that contribute to increased adiposity and metabolic comorbidities of obesity.

This body of work linking weight stigma to food intake, binge eating, physical activity, and stress indicates that stigmatizing experiences may lead to obesity-promoting responses and behaviors. Recent longitudinal studies confirm the predictive role of weight stigma on weight trajectories. A nationally representative longitudinal study (*N* = 6,157) from the Health and Retirement Study found that, regardless of baseline BMI, individuals who reported experiences of weight discrimination (but not other forms of discrimination, e.g., race or sexual orientation) were 2.5–3.0 times more likely to become obese or remain obese 4 years later compared to those who did not report weight discrimination (Sutin & Terracciano, 2013). Similarly, evidence from the English Longitudinal Study of Aging demonstrated that, independent of baseline BMI, adults (*N* = 2,944) who reported perceived weight discrimination had higher odds of becoming obese (OR = 6.67) and experienced significant increases in weight and waist circumference (Jackson, Beeken, & Wardle, 2014).

Taken together, evidence of the harmful psychological and physical health consequences associated with weight stigma suggests that this issue warrants attention as an important factor affecting psychosocial aspects of obesity, and may be a key mechanism linking body weight with psychosocial functioning and distress (see Figure 10.1). Although weight stigma can be considered a significant psychosocial consequence of obesity, it may also lead to health-risk behaviors that contribute to obesity and reinforce weight gain.

Implications for Clinical Practice

The longitudinal evidence highlighted in this chapter suggests that clinicians should not assume that individuals with obesity have mental disorders or impaired psychological functioning. Many individuals with obesity do not present with these problems, and there is insufficient evidence to conclude that psychological disorders definitively lead to obesity or weight gain. Still, effective clinical management of obesity requires an approach that recognizes the psychosocial factors that may adversely affect the emotional well-being of some patients with obesity. This approach includes an understanding of characteristics that may increase patient vulnerability to adverse psychosocial experiences. Patients with obesity at heightened risk for psychological distress include women and individuals who have severe obesity, those who are seeking treatment, and those who binge-eat. In addition, despite the co-occurrence of obesity with problems such as depression, these conditions are rarely treated concurrently (Faulconbridge, Wadden, Berkowitz, Pulcini, & Treadwill, 2011). Targeting symptoms of depression and stress as part of behavioral weight loss interventions may help improve treatment outcomes (Elder et al., 2012).

More broadly, the evidence to date signals a need for clinical attention to specific psy-

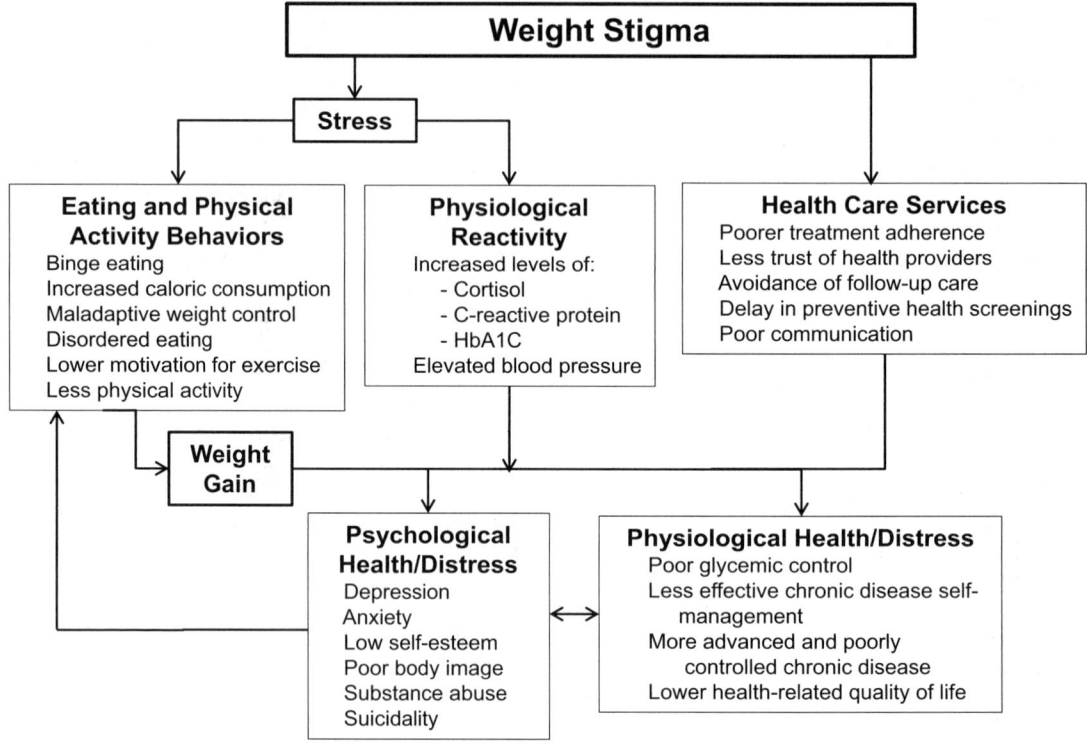

FIGURE 10.1. Health consequences resulting from experiences of weight stigma. From Puhl, Phelan, Nadglowski, and Kyle (2016). Overcoming weight bias in the management of patients with diabetes and obesity. *Clinical Diabetes, 34,* 44–50. Reprinted with permission from the American Diabetes Association, Inc. Copyright © 2016.

chosocial factors that should be assessed, monitored, and potentially integrated into interventions in the obesity management for some patients. Early detection and implementation of strategies to address depression, anxiety, stress, body dissatisfaction, and emotional or binge-eating patterns may help to reduce psychological distress and behaviors that could otherwise interfere with improved weight-related health. Obesity-focused interventions could be strengthened by screening and addressing these shared risk factors. Although more research is needed to clarify which psychosocial factors may be more or less detrimental for short-term weight loss versus long-term weight regulation, the evidence supports monitoring psychosocial symptoms during the course of treatment.

Given the deleterious consequences that weight stigma poses for emotional and physical health and its role as a likely mediator between obesity and psychological distress, we believe that weight stigma can interfere with effective obesity prevention and treatment. Accordingly, addressing experienced and internalized weight stigma of patients as part of clinical interventions for obesity could improve health outcomes and/or prevent weight regain by helping patients adopt strategies to cope with the impact of weight stigma and the associated emotional distress. To date, few obesity-focused clinical interventions have included components to help patients cope with weight stigma, but limited evidence suggests that doing so may have benefits for both emotional well-being and weight outcomes (Carels et al., 2014; Lillis, Hayes, Bunting, & Masuda, 2009). Given that weight stigma is a common experience for individuals with obesity and appears to hinder efforts to engage in behaviors that are necessary to achieve and sustain weight loss, including provisions of treatment that address stigma seems warranted. Research is needed to identify what types of clinical interventions are most effective at reducing the psychological impact of stigma and improving general functioning.

Finally, stigma expressed by health providers toward patients with obesity can negatively affect patient–provider interactions and reduce quality of patient care (Phelan et al., 2015). Even the terminology that clinicians use to discuss a patient's body weight can have negative implications for that patient's future health care utilization (Puhl, Peterson, & Luedicke, 2013). Thus, in addition to addressing negative psychological consequences resulting from weight stigma experienced by patients, it is important for clinicians (1) to be mindful of personal attitudes and biases that could unintentionally interfere with quality of care and (2) to implement strategies to avoid and reduce bias in clinical practice. Several stigma-reduction interventions have been tested and found to reduce weight biases among medical trainees (Dietz et al., 2015). Thus, increasing awareness and education about weight bias among health professionals through evidence-based methods and resources may help improve delivery of care to patients with obesity.

Conclusion

The evidence reviewed in this chapter suggests caution in assuming that psychological factors necessarily precipitate or result from obesity. Although a subset of individuals with obesity may be vulnerable to psychological distress (e.g., those with binge eating or severe obesity), it is important to acknowledge the heterogeneity of obesity and that the psychological status of individuals with obesity varies considerably. Pervasive societal weight stigmatization may contribute to and exacerbate adverse psychological and physical health outcomes for people with obesity. The deleterious effects of weight stigma deserve attention in research as an underlying mechanism linking psychosocial functioning and obesity, and in clinical settings as a psychosocial factor that may impede obesity prevention and treatment. Thus, it is important for the clinical management of obesity to be guided by an appreciation of the heterogeneous nature of obesity, an understanding of psychosocial vulnerabilities that may adversely affect some patients, and a recognition of the harmful impacts of stigmatization on individuals with obesity, underscoring the importance of providing compassionate, supportive care.

References

Alberga, A. S., Sigal, R. J., Goldfield, G., Prud'homme, D., & Kenny, G. P. (2012). Overweight and obese teenagers: Why is adolescence a critical period? *Pediatric Obesity, 7*(4), 261–273.

Ali, S., Stone, M. A., Peters, J. L., Davies, M. J., & Khunti, K. (2006). The prevalence of co-morbid depression in adults with type 2 diabetes: A systematic review and meta-analysis. *Diabetes Medicine, 23*(11), 1165–1173.

Alley, D. E., & Chang, V. W. (2007). The changing relationship between obesity and disability, 1988–2004. *Journal of the American Medical Association, 298*(17), 2020–2027.

Almeida, L., Savoy, S., & Boxer, P. (2011). The role of weight stigmatization in cumulative risk for binge eating. *Journal of Clinical Psychology, 67*(3), 278–292.

Anderson, L. A., Eyler, A. A., Galuska, D. A., Brown, D. R., & Brownson, R. C. (2002). Relationship of satisfaction with body size and trying to lose weight in a national survey of overweight and obese women aged 40 and older, United States. *Preventive Medicine, 35*(4), 390–396.

Anderson, S. E., Cohen, P., Naumova, E. N., Jacques, P. F., & Must, A. (2007). Adolescent obesity and risk for subsequent major depressive disorder and anxiety disorder: Prospective evidence. *Psychosomatic Medicine, 69*(8), 740–747.

Atlantis, E., & Baker, M. (2008). Obesity effects on depression: Systematic review of epidemiological studies. *International Journal of Obesity, 32*(6), 881–891.

Barnes, R. D., Blomquist, K. K., & Grilo, C. M. (2011). Exploring pretreatment weight trajectories in obese patients with binge eating disorder. *Comprehensive Psychiatry, 52*, 312–318.

Baum, C. L., & Ford, W. F. (2004). The wage effects of obesity: A longitudinal study. *Health Economics, 13*(9), 885–899.

Beck, A. T., Ward, C. H., Mendelson, M., Mock, J., & Erbaugh, J. (1961). An inventory for measuring depression. *Archives of General Psychiatry, 4*, 561–571.

Berkowitz, R. I., & Fabricatore, A. N. (2011). Obesity, psychiatric status, and psychiatric medications. *Psychiatric Clinics of North America, 34*(4), 747–764.

Berset, M., Semmer, N. K., Elfering, A., Jacobshagen, N., & Meier, L. L. (2011). Does stress at work make you gain weight?: A two-year longitudinal study. *Scandinavian Journal of Work, Environment and Health, 37*(1), 45–53.

Björntorp, P. (2001). Do stress reactions cause abdominal obesity and comorbidities? *Obesity Reviews, 2*(2), 73–86.

Bodenlos, J. S., Lemon, S. C., Schneider, K. L., August, M. A., & Pagoto, S. L. (2011). Associations of mood and anxiety disorders with obesity: Comparisons by ethnicity. *Journal of Psychosomatic Research, 71*(5), 319–324.

Brochu, P. M., & Dovidio, J. F. (2014). Would you like fries (380 calories) with that?: Menu labeling mitigates the impact of weight-based stereotype threat on food choice. *Social Psychological and Personality Science, 5,* 414–421.

Brumpton, B., Langhammer, A., Romundstad, P., Chen, Y., & Mai, X. M. (2013). The associations of anxiety and depression symptoms with weight change and incident obesity: The HUNT Study. *International Journal of Obesity, 37*(9), 1268–1274.

Bulik, C. M., Sullivan, P. F., & Kendler, K. S. (2002). Medical and psychiatric morbidity in obese women with and without binge eating. *International Journal of Eating Disorders, 32*(1), 72–78.

Calzo, J. P., Sonneville, K. R., Haines, J., Blood, E. A., Field, A. E., & Austin, S. B. (2012). The development of associations among BMI, body dissatisfaction, and weight and shape concern in adolescent boys and girls. *Journal of Adolescent Health, 51*(5), 517–523.

Carels, R. A., Burmeister, J. M., Koball, A. M., Oehlhof, M. W., Hinman, N., LeRoy, M., et al. (2014). A randomized trial comparing two approaches to weight loss: Differences in weight loss maintenance. *Journal of Health Psychology, 19*(2), 296–311.

Carpiniello, B., Pinna, F., Velluzzi, F., & Loviselli, A. (2012). Mental disorders in patients with metabolic syndrome: The key role of central obesity. *Eating and Weight Disorders, 17*(4), e259–e266.

Chao, Y. H., Yang, C. C., & Chiou, W. B. (2012). Food as ego-protective remedy for people experiencing shame: Experimental evidence for a new perspective on weight-related shame. *Appetite, 59*(2), 570–575.

Chiriboga, D. E., Ma, Y., Li, W., Olendzki, B. C., Pagoto, S. L., Merriam, P. A., et al. (2008). Gender differences in predictors of body weight and body weight change in healthy adults. *Obesity, 16*(1), 137–145.

Coffey, J. T., Brandle, M., Zhou, H., Marriott, D., Burke, R., Tabaei, B. P., et al. (2002). Valuing health-related quality of life in diabetes. *Diabetes Care, 25*(12), 2238–2243.

Dalrymple, K. L., Martinez, J., Rosenstein, L., Kneeland, E. T., & Zimmerman, M. (2015). Psychiatric disorder–weight associations and the moderative effect of sex in an outpatient psychiatric sample. *Annals of Clinical Psychiatry, 27*(2), 108–117.

Dawes, A. J., Maggard-Gibbons, M., Maher, A. R., Booth, M. J., Miake-Lye, I., Beroes, J. M., et al. (2016). Mental health conditions among patients seeking and undergoing bariatric surgery: A meta-analysis. *Journal of the American Medical Association, 315*(2), 150–163.

de Wit, L., Luppino, F., Straten, A. V., Penninx, B.,
Zitman, F., & Cuijpers, P. (2010). Depression and obesity: A meta-analysis of community-based studies. *Psychiatry Research, 178*(2), 230–235.

Derogatis, L. (1983). *SCL-90-R administration, scoring, and procedures manual.* Baltimore: Clinical Psychometric Research.

Dietz, W. H., Baur, L. A., Hall, K., Puhl, R. M., Taveras, E. M., Uauy, R., et al. (2015). Management of obesity: Improvement of healthcare training and systems for prevention and care. *Lancet, 385*(9986), 2521–2533.

Dong, C., Sanchez, L. E., & Price, R. A. (2004). Relationship of obesity to depression: A family-based study. *International Journal of Obesity, 28*(6), 790–795.

Durso, L. E., Latner, J. D., & Hayashi, K. (2012). Perceived discrimination is associated with binge eating in a community sample of non-overweight, overweight, and obese adults. *Obesity Facts, 5*(6), 869–880.

Durso, L. E., Latner, J. D., White, M. A., Masheb, R. M., Blomquist, K. K., Morgan, P. T., et al. (2012). Internalized weight bias in obese patients with binge eating disorder: Associations with eating disturbances and psychological functioning. *International Journal of Eating Disorders, 45*(3), 423–427.

Dutton, G. R., Lewis, T. T., Durant, N., Halanych, J., Kiefe, C. I, Sidney, S., et al. (2014). Perceived weight discrimination in the CARDIA study: Differences by race, sex, and weight status. *Obesity, 22*(2), 530–536.

Elder, C. R., Gullion, C. M., Funk, K. L., DeBar, L. L., Lindberg, N. M., & Stevens, V. J. (2012). Impact of sleep, screen time, depression and stress on weight change in the intensive weight loss phase of the LIFE study. *International Journal of Obesity, 36*(1), 86–92.

Faith, M. S., Butryn, M., Wadden, T. A., Fabricatore, A., Nguyen, A. M., & Heymsfield, S. B. (2011). Evidence for prospective associations among depression and obesity in population-based studies. *Obesity Reviews, 12*(5), e438–e453.

Faulconbridge, L. F., Wadden T. A., Berkowitz, R. I., Pulcini, M. E., & Treadwill, T. (2011). Treatment of comorbid obesity and major depressive disorder: A prospective pilot study for their combined treatment. *Journal of Obesity, 9,* 870385.

Field, A. E., Sonneville, K. R., Crosby, R. D., Swanson, S. A., Eddy, K. T., Camargo, C. A., et al. (2014). Prospective associations of concerns about physique and the development of obesity, binge drinking, and drug use among adolescent boys and young adult men. *JAMA Pediatrics, 168*(1), 34–39.

Fiske, L., Fallon, E. A., Blissmer, B., & Redding, C. A. (2014). Prevalence of body dissatisfaction among United States adults: Review and recommendations for future research. *Eating Behaviors, 15*(3), 357–365.

Fitzgibbon, M. L., Stolley, M. R., & Kirschenbaum, D. S. (1993). Obese people who seek treatment have different characteristics than those who do not seek treatment. *Health Psychology, 12*(5), 342–345.

Fontaine, K. R., & Barofsky, I. (2001). Obesity and health-related quality of life. *Obesity Reviews, 2*(3), 173–182.

Friedman, M. A., & Brownell, K. D. (1995). Psychological correlates of obesity: Moving to the next research generation. *Psychological Bulletin, 117*(1), 3–20.

Gariepy, G., Nitka, D., & Schmitz, N. (2010). The association between obesity and anxiety disorders in the population: A systematic review and meta-analysis. *International Journal of Obesity, 34*(3), 407–419.

Gariepy, G., Wang, J., Lesage, A. D., & Schmitz, N. (2010). The longitudinal association from obesity to depression: Results from the 12-year National Population Health Survey. *Obesity, 18*(5), 1033–1038.

Gavin, A. R., Simon, G. E., & Ludman, E. J. (2010). The association between obesity, depression, and educational attainment in women: The mediating role of body dissatisfaction. *Journal of Psychosomatic Research, 69*(6), 573–581.

Geoffroy, M. C., Li, L., & Power, C. (2014). Depressive symptoms and body mass index: Co-morbidity and direction of association in a British birth cohort followed over 50 years. *Psychological Medicine, 44*(12), 2641–2652.

Gibson-Smith, D., Bot, M., Paans, N. P. G., Visser, M., Brouwer, I., & Penninx, B. W. J. H. (2016). The role of obesity measures in the development and persistence of major depressive disorder. *Journal of Affective Disorders, 198*, 222–229.

Goldschmidt, A. B., Wall, M., Tse-Hwei, J. C., Becker, C., & Neumark-Sztainer, D. (2016). Shared risk factors for mood-, eating-, and weight-related health outcomes. *Health Psychology, 35*(3), 245–252.

Gormally, J., Black, S., Daston, S., & Rardin, D. (1982). The assessment of binge eating severity among obese persons. *Addictive Behaviors, 7*(1), 47–55.

Harding, J. L., Backholer, K., Williams, E. D., Peeters, A., Cameron, A. J., Hare, M. J., et al. (2014). Psychosocial stress is positively associated with body mass index gain over 5 years: Evidence from the longitudinal AusDiab study. *Obesity, 22*(1), 277–286.

Hassan, M. K., Joshi, A. V., Madhavan, S. S., & Amonkar, M. M. (2003). Obesity and health-related quality of life: A cross-sectional analysis of the US population. *International Journal of Obesity, 27*(10), 1227–1232.

Hatzenbuehler, M. L., Keyes, K. M., & Hasin, D. S. (2009). Associations between perceived weight discrimination and the prevalence of psychiatric disorders in the general population. *Obesity, 17*(11), 2033–2039.

Heiskanen, T. H., Niskanen, L. K., Hintikka, J. J., Koivumaa-Honkanen, H. T., Honkalampi, K. M., Haatainen, K. M., et al. (2006). Metabolic syndrome and depression: A cross-sectional analysis. *Journal of Clinical Psychiatry, 67*(9), 1422–1427.

Heo, M., Allison, D. B., Faith, M. S., Zhu, S., & Fontaine, K. R. (2003). Obesity and quality of life: Mediating effects of pain and comorbidities. *Obesity Research, 11*(2), 209–216.

Heo, M., Pietrobelli, A., Fontaine, K. R., Sirey, J. A., & Faith, M. S. (2006). Depressive mood and obesity in US adults: Comparison and moderation by sex, age, and race. *International Journal of Obesity, 30*(3), 513–519.

Hicken, M. T., Lee, H., Mezuk, B., Kershaw, K. N., Rafferty, J., & Jackson, J. S. (2013). Racial and ethnic differences in the association between obesity and depression in women. *Journal of Women's Health, 22*(5), 445–452.

Ibrahim, M., Thearle, M. S., Krakoff, J., & Gluck, M. E. (2016). Perceived stress and anhedonia predict short- and long-term weight change, respectively, in healthy adults. *Eating Behaviors, 21*, 214–219.

Ivezaj, V., Kalebjian, R., Grilo, C. M., & Barnes, R. D. (2014). Comparing weight gain in the year prior to treatment for overweight and obese patients with and without binge eating disorder in primary care. *Journal of Psychosomatic Research, 77*(2), 151–154.

Jackson, S. E., Beeken, R. J., & Wardle, J. (2014). Perceived weight discrimination and changes in weight, waist circumference, and weight status. *Obesity, 22*(12), 2485–2488.

Jia, H., & Lubetkin, E. I. (2010). Trends in quality-adjusted life-years lost contributed by smoking and obesity. *American Journal of Preventive Medicine, 38*(2), 138–144.

Kahl, K. G., Schweiger, U., Correll, C., Muller, C., Busch, M., Bauer, M., et al. (2015). Depression, anxiety disorders, and metabolic syndrome in a population at risk for type 2 diabetes mellitus. *Brain and Behavior, 5*(3), e00306.

Katz, D. A., McHorney, C. A., & Atkinson, R. L. (2000). Impact of obesity on health-related quality of life in patients with chronic illness. *Journal of General Internal Medicine, 15*(11), 789–796.

Klatzkin, R. R., Gaffney, S., Cyrus, K., Bigus, E., & Brownley, K. A. (2015). Binge eating disorder and obesity: Preliminary evidence for distinct cardiovascular and psychological phenotypes. *Physiology and Behavior, 142*, 20–27.

Kolotkin, R. L., Binks, M., Crosby, R. D., Ostbye, T., Gress, R. E., & Adams, T. D. (2006). Obesity and sexual quality of life. *Obesity, 14*(3), 472–479.

Kolotkin, R. L., Crosby, R. D., Kosloski, K. D., & Williams, G. R. (2001). Development of a brief measure to assess quality of life in obesity. *Obesity Research, 9*(2), 102–111.

Kolotkin, R. L., Crosby, R. D., & Williams, G. R. (2002). Health-related quality of life varies among obese subgroups. *Obesity Research, 10*(8), 748–756.

Kolotkin, R. L., Crosby, R. D., & Williams, G. R. (2003). Assessing weight-related quality of life in obese persons with type 2 diabetes. *Diabetes Research and Clinical Practice, 61*(2), 125–132.

Kolotkin, R. L., Meter, K., & Williams, G. R. (2001). Quality of life and obesity. *Obesity Reviews, 2*(4), 219–229.

Konttinen, H., Kiviruusu, O., Huurre, T., Haukkala, A., Aro, H., & Marttunen, M. (2014). Longitudinal associations between depressive symptoms and body mass index in a 20-year follow-up. *International Journal of Obesity, 38*(5), 668–674.

Labad, J., Price, J. F., Strachan, M. W. J., Fowkes, F. G. R., Ding, J., Deary, I. J., et al. (2010). Symptoms of depression but not anxiety are associated with central obesity and cardiovascular disease in people with type 2 diabetes: The Edinburgh Type 2 Diabetes Study. *Diabetologia, 53*(3), 467–471.

Lasserre, A. M., Glaus, J., Vandeleur, C. L., Marques-Vidal, P., Vaucher, J., Bastardot, F., et al. (2014). Depression with atypical features and increase in obesity, body mass index, waist circumference, and fat mass: A prospective, population-based study. *JAMA Psychiatry, 71*(8), 880–888.

Lillis, J., Hayes, S. C., Bunting, K., & Masuda, A. (2009). Teaching acceptance and mindfulness to improve the lives of the obese: A preliminary test of a theoretical model. *Annals of Behavioral Medicine, 37*(1), 58–69.

Loth, K. A., Watts, A. W., van den Berg, P., & Neumark-Sztainer, D. (2015). Does body satisfaction help or harm overweight teens?: A 10-year longitudinal study of the relationship between body satisfaction and body mass index. *Journal of Adolescent Health, 57*(5), 559–561.

Luppino, F. S., Wit, L. M. D., Bouvy, P. F., Stijnen, T., Cuijpers, P., Penninx, B. W. J. H., et al. (2010). Overweight, obesity, and depression: A systematic review and meta-analysis of longitudinal studies. *Archives of General Psychiatry, 67*(3), 220–229.

Ma, J., & Xiao, L. (2010). Obesity and depression in US women: Results from the 2005–2006 National Health and Nutritional Examination Survey. *Obesity, 18*(2), 347–353.

Major, B., Hunger, J. M., Bunyan, D. P., & Miller, C. T. (2014). The ironic effects of weight stigma. *Journal of Experimental Social Psychology, 51*, 74–80.

Manzato, E., Bolognesi, A., Simoni, M., & Cuzzolaro, M. (2015). Risk factors for weight gain: A longitudinal study in non-weight loss treatment-seeking overweight adults. *Eating and Weight Disorders—Studies on Anorexia, Bulimia and Obesity, 20*(3), 371–378.

Mather, A. A., Cox, B. J., Enns, M. W., & Sareen, J. (2009). Associations of obesity with psychiatric disorders and suicidal behaviors in a nationally representative sample. *Journal of Psychosomatic Research, 66*(4), 277–285.

McHorney, C. A., Ware, J. E., Lu, J. F., & Sherbourne, C. D. (1994). The MOS 36-item Short-Form Health Survey (SF-36): III. Tests of data quality, scaling assumptions, and reliability across diverse patient groups. *Medical Care, 32*(1), 40–66.

Meany, G., Conceição, E., & Mitchell, J. E. (2014). Binge eating, binge eating disorder and loss of control eating: Effects on weight outcomes after bariatric surgery. *European Eating Disorders Review, 22*(2), 87–91.

Mintem, G. C., Gigante, D. P., & Horta, B. L. (2015). Change in body weight and body image in adults: A longitudinal study. *BMC Public Health, 15*, 222–228.

Morris, S. (2006). Body mass index and occupational attainment. *Journal of Health Economics, 25*(2), 347–364.

Mouchacca, J., Abbott, G. R., & Ball, K. (2013). Associations between psychological stress, eating, physical activity, sedentary behaviours and body weight among women: A longitudinal study. *BMC Public Health, 13*(1), 828.

Needham, B. L., Epel, E. S., Adler, N. E., & Kiefe, C. (2010). Trajectories of change in obesity and symptoms of depression: The CARDIA study. *American Journal of Public Health, 100*(6), 1040–1046.

Onyike, C. U., Crum, R. M., Lee, H. B., Lyketsos, C. G., & Eaton, W. W. (2003). Is obesity associated with major depression?: Results from the Third National Health and Nutrition Examination Survey. *American Journal of Epidemiology, 158*(12), 1139–1147.

Pan, A., Keum, N., Okereke, O. I., Sun, Q., Kivimaki, M., Rubin, R. R., et al. (2012). Bidirectional association between depression and metabolic syndrome. *Diabetes Care, 35*(5), 1171–1180.

Pan, A., Sun, Q., Czernichow, S., Kivimaki, M., Okereke, O. I., Lucas, M., et al. (2012). Bidirectional association between depression and obesity in middle-aged and older women. *International Journal of Obesity, 36*(4), 595–602.

Papadopoulos, S., & Brennan, L. (2015). Correlates of weight stigma in adults with overweight and obesity: A systematic literature review. *Obesity, 23*(9), 1743–1760.

Paraponaris, A., Saliba, B., & Ventelou, B. (2005). Obesity, weight status and employability: Empirical evidence from a French national survey. *Economics and Human Biology, 3*(2), 241–258.

Pearl, R. L., Puhl, R. M., & Dovidio, J. F. (2014). Differential effects of weight bias experiences and internalization on exercise among women with overweight and obesity. *Journal of Health Psychology, 20*(12), 1626–1632.

Peeters, A., Bonneux, L., Nusselder, W. J., DeLaet, C., & Barendregt, J. J. (2004). Adult obesity and the burden of disability throughout life. *Obesity Research, 12*(7), 1145–1151.

Perez, M., & Warren, C. S. (2012). The relationship between quality of life, binge-eating disorder, and obesity status in an ethnically diverse sample. *Obesity, 20*(4), 879–885.

Petry, N. M., Barry, D., Pietrzak, R. H., & Wagner, J. A. (2008). Overweight and obesity are associated with psychiatric disorders: Results from the National Epidemiologic Survey on Alcohol and Related Conditions. *Psychosomatic Medicine, 70*(3), 288–297.

Phelan, S. M., Burgess, D. J., Yeazel, M. W., Hellerstedt, W. L., Griffin, J. M., & van Ryn, M. (2015). Impact of weight bias and stigma on quality of care and outcomes for patients with obesity. *Obesity Reviews, 16*(4), 319–326.

Pickering, R. P., Goldstein, R. B., Hasin, D. S., Blanco, C., Smith, S. M., Huang, B., et al. (2011). Temporal relationships between overweight and obesity and

DSM-IV substance use, mood, and anxiety disorders: Results from a prospective study. *Journal of Clinical Psychiatry, 72*(11), 1494–1502.

Preiss, K., Brennan, L., & Clarke, D. (2013). A systematic review of variables associated with the relationship between obesity and depression. *Obesity Reviews, 14*(11), 906–918.

Puhl, R., Andreyeva, T., & Brownell, K. (2008). Perceptions of weight discrimination: Prevalence and comparison to race and gender discrimination in America. *International Journal of Obesity, 32*(6), 992–1000.

Puhl, R. M., & Heuer, C. A. (2009). The stigma of obesity: A review and update. *Obesity, 17*(5), 941–964.

Puhl, R. M., Peterson, J. L., & Luedicke, J. (2013). Motivating or stigmatizing?: Public perceptions of language about weight used by health providers. *International Journal of Obesity, 37*(4), 612–619.

Puhl, R. M., Phelan, S., Nadglowski, J., & Kyle, T. (2016). Overcoming weight bias in the management of patients with diabetes and obesity. *Clinical Diabetes, 34*, 44–50.

Puhl, R. M., & Suh, Y. (2015). Health consequences of weight stigma: Implications for obesity prevention and treatment. *Current Obesity Reports, 4*(2), 182–190.

Quick, V., Wall, M., Larson, N., Haines, J., & Neumark-Sztainer, D. (2013). Personal, behavioral and socio-environmental predictors of overweight incidence in young adults: 10-yr longitudinal findings. *International Journal of Behavior, Nutrition, and Physical Activity, 10*(1), 37.

Redekop, W. K., Koopmanschap, M. A., Stolk, R. P., Rutten, G. E. H. M., Wolffenbuttel, B. H. R., & Niessen, L. W. (2002). Health-related quality of life and treatment satisfaction in Dutch patients with type 2 diabetes. *Diabetes Care, 25*(3), 458–463.

Rosenberg, M. (1965). *Society and the adolescent self-image*. Princeton, NJ: University Press.

Rosenberger, P. H., Henderson, K. E., & Grilo, C. M. (2006). Psychiatric disorder comorbidity and association with eating disorders in bariatric surgery patients: A cross-sectional study using structured interview-based diagnosis. *Journal of Clinical Psychiatry, 67*(7), 1080–1085.

Rosen-Reynosos, M., Alegria, M., Chen, C., Laderman, M., & Roberts, R. (2011). The relationship between obesity and psychiatric disorders across ethnic and racial minority groups in the United States. *Eating Behaviors, 12*(1), 1–8.

Roy, M., Shatenstein, B., Gaudreau, P., Morais, J., & Payette, H. (2014). Seniors' body weight dissatisfaction and longitudinal associations with weight changes, anorexia of aging, and obesity: Results from the NuAge study. *Journal of Aging and Health, 27*(2), 220–238.

Sarwer, D. B., Lavery, M., & Spitzer, J. C. (2012). A review of the relationship between extreme obesity, quality of life, and sexual function. *Obesity Surgery, 22*(4), 668–676.

Sarwer, D. B., Wadden, T. A., & Foster, G. D. (1998). Assessment of body dissatisfaction in obese women: Specificity, severity, and clinical significance. *Journal of Consulting and Clinical Psychology, 66*(4), 651–654.

Schmalz, D. L. (2010). "I feel fat": Weight-related stigma, body esteem, and BMI as predictors of perceived competence in physical activity. *Obesity Facts, 3*(1), 15–21.

Schmitt, M. T., Branscombe, N. R., Postmes, T., & Garcia, A. (2014). The consequences of perceived discrimination for psychological well-being: A meta-analytic review. *Psychological Bulletin, 140*(4), 921–948.

Schvey, N. A., Puhl, R. M., & Brownell, K. D. (2011). The impact of weight stigma on caloric consumption. *Obesity, 19*(10), 1957–1962.

Schvey, N. A., Puhl, R. M., & Brownell, K. D. (2014). The stress of stigma: Exploring the effect of weight stigma on cortisol reactivity. *Psychosomatic Medicine, 76*(2), 156–162.

Schwartz, M. B., & Brownell, K. D. (2004). Obesity and body image. *Body Image, 1*(1), 43–56.

Scott, K. M., Bruffaerts, R., Simon, G. E., Alonso, J., Angermeyer, M., deGirolamo, G., et al. (2008). Obesity and mental disorders in the general population: Results from the World Mental Health Surveys. *International Journal of Obesity, 32*(1), 192–200.

Simon, G. E., VonKorff, M., Saunders, K., Miglioretti, D. L., Crane, P. K., vanBelle, G., et al. (2006). Association between obesity and psychiatric disorders in the US adult population. *Archives of General Psychiatry, 63*(7), 824–830.

Skilton, M. R., Moulin, P., Terra, J., & Bonnet, F. (2007). Associations between anxiety, depression, and the metabolic syndrome. *Biological Psychiatry, 62*(11), 1251–1257.

Slade, P. D., Dewey, M. E., Newton, T., Brodie, D., & Kiemle, G. (1990). Development and preliminary validation of the Body Satisfaction Scale (BSS). *Psychology and Health, 4*(3), 213–220.

Snih, S. A., Ottenbacher, K. J., Markides, K. S., Kuo, Y., Eschbach, K., & Goodwin, J. S. (2007). The effect of obesity on disability vs mortality in older adults. *Archives of Internal Medicine, 167*(8), 774–780.

Sonneville, J. R., Calzo, J. P., Horton, N. J., Haines, J., Austin, S. B., & Field, A. E. (2013). Body satisfaction, weight gain, and binge eating among overweight and adolescent girls. *International Journal of Obesity, 36*(7), 944–949.

Stevens, S. D., Herbozo, S., Morrell, H. E. R., Schaefer, L. M., & Thompson, J. K. (2017). Adult and childhood weight influence body image and depression through weight stigmatization. *Journal of Health Psychology, 22*(8), 1084–1093.

Stunkard, A. J., & Wadden, T. A. (1992). Psychological aspects of severe obesity. *American Journal of Clinical Nutrition, 55*(2), 524S–532S.

Sturm, R., Ringel, J. S., & Andreyeva, T. (2004). Increasing obesity rates and disability trends. *Health Affairs, 23*(2), 199–205.

Sutin, A. R., & Terracciano, A. (2013). Perceived weight discrimination and obesity. *PLOS ONE, 8*(7), e70048.

Tomiyama, A. J. (2014). Weight stigma is stressful: A review of evidence for the cyclic obesity/weight-based stigma model. *Appetite, 82,* 8–15.

Tomiyama, A. J., Epel, E. S., McClatchey, T. M., Poelke, G., Kemeny, M. E., McCoy, S. K., et al. (2014). Associations of weight stigma with cortisol and oxidative stress independent of adiposity. *Health Psychology, 33*(8), 862–867.

Tsai, A. G., Wadden, T. A., Sarwer, D. B., Berkowitz, R. I., Womble, L. G., Hesson, L. A., et al. (2008). Metabolic syndrome and health-related quality of life in obese individuals seeking weight reduction. *Obesity, 16*(1), 59–63.

Tsenkova, V. K., Carr, D., Schoeller, D. A., & Ryff, C. D. (2011). Perceived weight discrimination amplifies the link between central adiposity and nondiabetic glycemic control (HbA1c). *Annals of Behavioral Medicine, 41*(2), 243–251.

Tunceli, K., Li, K., & Williams, L. K. (2006). Long-term effects of obesity on employment and work limitations among U.S. adults from 1986 to 1999. *Obesity, 14*(9), 1637–1646.

van Reedt Dortland, A., Giltay E. J., van Veen, R., Zitman, F. G., & Penninx, B. (2013). Longitudinal relationship of depressive and anxiety symptoms with dyslipidemia and abdominal obesity. *Psychosomatic Medicine, 75*(1), 83–89.

van Strien, T., Konttinen, H., Homberg, J. R., Engels, R. C., & Winkens, L. H. (2016). Emotional eating as a mediator between depression and weight gain. *Appetite, 100,* 216–224.

van Zutven, K., Mond, J., Latner, J., & Rodgers, B. (2015). Obesity and psychosocial impairment: Mediating roles of health status, weight/shape concerns and binge eating in a community sample of women and men. *International Journal of Obesity, 39*(2), 346–352.

Vartanian, L. R., & Novak, S. A. (2011). Internalized societal attitudes moderate the impact of weight stigma on avoidance of exercise. *Obesity, 19*(4), 757–762.

Vartanian, L. R., & Porter, A. M. (2016). Weight stigma and eating behavior: A review of the literature. *Appetite, 105*(2), 3–14.

Vetter, M. L., Wadden, T. A., Lavenberg, J., Moore, R. H., Volger, S., Perez, J. L., et al. (2011). Relation of health-related quality of life to metabolic syndrome, obesity, depression, and comorbid illnesses. *International Journal of Obesity, 35*(8), 1087–1094.

Vinai, P., DaRos, A., Speciale, M., Gentile, N., Tagliabule, A., Vinai, P., et al. (2015). Psychopathological characteristics of patients seeking for bariatric surgery, either affected or not by binge eating disorder following the criteria of the DSM IV TR and of the DSM 5. *Eating Behaviors, 16,* 1–4.

Vincent, H. K., Vincent, K. R., & Lamb, K. M. (2010). Obesity and mobility disability in the older adult. *Obesity Reviews, 11*(8), 568–579.

Vogelzangs, N., Kritchevsky, S. B., Beekman, A. T. F., Brenes, G. A., Newman, A. B., Satterfield, S., et al. (2010). Obesity and onset of significant depressive symptoms: Results from a community-based cohort of older men and women. *Journal of Clinical Psychiatry, 71*(4), 391–399.

Wadden, T. A., Butryn, M. L., Sarwer, D. B., Fabriactore, A. N., Crerand, C. E., Lipschutz, P. E., et al. (2006). Comparison of psychosocial status in treatment-seeking women with class III vs. class I–II obesity. *Obesity, 14*(2, Suppl.), 90S–98S.

Wadden, T. A., Faulconbridge, L. F., Jones-Corneille, L. R., Sarwer, D. B., Fabricatore, A. N., Thomas, J. G., et al. (2011). Binge eating disorder and the outcome of bariatric surgery at one year: A prospective, observational study. *Obesity, 19*(6), 1220–1228.

Wadden, T. A., & Foster, G. D. (2006). Weight and lifestyle inventory (WALI). *Obesity, 14*(S3), 99S–118S.

Wadden, T. A., & Stunkard, A. J. (1985). Social and psychological consequences of obesity. *Annals of Internal Medicine, 103*(6), 1062–1072.

Wardle, J., Chida, Y., Gibson, E. L., Whitaker, K. L., & Steptoe, A. (2011). Stress and adiposity: A meta-analysis of longitudinal studies. *Obesity, 19*(4), 771–778.

Wardle, J., Waller, J., & Jarvis, M. J. (2002). Sex differences in the association of socioeconomic status with obesity. *American Journal of Public Health, 92*(8), 1299–1304.

Warkentin, L. M., Majumdar, S. R., Johnson, J. A., Agborsangaya, C. B., Rueda-Clausen, C. F., Sharma, A. M., et al. (2014). Predictors of health-related quality of life in 500 severely obese patients. *Obesity, 22*(5), 1367–1372.

Xu, Q., Anderson, D., & Lurie-Beck, J. (2011). The relationship between abdominal obesity and depression in the general population: A review and meta-analysis. *Obesity Research and Clinical Practice, 5*(4), e267–e278.

Zhao, G., Ford, E. S., Dhingra, S., Li, C., Strine, T. W., & Mokdad, A. H. (2009). Depression and anxiety among US adults: Associations with body mass index. *International Journal of Obesity, 33*(2), 257–266.

Zhao, G., Ford, E. S., Li, C., Tsai, J., Dhingra, S., & Balluz, L. S. (2011). Waist circumference, abdominal obesity, and depression among overweight and obese U.S. adults: National Health and Nutrition Examination Survey 2005–2006. *BMC Psychiatry, 11*(1), 130.

CHAPTER 11

Obesity, Eating Disorders, and Addiction

Courtney McCuen-Wurst
Kelly C. Allison

Obesity is now considered a disease by the American Medical Association, as described by others in this volume. It is not considered a psychiatric disorder, although there are forms of disordered eating that qualify as psychiatric conditions and appear to be associated with weight gain, thus potentially contributing to obesity. The two most common of these eating disorders are binge-eating disorder (BED) and night eating syndrome (NES), which are the focus of this chapter. Some mental health experts have suggested that obesity should be classified as a type of addiction. We examine this issue, as well as the similarities between compulsive eating and addiction, and the possible impact of an addiction diagnosis for persons with obesity.

Obesity as an Eating Disorder

If obesity causes distress and impairment in functioning for many, why would it not be considered a psychiatric condition? Diagnosing obesity as an eating disorder would be difficult, given many variables, including the fact that the definition of obesity does not include any emotional, behavioral, or cognitive features. In addition, obesity is influenced by many factors, such as genetics and environment, and many people who have obesity often maintain a stable weight, thus eating and exercising in an energy-balanced manner. Because eating patterns and weights vary tremendously among individuals at any given time and within individuals across time, establishing a fixed set of criteria, such as those typically used to diagnose psychiatric disorders, is impractical (Allison & Cirona-Singh, 2015). For example, not all persons with obesity engage in objective overeating episodes, daily grazing, or frequent eating out at fast-food or other restaurants. Only a minority displays these behaviors. Additionally, whereas some individuals with obesity are distressed about their weight status, many are not bothered by it and remain physically healthy. For all of these reasons, among many, obesity is not considered a psychiatric disorder.

BED

Diagnostic Criteria

BED is characterized by recurrent episodes of binge eating, which is described in the fifth edition of the *Diagnostic and Statistical Manual of Mental Disorders* (American Psychiatric Association, 2013) as eating an amount of food that is larger than what most people would eat in a similar situation in a discrete period of time (i.e., within 2 hours). A binge is also characterized by a sense of loss of control over eating during the time period in question (see Table 11.1). In addition, the binge episode must be accompanied by at least three of the following: eating much more rapidly than normal; eating until uncomfortably full; eating large amounts when not physically hungry; eating alone because of feeling embarrassed about how much one eats; and feeling disgusted, depressed, or guilty afterward. The recurrent episodes must also be marked by distress and occur at least once a week for 3 months (American Psychiatric Association, 2013).

Prevalence

Data from the World Health Organization Mental Health Survey Study indicate that BED is the most common of the eating disorders with an average lifetime prevalence of 1.4% in the general population; the lifetime risk is higher for women than men (Kessler et al., 2013). The data also show that BED is more common in upper-middle and high-income countries. In addition, individuals with BED have a significantly higher body mass index (BMI), on average, than respondents without an eating disorder. Among treatment-seeking adults with obesity, BED has a prevalence between 16% and 30% (de Zwaan, 2001; Kolotkin et al., 2004), with estimates varying depending on assessment method (interview vs. survey) and on which diagnostic criteria are used. Self-report data typically yield prevalence estimates two to three times greater than those determined by diagnostic interview.

Initially, BED was considered an adult disorder; however, recent research has suggested that the age of onset may be lower than first presumed. Findings suggest that the disorder occurs in children and adolescents, with the average age of onset ranging from the later teen years to earlier 20s (Kessler et al., 2013). Loss of control eating without eating an "objectively large amount" typically precedes onset of full BED when there is adolescent onset. Data also have shown that BED tends to be a steady condition in which patterns of binge eating are relatively stable, and the crossover rate to other eating disorders, such as anorexia nervosa and bulimia nervosa, is low in comparison to the crossover among those disorders (Peterson et al., 2012; Castellini et al., 2011).

Associated Features and Comorbidities

BED increases with increasing BMI (Hudson, Hiripi, Pope, & Kessler, 2007). Thus, BED frequently is seen in association with other complications of obesity, including musculoskeletal conditions, type 2 diabetes mellitus, asthma, cardiovascular disease, and obstructive sleep apnea (Kessler et al., 2013; Bulik, Sullivan, & Kendler, 2002). BED is also associated with an increased independent risk for various comorbidities,

TABLE 11.1. Defining the Core Aspects of a Binge: An "Objectively Large Amount of Food" and "Loss of Control"

There are two main guidelines for "objectively large amount of food":	1. The ingestion of two full meals (each including two or more courses). 2. The ingestion of three main courses. One's BMI and social context must also be taken into consideration.
Examples of descriptions of "loss of control" felt during binge-eating episodes:	1. You feel like you could not stop even if you wanted to stop. 2. It is like a ball that keeps rolling down a hill. Once it gets started, it is difficult to stop. 3. You would not stop eating to answer the telephone or the door. 4. You intend to only eat two or three pieces/items, but cannot stop until you eat the whole package. 5. You feel like there is no hope that you will be able to eat just one serving and resign yourself to the fact that you will eat until you are uncomfortably full.

including chronic pain, hypertension, and chronic headaches (Kessler et al., 2013). In a study conducted by Bulik et al. (2002), women with obesity and BED showed greater health dissatisfaction than women with obesity but without BED.

BED also is associated with elevated rates of psychiatric illnesses, including mood and substance use disorders. Data from the World Health Organization Mental Health Survey Study showed that 79% of respondents with BED also met criteria for other DSM-IV diagnoses (Kessler et al., 2013). Bulik et al. (2002) examined psychiatric comorbidity in women with obesity with and without BED, and found that lifetime binge eating was associated with significantly increased risks for major depression, phobia, alcohol dependence, and panic disorder. In addition, those with BED reported more symptoms of anxiety, psychomotor retardation/agitation, and insomnia, as well as negative personality characteristics, such as dependency and lower self-esteem.

Risk Factors

Research suggests that individuals with obesity and BED have an earlier onset of obesity than people with obesity but not BED; in addition, weight history tends to be more inconsistent (Spitzer et al., 1993). Findings are mixed with regard to the onset of binge eating in relation to dieting behavior, or dietary restriction, with some studies suggesting that dietary restraint most often precedes BED (Polivy & Herman, 1985; Polivy, 1996), and others suggesting that dietary restraint occurs prior to binge eating only about half the time (Stunkard & Allison, 2003). Wadden et al. (2004) prescribed moderate, mild, or no calorie restriction to women with obesity in a weight management trial and found little evidence that prolonged moderate restriction (i.e., 1,000 kcal/day for 12 weeks) precipitated binge-eating episodes compared with the two other interventions. In addition to binge episodes, studies examining the construct of cognitive restraint of eating have found that it results in preoccupation with food, as well as issues with concentration and mood disturbance, including dysphoria and irritability (Polivy, 1996). Low mood and negative feelings have also been suggested as risk factors for the development of BED.

Neurobiological processes related to self-regulation, which assist in the regulation of eating behaviors, are often highly influenced by emotions (Heatherton & Wagner, 2011). Different theories that have described the function of binge eating include the affect regulation model, which posits that binge eating reduces negative feelings (Womble, Williamson, & Martin, 2001). As indicated by Haedt-Matt and Keel (2011), the affect regulation model suggests that binge eating in response to negative emotion is maintained by negative reinforcement. Escape theory similarly suggests that binge eating is used as a strategy to avoid feeling negative emotions. Individuals with negative self-assessment and affect are motivated to decrease self-awareness in order to escape negative emotion. Binge eating may narrow awareness to simple actions and sensations, including rewarding tastes (Heatherton & Baumeister, 1991; Paxton & Diggens, 1997). These theories often include at least one of these two elements: negative emotions as a trigger for a binge-eating episode, or relief of a negative emotion through binge eating. Based on these theories, binge eating can be considered a form of "emotional eating" (Nicholls, Devonport, & Blake, 2016).

Treatment

A meta-analysis by Voks et al. (2010) concluded that psychotherapies and structured self-help programs are more effective in the treatment of BED than weight loss treatments and pharmacotherapy. In particular, cognitive-behavioral therapy (CBT) has been the most rigorously evaluated and developed of the psychotherapies (Amianto, Ottone, Daga, & Fassino, 2015). CBT is the best established treatment for BED, receiving a "grade of A" for strong empirical evidence based on a recommendation from NICE (National Institute for Health and Clinical Excellence, 2004; Grilo, Masheb, Wilson, Gueorguieva, & White, 2011). The CBT approach is based on the belief that eating patterns become problematic and, in addition to weight and shape concerns, result in extreme dietary restriction. The goal of treatment is to disrupt the cycle of restraint and binge eating by promoting healthier, more structured eating patterns and improving concerns about shape, weight, and self-esteem, as discussed by Grilo (Chapter 34, this volume). CBT utilizes self-monitoring and the promotion of flexible thinking to reduce binge eating (Iacovino, Gredysa, Altman, & Wilfley, 2012).

Interpersonal therapy (IPT) is a brief, focused treatment that has been examined as an alternate intervention that emphasizes interpersonal problems, which have been commonly observed in individuals with BED (Tanofsky-Kraff et al., 2007). This type of psychotherapy focuses on problem resolution in four domains: grief, interpersonal role disputes, role transitions, and interpersonal deficits (Wilfley et al., 2002). In a study conducted by Wilfley et al. (2002), 162 patients with overweight meeting criteria for BED were randomized into group CBT or group IPT for 20 weeks. The researchers found that, for the primary outcomes, results for the intention-to-treat analyses and the completer analyses did not differ by treatment at any time point (Wilfley et al., 2002). The authors reported analyses for the completers showing that 82% of CBT patients and 74% of IPT patients did not continue to have binge episodes posttreatment, and 72% and 70% were abstinent at the 12-month follow-up, respectively. In regard to improvement (binge eating less than 4 days per month), 94% of CBT and 90% of IPT patients improved; at a 12-month follow-up, 84% and 89%, respectively, were improved. Lastly, at posttreatment, 85% of the CBT and 75% of the IPT participants endorsed a global eating disorders psychopathology equal to or below a sample of patients with obesity without binge eating. At a 12-month follow-up, the rates were 28% and 27%, respectively (Wilfley et al. 2002). This study found little difference in effectiveness between CBT and IPT (Wilfley et al., 2002).

Although psychotherapies like CBT have been shown to be effective in reducing binge-eating episodes (40–60% remission rates), these therapies do not produce significant weight loss (Wilson, Grilo, & Vitousek, 2007). Behavioral weight loss (BWL) treatment, reviewed by Gomez-Rubalcava, Stabbert, and Phelan (Chapter 20, this volume), is successful in inducing a mean weight loss of 7–8 kg (7–8% of initial weight) in persons with obesity. It does so by prescribing a calorie deficit of 500–750 kcal/day and increasing physical activity (to 180 minutes/week) to promote weight loss. BWL appears to be more effective than CBT in producing short-term weight loss (Berkman et al., 2015; Wilson, Wilfley, Agras, & Bryson, 2010). In a study by Grilo et al. (2011), 125 participants with obesity and BED were randomly assigned to one of three conditions: CBT, BWL, or CBT plus BWL. All three treatments produced improvements in binge eating and psychopathology at the end of treatment. Binge-eating remission rates posttreatment were 44.4% for CBT, 37.8% for BWL, and 48.6% for the combination treatment. Mean BMI reductions were −0.5, −2.6, and −2.7 kg/m^2 for the CBT, BWL, and combination treatments, respectively, indicating that both BWL and CBT plus BWL had significantly greater reductions than CBT alone. However, CBT was superior to BWL in reducing binge-eating episodes through the 12-month follow-up, whereas BWL produced greater BMI reductions during treatment and posttreatment, with absolute differences of −0.9 and −2.0 kg/m^2, respectively. Participants who received the combined treatment had a BMI reduction of −1.5 kg/m^2. At the 12-month follow-up, the superiority of BWL over CBT for BMI reduction was no longer significant.

In a recent report by Berkman et al. (2015) that focused on the management and outcomes of BED, a summary of evidence-based treatments was provided based on a comparison of two systematic reviews that examined randomized controlled trials (see Table 11.2). The authors searched for additional evidence that would allow them to address the efficacy of specific treatment approaches more comprehensively. According to the report, various forms of CBT (therapist-led CBT was most significant, followed by structured self-help and partially therapist-led CBT) were superior to a wait-list control in achieving abstinence from and reducing frequency of binge-eating episodes. In addition, modest evidence exists for both IPT and dialectical behavior therapy (DBT) as alternative therapies for facilitating achieving abstinence from and reducing the frequency of binge-eating episodes, compared to wait-list controls. However, the evidence is limited due to the lack of rigorous

TABLE 11.2. Definitions of the Grades of Overall Strength of Evidence for BED Treatments According to Berkman et al. (2015)

Grade	Definition	Examples of interventions
High	Confidence that the estimate of effect lies close to the true effect for this outcome. The body of evidence has no or few deficiencies; the findings are stable.	1. Therapist-led CBT vs. wait list ☐ Increased abstinence ☐ Decreased frequency per week ☐ Decreased eating-related psychopathology 2. Lisdexamfetamine vs. placebo 3. Second-generation antidepressants vs. placebo
Moderate	Moderate confidence that the estimate of effect lies close to the true effect for this outcome. The body of evidence has some deficiencies; the findings are likely to be stable, but some doubt remains.	1. Therapist-led CBT vs. BWL ☐ BWL decreased BMI more than CBT at end of treatment. 2. Therapist-led CBT vs. wait list ☐ No differences were found in BMI or symptoms of depression topiramate vs. placebo
Low	Limited confidence that the estimate of effect lies close to the true effect for this outcome. The body of evidence has major or numerous deficiencies (or both). Additional evidence is needed before concluding either that the findings are stable or that the estimate of effect is close to the true effect.	1. Partially therapist-led CBT vs. structured self-help CBT 2. Partially therapist-led CBT vs. wait list 3. Structured self-help CBT vs. wait list 4. Guided self-help CBT vs. wait list 5. Therapist-led CBT vs. partially therapist-led CBT 6. Therapist-led CBT vs. structured self-help CBT
Insufficient	No evidence is available, or the body of evidence has unacceptable deficiencies, precluding reaching a conclusion.	1. IPT 2. DBT

studies on these approaches. In agreement with other research, the report notes that although BWL helps patients lose weight, it is less effective than CBT for helping patients reach and maintain abstinence from and reduce the frequency of binge-eating episodes over the long term.

Research also suggests that pharmacotherapy may be effective in reducing the frequency of binge eating. Berkman et al. (2015) found evidence for the effectiveness of second-generation antidepressants in the treatment of BED. The data suggest that antidepressants were 1.67 times more likely than placebo to help patients abstain from binge eating. Antidepressants were also found to reduce the weekly frequency of binge eating by two-thirds of a binge episode per week, while also decreasing binge-related obsessive thoughts and compulsions. Furthermore, the review observed evidence of the effectiveness (in reducing weekly binge eating) of topiramate, an anticonvulsant medication, as well as lisdexamfetamine, a medication originally approved for attention-deficit/hyperactivity disorder (ADHD). At this time, lisdexamfetamine is the only medication approved by the U.S. Food and Drug Association (FDA) for the treatment of BED (Berkman et al., 2015; McElroy et al., 2015).

NES

Diagnostic Criteria

NES is characterized by a delay in the circadian pattern of eating, evidenced by recurrent episodes of night eating, which is described as either excessive food consumption in the evening (after dinnertime) or eating after awakening from sleep (i.e., nocturnal ingestions). In order to be diagnosed with NES, the individual must be conscious during eating episodes and be able to recall the eating episodes. These symptoms and behaviors must also cause significant distress and not be better explained by external factors (e.g., noises waking the person) or another disorder, such as a sleeping disorder or other disordered-eating pattern (i.e., sleep-related eating disorder; American Psychiatric Association, 2013). NES is classified in DSM-5 as an "other specified feeding or eating disorder."

Boston and colleagues examined the disparities in energy intake between individuals with NES as compared to those without NES through mathematical modeling (Boston, Moate, Allison, Lundgren, & Stunkard, 2008). Figure 11.1 illustrates a lack of regular meals and a significant delay in food intake across 24 hours among night eaters as compared to the controls. The model also suggests that persons with NES may be grazing throughout the latter portion of the day, indicating a role for structuring regular meal patterns during treatment.

Prevalence and Demographics

The prevalence of NES is estimated to be about 1–6% based on general population samples (Rand, Macgregor, & Stunkard, 1997; Striegel-Moore et al., 2005; Lamerz et al., 2005; Tholin et al., 2009; Colles, Dixon, & O'Brien, 2007; de Zwaan, Muller, Allison, Brahler, & Hilbert, 2014), suggesting that it may be as common as BED and more common than bulimia nervosa and anorexia nervosa. Studies have found that the prevalence is higher in persons who are

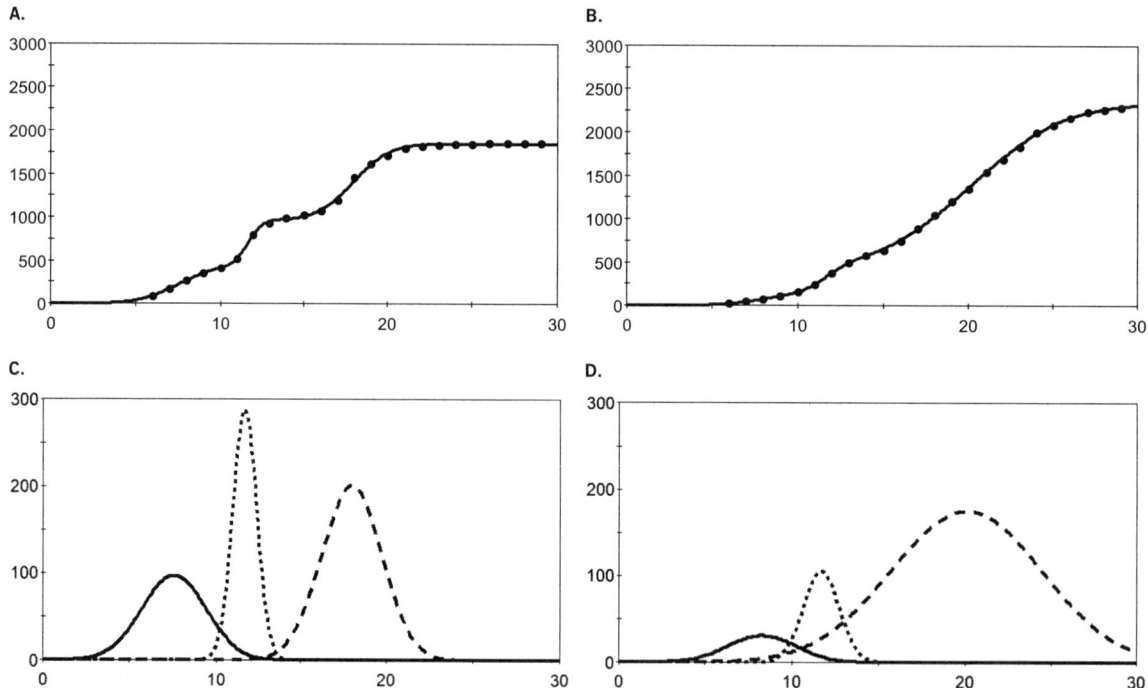

FIGURE 11.1. Modeling food intake for persons with night eating syndrome (NES) versus controls. (A and B) Cumulative caloric intake from 7-day food diaries for (B) participants with NES and (A) similar control participants. •, data; —, the model predictions. The top panels show that participants with NES (B; n = 148) have fewer distinct meals during the day, suggesting more grazing and less structured eating episodes, with eating continuing later in the day and calories surpassing similar control participants (A; n = 68) as the day progresses. (C and D) The bottom panels show use of the "Boston model" to illustrate the average cumulative caloric intake of individuals through estimations of the average rate of eating during a meal, peak intake rate, time of peak intake rate, and meal spread (i.e., intake duration). This model illustrates the disorganized nature—including fewer distinct meal episodes—and delayed pattern of food intake among those with NES (D) as compared to controls (C). From Boston, Moate, Allison, Lundgren, and Stunkard (2008). Modeling circadian rhythms of food intake by means of parametric deconvolution: Results from studies of the night eating syndrome. *American Journal of Clinical Nutrition, 87*(6), 1672–1677. Reprinted by permission.

overweight or obese, with up to 55% of individuals who seek bariatric surgery reporting some symptoms of NES (Gallant, Lundgren, & Drapeau, 2012). Interview-based studies, however, which carefully assessed diagnostic criteria for NES in surgery candidates, yielded much lower estimates; only 9% of patients in our bariatric surgery program met full criteria for NES (Allison et al., 2006).

NES typically begins during early adulthood (late teens to late 20s) and appears to be long-lasting, with periods of remission and relapse, often tied to life stressors (Marshall, Allison, O'Reardon, Birketvedt, & Stunkard, 2004; Napolitano, Head, Babyak, & Blumenthal, 2001). In one age and gender population survey, similar proportions of males and females reported waking at night to eat (Andersen, Stunkard, Sorensen, Petersen, & Heitmann, 2004). However, in an interview-based study of NES among Swedish Twin Registry participants, fewer men than women met full criteria for NES because they endorsed feeling distressed by their symptoms less often (Allison et al., 2014). This finding suggests that although this delayed eating pattern may be experienced fairly equally by men and women, women may be more affected psychologically.

Associated Features and Comorbidities

Although the prevalence of NES seems to increase with BMI, some studies suggest that there is no relationship between the two. Among the studies that have illustrated a positive link between NES and obesity, participants who screened positive for night eating in the Swedish Twin Registry's STAGE cohort showed an increased risk for obesity (2.5 times for men, 2.8 times for women; Tholin et al., 2009). In an outpatient clinical sample, psychiatric patients with NES were five times more likely to be obese than patients without NES (Lundgren et al., 2006). NES status also predicted weight gain in prospective studies. Over 6 years of follow-up, women with night eating (but not men) in the Danish MONICA study gained 5.2 kg more than women without night eating (Andersen et al., 2004). Finally, participants in an inpatient metabolic study who ate after 11 P.M. (considered night eating) were more likely to gain weight (mean 6.2 kg) over a 3.4-year follow-up period than were those without night eating habits (Gluck, Venti, Salbe, & Krakoff, 2008).

Some studies, however, observed no relationship between NES and higher BMI. Among samples of persons with obesity who sought treatment—including outpatient or inpatient BWL or bariatric surgery—at least five studies showed no differences in BMI between patients with and without NES (Adami, Campostano, Marinari, Ravera, Scopinaro, 2002; Allison et al., 2006; Cerú-Björk, Andersson & Rössner, 2001; Gluck, Geliebter, & Satov, 2001; Napolitano et al., 2001). One clinical sample recruited from general medical practices also showed no relationship between BMI and NES. Jarosz, Dobal, Wilson, and Schram (2007) showed that the prevalence of NES among a sample of black, urban women with obesity was 19%, substantially higher than figures cited from general population samples. However, BMI did not differ significantly in those with and without NES. Among general population samples, Striegel-Moore and colleagues studied samples from the National Health and Nutrition Examination Survey II and the Continuing Survey of Food Intakes by Individuals (Striegel-Moore, Franko, Thompson, Affenito, & Kraemer, 2006). They found no relationship between night eating (defined with various time parameters for late-night eating) and BMI. Striegel-Moore et al. (2005) also demonstrated that there was no relationship between BMI and night eating behaviors among a racially mixed sample of black and white young adult women.

There are a number of possible explanations for the inconsistent results regarding the relationship between NES and BMI. First, there could truly be no relationship between eating during the night and weight gain. This seems unlikely, but it would explain the absence of a clear correlation in the collective data. In our clinical experience, there are two presentations of NES. Many of our patients with NES who are of normal weight tend to restrict purposefully and/or over-exercise during the day to compensate for their night eating. This restriction increases the percentage of food they consume after dinner, and thus their night eating appears as more severe than the patients who do not engage in daytime compensation for their night eating. We see less of this compensatory behavior among our patients with overweight or obesity. Second, for samples that include only persons who have obesity, there may be a ceiling effect with BMI, such that no relationship would be observed. As there are many pathways to weight gain and obesity, NES would potentially represent just one of those pathways. Its influence may not contribute to obesity significantly more than other potential influences (e.g., BED, strong preferences for high-calorie foods). Finally, differences in the criteria used to define NES likely impact the nature of the relationship observed between weight status and NES.

Research demonstrates that NES has also been associated with psychiatric comorbidities, including mood and anxiety disorders. In addition, NES has been found to co-occur with other eating disorders, such as BED (de Zwaan et al., 2014; Tholin et al., 2009). In a study conducted by Tholin et al. (2009), male and female participants with NES had 3.4 and 3.6 times higher risk of binge eating compared to individuals without the syndrome. However, the genetic correlation between night eating and binge eating ($r = .66$) suggests that although there is significant overlap between these disorders, they are not genetically identical and do represent distinct disorders (Root et al., 2010).

Comorbidities with Sleep Disorders

One of the research diagnostic criteria for NES requires awareness and recall of the nocturnal eating episodes that occur. Sleep-related eating disorder (SRED) is a parasomnia in which patients sleepwalk and eat, typically with little to no awareness of their eating episodes. They may choose inedible substances to eat (e.g., shaving cream instead of ice cream) or cat food or frozen foods right out of the freezer. They may also injure themselves trying to prepare foods while in a somnolent state. The treatment is likely different for SRED as compared to NES, but patients have presented with mixed episodes—sometimes having awareness and sometimes not. Other times, patients report that their night eating episodes started as SRED, and although they gained awareness over the years, they were still unable to stop the behavior.

NES is also related to insomnia, as would be expected given that insomnia is part of the diagnostic criteria. In a study of the Swedish Twin Registry by Tholin et al. (2009), the risk of sleep-related problems was 1.6–3.4 times higher in men and 2.5–3.3 times higher in women with NES compared to those without NES.

Treatment

Research has suggested that NES has a serotonergic etiology, and as such, selective serotonin reuptake inhibitors (SSRIs) were the first agents tested in its treatment. Two open-label trials (O'Reardon, Stunkard, & Allison, 2004; Stunkard et al., 2006) and one randomized controlled trial of sertraline (O'Reardon et al., 2006) showed significant reductions in the number of nocturnal ingestions per night, percentage of food consumed after dinner, and a global measure of NES symptoms—the Night Eating Symptom Scale (Lundgren, Allison, Vinai, & Gluck, 2012). In the placebo-controlled trial, the sertraline group showed an 80% reduction in NES symptoms, compared to 14% in the placebo group. There also have been two studies with the SSRI escitalopram. Both the open-label study (Allison et al., 2013) and the randomized controlled trial with escitalopram (Vander Wal, Gang, Griffing, & Gadde, 2012) showed significant reductions in these same outcome measures, but the placebo-controlled trial did not show significant differences between the medication and placebo groups. The effect of the medication was weaker for black than for white participants.

Additional studies have found alternative treatments that may also reduce the symptoms of NES. In two case studies, bright light therapy was used to treat both seasonal depression and symptoms of NES. In one such study, a 51-year-old woman was being treated for depression with paroxetine; light therapy was added. After 14 daily sessions of white light for 30 minutes, the patient no longer met the DSM-IV criteria for depression or the core symptoms of NES. However, once the light treatment was discontinued, her symptoms of NES returned, although her depression remained in remission. After being treated for another 12 days with light therapy, her night eating symptoms remitted once more (Friedman, Even, Dardennes, & Guelfi, 2002).

Psychotherapy has also been shown to reduce night eating symptoms. Allison and colleagues developed a CBT approach that was administered in a pilot study to 25 patients over 12 weeks (Allison, Lundgren, Moore, O'Reardon, & Stunkard (2010). The intervention included building rapport, providing education about CBT, self-monitoring of sleep and eating disturbances and negative thoughts, development of coping skills, and, for those who were overweight or obese, behavioral weight management. At the end of the study, the participants showed significant reductions in caloric intake in the evening (after dinner), nocturnal ingestions, awakenings at night, and mood, as well as improvements in quality of life. They also lost a modest but significant amount of weight (3.1 kg).

Progressive muscle relaxation (PMR) has also been studied in an effort to determine alternative treatments for NES. PMR has been shown to reduce stress, which is often associated with NES. In a study conducted by Pawlow, O'Neil, and Malcolm (2003), 20 adults diagnosed with NES were randomized to either an abbreviated relaxation training group or a control group (sitting quietly for the same amount of time). Those in the treatment group displayed significantly less stress, anxiety, and salivary cortisol levels after 1 week of 20 minutes of muscle relaxation training per day, in addition to significantly higher morning and lower evening ratings of hunger. Those in the treatment condition also were more likely to eat breakfast and decrease nighttime eating. In a more recent study, Vander Wal and colleagues randomized 44 men and women to one of three groups: education, education plus PMR, or PMR plus exercise (Vander Wal, Maraldo, Vercellone, & Gagne, 2015). All three groups reported reduction in NES symptoms, as well as symptoms of depression, anxiety, and perceived stress. The only significant difference between groups was the percentage of food eaten after the evening meal, with the PMR group showing the greatest reduction, followed by the PMR plus exercise group and the educational group, respectively. Overall, more randomized controlled treatment trials of NES are needed to establish the same evidence-based literature for grading these treatment approaches as those describing treatments for BED.

Addiction

Investigators have debated whether food can be considered addictive to the extent that drugs such as cocaine and opioids are. Some literature suggests that this "addiction" to certain types of palatable foods may explain the obesity epidemic (Cocores & Gold, 2009). Although the DSM-5 has broadened the definition of addiction to be more inclusive of issues related to gambling, sex, and the Internet, no consensual definition of "food addiction" currently exists (Moreno & Tandon, 2011; Allison & Cirona-Singh, 2015).

A majority of the literature suggests that palatable foods have addictive potential based on findings that certain areas in the brain respond in similar ways when exposed to drugs of abuse and to highly palatable foods. For example, neuroimaging studies have shown that the dopaminergic system is involved in the motivation and processing of reward, among other behaviors (Lerma-Cabrera, Carvajal, & Lopez-Legarrea, 2016). Drugs of abuse increase the concentration of dopamine in the striatum and other associated areas of the mesolimbic region. Release of dopamine has also been associated with the reinforcing effects of food (Di Chiara, 2002; Wang, Volkow, Thanos, & Fowler, 2004). In addition to the involvement of the dopaminergic system in both food intake and drug use, Volkow and colleagues observed that individuals with obesity showed decreased activity in the frontal lobe areas of the brain that are associated with executive function (e.g., decision making) and control (Volkow, Wang, Tomasi, & Baler, 2013). This finding is also consistently described in persons with drug addiction.

In addition to the neurobiological underpinnings of both food and drug intake behaviors, other presenting symptoms such as cravings, withdrawal, and escalating patterns of eating may be evidence of increased tolerance, leading researchers to suggest that food addiction exists (Pelchat, 2002; Gearhardt, Corbin, & Brownell, 2009a). Similar to drug addiction, certain patterns of eating (e.g., binge eating) can be maladaptive, lead to distress, and continue despite these drawbacks (Moreno & Tandon, 2011).

Recent work on food addiction has described BED as a phenotype that can be conceptualized as an addiction, given that the eating behavior can be compulsive (Davis & Carter, 2009). The addiction model of eating disorders characterizes binge eating as a physiological addiction and treats the addiction by advocating abstinence from "addictive" foods (Ronel & Libman, 2003). In a study conducted by Cassin and von Ranson (2007), 94% of adults with BED described themselves as having a "food addiction" and met criteria for substance-dependence disorder in the DSM-IV when the term "substance" was substituted with "binge eating." Additionally, in a study conducted by Gearhardt et al. (2012), over 56% of a sample of 81 participants with BED met criteria for food addiction as measured by the Yale Food Addiction Scale (Gearhardt, Corbin, & Brownell, 2009b).

Although drug use and food intake behaviors share common features, other characteristics of drug addiction, such as engaging in the behavior in hazardous situations and failing to fulfill major role obligations, are not behaviors typically seen in eating patterns that may be considered maladaptive (Moreno & Tandon, 2011). In addition to the aforementioned markers of addiction, BMI may also be indicative of compulsive overeating. However, in a review of the available literature, Ziauddeen and Fletcher (2013) noted that, although binge eating is associated with obesity, a number of individuals who engage in this compulsive behavior are not obese, and most people with obesity do not have BED (Striegel-Moore et al., 2001) or "food addiction."

Treatment

With regard to treatment approaches, the previously mentioned treatment of complete abstinence from substances that is necessary for drug addiction is a questionable approach for "addictive" foods, as food is needed for survival (Wilson, Wilfley, Agras, & Bryson, 2010). In addition, with behavioral treatment, individuals with compulsive eating can successfully include a variety of foods in their diet (Wilson et al., 2010). CBT is considered to be an effective treatment for bulimia nervosa and BED. The intervention aims to increase flexibility in eating patterns, which is the opposite of an abstinence-based approach, and encourages more consistent eating (Fursland & Byrne, 2015). Although some models of Overeaters Anonymous espouse abstinence from white flour and sugar products, randomized controlled trials examining the efficacy of this approach are lacking, and one's ability to remain abstinent from these types of foods, given the current food environment, is typically quite limited. Subsequently, when these foods are inevitably consumed, skills for dealing with increased cravings have not been instilled, and relapse to binge eating is likely.

Conclusion and Future Directions

Obesity can be caused by multiple factors, including (but not limited to) the food environment, genetics, external stressors, and emotional dysregulation. Research has demonstrated that BED and NES are phenotypes associated with weight gain. However, not all people with obesity have these disorders, nor do all individuals diagnosed with NES and/or BED have obesity. Categorizing obesity as an eating disorder would be difficult due to multiple variations in eating patterns and weight within and between individuals with obesity. Taken together with these arguments, obesity is already a stigmatizing disease and shifting its classification to a psychiatric disorder would likely amplify this stigmatization to the detriment of afflicted individuals.

In regard to obesity as an addiction, drug use and food intake behaviors share common features, such as dopaminergic system involvement and cravings. However, other characteristics of drug addiction, such as engaging in the behavior in hazardous situations and failing to fulfill major role obligations, are not behaviors typically seen in eating disordered patterns (Moreno & Tandon,

2011). In addition, treatment approaches for drug use disorders would not be possible for those with a "food addiction," as it is not possible to maintain "sobriety" (avoidance of the substance) when food is necessary for survival. More research is needed to obtain a better understanding of food cravings and withdrawal and further explore the phenotype suggested by the term food addiction.

References

Adami, G. F., Campostano, A., Marinari, G. M., Ravera, G., & Scopinaro, N. (2002). Night eating in obesity: A descriptive study. *Nutrition, 18*(7–8), 587–589.

Allison, K. C., & Cirona-Singh, A. A. (2015). Is obesity an eating disorder? In L. Smolak & M. P. Levine (Eds.), *The Wiley handbook of eating disorders: Vol. 2. Assessment, prevention, treatment, policy, and future directions* (pp. 901–915). Chichester, UK: Wiley.

Allison, K. C., Lundgren, J. D., Moore, R. H., O'Reardon, J. P., & Stunkard, A. J. (2010). Cognitive behavior therapy for night eating syndrome: A pilot study. *American Journal of Psychotherapy, 64*(1), 91–106.

Allison, K. C., Lundgren, J. D., Stunkard, A. J., Bulik, C. M., Lindroos, A. K., Thornton, L. M., et al. (2014). Validation of screening questions and symptom coherence of night eating in the Swedish Twin Registry. *Comprehensive Psychiatry, 55*(3), 579–587.

Allison, K. C., Studt, S. K., Berkowitz, R. I., Hesson, L. A., Moore, R. H., Dubroff, J. G., et al. (2013). An open-label efficacy trial of escitalopram for night eating syndrome. *Eating Behaviors, 14*(2), 199–203.

Allison, K. C., Wadden, T. A., Sarwer, D. B., Fabricatore, A. N., Crerand, C. E., Gibbons, L. M., et al. (2006). Night eating syndrome and binge eating disorder among persons seeking bariatric surgery: Prevalence and related features. *Obesity, 14*(2, Suppl.), 77S–82S.

American Psychiatric Association. (2013). *Diagnostic and statistical manual of mental disorders* (5th ed.). Arlington, VA: Author.

Amianto, F., Ottone, L., Daga, G. A., & Fassino, S. (2015). Binge-eating disorder diagnosis and treatment: A recap in front of DSM-5. *BMC Psychiatry, 15*, 70–92.

Andersen, G. S., Stunkard, A. J., Sorensen, T. I. A., Petersen, L., & Heitmann, B. L. (2004). Night eating and weight change in middle-aged men and women. *International Journal of Obesity, 28*(10), 1338–1343.

Berkman, N. D., Brownley, K. A., Peat, C. M., Lohr, K. N., Cullen, K. E., Morgan, L. C., et al. (2015). Management and outcomes of binge-eating disorder (Comparative Effectiveness Review No. 160; AHRQ Publication No. 15(16)-EHC030-EF). Rockville, MD: Agency for Healthcare Research and Quality. Retrieved from *www.effectivehealthcare. ahrq.gov/reports/final.cfm*.

Boston, R. C., Moate, P. J., Allison, K. C., Lundgren, J. D., & Stunkard, A. J. (2008). Modeling circadian rhythms of food intake by means of parametric deconvolution: Results from studies of the night eating syndrome. *American Journal of Clinical Nutrition, 87*(6), 1672–1677.

Bulik, C. M., Sullivan, P. F., & Kendler, K. S. (2002). Medical and psychiatric morbidity in obese women with and without binge eating. *International Journal of Eating Disorders, 32*(1), 72–78.

Cassin, S. E., & von Ranson, K. M. (2007). Is binge eating experienced as an addiction? *Appetite, 49*(3), 687–690.

Castellini, G., Sauro, C. L., Mannucci, E., Ravaldi, C., Rotella, C. M., Faravelli, C., et al (2011). Diagnostic crossover and outcome predictors in eating disorders according to DSM-IV and DSM-V proposed criteria: A 6-year follow-up study. *Psychosomatic Medicine, 73*(3), 270–279.

Cerú-Björk, C., Andersson, I., & Rössner, S. (2001). Night eating and nocturnal eating: Two different or similar syndromes among obese patients? *International Journal of Obesity and Related Metabolic Disorders, 25*(3), 365–372.

Cocores, J. A., & Gold, M. S. (2009). The salted food addiction hypothesis may explain overeating and the obesity epidemic. *Medical Hypotheses, 73*(6), 892–899.

Colles, S. L., Dixon, J. B., & O'Brien, P. E. (2007). Night eating syndrome and nocturnal snacking: Association with obesity, binge eating and psychological distress. *International Journal of Obesity, 31*(11), 1722–1730.

Davis, C., & Carter, J. C. (2009). Compulsive overeating as an addiction disorder: A review of theory and evidence. *Appetite, 53*(1), 1–8.

de Zwaan, M. (2001). Binge eating disorder and obesity. *International Journal of Obesity, 25*(1, Suppl.), S51–S55.

de Zwaan, M., Muller, A., Allison, K. C., Brahler, E., & Hilbert, A. (2014). Prevalence and correlates of night eating in the German general population. *PLOS ONE, 9*(5), e97667.

Di Chiara, G. (2002). Nucleus accumbens shell and core dopamine: Differential role in behavior and addiction. *Behavioral Brain Research, 137*(1–2), 75–114.

Friedman, S., Even, C., Dardennes, R., & Guelfi, J. D. (2002). Light therapy, obesity, and night-eating syndrome. *American Journal of Psychiatry, 159*(5), 875–876.

Fursland, A., & Byrne, S. M. (2015). Cognitive-behavioral therapy for the treatment of eating disorders. In L. Smolak & M. P. Levine (Eds.), *The Wiley handbook of eating disorders: Vol. 2. Assessment, prevention, treatment, policy, and future directions* (pp. 773–787). Chichester, UK: Wiley.

Gallant, A. R., Lundgren, J., & Drapeau, V. (2012).

The night-eating syndrome and obesity. *Obesity Reviews, 13*(6), 528–536.

Gearhardt, A. N., Corbin, W. R., & Brownell, K. D. (2009a). Food addiction: An examination of the diagnostic criteria for dependence. *Journal of Addiction Medicine, 3*(1), 1–7.

Gearhardt, A. N., Corbin, W. R., & Brownell, K. D. (2009b). Preliminary validation of the Yale Food Addiction Scale. *Appetite, 52*(2), 430–436.

Gearhardt, A. N., White, M. A., Masheb, R. M., Morgan, P. T., Crosby, R. D., & Grilo, C. M. (2012). An examination of the food addiction construct in obese patients with binge eating disorder. *International Journal of Eating Disorders, 45*(5), 657–663.

Gluck, M. E., Geliebter, A., & Satov, T. (2001). Night eating syndrome is associated with depression, low self-esteem, reduced daytime hunger, and less weight loss in obese outpatients. *Obesity Research, 9*(4), 264–267.

Gluck, M. E., Venti, C. A., Salbe, A. D., & Krakoff, J. (2008). Nighttime eating: Commonly observed and related to weight gain in an inpatient food intake study. *American Journal of Clinical Nutrition, 88*(4), 900–905.

Grilo, C. M., Masheb, R. M., Wilson, G. T., Gueorguieva, R., & White, M. A. (2011). Cognitive-behavioral therapy, behavioral weight loss, and sequential treatment for obese patients with binge-eating disorder: A randomized controlled trial. *Journal of Consulting and Clinical Psychology, 79*(5), 675–685.

Haedt-Matt, A. A., & Keel, P. K. (2011). Revisiting the affect regulation model of binge eating: A meta-analysis of studies using ecological momentary assessment. *Psychological Bulletin, 137*(4), 660–681.

Heatherton, T. F., & Baumeister, R. F. (1991). Binge eating as escape from self-awareness. *Psychological Bulletin, 110*(1), 86–108.

Heatherton, T. F., & Wagner, D. D. (2011). Cognitive neuroscience of self-regulation failure. *Trends in Cognitive Sciences, 15*(3), 132–139.

Hudson, J. I., Hiripi, E., Pope, G., Jr., & Kessler, R. C. (2007). The prevalence and correlates of eating disorders in the national comorbidity survey replication. *Biological Psychiatry, 61*(3), 348–358.

Iacovino, J. M., Gredysa, D. M., Altman, M., & Wilfley, D. E. (2012). Psychological treatments for binge eating disorder. *Current Psychiatry Reports, 14*(4), 432–446.

Jarosz, P. A., Dobal, M. T., Wilson, F. L., & Schram, C. A. (2007). Disordered eating and food cravings among urban obese African American women. *Eating Behaviors, 8*(3), 374–381.

Kessler, R. C., Berglund, P. A., Chiu, W. T., Deitz, A. C., Hudson, J. I., Shahly, V., et al. (2013). The prevalence and correlates of binge eating disorder in the World Health Organization World Mental Health Surveys. *Biological Psychiatry, 73*(9), 904–914.

Kolotkin, R. L., Westman, E. C., Østbye, T., Crosby, R. D., Eisenson, H. J., & Binks, M. (2004). Does binge eating disorder impact weight-related quality of life? *Obesity Research, 12*(6), 999–1005.

Lamerz, A., Kuepper-Nybelen, J., Bruning, N., Wehle, C., Trost-Brinkhues, G., Brenner, H., et al. (2005). Prevalence of obesity, binge eating, and night eating in a cross-sectional field survey of 6-year-old children and their parents in a German urban population. *Journal of Child Psychology and Psychiatry, 46*(4), 385–393.

Lerma-Cabrera, J. M., Carvajal, F., & Lopez-Legarrea, P. (2016). Food addiction as a new piece of the obesity framework. *Nutrition Journal, 15*, 5.

Lundgren, J. D., Allison, K. C., Crow, S., O'Reardon, J. P., Berg, K. C., Galbraith, J., et al. (2006). Prevalence of the night eating syndrome in a psychiatric population. *American Journal of Psychiatry, 163*(1), 156–158.

Lundgren, J. D., Allison, K. C., Vinai, P., & Gluck, M. E. (2012). Assessment instruments for night eating syndrome. In J. D. Lundgren, K. C. Allison, & A. J. Stunkard (Eds.), *Night eating syndrome: Research, assessment, and treatment* (pp. 197–217). New York: Guilford Press.

Marshall, H. M., Allison, K. C., O'Reardon, J. P., Birketvedt, G., & Stunkard, A. J. (2004). Night eating syndrome among nonobese persons. *International Journal of Eating Disorders, 35*(2), 217–222.

McElroy, S. L., Hudson, J. I., Mitchell, J. E., Wilfley, D., Ferreira-Cornwell, M. C., Gao, J., et al. (2015). Efficacy and safety of lisdexamfetamine for treatment of adults with moderate to severe binge-eating disorder: A randomized clinical trial. *JAMA Psychiatry, 72*(3), 235–246.

Moreno, C., & Tandon, R. (2011). Should overeating and obesity be classified as an addictive disorder in DSM-5? *Current Pharmaceutical Design, 17*(12), 1128–1131.

Napolitano, M. A., Head, S., Babyak, M. A., & Blumenthal, J. A. (2001). Binge eating disorder and night eating syndrome: Psychological and behavioral characteristics. *International Journal of Eating Disorders, 30*(2), 193–203.

National Institute for Health and Clinical Excellence. (2004). *Eating disorders: Core interventions in the treatment and management of anorexia nervosa, bulimia nervosa, and related eating disorders* (NICE Clinical Guideline No. 9). London: Author.

Nicholls, W., Devonport, T. J., & Blake, M. (2016). The association between emotions and eating behavior in an obese population with binge eating disorder. *Obesity Reviews, 17*(1), 30–42.

O'Reardon, J. P., Allison, K. C., Martino, N. S., Lundgren, J. D., Heo, M., & Stunkard, A. J. (2006). A randomized, placebo-controlled trial of sertraline in the treatment of night eating syndrome. *American Journal of Psychiatry, 163*(5), 893–898.

O'Reardon, J. P., Stunkard, A. J., & Allison, K. C. (2004). Clinical trial of sertraline in the treatment of night eating syndrome. *International Journal of Eating Disorders, 35*(1), 16–26.

Pawlow, L. A., O'Neil, P. M., & Malcolm, R. J. (2003). Night eating syndrome: Effects of brief relaxation training on stress, mood, hunger, and eating patterns. *International Journal of Obesity, 27*(8), 970–978.

Paxton, S. J., & Diggens, J. (1997). Avoidance coping, binge eating, and depression: An examination of the escape theory of binge eating. *International Journal of Eating Disorders, 22*(1), 83–87.

Pelchat, M. L. (2002). Of human bondage: Food craving, obsession, compulsion, and addiction. *Physiology and Behavior, 76*(3), 347–352.

Peterson, C. B., Swanson, S. A., Crow, S. J., Mitchell, J. E., Agras, W. S., Halmi, K. A., et al. (2012). Longitudinal stability of binge-eating type in eating disorders. *International Journal of Eating Disorders, 45*(5), 664–669.

Polivy, J. (1996). Psychological consequences of food restriction. *Journal of the American Dietetic Association, 96*(6), 589–592.

Polivy, J., & Herman, C. P. (1985). Dieting and binging: A causal analysis. *American Psychologist, 40*(2), 193–201.

Rand, C. S., Macgregor, A. M., & Stunkard, A. J. (1997). The night-eating syndrome in the general population and among post-operative obesity surgery patients. *International Journal of Eating Disorders, 22*(1), 65–69.

Ronel, N., & Libman, G. (2003). Eating disorders and recovery: Lessons from Overeaters Anonymous. *Clinical Social Work Journal, 31*(2), 155–177.

Root, T. L., Thornton, L. M., Lindroos, A. K., Stunkard, A. J., Lichtenstein, P., Pedersen, N. L., et al. (2010). Shared and unique genetic and environmental influences on binge eating and night eating: A Swedish twin study. *Eating Behaviors, 11*(2), 92–98.

Spitzer, R. L., Yanovski, S., Wadden, T., Wing, R., Marcus, M. D., Stunkard, A., et al. (1993). Binge eating disorder: Its further validation in a multisite study. *International Journal of Eating Disorders, 13*(2), 137–153.

Striegel-Moore, R. H., Cachelin, F. M., Dohm, F., Pike, K. M., Wilfley, D. E., & Fairburn, C. G. (2001). Comparison of binge eating disorder and bulimia nervosa in a community sample. *International Journal of Eating Disorders, 29*(2), 157–165.

Striegel-Moore, R. H., Dohm, F., Hook, J. M., Schreiber, G. B., Crawford, P. B., & Daniels, S. R. (2005). Night eating syndrome in young adult women: Prevalence and correlates. *International Journal of Eating Disorders, 37*(3), 200–206.

Striegel-Moore, R. H., Franko, D. L., Thompson, D., Affenito, S., & Kraemer, H. C. (2006). Night eating: Prevalence and demographic correlates. *Obesity, 14*(1), 139–147.

Stunkard, A. J., & Allison, K. C. (2003). Binge eating disorder: Disorder or marker? *International Journal of Eating Disorders, 34*(1, Suppl.), S107–S116.

Stunkard, A. J., Allison, K. C., Lundgren, J. D., Martino, N. S., Heo, M., Etemad, B., et al. (2006). A paradigm for facilitating pharmacotherapy at a distance: Sertraline treatment of the night eating syndrome. *Journal of Clinical Psychiatry, 67*(10), 1568–1572.

Tanofsky-Kraff, M., Wilfley, D. E., Young, J. F., Mufson, L., Yanovski, S. Z., Glasofer, D. R., et al. (2007). Preventing excessive weight gain in adolescents: Interpersonal psychotherapy for binge eating. *Obesity, 15*(6), 1345–1355.

Tholin, S., Lindroos, A., Tynelius, P., Akerstedt, T., Stunkard, A. J., Bulik, C. M., et al. (2009). Prevalence of night eating in obese and nonobese twins. *Obesity, 17*(5), 1050–1055.

Vander Wal, J. S. (2012). Night eating syndrome: A critical review of the literature. *Clinical Psychology Review, 32*(1), 49–59.

Vander Wal, J. S., Gang, C. H., Griffing, G. T., & Gadde, K. M. (2012). Escitalopram for treatment of night eating syndrome: A 12-week, randomized, placebo-controlled trial. *Journal of Clinical Psychopharmacology, 32*(3), 341–345.

Vander Wal, J. S., Maraldo, T. M., Vercellone, A. C., & Gagne, D. A. (2015). Education, progressive muscle relaxation therapy, and exercise for the treatment of night eating syndrome: A pilot study. *Appetite, 89*, 136–144.

Voks, S., Tuschen-Caffier, B., Pietrowsky, R., Rustenbach, S. J., Kersting, A., & Herpertz, S. (2010). Meta-analysis of the effectiveness of psychological and pharmacological treatments for binge eating disorder. *International Journal of Eating Disorders, 43*(3), 205–217.

Volkow, N. D., Wang, G. J., Tomasi, D., & Baler, R. D. (2013). Obesity and addiction: Neurobiological overlaps. *Obesity Reviews, 14*(1), 2–18.

Wadden, T. A., Foster, G. D., Sarwer, D. B., Anderson, D. A., Gladis, M., Sanderson, R. S., et al. (2004). Dieting and the development of eating disorders in obese women: Results of a randomized controlled trial. *American Journal of Clinical Nutrition, 80*(3), 560–568.

Wang, G. J., Volkow, N., Thanos, P. K., & Fowler, J. S. (2004). Similarity between obesity and drug addiction as assessed by neurofunctional imaging. *Journal of Addictive Diseases, 23*(3), 39–53.

Wilfley, D. E., Welch, R. R., Stein, R. I., Spurrell, E. B., Cohen, L. R., Saelens, B. E., et al. (2002). A randomized comparison of group cognitive-behavioral therapy and group interpersonal psychotherapy for the treatment of overweight individuals with binge-eating disorder. *Archives of General Psychiatry, 59*(8), 713–721.

Wilson, G. T., Grilo, C. M., & Vitousek, K. M. (2007). Psychological treatments of eating disorders. *American Psychologist, 62*(3), 199–216.

Wilson, G. T., Wilfley, D. E., Agras, W. S., & Bryson, S. W. (2010). Psychological treatments of binge eating disorder. *Archives of General Psychiatry, 67*(1), 94–101.

Womble, L. G., Williamson, D. A., & Martin, C. K. (2001). Psychosocial variables associated with binge eating in obese males and females. *International Journal of Eating Disorders, 30*(2), 217–221.

Ziauddeen, H., & Fletcher, P. C. (2013). Is food addiction a valid and useful concept? *Obesity Reviews, 14*(1), 19–28.

PART III
Health Consequences of Weight Reduction

CHAPTER 12

The Impact of Intentional Weight Loss on Major Morbidity and Mortality

Edward W. Gregg
Marcela Rodriguez Flores

The increase in obesity prevalence over the past 30 years has had fundamental effects on a diverse spectrum of chronic conditions. As such, it is one of the most significant public health problems for the United States and much of the world. In the United States, increases in obesity prevalence accelerated in the 1980s. In recent data (2015–2016), obesity prevalence was 40% in U.S. adults and 18.5% in youth and adolescents (Flegal, Kruszon-Moran, Carroll, Fryar, & Ogden, 2016; Hales, Carroll, Fryar, & Ogden, 2017). The rise in obesity has been the most dramatic among the very obese categories, as about 9% of youth and adults have class 3 obesity. The increases in prevalence affect virtually all racial/ethnic and socioeconomic segments of the population (Wang & Beydoun, 2007; Flegal et al., 2016). Similar trends have occurred globally, with worldwide obesity prevalence more than doubling, from 5% to 12% between 1980 and 2015 (GBD 2015 Obesity Collaborators, 2017). Recent reports suggest that prevalence increases may have stabilized in some segments of the U.S. population, but such encouraging findings are tempered by the fact that prevalence of extreme obesity in 2013–2014 remained three times what it was 15 years earlier (Ogden, Carroll, Fryar, & Flegal, 2015; Ogden et al., 2016).

Obesity is notorious for its diverse acute and chronic morbidities and the increased risk for mortality that follow. Although debate continues about definitions of obesity and thresholds that signify increased or maximum risk, consistent evidence now associates obesity with diabetes, hypertension, renal disease, cardiovascular disease, arthritis, depression, certain cancers, disability, overall decreased quality of life, and mortality (National Heart, Lung, and Blood Institute [NHLBI], 1998). The most tangible effects of obesity have been seen in the increases in diabetes, for which obesity has been the dominant factor explaining the 60% increase in diabetes prevalence in the United States over the past 25 years (Gregg, Cheng, Narayan, Thompson, & Williamson, 2007; Geiss et al., 2014). This wide range of morbidity along with the care required to manage the associated risk factors have led to enormous costs for individuals, families, health systems, and societies (Hammond & Levine, 2010; Finkelstein, Trogdon, Cohen, & Dietz, 2009).

The role of weight loss in the public health response to obesity has been unclear for several reasons. First, the magnitude of weight loss, maintenance, and regain from weight loss interventions are heterogeneous across types and modalities of weight loss, leaving open questions of efficacy as well as questions of how to implement weight loss interventions at an adequate scale to influence public health (NHLBI, 2013). Second, many have argued that public health problems are best confronted through primary prevention aimed at the whole population, as opposed to treatment approaches aimed at subsegments of the population that have already succumbed to the risk (Rose, 2001). Third, weight loss is one of the most common health interventions undertaken by the public. In the United States, almost two-thirds of obese adults report trying to lose weight in a given year (Serdula et al., 1999; Kruger, Galuska, Serdula, & Jones, 2004; Nicklas, Huskey, Davis, & Wee, 2012), and about 10% of obese adults report engaging in structured or commercial weight loss programs (Nicklas et al., 2012). In addition, the number of people undergoing bariatric surgery has increased dramatically, with 179,000 surgeries performed in 2013 (Bariatric Surgery Source, 2017). The sheer number of people engaged in weight loss efforts of some sort means that the effectiveness or harm associated with weight loss has large potential ramifications for population health. Finally, the level of consensus about the role of weight loss in the clinical and public health response to obesity has been inconsistent, because epidemiological studies have yielded inconsistent findings and even adverse effects of weight loss, and findings from intervention studies have depended on the segment of the population and the outcomes being studied (Williamson & Pamuk, 1993; Harrington, Gibson, & Cottrell, 2009).

Chronic disease epidemics and public health problems generally respond best to a multicomponent set of strategies (Bauer, Briss, Goodman, & Bowman, 2014). This approach includes efforts in clinical systems to provide effective preventive care, health promotion efforts to alter health behaviors of individuals, and public policies to change the underlying environment, including the nutritional environment and opportunities and tendencies for physical activity (Rose, 2001; Manuel, Rosella, Tuna, Bennett, & Stukel, 2013). For this reason, it is important to understand the impact of weight loss efforts as implemented through different avenues, including clinical systems, community programs, and individually motivated behavior.

In this chapter, we review evidence for the impact of intentional weight loss on morbidity and mortality. We consider evidence of measured intentional weight loss of several types, including multicomponent lifestyle-based behavioral counseling with maintained support; medical management with pharmacological treatment and supportive behavioral counseling; surgical treatment; and self-directed behavior change to lose weight. We limit this evidence synthesis to longitudinal, observational, and intervention studies that essentially include cohort studies and registry-based studies of weight loss interventions and nonrandomized and randomized intervention trials. We exclude from this synthesis cross-sectional studies, uncontrolled case series, and uncontrolled intervention studies.

Short-Term and Intermediate Effects of Weight Loss

An extensive literature has documented the physiological health benefits of weight loss intervention over the short-term (6–12 months), which, if adequately maintained, should lead to diverse benefits on morbidity and mortality. As shown in Figure 12.1, weight loss leads to consistent, predictable benefits for parameters of insulin resistance and glucose tolerance, including fasting and post load insulin and glucose levels. One-year multicomponent lifestyle interventions with overweight and obese adults, focused on facilitating weight loss through healthy

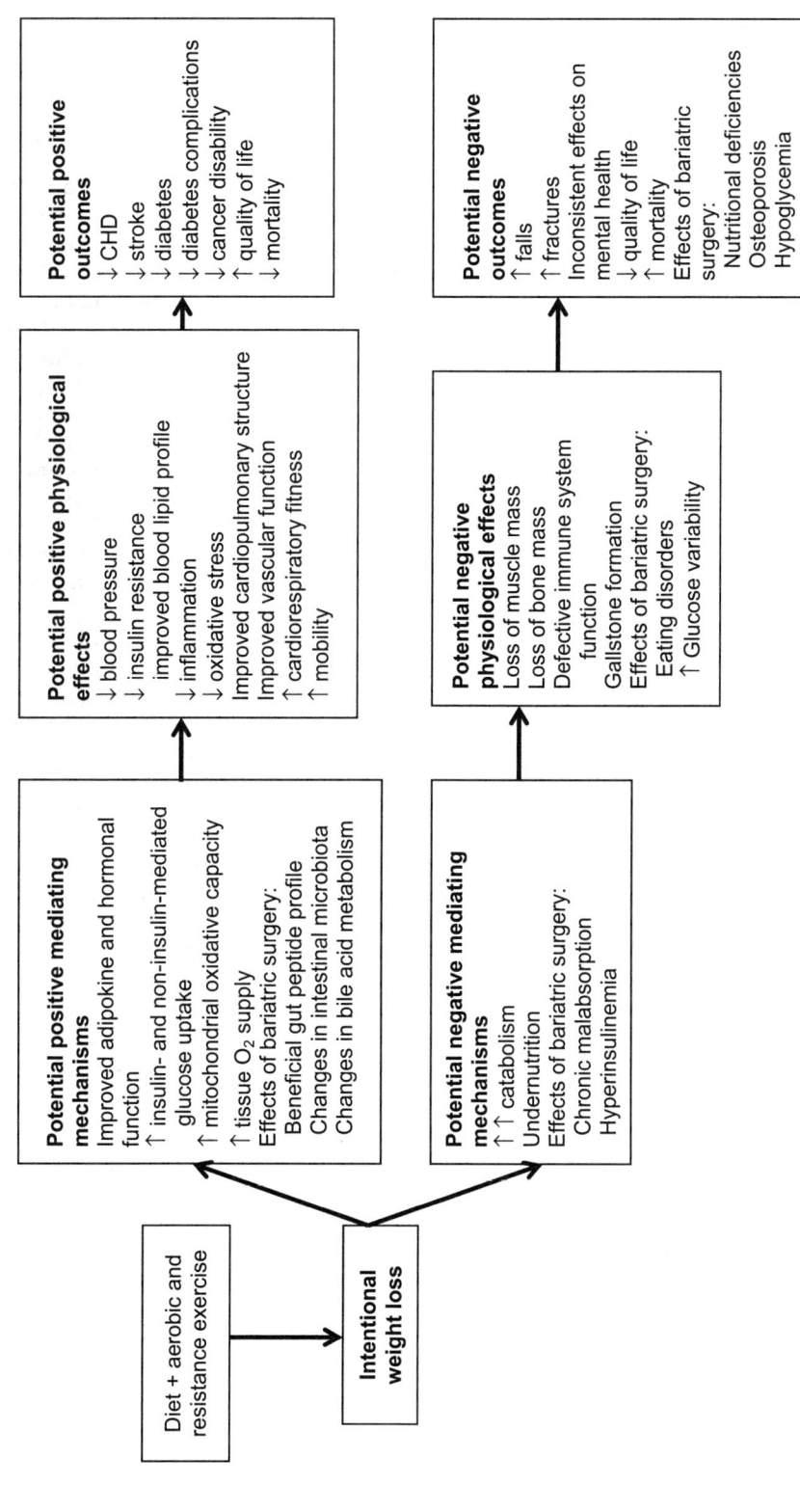

FIGURE 12.1. Putative pathways for the influence of weight loss on disease incidence and mortality. Adapted and modified from Gregg and Williamson (2002) and Ryan (2007).

diet and physical activity and achieving moderate weight loss (mean reductions of 2–5%), led to an average reduction of fasting plasma glucose of 2.6 mg/dL (Lin et al., 2014; Zhang, et al., 2017). Among adults with type 2 diabetes, interventions led to an average 0.3% reduction in glycated hemoglobin (HbA1C) (Norris et al., 2004; Jensen et al., 2014).

Meta-analyses also show that each 10 kg of weight loss over 1–2 years is associated with average reductions of 2 mmHg in systolic blood pressure, 4–5 mg/dL of total cholesterol, 3–4 mg/dL of low-density lipoprotein (LDL), 8–12 mg/dL of triglyceride, and 2 mg/dL increase in high-density lipoprotein (HDL) cholesterol (Jensen et al., 2014; Lin et al., 2014). In longer-term studies of 2–3 years, these reductions in blood pressure have resulted in a significant 20–30% reduced incidence of hypertension (Trials of Hypertension Prevention [TOHP II] Collaborative Research Group, 1997) and in a reduced need for antihypertensive medications (Stevens et al., 2001). Weight loss leads to improvements in cardiac function, including left ventricular hypertrophy, resting heart rate, increased stroke volume and cardiac output, and cardiorespiratory fitness (Hankey, Lean, Lowe, Rumley, & Woodward, 2002; Poirier et al., 2006). Weight loss also leads to improvements in systemic inflammation (Esposito et al., 2003; Ryan & Nicklas, 2004), chronic kidney disease, sleep apnea symptoms, and pulmonary function (Kuna et al., 2013; Rubin et al., 2014). Finally, several benefits in functional status occur with weight loss, particularly from programs involving physical activity. These benefits include improved mobility and lower extremity function, reduced arthritic pain, and reduced depressive symptoms (Messier et al., 2004; Rejeski et al., 2012; Rubin et al., 2014). In spite of the diverse benefits described above, adverse short-term effects of weight loss may also exist, including gallstone formation, fatigue, and loss of bone density and lean mass. The effect on lean mass has raised questions about the advisability of weight loss in older adults (Launer, Harris, Rumpel, & Maddins, 1994; Syngal et al., 1999; Ensrud et al., 2007).

Impact on Long-Term Morbidity and Mortality

Lifestyle Interventions

Intervention Trials and Diabetes Incidence

Over the past 20 years, more than 10 major intervention studies have examined the impact of lifestyle-based weight loss intervention on diabetes incidence. One of the earliest and most influential investigations in this line of research began in the late 1980s, with a study of diet and exercise conducted in Malmo, Sweden, with 260 men ages 47–49 who had impaired glucose tolerance. As summarized in Table 12.1, the study reported a 2.8% net weight loss and found a 63% reduced incidence of diabetes over 6 years (Eriksson & Lindgarde, 1991). Despite the modest weight loss and the nonrandomized design, the Malmo Prevention Study set the stage for a series of randomized trials demonstrating consistent effects of weight loss on diabetes incidence. A subsequent study conducted in Da Qing, China, a rapidly modernizing oil city in Heilongong Province in the far north of China, assigned 33 clinics of 577 men and women with impaired glucose tolerance (IGT) to one of four conditions: usual care, diet, exercise, or both diet and exercise. Although net weight loss was minimal (< 2%), the study found a 29–32% reduction in all three interventions among both lean and overweight adults (Pan et al., 1997).

Studies in Finland, the United States, and India followed, with more detailed quantification of the intervention components and benefits. In Finland, 522 overweight men and women with IGT were assigned to either usual care or group-based, tailored advice to reduce weight, reduce saturated and total fat intake, increase fiber intake, and increase physical activity levels (Tuomilehto et al., 2001). The intervention resulted in a 2.7% net weight loss (3.4% over the first year) and a 58% reduction in diabetes incidence over 4 years. The next year, the U.S. Diabetes Prevention Program (DPP) reported findings from the 3-year trial comparing multicomponent lifestyle intervention with metformin and usual care among more than 3,000 adults with IGT (Knowler et al., 2002). The study reported a net 7% weight loss at 1

TABLE 12.1. Summary of Controlled Trials of the Impact of Lifestyle-Based Weight Loss Interventions on Diabetes Incidence

Study/author	Population	Mean follow-up (years)	Intervention	Weight change	Effect of weight loss relative to control or referent group
Malmo Prevention Study (Eriksson & Lindgarde, 1991)	Swedish men ages 47–49 y with IGT ($n = 260$)	6	Diet, exercise, behavioral counseling	2.3% loss vs. 0.5% gain (net 2.8%)	63% ↓ diabetes incidence
Da Qing Diabetes Prevention Study (Pan et al., 1997)	Chinese men and women with IGT; mean age 45 y ($n = 577$)	6	Diet, exercise, diet + exercise vs. control; 14 contacts in first year	Net 2% loss among diet + exercise group	29% ↓ DM incidence for diet 32% ↓ DM incidence for exercise 33% ↓ DM incidence diet + exercise
Finnish Diabetes Prevention Study (Tuomilehto et al., 2001; Lindstrom et al., 2006, 2013)	Finnish men and women with IGT; mean age 55 y ($n = 522$)	3.2	Diet, exercise, behavioral counseling; 9 contacts first year	Net 3.4% loss at 3 y	58% ↓ DM incidence at 3 y 43% ↓ DM incidence at 7 y 38% ↓ DM incidence at 13 y
Diabetes Prevention Program (2015); Knowler et al. (2002)	U.S. men and women with IGT; mean age 50 y ($n = 3,234$)	2.8	Diet, exercise, behavioral counseling; 22 contacts first year	Net 4.5% loss at 3 y	58% ↓ DM incidence at 2.8 y 34% ↓ DM incidence at 10 y (7 years after end of intervention)
Kosaka et al. (2005)	Japanese men with IGT; mean age 52 y ($n = 458$)	4	Diet, exercise, behavioral counseling; < 6 contacts first year	Net 1.8 kg loss at 4 y	67% ↓ DM incidence at 4 y
Indian Diabetes Prevention Program (Ramachandran et al., 2006)	Indian men and women with IGT; mean age 46 y ($n = 531$)	3	Diet, exercise, behavioral counseling; 16 contacts first year	No net weight loss	29% ↓ DM incidence
Zensharen Study (Saito et al., 2011)	Japanese adults with IFG; mean age 49 y ($n = 642$)	3	Diet and exercise counseling; 9 contacts over 3 years	Net 1.9% loss at 1 y	44% ↓ diabetes incidence overall *Subgroup analyses* No difference in DM incidence among isolated IFG 33% ↓ DM incidence among low FPG (< 110) 50% ↓ DM among high FPG (> 110) No difference in DM among low A1C (<6.0) 76% ↓ DM among high A1C (> 6.0)
Weber et al. (2016)	578 overweight/obese Asian Indians with pre-diabetes	3	Diet, exercise, behavioral counseling; 16 contacts first year	Net 3% loss at 6 months	29% ↓ diabetes incidence overall *Subgroup analyses* 12% ↓ DM incidence among isolated IFG 31% ↓ DM among isolated IGT 36% ↓ DM among IFG and IGT 13% ↓ DM among low A1C (< 5.7) 50% ↓ DM among high A1C (5.7–6.2)

Note. FPG, fasting plasma glucose; IFG, impaired fasting glucose; IGT, impaired glucose tolerance; DM, diabetes mellitus.

year and a 4.5% weight loss at 4 years and found a 58% reduced incidence of diabetes. In a subsequent study in Japan, 4 years of regular behavioral support to improve diet and physical activity led to a modest reduction in weight (net 1.8 kg) and a 67% reduction in diabetes incidence (Kosaka, Noda, & Kuzuya, 2005). Finally, a randomized controlled trial (RCT) comparing lifestyle modification, metformin, and the combination with usual care among 502 Asian Indians resulted in 35–38% reductions in diabetes incidence among all three groups compared to usual care (Ramachandran et al., 2006).

Post-hoc analyses conducted on the Finnish and U.S. prevention trials suggest that the benefits of the trials were a result of multiple intervention components, as each of the study goals (achieving 5% weight loss, reducing fat intake to < 30%, reducing saturated fat to < 10%, increasing fiber intake to > 15g/day, and increasing physical activity levels to > 4 hours/week) was associated with substantial reductions in risk. In the U.S. DPP, post-hoc analyses suggested that weight loss was the most dominant of these factors and showed that each kilogram of weight loss was associated with a 16% reduction in diabetes incidence. Participants who met all three goals (7% weight loss, 150 minutes per week walking, < 30% of fat in the diet) had an 80% reduced risk of diabetes (Hamman et al., 2006). However, these post-hoc analyses should be interpreted cautiously because they are not randomized comparisons, and the weaker association of dietary and physical activity factors (i.e., vs. weight loss) may be partly a function of less accurate measurement and more measurement error.

The studies conducted in Asian populations raise other questions about the role of weight loss as the central mechanism of effect in these lifestyle interventions. The Da Qing study and the India Diabetes Prevention Study found little or no weight change in any of the intervention groups, yet found significant reductions in diabetes incidence (Pan et al., 1997; Ramachandran et al., 2006). This finding may reflect the limitations of using overall body weight as a marker of the specific effects on visceral adiposity and lean mass, which may be the most important factors affecting diabetes risk.

These variable effects also raise the question of the degree to which behavior changes, including increasing physical activity levels and qualitative components of the diet (e.g., healthy fats vs. saturated fats; whole grains and healthy carbohydrates vs. added sugar and refined carbohydrates), affect the risk of diabetes irrespective of weight loss (Mozaffarian, 2016).

Several of the diabetes prevention trials have examined the extended or "legacy" effects of the intervention on diabetes. The Finnish Diabetes Prevention Study (DPS) found a 43% reduction in diabetes incidence 3 years after the cessation of the lifestyle intervention (Uusitupa et al., 2009). In a 20-year follow-up (14 years after the cessation of the intervention), the Da Qing Diabetes Prevention Study also found that a significant 43% reduction in diabetes incidence remained (Li et al., 2008). In the Diabetes Prevention Program Outcomes Study (DPPOS), participants in the lifestyle intervention program had a 24% reduced incidence of diabetes 8 years after completion of a 10-year trial, even though the participants in the control group were offered lifestyle intervention after completion of the primary trial. The DPPOS also found that participants with IGT who regressed to normal glucose tolerance over 6 years had a reduced risk of progression to diabetes, compared to those who remained in the IGT category (Perreault et al., 2012).

The focus of almost all of the prevention studies on adults with IGT has led to an important gap in the literature, given that many contemporary settings quantify diabetes risk using different glycemic definitions, including fasting glucose or HbA1C. The few studies that have either stratified or recruited people with isolated impaired fasting glucose (IFG) or isolated, elevated HbA1C have yielded inconsistent findings on diabetes prevention. In post-hoc analyses of the Zensharen Study for the Prevention of Lifestyle Diseases, the benefit of lifestyle interventions (56% reduction in incidence) was limited to persons with IGT and HbA1C levels > 6%, with no prevention effect observed among those with isolated IFG or HbA1C levels < 6% (Saito et al., 2011). More recently, the Diabetes Community Lifestyle Improvement Program (D-CLIP) study found that the lifestyle intervention was less effective (12% reduction) in those with isolated IFG than in those with any evidence of IGT (31–36% reduction), consistent with the hypothesis that lifestyle interventions act more on insulin resistance than on insulin secretion (Weber et al., 2016). However, since race/ethnic variation in the pathogenesis of diabetes (i.e., differing influence of beta cell failure vs, peripheral insulin resistance on diabetes) may exist, follow-up prevention studies are needed to better quantify the heterogeneity of prevention effectiveness.

Taken as a whole, the studies of diabetes prevention clearly indicate that multidisciplinary, lifestyle-based weight loss interventions with goals of modest weight loss reduce diabetes incidence by 30–60% after 2–6 years. Such interventions work in diverse cultural settings and across both genders, diverse ages, and racial/ethnic groups. These trials have led to considerable activity in translating the positive findings into practical interventions and programs in communities, as well as using diverse modalities such as virtual support, social media, and telephone counseling. There have also been many short-term intervention studies examining the impact of these community-based programs on body weight, which have generally been favorable and encouraging. However, the impact of community-based programs on long-term outcomes has not been assessed yet and will be an important public health research challenge for the near future.

Cardiovascular Disease Incidence and Mortality

Despite the clear benefit of weight loss on diabetes incidence, the impact of lifestyle-based weight loss programs on cardiovascular health remains controversial, as reflected by the results of selected studies summarized in Table 12.2. In theory, the diverse benefits of weight loss in hypertension, lipids, inflammatory factors, and insulin resistance should lead to reductions in cardiovascular disease (Wing, 2010). Early observational studies of the effects of intentional weight loss on cardiovascular disease incidence and mortality reported inconsistent findings. Many were unable to rule out reverse causality or the confounding of unintentional weight loss (Williamson, 1998), indicating that intervention studies would be a preferable approach. One of the first such analyses was a follow-up of the Malmo Prevention Study, a nonrandomized lifestyle intervention trial that found a 56% reduction in cardiovascular disease (CVD) mortality, but could have been confounded by the large difference in levels of hypertension at baseline (Eriksson & Lindgarde, 1998). Subsequent studies of intensive, cardioprotective interventions focused on saturated fat reduction, increasing vegetable intake, and increasing physical activity levels found significant reductions in cardiac events and a slower rate of progression of coronary artery stenosis (Ornish, 1993; Haskell et al., 1994; Ornish et al., 1998). Weight loss in these studies ranged from 4 to 8%, but as these studies were conducted using persons with prior CVD and the interventions were accompanied by lipid-lowering and antihypertensive drugs, it is difficult to know how much the effects in these relatively small studies were really driven by weight loss.

Follow-up analyses of the diabetes prevention trials have also generated ambiguous findings related to the impact of lifestyle-based weight loss interventions on CVD incidence. In the Finnish DPS, adults assigned to the lifestyle intervention had no difference in rate of CVD incidence relative to adults in the control condition (Uusitupa et al., 2009). Similarly, the DPPOS found no overall difference in the prevalence of aggregate microvascular complications (neuropathy, nephropathy, retinopathy) between intervention conditions but found a 22% reduced risk of microvascular complications in women participating in the lifestyle intervention (Diabetes Prevention Program Outcomes Study Research Group, 2015). In contrast with the Finnish DPS and the U.S. DPPOS, the Da Qing Diabetes Prevention Study found a 47% reduced incidence of severe diabetes retinopathy and a 41% reduced incidence of CVD mortality (Gong et al., 2011; Li et al., 2014). However, reductions in CVD mortality were fully driven by reductions in women, and there was no impact on other diabetes-related complications. The lack of a benefit in men may have been affected by the very large prevalence of smoking among study participants.

TABLE 12.2. Summary of Controlled Trials of the Impact of Lifestyle-Based Weight Loss Interventions on Long-Term Morbidity

Study/author	Population	Mean follow-up (years)	Intervention	Weight change	Effect of weight loss relative to control or referent group
CVD or mortality incidence					
Malmo Prevention Study (Eriksson & Lindgarde, 1998)	423 men with IGT, ages 47–49	12	Diet, exercise, behavioral counseling	2.3% loss vs. 0.5% gain (net 2.8%) at 6 y	51% ↓ ischemic heart disease incidence; 55% ↓ all-cause mortality
Whelton et al. (1998)	U.S. men and women with obesity, hypertension, ages 60–80 y ($n = 585$)	2.5	Diet, exercise, behavioral counseling; 28 contacts in first year	Net 4% loss	30% ↓ combined hypertension and CVD outcomes
Lifestyle Heart Study (Ornish et al., 1998)	Adults with moderate to severe CVD ($n = 48$)	5	Cardioprotective diet and exercise prescription with twice weekly counseling sessions	Net 8% at 5 y	40% ↓ cardiovascular events; significant reduction in coronary artery stenosis
Finnish Diabetes Prevention Study (Uusitupa et al., 2009)	Finnish men and women with IGT, ages 55 ± 7 ($n = 522$)	10	Diet, exercise, behavioral counseling; 9 contacts first year	Net 3.4% at 3 y	No association with CVD events; nonsignificant 42% lower total mortality rate
Japan Diabetes Complications Study (Sone et al., 2010)	Japanese men and women with IGT, mean age 45 y ($n = 542$)		10-minute counseling added to usual care + 15-minute counseling twice per month	No net weight loss	47% ↓ diabetic retinopathy; no effect on diabetic nephropathy
Look AHEAD study (2013)	U.S. men and women with diabetes, ages 45–74 y ($n = 5,145$)	9.6	Diet, exercise, behavioral support	Net 7.9% at 1 y and 2.5% at 9.6 y	No association with cardiovascular disease events.
Disability incidence					
Look AHEAD study (Rejeski et al., 2012)	U.S. adults with diabetes, ages 45–74 ($n = 5,145$)	RCT, 4	Diet, exercise, behavioral counseling; 44 visits first year	Net 5.3% loss vs. control at 4 y	48% ↓ incidence of mobility loss

Among the chain of research studies just described, ranging from observational studies of weight loss to the diabetes prevention studies, none were designed or statistically powered to test the impact of weight loss on the risk of CVD incidence. Initiated in 2001, the Look AHEAD study provided the largest test to date of structured weight loss intervention results for reduced CVD incidence (Wing et al., 2013). The study randomized more than 5,000 adults with type 2 diabetes to compare the effect of intensive weight loss intervention to a control condition consisting of modest diabetes support and education. The lifestyle intervention group in Look AHEAD received extensive support (44 visits per year during the first year, 24 visits during years 2–4, and at least quarterly visits thereafter from a multidisciplinary team, whereas the diabetes support and education (DSE) group received three visits during the first year. The lifestyle intervention group achieved a net weight loss of 7.9% at year 1 and 2.6% at year 8, with 27% maintaining a 10% weight loss (vs. 17% in DSE group)—results that were unprecedented for a major intervention trial (Look AHEAD Study, 2014). The lifestyle intervention group also achieved 15% and 12% net improvements in treadmill walking capacity at years 1 and 4, respectively. The weight loss and fitness gains were paralleled by large, first-year reductions in blood pressure (6.8/3.0 mmHg), triglyceride (−30 mg/dL), HbA1C (−5.0%), and fasting plasma glucose (−21 mg/dL). However, there was no significant effect on LDL cholesterol, perhaps because there was a slightly lower proportion taking lipid-lowering medications among lifestyle intervention group participants relative to the control condition (Wing et al., 2013). The risk factor reductions remained significant after 4 years, but the magnitude of differences in risk factors between groups had diminished to 2.4/0.4 mmHg for blood pressure, 5 mg/dL class for triglycerides, and 0.3% for HbA1c.

Despite the large weight loss and risk factor reductions achieved in Look AHEAD, the study ultimately found no significant effect on the primary outcome of CVD incidence, defined by a composite of fatal and nonfatal heart attacks and stroke, CVD death, or hospitalization for angina. There was a tendency for a more favorable effect among those without preexisting CVD than those with CVD, but the differences in risk between the intervention and control group were not significant in either stratum. Several hypotheses were raised to explain the unexpected, null findings of Look AHEAD, including factors related to the study population (previously diagnosed with diabetes), inclusion of participants with prior CVD, and the midtrial protocol change to incorporate hospitalized angina as an outcome. However, none of the subgroup analyses or tests of interaction uncovered major effects of the factors.

Nevertheless, a post-hoc epidemiological analysis suggests that the magnitude of weight loss and response to the intervention may be an important factor. In analyses combining intervention and control groups, persons with at least a 10% weight loss over the first year had a 21% reduced CVD incidence compared to persons with no weight change or weight gain. Similarly, those with large fitness change had a 22% reduced CVD incidence compared to those with no fitness gain, adjusting for differences in baseline risk factors. In a second analysis akin to a per-protocol or on-treatment analysis, participants who were assigned to the intensive lifestyle intervention (ILI) condition and met the 10% weight loss goal at year 1 had a 20% reduced CVD incidence compared to the control condition, adjusting for baseline risk factors (Look AHEAD Study Group, 2016a). These findings suggest that the structured weight loss interventions may have had a positive impact on CVD among the subset of participants with high levels of adherence and strong weight loss responses to the intervention.

Disability and Quality of Life

The association of obesity with disability and diverse domains of quality of life, including physical, psychological, and social functioning, have raised the question of whether weight loss interventions could reduce disability and improve quality of life (Alley & Chang, 2007). The association of obesity with disability is thought to be multifactorial, with obesity having direct effects on physical function and fatigue as well as indirect effects through multiple comorbid conditions, including diabetes, arthritis, coronary heart disease, stroke, and depression. It is less obvious whether weight loss, in turn, reduces disability in older adults, as observational studies of weight change and disability have actually associated weight loss with decreased physical functioning. However, the relationship may be explained by confounding due to underlying health status or reverse causality (Launer et al., 1994; Lee et al., 2005), underscoring the importance of controlled trials for the examination of the impact of weight loss on disability.

Initial trials of the impact of weight loss on functional impairment have focused on older, overweight adults with arthritis. The Arthritis, Diet, and Activity Promotion Trial (ADAPT) study randomized 316 people ages > 60 years with body mass index (BMI) > 28 kg/m² and knee pain and disability to an 18-month diet and exercise program that achieved a 5–6% weight loss, with significant improvements in lower extremity and physical functioning, 6-minute walking distance, and knee pain. A subsequent study randomized adults to dietary, exercise, diet plus exercise, or usual care conditions and found a net 9–10% weight loss, large decreases in fat mass as well as lean mass, and improvements in several metrics of strength, balance, and gait (Messier et al., 2004). The greatest overall improvements in function were associated with weight loss that resulted from exercise and diet combined. The exercise condition had no effect on weight but preserved bone mineral density and muscle mass relative to the diet condition.

The Look AHEAD Study has provided the most extensive long-term examination of the effects of weight loss on disability and quality of life to date (Rejeski et al., 2012, 2015). After 4 years of follow-up, the intensive lifestyle condition was associated with a 48% reduction in incidence of mobility loss. These improvements were most pronounced in the incidence of severe mobility-related disability, which occurred in 21% of ILI participants after 4 years, compared to 26% of those in the DSE control condition. Secondary analyses indicated that the reductions in mobility loss were explained both by reductions in body weight and improvements in physical fitness. In a subsequent analysis, the advantage of the intervention on physical function was maintained through 8 years of follow-up. However, this difference was primarily driven by older adults (ages 60–76 at baseline) and those without CVD, as the intervention-related differences gradually diminished over 8 years in the younger adults (ages 45–59 at baseline) and those with prior CVD (Rejeski et al., 2015). In a more recent analysis of the impact of the Look AHEAD intervention, the lifestyle intervention was associated with a significant, 1-year average delay in the onset of disability and a significant increase in the number of active years of life. For an average 60-year-old, ILI was associated with an increase in the number of active years of life (12.0 vs. 11.1 years), leading to a delay in disability onset (age 72.0 vs. 71.1 years) followed by a decrease in the number of years of life spent disabled (15.2 vs. 15.7 years; $p < .01$; Gregg et al., 2018).

Mortality

A long history of observational studies have raised questions about whether weight loss decreases or even increases mortality risk (Williamson, 1998). This literature is difficult to interpret due to the lack of assessment of intentionality of weight loss, leading to subsequent analyses of intentional weight loss based on self-report from cohort studies. Analyses of the Cancer Prevention Studies I and II from the late 1990s and early 2000s found reductions in mortality associated with weight loss among middle-age women and with obesity-related conditions among low-risk women (Williamson et al., 1995), but no association between the magnitude of weight loss and mortality among women without obesity-related conditions. Among men, reductions in mortality were observed only among those with preexisting disease (Williamson et al., 1995, 1999). However, subsequent analysis of adults with diagnosed diabetes in the Cancer Prevention Study and the National Health Interview Survey (NHIS) found roughly 25% reduced mortality risk compared to those who were not losing weight (Williamson, Thompson, Thun, Flanders, & Pamuk, 2000; Gregg, Gerzoff, Thompson, & Williamson, 2004). However, in the NHIS, mortality rates were 20% lower among persons who were trying to lose weight but reported no weight change during the previous year. Thus, trying to lose weight appeared to be as important as weight loss itself. This could be attributed to health benefits associated with weight loss attempts or, alternatively, an indication that people who report trying to lose weight engage in other healthier behaviors.

A study of 5,000 British men provided yet another insight into the potential role of intentional weight loss (Wannamethee, Shaper, & Lennon, 2005). Intentional weight loss was associated with a 41% reduced risk of all-cause mortality and a 64% reduced risk of non-CVD-related mortality if the weight loss resulted from personal choice. However, intentional weight loss that was attributed to ill health or a physician's advice was associated with a 37% increased mortality risk. Other observational studies have been less encouraging about the benefits of intentional weight loss on mortality. There was no association of weight loss with mortality among women in the Iowa Women's Health Study, and in the 18-year follow-up of the Finnish Twin Cohort Study, intentional weight loss was associated with increased mortality risk (French, Folsom, Jeffrey, & Williamson, 1999; Sorensen, Rissanen, Korkeila, & Kaprio, 2005). A meta-analysis quantified that these observational studies found no significant overall association of weight loss with mortality risk. However, there was a modest (19%) risk reduction among those with prior comorbid conditions and a modest (11%) increased mortality risk among healthy individuals (Harrington et al., 2009). Taken as a whole, these reviews dispel the notion that weight loss is detrimental to longevity but leave the question of benefit somewhat unclear, underscoring the importance of intervention trials to accurately assess the impact of weight loss on morbidity and mortality.

Unfortunately, RCTs of lifestyle interventions have not been adequately powered to test the impact of weight loss on mortality. As described above, the Malmo Prevention Study and the Da Qing Diabetes Prevention Study are the only lifestyle-based weight loss studies of which we are aware to report a reduction in CVD-related mortality, and the Look AHEAD study found no effect on CVD incidence. However, studies of bariatric surgery (described later) represent the one segment of the human weight loss literature suggesting that weight loss increases longevity. Finally, an ecological study explored the impact of populationwide weight change on health trends associated with the Cuban economic crisis that followed the dissolution of the Soviet Union (Franco et al., 2007). Between 1988 and 1993, average per capita daily energy intake decreased by over 1,000 calories, the proportion of citizens considered physically active doubled, obesity prevalence declined from 14 to 7%, and the prevalence of overweight remained relatively stable. During the same period, mortality due to diabetes, coronary heart disease mortality, and all-cause mortality declined by 51%, 35%, and 18%, respectively, with no change in cancer mortality rates. By 2000, the economic crisis had subsided and energy intake and obesity returned to precrisis levels. Mortality rates plateaued about 2 years later.

Medical and Surgical Interventions

Pharmacological Treatment

Following a long period of limited pharmacological options for weight loss, several new agents have been approved by the FDA in recent years. As of 2016, a total of five weight loss medications are now available. Of these, five (orlistat, phentermine/topiramate, liraglutide, naltrexone/pupropion) have been tested in randomized controlled trials of adequate size and follow-up to examine the incidence of morbidity. In 2004, the Xendos study found a net 2.8-kg weight loss with orlistat versus a placebo and a 37% reduced diabetes incidence in 3,305 obese adults with and without pre-diabetes and a 45% reduced incidence in those with IGT (see Table 12.3). As in other studies involving pharmacotherapy for obesity, the study suffered from a loss to follow-up of 66% in the placebo group and 48% in the orlistat group (Torgerson, Hauptman, Boldrin, & Sjöström, 2004). More recently, the SEQUEL trial found a net 8–9% weight loss and a 54% and 76% reduced diabetes incidence with moderate and high doses of phentermine/topiramate (Garvey et al., 2014). However, diabetes was assessed only for two-thirds of the participants due to a

TABLE 12.3. Summary of RCTs of Pharmacological Interventions: Effects on Disease Incidence and Mortality

Author(s)	Design/mean follow-up	Population	Intervention	Weight change	Lost to follow-up	Effect of weight loss relative to control
XENDOS study (Torgerson et al., 2004)	RCT, 4 y	3,305 men and women with BMI ≥ 30 kg/m^2, w/ and w/o pre-diabetes, age 43	LS changes plus orlistat 120 mg three times daily or placebo	5.8 kg vs. 3.0 kg WL	48% in the orlistat group and 66% in the placebo group	37.3% ↓ diabetes incidence
SEQUEL trial (Garvey et al., 2014)	RCT, 108 weeks	675 men and women with BMI ≥ 27 kg/m^2 and pre-diabetes, age 52	LS modification plus phentermine/topiramate 7.5/46 mg, 15/92 mg, or placebo	10.9%, 12.1%, and 2.5% WL	17% in the 7.5/46 group; 17.9% in the 15/92 group; and 17% in the placebo group	7.5/46 mg group, 54% ↓ diabetes incidence; 15/92 mg group, 76% ↓ diabetes incidence
SCALE Obesity and Prediabetes trial (Pi-Sunyer et al., 2015)	RCT, 56 weeks	3,731 men and women w/o diabetes + untreated comorbidities, with BMI ≥ 30 kg/m^2 or ≥ 27 kg/m^2, age 45	LS modification plus liraglutide 3.0 mg once daily, or placebo	8.0% vs. 2.6% WL	28.1% in the liraglutide group; 55.6% in the placebo group	65% ↓ pre-diabetes incidence 90% ↓ diabetes incidence
SCALE Obesity and Prediabetes trial (le Roux et al., 2017)	RCT, 3 y	2,254 men and women, with BMI ≥ 30 kg/m^2 or ≥ 27 kg/m^2 and pre-diabetes + comorbidities, age 47	LS modification plus liraglutide 3.0 mg once daily, or placebo	7.1% vs. 2.7% WL	47.4% in the liraglutide group; 55.0% in the placebo group	67% ↓ diabetes incidence
LEADER trial (Marso et al., 2016)	RCT, 3.8 y	9,340 men and women with mean BMI 32 kg/m^2, diabetes, and high cardiovascular risk, age 64	SDC plus liraglutide 1.8 mg once daily, or placebo	2.3 kg higher WL	3.0% in the liraglutide group; 3.4% in the placebo group	13% ↓ death from cardiovascular causes, nonfatal MI, or nonfatal stroke 22% ↓ death from cardiovascular causes 15% ↓ death from any cause 14% ↓ MI incidence 21% ↓ diabetic nephropathy incidence
Nissen et al. (2016)	RCT, 2.5 y	4,455 men and women with mean BMI 36.6 kg/m^2, 85% with diabetes, age 61	Internet-based weight management program, personal weight-loss coach, tracking programs, meal plans plus naltrexone-buproprion, or placebo	5–9 kg	9% in the naltrexone-bupropion group; 9% in the placebo group	16% ↓ death from all causes 12% ↓ MACE (cardiovascular death, nonfatal stroke, nonfatal MI)

Note. RCT, randomized controlled trial; BMI, body mass index; LS, lifestyle; WL, weight loss; SDC, standard diabetes care; MACE, major adverse cardiovascular events; MI, myocardial infarction.

combination of loss to follow-up and a study design that consisted of a 1-year extension with an opt-out for participants.

Three RCTs have tested the impact of liraglutide, a long-acting glucagon-like peptide-1 (GLP-1) receptor agonist, on weight loss and morbidity. The SCALE Obesity and Prediabetes trial tested the impact in 3,731 men and women with pre-diabetes and found a 5.4% net weight loss and 90% reduced diabetes incidence. A 3-year follow-up for those with pre-diabetes found a 67% reduced diabetes incidence (le Roux et al., 2016). However, the SCALE study also had substantial loss to follow-up (28–47%) in the liraglutide group and 67–90% in the control group, leaving open the possibility that both the tolerability of the drug and the effect on diabetes incidence were overestimated. Finally, the LEADER study randomized more than 9,000 obese men and women to 1.8 mg liraglutide or placebo. The study observed a 2.3-kg weight loss over almost 4 years and a significant 13–21% relative reduction in myocardial infarction, overall CVD and related deaths, and nephropathy. This trial, despite not having been designed to evaluate weight loss, provided the first test of a weight loss drug on CVD incidence (Marso et al., 2016). The most recent study to have evaluated multiple morbidity and mortality with an anti-obesity drug evaluated the effect of Naltrexone-bupropion added to weight management. They found a 16% death reduction from all causes, and 12% reduction of major cardiovascular events after a mean follow-up of 2.5 years.

Bariatric Surgery

The proliferation of bariatric surgery in obesity treatment in recent decades has been accompanied by a large increase in the number of studies examining long-term outcomes. Most studies have been registry-based cohorts comparing the rates of diabetes incidence, remission, CVD, and other forms of morbidity and mortality between surgical patients and nonrandom or matched controls. These studies have demonstrated large weight loss, averaging 30% over 1 or 2 years and 25% over 5 years (Maciejewski et al., 2016). As summarized in Table 12.4, the impact of surgery on diabetes incidence has been consistent and substantial, with estimates of 65–90% reductions in diabetes incidence (Adams et al., 2012; Sjoholm et al., 2013; Wentworth et al., 2014).

Much of the evidence for the benefit of bariatric surgery has been derived from the Swedish Obese Subjects (SOS) study, a long-term study of 2,010 bariatric surgery patients with 2,037 control subjects over a 20-year period. The study population ranged in age from 37 to 60 years at baseline (average age 46 for intervention, 47 for control) and had minimum BMIs of 34 for men and 37 for women (average of 41, kg/m^2). Average weight loss after 10 years ranged from 32% for gastric bypass to 20% for banding. Analyses from the SOS trial have reported 53% reductions in mortality and 33–47% reductions in CVD incidence and macrovascular and microvascular complications of diabetes (Sjöström et al., 2012). These findings have been supported by other registry-based cohorts that have observed substantial reductions in other vascular outcomes, including microvascular and macrovascular complications among patients with type 2 diabetes (Sampalis, Sampalis, & Christou, 2006; Romeo et al., 2012; Johnson et al., 2013; Sjöström et al., 2014; Coleman et al., 2016).

Four studies also observed reductions in the incidence of obesity-related cancers, breast cancer, and cancer mortality (Christou, Lieberman, Sampalis, & Sampalis, 2008; Adams et al., 2009; Sjöström et al., 2009; Aravani et al., 2018). However, a study of more than 15,000 men and women found an increased risk of colorectal cancer among surgery patients, a finding that warrants examination in additional studies. The impact of bariatric surgery on mortality has also been consistent and substantial, with reductions in mortality rates ranging from about 25 to 90% relative reductions across more than 10 studies (Derogar et al., 2013). The primary limitation of these studies is the lack of randomization, leaving open the possibility that surgical patients are somehow healthier in other ways due to selection biases that favor their referral for surgery or inherent differences in health behaviors in individuals willing to undergo surgery. Nevertheless, the health benefits of obesity surgery on diabetes incidence, diabetes re-

TABLE 12.4. Summary of Controlled Trials of Surgical Interventions: Effects on Disease Incidence and Mortality

Author(s)	Design, mean follow-up	Population	Definition of weight loss	Weight change comparison	Lost to follow-up	Effect of weight loss relative to control
Diabetes incidence						
Swedish Obese Subjects study (Sjöholm et al., 2013)	RCS, 10 y	1,540 men and women with bariatric surgery, age 45; 1,591 controls, age 47	Bariatric surgery (VBG, GB, RYGB) vs. UOC	21.2 kg/m² WL in the bariatric surgery group vs. 0.4 kg/m² in controls	77% in the bariatric surgery group; 65% in the control group	66% ↓ diabetes incidence
Wentworth et al. (2014)	RCS, 6.1 y	281 patients with LAGB, 322 controls, all age 46	LAGB vs. community-dwelling Australians	19% WL in LAGB group	16% in the LAGB group	75% ↓ diabetes incidence 19.1, 3.4, 1.8, and 20.5 cases/1,000 persons/y according with 6 ± 9% WL, 19 ± 3% WL, 32 ± 8% WL, and controls
Diabetes complications						
Johnson et al. (2013)	RCS, 5 y	Men and women with diabetes; 2,580 undergoing bariatric surgery, age 47; 13,371 controls, age 52	Bariatric surgery (GB, RYGB, VBG, BPD, SG)	NR	0.3% in the surgery group; 0.4% in the control group	79% ↓ in any major macro- (MI, stroke, all-cause death) or microvascular (new diagnosis of blindness, laser eye or retinal surgery, nontraumatic amputation, creation of permanent AV access for hemodialysis) event 78% ↓ in macrovascular events 90% ↓ in microvascular events 83% ↓ in other vascular events
Swedish Obese Subjects study (Sjöström et al., 2014)	RCS, 18.1 y	Men and women with diabetes: 343 w/bariatric surgery, age 48; 260 controls, age 50	Bariatric surgery (GB, VBG, RYGB) vs. UOC	At 10 y, 18% WL in the surgery group and 3.6% in the control group	68% in the surgery group; 82% in the control group	57% and 26% ↓ in microvascular and macrovascular disease incidence Microvascular disease: 20.6 vs. 41.8 cases/1,000 persons/y in surgical vs. control Macrovascular disease: surgery 31.7 vs. 44.2 cases/1,000 persons/y in surgical vs. control
Coleman et al. (2016)	RCS, 7 y	4,683 men and women with diabetes, age 46.7	Bariatric surgery (GB, SG, RYGB)	NR	31% at 5 years	29% ↓ microvascular disease incidence in patients with diabetes remission 37% ↓ retinopathy incidence 19% ↓ microvascular disease for each y spent in remission

Study	Design, duration	Sample	Intervention	Weight loss		Outcomes

Cardiovascular outcomes

Study	Design, duration	Sample	Intervention	Weight loss		Outcomes
Sampalis et al. (2006)	RCS, 2.5 y	1,035 men and women w/ bariatric surgery, age 45; 5,746 controls, age 47	Bariatric surgery (RYGB, VBG) vs. no surgery	62% WL in the surgery group	NR	29% ↓ MI incidence 47% ↓ angina 58% ↓ heart failure
Swedish Obese Subjects study (Romeo et al., 2012)	RCS, 13.3 y	Men and women with diabetes: 345 in surgery group, age 49; 262 controls, age 50	Bariatric surgery (VBG, GB, RYGB) vs. SODT	At 10 y, 18% WL in the surgery group and 3.6% in the control group	23% in the surgery group; 26% in the control group	47% ↓ in CV events incidence 44% ↓ in MI incidence No ↓ in stroke incidence
Swedish Obese Subjects study (Sjöström et al., 2012)	NCT, 14.7 y	2,010 men and women w/ bariatric surgery, age 46; 2,037 controls, age 47	Bariatric surgery (GB, VBG, RYGB) vs. LS intervention	16% WL in the surgery group and 1% in the control group	23% in the surgery group; 30% in the control group	33% ↓ CV events incidence 53% ↓ CV death

Cancer

Study	Design, duration	Sample	Intervention	Weight loss		Outcomes
Adams et al. (2009)	RCS, 12.5 y	6,596 men and women w/ bariatric surgery, age 38; 9,442 controls, age 39	RYGB vs. no surgery	NR	NR	24% ↓ any type of cancer incidence in women, no ↓ in men 38% ↓ obesity-related cancer incidence No ↓ in non-obesity-related cancer incidence 46% ↓ cancer mortality
Derogar et al. (2013)	RCS, 7 y	15,095 men and women w/bariatric surgery, age 39; 62,016 controls age 49	Bariatric surgery (VBG, GB, RYGB) vs. no surgery	NR	2% in the surgery group; 0% in the control group	↑ colorectal cancer incidence 10-year SIR: 3.11 and 1.63 in men and women w/surgery vs. 1.48 and 1.16 in men and women w/obesity w/o surgery
Swedish Obese Subjects study (Sjöström et al., 2009)	NCT, 10.9 y	2,010 men and women w/ bariatric surgery, age 46; 2,037 controls, age 47	Bariatric surgery (GB, VBG, RYGB) vs. LS intervention	19.9 kg WL in the surgery group vs. 1.3 kg gain in the control group	0.2% in the surgery group, 0.05% in the control group	33% ↓ cancer incidence
Aravani et al. (2018)	RCS, 3 y	39,747 men and women w/bariatric surgery age 45 y; 962,860 controls aged 53 y	Bariatric surgery vs. no surgery	NR	NR	30% ↓ breast cancer incidence 42% ↑ kidney cancer Nonsignificant for uterus cancer 36% ↓ lung cancer

(continued)

TABLE 12.4. (continued)

Author(s)	Design, mean follow-up	Population	Definition of weight loss	Weight change comparison	Lost to follow-up	Effect of weight loss relative to control
Mortality						
MacDonald et al. (1997)	RCS, 9 y in the surgery group, 6.2 y in controls	232 men and women w/ diabetes: 154 w/bariatric surgery, age 41; 78 controls, age 43	RYGB vs. no surgery	50% excess WL in the surgery group	1% in the control group	↓ mortality; 9% in the surgery group vs. 28% in the control group
Flum et al. (2004)	RCS, 15 y	3,328 men and women w/ bariatric surgery, age 43; 62,781 controls, age 47	Gastric bypass vs. no surgery	NR	75% overall	19% ↓ 5-year mortality; 33% ↓ 15-year mortality
Christou et al. (2004)	RCS, 5 y	1,035 men and women w/ bariatric surgery, age 45; 5,746 controls, age 46	Bariatric surgery (RYGB, VBG) vs. no surgery	67% excess WL in the surgery group	0% overall	89% ↓ mortality
Swedish Obese Subjects study (Sjöström et al., 2007)	NCT, 10.9 y	2,010 men and women w/ bariatric surgery, age 46; 2,037 controls, age 47	Bariatric surgery (RYGB, VBG, GB) vs. LS intervention	25%, 16%, and 14% WL in the RYGB, VBG, and GB groups, respectively	0.1% for vital status; 16% and 25% in the surgery and control groups, respectively, for examination	29% ↓ mortality
Sowemimo et al. (2007)	RCS, 9 y	908 men and women w/ bariatric surgery, age 47; 112 controls, age 43	Bariatric surgery (RYGB, LAGB) vs. no surgery	NR	48% and 66% at 5 years; 91% and 94% at 9 years in the surgery and control groups, respectively	82% ↓ mortality
Peeters et al. (2007)	RCS, median of 4 y	966 men and women w/ bariatric surgery, age 47; 2,119 controls, age 55	LAGB vs. no surgery	23% at 2 years and 22% at 5 years in the surgery group	2% for vital status; 16% at 2 years and 63% at 5 years for examination in the surgery group	72% ↓ mortality
Busetto et al. (2007)	RCS, 5.6 and 7.2 y in the surgery and reference groups, respectively	821 men and women w/ bariatric surgery, age 38; 821 controls, age 42	LAGB vs. no surgery	23% excess WL at 2 years and 22% excess WL at 5 years in the surgery group	2.4% and 2.6% for vital status; 40% at 1 year and 37% at 5 years for examination in the surgery and reference groups, respectively	64% ↓ mortality

Study	Design, follow-up	Sample	Intervention	Weight loss	Diabetes	Mortality/Other outcomes
Adams et al. (2007)	RCS, 7.1 y	9,949 men and women w/ bariatric surgery, age 39; 9,628 controls, age 39	RYGB vs. no surgery	NR	NR	40% ↓ any-cause mortality; 37.6 vs. 57.1 deaths/10,000 persons/y in surgical vs. control; 56% ↓ CAD mortality; 92% ↓ diabetes-related mortality; 60% ↓ cancer-related mortality; 58% ↑ accidents/suicide-related mortality
Perry et al. (2008)	RCS, 2 y	11,903 men and women w/bariatric surgery, 11,904 controls	Bariatric surgery (RYGB, VBG, GB) vs. no surgery	NR	NR	48% ↓ mortality for patients < 65 y and 34% ↓ mortality for patients ≥65 y
Miranda et al. (2012)	RCS, 7.4 y	2,020 men and women w/ bariatric surgery, age 54; 2,907 controls, age 58	RYGB surgery vs. no surgery	NR	NR	24% ↓ mortality
Arterburn et al. (2013)	RCS, 2 y	Men and women w/ diabetes: 1,395 w/ bariatric surgery, age 48; 62,322 controls, age 49	Bariatric surgery (RYGB, LAGB, SG) vs. medical treatment	NR	NR	No difference in mortality
Arterburn et al. (2015)	RCS, 6.6 y	2,500 men and women w/ bariatric surgery, age 52; 7,462 controls, age 53	Bariatric surgery vs. no surgery	NR	44% in the surgery group and 48% in the control group	55%, 53% ↓ mortality at 1–5 y and 5–14 y, respectively
Reges et al. (2018)	RCS, 4.5 y	8,385 men and women who underwent bariatric surgery age 46 y; 25,155 controls age 46 y	Bariatric surgery (GB, RYGB, LSG) vs. UOC	Mean BMI reduction of 9.3 vs. 1.2 kg/m²	NR	45% ↓ mortality; 90% ↓ diabetes incidence; 60% ↓ hypertension incidence; 45% ↓ hyperlipidemia incidence; 3% ↓ MACE incidence
Combined outcomes						
Adams et al. (2012)	PCS, median of 5.8 y	418 men and women w/ bariatric surgery, age 42; 417 controls seeking surgery (1) age 43; 321 controls not seeking surgery (2) age 49	RYGB vs. no surgery	28% WL vs. 0.2% in controls (1) vs. 0% in controls (2)	7% in the RYGB group; 27% in controls (1); 3% in controls (2)	88% ↓ diabetes incidence; 60% ↓ hypertension incidence; No effect in mortality

Note. NCT, non-randomized controlled trials; PCS, prospective cohort studies; RCS, retrospective cohort studies; CV, cardiovascular; VBG, vertical banded gastroplasty; GB, gastric banding; RYGB, gastric bypass; SODT, standard obesity and diabetes treatment; LAGB, laparoscopic adjustable gastric banding; UOC, usual obesity care; SG, sleeve gastrectomy; AV, arteriovenous; BPD, biliopancreatic diversion; LS, lifestyle; NR, not reported; NS, nonsignificant; SIR, standardized incidence ratio; CAD, coronary artery disease; and WL, weight loss.

mission, and mortality are consistent. The key questions that remain concern gaining a better understanding of how to identify patients who will benefit most and have the least adverse health outcomes.

Summary and Conclusions

This synthesis of the literature demonstrates clear evidence of the health benefits of intentional weight loss, except that the benefits depend on the modality of the weight loss, the target population for intervention, and the outcome of interest. Evidence is strongest for structured lifestyle interventions and bariatric surgery, particularly when applied to populations who have IGT and/or are very obese. The effects are most evident for diabetes, disability, and mortality. Benefits on other major outcomes such as CVD and cancer are less clear, as few studies exist. Specific conclusions from this synthesis, categorized according to modality of weight loss, suggest the following:

Lifestyle Interventions

1. Structured lifestyle-based weight loss interventions of at least 2 years are consistently associated with a 30–60% decreased incidence of diabetes among high-risk individuals. These findings appear strongest for overweight and obese persons with IGT. Key questions remain, including the magnitude of benefit in low-risk populations as well as the impact of less intensive, community-based approaches.

2. Lifestyle interventions have favorable effects on disability risk and active and disabled life expectancy, but more studies are needed to confirm these findings and clarify which population subgroups can expect to benefit.

3. Lifestyle-based weight loss interventions do not appear to affect CVD incidence among people with type 2 diabetes, but this may depend on the magnitude of weight loss.

4. Lifestyle-based weight loss interventions may have several other additional long-term benefits on morbidity, including decreases in chronic kidney disease, depression, and cancer, but these benefits have been dominated by findings from the Look AHEAD study and warrant replication.

Medical and Surgical Interventions

5. Bariatric surgery leads to substantial reductions in diabetes incidence and mortality and has shown promising associations with CVD incidence, diabetes-related complications, and cancer. However, these findings are limited to nonrandomized studies; RCTs would help clarify the true magnitude of effect as well as how benefits vary across segments of the population.

6. Newly approved weight loss medications have shown promising effects on both diabetes and CVD incidence, but the large loss to follow-up in many of these studies, along with the small number of studies, leaves the impact on morbidity unclear.

The growing evidence base supporting the benefit of intentional weight loss on long-term morbidity has led to an expansion of community-based interventions for overweight and obese adults with cardiometabolic risk factors, including the National Diabetes Prevention Program (Ely et al., 2017). This translation of the science into practice is an encouraging and important step in limiting the burden of morbidity caused by overweight and obesity in the United States. However, the size of the population at risk due to overweight and obesity, in part due to expanding longevity in the U.S. population, is too large to rely fully on clinical interventions and structured lifestyle programs. This problem will ultimately call upon a stronger science base to bolster the effectiveness of policy-level approaches to enhance weight loss, maintenance, and prevention of obesity. As such, there will be a continued need for rigorous trials of diverse weight loss interventions. There will also be a need for a new generation of observational studies and natural experiments to more rigorously examine the effectiveness of the diverse approaches to weight loss carried out in communities, as well as the impact of health policies aimed at managing and preventing obesity.

References

Adams, T. D., Davidson, L. E., Litwin, S. E., Kolotkin, R. L., LaMonte, M. J., Pendleton, R. C., et al (2012). Health benefits of gastric bypass surgery after 6 years. *Journal of the American Medical Association, 308*(11), 1122–1131.

Adams, T. D., Gress, R. E., Smith, S. C., Halverson, R. C., Simper, S. C., Rosamond, W. D., et al. (2007). Long-term mortality after gastric bypass surgery. *New England Journal of Medicine, 357*(8), 753–761.

Adams, T. D., Stroup, A. M., Gress, R. E., Adams, K. F., Calle, E. E., Smith, S. C., et al. (2009). Cancer incidence and mortality after gastric bypass surgery. *Obesity (Silver Spring), 17*(4), 796–802.

Alley, D. E., & Chang, V. W. (2007). The changing relationship of obesity and disability, 1988–2004. *Journal of the American Medical Association, 298*(17), 2020–2027.

Aravani, A., Downing, A., Thomas, J. D., Lagergren, J., Morris, E. J. A., & Hull, M. A. (2018). Obesity surgery and risk of colorectal and other obesity-related cancers: An English population-based cohort study. *Cancer Epidemiology, 53*, 99–104.

Arterburn, D. E., Bogart, A., Coleman, K. J., Haneuse, S., Selby, J. V., Sherwood, N. E., et al. (2013). Comparative effectiveness of bariatric surgery vs. nonsurgical treatment of type 2 diabetes among severely obese adults. *Obesity Research in Clinical Practice, 7*(4), e258–e268.

Arterburn, D. E., Olsen, M. K., Smith, V. A., Livingston, E. H., Van Scoyoc, L., Yancy, W. S., et al. (2015). Association between bariatric surgery and long-term survival. *Journal of the American Medical Association, 313*(1), 62–70.

Bariatric Surgery Source. (2017). Obesity United States Statistics: Updated. Retrieved November 21, 2016, from *www.bariatric-surgery-source.com/obesity-united-states-statistics.html*.

Bauer, U. E., Briss, P. A., Goodman, R. A., & Bowman, B. A. (2014). Prevention of chronic disease in the 21st century: Elimination of the leading preventable causes of premature death and disability in the USA. *Lancet, 384*(9937), 45–52.

Busetto, L., Mirabelli, D., Petroni, M. L., Mazza, M., Favretti, F., Segato, G., et al. (2007). Comparative long-term mortality after laparoscopic adjustable gastric banding versus nonsurgical controls. *Surgery for Obesity and Related Diseases, 3*(5), 496–502; discussion 502.

Christou, N. V., Lieberman, M., Sampalis, F., & Sampalis, J. S. (2008). Bariatric surgery reduces cancer risk in morbidly obese patients. *Surgery for Obesity and Related Diseases, 4*(6), 691–695.

Christou, N. V., Sampalis, J. S., Liberman, M., Look, D., Auger, S., & McLean, A. P. (2004). Surgery decreases long-term mortality, morbidity, and health care use in morbidly obese patients. *Annals of Surgery, 240*(3), 416–423; discussion 423–414.

Coleman, K. J., Haneuse, S., Johnson, E., Bogart, A., Fisher, D., O'Connor, P. J., et al. (2016). Long-term microvascular disease outcomes in patients with type 2 diabetes after bariatric surgery: Evidence for the legacy effect of surgery. *Diabetes Care, 39*(8), 1400–1407.

Derogar, M., Hull, M. A., Kant, P., Ostlund, M., Lu, Y., & Lagergren, J. (2013). Increased risk of colorectal cancer after obesity surgery. *Annals of Surgery, 258*(6), 983–988.

Diabetes Prevention Program Outcomes Study Research Group. (2015). Long-term effects of lifestyle intervention or metformin on diabetes development and microvascular complications over 15-year follow-up: The Diabetes Prevention Program Outcomes Study. *Lancet Diabetes and Endocrinology, 3*(11), 866–875.

Ely, E. K., Gruss, S. M., Luman, E. T., Gregg, E. W., Ali, M. K., Nhim, K., et al. (2017). A national effort to prevent type 2 diabetes: Participant-level evaluation of CDC's National Diabetes Prevention Program. *Diabetes Care, 40*(10), 1331–1341.

Ensrud, K. E., Ewing, S. K., Taylor, B. C., Fink, H. A., Stone, K. L., & Cauley, J. A. (2007). Frailty and risk of falls, fracture, and mortality in older women: The study of osteoporotic fractures. *Journals of Gerontology: Biological Sciences and Medical Sciences, 62*(7), 744–751.

Eriksson, K. F., & Lindgarde, F. (1991). Prevention of type 2 (non-insulin-dependent) diabetes mellitus by diet and physical exercise: The 6-year Malmo feasibility study. *Diabetologia, 34*(12), 891–898.

Eriksson, K. F., & Lindgarde, F. (1998). No excess 12-year mortality in men with impaired glucose tolerance who participated in the Malmo Preventive Trial with diet and exercise. *Diabetologia, 41*(9), 1010–1016.

Esposito, K., Pontillo, A., Di, P. C., Giugliano, G., Masella, M., Marfella, R., et al.(2003). Effect of weight loss and lifestyle changes on vascular inflammatory markers in obese women: A randomized trial. *Journal of the American Medical Association, 289*(14), 1799–1804.

Finkelstein, E. A., Trogdon, J. G., Cohen, J. W., & Dietz, W. (2009). Annual medical spending attributable to obesity: Payer- and service-specific estimates. *Health Affairs (Millwood), 28*(5), w822–w831.

Flegal, K. M., Kruszon-Moran, D., Carroll, M. D., Fryar, C. D., & Ogden, C. L. (2016). Trends in obesity among adults in the United States, 2005 to 2014. *Journal of the American Medical Association, 315*(21), 2284–2291.

Flum, D. R., & Dellinger, E. P. (2004). Impact of gastric bypass operation on survival: A population-based analysis. *Journal of the American College of Surgery, 199*(4), 543–551.

Franco, M., Ordunez, P., Caballero, B., Tapia Granados, J. A., Lazo, M., Bernal, J. L., et al. (2007). Impact of energy intake, physical activity, and population-wide weight loss on cardiovascular disease and diabetes mortality in Cuba, 1980–2005. *American Journal of Epidemiology, 166*(12), 1374–1380.

French, S. A., Folsom, A. R., Jeffery, R. W., & Williamson, D. F. (1999). Prospective study of intentionality of weight loss and mortality in older women: The

Iowa Women's Health Study. *American Journal of Epidemiology, 149*(6), 504–514.

Garvey, W. T., Ryan, D. H., Bohannon, N. J., Kushner, R. F., Rueger, M., Dvorak, R. V., et al. (2014). Weight-loss therapy in type 2 diabetes: Effects of phentermine and topiramate extended release. *Diabetes Care, 37*(12), 3309–3316.

GBD 2015 Obesity Collaborators. (2017). Health effects of overweight and obesity in 195 countries over 25 years. *New England Journal of Medicine, 377,* 13–27.

Geiss L. S., Wang, J., Cheng, Y. J., Thompson, T. J., Barker, L., Li, Y., et al. (2014). Prevalence and incidence trends for diagnosed diabetes among adults aged 20 to 79 years, United States, 1980–2012: Trends in diabetes incidence of diagnosed diabetes—Is the diabetes epidemic abating? *Journal of the American Medical Association, 312,* 1218–1226.

Gong, Q., Gregg, E. W., Wang, J., An, Y., Zhang, P., Yang, W., et al. (2011). Long-term effects of a randomised trial of a 6-year lifestyle intervention in impaired glucose tolerance on diabetes-related microvascular complications: The China Da Qing Diabetes Prevention Outcome Study. *Diabetologia, 54*(2), 300–307.

Gregg, E. W., Bardenheier, L., Chen, H., Rejeski, W. J., Zhuo, X., Hergenroeder, A. L., et al. (2018). Impact of intensive lifestyle intervention on disability-free life expectancy: The Look AHEAD Study. *Diabetes Care, 41,* 1–9.

Gregg, E. W., Cheng, Y. J., Narayan, K. M., Thompson, T. J., & Williamson, D. F. (2007). The relative contributions of different levels of overweight and obesity to the increased prevalence of diabetes in the United States: 1976–2004. *Preventive Medicine, 45,* 348–352.

Gregg, E. W., Gerzoff, R. B., Thompson, T. J., & Williamson, D. F. (2004). Trying to lose weight, losing weight, and 9-year mortality in overweight U.S. adults with diabetes. *Diabetes Care, 27*(3), 657–662.

Gregg, E. W., & Williamson, D. F. (2002). The relationship of intentional weight loss to disease incidence and mortality. In T. A. Wadden & A. J. Stunkard (Eds.), *Handbook of obesity treatment* (pp. 125–143). New York: Guilford Press.

Hales, C. M., Carroll, M. D., Fryar, C. D., & Ogden, C. L. (2017). Prevalence of obesity among adults and youth: United States, 2015–2016. *NCHS Data Brief, 288,* 1–8.

Hamman, R. F., Wing, R. R., Edelstein, S. L., Lachin, J. M., Bray, G. A., Delahanty, L., et al. (2006). Effect of weight loss with lifestyle intervention on risk of diabetes. *Diabetes Care, 29*(9), 2102–2107.

Hammond, R. A., & Levine, R. (2010). The economic impact of obesity in the United States. *Diabetes, Metabolic Syndrome and Obesity, 3,* 285–295.

Hankey, C. R., Lean, M. E., Lowe, G. D., Rumley, A., & Woodward, M. (2002). Effects of moderate weight loss on anginal symptoms and indices of coagulation and fibrinolysis in overweight patients with angina pectoris. *European Journal of Clinical Nutrition, 56*(10), 1039–1045.

Harrington, M., Gibson, S., & Cottrell, R. C. (2009). A review and meta-analysis of the effect of weight loss on all-cause mortality risk. *Nutrition Research and Reviews, 22*(1), 93–108.

Haskell, W. L., Alderman, E. L., Fair, J. M., Maron, D. J., Mackey, S. F., & Superko, H. R. (1994). Effects of intensive multiple risk factor reduction on coronary atherosclerosis and clinical cardiac events in men and women with coronary artery disease: The Stanford Coronary Risk Intervention Project (SCRIP). *Circulation, 89*(3), 975–990.

Jensen, M. D., Ryan, D. H., Apovian, C. M., Ard, J. D., Comuzzie, K. A., Donato, K. A., et al. (2014). 2013 AHA/ACC/TOS guideline for the management of overweight and obesity in adults: A report of the American College of Cardiology/American Heart Association Task Force on Practice Guidelines and The Obesity Society. *Circulation, 129*(25, Suppl. 2), S102–S138.

Johnson, B. L., Blackhurst, D. W., Latham, B. B., Cull, D. L., Bour, E. S., Oliver, T. L., et al. (2013). Bariatric surgery is associated with a reduction in major macrovascular and microvascular complications in moderately to severely obese patients with type 2 diabetes mellitus. *Journal of the American College of Surgery, 216*(4), 545–556; discussion 556–558.

Knowler, W. C., Barrett-Connor, E., Fowler, S. E., Hamman, R. F., Lachin, J. M., Walker, E. A., et al. (2002). Reduction in the incidence of type 2 diabetes with lifestyle intervention or metformin. *New England Journal of Medicine, 346*(6), 393–403.

Kosaka, K., Noda, M., & Kuzuya, T. (2005). Prevention of type 2 diabetes by lifestyle intervention: A Japanese trial in IGT males. *Diabetes Research and Clinical Practice, 67*(2), 152–162.

Kruger, J., Galuska, D. A., Serdula, M. K., & Jones, D. A. (2004). Attempting to lose weight: Specific practices among U.S. adults. *American Journal of Preventive Medicine, 26*(5), 402–406.

Kuna, S. T., Reboussin, D. M., Borradaile, K. E., Sanders, M. H., Millman, R. P., Zammit, G., et al. (2013). Long-term effect of weight loss on obstructive sleep apnea severity in obese patients with type 2 diabetes. *Sleep, 36*(5), 641A–649A.

Launer, L. J., Harris, T., Rumpel, C., & Madans, J. (1994). Body mass index, weight change, and risk of mobility disability in middle-aged and older women: The epidemiologic follow-up study of NHANES I. *Journal of the American Medical Association, 271*(14), 1093–1098.

Lee, J. S., Kritchevsky, S. B., Tylavsky, F., Harris, T., Simonsick, E. M., Rubin, S. M., et al. (2005). Weight change, weight change intention, and the incidence of mobility limitation in well-functioning community-dwelling older adults. *Journals of Gerontology A: Biological Sciences and Medical Sciences, 60*(8), 1007–1012.

le Roux, C. W., Astrup, A., Fujioka, K., Greenway, F., Lau, D. C. W., van Gaal, L., et al. (2017). 3 years of liraglutide versus placebo for type 2 diabetes risk reduction and weight management in individuals with prediabetes: A randomized, double-blind study. *Lancet, 389,* 1399–1409.

Li, G., Zhang, P., Wang, J., An, Y., Gong, Q., Gregg,

E. W., et al. (2014). Cardiovascular mortality, all-cause mortality, and diabetes incidence after lifestyle intervention for people with impaired glucose tolerance in the Da Qing Diabetes Prevention Study: A 23-year follow-up study. *Lancet Diabetes and Endocrinology, 2*(6), 474–480.

Li, G., Zhang, P., Wang, J., Gregg, E. W., Yang, Q., Gong, Q., et al. (2008). The long-term effect of lifestyle interventions to prevent diabetes in the China Da Qing Diabetes Prevention Study: A 20-year follow-up study. *Lancet, 371*(9626), 1783–1789.

Lin, J. S., O'Connor, E., Evans, C. V., Sengar, C. A., Rowland, M. G., & Groom, H. C. (2014). Behavioral counseling to promote a healthy lifestyle in persons with cardiovascular risk factors: A systematic review for the U.S. Preventive Services Task Force. *Annals of Internal Medicine, 161*(8), 568–578.

Lindström, J., Ilanne-Parikka, P., Peltonen, M., Aunola, S., Eriksson, J. G., Hemiö, K., et al. (2006). Sustained reduction in the incidence of type 2 diabetes by lifestyle intervention: Follow-up of the Finnish Diabetes Prevention Study. *Lancet, 368*(9548), 1673–1679.

Lindström, J., Peltonen, M., Eriksson, J. G., Ilanne-Parikka, P., Aunola, S., Keinänen-Kiukaanniemi, S., et al. (2013). Improved lifestyle and decreased diabetes risk over 13 years: Long-term follow-up of the randomised Finnish Diabetes Prevention Study (DPS). *Diabetologia, 56*(2), 284–293.

Look AHEAD Research Group. (2013). Cardiovascular effects of intensive lifestyle intervention in type 2 diabetes. *New England Journal of Medicine, 369*(2), 145–154.

Look AHEAD Research Group. (2014). Eight-year weight losses with an intensive lifestyle intervention: The Look AHEAD Study. *Obesity (Silver Spring), 22*(1), 5–13.

Look AHEAD Research Group. (2016). Association of the magnitude of weight loss and changes in physical fitness with long-term cardiovascular disease outcomes in overweight or obese people with type 2 diabetes: A post-hoc analysis of the Look AHEAD randomised clinical trial. *Lancet Diabetes Endocrinology, 4*(11), 913–921.

MacDonald, K. G., Long, S. D., Jr., Swanson, M. S., Brown, B. M., Morris, P., Dohm, G. L., et al. (1997). The gastric bypass operation reduces the progression and mortality of non-insulin-dependent diabetes mellitus. *Journal of Gastrointestinal Surgery, 1*(3), 213–220; discussion 220.

Maciejewski, M. L., Arterburn, D. E., Van Scoyoc, L., Smith, V. A., Yancy, W. S., Jr., Weidenbacher, H. J., et al. (2016). Bariatric surgery and long-term durability of weight loss. *Journal of the American Medical Association Surgery, 151*(11), 1046–1055.

Manuel, D. G., Rosella, L. C., Tuna, M., Bennett, C., & Stukel, T. A. (2013). Effectiveness of community-wide and individual high-risk strategies to prevent diabetes: A modelling study. *PLOS ONE, 8*(1), e52963.

Marso, S. P., Daniels, G. H., Brown-Frandsen, K., Kristensen, P., Mann, J. F., Nauck, M. A., et al. (2016). Liraglutide and cardiovascular outcomes in type 2 diabetes. *New England Journal of Medicine, 375*(4), 311–322.

McCarty, T. R., Echouffo-Tcheugui, J. B., Lange, A., Haque, L., & Njei, B. (2018). Impact of bariatric surgery on outcomes of patients with nonalcoholic fatty liver disease: A nationwide inpatient sample analysis, 2004–2012. *Surgery for Obesity and Related Disease, 14*(1), 74–80.

Messier, S. P., Loeser, R. F., Miller, G. D., Morgan, T. M., Rejeski, W. J., Sevick, M. A., et al. (2004). Exercise and dietary weight loss in overweight and obese older adults with knee osteoarthritis: The Arthritis, Diet, and Activity Promotion Trial. *Arthritis and Rheumatism, 50*(5), 1501–1510.

Miranda, W. R., Goel, K., Batsis, J. A., Rodriguez-Escudero, J. P., Sarrollazo-Clavell, M. L., et al. (2012). Long-term mortality in patients undergoing bariatric surgery compared to patients managed non-operatively for morbid obesity. *European Heart Journal, 33,* 494.

Mozaffarian, D. (2016). Dietary and policy priorities for cardiovascular disease, diabetes, and obesity: A comprehensive review. *Circulation, 133*(2), 187–225.

NHLBI. (1998). Clinical guidelines on the identification, evaluation, and treatment of overweight and obesity in adults: The evidence report. *Obesity Research, 6*(Suppl. 2), 51S–209S.

NHLBI. (2013). *Managing overweight and obesity in adults: Systematic evidence review from the obesity expert panel*. Washington, DC: National Institutes of Health.

Nicklas, J. M., Huskey, K. W., Davis, R. B., & Wee, C. C. (2012). Successful weight loss among obese U.S. adults. *American Journal of Preventive Medicine, 42*(5), 481–485.

Nissen, S. E., Wolski, K. E., Prcela, L., Wadden, T., Buse, J. B., Bakris, G., et al. (2016). Effect of naltrexone-bupropion on major adverse cardiovascular events in overweight and obese patients with cardiovascular risk factors: A randomized clinical trial. *JAMA, 315*(10), 990–1004.

Norris, S. L., Zhang, X., Avenell, A., Gregg, E., Bowman, B., Serdula, M., et al. (2004). Long-term effectiveness of lifestyle and behavioral weight loss interventions in adults with type 2 diabetes: A meta-analysis. *American Journal of Medicine, 117*(10), 762–774.

Ogden, C. L., Carroll, M. D., Fryar, C. D., & Flegal, K. M. (2015). Prevalence of obesity among adults and youth: United States, 2011–2014. *NCHS Data Brief, 219,* 1–8.

Ogden, C. L., Carroll, M. D., Lawman, H. G., Fryar, C. D., Kruszon-Moran, D., Kit, B. K., et al. (2016). Trends in obesity prevalence among children and adolescents in the United States, 1988–1994 through 2013–2014. *Journal of the American Medical Association, 315*(21), 2292–2299.

Ornish, D. (1993). Can lifestyle changes reverse coronary heart disease? *World Review of Nutrition and Diet, 72,* 38–48.

Ornish, D., Scherwitz, L. W., Billings, J. H., Brown, S. E., Gould, K. L., & Merritt, T. A. (1998). Intensive lifestyle changes for reversal of coronary heart disease. *Journal of the American Medical Association, 280*(23), 2001–2007.

Pan, X. R., Li, G. W., Hu, Y. H., Wang, J. X., Yang, W. Y., An, Z. X., et al. (1997). Effects of diet and exercise in preventing NIDDM in people with impaired glucose tolerance: The Da Qing IGT and Diabetes Study. *Diabetes Care, 20*(4), 537–544.

Peeters, A., O'Brien, P. E., Laurie, C., Anderson, R., Wolfe, R., Flum, D., et al. (2007). Substantial intentional weight loss and mortality in the severely obese. *Annals of Surgery, 246*(6), 1028–1033.

Perreault, L., Pan, Q., Mather, K. J., Watson, K. E., Hamman, R. F., & Kahn, S. E. (2012). Effect of regression from prediabetes to normal glucose regulation on long-term reduction in diabetes risk: Results from the Diabetes Prevention Program Outcomes Study. *Lancet, 379*(9833), 2243–2251.

Perry, C. D., Hutter, M. M., Smith, D. B., Newhouse, J. P., & McNeil, B. J. (2008). Survival and changes in comorbidities after bariatric surgery. *Annals of Surgery, 247*(1), 21–27.

Pi-Sunyer, X., Astrup, A., Fujioka, K., Greenway, F., Halpern, M., Krempf, M., et al. (2015). A randomized, controlled trial of 3.0 mg of liraglutide in weight management. *New England Journal of Medicine, 373*(1), 11–22.

Poirier, P., Giles, T. D., Bray, G. A., Hong, Y., Stern, J. S., Pi-Sunyer, F. X., et al. (2006). Obesity and cardiovascular disease: Pathophysiology, evaluation, and effect of weight loss—An update of the 1997 American Heart Association Scientific Statement on Obesity and Heart Disease from the Obesity Committee of the Council on Nutrition, Physical Activity, and Metabolism. *Circulation, 113*(6), 898–918.

Ramachandran, A., Snehalatha, C., Mary, S., Mukesh, B., Bhaskar, A. D., & Vijay, V. (2006). The Indian Diabetes Prevention Programme shows that lifestyle modification and metformin prevent type 2 diabetes in Asian Indian subjects with impaired glucose tolerance (IDPP-1). *Diabetologia, 49*(2), 289–297.

Reges, O., Greenland, P., Dicker, D., Leibowitz, M., Hoshen, M., Gofer, I., et al. (2018). Association of bariatric surgery using laparoscopic banding, roux-en-Y gastric bypass, or laparoscopic sleeve gastrectomy vs. usual care obesity management with all-cause mortality. *Journal of the Amerian Medical Association, 319*(3), 279–290.

Rejeski, W. J., Bray, G. A., Chen, S. H., Clark, J. M., Evans, M., Hill, J. O., et al. (2015). Aging and physical function in type 2 diabetes: 8 years of an intensive lifestyle intervention. *Journals of Gerontology A: Biological Sciences and Medical Sciences, 70*(3), 345–353.

Rejeski, W. J., Isp, E. H., Bertoni, A. G., Bray, G., Evans, G., Gregg, E. W., et al. (2012). Lifestyle change and mobility in obese adults with type 2 diabetes. *New England Journal of Medicine, 366*(13), 1209–1217.

Romeo, S., Maglio, C., Burza, M. A., Pirazzi, C., Sjoholm, K., Jacobson, P., et al. (2012). Cardiovascular events after bariatric surgery in obese subjects with type 2 diabetes. *Diabetes Care, 35*(12), 2613–2617.

Rose, G. (2001). Sick individuals and sick populations. *International Journal of Epidemiology, 30*(3), 427–432.

Rubin, R. R., Wadden, T. A., Bahnson, J. L., Blackburn, G. L., Brancati, F. L., & Bray, G. A. (2014). Impact of intensive lifestyle intervention on depression and health-related quality of life in type 2 diabetes: The Look AHEAD Trial. *Diabetes Care, 37*(6), 1544–1553.

Ryan, A. S., & Nicklas, B. J. (2004). Reductions in plasma cytokine levels with weight loss improve insulin sensitivity in overweight and obese postmenopausal women. *Diabetes Care, 27*(7), 1699–1705.

Ryan, D. (2007). Risks and benefits of weight loss: Challenges to obesity research. *European Heart Journal Supplements, 7*, L27–L31.

Saito, T., Watanabe, M., Nishida, J., Izumi, T., Omura, M., Takagi, T., et al. (2011). Lifestyle modification and prevention of type 2 diabetes in overweight Japanese with impaired fasting glucose levels: A randomized controlled trial. *Archives of Internal Medicine, 171*(15), 1352–1360.

Sampalis, J. S., Sampalis, F., & Christou, N. (2006). Impact of bariatric surgery on cardiovascular and musculoskeletal morbidity. *Surgery of Obesity Related Disorders, 2*(6), 587–591.

Serdula, M. K., Mokdad, A. H., Williamson, D. F., Galuska, D. A., Mendlein, J. M., & Heath, G. (1999). Prevalence of attempting weight loss and strategies for controlling weight. *Journal of the American Medical Association, 282*(14), 1353–1358.

Sjoholm, K., Anveden, A., Peltonen, M., Jacobson, P., Romeo, S., Svensson, P. A., et al. (2013). Evaluation of current eligibility criteria for bariatric surgery: Diabetes prevention and risk factor changes in the Swedish Obese Subjects (SOS) study. *Diabetes Care, 36*(5), 1335–1340.

Sjöström, L., Gummesson, A., Sjöström, C. D., Narbro, K., Peltonen, M., Wedel, H., et al. (2009). Effects of bariatric surgery on cancer incidence in obese patients in Sweden (Swedish Obese Subjects study): A prospective, controlled intervention trial. *Lancet Oncology, 10*(7), 653–662.

Sjöström, L., Narbro, K., Sjöström, C. D., Karason, B., Larsson, H., Wedel, H., et al. (2007). Effects of bariatric surgery on mortality in Swedish obese subjects. *New England Journal of Medicine, 357*(8), 741–752.

Sjöström, L., Peltonen, M., Jacobson, P., Ahlin, S., Andersson-Assarsson, J., Anveden, A., et al. (2014). Association of bariatric surgery with long-term remission of type 2 diabetes and with microvascular and macrovascular complications. *Journal of the American Medical Association, 311*(22), 2297–2304.

Sjöström, L., Peltonen, M., Jacobson, P., Sjöström, C. D., Karason, K., Wedel, H., et al. (2012). Bariatric surgery and long-term cardiovascular events. *Journal of the American Medical Association, 307*(1), 56–65.

Sone, H., Tanka, S., Limuro, S., Tanaka, S., Oida, K. , Yamasaki, Y., et al. (2010). Long-term lifestyle intervention lowers the incidence of stroke in Japanese patients with diabetes: A nationwide multicentre randomised controlled trial (the Japan Diabetes Complications Study). *Diabetologia, 53*(3), 419–428.

Sorensen, T. I., Rissanen, A., Korkeila, M., & Kaprio, J. (2005). Intention to lose weight, weight changes, and 18-y mortality in overweight individuals without co-morbidities. *PLOS Medicine, 2*(6), e171.

Sowemimo, O. A., Yood, S. M., Courtney, J., Moore, J., Huang, M., Ross, R., et al. (2007). Natural history of morbid obesity without surgical intervention. *Surgery for Obesity and Related Diseases, 3*(1), 73–77; discussion 77.

Stevens, V. J., Obarzanek, E., Cook, N. R., Lee, I. M., Appel, L. J., Smith, D. D., et al. (2001). Long-term weight loss and changes in blood pressure: Results of the Trials of Hypertension Prevention, phase II. *Annals of Internal Medicine, 134*(1), 1–11.

Syngal, S., Coakley, E. H., Willett, W. C., Byers, T., Williamson, D. F., & Colditz, G. A. (1999). Long-term weight patterns and risk for cholecystectomy in women. *Annals of Internal Medicine, 130*(6), 471–477.

Torgerson, J. S., Hauptman, J., Boldrin, M. N., & Sjöström, L. (2004). XENical in the prevention of diabetes in obese subjects (XENDOS) study: A randomized study of orlistat as an adjunct to lifestyle changes for the prevention of type 2 diabetes in obese patients. *Diabetes Care, 27*(1), 155–161.

Trials of Hypertension Prevention Collaborative Research Group. (1997). Effects of weight loss and sodium reduction intervention on blood pressure and hypertension incidence in overweight people with high-normal blood pressure: The Trials of Hypertension Prevention, phase II. *Archives of Internal Medicine, 157*(6), 657–667.

Tuomilehto, J., Lindstrom, J., Eriksson, J. G., Valle, T. T., Hamalainen, H., Ilanne-Parikka, P., et al. (2001). Prevention of type 2 diabetes mellitus by changes in lifestyle among subjects with impaired glucose tolerance. *New England Journal of Medicine, 344*(18), 1343–1350.

Uusitupa, M., Peltonen, M., Lindstrom, J., Aunola, S., Ilanne-Parikka, P., Keinanen-Kiukaanniemi, S., et al. (2009). Ten-year mortality and cardiovascular morbidity in the Finnish Diabetes Prevention Study: Secondary analysis of the randomized trial. *PLOS ONE, 4*(5), e5656.

Wang, Y., & Beydoun, M. A. (2007). The obesity epidemic in the United States—gender, age, socioeconomic, racial/ethnic, and geographic characteristics: A systematic review and meta-regression analysis. *Epidemiologic Reviews, 29*, 6–28.

Wannamethee, S. G., Shaper, A. G., & Lennon, L. (2005). Reasons for intentional weight loss, unintentional weight loss, and mortality in older men. *Archives of Internal Medicine, 165*(9), 1035–1040.

Weber, M. B., Ranjani, H., Staimez, L. R., Amnjana, R. M., Ali, M. K., Narayan, K. M., et al., (2016). The stepwise approach to diabetes prevention: Results from the D-CLIP randomized controlled trial. *Diabetes Care, 39*(10), 1760–1767.

Wentworth, J. M., Hensman, T., Playfair, J., Laurie, C., Ritchie, M. E., Brown, W. A., et al. (2014). Laparoscopic adjustable gastric banding and progression from impaired fasting glucose to diabetes. *Diabetologia, 57*(3), 463–468.

Whelton, P., Appel, L. J., Espeland, M. A., Applegate, W. B., Ettinger, W. H., Kostis, J. B., et al. (1998). Sodium reduction and weight loss in the treatment of hypertension in older persons: A randomized controlled trial of nonpharmacologic interventions in the elderly (TONE). TONE Collaborative Research Group. *Journal of the American Medical Association, 279*(11), 839–846.

Williamson, D. F. (1998). Weight loss and mortality in persons with type-2 diabetes mellitus: A review of the epidemiological evidence. *Experimental and Clinical Diabetes and Endocrinology, 106*(Suppl. 2), 14–21.

Williamson, D. F., & Pamuk, E. R. (1993). The association between weight loss and increased longevity: A review of the evidence. *Annals of Internal Medicine, 119*(7, Pt. 2), 731–736.

Williamson, D. F., Pamuk, E. R., Thun, D., Flanders, D., Byers, T., & Heath, C. (1995). Prospective study of intentional weight loss and mortality in never-smoking overweight U.S. white women aged 40–64 years. *American Journal of Epidemiology, 141*(12), 1128–1141.

Williamson, D. F., Pamuk, E. R., Thun, D., Flanders, D., Byers, T., & Heath, C. (1999). Prospective study of intentional weight loss and mortality in overweight white men aged 40–64 years. *American Journal of Epidemiology, 149*(6), 491–503.

Williamson, D. F., Thompson, T. J., Thun, M., Flanders, D., & Pamuk, E. R. (2000). Intentional weight loss and mortality among overweight individuals with diabetes. *Diabetes Care, 23*(10), 1499–1504.

Wing, R. R. (2010). Long-term effects of a lifestyle intervention on weight and cardiovascular risk factors in individuals with type 2 diabetes mellitus: Four-year results of the Look AHEAD trial. *Archives of Internal Medicine, 170*(17), 1566–1575.

Wing, R. R., Bolin, P., Brancatie, F. L., Bray, G. A., Clark, J. M., Coday, M., et al. (2013). Cardiovascular effects of intensive lifestyle intervention in type 2 diabetes. *New England Journal of Medicine, 369*(2), 145–154.

Zhang, X., Imperatore, G., Thomas, W., Cheng, Y. J., Lobelo, F., Norris, K., et al. (2017). Effect of Lifestyle Interventions on Glucose Regulation among Adults without Impaired Glucose Tolerance or Diabetes: A Systematic Review and Meta-Analysis Diabetes Research and Clinical Practice. *Diabetes Research and Clinical Practice, 123*, 149—164.

CHAPTER 13

Weight Loss and Changes in Psychosocial Status and Cognitive Function

Candice A. Myers
Corby K. Martin

Current guidelines for treating overweight and obesity in adults recommend that patients receive a comprehensive lifestyle intervention comprised of diet, exercise, and behavior therapy to improve weight and health (Jensen et al., 2014). These recommendations are based on evidence from randomized controlled trials (RCTs) that demonstrate that weight loss improves several cardiovascular risk factors (Warkentin, Das, Majumdar, Johnson, & Padwal, 2014). Weight loss can also improve health-related quality of life (HRQoL) (see Rejeski & Williamson, Chapter 14, this volume). For example, weight loss has been shown to significantly improve physical components of HRQoL, such as physical functioning and bodily pain, in adults who are overweight or obese and have type 2 diabetes (Williamson et al., 2009). However, weight loss often does not produce similar improvements in mental or psychological aspects of HRQoL (Warkentin et al., 2014; Williamson et al., 2009; Yancy et al., 2009). This chapter reviews the literature on how weight loss in adults influences psychosocial status and cognitive function. The literature review focuses on RCTs that investigated weight loss or calorie restriction, and, importantly, includes studies that promoted weight loss or calorie restriction among both persons who were overweight or obese and persons of normal weight.

Effects of Weight Loss on Mood

Severe calorie restriction negatively affected mood and psychological well-being in Ancel Keys's Minnesota Starvation Experiment, which enrolled normal-weight volunteers as an alternative to military service during World War II (Keys, Brozek, Henschel, Mickelsen, & Taylor, 1950). The study was designed to quantify the effects of prolonged severe calorie restriction and to identify methods of refeeding individuals who experienced prolonged starvation as a result of World War II. Volunteers in the study were subjected to 24 weeks of severe calorie restriction (i.e., 50% decrease in baseline intake) and a low-fat, lower-protein monotonous diet while maintaining an active lifestyle (i.e., walking 22 miles/week). After losing 24% of their starting body weight, the men displayed significant psychiatric complications, including major depression and symptoms of binge eating. These complications gradually remitted with the restoration of body weight, which had been reduced during the experiment to levels observed in patients with anorexia nervosa.

Although this study improved our understanding of the physiological and psychological effects of prolonged severe calorie restriction (and refeeding), the generalizability of the findings are limited, particularly when considering the effects of modest levels of nutritionally adequate calorie restriction in individuals who are overweight or obese. In the latter case, a review and meta-analysis by Maciejewski, Patrick, and Williamson (2005) concluded that HRQoL, including depression, was not negatively affected by weight loss, although it also did not consistently improve, in participants in weight loss RCTs. However, a number of studies conducted in recent years have shown that symptoms of depression in patients with obesity declined significantly during intentional weight loss (Fabricatore et al., 2011; Faulconbridge, 2017).

Among these recent investigations of the psychosocial effects of weight loss are the comprehensive assessment of long-term effect of reducing intake of energy (CALERIE) studies. The researchers examined the short-term (CALERIE 1, 6 months; Heilbronn et al., 2006) and long-term (CALERIE 2, 2 years; Ravussin et al., 2015) effects of calorie restriction on physical and psychological outcomes in adults who were non-obese.

Phase I of the CALERIE trial (CALERIE 1) included three separate RCTs conducted at the Pennington Biomedical Research Center in Baton Rouge, Louisiana, Washington University, in St. Louis, Missouri, and Tufts University, in Boston, with Duke University, in Durham, North Carolina, serving as the Coordinating Center. In CALERIE 1 at Pennington, 48 men and women who were overweight were randomized to one of four treatment arms: (1) calorie restriction, which targeted 25% calorie restriction of weight maintenance energy requirements; (2) calorie restriction plus exercise; (3) low-calorie diet, in which participants consumed 890 kcal/day to achieve 15% weight loss and then followed a weight maintenance diet; and (4) a healthy diet control group (Heilbronn et al., 2006). Change in mood was assessed using the Beck Depression Inventory–II (BDI-II; Beck, Steer, & Brown, 1996) and the Multifactorial Assessment of Eating Disorder Symptoms (MAEDS; Anderson, Williamson, Duchmann, Gleaves, & Barbin, 1999) depression subscale. Results demonstrated no negative effect of calorie restriction on mood, with improvements in depression in the calorie restriction group, despite the small sample size and consequent limitations in statistical power (Redman, Martin, Williamson, & Ravussin, 2008). CALERIE 2 was a multisite trial conducted at the same three locations as CALERIE 1, with Duke University again serving as the Coordinating Center. This trial tested the effect of 2 years of 25% calorie restriction on a number of outcomes compared to an *ad libitum* control group. The study sample consisted of 220 healthy adults who were normal weight to mildly overweight. The BDI-II and the Profile of Mood States (POMS; McNair, Heuchert, Droppleman, & Lorr, 2003) were used to assess the effect of calorie restriction on mood. Compared to the control group, the calorie restriction group reported improvements in mood over the 2-year period, although the effect size was modest, and the improvement in mood was not clinically meaningful, primarily due to the sample being healthy and having low levels of mood disturbance at baseline (Martin et al., 2016).

In the Look AHEAD clinical trial, over 5,000 adults who were overweight or obese and had been diagnosed with type 2 diabetes were randomized to one of two treatment arms—(1) intensive lifestyle intervention or (2) diabetes support and education—to investigate the long-term (10 years) impact of weight loss on cardiovascular health (Ryan et al., 2003). Improvements in depression (BDI-II) were observed in both treatment arms, with the effect being greater for those randomized to the intensive lifestyle intervention (Williamson et al., 2009). Importantly, improvements in depression were greatest for lifestyle intervention participants who began the study with higher levels of depression. This positive effect of weight loss on mood was maintained through 8 years of follow-up; participants in the intensive lifestyle intervention had a significantly lower incidence of depression than did participants in the diabetes support and education arm (Pi-Sunyer, 2014; Rubin et al., 2014).

Similar results were found in the Diabetes Prevention Program study, which examined the effects of an intensive lifestyle intervention or pharmacotherapy (metformin) versus a control condition on the development of type 2 diabetes in a large sample of adults with impaired glucose tolerance (Ackermann et al., 2009). This study found a reduction in depression in all three study groups from baseline to year 1; all reductions were clinically small (Ackermann et al., 2009; Florez et al., 2012).

Diet Type

Weight loss diets vary in their macronutrient composition and glycemic index. Researchers have examined if these aspects of weight loss diets affect changes in mood. In a 6-month study, 46 healthy adults who were overweight were randomized to a high-glycemic-load or low-glycemic-load diet. The two groups achieved similar weight losses that were not significantly different. Patients assigned to the high-glycemic load diet reported a worsening of mood, measured with the depression subscale of POMS, compared to those randomized to the low-glycemic-load diet (Cheatham et al., 2009). In addition to glycemic load, researchers have also focused on the carbohydrate and fat composition of weight loss diets. For example, in an 8-week study, Halyburton et al. (2007) randomized 93 adults who were overweight or obese to a low-carbohydrate, high-fat diet or a high-carbohydrate, low-fat, energy-restricted diet. Both diets reduced body weight and were shown to improve psychological well-being, specifically mood (POMS) and depression (BDI; Halyburton et al., 2007).

However, in at least one study, a low-fat diet was found to have a more beneficial effect on mood compared to a low-carbohydrate diet. This was a 52-week study of 106 adults with overweight and obesity randomly assigned to either a low-carbohydrate or a low-fat, energy-restricted diet. Those assigned to the low-fat diet reported improvements in mood, compared to those in the low-carbohydrate diet, which included improvements in depression (BDI), mood disturbance, anger, depression, and confusion (POMS; Brinkworth, Buckley, Noakes, Clifton, & Wilson, 2009). However, a similar study failed to support the superior effects of a low-fat diet. That study included 115 adults with obesity and type 2 diabetes who were assigned to 1 year of a low-carbohydrate or a low-fat, energy-restricted diet. Both diets improved depression (BDI), diabetes-specific emotional distress (Problem Areas in Diabetes [PAID] questionnaire; Polonsky et al. 1995), and various aspects of mood (POMS), including total mood disturbance, anger–hostility, confusion–bewilderment, depression–dejection, fatigue–inertia, vigor–activity, and tension–anxiety (Brinkworth et al., 2016).

The failure to consistently identify aspects of diets that more favorably affect mood suggests one of two conclusions: (1) that there truly is no relation between diet type and improvements in mood; or (2) that the effect of diet type on mood is sufficiently small that it is difficult to detect, particularly when mood is more strongly affected by other variables, such as the amount of weight loss. Indeed, in a recent review, El Ghoch, Calugi, and Dalle Grave (2016) comprehensively assessed studies that investigated the effect of low-carbohydrate diets on psychosocial outcomes. Their review concluded that the psychosocial improvement observed in patients who participated in these studies was the result of weight loss independent of diet composition.

Sex Differences

There may also be sex differences in changes in mood in response to weight loss. A short-term study (3 weeks) with women found that diet monitoring increased perceived psychological stress, and calorie restriction increased cortisol levels, suggesting that dieting may have induced a stress response (Tomiyama et al., 2010). Conversely, the fasting and calorie restriction dietary regime, which consisted of a calorie-restricted diet and 2 days of Muslim Sunnah fasting per week for 3 months, was demonstrated to significantly reduce negative mood, including tension, anger, confusion, and total mood disturbance. The intervention also improved mood among aging men compared to a control group (Hussin, Shahar, Teng, Hgah, & Das, 2013). This study found no effect for depression assessed with the BDI-II. Turning again to the CALERIE 2 study, men in the *ad libitum* group experienced significantly higher depression scores compared to the calorie restriction groups, whereas no significant relationship was formed between treatment group and depression in women (Martin et al., 2016). Results from these studies set the stage for further research to better elucidate the possible role of sex differences in the relationship between weight loss and changes in mood.

Effects of Weight Loss on Cognitive Function

Dieting to lose weight has been reported to have deleterious effects on working memory and central executive functioning (Kemps & Tiggemann, 2005; Kemps, Tiggemann, & Marshall, 2005; Vreugdenburg, Bryan, & Kemps, 2003), leading to further examination of the effects of weight loss on cognitive function. In the CALERIE 1 study at the Pennington Biomedical Research Center, a battery of tests was administered to participants to understand if calorie restriction affected cognitive function (Martin et al., 2007). Tests included assessments of verbal memory, visual memory, and attention/concentration. In this sample of adults who were overweight, calorie restriction that induced a weight loss of ~10% was not found to be associated with deficits in verbal and visual memory or attention/concentration performance (Martin et al., 2007; Redman et al., 2008). Similarly, Cheatham et al. (2009) found no significant association between cognitive performance and weight loss via energy-restricted low- and high-glycemic-load diets.

Whereas CALERIE 1 and Cheatham et al. (2009) found no effect of weight loss on cognitive function, other weight loss studies have found significant positive effects of weight loss on working memory and processing speed. Halyburton et al. (2007) examined weight loss induced by two diets (i.e., low-carbohydrate, high-fat diet or high-carbohydrate, low-fat diet) and found improvements in both working memory and speed of processing over the 8-week study. Moreover, the change in speed of processing was greater for participants in the high-carbohydrate, low-fat diet versus the low-carbohydrate, high-fat diet. In a longer-term study by Brinkworth et al. (2009), working memory improved over the course of 1 year, with no significant differences between the low-carbohydrate and low-fat weight loss diets. However, speed of processing was not significantly altered during the study.

A systematic review of studies that assessed the impact of weight loss on cognitive function was undertaken by Siervo et al. (2011). Their meta-analysis found low-order improvements in attention/executive functioning and memory in individuals with obesity who lost weight. In a subsequent pilot study, Siervo et al. (2012) examined the effect of weight loss on cognitive function (i.e., global cognitive function, memory, executive function, and speed of processing) in middle-age and older adults with obesity. They found a beneficial effect of weight loss (of approximately 10%) on cognitive function, including global cognitive function, executive functions, and speed of processing.

In addition to weight loss achieved through dieting and calorie restriction, studies have also examined how weight loss induced by bariatric surgery affects cognitive function. The Longitudinal Assessment of Bariatric Surgery (LABS) project is a prospective longitudinal study of bariatric surgery patients and similar control participants with obesity (Spitznagel et al., 2015). This study found improvements in memory function at 12 months following weight loss surgery, compared to a control group of participants with obesity that did not undergo surgery (Gunstad et al., 2011). Similar results were also observed at 24 months (Alosco, Spitznagel, et al., 2014). At 36 months postoperative, the bariatric surgery patients in the LABS project showed improvements in attention, executive function, and memory (Alosco, Galioto, et al., 2014).

Although concern has been expressed over the potential for calorie restriction and weight loss to impair cognitive function (French & Jeffery, 1994), research findings to date do not support this concern. The evidence indicates no detrimental and some positive effects of calorie restriction and modest weight loss on cognitive function. We recognize, of course, that these conclusions do not extend beyond the evidence and that cognitive deficits could occur with severe weight loss, particularly if achieved with a diet that is not nutritionally adequate.

Effects of Weight Loss on Sexual Function

Kolotkin, Zunker, and Ostbye (2012) reviewed studies that examined obesity and sexual function and concluded that a robust association existed between obesity and reduced sexual functioning. They proceeded to review studies that assessed whether weight loss improved sexual functioning. Of these studies, three found no significant effect of weight loss on sexual activity in men (Kaukua, Pekkarinen, Sane, & Mustajoki, 2003) or on sexual functioning in women (Huang, Stewart, Henandez, Shen, & Subak, 2009; Kaukua et al., 2003). However, one study of diabetic and nondiabetic men with obesity found that weight loss was associated with increases in erectile function and sexual desire (Khoo, Piantadosi, Worthley, & Wittert, 2010).

Since the review by Kolotkin et al. (2012), a number of additional studies have been undertaken to more thoroughly explore the effects of weight loss on sexual function in females and males, and in people diagnosed with diabetes. These studies have demonstrated that weight loss is associated with improved sexual function. Aversa et al. (2013) investigated the impact of weight loss on sexual function in a sample of young fertile women who were obese. Using the Female Sexual Function Index–6 (FSFI-6; Isidori et al., 2010) to measure female sexual dysfunction as a primary outcome, they randomized 44 women to either 8 weeks of an intensive residential program or 8 weeks of a nonintensive outpatient clinic program. Both groups were prescribed a hypocaloric diet for weight loss. When assessed 8 weeks after completing their respective programs, women who had been randomized to the intensive residential program demonstrated increases in sexual function and frequency of sexual activity compared to women in the nonintensive program. In a sample of men with obesity and diabetes, Khoo et al. (2011) examined how diet-induced weight loss influenced sexual function. The researchers found that weight loss over an 8-week period, achieved with either a meal-replacement-based low-calorie diet (LCD) or a low-fat, high-protein, reduced-carbohydrate diet, resulted in improvements in erectile function (International Index of Erectile Function–5 [IIEF-5]; Rhoden, Telöken, Sogari, & Vargas Souto, 2002), sexual desire (Sexual Desire Inventory [SDI]; Spector, Carey, & Steinberg, 1996), and lower urinary tract symptoms (LUTS). Khoo et al. (2014) found similar improvements in sexual function (i.e., erectile function, sexual desire) in a sample of Asian men with obesity who lost weight loss during 12 weeks of either meal replacement or a conventional reduced-fat diet.

In a sample of 46 participants with type 2 diabetes randomized to either a low-carbohydrate or low-fat diet for 12 months, improvements in sexual function (Diabetes–39 questionnaire—sexual functioning domain; Boyer & Earp, 1997) were reported, with no between-diet differences (Davis, Tomuta, Isasi, Leung, & Wylie-Rosett, 2012). Similarly, sexual function was improved in a sample of 115 adults with obesity and type 2 diabetes who completed a weight loss study with two energy-restricted diets (Brinkworth et al., 2016). In CALERIE 2, participants in the calorie restriction group reported improved sexual drive and relationships (Derogatis Interview for Sexual Function-Self-Report [DISF-SR]; Derogatis, 1997) at the end of the study, compared to the *ad libitum* control group (Martin et al., 2016).

In addition, Kolotkin et al. (2012) reviewed a weight loss study that assessed erectile dysfunction following gastric bypass surgery. This trial found significant improvements in erectile function in men postoperatively, compared to a control group (Reis et al., 2010). In a prospective observational case series of 39 men who underwent bariatric surgery, Mora et al. (2013) assessed erectile function 1 year after surgery.

Weight loss following gastric bypass surgery was a significant predictor of improved sexual function. Similar improvements in sexual function were observed in women who underwent bariatric surgery (Sarwer et al., 2014). Given this evidence, it appears that weight loss improves sexual function in women and men, in adults with obesity and type 2 diabetes, and in individuals who undergo gastric bypass surgery.

Effects of Weight Loss on Symptoms Associated with Eating Disorders

High dietary restraint scores in adolescent females are associated with eating disorder symptoms, yet only a small percentage of adolescent females with high restraint scores develop clinically significant symptoms of an eating disorder, and adolescent females with high restraint scores do not eat less than those with low restraint scores (Stice, Davis, Miller, & Marti, 2008). Hence, chronic calorie restriction does not appear to be driving the association between restraint scores and eating disorder symptomatology. Instead, more severe behaviors, such as fasting for 24 hours to manage weight, are better predictors of binge-eating pathology in adolescent females (Stice, et al., 2008). Additionally, evidence from studies in other populations does not support a relationship between dieting and the development of eating disorder symptoms, particularly when dieting is defined by calorie restriction and subsequent weight loss rather than by self-reported dietary restraint. In one of the first randomized trials to assess whether weight loss achieved by dieting (calorie restriction) induced eating disorder symptoms, Wadden et al. (2004) randomized 123 women who were obese (and free of binge eating at baseline) to one of three groups for 40 weeks of treatment, with follow-up at 52 and 65 weeks. The groups included (1) a 1,000 kcal/day diet that included a liquid meal replacement; (2) a 1,200–1,500 kcal/day balanced deficit diet; and (3) a nondieting control group. The Eating Disorder Examination (Fairburn, 1993) was used to measure binge eating and other eating disorder symptoms at multiple time points during the study. With the exception of a single time point, no evidence of binge eating or disordered eating was found in any of the treatment groups (see Figure 13.1).

In the CALERIE 1 study at Pennington, eating disorder symptoms were assessed using the MAEDS, and concern about body size and shape was assessed with the Body Shape Questionnaire (Cooper, Taylor, Cooper, & Fairburn, 1987; Williamson et al., 2008). Dietary restraint increased over the course of the study in all three dietary restriction groups, compared to the control group, which is expected with an intervention to increase restraint and restrict energy intake. Disinhibition decreased in each of the dietary restriction groups, and binge eating decreased in all four study groups. Concern about body size and shape also decreased in all three dietary restriction groups, whereas fear of fatness and purgative behavior did not change. These results demonstrated that dieting marked by significant caloric restriction and weight loss was not associated with increased eating disorder symptoms. Similar assessments were undertaken in the CALERIE 2 study, in which calorie restriction was not associated with the development of eating disorder symptoms or cognitive biases for food- and body-shape-related information over 2 years. The study results indicated that calorie restriction did not cause eating disorder symptoms in adults who were normal weight or mildly overweight (Stewart et al., 2014).

Niego and colleagues reviewed the literature on binge eating and bariatric surgery and found that most studies observed an association between presurgery and postsurgery binge eating (Niego, Kofman, Weiss, & Geliebter, 2007). If binge eating was present prior to surgery, it most likely persisted following surgery. A follow-up review by Meany, Conceição, and Mitchell (2014) concluded that presurgery binge eating was largely improved after bariatric surgery, and that the prevalence of postoperative binge eating ranged from 0 to 46% in the studies examined. Further, postoperative eating disorders, such as binge eating and loss of control of eating, were associated with poorer weight outcomes following surgery (Conceição, Utzinger, & Pisetsky, 2015).

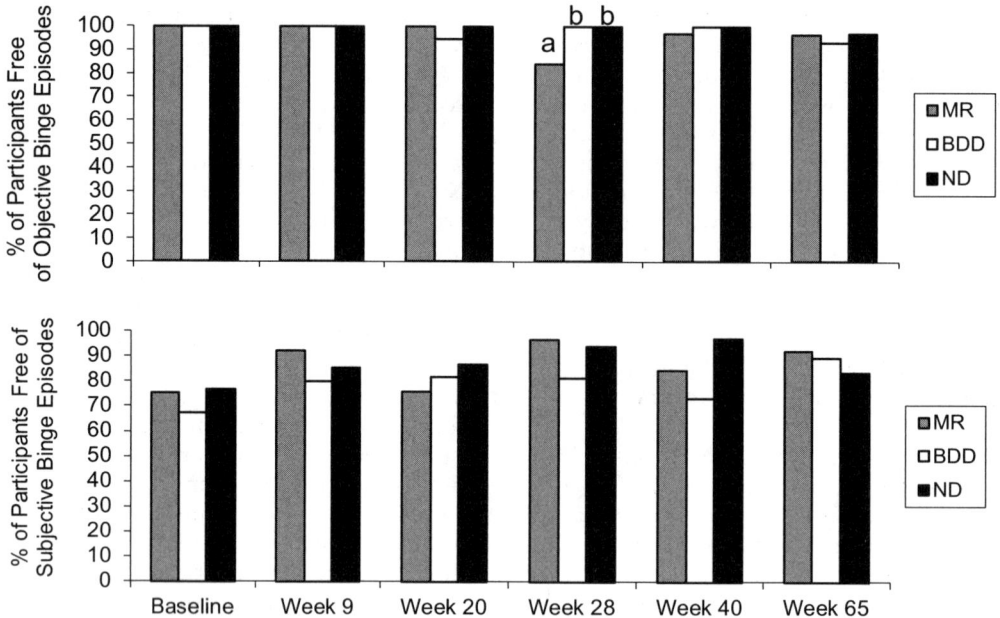

FIGURE 13.1. The percentages of participants in the meal replacement (MR), balanced deficit diet (BDD), and nondieting (ND) groups who were free of objective binge episodes at different times (A) and free of subjective binge episodes at each period (B). (A) Significant differences ($p < .003$), as determined by Fisher's exact test, were observed between groups at week 28 in the number of participants who reported one or more binge episodes. No other differences were observed among groups at any time. (B) Differences among groups did not reach statistical significance (with Bonferroni's adjustment, $p \leq .01$) at any time, although they approached significance at Week 40. From Wadden et al. (2004).

Effects of Weight Loss on Body Image

As reviewed by Chao (2015) and by Sarwer, Tewksbury, and Polonsky (Chapter 35, this volume), body image improves following weight loss, especially in individuals who are overweight or obese. Teixeira et al. (2010) randomized 225 women who were overweight or obese to a control condition or a 1-year weight loss intervention. The Body Shape Questionnaire was used to assess changes in multiple dimensions of body image. Women in the intervention reported significantly greater decreases in body shape concern and body shape dissatisfaction than those in the control group. Similarly, Annesi (2010) randomly assigned 150 women who were obese to either a treatment group consisting of exercise and behavioral instruction or a control group. The Body Areas Satisfaction Scale (Cash, 2000) was used to evaluate body satisfaction. After 24 weeks, the treatment group demonstrated greater improvement in body satisfaction than the control participants. In a study of both women and men, greater improvements in body image (e.g., attractiveness/self-confidence) were observed in the treatment group, which received nutrition and lifestyle instruction, than in the control group (Munsch, Biedert, & Keller, 2003). CALERIE 2 also found that calorie restriction was associated with improved body image in healthy adults who were not obese (Stewart et al., 2014).

In their weight loss study, Wadden et al. (2004) also found large reductions in negative body image in both weight loss groups and in the nondieting control group. This led them to conclude that improvements in body image satisfaction could be achieved with cognitive behavioral treatment, provided to nondieting participants, regardless of body weight, dieting, and weight loss. Results of this study indicate that increases in body image satisfaction can result from psychological intervention alone without the need for weight loss (Crerand et al., 2007).

In a review of studies that examined the impact of bariatric surgery on body image, Sarwer and Steffen (2015) found that many studies have reported improvements in body image following bariatric surgery among both men and women. However, bodily changes (e.g., loose skin) that occur after drastic weight loss often lead to body dissatisfaction and the pursuit of additional surgery for body contouring (Ellison, Steffen, & Sarwer, 2015).

Effects of Weight Loss on Appetite, Food Cravings, and Food Preference

In an older study that examined how calorie restriction influenced appetite, Wadden and colleagues showed that less food intake was associated with less reported hunger (Wadden, Stunkard, Day, Gould, & Rubin, 1987). They randomized 28 participants with obesity to either a very-low-calorie diet or a low-calorie diet. Greater decreases in hunger were reported with the very-low-calorie diet relative to the low-calorie diet. In the Wadden et al. (2004) study that assessed the impact of dieting on eating disorders in women, the researchers also examined measures of appetite. Cognitive restraint, disinhibition, and hunger were measured throughout the study using the Eating Inventory (EI; Stunkard & Messick, 1988). The results revealed that women in all three treatment groups, including the nondieting control group, experienced decreases in hunger and disinhibition. Similarly, in CALERIE 1, calorie restriction in healthy men and women who were overweight produced significant weight loss, but this weight loss did not alter appetite ratings (hunger, fullness, desire to eat, satisfaction, and prospective food consumption) in the three dietary restriction groups compared to the control group (Anton et al., 2009; Redman et al., 2008). In addition, weight loss diets have been shown to reduce food cravings. In a study that examined how a food-based LCD and a supplement-based very-low-calorie diet affected food cravings, Martin, O'Neil, and Pawlow (2006) found that more restrictive diets resulted in larger reductions in food cravings, as illustrated in Figure 13.2. Other studies have also found that people who lost more weight during a diet did not indulge in cravings as frequently as those who lost less weight (Gilhooly et al., 2007). Together, the results indicate that appetite ratings change even in nondieting control groups and that changes in appetite ratings are frequently similar among dieting and control groups.

Recent evidence also suggests that the macronutrient content of the diet affects changes in cravings for specific types of foods. Over 2 years, a low-fat diet reduced cravings for high-fat foods, and a low-carbohydrate diet reduced cravings and preferences for foods

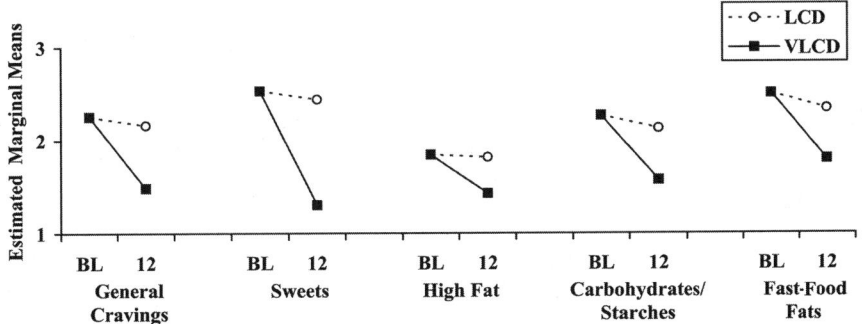

FIGURE 13.2. Estimated marginal means for cravings change scores from baseline (BL) to Week 12 for the low-calorie diet (LCD; $n = 19$) and very-low-calorie diet (VLCD; $n = 39$) groups. The VLCD group demonstrated significantly larger decreases on all cravings scores compared to the LCD group ($p < .01$). From Martin, O'Neil, and Pawlow (2006).

high in carbohydrate (Martin et al., 2011). Dieting was also associated with decreased cravings and preferences for restricted foods, with the effect being more pronounced in men than women (Martin et al., 2011). These results indicate that restricting consumption of certain types of foods results in decreased cravings and preferences for the restricted foods (see Figure 13.3). These findings are relevant to dieters, as food cravings and food preferences are appetitive forces that influence eating behavior, and the results indicate that dieting, in fact, reduces the drive to eat restricted food.

Effects of Weight Loss on Sleep

Sleep duration, a facet of sleep quality, has been linked to body weight; short sleep duration is related to greater body weight (Chaput, Despres, Bouchard, & Tremblay, 2008; Patel, 2009; Spaeth & Dinges, Chapter 8, this volume). Moreover, there has been a recent increase in awareness of sleep as an important factor in quality of life and overall health, with a specific focus on health disparities in sleep (Jean-Louis & Grandner, 2016; Laposky, Van Cauter, & Diez-Roux, 2016). Several studies have assessed how weight loss affects sleep. In a 3-month clinical trial of calorie restriction in aging men, Teng et al. (2011) used the Pittsburgh Sleep Quality Index (PSQI; Buysse, Reynolds, Monk, Berman, & Kupfer, 1989) to test how a fasting calorie restriction model affected quality of life. They found that sleep quality was poor for all study participants at baseline, but improved significantly during the study. Verhoef and colleagues investigated

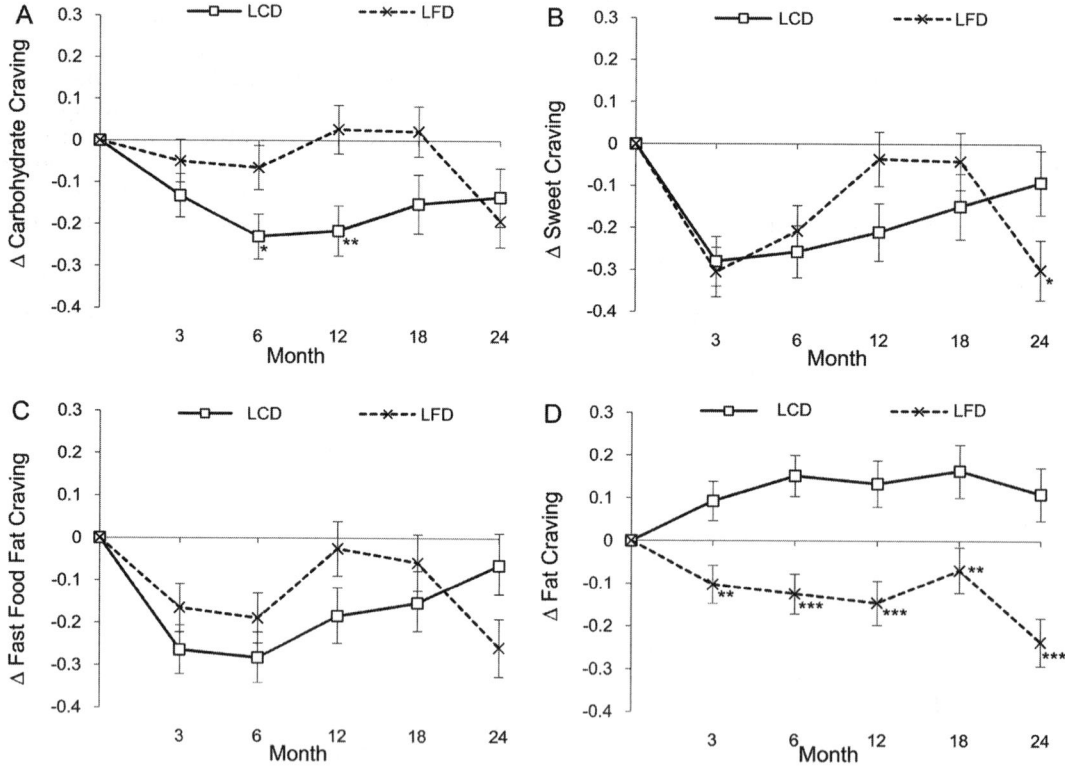

FIGURE 13.3. Change in cravings is illustrated for (A) carbohydrates, (B) sweets, (C) fast-food fats, and (D) high fats by group (low-carbohydrate diet [LCD] and low-fat diet [LFD]). Asterisks indicate the time points at which significant differences were found between groups with post-hoc tests (*$p < .05$, **$p < .01$, ***$p < .0001$). From Martin et al. (2011).

sleep duration during a 2-month weight loss diet and 10-month weight maintenance period in 98 men and women (Verhoef, Camps, Gonissen, Westerterp, & Westerterp-Plantenga, 2013). They observed improvements in sleep duration at the end of the study. Turning again to CALERIE 2, Martin et al. (2016) observed worsened sleep duration in the *ad libitum* control group compared to the calorie restriction group at 12 months. At the end of the study, participants in the calorie restriction group reported improvements in overall sleep quality.

Taken together, these few studies do not paint a complete picture of how weight loss influences sleep. In their review of studies investigating sleep duration and obesity, Marshall, Glozier, and Grunstein (2008) concluded that more research was needed to further explicate the role of sleep duration as a risk factor for obesity. Undoubtedly, the same is true for the relationship between weight loss and sleep quality: More research is needed to further elucidate this association.

Weight Cycling

Weight regain is common following weight loss, and "weight cycling" may have potential consequences for psychosocial functioning and quality of life. Engel et al. (2003) examined 122 women and men who were overweight or obese and had lost 5% or more initial weight in a structured program, and who then regained at least 5% during a follow-up period. They found that weight cycling produced a "mirror image" in HRQoL, measured with the Impact of Weight on Quality of Life—Lite (Kolotkin, Crosby, Kosloski, & Williams, 2001). The degree of improvement observed in the HRQoL with weight loss was equivalent to the degree of decline in the HRQoL that occurred with weight regain, with patients returning to their baseline values. Alternatively, Yankura et al. (2008) examined how weight regain after weight loss influenced responses on the HRQoL in 508 postmenopausal women with overweight and obesity who had lost at least 5 pounds (2.3 kg) during a weight loss RCT. They found that women who re-gained weight did not report any significant changes in mental health (Rand 36-Item Short Form [SF-36]: Mental Health composite scale; Ware, Kosinski, & Gandek, 2002) and actually reported improvements in social functioning (Social Functioning subscale of SF-36). Given the increasing prevalence of weight cycling (Montani, Schutz, & Dulloo, 2015), continued research is needed to understand the effects of weight loss and subsequent regain on psychological status and cognitive function.

Summary and Conclusions

In this chapter, we reviewed the literature concerning the effect of weight loss on changes in a wide range of quality-of-life indicators, including psychosocial and cognitive status. Our review highlights a number of important findings in the literature. Regarding the effect of weight loss on mood, individuals with greater body weight and higher baseline depression levels experienced the greatest improvements in mood with weight loss. Studies have also detected improved mood even in individuals who are normal weight to mildly overweight and have very low levels of baseline mood disturbance. Improvements in mood last over the long term (i.e., 2 years), as seen in the Look AHEAD and Diabetes Prevention Program studies. Although early concerns existed about weight loss negatively affecting various facets of cognitive function, there is no current evidence of decrements, even when calorie restriction is documented, with some improvements reported in the research literature. Poor sexual function and excess weight are associated; however, recent studies have shown that weight loss improves sexual function in men and women with and without obesity-related conditions (e.g., diabetes).

Research findings indicate that eating disorder symptoms actually decrease with calorie restriction and weight loss, although in a small percent of adolescent females, drastic weight loss efforts (i.e., fasting) are associated with eating disorder symptomology. As expected, body image improves with weight loss. Surprisingly, there is no evidence of increases in hunger with weight loss, especially in studies that use control groups. During very-low-calorie diets, shake and meal replacement programs dramatically reduce appetite, despite limited energy intake and rapid weight loss. This finding suggests that restricting foods decreases cravings and preferences for those foods, which is good news for dieters. Although weight loss is a primary target for treating overweight and obesity, avoiding weight regain is also important to ensure the maintenance of psychosocial benefits. This point is demonstrated by research revealing a "mirror image" in relation to weight loss and HRQoL benefits and subsequent weight regain and deterioration in HRQoL. Furthermore, this research and other RCTs support the causality of weight loss in improving HRQoL, although not all of the research has found that HRQoL worsens with weight regain.

Whereas understanding that weight loss induces significant physiological improvements, it is also important for researchers and practitioners to fully grasp the range of physical and psychological outcomes resulting from weight loss, including psychosocial status, cognitive function, and quality of life. Our review found that positive psychosocial and cognitive benefits accrued with weight loss, and these conclusions are similar to those reached by other researchers (e.g., Lasikiewicz, Myrissa, Hoyland, & Lawton, 2014). However, our review also points to a number of directions for future research that are worthy of further examination in order to better elucidate the complexities underlying how weight loss affects nonphysiological outcomes. These directions for future research are outlined in Table 13.1.

TABLE 13.1. Directions for Future Research

- Investigation of sex differences in how weight loss affects psychosocial status and cognitive function.
- Examination of potential health disparities in the relationship between weight loss and psychosocial, cognitive, and quality of life benefits, based upon race/ethnicity and socioeconomic status.
- Further research into the relationship between weight loss and sleep and potential causality in this relationship.
- Continued research assessing psychosocial status and quality of life during weight maintenance and weight cycling.
- Examination of the relationship between the amount of weight loss (and weight regain) and the degree/magnitude of improvement (and decrement) in psychosocial status, cognitive function, and quality of life.

References

Ackermann, R. T., Edelstein, S. L., Narayan, K. M., Zhang, P., Engelgau, M. M., Herman, W. H., et al. (2009). Changes in health state utilities with changes in body mass in the Diabetes Prevention Program. *Obesity (Silver Spring), 17*(12), 2176–2181.

Alosco, M. L., Galioto, R., Spitznagel, M. B., Strain, G., Devlin, M., Cohen, R., et al. (2014). Cognitive function after bariatric surgery: Evidence for improvement 3 years after surgery. *American Journal of Surgery, 207*(6), 870–876.

Alosco, M. L., Spitznagel, M. B., Strain, G., Devlin, M., Cohen, R., Paul, R., et al. (2014). Improved memory function two years after bariatric surgery. *Obesity (Silver Spring), 22*(1), 32–38.

Anderson, D. A., Williamson, D. A., Duchmann, E. G., Gleaves, D. H., & Barbin, J. M. (1999). Development and validation of a multifactorial treatment outcome measure for eating disorders. *Assessment, 6,* 7–20.

Annesi, J. J. (2010). Relations of changes in self-regulatory efficacy and physical self-concept with improvements in body satisfaction in obese women initiating exercise with cognitive-behavioral support. *Body Image, 7*(4), 356–359.

Anton, S. D., Han, H., York, E., Martin, C. K., Ravussin, E., & Williamson, D. A. (2009). Effect of calorie restriction on subjective ratings of appetite. *Journal of Human Nutrition and Dietetics, 22*(2), 141–147.

Aversa, A., Bruzziches, R., Francomano, D., Greco, E. A., Violi, F., Lenzi, A., et al. (2013). Weight loss by multidisciplinary intervention improves endothelial and sexual function in obese fertile women. *Journal of Sexual Medicine, 10*(4), 1024–1033.

Beck, A. T., Steer, R. A., & Brown, G. K. (1996). *Beck Depression Inventory—Second Edition: Manual.* San Antonio, TX: Psychological Corporation.

Boyer, J. G., & Earp, J. A. (1997). The development of an instrument for assessing the quality of life of people with diabetes. Diabetes-39. *Medical Care, 35*(5), 440–453.

Brinkworth, G. D., Buckley, J. D., Noakes, M., Clifton, P. M., & Wilson, C. J. (2009). Long-term effects of a very low-carbohydrate diet and a low-fat diet on mood and cognitive function. *Archives of Internal Medicine, 169*(20), 1873–1880.

Brinkworth, G. D., Luscombe-Marsh, N. D., Thompson, C. H., Noakes, M., Buckley, J. D., Wittert, G., et al. (2016). Long-term effects of very low-carbohydrate and high-carbohydrate weight-loss diets on psychological health in obese adults with type 2 diabetes: Randomized controlled trial. *Journal of Internal Medicine, 280*(4), 388–397.

Buysse, D. J., Reynolds, C. F., III, Monk, T. H., Berman, S. R., & Kupfer, D. J. (1989). Pittsburgh Sleep Quality Index: A new instrument for psychiatric practice and research. *Psychiatry Research, 28*(2), 193–213.

Cash, T. F. (2000). *The Multidimensional Body-Self Relations Questionnaire User's Manual.* Norfolk, VA: Body Images.

Chao, H. L. (2015). Body image change in obese and overweight persons enrolled in weight loss intervention programs: A systematic review and meta-analysis. *PLOS ONE, 10*(5), e0124036.

Chaput, J. P., Despres, J. P., Bouchard, C., & Tremblay, A. (2008). The association between sleep duration and weight gain in adults: A 6-year prospective study from the Quebec Family Study. *Sleep, 31*(4), 517–523.

Cheatham, R. A., Roberts, S. B., Das, S. K., Gilhooly, C. H., Golden, J. K., Hyatt, R., et al. (2009). Long-term effects of provided low and high glycemic load low energy diets on mood and cognition. *Physiology and Behavior, 98*(3), 374–379.

Conceição, E. M., Utzinger, L. M., & Pisetsky, E. M. (2015). Eating disorders and problematic eating behaviours before and after bariatric surgery: Characterization, assessment and association with treatment outcomes. *European Eating Disorders Review, 23*(6), 417–425.

Cooper, P. J., Taylor, M. J., Cooper, Z., & Fairburn, C. G. (1987). The development and validation of the Body Shape Questionnaire. *International Journal of Eating Disorders, 6*, 485–494.

Crerand, C. E., Wadden, T. A., Foster, G. D., Sarwer, D. B., Paster, L. M., & Berkowitz, R. I. (2007). Changes in obesity-related attitudes in women seeking weight reduction. *Obesity (Silver Spring), 15*(3), 740–747.

Davis, N. J., Tomuta, N., Isasi, C. R., Leung, V., & Wylie-Rosett, J. (2012). Diabetes-specific quality of life after a low-carbohydrate and low-fat dietary intervention. *The Diabetes Educator, 38*(2), 250–255.

Derogatis, L. R. (1997). The Derogatis Interview for Sexual Functioning (DISF/DISF-SR): An introductory report. *Journal of Sex and Marital Therapy, 23*(4), 291–304.

El Ghoch, M., Calugi, S., & Dalle Grave, R. (2016). The effects of low-carbohydrate diets on psychosocial outcomes in obesity/overweight: A systematic review of randomized, controlled studies. *Nutrients, 8*(7), 402.

Ellison, J. M., Steffen, K. J., & Sarwer, D. B. (2015). Body contouring after bariatric surgery. *European Eating Disorders Review, 23*(6), 479–487.

Engel, S. G., Crosby, R. D., Kolotkin, R. L., Hartley, G. G., Williams, G. R., Wonderlich, S. A., et al. (2003). Impact of weight loss and regain on quality of life: Mirror image or differential effect? *Obesity Research, 11*(10), 1207–1213.

Fabricatore, A. N., Wadden, T. A., Higginbotham, A. J., Faulconbridge, L. F., Nguyen, A. M., Heymsfield, S. B., et al. (2011). Intentional weight loss and change in symptoms of depression: A systematic review and meta-analysis. *International Journal of Obesity (London), 35*(11), 1363–1376.

Fairburn, C. G. (1993). The Eating Disorder Examination (12th ed.). In C. G. Fairburn & G. T. Wilson (Eds.), *Binge eating: Nature, assessment, and treatment* (pp. 317–360). New York: Guilford Press.

Faulconbridge, L. F. (2017). Social and psychological effects of weight loss. In K. D. Brownell & B. T. Walsh (Eds.), *Eating disorders and obesity* (pp. 664–672). New York: Guilford Press.

Florez, H., Pan, Q., Ackermann, R. T., Marrero, D. G., Barrett-Connor, E., Delahanty, L., et al. (2012). Impact of lifestyle intervention and metformin on health-related quality of life: The diabetes prevention program randomized trial. *Journal of General Internal Medicine, 27*(12), 1594–1601.

French, S. A., & Jeffery, R. W. (1994). Consequences of dieting to lose weight: Effects on physical and mental health. *Health Psychology, 13*(3), 195–212.

Gilhooly, C. H., Das, S. K., Golden, J. K., McCrory, M. A., Dallal, G. E., Saltzman, E., et al. (2007). Food cravings and energy regulation: The characteristics of craved foods and their relationship with eating behaviors and weight change during 6 months of dietary energy restriction. *International Journal of Obesity (London), 31*(12), 1849–1858.

Gunstad, J., Strain, G., Devlin, M. J., Wing, R., Cohen, R. A., Paul, R. H., et al. (2011). Improved memory function 12 weeks after bariatric surgery. *Surgery for Obesity and Related Diseases, 7*(4), 465–472.

Halyburton, A. K., Brinkworth, G. D., Wilson, C. J., Noakes, M., Buckley, J. D., Keogh, J. B., et al. (2007). Low- and high-carbohydrate weight-loss diets have similar effects on mood but not cognitive performance. *American Journal of Clinical Nutrition, 86*(3), 580–587.

Heilbronn, L. K., de Jonge, L., Frisard, M. I., DeLany, J. P., Larson-Meyer, D. E., Rood, J., et al. (2006). Effect of 6-month calorie restriction on biomarkers of longevity, metabolic adaptation, and oxidative stress in overweight individuals: A randomized controlled trial. *Journal of the American Medical Association, 295*(13), 1539–1548.

Huang, A. J., Stewart, A. L., Henandez, A. L., Shen, H. C., & Subak, L. L. (2009). Sexual function among overweight and obese women with urinary incontinence in a randomized controlled trial of an intensive behavioral weight loss intervention. *Journal of Urology, 181*(5), 2235–2242.

Hussin, N. M., Shahar, S., Teng, N. I. M. F., Hgah, W. Z. W., & Das, S. K. (2013). Efficacy of fasting and calorie restriction (FCR) on mood and depression among aging men. *Journal of Nutrition, Health, and Aging, 17*(8), 674–680.

Isidori, A. M., Pozza, C., Esposito, K., Giugliano, D., Morano, S., Vignozzi, L., Corona, G., et al. (2010). Development and validation of a 6-item version of the Female Sexual Function Index (FSFI) as a diagnostic tool for female sexual dysfunction. *Journal of Sexual Medicine, 7,* 1139–1146.

Jean-Louis, G., & Grandner, M. (2016). Importance of recognizing sleep health disparities and implementing innovative interventions to reduce these disparities. *Sleep Medicine, 18,* 1–2.

Jensen, M. D., Ryan, D. H., Apovian, C. M., Ard, J. D., Comuzzie, A. G., Donato, K. A., et al. (2014). 2013 AHA/ACC/TOS guideline for the management of overweight and obesity in adults: A report of the American College of Cardiology/American Heart Association Task Force on Practice Guidelines and The Obesity Society. *Journal of the American College of Cardiology, 63*(25, Pt. B), 2985–3023.

Kaukua, J., Pekkarinen, T., Sane, T., & Mustajoki, P. (2003). Sex hormones and sexual function in obese men losing weight. *Obesity Research, 11*(6), 689–694.

Kemps, E., & Tiggemann, M. (2005). Working memory performance and preoccupying thoughts in female dieters: Evidence for a selective central executive impairment. *British Journal of Clinical Psychology, 44*(Pt. 3), 357–366.

Kemps, E., Tiggemann, M., & Marshall, K. (2005). Relationship between dieting to lose weight and the functioning of the central executive. *Appetite, 45*(3), 287–294.

Keys, A., Brozek, J., Henschel, A., Mickelsen, O., & Taylor, H. L. (1950). *The biology of human starvation.* Minneapolis: University of Minnesota Press.

Khoo, J., Ling, P. S., Tan, J., Teo, A., Ng, H. L., Chen, R. Y., et al. (2014). Comparing the effects of meal replacements with reduced-fat diet on weight, sexual and endothelial function, testosterone and quality of life in obese Asian men. *International Journal of Impotence Research, 26*(2), 61–66.

Khoo, J., Piantadosi, C., Duncan, R., Worthley, S. G., Jenkins, A., Noakes, M., et al. (2011). Comparing effects of a low-energy diet and a high-protein low-fat diet on sexual and endothelial function, urinary tract symptoms, and inflammation in obese diabetic men. *International Society for Sexual Medicine, 8*(10), 2868–2875.

Khoo, J., Piantadosi, C., Worthley, S., & Wittert, G. A. (2010). Effects of a low-energy diet on sexual function and lower urinary tract symptoms in obese men. *International Journal of Obesity (London), 34*(9), 1396–1403.

Kolotkin, R. L., Crosby, R. D., Kosloski, T., & Williams, G. T. (2001). Development of a brief measure to assess quality of life in obesity. *Obesity Research, 9,* 102–111.

Kolotkin, R. L., Zunker, C., & Ostbye, T. (2012). Sexual functioning and obesity: A review. *Obesity (Silver Spring), 20*(12), 2325–2333.

Laposky, A. D., Van Cauter, E., & Diez-Roux, A. V. (2016). Reducing health disparities: The role of sleep deficiency and sleep disorders. *Sleep Medicine, 18,* 3–6.

Lasikiewicz, N., Myrissa, K., Hoyland, A., & Lawton, C. L. (2014). Psychological benefits of weight loss following behavioural and/or dietary weight loss interventions: A systematic research review. *Appetite, 72,* 123–137.

Maciejewski, M. L., Patrick, D. L., & Williamson, D. F. (2005). A structured review of randomized controlled trials of weight loss showed little improvement in health-related quality of life. *Journal of Clinical Epidemiology, 58*(6), 568–578.

Marshall, N. S., Glozier, N., & Grunstein, R. R. (2008). Is sleep duration related to obesity?: A critical review of the epidemiological evidence. *Sleep Medicine Review, 12*(4), 289–298.

Martin, C. K., Anton, S. D., Han, H., York-Crowe, E., Redman, L. M., Ravussin, E., et al. (2007). Examination of cognitive function during six months of calorie restriction: Results of a randomized controlled trial. *Rejuvenation Research, 10*(2), 179–190.

Martin, C. K., Bhapkar, M., Pittas, A. G., Pieper, C. F., Das, S. K., Williamson, D. A., et al. (2016). Effect of calorie restriction on mood, quality of life, sleep, and sexual function in healthy nonobese adults: The calorie 2 randomized clinical trial. *JAMA Internal Medicine, 176*(6), 743–752.

Martin, C. K., O'Neil, P. M., & Pawlow, L. (2006). Changes in food cravings during low-calorie and very-low-calorie diets. *Obesity (Silver Spring), 14*(1), 115–121.

Martin, C. K., Rosenbaum, D., Han, H., Geiselman, P. J., Wyatt, H. R., Hill, J. O., et al. (2011). Change in food cravings, food preferences, and appetite during a low-carbohydrate and low-fat diet. *Obesity (Silver Spring), 19*(10), 1963–1970.

McNair, D. M., Heuchert, J. W. P., Droppleman, L. F., & Lorr, J. (2003). *Profile of mood states: Technical update.* North Tonawanda, NY: Multi-Health Systems.

Meany, G., Conceição, E., & Mitchell, J. E. (2014). Binge eating, binge eating disorder and loss of control eating: Effects on weight outcomes after bariatric surgery. *European Eating Disorders Review, 22*(2), 87–91.

Montani, J. P., Schutz, Y., & Dulloo, A. G. (2015). Dieting and weight cycling as risk factors for cardiometabolic diseases: Who is really at risk? *Obesity Review, 16*(Suppl. 1), 7–18.

Mora, M., Aranda, G. B., de Hollanda, A., Flores, L., Puig-Domingo, M., & Vidal, J. (2013). Weight loss is a major contributor to improved sexual function after bariatric surgery. *Surgical Endoscopy, 27*(9), 3197–3204.

Munsch, S., Biedert, E., & Keller, U. (2003). Evaluation of a lifestyle change programme for the treatment of obesity in general practice. *Swiss Medical Weekly, 133*(9–10); discussion 148–154.

Niego, S. H., Kofman, M. D., Weiss, J. J., & Geliebter, A. (2007). Binge eating in the bariatric surgery population: A review of the literature. *International Journal of Eating Disorders, 40*(4), 349–359.

Patel, S. R. (2009). Reduced sleep as an obesity risk factor. *Obesity Review, 10*(Suppl. 2), 61–68.

Pi-Sunyer, X. (2014). The Look AHEAD Trial: A review and discussion of its outcomes. *Current Nutrition Reports, 3*(4), 387–391.

Polonsky, W. H., Anderson, B. J., Lohrer, P. A., Welch, G., Jacobson, A. M., Aponte, J. E., et al. (1995). Assessment of diabetes-related distress. *Diabetes Care, 18*(6), 754–760.

Ravussin, E., Redman, L. M., Rochon, J., Das, S. K., Fontana, L., Kraus, W. E., et al. (2015). A 2-year randomized controlled trial of human caloric restriction: Feasibility and effects on predictors of health span and longevity. *Journals of Gerontology Series A: Biological Sciences and Medical Sciences, 70*(9), 1097–1104.

Redman, L. M., Martin, C. K., Williamson, D. A., & Ravussin, E. (2008). Effect of caloric restriction in non-obese humans on physiological, psychological and behavioral outcomes. *Physiology and Behavior, 94*(5), 643–648.

Reis, L. O., Favaro, W. J., Barreiro, G. C., de Oliveira, L. C., Chaim, E. A., Fregonesi, A., et al. (2010). Erectile dysfunction and hormonal imbalance in morbidly obese males is reversed after gastric bypass surgery: A prospective randomized controlled trial. *International Journal of Andrology, 33*(5), 736–744.

Rhoden, E. L., Telöken, C., Sogari, P. R., & Vargas Souto, C. A. (2002). The use of the simplified International Index of Erectile Function (IIEF-5) as a diagnostic tool to study the prevalence of erectile dysfunction. *International Journal of Impotence Research, 14*(4), 245–250.

Rubin, R. R., Wadden, T. A., Bahnson, J. L., Blackburn, G. L., Brancati, F. L., Bray, G. A., et al. (2014). Impact of intensive lifestyle intervention on depression and health-related quality of life in type 2 diabetes: The Look AHEAD Trial. *Diabetes Care, 37*(6), 1544–1553.

Ryan, D. H., Espeland, M. A., Foster, G. D., Haffner, S. M., Hubbard, V. S., Johnson, K. C., et al. (2003). Look AHEAD (Action for Health in Diabetes): Design and methods for a clinical trial of weight loss for the prevention of cardiovascular disease in type 2 diabetes. *Controlled Clinical Trials, 24*(5), 610–628.

Sarwer, D. B., Spitzer, J. C., Wadden, T. A., Mitchell, J. E., Lancaster, K., Courcoulas, A., et al. (2014). Changes in sexual functioning and sex hormone levels in women following bariatric surgery. *JAMA Surgery, 149*(1), 26–33.

Sarwer, D. B., & Steffen, K. J. (2015). Quality of life, body image and sexual functioning in bariatric surgery patients. *European Eating Disorders Review, 23*(6), 504–508.

Siervo, M., Arnold, R., Wells, J. C., Tagliabue, A., Colantuoni, A., Albanese, E., et al. (2011). Intentional weight loss in overweight and obese individuals and cognitive function: A systematic review and meta-analysis. *Obesity Review, 12*(11), 968–983.

Siervo, M., Nasti, G., Stephan, B. C., Papa, A., Muscariello, E., Wells, J. C., et al. (2012). Effects of intentional weight loss on physical and cognitive function in middle-aged and older obese participants: A pilot study. *Journal of the American College of Nutrition, 31*(2), 79–86.

Spector, I. P., Carey, M. P., & Steinberg, L. (1996). The Sexual Desire Inventory: Development, factor structure, and evidence of reliability. *Journal of Sex and Marital Therapy, 22*(3), 175–190.

Spitznagel, M. B., Hawkins, M., Alosco, M., Galioto, R., Garcia, S., Miller, L., et al. (2015). Neurocognitive effects of obesity and bariatric surgery. *European Eating Disorders Review, 23*(6), 488–495.

Stewart, T. M., Williamson, D. A., Martin, C. K., Gilhooly, C. H., Robinson, L., Scott, T. M., et al. (2014, November). *Is calorie restriction associated with the development of eating disorders in non-obese adults?* Paper presented at the annual meeting of the Obesity Society, Boston, MA.

Stice, E., Davis, K., Miller, N. P., & Marti, C. N. (2008). Fasting increases risk for onset of binge eating and bulimic pathology: A 5-year prospective study. *Journal of Abnormal Psychology, 117*(4), 941–946.

Stunkard, A. J., & Messick, S. (1988). *The eating inventory.* San Antonio, TX: Psychological Corporation.

Teixeira, P. J., Silva, M. N., Coutinho, S. R., Palmeira, A. L., Mata, J., Vieira, P. N., et al. (2010). Mediators of weight loss and weight loss maintenance in middle-aged women. *Obesity (Silver Spring), 18*(4), 725–735.

Teng, N. I. M. F., Shahar, S., Manaf, Z. A., Das, S. K., Taha, C. S. C., & Ngah, W. Z. (2011). Efficacy of fasting calorie restriction on quality of life among aging men. *Physiology and Behavior, 104,* 1059–1064.

Tomiyama, A. J., Mann, T., Vinas, D., Hunger, J. M., Dejager, J., & Taylor, S. E. (2010). Low calorie dieting increases cortisol. *Psychosomatic Medicine, 72*(4), 357–364.

Verhoef, S., Camps, S., Gonissen, H., Westerterp, K., & Westerterp-Plantenga, M. (2013). Concomitant changes in sleep duration and body weight and body composition during weight loss and 3-mo weight maintenance. *American Society for Nutrition, 98*(1), 25–31.

Vreugdenburg, L., Bryan, J., & Kemps, E. (2003). The effect of self-initiated weight-loss dieting on working memory: The role of preoccupying cognitions. *Appetite, 41*(3), 291–300.

Wadden, T. A., Foster, G. D., Sarwer, D. B., Anderson, D. A., Gladis, M., Sanderson, R. S., et al. (2004). Dieting and the development of eating disorders in obese women: Results of a randomized controlled trial. *American Journal of Clinical Nutrition, 80*(3), 560–568.

Wadden, T. A., Stunkard, A. J., Day, S. C., Gould, R. A., & Rubin, C. J. (1987). Less food, less hunger: Reports of appetite and symptoms in a controlled study of a protein-sparing modified fast. *International Journal of Obesity, 11*(3), 239–249.

Ware, J. E., Kosinski, M., & Gandek, B. (2002). *SF-36 Health Survey: Manual and interpretation guide.* Lincoln, RI: Quality Metric.

Warkentin, L. M., Das, D., Majumdar, S. R., Johnson, J. A., & Padwal, R. S. (2014). The effect of weight loss on health-related quality of life: Systematic review and meta-analysis of randomized trials. *Obesity Review, 15*(3), 169–182.

Williamson, D. A., Martin, C. K., Anton, S. D., York-Crowe, E., Han, H., Redman, L., et al. (2008). Is caloric restriction associated with development of eating-disorder symptoms?: Results from the CALERIE trial. *Health Psychology, 27*(1, Suppl.), S32–S42.

Williamson, D. A., Rejeski, J., Lang, W., Van Dorsten, B., Fabricatore, A. N., & Toledo, K. (2009). Impact of a weight management program on health-related quality of life in overweight adults with type 2 diabetes. *Archives of Internal Medicine, 169*(2), 163–171.

Yancy, W. S., Jr., Almirall, D., Maciejewski, M. L., Kolotkin, R. L., McDuffie, J. R., & Westman, E. C. (2009). Effects of two weight-loss diets on health-related quality of life. *Quality of Life Research, 18*(3), 281–289.

Yankura, D. J., Conroy, M. B., Hess, R., Pettee, K. K., Kuller, L. H., & Kriska, A. M. (2008). Weight regain and health-related quality of life in postmenopausal women. *Obesity (Silver Spring), 16*(10), 2259–2265.

CHAPTER 14

Effects of Lifestyle Interventions on Health-Related Quality of Life and Physical Functioning

W. Jack Rejeski
Donald A. Williamson

The health consequences of obesity are far-reaching, adversely influencing multiple organ systems and contributing significantly to the increase in morbidity that people experience as they age across the lifespan. This chapter focuses on an equally important, yet often ignored, consequence of obesity: its effect on quality of life and physical function. Because depression is such a central feature of mental health and quality of life, we also include data from the Beck Depression Inventory–II (BDI-II; Beck, Ward, Mendelson, Mock, & Erbaugh, 1961) under the umbrella of health-related quality of life (HRQoL).

In the first section of this chapter, we review evidence concerning the effects of intensive lifestyle interventions (ILIs) involving caloric restriction and physical activity on HRQoL and physical functioning. There is benefit in considering these joint outcomes, since, as our review demonstrates, obesity has a stronger effect on facets of HRQoL that involve physical as opposed to mental health. Whereas HRQoL assesses self-reported limitations in physical and mental health, physical functioning encompasses objective measures of physical capacities, such as strength and walking tests that assess mobility. In the second section of this chapter, we explore several issues that are important to consider for a complete understanding of how obesity and ILIs may be related to HRQoL, physical functioning, and potential mediators of change.

While HRQoL and physical functioning are obviously important at the individual level, it is well known that they also place a burden on the health care system and eventually on society at-large. For example, the self-reported inability to walk one-fourth of a mile or to climb stairs is a major risk factor for both assisted living and nursing home care. Moreover, with the "Graying of America," these outcomes will become increasingly important due their burden on Medicare.

Consistent with the SF-36 Physical and Mental Component Summary subscales of the Medical Outcome Study 36-Item Short-Form Health Survey (SF-36; Ware, Kosinski, & Keller, 1994), a generic index of HRQoL, we embrace the view that HRQoL consists of two broad dimensions: physical and mental health. These two dimensions are captured by eight subscales of the SF-36 that assess limitations in (1) physical functioning, (2) role functioning that is dependent upon physical health, (3) bodily pain, (4) energy and fatigue, (5) emotional well-being, (6) role functioning dependent upon emotional health, (7) social functioning, and (8) general health perceptions. At the onset, it is worth mentioning that most studies simply report data on the composite dimensions of physical and mental health. Although we recognize that there are other measures of HRQoL, both generic and disease-specific in use in the field of behavioral medicine, we felt that there were insufficient data to integrate these findings with what is known from the SF-36. The SF-36 also has extensive psychometric support (Ware et al., 1994). As noted above, we do supplement data on the SF-36 with research on the BDI-II and objective measures of physical function.

Effects of ILIs on HRQoL and Physical Functioning

In a 2005 review, Maciejewski, Patrick, and Williamson concluded that weight loss was not associated with improved HRQoL. Since that publication, several reviews have modified this broad, sweeping conclusion, noting that ILIs have positive effects on some components of HRQoL but not others (Lasikiewicz, Myrissa, Hoyland, & Lawton, 2014; Williamson & Rejeski, 2014). In particular, Williamson and Rejeski (2014) concluded that ILIs generally improve HRQoL related to physical health but have less robust effects on mental health. All of these reviews focused on face-to-face clinic-based delivery of ILIs. We note that Raaijmakers and colleagues, after reviewing the technology-based delivery of weight loss interventions, concluded that e-health programs do not significantly improve HRQoL (Raaijmakers, Pouwels, Berghuis, & Nienhuijs, 2015).

General Findings on the Effects of ILIs on HRQoL

Table 14.1 summarizes the results of 13 studies that were selected to represent the effects of different types of ILIs on HRQoL for a diverse set of adults from a variety of countries. Of these studies, 11 were randomized controlled trials (RCTs), one was a 2-year observational study (Kaukua, Pekkarinen, Sane, & Mustajoki, 2003), and another was a posttreatment cross-sectional study of adults who lost weight, were weight stable, or gained weight (Yankura et al., 2008). Most studies were conducted in the United States, but three were from Europe; 10 of 13 included follow-up periods lasting at least 1 year, with 7 of 13 lasting 2 years or more. Retention was high, ranging from 47% (Pekkarinen, Kaukua, & Mustajoki, 2015) to 99% (Marrero et al., 2014), with 11 of the 13 studies reporting levels above 75%. Thus, most studies used RCT methodology, had good retention, and were of sufficient length to allow adequate tests of the long-term effects of weight loss and weight regain on HRQoL.

Figure 14.1 displays the 1-year effects on the Physical Component Summary (PCS) and Mental Component Summary (MCS) subscales of the SF-36 for the Look AHEAD trial (Williamson et al., 2009). As compared to a diabetes support and education (DSE) control group, the PCS of the SF-36 of the ILI improved, but the MCS remained unchanged. This same result was observed in four of the other 13 studies that included the SF-36 as a measure of HRQoL (Marrero et al., 2014; Rejeski et al., 2002; Rubin et al., 2014; Villareal et al., 2011). Two additional studies reported improvement after ILI treatment on both the PCS and MCS (Kaukua et al., 2003; Yancey et al., 2009). One study (Blissmer et al., 2006) reported the opposite pattern of results: That is, MCS but not PCS scores were improved at a 2-year follow-up, although both scores were improved after 6 months of ILI. Two studies reported no beneficial effects of ILI on either scale of the SF-36, but as noted later in this chapter, both of these studies tested ILIs that were relatively brief in duration (Pekkarinen et al., 2015; van Gemert et al., 2015). Thus, a preponderance of evidence suggests that HRQoL improves after at least 1 year of an ILI and that this improvement is most notable for the PCS. Furthermore, Rejeski et al. (2015), focusing on a subset of items from the PCS that target mobility, showed that the ILI in Look AHEAD resulted in statistically significant differences between the ILI and DSE throughout the first 8 years of the study and that the effects were strongest for older participants (Figure 14.2).

TABLE 14.1. Effects of ILIs on Weight Loss and Maintenance per SF-36 HRQoL

Author; country	Sample	Design	Primary results related to SF-36
Blissmer et al. (2006); USA	144 adults; 78% women; mean age = 50; mean BMI = 32.5	2-year RCT testing two weight maintenance approaches; all participants were part of a 6-month weight loss ILI and were then randomized to two follow-up arms. SF-36 was administered at 6, 12, and 24 months.	Retention = 63%. At 6 months improvement for Physical Component Summary (PCS) and Mental Component Summary (MCS) observed. During follow-up, the two arms did not differ and the improved MCS was maintained, but PCS worsened to baseline levels.
Kaukua, Pekkarinen, Sane, & Mustajoki (2003); Finland	126 adults; 61% women; mean age = 48.2; mean BMI = 42.8	2-year observational weight loss and weight maintenance/regain study; ILI involved 4-month lifestyle modification program that included a 10-week VLCD; participants were followed for 2 years.	Retention = 79%. After 4-month ILI, all subscales of the SF-36 were improved. However, at 2-year follow-up, most participants had regained weight lost and only the physical functioning subscale was improved relative to baseline.
Marrero et al. (2014); USA	3,234 adults; 68% women; mean age = 50.6; mean BMI = 34	6-year RCT; follow-up study of the DPP; participants were randomized to three arms: ILI, metformin, or placebo. SF-36 was used to measure HRQoL.	Retention = 99%. At the end of one year, ILI was associated with improved PCS scores, but this improvement gradually diminished over 6 years. No difference between arms was observed for MCS.
Martin, Church, Thompson, Earnest, & Blair (2009); USA	464 sedentary postmenopausal women; mean age = 57.4; mean BMI = 31.8	6-month RCT; participants were randomized to four arms: control and three levels of physical activity: 4 kcal/kg/week, 8 kcal/kg/week, 12 kcal/kg/week. SF-36 subscales were used to measure HRQoL.	Retention = 93%. A dose–response relationship existed between physical activity and all subscales of the SF-36. Weight loss was unrelated to improved scores on the SF-36.
Martin et al. (2016); USA	220 adults; 69% women; mean age = 37.9; mean BMI = 25.1	2-year RCT; participants were randomized to two arms: calorie restriction (ILI) or *ad libitum* eating (control). Subscales of the SF-36 and the BDI-II were used to measure HRQoL. HRQoL measures were administered at 12-month intervals.	Retention = 85%. ILI was associated with lower BDI scores and higher general health scores in comparison to the control group. The arms did not differ on any other measures of HRQoL.
Pekkarinen, Kaukua, & Mustajoki (2015); Finland	201 adults; 71% women; mean age = 47; mean BMI = 42	2-year RCT; participants were randomized to two arms: 17-week ILI with a 1-year maintenance (12 sessions) or 17-week ILI with no maintenance program. HRQoL was measured using the SF-36 1 and 2 years following the ILI treatment.	Retention = 47%. Treatment arms did not differ for any subscales of the SF-36 at the end of 2-year follow-up. Improved HRQoL observed after ILI deteriorated over the 2-year follow-up. Most weight loss was regained over the 2-year follow-up.
Rejeski et al. (2002); USA	316 older adults with knee OA; 78% women; mean age = 68.5; mean BMI = 34.5	18-month RCT; participants were randomized to four arms: control (C), weight loss only (WL), exercise only (E), and weight loss plus exercise (WL + E).	Retention = 80%. Across the 18 months, only the WL + E differed from C on PCS. The other two arms (WL and E) showed improved PSC that was intermediate. No differences for MCS were observed.

(continued)

TABLE 4.1. *(continued)*

Author; country	Sample	Design	Primary results related to SF-36
Rubin et al. (2014); USA	5,145 adults diagnosed with type 2 diabetes; 60% women; mean age = 58.7; mean BMI = 36	10-year RCT; 10-year follow-up for the Look AHEAD study; participants were randomized to ILI or DSE control arm and followed for 10 years. ILI included periodic booster sessions throughout the 10 years. SF-36 and BDI-II were used to measure HRQoL at yearly intervals.	Retention = 97%. The ILI had higher scores on PCS for the first 8 years. PCS scores for both arms deteriorated over the 10-year period. Differences for the MCS were not observed at any measurement point. The incidence of elevated (≥ 10) scores on the BDI-II was reduced for 8 years of ILI in comparison to DSE.
van Gemert et al. (2015); The Netherlands	243 women; mean age = 60; mean BMI = 29	16-week RCT; participants were randomized to three arms: diet, exercise, or control. The SF-36 was used to measure HRQoL at baseline and at the end of the study (16 weeks).	Retention = 89%. Treatment arms did not differ on PCS, MCS, or any subscale of the SF-36.
Villareal et al. (2011); USA	93 obese, prefrail older adults; mean age = 69; mean BMI = 37.3	1-year RCT; participants were randomized to four arms: control (C), weight loss (WL), exercise (E), WL + E. The SF-36 assessed HRQoL at baseline, 6 months, and 1 year.	Retention = 87%. At 1-year follow-up, scores for PCS improved for the three treatment arms (WL, E, and WL + E) in comparison to the control arm.
Williamson et al. (2009); USA	5,145 men and women with diabetes; 60% women; mean age = 58.7; mean BMI 36	1-year RCT; first year of the Look AHEAD study. Participants were randomized to ILI for weight loss or DSE; SF-36 and BDI-II assessed at baseline and 1 year. This study reported on HRQoL results after the first year of the Look AHEAD study.	Retention = 97%. ILI improved more across 1 year than DSE on SF-36 PCS and BDI-II; greatest improvement for PCS seen in those with the lowest PCS scores at baseline; reduced weight, improved fitness, and improved physical symptoms mediated treatment effects for both PCS and BDI-II at 1 year.
Yankura et al. (2008); USA	248 postmenopausal women who lost ≥ 5 lbs. in first 6 months of treatment; mean age = ~57; mean BMI = ~31	Report from the WOMAN study, restricted to women who initially lost weight in 6-month ILI. Based on weight change status from 6 to 18 months, participants were divided into three groups: weight loss ≥ 5 lbs (21%); weight stable $< \pm 5$ lbs (51%); weight regain > 5 lb gain (28%).	Retention = 100% (post-hoc analysis). Groups based on WL vs. weight stable vs. WR did not differ at 18-month follow-up on PCS or MCS. The only SF-36 scale that differed across groups was the Vitality subscale.
Yancy et al. (2009); USA	119 adults; 76% women; mean age = 45; mean BMI = 34	24-week RCT; participants were randomized to LCKD or LFD; both arms were instructed to exercise 30 minutes at least 3x/week; HRQoL was measured using the SF-36 every 4 weeks for 24 weeks.	At 24 weeks, physical function, role physical health, general health, vitality, social functioning, and PCS improved in both groups; body pain improved in LFD only. Role emotional health, mental health, and MCS improved in LCKD only; MCS improved in LCKD improved more than in LFD.

Note. BDI-II, Beck Depression Inventory–II; BMI, body mass index; C, control; DPP, Diabetes Prevention Program; DSE, diabetes support and education; E, exercise only; HRQoL, health-related quality of life; ILI, intensive lifestyle intervention; LCKD, low-carbohydrate ketogenic diet; LFD, low-fat diet; MCS, mental health component score; OA, osteoarthritis; PCS, physical health component score; RCT, randomized controlled trial; VLCD, very-low-calorie diet; WL, weight loss only; WL + E, weight loss plus exercise.

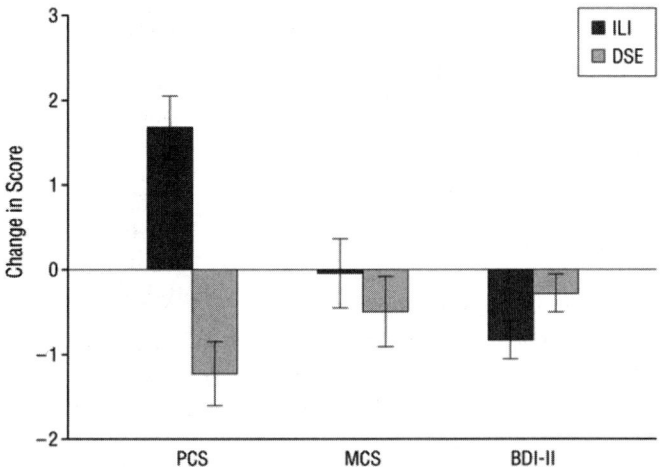

FIGURE 14.1. Changes in measures of HRQoL as a function of treatment arm (ILI vs. diabetes support and education [DSE]). This figure depicts the changes for the physical health component score (PCS), mental health component score (MCS), and Beck Depression Inventory–II (BDI-II) score. Error bars reflect 99% confidence intervals. Adapted with permission from Williamson, Rejeski, Lang, Van Dorsten, Fabricatore, and Toledo (2009). Impact of a weight management program on health-related quality of life in overweight adults with type 2 diabetes. *Archives of Internal Medicine, 169*(2), 163–171. Copyright © 2009 the American Medical Association. All rights reserved.

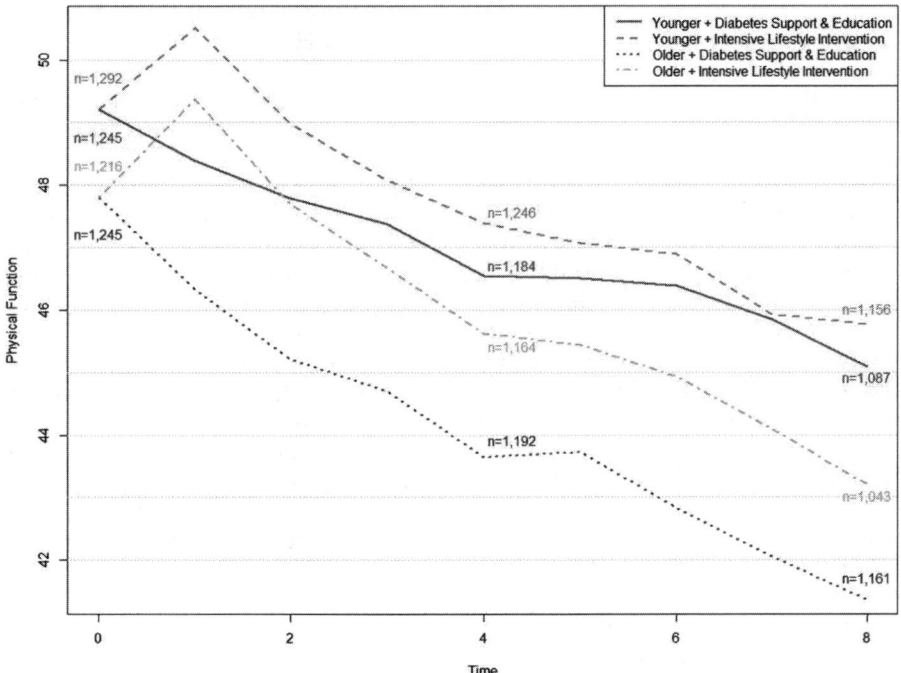

FIGURE 14.2. Plot of the SF-36 physical functioning subscale by treatment group for younger and older participants across 8 years of the Look AHEAD study. From Rejeski, Bray, Chen, Clark, Evans, Hill, et al. (2015). Aging and physical function in type 2 diabetes: 8 years of an intensive lifestyle intervention. *Journals of Gerontology Series A: Biological Sciences and Medical Sciences, 70*(3), 343–353. Reprinted by permission of Oxford University Press.

Effects on Depression

In addition to 1-year results from Look AHEAD on the SF-36, Figure 14.1 also provides data on BDI-II scores (Williamson et al., 2009). Of considerable importance is the fact that most overweight/obese people are not depressed and have quite low scores on the BDI-II. Thus, the modest yet statistically significant reductions in BDI scores in the ILI arm are impressive in the context of a potential floor effect. The most clinically important effect of ILIs is the beneficial effect in persons with mild or greater symptoms of depression (i.e., BDI score $\geq$ 10). During the first 4 years of the Look AHEAD trial, BDI scores fell by 5 or more points in ILI participants who began the study with mild or more intense symptoms of depression. In addition, in participants who were not depressed at baseline, the ILI, compared with the DSE, reduced the risk of new cases of depression by 15% over the approximately 10 years of intervention.

The Independent Effects of Caloric Restriction or Exercise on HRQoL

As evident from the studies reviewed in Table 14.1, most ILIs have included components that address both caloric restriction and exercise training. However, several trials have examined the independent effects of either caloric restriction or exercise on HRQoL. The CALERIE Phase 2 study (Ravussin et al., 2015) was an RCT that compared 2 years of caloric restriction, without an exercise program, to an ad libitum eating control group. Participants in the study were not obese and were relatively healthy young adults with an average body mass index (BMI) of 25 kg/m^2. A publication from this trial by Martin et al. (2016) reported that caloric restriction had no significant adverse effects on HRQoL when compared to the control group and led to improved scores on the General Health scale of the SF-36, as well as on the BDI-II. Villareal et al. (2011) also reported that a weight loss program without an exercise component was associated with improved PCS scores in comparison to a control group. Thus, based on this limited evidence, it appears that the caloric restriction component of ILIs can lead to some improvement in HRQoL, albeit not as great as that reported when caloric restriction is combined with exercise.

How about exercise? Perhaps the most comprehensive study to address whether exercise affects HRQoL was conducted by Martin, Church, Thompson, Earnest, and Blair (2009). In this study, three levels of exercise training (4 kcal/kg/week, 8 kcal/kg/week, and 12 kcal/kg/week) were compared to a control group. HRQoL was assessed using the eight subscales of the SF-36. The overall pattern of results suggested an exercise dose–response relationship, with increased exercise associated with stepwise improvement in HRQoL. Secondary analyses found that this dose–response relationship of exercise level on HRQoL was not related to change in weight. Two other studies tested the independent and combined effects of caloric restriction and exercise on HRQoL. In a study of older adults with knee osteoarthritis, Rejeski et al. (2002) examined the effects of exercise only, weight loss only, the combination of exercise and weight loss, and a health education control group on HRQoL. They found that only the combination of weight loss and exercise differed from the control group, with effects observed on the PCS but not the MCS. The previously discussed study by Villareal et al. (2011), also of older adults, reported that all three active treatment arms—weight loss, exercise, and the combination of weight loss and exercise—improved PCS scores when compared to a control group. Given the small number of studies, it is difficult to draw firm conclusions about the effects of exercise on HRQoL. Clearly, exercise combined with caloric restriction has positive effects on the physical domain of HRQoL. At least one study (Martin et al., 2009) suggests that the independent effects of intense exercise may be sufficient to improve HRQoL.

Moderators of the Effects of ILIs on HRQoL

Sex does not appear to moderate the effects of ILIs on HRQoL (Rejeski et al., 2002; Williamson et al., 2009). However, as noted earlier, Rejeski et al. (2015) found that older participants in Look AHEAD derived more benefit in self-reported physical functioning from the ILI than did younger participants.

This effect is likely due to the fact that the older adults were more compromised to begin with, making change in physical functioning highly salient. In addition, duration of treatment appears to be an important consideration, since the two studies that reported no significant effects of ILIs on HRQoL (van Gemert et al., 2015; Pekkarinen et al., 2015) were relatively brief (16–17 weeks). Two large scale RCTs, the Diabetes Prevention Program (DPP; Marrero et al., 2014) and Look AHEAD (Rubin et al., 2014), included ILIs during the first year of treatment, coupled with intensive weight loss maintenance programs. Figure 14.3 depicts the effects of the DPP ILI on three aspects

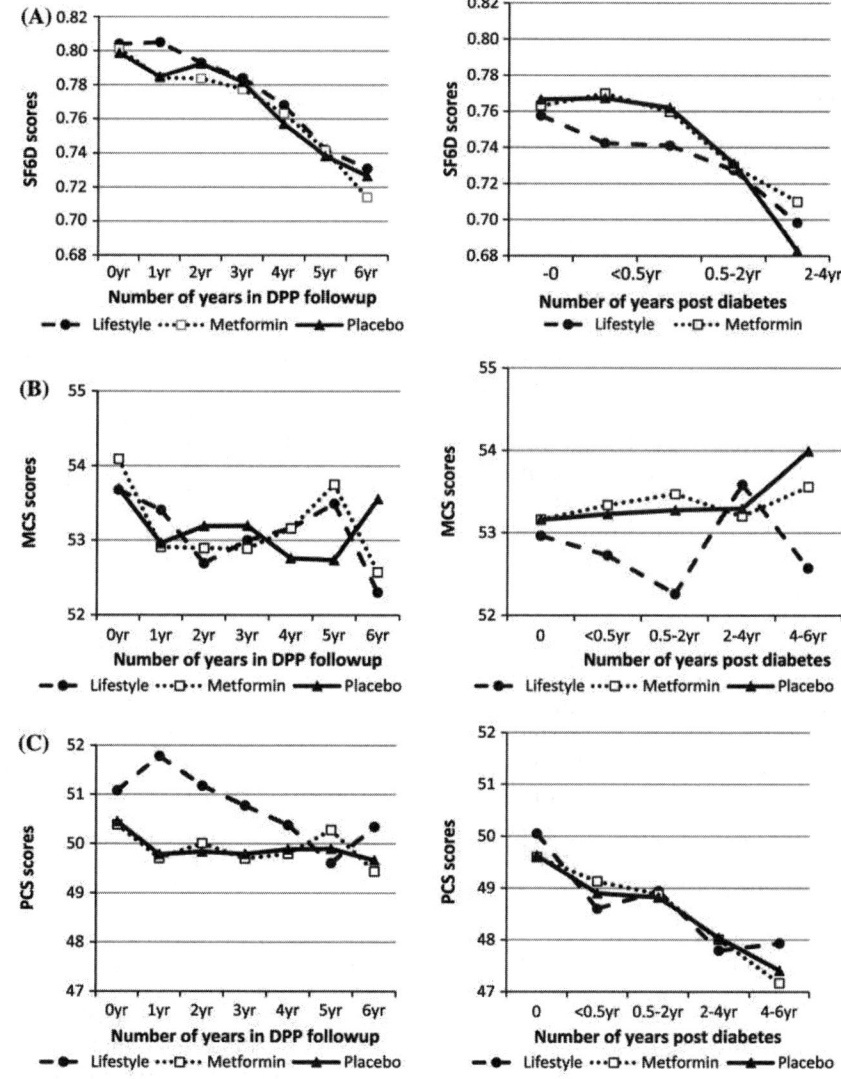

FIGURE 14.3. Left: Average treatment-specific HRQoL scores over the Diabetes Prevention Program (DPP) follow-up among diabetes-free participants. Right: Predicted average treatment-specific HRQoL scores postdiabetes. MCS, Mental Component Summary; PCS, Physical Component Summary. From Marrero, Pan, Barrett-Connor, de Groot, Zhang, Percy, et al. (2014). Impact of diagnosis of diabetes on health-related quality of life among high risk individuals: The Diabetes Prevention Program outcomes study. *Quality of Life Research, 23*(1), 75–88. Reprinted with permission of Springer.

of HRQoL. Examination of panel C reveals the immediate positive impact of ILI on the PCS, a benefit that persisted for at least 3 years. Figure 14.4 illustrates the impact of the Look AHEAD ILI on the PCS and MCS of the SF-36. Whereas initial differences on the PCS between the ILI and DSE deteriorated over the course of the 10-year study, ILI had a statistically significant benefit on PCS scores, as compared to DSE, through the first 8 years of treatment. In contrast, ILI was not different from DSE on MCS scores.

Effects of ILIs on Physical Functioning

An increasing number of studies involving ILIs for weight loss have chosen to employ objective measures of physical function as study outcomes. Of those reviewed, the largest have been the Arthritis, Diet, and Activity Promotion Trial (ADAPT; Messier et al., 2004), the Cooperative Lifestyle Intervention Program (CLIP; Rejeski et al., 2011), and a study conducted on an older frail population (Villareal et al., 2011). ADAPT was an 18-month RCT involving 316 older adults who had documented evidence of disability and BMI ≥ 28 kg/m². They were randomized to one of four groups: exercise only, diet only, diet plus exercise, or a control group. The objective measures of physical function included the 6-minute walk and stair climbing tests. The exercise-only and combined-treatment groups experienced significant improvement in their 6-minute walk time across the 18 months of the study; however, the combined group had the greatest improvement in stair-climbing performance (Messier et al., 2004). This pattern in the data suggests that the benefits of weight loss on physical disability are most likely to appear on tasks that require moving the center of gravity in a vertical direction as occurs when climbing stairs or walking up a hill.

CLIP was an 18-month RCT involving 288 men and women who were overweight or obese and had either cardiovascular disease or the metabolic syndrome. Participants were assigned to one of three treatment groups: (1) successful aging, (2) physical activity (PA) only, or (3) weight loss plus PA with the primary outcome consisting of time to complete a 400-meter fast walk. The successful aging intervention was designed as

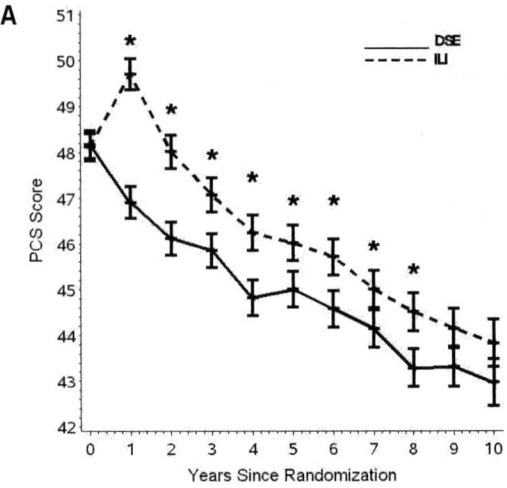

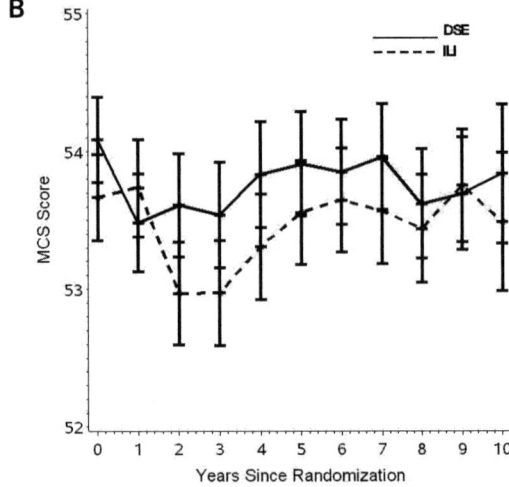

FIGURE 14.4. (A) Mean PCS scores over 10 years by treatment arm. The sample size for diabetes support and education (DSE) appears above the sample size for the intensive lifestyle intervention (ILI). Asterisks indicate significant differences between groups ($p < .005$). (B) Mean mental health component scores (MCS) over 10 years by treatment arm. The sample size for DSE appears above the sample size for ILI. From Rubin, Wadden, Bahnson, Blackburn, Brancati, Bray, et al. (2014). Impact of intensive lifestyle intervention on depression and health-related quality of life in type 2 diabetes: The Look AHEAD Trial. *Diabetes Care, 37*(6), 1544–1553. Copyright and all rights reserved. Material from this publication has been used with the permission of the American Diabetes Association.

an attention control condition that involved group education on health topics relevant to aging, whereas the physical activity intervention involved a moderate intensity walking program with a target activity level of ≥ 150 minutes/week. As shown in Figure 14.5, the combined condition produced improved and sustained changes in the 400-meter walk time over the 18 months of the study. Also of note was the finding that participants who had the poorest function at baseline benefited the most from the combined treatment.

The study conducted by Villareal et al. (2011) was a 1-year RCT of 107 obese, older adults who had mild to moderate levels of frailty at baseline. Participants were randomized to one of four treatment conditions: (1) a general education control group that met monthly, (2) an exercise only group, (3) a weight loss only group, or (4) an exercise plus weight loss group. The primary outcome was a composite score from a multicomponent physical performance test that included walking, two stair-climbing tasks, two fine motor tasks, rising from a chair, balance, and lifting a book. The three active interventions led to improved physical performance, as compared to the control group. However, the combined treatment group had a superior performance compared to any of the other treatment conditions: a 21% improvement over baseline. Participants in the weight loss only group improved 12%, and those in the exercise only group improved 15%. The control group participants increased their performance over baseline by only 1%.

Two other small RCTs have replicated the benefits of a weight loss plus exercise intervention on the functional health of obese older adults (Miller et al., 2006; Villareal, Banks, Sinacore, Siener, & Klein, 2006). In both of these studies, the exercise involved a combination of aerobic and resistance exercise. Miller et al. (2006) conducted a 6-month study that was similar to ADAPT, with the exception that the weight loss goal was much more ambitious: a 10% as opposed to ~5% reduction in weight. The second 6-month study by Villareal et al. (2006) compared diet plus exercise to a control group but employed physically frail, obese, older adults. In addition, the study by Villareal et al. employed high-intensity resistance training as part of the exercise intervention. These two investigations found that diet plus exercise produced significant improvements in performance-based measures of physical function.

Finally, Dunstan et al. (2002) and Frimel, Sinacore, and Villareal (2008) conducted

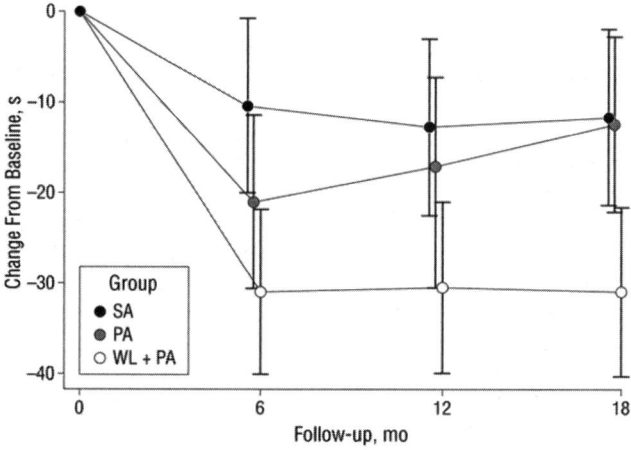

FIGURE 14.5. Adjusted means of the change from baseline in 400-meter walk time, and 95% confidence intervals by treatment condition (SA, successful aging; PA, physical activity; WL + PA, weight loss + physical activity). From Rejeski, Brubaker, Goff, Jr., Bearon, McClelland, Perri, et al. (2011). Translating weight loss and physical activity programs into the community to preserve mobility in older, obese adults in poor cardiovascular health. *Archives of Internal Medicine, 171*(10), 880–886. Copyright © 2011 the American Medical Association. All rights reserved.

6-month investigations on the effect of high-intensity resistance exercise in combination with dietary therapy on the strength and lean body mass of older adults. The study by Dunstan and colleagues studied patients with type 2 diabetes and a comparison group in a protocol that involved flexibility training combined with dietary weight loss, whereas Frimel and colleagues employed older adults who had mild-to-moderate frailty and a weight loss only comparison group. Dunstan et al. found that those in the resistance training arm had greater increases in strength than those in the flexibility plus weight loss arm. In addition, lean body mass increased in the resistance training plus weight loss arm, whereas it decreased in the comparison group. Frimel et al. also found that the addition of exercise training to dietary therapy resulted in increases in strength relative to the dietary only arm and that resistance training attenuated losses in fat-free mass when compared to dietary weight loss only.

We note that of the above studies (Dunstan et al., 2002; Frimel et al., 2008; Miller et al., 2006; Villareal et al., 2006), the only one to report an increase of fat-free mass with weight loss was the investigation by Dunstan et al. (2002). A factor that may account for this result is that their daily weight training regimen was the most intense and lengthy of all four studies; participants exercised for 45 minutes each session and did so at an intensity of ~80% of maximum.

Obesity, HRQoL, and Physical Functioning: Considerations Moving Forward

Data from the previously reviewed studies suggest that ILIs can mitigate the adverse effect of obesity on HRQoL, particularly on those roles or activities that are based on self-reported physical capacities, a finding corroborated by research using objective markers of physical function. At this point, we examine several important questions and concerns that warrant attention when considering this literature, particularly as we look toward the future. First, the trials reviewed in this chapter have, for the most part, studied overweight or obese individuals as a group without any consideration of whether the effects of ILIs might differ for someone who is mildly overweight versus excessively obese. Interestingly, this has been a topic that has drawn increasing attention in the aging literature.

HRQoL and Physical Functioning: Does the Degree of Obesity Matter?

Jensen and colleagues have argued that BMI levels ≥ 35 kg/m^2 constitute a risk for functional decline with aging. For example, in a 3- to 4-year follow-up of older men and women, class 1 obesity was not a risk factor for an increased need of assistance in performing either basic activities of daily living or instrumental activities of daily living, with odds ratios of 0.77 for men and 0.82 for women. However, BMIs ≥ 35 kg/m^2 yielded risk ratios of 3.32 for men and 2.61 for women (Jensen & Friedmann, 2002). In a more recent study, Jensen et al. (2006) reported that class 2 obesity or higher (BMIs ≥ 35 kg/m^2), but not class 1 obesity, predicted older men and women, ages 65–97, becoming homebound. Interestingly, Al Snih and colleagues reported that older adults with a BMI ≥ 30 kg/m^2 were three times as likely to recover from disability in basic activities of daily living over a 2-year period than those with a BMI < 30 kg/m^2, suggesting that class 1 obesity may provide some resilience to physical insults as people age (Al Snih, Markides, Ostir, Ray, & Goodwin, 2003).

We note that the BMI cutpoint that constitutes an increased risk for physical disability in aging may depend on race. Mendes de Leon and colleagues found that for either self-reported or performance-related measures of mobility, the maximum predicted scores occurred at a higher level of BMI for blacks than whites (Mendes de Leon, Hansberry, Bienias, Morris, & Evans, 2006). We also note the obvious main effects for both race and sex in these data. In general, women experienced higher rates of disability with aging than men (Friedmann, Elasy, & Jensen, 2001; Jenkins, 2004; Jensen & Friedmann, 2002; Reynolds, Saito, & Crimmins, 2005; Wray & Blaum, 2001), and blacks were at a greater risk for disability than whites (Clark, 1997; Kelley-Moore & Ferraro, 2004; Mendes de Leon, Barnes, Bienias, Skarupski, & Evans, 2005). Whereas clinical research data are unclear as to whether class 1 obesity constitutes a risk for functional decline in geriatric medicine, the evidence clearly indicates that being overweight—having a BMI from 25–30 kg/m^2—is not a cause for concern; in fact, as suggested above, it could confer some protection against functional decline. We also note that obesity does not appear to constitute a risk for mortality among older adults (Al Snih et al., 2007). An informative analysis of large datasets such as Look AHEAD could reexamine treatment effects on HRQoL as a function of categories of obesity and also explore race and ethnicity as potential moderating variables.

A related question is whether the effect of obesity on HRQoL and physical function is a linear phenomenon. Again, the most relevant data on this topic can be found in the aging literature, since there has been a steady increase in the number of prospective epidemiological studies that have addressed the relationship between body weight and the subsequent risk for physical disability as people age (Al Snih et al., 2007; Brach, Simonsick, Kritchevsky, Yaffe, & Newman, 2004; Ferraro, Su, Gretebeck, Black, & Badylak, 2002; Fine et al., 1999; Houston, Stevens, & Cai, 2005; Jensen & Friedmann, 2002; Jensen et al., 2006; Koster et al., 2008; Koster et al., 2007; Launer, Harris, Rumpel, & Madans, 1994; Ohmori et al., 2005; Stenholm et al., 2007; Visscher et al., 2004). While some studies have reported a linear association between BMI and disability (Houston et al., 2005; Sharkey, Branch, Giuliani, Zohoori, & Haines, 2004), a number of studies had adequate sampling to examine the BMI–disability relationship across the entire spectrum of BMI, from underweight (BMI < 18 kg/m^2) to morbid obesity (BMI ≥ 40 kg/m^2) (Al Snih et al., 2007; Mendes de Leon et al., 2006). Figure 14.6 displays data presented by Al Snih et al. (2007) for older adults who were free of disability at baseline. Panel B provides data on mortality. Across a 7-year follow-up period, the relationship between body weight as assessed by BMI and subsequent disability in activities of daily living was curvilinear, with the lowest risk at a BMI of 24 kg/m^2. This effect held true in an adjusted model (model 2), in an adjusted model controlling for baseline comorbidities (model 1), and in a model that adjusted for comorbidities and also excluded current smokers or those who died during the first 2 years of follow-up (model 3). In fact, these authors found that the most favorable hazard's ratio for disability-free life expectancy was among participants with a BMI of 25 kg/m^2 to less than 30 kg/m^2 (i.e., overweight). This finding is consistent with earlier studies that reported that the extremes of the BMI distribution in older adult populations are associated with higher disability (Ferraro & Booth, 1999; Ferraro et al., 2002; Galanos, Pieper, Cornoni-Huntley, Bales, & Fillenbaum, 1994; Launer et al., 1994). As Rejeski and colleagues have shown in a large prospective trial of older adults with knee pain, people with BMIs of ≥ 35 kg/m^2 have an increased probability of transitioning to more severe states of physical disability over time and are less likely to recover from severe states of physical disability, such as functional decline following a period of hospitalization (Rejeski, Ip, Marsh, Zhang, & Miller, 2008).

The Influence of Fitness and Physical Activity on Obesity and Functional Decline

An important question when examining the relationship between obesity and functional decline in the presence of excessive weight is the role played by physical fitness and physical activity. In other words, is the negative effect of obesity on functional decline in aging buffered by strength, cardiovascular fitness, and/or level of physical activity? There is both indirect and direct evidence to suggest that being fit when one is fat is beneficial. Stenholm et al. (2007), in a 22-year longitudinal study of a Finnish population of predominately middle-age adults, examined the combined effects of BMI and fitness—grip strength, a performance measure of squatting, and self-reported difficulty running 500 meters—on walking speed over a 6.1 meter course 22 years later. The age- and sex-adjusted risk of walking limitation among those at baseline who were in the highest tertile of BMI and had two or more fitness impairments was 6.4 times that of participants who were neither overweight nor had evidence of a fitness-related impair-

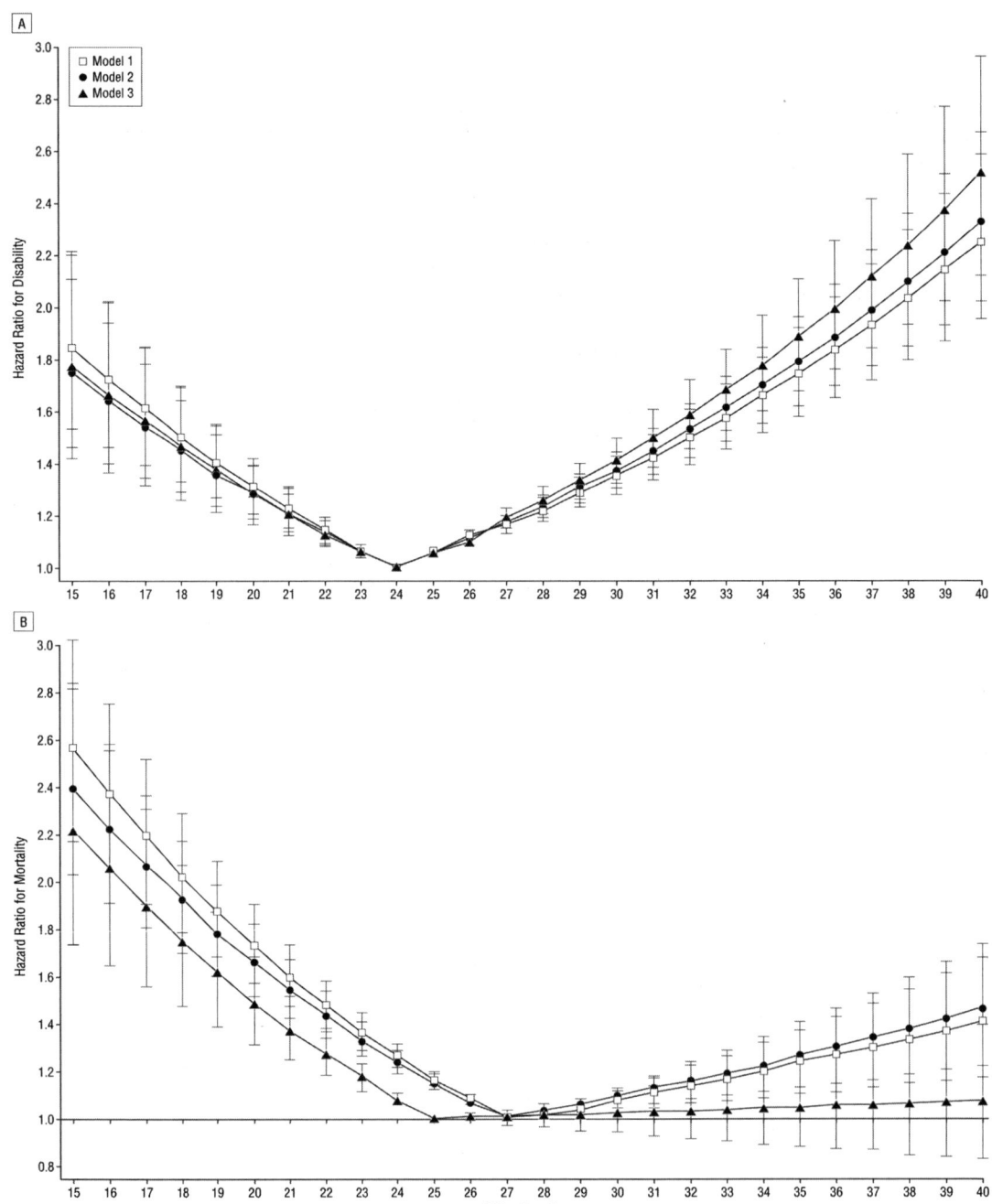

FIGURE 14.6. Hazard ratios predicting disability in ADLs (A) and mortality (B) during 7 years of follow-up as a function of BMI, calculated as weight in kilograms divided by height in meters squared, among nondisabled older Americans at baseline. Values are given as mean (95% confidence interval). Model 1 was adjusted for baseline comorbidity, model 2 was not adjusted for comorbidity, and model 3 excluded current smokers and subjects who died during the first 2 years of follow-up and controlled for comorbidity. From Al Snih, Ottenbacher, Markides, Kuo, Eschbach, and Goodwin (2007). The effect of obesity on disability vs. mortality in older Americans. *Archives of Internal Medicine, 167*(8), 774–780. Copyright © 2007 the American Medical Association. All rights reserved.

ment. The BMI cutpoint for the third tertile was 26.5 kg/m² for men and 26.1 kg/m² for women. The risk was attenuated some when adjusting for socioeconomic position, co-morbidities, and lifestyle behaviors, yielding an odds ratio of 4.4. Thus, whereas being overweight does appear to afford some protection against disability among older adults, these data suggest that being overweight at middle age may be a risk factor for disability in late life.

McDermott et al. (2006) followed older patients (mean age ~72) with peripheral artery disease for a period of 48 months and examined the relationship between obesity and performance measures of functional decline. In fully adjusted models that controlled for demographic and comorbid conditions, they observed that, compared to a reference group with BMIs between 20 and 25 kg/m², those with a BMI > 30 kg/m² had significantly greater average declines in 6-minute walk performance, usual-paced 4-meter walking velocity, and the fast-paced 4-meter walking velocity (~0.03 m/sec). Of particular interest in their study was the interaction effect for associations between weight change, exercise, and declines in 6-minute walking performance. Relevant to the topic of this section was the finding that regular exercise buffered the negative effects that a ≥ 5 to < 10 pounds (4.5 kg) annual weight gain had on decrements in the 6-minute walking performance. However, exercise did not buffer weight gain when it was in excess of 10 pounds (4.5 kg). Related to this work is a 14-year follow-up of 171 women who had participated in a physical activity trial (Brach et al., 2004). At the final assessment in 1999, women who had reported > 1,000 kcal of physical activity each week in 1982, 1985, and 1995, and who had a BMI < 25 kg/m² at each of these time points, reported less difficulty with activities of daily living (ADLs) and had a faster gait speed than those who were either inactive or who had been overweight or obese at any of the assessments. Women who were never active and were overweight or obese had the greatest disability in both ADLs and gait speed. This effect was tempered in overweight and obese women who were physically active.

Lang, Guralnik, and Melzer (2007) reported that although excess body weight, assessed by BMI, was a risk factor for impaired physical function, physical activity was protective across all categories of BMI. Similarly, Bruce, Fries, and Hubert (2008) reported that being physically active was protective against disability, largely independent of BMI. Finally, Koster et al. (2008) reported on the joint effects of adiposity and self-reported physical activity on incident mobility disability among older adults in the Health, Aging, and Body Composition (ABC) study. During two consecutive semiannual visits over 6.5 years, they measured mobility disability as self-reported difficulty walking one-quarter of a mile or climbing 10 steps. Level of physical activity, assessed at baseline, was split into quartiles based on energy expended in all types of work and exercise, using a 7-day recall instrument. The high-activity group was represented by the fourth quartile, whereas the low-activity group consisted of those in the first quartile. The moderate-activity group was represented by those in the second and third quartiles. With the exception of black women, high levels of physical activity offset the negative effect that obesity (BMI > 30 kg/m²) had on mobility disability. In general, this was not the case for moderate or low levels of physical activity. However, the authors have emphasized that physical activity and other positive health behaviors (e.g., being a nonsmoker and consuming a high-quality diet) do not overcome the detrimental effect that obesity has on physical functioning at an advanced age (Koster et al., 2007).

Mediating Variables

Within the context of RCTs related to ILIs, it is logical to hypothesize that improvements in HRQoL and depression associated with ILIs for weight loss are mediated by reduced body weight. Oddly, however, there is a lack of evidence supporting this hypothesis. Correlational data offer support for the notion that improved HRQoL is related to weight loss (Kaukua et al., 2003), but the only direct test of weight loss as a mediator of change in HRQoL has been provided by Williamson et al. (2009). Based on analyses from the Look AHEAD study, they reported that reduced weight, in addition to improved fitness and reduced physical symptoms, mediated improved PCS and BDI-II scores. Thus, although weight loss appears to provide a partial explanation for why ILIs have a positive effect on HRQoL, clearly there are other important variables that deserve consideration. As an example, Rejeski et al. (2002), in a weight loss study of older adults with knee osteoarthritis, found that reduction in pain and improved satisfaction with function mediated change in PCS scores. Finally, Brawley and colleagues, in a secondary analyses of an ILI involving older adults from the CLIP study, reported that change in self-efficacy for walking ability from baseline to 6 months mediated the baseline-adjusted 18-month change in the 400-meter walk time (Brawley, Rijeski, Gaukstern, & Ambrosius, 2012).

Although the intent of existing longitudinal study designs has not been to test potential mediators of the effect that obesity may have on physical disability in aging, three general focal points of study have evolved. The first is the impact that obesity may have on pathophysiological processes that directly influence markers of disability. This category includes the role that body fat plays in inflammation and the mechanical stress that excessive weight places on the joints. For example, the study of peripheral artery disease patients by McDermott et al. (2006) reported that obesity was related to decline in 6-minute walk performance. When these authors controlled for the effect of cytokines in their analyses, the performance deficits attributed to obesity were eliminated. Although their study design and analytical approach did not allow for an actual statistical test of mediation (Kraemer, Wilson, Fairburn, & Agras, 2002), these results remain provocative, albeit controversial (Huffman, Slentz, Bales, Houmard, & Kraus, 2008).

The notion that obesity places excessive loads on joints in the lower extremities is yet another plausible cause for declining physical function. For some time, obesity has been linked to knee osteoarthritis (Felson, 1995; Guccione, Felson, & Anderson, 1990; Hartz et al., 1986). Not only are knee joint loads higher in obese individuals (Baliunas et al., 2002), but gait changes associated with obesity compound the problem by also increasing the loading rate in these joints (Mundermann, Dyrby, & Andriacchi, 2005). Of interest are data from Messier and colleagues, who observed a reduction in knee joint loading following weight loss in overweight and obese older adults (Messier, Gutekunst, Davis, & DeVita, 2005).

Second, physical inactivity is widely recognized as a risk factor for obesity (Brown & Siahpush, 2007; Kaplan, Huguet, Newsom, McFarland, & Lindsay, 2003), and obese individuals are more inactive (Kaplan, Newsom, McFarland, & Lu, 2001). Physical inactivity undermines strength, cardiorespiratory function, balance, and flexibility—parameters of fitness that determine one's functional abilities. In particular, strength is related to muscle mass, and muscle mass is related to functional limitations later in life (Janssen, Baumgartner, Ross, Rosenberg, & Roubenoff, 2004; Visser et al., 2005). Interestingly, data from studies that have examined the interplay between muscle mass and fat mass suggest that fat mass may play a more important role in limiting function than muscle mass (Lebrun, van der Schouw, de Jong, Grobbee, & Lamberts, 2006; Visser, Fuerst, Lang, Salamone, & Harris, 1999; Zoico et al., 2004). As an example, Visser et al. (1998), using data from the Cardiovascular Health Study, reported in longitudinal analyses that fat mass at baseline, but not lean mass, was a predictor of future mobility disability. LeBrun and colleagues reported that in spite of a positive association between fat mass and lean mass, increasing BMI had a detrimental effect on Short Physical Performance Battery scores (Lebrun et al., 2006). In other words, the increase in lean mass associated with increases in BMI did not counteract the concomitant increase in fat mass. Finally, Baumgartner (2000) observed that older men and women who were obese and had low muscle mass, as compared to nonobese older adults with normal muscle mass, had an 8- and 11-fold higher risk of having three or more physical disabilities, respectively.

General Discussion

There are compelling data that ILIs that combine caloric restriction with exercise training mitigate the adverse effects of obesity on physical roles and activities that contribute significantly to HRQoL and on objective measures of physical functioning. Whereas some evidence shows that ILIs positively affect mild depression, there is no support that they improve mental health when assessed as a composite index of HRQoL. The effects of ILIs on the PCS of the SF-36 and on various indices of physical function have been found to be robust in that they are not moderated by sex or age. However, future research should examine whether baseline levels of obesity status may interact with ILIs, since the benefit that ILIs have on HRQoL and physical functioning, particularly among older adults, may be limited to individuals with class 2 obesity or higher. In fact, there is growing concern that ILIs are ill advised for elderly individuals who are overweight or barely meet the criterion for class 1 obesity. Whereas prospective epidemiological studies suggest that relatively high levels of physical activity may buffer the adverse effects of obesity on HRQoL and physical functioning, evidence from controlled clinical trials of ILIs that have compared physical activity alone to ILIs does not strongly support this position. It is possible that the prospective studies have just observed the benefit that being physically active earlier in life has on delaying the decline of physical function for older people who are moderately obese. Finally, a topic that deserves increased attention in the future is the study of mediation. For example: Why is adiposity a risk factor for the decline that is frequently observed in physical health scales of HRQoL and objective measures of physical functioning? Also, when participants in ILIs lose weight and become more physically active, what is responsible for the improvements observed in HRQoL and physical function?

References

Al Snih, S., Markides, K. S., Ostir, G. V., Ray, L., & Goodwin, J. S. (2003). Predictors of recovery in activities of daily living among disabled older Mexican Americans. *Aging Clinical and Experimental Research*, 15(4), 315–320.

Al Snih, S., Ottenbacher, K. J., Markides, K. S., Kuo, Y. F., Eschbach, K., & Goodwin, J. S. (2007). The effect of obesity on disability vs. mortality in older Americans. *Archives of Internal Medicine*, 167(8), 774–780.

Baliunas, A. J., Hurwitz, D. E., Ryals, A. B., Karrar, A., Case, J. P., Block, J. A., et al. (2002). Increased knee joint loads during walking are present in subjects with knee osteoarthritis. *Osteoarthritis Cartilage*, 10(7), 573–579.

Baumgartner, R. N. (2000). Body composition in healthy aging. *Annals of the New York Academy of Sciences*, 904, 437–448.

Beck, A. T., Ward, C. H., Mendelson, M., Mock, J., & Erbaugh, J. (1961). An inventory for measuring depression. *Archives of General Psychiatry*, 4, 561–571.

Blissmer, B., Riebe, D., Dye, G., Ruggiero, L., Greene, G., & Caldwell, M. (2006). Health-related quality of life following a clinical weight loss intervention among overweight and obese adults: Intervention and 24-month follow-up effects. *Health and Quality of Life Outcomes*, 4, 43.

Brach, J. S., Simonsick, E. M., Kritchevsky, S., Yaffe, K., & Newman, A. B. (2004). The association between physical function and lifestyle activity and exercise in the health, aging and body composition study. *Journal of the American Geriatrics Society*, 52(4), 502–509.

Brawley, L., Rejeski, W. J., Gaukstern, J. E., & Ambrosius, W. T. (2012). Social cognitive changes following weight loss and physical activity interventions in obese, older adults in poor cardiovascular health. *Annals of Behavioral Medicine*, 44(3), 353–364.

Brown, A., & Siahpush, M. (2007). Risk factors for overweight and obesity: Results from the 2001 National Health Survey. *Public Health*, 121(8), 603–613.

Bruce, B., Fries, J. F., & Hubert, H. (2008). Regular vigorous physical activity and disability development in healthy overweight and normal-weight seniors: A 13-year study. *American Journal of Public Health*, 98(7), 1294–1299.

Clark, D. O. (1997). Physical activity efficacy and effectiveness among older adults and minorities. *Diabetes Care*, 20(7), 1176–1182. [See comments.]

Dunstan, D. W., Daly, R. M., Owen, N., Jolley, D., Courten, D., Shaw, J., et al. (2002). High-intensity resistance training improves glycemic control in older patients with type 2 diabetes. *Diabetes Care*, 25(10), 1729–1736.

Felson, D. T. (1995). Weight and osteoarthritis. *Journal of Rheumatology*, 43(Suppl.), 7–9.

Ferraro, K. F., & Booth, T. L. (1999). Age, body mass index, and functional illness. *Journal of Gerontology Series B: Psychological Sciences and Social Sciences*, 54(6), S339–S348.

Ferraro, K. F., Su, Y. P., Gretebeck, R. J., Black, D. R., & Badylak, S. F. (2002). Body mass index and disability in adulthood: A 20-year panel study. *American Journal of Public Health*, 92(5), 834–840.

Fine, J. T., Colditz, G. A., Coakley, E. H., Moseley, G., Manson, J. E., Willett, W. C., et al. (1999). A prospective study of weight change and health-related quality of life in women. *Journal of the American Medical Accociation*, 282(22), 2136–2142.

Friedmann, J. M., Elasy, T., & Jensen, G. L. (2001). The relationship between body mass index and self-reported functional limitation among older adults: A gender difference. *Journal of the American Geriatrics Society, 49*(4), 398–403.

Frimel, T. N., Sinacore, D. R., & Villareal, D. T. (2008). Exercise attenuates the weight-loss-induced reduction in muscle mass in frail obese older adults. *Medicine and Science in Sports and Exercise, 40*(7), 1213–1219.

Galanos, A. N., Pieper, C. F., Cornoni-Huntley, J. C., Bales, C. W., & Fillenbaum, G. G. (1994). Nutrition and function: Is there a relationship between body mass index and the functional capabilities of community-dwelling elderly? *Journal of the American Geriatrics Society, 42*(4), 368–373.

Guccione, A. A., Felson, D. T., & Anderson, J. J. (1990). Defining arthritis and measuring functional status in elders: Methodological issues in the study of disease and physical disability. *American Journal of Public Health, 80*(8), 945–949.

Hartz, A. J., Fischer, M. E., Bril, G., Kelber, S., Rupley, D., Jr., Oken, B., et al. (1986). The association of obesity with joint pain and osteoarthritis in the HANES data. *Journal of Chronic Diseases, 39*(4), 311–319.

Houston, D. K., Stevens, J., & Cai, J. (2005). Abdominal fat distribution and functional limitations and disability in a biracial cohort: The Atherosclerosis Risk in Communities Study. *International Journal of Obesity, 29*(12), 1457–1463.

Huffman, K. M., Slentz, C. A., Bales, C. W., Houmard, J. A., & Kraus, W. E. (2008). Relationships between adipose tissue and cytokine responses to a randomized controlled exercise training intervention. *Metabolism, 57*(4), 577–583.

Janssen, I., Baumgartner, R. N., Ross, R., Rosenberg, I. H., & Roubenoff, R. (2004). Skeletal muscle cutpoints associated with elevated physical disability risk in older men and women. *American Journal of Epidemiology, 159*(4), 413–421.

Jenkins, K. R. (2004). Obesity's effects on the onset of functional impairment among older adults. *Gerontologist, 44*(2), 206–216.

Jensen, G. L., & Friedmann, J. M. (2002). Obesity is associated with functional decline in community-dwelling rural older persons. *Journal of the American Geriatrics Society, 50*(5), 918–923.

Jensen, G. L., Silver, H. J., Roy, M. A., Callahan, E., Still, C., & Dupont, W. (2006). Obesity is a risk factor for reporting homebound status among community-dwelling older persons. *Obesity (Silver Spring), 14*(3), 509–517.

Kaplan, M. S., Huguet, N., Newsom, J. T., McFarland, B. H., & Lindsay, J. (2003). Prevalence and correlates of overweight and obesity among older adults: Findings from the Canadian National Population Health Survey. *Journals of Gerontology Series A: Biological Sciences and Medical Sciences, 58*(11), 1018–1030.

Kaplan, M. S., Newsom, J. T., McFarland, B. H., & Lu, L. (2001). Demographic and psychosocial correlates of physical activity in late life. *American Journal of Preventive Medicine, 21*(4), 306–312.

Kaukua, J., Pekkarinen, T., Sane, T., & Mustajoki, P. (2003). Health-related quality of life in obese outpatients losing weight with very-low-energy diet and behaviour modification: A 2-y follow-up study. *Internal Journal of Obesity and Related Metabolic Disorders, 27*(10), 1233–1241.

Kelley-Moore, J. A., & Ferraro, K. F. (2004). The black/white disability gap: Persistent inequality in later life? *Journals of Gerontology Series B: Psychological Sciences and Social Sciences, 59*(1), S34–S43.

Koster, A., Patel, K. V., Visser, M., van Eijk, J. T. M., Kanaya, A. M., de Rekeneire, N., et al. (2008). Joint effects of adiposity and physical activity on incident mobility limitation in older adults. *Journal of the American Geriatrics Society, 56*(4), 636–643.

Koster, A., Penninx, B. W., Newman, A. B., Visser, M., van Gool, C. H., Harris, T. B., et al. (2007). Lifestyle factors and incident mobility limitation in obese and non-obese older adults. *Obesity (Silver Spring), 15*(12), 3122–3132.

Kraemer, H. C., Wilson, G. T., Fairburn, C. G., & Agras, W. S. (2002). Mediators and moderators of treatment effects in randomized clinical trials. *Archives of General Psychiatry, 59*(10), 877–883.

Lang, I. A., Guralnik, J. M., & Melzer, D. (2007). Physical activity in middle-aged adults reduces risks of functional impairment independent of its effect on weight. *Journal of the American Geriatrics Society, 55*(11), 1836–1841.

Lasikiewicz, N., Myrissa, K., Hoyland, A., & Lawton, C. L. (2014). Psychological benefits of weight loss following behavioural and/or dietary weight loss interventions: A systematic research review. *Appetite, 72*, 123–137.

Launer, L. J., Harris, T., Rumpel, C., & Madans, J. (1994). Body mass index, weight change, and risk of mobility disability in middle-aged and older women: The epidemiologic follow-up study of NHANES I. *Journal of the American Medical Association, 271*(14), 1093–1098.

Lebrun, C. E., van der Schouw, Y. T., de Jong, F. H., Grobbee, D. E., & Lamberts, S. W. (2006). Fat mass rather than muscle strength is the major determinant of physical function and disability in postmenopausal women younger than 75 years of age. *Menopause, 13*(3), 474–481.

Maciejewski, M. L., Patrick, D. L., & Williamson, D. F. (2005). A structured review of randomized controlled trials of weight loss showed little improvement in health-related quality of life. *Journal of Clinical Epidemiology, 58*(6), 568–578.

Marrero, D., Pan, Q., Barrett-Connor, E., de Groot, M., Zhang, P., Percy, C., et al. (2014). Impact of diagnosis of diabetes on health-related quality of life among high risk individuals: The Diabetes Prevention Program outcomes study. *Quality of Life Research, 23*(1), 75–88.

Martin, C. K., Bhapkar, M., & Pittas, A. G., Pieper, C. F., Das, S. K., Williamson, D. A., et al. (2016). Effect of calorie restrcition on mood, quality of life, sleep and sexual function in healthy nonobese women. *JAMA Internal Medicine, 176*(6), 743–752.

Martin, C. K., Church, T. S., Thompson, A. M., Earnest, C. P., & Blair, S. N. (2009). Exercise dose and quality of life: A randomized controlled trial. *Archives of Internal Medicine, 169*(3), 269–278.

McDermott, M. M., Criqui, M. H., Ferrucci, L., Guralnik, J. M., Tian, L., Liu, K., et al. (2006). Obesity, weight change, and functional decline in peripheral arterial disease. *Journal of Vascular Surgery, 43*(6), 1198–1204.

Mendes de Leon, C. F., Barnes, L. L., Bienias, J. L., Skarupski, K. A., & Evans, D. A. (2005). Racial disparities in disability: Recent evidence from self-reported and performance-based disability measures in a population-based study of older adults. *Journals of Gerontology Series B: Psychological Sciences and Social Sciences, 60*(5), S263–S271.

Mendes de Leon, C. F., Hansberry, M. R., Bienias, J. L., Morris, M. C., & Evans, D. A. (2006). Relative weight and mobility: A longitudinal study in a biracial population of older adults. *Annals of Epidemiology, 16*(10), 770–776.

Messier, S. P., Gutekunst, D. J., Davis, C., & DeVita, P. (2005). Weight loss reduces knee-joint loads in overweight and obese older adults with knee osteoarthritis. *Arthritis and Rheumatology, 52*(7), 2026–2032.

Messier, S. P., Loeser, R. F., Miller, G. D., Morgan, T. M., Rejeski, W. J., Sevick, M. A., et al. (2004). Exercise and dietary weight loss in overweight and obese older adults with knee osteoarthritis: The arthritis, diet, and activity promotion trial. *Arthritis and Rheumatology, 50*(5), 1501–1510.

Miller, G. D., Nicklas, B. J., Davis, C., Loeser, R. F., Lenchik, L., & Messier, S. P. (2006). Intensive weight loss program improves physical function in older obese adults with knee osteoarthritis. *Obesity (Silver Spring), 14*(7), 1219–1230.

Mundermann, A., Dyrby, C. O., & Andriacchi, T. P. (2005). Secondary gait changes in patients with medial compartment knee osteoarthritis: Increased load at the ankle, knee, and hip during walking. *Arthritis and Rheumatology, 52*(9), 2835–2844.

Ohmori, K., Kuriyama, S., Hozawa, A., Ohkubo, T., Tsubono, Y., & Tsuji, I. (2005). Modifiable factors for the length of life with disability before death: Mortality retrospective study in Japan. *Gerontology, 51*(3), 186–191.

Pekkarinen, T., Kaukua, J., & Mustajoki, P. (2015). Long-term weight maintenance after a 17-week weight loss intervention with or without a one-year maintenance program: A randomized controlled trial. *Journal of Obesity, 2015*, 651460.

Raaijmakers, L. C., Pouwels, S., Berghuis, K. A., & Nienhuijs, S. W. (2015). Technology-based interventions in the treatment of overweight and obesity: A systematic review. *Appetite, 95*, 138–151.

Ravussin, E., Redman, L. M., Rochon, J., Das, S. K., Fontana, L., Kraus, W. E., et al. (2015). A 2-year randomized controlled trial of human caloric restriction: Feasibility and effects on predictors of health span and longevity. *Journals of Gerontology Series A: Biological Sciences and Medical Sciences, 70*(9), 1097–1104.

Rejeski, W. J., Bray, G. A., Chen, S. H., Clark, J. M., Evans, M., Hill, J. O., et al. (2015). Aging and physical function in type 2 diabetes: 8 years of an intensive lifestyle intervention. *Journals of Gerontology Series A: Biological Sciences and Medical Sciences, 70*(3), 343–353.

Rejeski, W. J., Brubaker, P. H., Goff, D. C., Jr., Bearon, L. B., McClelland, J. W., Perri, M. G., et al. (2011). Translating weight loss and physical activity programs into the community to preserve mobility in older, obese adults in poor cardiovascular health. *Archives of Internal Medicine, 171*(10), 880–886.

Rejeski, W. J., Focht, B. C., Messier, S. P., Morgan, T., Pahor, M., & Penninx, B. (2002). Obese, older adults with knee osteoarthritis: Weight loss, exercise, and quality of life. *Health Psychology, 21*(5), 419–426.

Rejeski, W. J., Ip, E. H., Marsh, A. P., Zhang, Q., & Miller, M. E. (2008). Obesity influences transitional states of disability in older adults with knee pain. *Archives of Physical Medicine and Rehabilitation, 89*(11), 2102–2107.

Reynolds, S. L., Saito, Y., & Crimmins, E. M. (2005). The impact of obesity on active life expectancy in older American men and women. *Gerontologist, 45*(4), 438–444.

Rubin, R. R., Wadden, T. A., Bahnson, J. L., Blackburn, G. L., Brancati, F. L., Bray, G. A., et al. (2014). Impact of intensive lifestyle intervention on depression and health-related quality of life in type 2 diabetes: The Look AHEAD Trial. *Diabetes Care, 37*(6), 1544–1553.

Sharkey, J. R., Branch, L. G., Giuliani, C., Zohoori, M., & Haines, P. S. (2004). Nutrient intake and BMI as predictors of severity of ADL disability over 1 year in homebound elders. *Journal of Nutrition Health and Aging, 8*(3), 131–139.

Stenholm, S., Rantanen, T., Alanen, E., Reunanen, A., Sainio, P., & Koskinen, S. (2007). Obesity history as a predictor of walking limitation at old age. *Obesity (Silver Spring), 15*(4), 929–938.

van Gemert, W., van der Palen, J., Monninkhof, E., Rozeboom, A., Peters, R., Wittink, H., et al. (2015). Quality of life after diet or exercise-induced weight loss in overweight to obese postmenopausal women: The SHAPE-2 randomized controlled trial. *Public Library of Science ONE, 10*(6), 1–13.

Villareal, D. T., Banks, M., Sinacore, D. R., Siener, C., & Klein, S. (2006). Effect of weight loss and exercise on frailty in obese older adults. *Archives of Internal Medicine, 166*(8), 860–866.

Villareal, D. T., Chode, S., Parimi, N., Sinacore, D. R., Hilton, T., Armamento-Villareal, R., et al. (2011). Weight loss, exercise, or both and physical function in obese older adults. *New England Journal of Medicine, 364*(13), 1218–1229.

Visscher, T. L. S., Rissanen, A., Seidell, J. C., Heliovaara, M., Knekt, P., Reunanen, A., et al. (2004). Obesity and unhealthy life-years in adult Finns: An empirical approach. *Archives of Internal Medicine, 164*(13), 1413–1420.

Visser, M., Fuerst, T., Lang, T., Salamone, L., & Harris, T. B. (1999). Validity of fan-beam dual-energy X-ray absorptiometry for measuring fat-free mass and leg muscle mass. *Journal of Applied Physiology, 87*(4), 1513–1520.

Visser, M., Goodpaster, B. H., Kritchevsky, S. B., Newman, A. B., Nevitt, M., Rubin, S. M., et al. (2005). Muscle mass, muscle strength, and muscle fat infiltration as predictors of incident mobility limitations in well-functioning older persons. *Journals of Gerontology Series A: Biological Sciences and Medical Sciences, 60*(3), 324–333.

Visser, M., Harris, T. B., Langlois, J., Hannan, M. T., Roubenoff, R., Felson, D. T., et al. (1998). Body fat and skeletal muscle mass in relation to physical disability in very old men and women of the Framingham Heart Study. *Journals of Gerontology Series A: Biological Sciences and Medical Sciences, 53*(3), M214–M221.

Ware, J. E., Kosinski, M., & Keller, S. K. (1994). *SF-36 Physical and Mental Health Summary Scales: A user's manual*. Boston: Health Institute.

Williamson, D. A., & Rejeski, W. J. (2014). Obesity and quality of life. In G. A. Bray & C. Bouchard (Eds.), *Handbook of obesity* (Vol. 1, pp. 645–655). New York: CRC Press.

Williamson, D. A., Rejeski, W. J., Lang, W., Van Dorsten, B., Fabricatore, A. N., & Toledo, K. (2009). Impact of a weight management program on health-related quality of life in overweight adults with type 2 diabetes. *Archives of Internal Medicine, 169*(2), 163–171.

Wray, L. A., & Blaum, C. S. (2001). Explaining the role of sex on disability: A population-based study. *Gerontologist, 41*(4), 499–510.

Yancey, A. K., Cole, B. L., Brown, R., Williams, J. D., Hillier, A., Kline, R. S., et al. (2009). A cross-sectional prevalence study of ethnically targeted and general audience outdoor obesity-related advertising. *Milbank Quarterly, 87*(1), 155–184.

Yancy, W. S., Jr., Almirall, D., Maciejewski, M. L., Kolotkin, R. L., McDuffie, J. R., & Westman, E. C. (2009). Effects of two weight-loss diets on health-related quality of life. *Quality Life Research, 18*(3), 281–289.

Yankura, D. J., Conroy, M. B., Hess, R., Pettee, K. K., Kuller, L. H., & Kriska, A. M. (2008). Weight regain and health-related quality of life in postmenopausal women. *Obesity (Silver Spring), 16*(10), 2259–2265.

Zoico, E., Di Francesco, V., Guralnik, J. M., Mazzali, G., Bortolani, A., Guariento, S., et al. (2004). Physical disability and muscular strength in relation to obesity and different body composition indexes in a sample of healthy elderly women. *International Journal of Obesity and Related Metabolic Disorders, 28*(2), 234–241.

PART IV
Assessment of Patients with Obesity

CHAPTER 15

Medical Evaluation of Patients with Obesity

Rekha B. Kumar
Louis J. Aronne

Over the past decade there has been an increase in awareness among both adult and pediatric primary care doctors of the value of being formally trained in evaluating patients with obesity. This increased awareness can be attributed to several factors, ranging from scientific advances in the field of obesity medicine to policy efforts made by government and nonprofit medical societies. The increasing body of literature on neurohormonal aberrations in the condition of excess adiposity (Thaler et al., 2012) and metabolic adaptions after weight loss (Sumithran et al., 2011) has led physicians to look beyond the notion that diet and exercise alone will solve the obesity epidemic. The American Medical Association's (AMA) classification of obesity as a disease state ("AMA Adopts New Policies," 2013), the creation of the American Board of Obesity Medicine ("History of American Board of Obesity Medicine," 2011), and the coverage of doctors' visits for obesity care by the Centers for Medicare and Medicaid Services ("Intensive behavioral therapy," 2012) are just a few examples of broader efforts encouraging appropriate medical evaluation of patients with obesity. On the patient care level, physicians are witnessing increases in the prevalence of extreme obesity (Flegal, Kruszon-Moran, Carroll, Fryar, & Ogden, 2016), and an increasing portion of U.S. health care spending is devoted to comorbidities of excess adiposity ("Adult Obesity Facts," 2015). Despite these developments, only 2,000 physicians have been credentialed in obesity medicine. The majority of physicians, nurse practitioners, and physician assistants are not comfortable treating obesity.

The medical evaluation of patients with obesity can follow an algorithmic approach in the same way that physicians evaluate other chronic diseases. The 2013 American Heart Association (AHA)/American College of Cardiology (ACC)/Obesity Society (TOS) guidelines by Jensen et al. (2014) propose assessing body mass index (BMI) to screen for overweight and obesity at each patient encounter (Figure 15.1). Assessment should include height, weight, and calculation of BMI. If a patient is found to have a normal BMI ($\geq 18.5- < 25$ kg/m^2), he or she should be advised to avoid weight gain, and potential risk factors for weight gain in their history should be addressed. If a patient meets criteria for overweight or obesity, the patient should be screened and treated

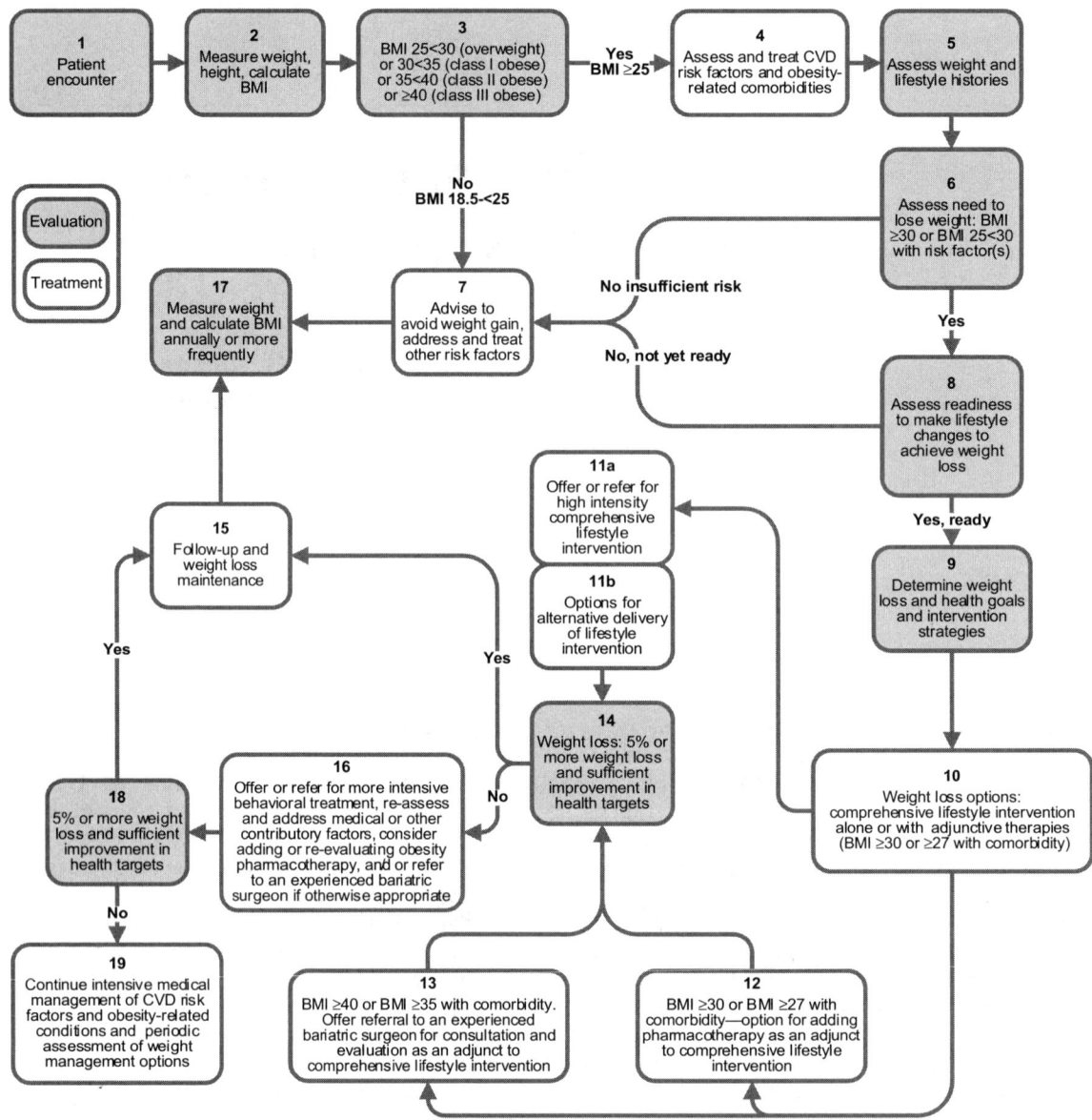

FIGURE 15.1. 2013 American Heart Association/American College of Cardiology/Obesity Society Guideline for Management of Overweight and Obesity in Adults. CVD, cardiovascular disease.

for cardiovascular comorbidities, including diabetes, hypertension, and hyperlipidemia. The severity of obesity determined by BMI class and comorbidities should further lead the physician through the algorithm toward offering behavioral intervention for weight management or behavioral intervention with anti-obesity pharmacotherapy: if BMI is 30 or greater, or if BMI is 27 or greater with comorbidities. Individuals with refractory class 2 obesity (BMI 35– < 40 kg/m^2) with medical complications, as well as with class 3 obesity (BMI ≥ 40 kg/m^2), should be offered bariatric surgical options.

In addition to identifying patients with obesity based on BMI classification, further health risks can be assessed through staging. An example of an obesity staging system is the Edmonton Obesity Staging System (EOSS) (Table 15.1) devised by Arya Sharma, Robert Kushner, and colleagues (Sharma & Kushner, 2009). This system identifies the presence of physical, functional, and mental comorbidities, assigning a stage to the total of all comorbidities. For example, a patient with a BMI of 31 kg/m² with no physical, functional, or mental weight-related complications would be considered class 1, stage 0, whereas another patient with a BMI of 31 kg/m² with nonalcoholic steatohepatitis (NASH) and type 2 diabetes would be staged as class 2.

TABLE 15.1. Edmonton Obesity Staging System

Stage 0	No complications of obesity (no laboratory, psychological, or functional limitations)
Stage 1	Subclinical factors (pre-diabetes, borderline hypertension, mild distress over weight, mild aches and pains)
Stage 2	Established comorbidity (type 2 diabetes, hypertension, hyperlipidemia, distress over weight)
Stage 3	End-organ damage (coronary artery disease, neuropathy), fatty liver
Stage 4	End-stage disease (congestive heart failure, diabetic nephropathy requiring hemodialysis, significant physical limitations, immobility)

History and Physical Examination

Taking a history in a patient with obesity is complicated due to the multifactorial nature of the disease that can span an entire lifetime from in utero factors to job-related stressors and hormonal changes that occur as people progress through life. It is imperative that the history not be taken in a biased or judgmental way that implicitly blames the patient for his or her condition. The history should address age of onset of obesity, minimum adult weight maintained for over a year, and notable events associated with weight gain (e.g., cessation of smoking, pregnancy, menopause, medication use; see Figure 15.2). Details on prior weight loss attempts and which modalities were used to obtain successful weight loss should be investigated. A history of eating disorders, such as anorexia, bulimia, or binge-eating disorder, usually requires close follow-up with a mental health practitioner in addition to the obesity medicine specialist. The care of significant alcohol and substance abuse should take precedence over obesity treatment. Cigarette smoking can complicate treatment history because weight is often gained upon stopping smoking. The average weight gain after smoking cessation is approximately 4.5 kg (Aubin, Farley, Lycett, Lahmek, & Aveyard, 2012). It would be prudent to encourage smoking cessation and to manage a patient with medical/nutri-

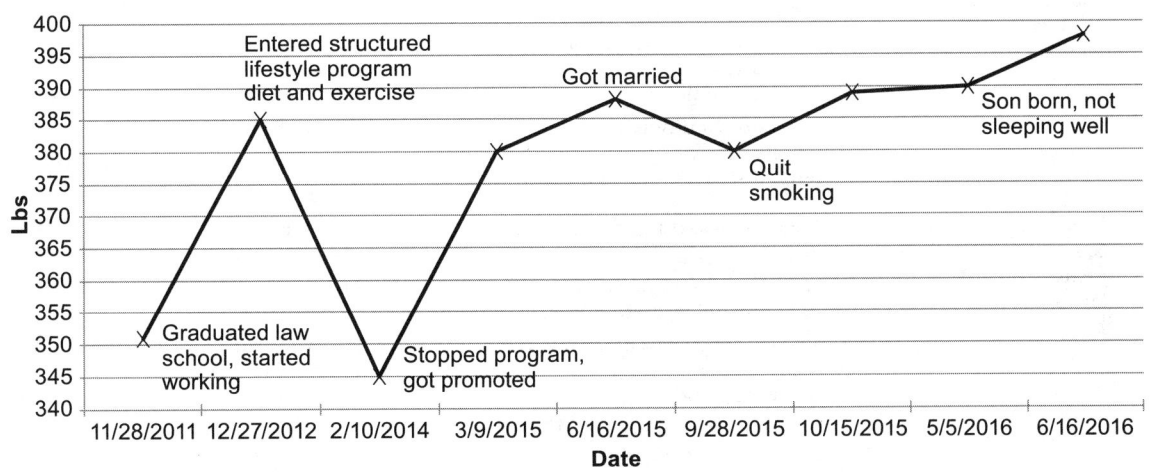

FIGURE 15.2. Sample graph of weight and life events.

tional therapy for weight control, in order to avoid or mitigate weight gain after smoking cessation. (Bupropion, a medicine that is FDA approved for smoking cessation, can also aid in weight loss and can be considered for patients who are obese and would like to stop smoking [Patel & Steinberg 2016].)

Although monogenic causes of obesity such as defects in leptin, melanocortin-4 receptor, and pro-opiomelanocortin (POMC) deficiency are very rare, it is important to document whether there is a family history of obesity and obesity-related comorbidities in first- and second-degree relatives. Having a family history of obesity substantially increases an individual's likelihood of developing obesity. The biggest risk factor for obesity in a child is having a parent or first-degree relative with obesity (Parrino et al., 2016). Having a first- or second-degree relative with type 2 diabetes is an independent risk factor for insulin resistance (Ferry, 2011).

A detailed history of a patient's current level of physical activity, including lifestyle, physical activity, and structured exercise, should be documented prior to initiating an exercise program. This information will help to determine what level of activity should be prescribed and whether any testing or medical supervision is necessary (Thompson, Arena, Riebe, & Pescatello, 2013; Table 15.2).

Evaluation of Weight-Related Disorders

Medical conditions that lead to abnormal weight gain should not be overlooked by the clinician and should be screened for if a patient exhibits signs and symptoms of these diseases (Table 15.3). Examples include polycystic ovarian syndrome, Cushing syndrome, hypothyroidism, and acromegaly. Insulin resistance and hyperinsulinemia in the months or years before developing overt type 2 diabetes can lead to significant weight gain (Kronenberg, Melmed, Polonsky, & Larsen, 2007).

Evaluation of Complications of Obesity

When overt complications of obesity, such as hypertension, type 2 diabetes, hyperlip-

TABLE 15.2. Recommendations for Medical Clearance for Exercise

Exercise history	Medical history	Medical clearance from a health care professional
Not participating in regular exercise at a moderate intensity on at least 3 days/week for at least the past 3 months	• No cardiovascular, metabolic, or renal disease	Not necessary
	• No signs or symptoms suggestive of cardiovascular, metabolic, or renal disease	Not necessary
	• Known cardiovascular, metabolic, or renal disease • Asymptomatic	Recommended
	• Signs or symptoms suggestive of cardiovascular disease, metabolic, or renal disease	Recommended
Participating in regular exercise at a moderate intensity on at least 3 days/week for at least the past 3 months	• No cardiovascular, metabolic, or renal disease	Not necessary
	• No signs or symptoms suggestive of cardiovascular, metabolic, or renal disease	Not necessary
	• Known cardiovascular, metabolic, or renal disease • Asymptomatic	Not necessary for moderate-intensity exercise; recommended for vigorous-intensity exercise
	• Signs or symptoms suggestive of cardiovascular disease, metabolic, or renal disease	Discontinue exercise and seek medical clearance

Note. Data from the American College of Sports Medicine (2015).

TABLE 15.3. Medical Conditions That Can Contribute to Weight Gain and Obesity

Disease	Diagnostic tests
Hypothyroidism	Thyroid-stimulating hormone, free thyroxine, thyroid peroxidase antibodies for autoimmune etiology, triiodothyronine
Cushing disease	24-hour urine cortisol, 1 mg dexamethasone suppression test
Acromegaly	Insulin-like growth factor 1 and growth hormone levels
Insulinoma	Fasting insulin, c-peptide, glucose
Polycystic ovarian syndrome	Clinical diagnosis using Rotterdam criteria for hyperandrogenism, oligomenorrhea, and polycystic ovaries; A.M. blood draw for total testosterone, free testosterone, dehydroepiandrosterone, prolactin, thyroid-stimulating hormone, and early-morning 17-hydroxyprogesterone levels; testing should be done when the patient is off oral contraceptives

idemia, or coronary heart disease, are diagnosed, these conditions should be treated concomitantly with medically supervised weight loss. Certain conditions such as osteoarthritis will get better as the patient loses weight, unless the severity requires joint replacement. All patients should have up-to-date cancer screening in light of the fact that obesity increases the risk of several cancers, including breast, colon, and uterine cancers (Bray, 2003). These cancers may be more difficult to detect in the patient with obesity (Printz, 2015), and individuals with obesity may be less likely to seek out screening. Patients with daytime fatigue, sleepiness, and/or morning headaches should be screened with a diagnostic sleep study for obstructive sleep apnea (OSA). Increased neck circumference (≥ 17 inches in men and ≥ 16 in women), enlarged floppy uvula, and tonsillar hypertrophy are predictors of OSA (Onat et al., 2009). Associated findings may include reports of snoring, disturbed sleep, irritability, and decreased libido. Laboratory studies may show polycythemia. OSA can be associated with further weight gain, and treating it can facilitate weight loss (Blackman et al., 2016).

Medication-Induced Weight Gain

Several commonly prescribed medicines can contribute to abnormal weight gain or interfere with patients' ability to lose weight (Table 15.4). These medications include antipsychotics, antidepressants, anitepileptics, insulin and insulin secretagogues (e.g., thiazolidinediones), glucocorticoids, progestational hormones and implants, oral contraceptives, beta-blockers, and others (Apovian, Aronne, & Powell, 2015). If possible, these medications should be substituted for other medications that are weight neutral, or agents that can treat the underlying condition and cause weight loss at the same time. Use of over-the-counter medications and supplements should be reviewed. Medications that could interact with anti-obesity pharmacotherapy, such as the pseudoephedrine in cold remedies, should be discontinued if stimulants are used for weight loss.

Physical Exam

A comprehensive physical exam should be performed to evaluate the etiologies of obesity, as well as the complications of this disease. Height and weight should be measured and the BMI calculated in order to categorize the class and severity of obesity. Waist circumference should be measured with the proper technique at the level directly above the iliac crests (Akabas, Lederman, & Moore, 2012), especially in patients with a BMI > 25–35 kg/m^2 who need further risk stratification (Bray, 2003; Table 15.5). Blood pressure should be checked with an appropriately sized cuff to avoid mismeasurement (by cuffs that are too tight or too loose). Other exam findings to note are the presence of acanthosis nigricans and skin tags indicative of insulin resistance, violaceous striae and dorsocervial fat pads indicative of hypercortisolism, and thyromegaly and delayed reflexes as signs of hypothyroidism. Some findings such as fungal skin infections, lower extremity edema, and foot

TABLE 15.4. Drugs That May Promote Weight Gain and Alternatives

Drug class	Associated with weight gain	Alternatives associated with less weight gain, weight neutral, or inducing weight loss
Antidepressants	Nortriptyline, amitriptyline, paroxetine, citalopram, mirtazapine, fluoxentine (>1 year), sertraline (>1 year)	Fluoxetine (< 1 year), sertraline (< 1 year), bupropion (can induce weight loss)
Antipsychotics	Clozapine, olanzapine, risperidone, quetiapine, lithium	Ziprasidone, aripiprazole
Antiepileptics	Gabapentin, pregabalin, valproate, carbamazepine	Topiramate, zonisamide, lamotrigine, levetiracetam, phenytoin
Antidiabetic agents	Insulin, sulfonylureas, thiazoladinediones	Acarbose, metformin, glucagon-like peptide-1 receptor agonists, dipeptidyl peptidase-4 inhibitors, sodium–glucose cotransporter 2 inhibitors, pramlintide
Steroids	Glucocorticoids, progestins	Use lowest dose of glucocorticoids needed to control underlying disease
Contraceptives	Depomedroxyprogesterone acetate, combination oral contraceptive pills (older generation)	Copper intrauterine device (IUD), low-dose combination oral contraceptive pill
Antihypertensives	Prazosin, doxazosin, terazosin, metoprolol tartrate, propranolol	Carvedilol, nebivolol
Antihistamines: over-the-counter allergy remedies and sleep remedies used chronically	Diphenhydramine, other antihistamines	Use for as short of a duration as needed

TABLE 15.5. Classification of Overweight and Obesity by BMI, Waist Circumference, and Associated Disease Risk

			Disease risk (relative to normal weight and waist circumference)[a]	
	BMI (kg/m^2)	Obesity class	Men ≤ 40 in. (≤ 102 cm) Women ≤ 35 in. (≤ 88 cm)	> 40 in. (> 102 cm) > 35 in. (> 88 cm)
Underweight	< 18.5	—	—	
Normal[b]	18.5–24.9	—	—	
Overweight	25.0–29.9		Increased	High
Obesity	30.0–34.9	1	High	Very high
	35.0–39.9	2	Very high	Very high
Extreme obesity	≥ 40	3	Extremely high	Extremely high

[a]Disease risk for type 2 diabetes mellitus, hypertension, and cardiovascular disease.
[b]Increased waist circumference can also be a marker for increased risk, even in persons of normal weight.

deformities may occur in patients with long-standing obesity.

Laboratory Evaluation

Certain obesity complications may manifest only with laboratory and investigational testing. A hemoglobin A1C, fasting blood glucose, or 75 g oral glucose tolerance test can be done to screen for type 2 diabetes (American Diabetes Association, 2003). A full lipid panel, including fractionated lipoprotein levels, would be required to assess for genetic disorders of lipid metabolism such as familial hypercholesterolemia. Often hyperuricemia, hepatic steatosis, and cholestasis are only discovered upon further lab testing (Table 15.6). A complete laboratory evaluation includes blood glucose, uric acid, blood urea nitrogen (BUN), creatinine, alanine aminotransferase (ALT), aspartate aminotransferase (AST), total and direct bilirubin, alkaline phosphatase, total cholesterol, high-density lipoprotein cholesterol (HDL) and low-density lipoprotein (LDL) cholesterol, triglycerides, complete blood count, thyroid-stimulating hormone (TSH) test, and urinalysis. A fasting insulin and glucose can be used to calculate homeostatic model assessment levels of insulin resistance (HOMA-IR; Matthews et al., 1985).

Measurements of body composition utilizing accessible methods such as bioelectrical impedance or dual-energy X-ray absorptiometry (DXA) can provide more information on body fat percentage, sarcopenic obesity, and lean body mass, and can be tracked longitudinally with a patient's progress.

Formulating a Treatment Plan

Formulating a reasonable and safe treatment plan should be done by sharing all results of the physical exam and investigational studies with the patient. Realistic targets for weight loss should be set with the goal of improvement in comorbidities. For example, informing patients that clinically significant weight loss is defined as a loss of 5% or more of total body weight, because of improvements in health with this degree of loss, can be motivating to them. Emphasis should be placed on any findings associated with obesity that would be expected to improve with weight loss, rather than stressing arbitrary goal weights or cosmetic endpoints. Figure 15.3 depicts how much weight loss is required to produce improvements in various medical conditions (Wing et al., 2011). Weight maintenance, achieved through combined changes in diet, physical activity, and behavior, should be the priority following the first 6 months of weight loss.

Assessing Readiness

The decision to start a medically supervised weight loss regimen should consider patients' motivation to lose weight, as well as their prior experiences with weight loss attempts, available support systems, financial resources, and time constraints (Wadden, Butryn,

TABLE 15.6. Laboratory and Diagnostic Evaluation of the Obese Patient Based on Presentation of Symptoms, Risk Factors, and Index of Suspicion

Suspicion of obesity comorbidity	Testing
Sleep apnea and alveolar hypoventilation (Pickwickian syndrome) (hypersomnolence, possible right-sided heart failure)	Polysomnography for oxygen desaturation, apneic and hypopneic events; ear, nose, and throat examination for upper airway obstruction
	Complete blood count (to rule out polycythemia); pulmonary function tests (reduced lung volume); blood gases (partial pressure of carbon dioxide often elevated); electrocardiogram (to rule out right-sided heart strain)
Gallstones	Ultrasonography of gallbladder
Hepatomegaly/nonalcoholic steatohepatitis	Liver function tests, liver sonogram

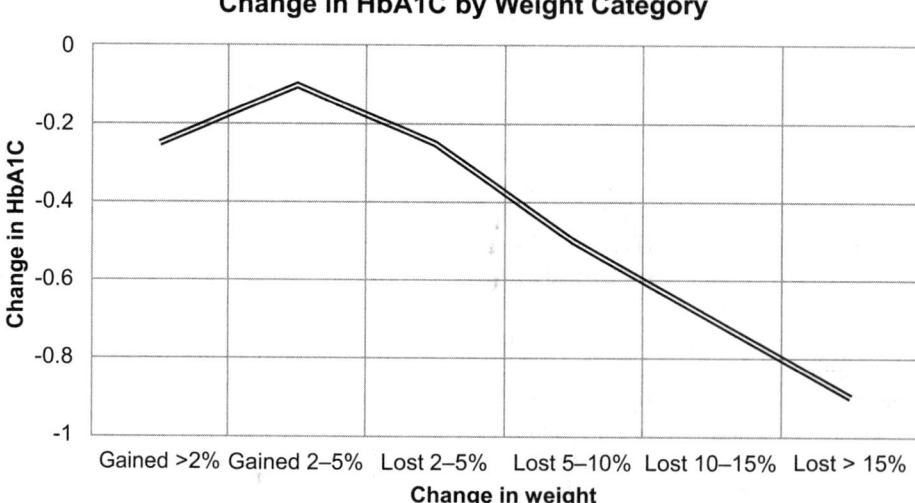

FIGURE 15.3. Improvement in comorbidities with weight loss. Adapted from Wing et al. (2011). HbA1C, glycated hemoglobin; BP, blood pressure; SBP, systolic blood pressure; DBP, diastolic blood pressure.

Hong, & Tsai, 2014). At the present time, the data indicate that an unmotivated patient will not succeed in the long run. If the patient does not wish to lose weight and is not at high risk, weight maintenance should be encouraged. If the patient is at high risk as a result of obesity but unmotivated, the clinician can raise awareness of the medical consequences of continued obesity.

Special Considerations and Contraindications to Treatment

Obesity treatment is relatively contraindicated in patients who are pregnant. Although extreme weight loss, anti-obesity pharmacotherapy, and bariatric procedures are contraindicated in the pregnant patient with obesity, a patient who is at high risk of excess weight gain and gestational diabetes can be managed conservatively to control weight gain while pregnant (Thangaratinam et al., 2012). Other contraindications for medical weight loss include active anorexia nervosa, terminal illness, and patients receiving chemotherapy that can result in malnutrition and cachexia. Medical or psychiatric illnesses, including cardiovascular disease, depression, and anxiety, should be stable and concomitantly managed as weight reduction begins and may influence the choice of weight loss medications (if they are used). Patients with cholelithiasis or osteoporosis should be counseled that these conditions might be exacerbated with weight loss.

Summary

There has been increasing effort over the past decade to raise awareness among health care providers about the proper diagnosis and treatment of obesity. The paucity of physicians trained to treat obesity, the prevalence of weight bias among providers, and poor reimbursement for weight-related care has led the medical community to lag behind in combatting the obesity epidemic. A place to begin addressing this epidemic is to educate health care providers on proper medical evaluation of the patient with obesity. Obesity treatment requires physicians, nurse practitioners, and physician assistants to have comprehensive knowledge of the various etiologies of obesity, as well as the skills to treat complications of the disease. In evaluating patients with obesity, it is important to understand the influence of genetics, environment, the natural aging process, and the effects of other medications. The measurement of height, weight, BMI, and waist circumference should be documented and tracked. Noted changes in these parameters should be addressed with patients in a nonbiased way. Physical exam findings and laboratory abnormalities concerning specific endocrine causes of obesity should be pursued and might require referral to a specialist. Staging the degree of obesity will help the provider be aware of anticipated complications and will assist him or her in using formal guidelines that outline treatment algorithms and options for care.

References

Adult obesity facts. (2015). Retrieved from *www.cdc.gov/obesity/data/adult.html*.

Akabas, S. R., Lederman, S. A., & Moore, B. J. (Eds.). (2012). *Textbook of obesity: Biological, psychological and cultural influences*. Hoboken, NJ: Wiley-Blackwell.

AMA adopts new policies on second day of voting at annual meeting. (2013, June). Retrieved from *www.ama-assn.org/ama/pub/news/news/2013/2013-06-18-new-ama-policies-annual-meeting.page*.

American Board of Obesity Medicine Statistics. (2016). Retrieved from *http://abom.org/stats*.

American College of Sports Medicine. (2015). *ACSM's Guidelines for Exercise Testing and Prescription* (10th ed.). Alphen aan den Rijn, The Netherlands: Wolters Kluwer.

American Diabetes Association. (2003). Screening for type 2 diabetes. *Diabetes Care, 26*(1, Suppl.), S21–S24.

Apovian, C. M., Aronne, L. J., & Powell, A. G. (Eds.). (2015). *Clinical management of obesity*. West Islip, NY: Professional Communications.

Aubin, H. J., Farley, A., Lycett, D., Lahmek, P., & Aveyard, P. (2012). Weight gain in smokers after quitting cigarettes: Meta-analysis. *British Medical Journal, 345*, e4439.

Blackman, A., Foster, G. D., Zammit, G., Rosenberg, R., Aronne, L., Wadden, T., et al. (2016). Effect of liraglutide 3.0μmg in individuals with obesity and moderate or severe obstructive sleep apnea: The SCALE Sleep Apnea randomized clinical trial. *International Journal of Obesity (London), 40*(8), 1310–1319.

Bray, G. A. (2003). *Contemporary diagnosis and management of obesity and the metabolic syndrome*. Longboat Key, FL: Handbooks in Healthcare.

Ferry, R. J. (Ed.). (2011). *Management of pediatric obesity and diabetes (nutrition and health)*. Totowa, NJ: Humana Press.

Flegal, K. M., Kruszon-Moran, D., Carroll, M. D., Fryar, C. D., & Ogden, C. L. (2016). Trends in obesity among adults in the United States, 2005 to 2014. *Journal of the American Medical Association, 315*(21), 2284–2291.

History of American Board of Obesity Medicine. (2011). Retrieved from *http://abom.org/history*.

Intensive Behavioral Therapy (IBT) for Obesity. (2012, March). Retrieved from *www.cms.gov/Outreach-and-Education/Medicare-Learning-Network-MLN/MLNMattersArticles/downloads/MM7641.pdf*.

Jensen, M. D., Ryan, D. H., Apovian, C. M., Ard, J. D., Comuzzie, A. G., Donato, K. A., et al. (2014). 2013 AHA/ACC/TOS guideline for the management of overweight and obesity in adults: A report of the American College of Cardiology/American Heart Association Task Force on Practice Guidelines and The Obesity Society. *Circulation, 129*(25, Suppl. 2), S102–S138.

Kronenberg, H. M., Melmed, S., Polonsky, K., &

Larsen, P. R. (Eds.). (2007). *Williams textbook of endocrinology.* Philadelphia: Saunders.

Matthews, D. R., Hosker, J. P., Rudenski, A. S., Naylor, B. A., Treacher, D. F., & Turner, R. C. (1985). Homeostasis model assessment: Insulin resistance and beta-cell function from fasting plasma glucose and insulin concentrations in man. *Diabetologia, 28*(7), 412–419.

Onat, A., Hergenç, G., Yüksel, H., Can, G., Ayhan, E., Kaya, Z., et al. (2009). Neck circumference as a measure of central obesity: Associations with metabolic syndrome and obstructive sleep apnea syndrome beyond waist circumference. *Clinical Nutrition, 28*(1), 46–51.

Parrino, C., Vinciguerra, F., La Spina, N., Romeo, L., Tumminia, A., Baratta, R., et al. (2016). Influence of early-life and parental factors on childhood overweight and obesity. *Journal of Endocrinology Investigation, 39*(11), 1315–1321.

Patel, M. S., & Steinberg, M. B. (2016). In the clinic: Smoking cessation. *Annals of Internal Medicine, 164*(5), ITC33–ITC48.

Printz, C. (2015). ACS report: Progress lags in some cancer control efforts. *Cancer, 121*(15), 2478–2479.

Sharma, A. M., & Kushner, R. F. (2009). A proposed clinical staging system for obesity. *International Journal of Obesity (London), 33*(3), 289–295.

Sumithran, P., Prendergast, L. A., Delbridge, E., Purcell, K., Shulkes, A., Kriketos, A., et al. (2011). Long-term persistence of hormonal adaptations to weight loss. *New England Journal of Medicine, 365*(17), 1597–1604.

Thaler, J. P., Yi, C. X., Schur, E. A., Guyenet, S. J., Hwang, B. H., Dietrich, M. O., et al. (2012). Obesity is associated with hypothalamic injury in rodents and humans. *Journal of Clinical Investigation, 122*(1), 153–162.

Thangaratinam, S., Rogozinska, E., Jolly, K., Glinkowski, S., Roseboom, T., Tomlinson, J. W., et al. (2012). Effects of interventions in pregnancy on maternal weight and obstetric outcomes: Meta-analysis of randomised evidence. *British Medical Journal, 344,* e2088

Thompson, P. D., Arena, R., Riebe, D., & Pescatello, L. S. (2013). ACSM's new preparticipation health screening recommendations from ACSM's guidelines for exercise testing and prescription, ninth edition. *Current Sports Medicine Reports, 12*(4), 215–217.

Wadden, T. A., Butryn, M. L., Hong, P. S., & Tsai, A. G. (2014). Behavioral treatment of obesity in patients encountered in primary care settings: A systematic review. *Journal of the American Medical Association, 312*(17), 1779–1791.

Wing, R. R., Lang, W., Wadden, T. A., Safford, M., Knowler, W. C., Bertoni, A. G., et al. (2011). Benefits of modest weight loss in improving cardiovascular risk factors in overweight and obese individuals with type 2 diabetes. *Diabetes Care, 34*(7), 1481–1486.

CHAPTER 16

Behavioral Assessment of Patients with Obesity

Jena Shaw Tronieri
Thomas A. Wadden

The medical evaluation of an individual with obesity, described by Kumar and Aronne (Chapter 15, this volume), should be complemented whenever possible by a behavioral assessment. The goals of this assessment are to (1) obtain a fuller understanding of biological and behavioral factors that may contribute to a patient's obesity; (2) assess the psychosocial consequences of excess weight; and (3) examine the individual's goals and expectations for weight reduction (if it is desired). Another key objective is to provide patients with an opportunity to discuss their personal experiences with their weight and to have someone listen attentively and respectfully. As Stunkard (1993) has noted, "Such an experience may be the greatest gift that a doctor can give an obese patient; it compares favorably with the modest benefits of our programs of weight reduction" (p. 356).

Guidelines for working with individuals with overweight or obesity recommend that clinicians assess patients' weight and lifestyle histories (Jensen et al., 2014). However, few assessment models are available. The assessment described in this chapter has been developed by our research team over the past 30 years. It is organized around five major areas, summarized by the acronym "BEST Treatment." *B* captures biological factors that may contribute to the patient's obesity; *E* stands for environmental influences; *S* represents social/psychological status; and *T* describes the timing of the present weight loss effort. Following a review of these four components, patient and provider select the best *Treatment* option.

Prior to their behavioral assessment, we ask patients to complete the Beck Depression Inventory–II (BDI-II; Beck, Steer, & Brown, 1996) and the Weight and Lifestyle Inventory (WALI; Wadden & Foster, 2006). The latter is a questionnaire that inquires about the four areas described above. (The WALI is available to purchasers of this book; see the box at the end of the table of contents.) The patient's completion of these materials prior to the assessment allows the health care provider to identify the points of greatest interest and to focus the interview accordingly. The BDI-II has excellent reliability, as well as criterion and predictive validity (Beck et al., 1996). Items on the WALI have good test–retest reliability (e.g., Crerand et al., 2006; Wadden et al., 2006). WALI items also have been found to have good convergent validity with established psychological and behavioral measures (Wadden et al., 2006). However, we have no data on the predictive validity of this inventory in, for example, identifying patients who will or will not lose weight. Further research of this kind is needed. At present, the WALI is best viewed as a method of eliciting and organizing patient information.

Members of our staff usually take 60 minutes to conduct the behavioral assessment, which makes it most appropriate for use in a specialty clinic. Such an assessment is probably best conducted by a mental health professional who specializes in obesity or by a registered dietitian who has a consultative relationship with a psychologist or psychiatrist. These personnel usually have more time to meet with patients than do primary care professionals (e.g., physicians, nurse practitioners). Primary care providers, however, may want their patients to complete the questionnaires, which practitioners can then quickly review for problem areas. Similarly, familiarity with the assessment will sensitize primary care providers to problems such as binge eating or mood disorders, which are encountered in a significant minority of individuals with obesity. Providers who interact with patients with obesity in a context where questionnaires cannot be completed prior to the appointment might still use the WALI or BEST Treatment model as a guide for discussion.

Minor adjustments in this assessment are necessary when it is applied to the behavioral evaluation of individuals seeking bariatric surgery. Considerations relevant to this population are discussed at the end of the chapter.

Initiating the Interview

In our experience, practitioners frequently initiate weight reduction therapy without adequately knowing the person they plan to treat. Thus, the first 5–10 minutes of the interview should be devoted to getting to know the patient. The interview should provide an overview of the patient's (1) intimate relationships (i.e., with parents, spouse/partner, children, and friends); (2) satisfaction with work and leisure activities; and (3) current life goals. From the beginning, the practitioner should seek to understand how weight affects and is affected by these factors, and what life changes the patient anticipates with weight loss.

We usually begin the assessment by thanking patients for completing the questionnaires and explaining that we will review them to get a better sense of "your weight and dieting history, eating and activity habits, and mood. We will then discuss your interest in losing weight and the goals you hope to achieve. We will finish by talking about treatment options." We then speak briefly with patients about some aspect of their work or leisure activities before proceeding to review the questionnaire items. We select what appears to be a conflict-free topic that a patient can discuss comfortably. For instance, we might remark, "I read that you are a teacher. What do you teach?" This discussion may resemble social chitchat, but it provides an opportunity to observe the patient's mood and verbal behavior, particularly if the patient is going to participate in a group program. It also provides an initial opportunity to learn about the patient's satisfaction with work and the degree of stress associated with it.

Primary Care Practice

Primary care professionals will probably need to take a different approach to initiate a conversation about weight control with patients whom they already know. The question is how best to broach this topic with individuals who have not asked for assistance. A physician's acknowledgment of a patient's obesity may increase the individual's desire to lose weight (Post et al., 2011). However, most practitioners have had limited training in obesity care (Kushner & Kahan, Chapter 24, this volume), and patients may be upset by practitioners' comments about their weight if the topic is not introduced in a respectful manner (Wadden et al., 2000). Instead of either avoiding discussion of weight or admonishing patients that they need to lose weight, a practitioner can use open-ended questions to invite patients to discuss their possible concerns—for example: "We have not talked about your weight in a while. What are your thoughts about your weight at this time?" Another option is to summarize the results of the physical examination to include a discussion of weight control.

The practitioner might state, "Your blood pressure today was 146/90 mmHg, and your weight was 215 pounds. I bet you could bring your blood pressure into the normal range by losing just 10–15 pounds. Would you like to consider this?" These approaches show respect for the patient and underscore the importance of inviting the individual's participation in treatment.

Reviewing BEST Treatment

In this chapter, we review biological, environmental, social, and timing factors, in that order (the same in which they are assessed by the WALI), and then discuss the selection of the best treatment option. Of course, practitioners may cover the BEST items however they wish, particularly if a patient is eager to discuss a particular topic at the outset of the interview.

Biological Factors

Classification

Obesity guidelines (reviewed by Kumar & Aronne, Chapter 15, this volume) classify patients into different categories of overweight and obesity based on body mass index (BMI). In addition, waist circumference may be used to assess whether the individual has upper-body fat distribution. These two simple measures provide an estimate of the patient's risk of weight-related health complications.

Genetic Factors

As reviewed by Farooqi (Chapter 4, this volume), recent twin and adoption studies suggest that genetic factors account for an estimated 45–75% of the variance in body weight (Farooqi & O'Rahilly, 2007). Body fat distribution (e.g., waist circumference) also appears to be highly heritable (Chaput, Pérusse, Després, Tremblay, & Bouchard, 2014). Although monogenic mutations, particularly those affecting the leptin–melanocortin pathway, have been shown to produce severe early-onset obesity, these genetic alterations are rare in humans and are present in fewer than 5% of individuals with severe obesity (Walley, Blakemore, & Froguel, 2006). In most cases, the heritability of obesity appears to be polygenetic, with over 127 genes having been identified as potentially linked to overweight, though only a minority of these associations ($n = 22$) have been replicated by five or more studies (Walley et al., 2006).

Currently, there are no simple, inexpensive tests that can be used in clinical practice to assess an individual's genetic predisposition to obesity. However, several factors are likely to suggest an increased role of biological, as compared to environmental, influences in the etiology of obesity. These variables can be assessed by obtaining a detailed weight and dieting history:

1. *Age of onset of obesity.* Childhood and adolescent onset of obesity are generally associated with greater body weight as an adult. Among adults with obesity, those with a relatively higher BMI and waist circumference report relatively younger ages of overweight/obesity onset (Gordon-Larsen, Adair, & Suchindran, 2007). Obesity in childhood doubles the risk of obesity in adulthood, and the risk increases further if an individual is obese as an adolescent (Rooney, Mathiason, & Schauberger, 2011; Whitaker, Wright, Pepe, Seidel, & Dietz, 1997). These differences may be attributed to the more rapid proliferation of adipose cells in children and adolescents with obesity, resulting in greater fat cell number in adulthood (Spalding et al., 2008). Earlier age of onset also appears to be associated with a stronger familial history of overweight (Gordon-Larsen et al., 2007; Rooney et al., 2011). Age of onset of overweight/obesity can be assessed by taking a careful weight history, as captured by items B1 and B4 of the WALI. Persons with childhood or adolescent onset of obesity can lose large amounts of weight but may be less likely to reach statistically average weight (Spalding et al., 2008).

2. *Family history.* As noted above, obesity runs in families, an occurrence due in part to shared genetic characteristics (Farooqi & O'Rahilly, 2007). Obesity in one parent more than doubles the risk that a child will be obese as an adult (Pachucki, Lovenheim, & Harding, 2014; Rooney et al., 2011), and the risk is even greater if both parents are

obese (Whitaker et al., 1997). Sibling obesity status is also associated with increased risk of obesity in childhood (Pachucki et al., 2014), and obese adults with relatively higher BMIs report higher levels of obesity in both their siblings and parents (Crerand et al., 2006). The strongest predictor of adult obesity is the combination of childhood or adolescent onset with a family history of obesity; 65–70% of children with these two risk factors become obese as adults (Whitaker et al., 1997).

Family history may be assessed by obtaining patients' reports of the weights and heights of their mother, father, and siblings (items C1, C3, and C4 of the WALI), which have been shown to be highly correlated with measured familial weights (Paradis, Pérusse, Godin, & Vohl, 2008). Weights of maternal and paternal grandparents also should be assessed. The use of figure size silhouettes, included in the WALI, helps to confirm the presence of overweight and obesity in relatives. These ratings also correlate highly with actual BMI (e.g., Cardinal, Kaciroti, & Lumeng, 2006), and provide a useful alternative for patients who have difficulty recalling familial measurements.

3. *Weight loss history.* Two-thirds of American adults and 89% of adults who consider themselves to be overweight have attempted to lose weight (Carroll, 2005). Patients with obesity who present to a specialty clinic such as ours frequently report a history of numerous weight loss attempts, usually followed by weight regain, as illustrated by Figures 16.1 and 16.2. Figure 16.1 shows the weight histories of patients who presented for behavioral weight loss and Figure 16.2 shows the weight histories of individuals who sought bariatric surgery. Frequent weight cycling may indicate that the body is defending an elevated body weight set point, resulting in rapid regain after weight loss (MacLean, Bergouignan, Cornier, & Jackman, 2011). Weight cycling may be a marker of a biological predisposition toward obesity.

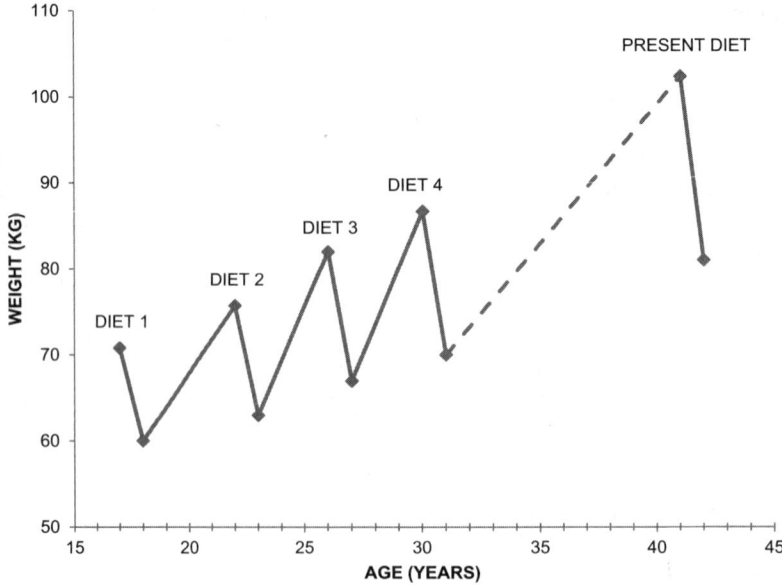

FIGURE 16.1. Weight and dieting histories of 31 women seeking behavioral weight loss who had engaged in a minimum of four diets. Overall, the 50 women surveyed reported 4.9 ± 0.5 diets on which they had lost 5 kg or more and lost a lifetime total of 55.9 ± 6.0 kg. Data were collected at the time of the "present diet," with subsequent weight loss for this diet shown. From Wadden and Letizia (1992). Copyright © 1992 The Guilford Press. Reprinted by permission.

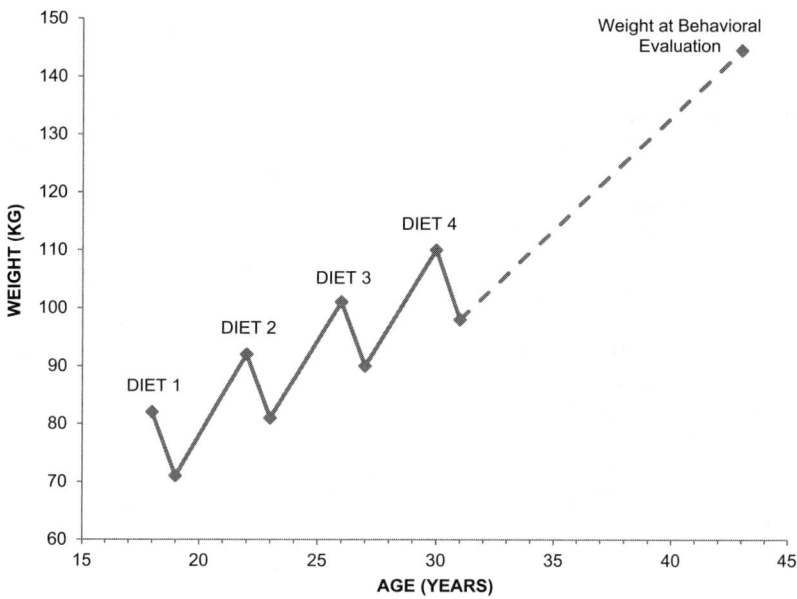

FIGURE 16.2. Weight and dieting histories of 77 women seeking bariatric surgery who had engaged in a minimum of four diets. Overall, the 83 women surveyed reported 4.7 ± 2.9 diets on which they had lost 5 kg or more and lost a lifetime total of 61.1 ± 41.3 kg. Data were collected at the time of the "behavioral evaluation" for bariatric surgery. From Gibbons, Sarwer, Crerand, Fabricatore, Kuehnel, Lipschutz, et al. (2006). Previous weight loss experiences of bariatric surgery candidates: How much have patients dieted prior to surgery? *Obesity, 14*(Suppl. 3), 70S–76S. Copyright © 2016 Wiley. Reprinted by permission.

Practitioners should know what weight loss methods a patient has tried before prescribing a new course of treatment. Weight loss history may be assessed by item E1 of the WALI, which inquires about the number of diets that resulted in a weight loss of 10 pounds (4.2 kg) or more, as well as less successful dieting attempts (E3 and E4 of the WALI). We also encourage practitioners to acknowledge the sincere efforts (and frequently expense) that patients have devoted to weight loss. Statements such as "You have really worked hard to control your weight, and I admire your efforts" are greatly appreciated by most individuals.

Medical Conditions and Medication Use

In addition to genetic factors, certain medical conditions and medications may produce weight gain. Hypothyroidism, polycystic ovarian syndrome, Cushing syndrome, Hashimoto disease, and acromegaly can all cause rapid increases in weight. Certain antipsychotics, antidepressants, antiepileptics, insulins, glucocorticoids, progestational hormones, oral contraceptives, and beta-blockers also have been associated with weight gain (for a review, see Kumar & Aronne, Chapter 15, this volume), as is smoking cessation (Tian, Venn, Otahal, & Gall, 2015). In addition to reviewing the patient's medical history, the provider should discuss factors that the patient believes contributed to weight gain (included in B4 of the WALI), particularly during periods marked by rapid increases in weight.

Summarizing the Role of Biological Factors

Some patients will present histories that clearly suggest a biological predisposition to obesity, but other cases will be less clear. For example, a patient with a BMI of 40 kg/m^2, childhood onset of obesity, and a positive family history is likely to have a genetic predisposition to this disorder. The presence of a biological predisposition is harder to determine in a patient with a similar BMI who became obese as an adult, has lost and regained weight only once, and, as a result of adoption, knows nothing about the weights of his or her biological parents.

At least three issues should be discussed with patients in whom a marked biological predisposition to obesity is suspected. The first is that even though obesity is a heritable disorder, it is not inherited in the same manner as eye color (in which a person is born with blue, green, or brown eyes, with little influence of the environment). By contrast, genes may confer the potential for obesity, but it is the environment that determines the extent to which this potential is realized (Swinburn et al., 2011). A second point is that by changing their behavior and environment, patients with obesity can lose weight, even if they are not likely to achieve a statistically average weight. Third, information about biological contributions to obesity can be used to assuage feelings of guilt and shame that burden some patients. Studies such as those by Bouchard et al. (1990) have shown clearly that some people gain more weight than others when overfed by the same number of calories. This finding resonates with the experience of many persons with obesity who are perplexed by their body weight when they compare their eating and activity habits with those of lean friends. The overall message is that patients with obesity are not to blame for their excess weight, and they may be able to improve their weight and health by adopting new eating and activity habits.

We might summarize findings in the following manner: "You have been overweight since you were 12 years old, and you noted that your mother had a weight problem all of her life, as did her mother. In addition, you have lost and regained weight on several occasions. These factors suggest that you have a biological (or genetic) tendency toward obesity—a tendency that probably makes weight control more difficult for you than the next person. This does not mean that you cannot lose weight; you certainly can. We'll look at ways that you can change your eating and activity habits to help you achieve a lower weight."

Environmental Factors

Environmental factors are clearly more responsible than genetic influences for the increased prevalence of obesity observed in industrialized nations in the past 30–40 years (Hill, Wyatt, Reed, & Peters, 2003). This fact makes it imperative to assess eating and activity habits to determine their possible contribution to a patient's obesity. Such an assessment will also reveal areas for intervention. This portion of the assessment should provide a sketch of the patient's daily eating pattern, approximate calorie intake, problem eating, and physical activity. Assessment of these variables typically continues throughout treatment.

Food Intake

Number of Meals and Snacks per Day

A key task is to determine the number of meals and snacks that the patient consumes each day (item H2 of the WALI). This includes assessing when meals and snacks are typically consumed and the consistency of the meal pattern. Individuals who skip meals (Levitsky & Pacanowski, 2013) or have highly variable eating patterns (Rogers, 1999) report greater hunger and dietary disinhibition (i.e., loss of control over dieting). Meal skipping has been associated with obesity (Mesas, Muñoz-Pareja, López-García, & Rodríguez-Artalejo, 2012) and meal regularity with successful weight loss maintenance (Fuglestad, Jeffery, & Sherwood, 2012). A principal goal of treatment is therefore to establish a structured eating plan.

Calorie Intake

A rough estimate of the patient's calorie intake can be obtained by reviewing food intake for a typical day (section I of the WALI). Diet composition can be assessed more fully by a registered dietitian, a 24-hour food recall, or the use of a food frequency questionnaire, such as that developed by Block, Woods, Potosky, and Clifford (1990). As treatment progresses, daily food records can be used to further assess intake and identify targets of intervention. Paper-and-pencil diaries are increasingly being replaced by online monitoring or the use of smartphone apps (e.g., myfitnesspal, Lose It!), which simplify calorie counting (Hutchesson, Rollo, Callister, & Collins, 2015).

No self-report measure of dietary intake has adequate reliability or validity compared to doubly labeled water, the preferred method of assessing energy requirements; however, this latter method is too expensive for use in clinical practice (see Marlatt & Ravussin, Chapter 3, this volume). On average, individuals with obesity underestimate their calorie intake by 30–50%, as compared with estimates from doubly labeled water; persons of average weight underestimate by 20–30% (Hutchesson et al., 2015; Lichtman et al., 1992). The underestimation does not appear to be intentional, but reflects the difficulty in remembering all foods eaten and estimating their quantities and calories. Emerging technological innovations that involve the use of smartphone cameras to capture food images may lead to improvements in recording accuracy, but at this time these methods are still under development (Stumbo, 2013).

The initial goal of dietary assessment is to determine whether the patient's reported calorie intake is consistent with elevated body weight or is lower than would be expected. Patients who report, often with embarrassment, that they eat a high-calorie diet can be told that this is actually good news, because treatment can help them reduce their intake. By contrast, those who report an unexpectedly low energy intake can be told that their estimate may be accurate; however, it is difficult to count portion sizes and to keep track of calories. Failure to lose weight while reportedly adhering to a calorie-restricted diet is often associated with substantial underreporting of calorie intake rather than with metabolic abnormality (Lichtman et al., 1992). In treatment, such individuals may benefit from increased attention to recording accuracy or from the use of meal replacements or portion-controlled entrées to facilitate calorie counting (see Wadden, Bakizada, Wadden, & Alamuddin, Chapter 17, this volume). Measurement of resting energy expenditure by indirect calorimetry is an option when patient and provider believe that the patient's energy requirements are abnormally low. In many hospitals, the pulmonary medicine service can measure resting energy expenditure following an overnight fast.

Diet Composition

The prevalence of high-calorie, high-fat, and high-sugar foods in the diet should also be assessed. Systematic reviews suggest an association between weight gain and greater intake of fast food (Rosenheck, 2008) and sugar-sweetened beverages (Malik, Schulze, & Hu, 2006). Reducing consumption of these items is a straightforward target for intervention. Patients generally should be encouraged to follow a balanced diet consistent with the 2015–2020 Dietary Guidelines (U.S. Department of Health and Human Services & U.S. Department of Agriculture, 2015). MyPlate provides resources for translating these guidelines into daily food choices (U.S. Department of Agriculture, 2017). However, a variety of different diets of markedly different macronutrient composition may be used, provided they induce an adequate energy deficit (Jensen et al., 2014).

Portion Sizes

In addition to dietary composition, portion size can be another source of excess calories in the diet. The consumption of larger self-reported portion sizes at mealtimes is associated with obesity (Berg et al., 2009). Many individuals are not aware that they eat larger portions than required for their calorie needs because of the role of large restaurant portions, packaged products, and larger plates and bowls in expanding our consumption norms (Wansink, 2007). A patient's tendency to consume larger portions can be assessed through examining the amounts of food listed in the WALI (section I, although individuals may omit or underestimate these amounts without training) and by their endorsement of overeating items listed under H1. We also frequently ask, "How much food do you typically eat compared to persons of average weight whom you know? About the same amount, more, or less?" For patients who endorse frequent overeating, we again emphasize that this habit provides a straightforward opportunity for intervention.

Environmental Cues

Environmental cues—including times, people, places, emotions, and activities—have been shown to influence the eating decisions of individuals across the weight spectrum (Wansink, 2004). Practitioners should attempt to identify cues that are reliably associated with overeating for the individual. Environmental cues are covered by item H1 (L–X) of the WALI, and should be assessed on an ongoing basis during treatment.

Appetite

Some individuals who report eating larger amounts of food indicate that they have trouble feeling full at mealtimes. Such individuals appear to have impaired satiation, a problem that may be treated by behavioral intervention or by pharmacological agents such as phentermine, phentermine/topiramate, lorcaserin, and liraglutide (Mordes, Liu, & Xu, 2015), or by bariatric surgery (Pournaras & Le Roux, 2009), as appropriate. Similarly, the practitioner may ask whether the individual experiences significant hunger or cravings and, if so, what times and places are associated with these sensations. These variables are assessed by item H1 (G–J) of the WALI. Several questionnaires can be used to provide a more in-depth assessment, including the Eating Inventory (Stunkard & Messick, 1988), which provides an assessment of hunger, disinhibition, and dietary restraint. The Food Craving Inventory (White, Whisenhunt, Williamson, Greenway, & Netemeyer, 2002) assesses the frequency of general and specific food cravings, and the Power of Food Scale (Lowe et al., 2009) is useful for assessing drive to eat palatable foods.

Problem Eating

A minority of individuals with obesity report symptoms of eating disorders, including binge-eating disorder (BED) and night eating syndrome (NES). As reviewed by McCuen-Wurst and Allison (Chapter 11, this volume), 20–50% of patients seeking weight reduction report symptoms of binge eating, and 10–15% meet criteria for BED as confirmed by a diagnostic interview. BED is characterized by the consumption of an objectively large amount of food in a short period of time (i.e., 2 hours) with an accompanying subjective loss of control (American Psychiatric Association, 2013) that has occurred at least once weekly over the prior 3 months. Individuals with BED are more likely to report symptoms of depression and other psychopathology, as discussed by McCuen-Wurst and Allison (Chapter 11, this volume).

NES is currently included as an "other specified feeding or eating disorder" in the fifth edition of the *Diagnostic and Statistical Manual of Mental Disorders* (DSM-5; American Psychiatric Association, 2013). Proposed diagnostic criteria include significantly increased intake in the evening or nighttime, as characterized by either consumption of at least 25% of daily intake after the evening meal or by at least two episodes of nocturnal eating per week. NES may co-occur with BED and, like BED, is associated with an increased prevalence of mood and anxiety disorders (see McCuen-Wurst & Allison, Chapter 11, this volume).

The Questionnaire on Eating and Weight Patterns—Revised (QEWP-R; Yanovski, Marcus, Wadden, & Walsh, 2015) and the Night Eating Questionnaire (NEQ; Allison, Stunkard, & Thier, 2004) are contained within the WALI (sections J and K) and serve as screening measures for BED and NES, respectively. The QEWP-R also provides items for differentiating BED from bulimia nervosa and related eating disorders. The Eating Disorder Examination Questionnaire (EDE-Q; Fairburn & Beglin, 2008) also can be used to assess behavioral symptoms of binge eating and other eating disorders. The practitioner should confirm reports of binge eating by having patients describe two or more recent binge episodes to determine that they ate an objectively large amount of food and experienced loss of control. We have observed that patients may endorse questionnaire items related to loss of control if they recall overeating episodes in which they determined, after mindlessly overeating, that they had eaten too much. Patients may describe feeling sad, guilty, or uncomfortably full after such episodes, but these occurrences should be distinguished from true loss of control eating in making a diagnosis of BED.

Both binge-eating and night eating episodes decline with weight loss treatment (Gallant, Lundgren, & Drapeau, 2012). However, recent systematic reviews suggest that cognitive-behavioral therapy (CBT) and other psychological treatments are superior for achieving long-term abstinence from disordered eating (see McCuen-Wurst & Allison, Chapter 11, and Grilo, Chapter 34, this volume). Although individuals with BED and/or NES may need additional treatments, these disorders should not be considered contraindications to weight loss. Most studies have found no differences in weight loss between obese individuals with and without BED who received behavioral weight control (Sherwood, Jeffery, & Wing, 1999), particularly if BED resolves during treatment (Gorin et al., 2008). Fewer studies have been conducted, but the same appears to be true of NES (Gallant et al., 2012).

Physical Activity

Frequent sedentary behavior and infrequent leisure-time physical activity are independent risk factors for increased weight, cardiovascular disease, and type 2 diabetes (e.g., Thorp et al., 2010; Wahid et al., 2016). A lower amount of physical activity also has been associated with increased all-cause mortality, independent of the effect of BMI, in large population-based cohorts (Arem et al., 2015). Increased physical activity improves initial weight losses only slightly (i.e., 1–2 kg in 16 weeks) but is the single best predictor of the maintenance of weight loss (Swift, Johannsen, Lavie, Earnest, & Church, 2014).

The goal in assessing physical activity is to locate patients on a continuum that ranges from completely sedentary to "marathon athlete." Assessing the typical amount of time a person spends engaging in sedentary activity (e.g., television, computer, or other "screen time"), lifestyle activity (e.g., number of blocks walked or flights of stairs climbed; Andersen et al., 1999), and programmed or purposeful activity (e.g., walking, jogging, and other aerobic or anaerobic activities) can provide an indication of his or her activity level. Physical activity and sedentary behaviors are covered in section L of the WALI. Other self-report measures, such as the Paffenbarger Physical Activity Questionnaire (Paffenbarger, Wing, & Hyde, 1995) and the Minnesota Leisure Time Physical Activity Questionnaire (Folsom, Jacobs, Caspersen, Gomez-Marin, & Knudsen, 1986), focus on the frequency, intensity, duration, and/or total amount of activity performed. Most self-report measures have only limited to moderate reliability and validity (Shephard, 2003). Wearable motion sensors provide a more accurate assessment of physical activity; they include pedometers, accelerometers, heart-rate monitors, and other multisensor devices (Ainsworth, Cahalin, Buman, & Ross, 2015; Shephard, 2003). With the proliferation of commercially marketed step-tracking devices (e.g., Fitbit, Jawbone, and Misfit) and phone applications, some patients may have such measurements available at the time of their assessment.

Some of our patients indicate that they are quite physically active, but most report that they are very sedentary. Limited physical activity can be reframed positively as a potential treatment target. To support later goal setting, we also inquire about exercise preferences, including type of activity (e.g., walking, swimming, aerobics) and whether the individual prefers to exercise alone or with others. Barriers that prevent the patient from exercising regularly should also be examined (see Jakicic, Rogers, Sherman, & Kovacs, Chapter 19, this volume). A common belief is that one must enjoy vigorous activity in order to be active, and that physical activity must be vigorous in order to benefit weight or health. Findings, however, indicate that moderate physical activity (equivalent to a brisk walk) is sufficient to improve cardiovascular and overall health (Shiroma, Sesso, Moorthy, Buring, & Lee, 2014). Individuals with obesity also may welcome news that increased lifestyle activity, without regard to intensity, is as effective as programmed activity in inducing and maintaining weight loss (Andersen et al., 1999). Practitioners should emphasize that any increase in physical activity, or reduction in sedentary activity, can benefit fitness, health, and long-term weight control.

Summarizing the Role of Environmental (Behavioral) Factors

This section of the interview concludes with a brief summary of the extent to which dietary intake and physical activity appear to contribute to the patient's weight problem. Clearly this assessment is impressionistic; in most cases, however, the practitioner can determine whether there is opportunity to modify the patient's food intake, physical activity, or both.

We usually summarize findings in the following manner: "You indicated that you don't enjoy exercising and are very sedentary. In some ways, I'm glad to hear that. If you were already running marathons, we wouldn't have much room for change. In terms of your eating habits, you said that you do not overeat at mealtimes, but often snack after dinner while watching television. Sometimes you eat as late as 11:00 P.M. We'll need to determine how many calories you consume in this fashion and find ways to help you control your evening snacking."

Social/Psychological Factors

The psychosocial assessment should address several topics, including the patient's living arrangements, satisfaction with personal relationships, and expected social support when attempting to lose weight (section M of the WALI). The patient's mood and psychosocial status also should be evaluated (sections N and O of the WALI).

Social Context of Weight Loss

"What is the social context in which the patient will lose weight?" Weight loss does not occur in a vacuum. The weights, eating habits, and attitudes of a patient's family members, friends, and coworkers are likely to affect his or her weight control efforts. For example, studies have shown that social influence can lead to increasing degrees of overweight among friends (Christakis & Fowler, 2007) and that having more social contacts who are attempting weight loss can enhance motivation to lose weight (Leahey, Larose, Fava, & Wing, 2011). We frequently ask, "What did you partner [or family/friends] do that helped you lose weight the last time you tried? What did your partner [or family/friends] do that hindered your weight control efforts?" The practitioner and patient might later invite family members to a session if such individuals are identified as significant barriers to weight control.

Psychosocial Effects of Obesity

Weight Stigma and Quality of Life

"What effect does weight have on the patient's social functioning, self-esteem, body image, and general quality of life?" Overweight and obese individuals are subjected to significant stigma and discrimination in the United States and other industrialized nations. Weight-related stigmatization can occur across a wide variety of life domains and may negatively affect an individual's psychological functioning, body image, weight-related health behaviors, and stress levels (see Puhl & Pearl, Chapter 10, this volume). Experiences of weight stigma can be assessed using the Experiences of Weight Bias questionnaire (Puhl, Heuer, & Sarda, 2011), which is found in section N of the WALI (items 5–7). Weight bias internalization may be associated with the greatest negative psychological outcomes and can be assessed using the Weight Bias Internalization Scale (WBIS; Durso & Latner, 2008).

Practitioners also may wish to obtain a measure of general health-related quality of life. The most widely used instrument is the Medical Outcome Study 36-Item Short-Form Health Survey (SF-36), which includes eight scales that measure domains including mental health, energy level, and role and social functioning (Ware & Sherbourne, 1992). The SF-36 is easily scored and has excellent validity and reliability. An obesity-specific quality-of-life measure also is available, the Impact of Weight on Quality of Life (IWQOL; Kolotkin, Head, Hamilton, & Tse, 1995), which is now more commonly used in its abbreviated form, the IWQOL—Lite (Kolotkin & Crosby, 2002). Both versions have excellent validity and reliability. Higher BMI levels are associated with lower quality of life on all three of these measures (Kolotkin & Crosby, 2002). Physical complications associated with obesity (e.g., pain, type 2 diabetes, sleep apnea) predict

Mood Disorder

"Does the individual have a mood disorder or other psychiatric condition?" Obesity is associated with an increased risk of depression, particularly among women and those with severe (class 3) obesity (see Puhl & Pearl, Chapter 10, this volume). Approximately 20% of obese women who seek weight reduction report significant symptoms of depression (Carey et al., 2014; Wadden et al., 2000), although fewer than 10% are likely to meet full criteria for a major depressive episode as defined by DSM-5 (American Psychiatric Association, 2013) and shown in Table 16.1.

We routinely assess mood with the BDI-II, although the Patient Health Questionnaire–9 (PHQ-9) mood scale (Kroenke, Spitzer, & Williams, 2001) may also be used and is shorter. Scores of 13 or less on the BDI-II are generally not of clinical concern unless the patient reports suicidal ideation (Beck et al., 1996). With scores of 14 or more, we review some of the individual items to assess more fully the patient's affect, behavior, and cognition and the extent to which symptoms of depression may be attributable to excess weight or recent life events (e.g., the loss of a relative). Scores of 29 or more indicate severe depression that requires professional attention. Figure 16.3 shows the distribution of BDI scores (at baseline) for 90 women with classes 1 and 2 obesity (mean BMI = 33.8 kg/m^2) who sought behavioral weight loss in a research trial at our clinic, as well as for 149 women with class 3 obesity (mean BMI = 52.6 kg/m^2) who sought bariatric surgery (Wadden et al., 2006). Approximately 30% of those with class 3 obesity reported moderate to severe symptoms of depression that potentially would benefit from CBT and/or pharmacotherapy, as compared to fewer than 10% of those with class 1 obesity.

Individuals with significant depressive symptoms typically have been excluded from behavioral weight loss trials because of concerns about their potential for increased attrition from treatment (e.g., Trief, Cibula, Delahanty, & Weinstock, 2014) and poorer weight loss outcomes. Although some studies have confirmed these associations (Pagoto et al., 2013; Trief et al., 2014), others have not (e.g., Elder et al., 2012). Further, depressive symptoms improve following weight loss treatment (Fabricatore et al., 2011; Pagoto et al., 2013), although these improvements may decline with weight regain over long-term follow-up (Dawes et al., 2016).

As a whole, these findings suggest that depression, including major depressive disorder, is not an absolute contraindication to weight loss treatment. However, weight loss is not an evidence-based treatment for significant depression, comparable to CBT or pharmacotherapy. We believe that best practice is to provide appropriate mental health referrals to patients who report clinically significant depressive symptoms, and to discuss with patients the potential benefits of treating their mood symptoms prior to undertaking weight loss. Depression that significantly impairs a person's day-to-day functioning (e.g., basic self-care, attendance at work or school) or is accompanied by suicidal ideation should be treated prior to initiating weight loss treatment. With individuals who report moderate or less severe symptoms of depression and who attribute their mood to distress about their weight, mood often improves substantially with weight loss alone. Treatments that combine behavioral weight loss and CBT for depression may further improve mood outcomes, but they do not enhance weight loss outcomes (Pagoto et al., 2013).

Obesity is also associated with an increased risk of anxiety disorders, although this relationship is less consistent than that for depression (see Puhl & Pearl, Chapter 10, this volume). Anxiety may be less likely than depression to improve with weight loss treatment, but further study is needed (de Zwaan et al., 2011). Anxiety can be assessed informally when discussing a patient's psychological functioning and current stressors (Items O1–O2 and P1–P4 of the WALI). It also may be evaluated using measures such as the Generalized Anxiety Disorder–7 (GAD-7; Spitzer, Kroenke, Williams, & Löwe, 2006), Beck Anxiety Inventory (BAI; Beck & Steer, 1990) or Hamilton Anxiety Rating Scale (HAM-A; Hamilton, 1959). Individuals with clinically significant anxiety should be provided with appropriate treatment referrals.

TABLE 16.1. DSM-5 Diagnostic Criteria for Major Depressive Disorder (Single Episode 296.2X/F32.X; Recurrent Episode 296.3X/F33.X)

A. Five (or more) of the following symptoms have been present during the same 2-week period and represent a change from previous functioning; at least one of the symptoms is either (1) depressed mood or (2) loss of interest or pleasure.

   Note: Do not include symptoms that are clearly attributable to another medical condition.

   1. Depressed mood most of the day, nearly every day, as indicated by either subjective report (e.g., feels sad, empty, hopeless) or observation made by others (e.g., appears tearful). (*Note*: In children and adolescents, can be irritable mood.)
   2. Markedly diminished interest or pleasure in all, or almost all, activities most of the day, nearly every day (as indicated by either subjective account or observation).
   3. Significant weight loss when not dieting or weight gain (e.g., a change of more than 5% of body weight in a month), or decrease or increase in appetite nearly every day. (*Note*: In children, consider failure to make expected weight gain.)
   4. Insomnia or hypersomnia nearly every day.
   5. Psychomotor agitation or retardation nearly every day (observable by others, not merely subjective feelings of restlessness or being slowed down).
   6. Fatigue or loss of energy nearly every day.
   7. Feelings of worthlessness or excessive or inappropriate guilt (which may be delusional) nearly every day (not merely self-reproach or guilt about being sick).
   8. Diminished ability to think or concentrate, or indecisiveness, nearly every day (either by subjective account or as observed by others).
   9. Recurrent thoughts of death (not just fear of dying), recurrent suicidal ideation without a specific plan, or a suicide attempt or a specific plan for committing suicide.

B. The symptoms cause clinically significant distress or impairment in social, occupational, or other important areas of functioning.

C. The episode is not attributable to the physiological effects of a substance or to another medical condition.

   Note: Criteria A–C represent a major depressive episode.

   Note: Responses to a significant loss (e.g., bereavement, financial ruin, losses from a natural disaster, a serious medical illness or disability) may include the feelings of intense sadness, rumination about the loss, insomnia, poor appetite, and weight loss noted in Criterion A, which may resemble a depressive episode. Although such symptoms may be understandable or considered appropriate to the loss, the presence of a major depressive episode in addition to the normal response to a significant loss should also be carefully considered. This decision inevitably requires the exercise of clinical judgment based on the individual's history and the cultural norms for the expression of distress in the contest of loss.

D. The occurrence of the major depressive episode is not better explained by schizoaffective disorder, schizophrenia, schizophreniform disorder, delusional disorder, or other specified and unspecified schizophrenia spectrum and other psychotic disorders.

E. There has never been a manic episode or a hypomanic episode.

   Note: This exclusion does not apply if all of the manic-like or hypomanic-like episodes are substance-induced or are attributable to the physiological effects of another medical condition.

Note. Reprinted with permission from the *Diagnostic and Statistical Manual of Mental Disorders, Fifth Edition.* Copyright © 2013 American Psychiatric Association. All rights reserved.

History of Substance Abuse/Dependence

"*Does the patient have a history of a substance use disorder?*" The prevalence of substance use disorders appears to be lower among individuals with obesity than in the general population, particularly among women and minority patients (see Puhl & Pearl, Chapter 10, this volume). Patients with obesity who seek treatment generally report a very low alcohol intake, and fewer than 10% have a history of alcohol or other substance abuse or dependence (Items G3–G4 of the WALI; King et al., 2012; Svensson et al., 2013; Wadden et al., 2006).

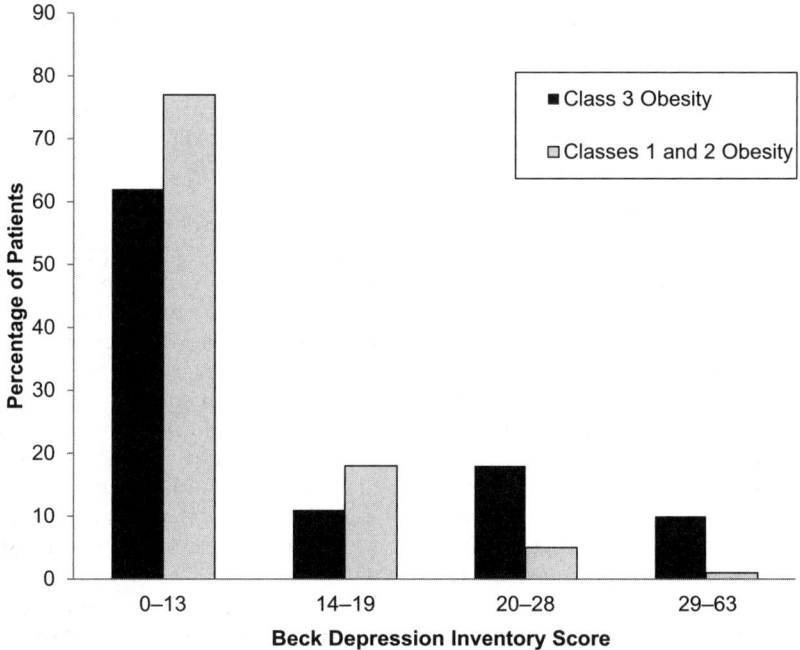

FIGURE 16.3. Depression among women with class 3 versus classes 1 and 2 obesity. The figure shows the percentage of women with class 3 versus classes 1 and 2 obesity who reported minimal (0–13), mild (14–19), moderate (20–28), and severe (29–63) symptoms of depression, based on BDI-II score. Data from Wadden et al. (2006).

Correlational evidence examining the relationship between alcohol consumption and weight has been inconsistent; data suggest that only heavy or frequent alcohol consumption is likely to contribute to overweight (Traversy & Chaput, 2015). Among individuals without current alcohol abuse, weight loss in behavioral programs is associated with reduced alcohol intake (Kase, Piers, Schaumberg, Forman, & Butryn, 2016). Alcohol and other substance use problems are uncommon in persons with obesity but, when identified, they should be treated prior to weight reduction.

Physical/Sexual Abuse

"Does the patient have a history of physical/sexual abuse?" Both retrospective (e.g., Mason et al., 2015) and prospective longitudinal studies (e.g., Bentley & Widom, 2009) suggest a relationship between abuse in childhood or adolescence and higher adult body weight. Few data are available concerning the effect of an abuse history on behavioral weight loss outcomes. Felitti (1993) found that women with a history of sexual abuse were more likely to terminate weight reduction therapy prematurely, and King, Clark, and Pera (1996) found that such individuals reported more episodes of dietary nonadherence, and they lost less weight. These effects may occur because some individuals with an abuse history perceive excess weight as a protective factor and feel anxious or vulnerable as a result of weight loss (Felitti, 1993). The impact of abuse history on weight loss has been investigated more extensively in individuals seeking bariatric surgery. Individuals with such a history, compared to those without, lose less weight, but this effect is small and does not prevent these patients from benefiting from the surgery (Steinig, Wagner, Shang, Dölemeyer, & Kersting, 2012).

The WALI includes two items that inquire about a history of sexual or physical abuse (see items 08–09). More comprehensive measures such as the Childhood Trauma Questionnaire (CTQ; Bernstein & Fink, 1998), and its abbreviated form (CTQ-SF; Bernstein et al., 2003), have demonstrated good psychometric properties for assessing diverse forms of childhood maltreatment. When patients respond "yes" on the questionnaire to having been abused, we usually state, "You indicated that you have been sexually/physically abused. Did you receive any counseling or other help?" With patients who have received treatment, we ask the extent to which they feel that they have recovered from the abuse. Those who report that they have never received counseling require greater attention. A small minority of patients report that they have never discussed their abuse with anyone over the course of many years. Some experience great sadness, pain, remorse, anger, or resentment as they describe what had happened. We always encourage these patients to obtain counseling. Some decline, stating that they have moved on and do not wish to revisit those events. Others express the belief that treatment will not help or may create problems if family members find out. We acknowledge these concerns, but reiterate that professional assistance can be helpful. We provide appropriate referrals and encourage patients to take a few days to think things over. We also encourage patients to call us if they find that they remain upset as a result of their disclosure.

Physical or sexual abuse is not a contraindication to weight reduction, although it is possible that this history may affect patients' experiences in treatment, as described above. The key concern with sexual abuse, as it is with depression or other psychiatric conditions, is to ensure that individuals with obesity receive the care they need. This is the same care that would be provided to people of average weight.

Summarizing Social/Psychological Factors

The great majority of individuals with obesity in the general population have essentially normal psychological functioning (see Puhl & Pearl, Chapter 10, this volume). A minority of patients who seek weight reduction have a psychiatric condition that may benefit from psychological intervention. For most patients with BED, depressive disorders, anxiety disorders, or body image disturbance, we discuss the potential benefits of psychological or pharmacological intervention. However, weight reduction usually is possible in the absence of adjunctive psychiatric care.

For the small minority of patients with severe depressive symptoms, current substance abuse, or other problems that present a safety risk or may interfere with successful weight loss, we recommend psychiatric treatment prior to attempting weight loss. In talking with such a patient, the practitioner might explain, "You seem to be having a hard time now. Your mood is blue. You are having trouble sleeping and concentrating. Activities that used to be pleasurable no longer are, and you are having trouble getting up the energy to do everyday things like taking care of the house and going to work. These are symptoms of depression." The practitioner should check the patient's response to this feedback and continue: "I know you want to lose weight, and you will be able to. But it will be much easier to lose weight, and to start enjoying life again, if we first help you feel better. There are effective treatments for symptoms of depression that include talking with someone or taking medicine." Patients often are disappointed when informed that weight reduction should be delayed until they receive treatment for their mood or other disorder. We communicate our belief that they will be more successful with weight control, as well as with other aspects of daily life, after getting the care they need.

Temporal Factors

This section of the assessment is an extension of the social/psychological evaluation and inquires about the timing of the planned weight loss effort. It seeks to answer two principal questions.

Timing of Weight Loss

"Why has the patient decided to lose weight now?" Although this question may be answered perfunctorily (e.g., "Because I'm overweight and want to weigh less"), the

practitioner should remember that the patient probably has been obese for many months, if not years. In all likelihood, something has happened recently to motivate the individual to lose weight. Individuals who are overweight seek weight loss for a variety of reasons. These include physical health concerns, distress about their appearance, feeling that their eating is out of control, prompting by a partner or employer, or the desire to reclaim aspects of their identity that had been submerged by the demands of raising a family. In some cases, patients have experienced disappointment, sadness, anger, or other feelings, which should be examined before weight loss is initiated. Discussion of these experiences will illuminate such patients' psychosocial goals for weight reduction, as discussed previously.

Favorable Time for Weight Loss

"Is this a favorable time to lose weight?" Successful weight reduction requires time, effort, and sustained concentration and motivation. Ideally, a patient should be relatively free of major life stressors. We have found that protracted stress in intimate or professional relationships, as well as life crises (e.g., death of a parent, financial or legal problems), may disrupt patients' weight reduction efforts (Wadden & Letizia, 1992). In one study, patients who discontinued treatment during the first 2 months of a multicenter trial endorsed more stressors at baseline (as measured by items P1–P4 of the WALI) than persons who remained in treatment. The distinguishing stressors were "relationship with significant other," "events related to parents," and "financial or legal difficulties" (Wadden & Letizia, 1992). Two recent studies found that individuals who scored high on the Perceived Stress Scale (PSS; Cohen, Kamarck, & Mermelstein, 1983), which measures the subjective level of stress in the past month, lost less weight than those with lower scores (Elder et al., 2012; Trief et al., 2014).

Persons who report that they are experiencing high stress, as compared to their usual levels, should consider delaying weight reduction until the stressor has passed. For example, an accountant might wait until after tax season to lose weight, or a parent of three young children might wait until after his or her kitchen remodeling has been completed. The goal during the interlude is to maintain a stable body weight. If, however, patients with stressful lives insist that they can meet the demands of treatment, we usually defer to their judgment. Some report that weight is the one thing they can control in a life that otherwise feels out of control. Interventions that combine behavioral weight loss with stress management may be of particular benefit to such patients (e.g., Cox et al., 2013).

The patient's travel and vacation schedules should also be considered. Preferably, the individual should have a 2- to 3-month block of time in which to participate in treatment regularly. If a behavioral intervention is to be used, the individual should be able to participate in counseling sessions in person or by phone at least every other week and preferably on a weekly basis. It is critical that patients get off to a successful start, which is facilitated by continuity of care during the first few months. Initial success (with weight loss) is associated with long-term success (e.g., Unick et al., 2015). False starts are demoralizing to both patients and providers and are often the result of missed visits early in treatment.

Summarizing Temporal Factors

Patients who seek weight reduction are usually "ready" for treatment, as reflected by their having taken the initiative to contact a health care provider. Thus it is not surprising, in this self-selected sample, that self-report measures of weight loss readiness generally do not predict attrition or weight loss (Casazza et al., 2013). Behavioral indicators, such as completion of food records during the first weeks, may be a better marker of future success (Tsai et al., 2014). Practitioners should determine that a patient has selected a propitious time to lose weight. In the minority of cases in which timing does not appear favorable, the practitioner might remark, "You clearly are motivated to lose weight and have given this a lot of thought. As we look at the next month, however, it seems that you're going to be very busy. What do you think about waiting until after your business trip to begin your program?

Your goal until that time would be to maintain a stable weight."

A greater challenge, particularly for primary care practitioners, is to motivate patients who appear to be uninterested in weight control, either because they have made previous unsuccessful attempts or because they do not believe that obesity is a serious problem. Motivational interviewing, in comparison to usual care, has been shown to enhance weight loss (Armstrong et al., 2011), and practitioners can borrow from this approach to elicit patients' curiosity about their inconsistent or contradictory behavior. With those who feel frustrated with weight loss, the practitioner might acknowledge, "I know how frustrated you are with your weight. You have worked so hard on it. I admire your efforts to improve your weight and health. There are some new approaches that could be of help to you. I would be pleased to discuss them, if you would like." With individuals who appear unconcerned about their weight, a different approach may be useful: "You seem like a person who's determined to be successful in life. I'm sure you've heard that carrying extra weight can affect your health and get in the way of your goals. Tell me why you're not more interested in your weight." As the patient describes the reasons for his or her ambivalence, the practitioner can look for opportunities to highlight the patient's own reasons for changing behaviors that affect his or her weight.

Identifying Treatment Goals

We conclude the behavioral assessment by briefly summarizing what we have learned about contributors to the patient's obesity, about the individual's psychosocial status, and concerning the timing of the current weight loss effort. In summarizing the interview, we might highlight the biological and environmental factors that potentially have contributed to the patient's obesity and indicate (when applicable) that the individual has previously worked hard to change eating and activity habits and has lost weight. We also highlight the potential influence of psychosocial and health factors on pursuing weight loss at this time. Patients should be encouraged to ask questions or to comment.

Identifying Goals of Treatment

Patient and practitioner are likely to have discussed the patient's goals of treatment throughout the interview. However, these should be clarified. Many individuals with obesity seek weight loss as a means to another goal, and patients may have implicit assumptions or desires that need to be articulated. The most commonly cited goals for pursuing weight loss are to improve health and/or appearance (e.g., LaRose, Leahey, Hill, & Wing, 2013). Many individuals specify that they seek to improve a particular health condition, their mobility, or their energy level. Others hope that weight loss will improve their social life, self-esteem, body image, or a failing marriage. If these goals are articulated at the outset of treatment, the patient and practitioner can evaluate whether they are realistic. If necessary, additional interventions can be planned to achieve these goals.

We often ask patients to rate (on a 1–10 scale) the likelihood that they will obtain the desired psychosocial outcomes if they lose weight. We also ask how much weight they think they need to lose to achieve these outcomes, and whether weight loss on previous occasions yielded the benefits desired. We inform patients that weight loss typically does not change personality or intimate relationships. It may improve body image, self-esteem, or mood, but these events are also influenced by factors other than weight (Blaine, Rodman, & Newman, 2007). Thus, if changes in these areas are the principal ones desired, the patient should consider the benefits of CBT, interpersonal psychotherapy, or other interventions. Body image, for example, improves with CBT in the absence of weight loss (Jarry & Ip, 2005).

By contrast, weight loss reliably improves health complications of obesity, including hypertension, hyperlipidemia, and type 2 diabetes (Jensen et al., 2014). Losses of 5–10% of initial weight are sufficient to improve these disorders, although larger losses usually have a greater impact (Gloy et al., 2013; Jensen et al., 2014; Wing et al., 2011). Patients also achieve improvements in physical function (Herring et al., 2016) and reductions in medication use (Gloy et al., 2013). In addition to health changes, we ask patients to think of changes in quality of life that they seek as a result of weight loss. These might include climbing stairs more easily, having more energy to play with children or grandchildren, or being able to enjoy tennis, swimming, or other sports again. Weight loss reliably improves health-related quality of life (Jensen et al., 2014). We suggest that patients measure their success, in large part, by the extent to which they reach these lifestyle goals.

Weight Loss Goals

The approach described above encourages patients to focus on non-weight-related outcomes in lieu of a particular goal weight. Nevertheless, it is important to discuss patients' weight loss goals; almost all patients have them, even if they do not make them explicit. In a memorable study, Foster, Wadden, Vogt, and Brewer (1997) first described women's goals of losing approximately one-third of their initial body weight (from a BMI of 36 kg/m^2). Weight loss goals have decreased in recent years, but individuals still wish to lose 20–25% of starting weight with nonsurgical interventions (Lent et al., 2016), even when they are informed that they should expect to lose 5–15% (Fabricatore et al., 2007). These elevated goals do not appear to be harmful, with most studies showing no relationship between patients' goals and actual weight lost. Some studies suggest that individuals with larger goals may lose more weight (Lent et al., 2016). In addition, after moderate weight loss (i.e., 5–15%), patients report experiencing greater physical, social, and psychological benefits than they had anticipated (Fabricatore et al., 2007; Foster et al., 1997).

Practitioners should underscore that a weight loss of 5–15% of initial weight—the amount the great majority of patients will lose—is a treatment success and is sufficient to improve both health and appearance concerns. We might remark, "Typically, people participating in a program like this one will lose 5–15% of their initial weight. At your weight of 260 pounds, that would be a loss of 13–39 pounds. What do you think of a loss of that amount?" Some patients may be discouraged by the practitioner's suggestion of a relatively modest weight loss. Others may simply insist that they plan to lose much more. As indicated, there is no need to convince the patient that a weight loss of greater than 15% is not possible. Indeed, some individuals can achieve and maintain losses of 20–30% of initial weight, as shown by the National Weight Control Registry (Thomas, Bond, Phelan, Hill, & Wing, 2014). We often say to patients that if they are to achieve a larger weight loss, they will first need to lose 5%, and that focusing on that amount will be a good start.

Selecting the Best Treatment

Reviewing Treatment Options

Following the discussion of the patient's goals of weight reduction, we review treatment options. This discussion is guided by an algorithm provided by the 2013 AHA/ACC/TOS guidelines, which recommends treatment based upon the patient's BMI, associated risk factors, and history of weight control efforts (Jensen et al., 2014). As a general rule, more intensive therapy is recommended for individuals with higher BMIs and with greater risk of health complications. Thus we might discuss the option of bariatric surgery with persons whose BMI is above 40 kg/m^2 (or ≥ 35 kg/m^2 with comorbid conditions) and who have lost and regained weight repeatedly. A portion-controlled diet, followed by long-term pharmacotherapy for obesity, may be appropriate for people who are uncomfortable with bariatric surgery. At the other end of the continuum, patients with BMIs under 30 kg/m^2 who are free of health complications may be advised to eat more fruits and vegetables, reduce sweets or salty snacks, and increase their physical activity. Depending on the individual's wishes, the goal for such patients will either be to prevent weight gain or to lose weight. Selection of treatment is discussed more fully in Wadden et al. (Chapter 17, this volume).

Overview of the Course of Treatment

This section of the interview concludes by providing patients with an overview of the course of treatment selected. This includes discussing the duration and frequency of treatment visits during the first 6 months;

the assignments patients will be asked to complete (e.g., keeping food and activity logs); and the expected results of therapy, including weight loss and improvements in physical and psychosocial status. If a lifestyle intervention is selected, patients are informed that they will need to devote about 30 minutes a day to their weight control regimen. Patients are encouraged to ask questions about the proposed course of treatment. At the conclusion, we ask, "Knowing what you do about the proposed treatment, how confident are you that you can adhere to the program?" Patients give a number from 1 to 10 in which 1 is "not at all confident" and 10 is "extremely confident." For numbers less than 8, we inquire, "What skills do you need to acquire to feel more confident?" In short, we want to ensure that patients begin treatment with adequate weight loss self-efficacy, given that self-efficacy is one of the few consistent predictors of weight loss (Burke et al., 2015).

Evaluation of Bariatric Surgery Patients

A 1991 consensus conference recommended that bariatric surgery candidates undergo a behavioral (psychological/psychiatric) assessment (NIH Conference, 1991), which is now required by many insurance companies. There is no standardized procedure for this assessment (Fabricatore et al., 2006), although several groups have described their approaches (e.g., Mechanick et al., 2013; Sogg, Lauretti, & West-Smith, 2016; Wadden & Sarwer, 2006).

Our assessment of bariatric surgery candidates follows the BEST Treatment model described previously, with minor modifications (Wadden & Sarwer, 2006). For many patients, this assessment represents their first meeting with a mental health provider, and some report (often with relief at the end of the assessment) that they had been quite nervous about the appointment. We therefore take time from the outset to describe the purpose of the meeting: "Today we'll talk with you about your weight and dieting histories, why you have decided to seek bariatric surgery, and what you are doing now to prepare for surgery. We want to help you decide whether the surgery is the right choice for you and to make sure that you have the support you'll need to be successful if you choose to move forward." We often begin the interview by asking which surgical procedure the patient plans to undergo and use this discussion as a means of assessing the patient's understanding of the procedure and his or her knowledge of its risks and benefits.

Biological Considerations

Most bariatric surgery candidates have an early age of onset of their obesity and a marked family history of obesity (Crerand et al., 2006), suggesting a significant genetic predisposition to this condition. We discuss this predisposition with patients, trying to allay feelings of shame or blame in candidates who believe their obesity is attributable solely to lack of willpower or poor eating and activity habits.

Because bariatric surgery is considered a last option when other treatments have failed, we pay particular attention to whether the patient has participated in organized weight loss programs or received pharmacotherapy. For the minority of individuals who have made no significant previous attempts to lose weight—and do not present with significant comorbidity—we recommend lifestyle intervention or pharmacotherapy prior to pursuing surgery. However, in cases in which patients report that they cannot afford these treatments, we recommend that they practice postoperative dietary changes for several months before surgery, ideally resulting in weight loss (Wadden & Sarwer, 2006).

Environmental Considerations

Assessment of environmental factors includes both the patients' typical eating patterns and their progress in practicing the eating behaviors required after surgery. The latter may include making healthier choices, eating five small meals per day, separating eating from drinking, eating slowly, and chewing food thoroughly (Laurenius et al., 2012; Sarwer et al., 2008). We review the rationales behind these behaviors with the patient, emphasizing their importance to postsurgical success, and refer the patient to

Social/Psychological Considerations

Psychiatric problems such as depression and BED are more prevalent among individuals seeking bariatric surgery than in the general population of individuals with obesity. A recent meta-analysis reported that 19% (95% CI: 15–31%) of these individuals had a depressive disorder and 17% (95% CI: 13–21%) had BED (Dawes et al., 2016). There does not appear to be a consistent relationship between preoperative depression or BED and postoperative weight loss at follow-up ranging from 6 to 60 months (Dawes et al., 2016; Livhits et al., 2012). The prevalence of both conditions is significantly reduced after bariatric surgery, although symptoms may increase at later follow-up assessments (Dawes et al., 2016).

We note that the risk of suicide and other self-harm behaviors in these patients is very low in absolute numbers, but may increase in the years after bariatric surgery (Bhatti et al., 2016; Dawes et al., 2016). The data on risk factors for suicide are very limited because of the low prevalence of these behaviors, and because the majority of studies have relied on state or medical records that do not include relevant covariates. One study found that a history of psychiatric diagnosis was associated with incidence of self-harm after bariatric surgery (Bhatti et al., 2016).

Substance and alcohol use disorders are rare among patients seeking bariatric surgery (e.g., 1% to 4%, Dawes et al., 2016). Moderate alcohol consumption prior to surgery does not reduce postoperative weight loss (Livhits et al., 2012). Some investigators have raised concerns that alcohol consumption may increase after surgery, a purported form of addiction transfer (Steffen, Engel, Wonderlich, Pollert, & Sondag, 2015). Current data suggest minimal risk of this occurrence for most patients, with over 93% consistently reporting low-risk alcohol consumption over a 10-year follow-up period (Svensson et al., 2013). For a small minority of individuals, alcohol consumption may increase after bariatric surgery, particularly with gastric bypass (King et al., 2012; Svensson et al., 2013). However, one study highlighted that this is a mixed effect, with as many individuals discontinuing high-risk drinking following surgery as are developing new onset of this behavior (Wee et al., 2014). Patients who are male, younger in age, smokers, or who regularly drink alcohol prior to surgery have a higher risk of developing an alcohol use disorder after surgery (King et al., 2012; Svensson et al., 2013). They should be cautioned to limit postsurgical alcohol consumption, particularly with gastric bypass.

Most psychiatric conditions are not absolute contraindications to surgery. However, we discuss their potential effect on patients' general well-being, as well as on their adherence to the postoperative diet, and provide treatment referrals as appropriate. About one-third of candidates receive recommendations for adjunctive psychiatric care, which is considered to be of potential benefit but optional for patients (Wadden & Sarwer, 2006). There is not a sufficient evidence base to show that such care is integral to a successful surgical outcome. Patients may decline our recommendations and proceed to surgery. By contrast, for the minority of individuals who report recent suicidal ideation, active symptoms of severe depression, bulimia, psychosis, or substance abuse—about 5–10% of our surgery candidates (Wadden & Sarwer, 2006)—we refer them to mental health services and schedule a follow-up assessment after 3–6 months of psychiatric treatment. For persons who are receiving mental health treatment at the time of their assessment, we obtain permission to contact their practitioner to obtain the provider's impressions of the patient's mental health and ability to adhere to the behavior changes required with surgery. As discussed above, we also caution patients regarding postsurgical consumption of alcohol and direct those with a history of psychiatric disorder to contact their medical or mental health providers if they experience a deterioration in mood after the surgery.

Timing Considerations

As with behavioral weight loss, the timing of a patient's surgery can be important to his or her success. In addition to the factors described previously, we discuss whether the patient will be able to take time off from work (ideally 3–6 weeks) to undergo and recover from the operation and establish new lifestyle habits. We also assess whether family members and friends are supportive of the patient's desire to have surgery and can assist him or her with transportation, child care, or other activities of daily living during recovery from the surgery.

Concluding the Presurgical Behavioral Assessment

After summarizing what we have learned about the patient, we review our findings and provide a written list of our recommendations, many of which will have been discussed during the assessment. We also indicate that we will provide the surgical team with a letter that summarizes our findings and recommendations (sample copies are included at the end of this chapter in Appendix 16.1). We encourage patients to contact us (or their surgical team) if they are in need of assistance and wish them success with their treatment.

Conducting the Behavioral Assessment

The behavioral assessment requires a practitioner to obtain a formidable amount of information in a brief period. In addition, the clinician must convey interest in the patient by giving the individual ample opportunity to raise questions and concerns. As noted above, we send patients (by mail or email) the BDI-II and WALI prior to the behavioral assessment and have them bring the completed materials to the appointment. In as few as 2 minutes, prior to meeting a patient, we can review the materials and determine the areas that need significant attention. We have observed informally that patients' completion of questionnaires and punctual attendance at the initial interview are markers for adherence and attendance during behavioral weight loss treatment. Persons who do not complete the questionnaires satisfactorily often dislike and do not complete the diet diaries and other homework assignments. This potential problem should be addressed with patients during the behavioral assessment.

Some patients come to the behavioral assessment feeling anxious. They feel ashamed of their inability to control their weight and worry that they will fail in treatment again. They also may wonder whether a practitioner will be sensitive to their problems and treat them respectfully, or instead will be critical of their apparent shortcomings. Thus, the health care provider should be aware that patients use the interview to conduct their own assessments of the practitioner.

We try to ensure that patients leave the behavioral assessment having learned something new about the nature and causes of their weight problem. They should also leave with a clear understanding of the course of the proposed treatment, if weight reduction is to be undertaken, and what they will need to do to be successful.

Finally, we hope that patients leave feeling that they have been treated with respect and understanding. It is hard to grasp, in only 60 minutes, the many years of effort that most persons with obesity have already devoted to weight control. So many have experienced sadness and frustration each time they lost and regained weight, in full view of family, friends, and coworkers. Few health problems are as public as obesity. Practitioners must look to the future to renew their patients' hope with the promise of new treatments. But they must also look to the past with respect and admiration for the individuals' previous efforts.

References

Ainsworth, B., Cahalin, L., Buman, M., & Ross, R. (2015). The current state of physical activity assessment tools. *Progress in Cardiovascular Diseases, 57*(4), 387–395.

Allison, K. C., Stunkard, A. J., & Thier, S. L. (2004). *Overcoming night eating syndrome: A step-by-step guide to breaking the cycle*. Oakland, CA: New Harbinger.

American Psychiatric Association. (2013). *Diagnostic and statistical manual of mental disorders* (5th ed.). Arlington, VA: Author.

Andersen, R. E., Wadden, T. A., Bartlett, S. J., Zemel, B. S., Verde, T. J., & Franckowiak, S. C. (1999). Effects of lifestyle activity vs. structured aerobic exercise in obese women: A randomized trial. *Journal of the American Medical Association, 287*, 335–340.

Arem, H., Moore, S., Patel, A., Hartge, P., de Gonzalez, A., Visvanathan, K., et al. (2015). Leisure time physical activity and mortality: A detailed pooled analysis of the dose–response relationship. *JAMA Internal Medicine, 175*(6), 959–967.

Armstrong, M., Mottershead, T., Ronksley, P., Sigal, R., Campbell, T., & Hemmelgarn, B. (2011). Motivational interviewing to improve weight loss in overweight and/or obese patients: A systematic review and meta-analysis of randomized controlled trials. *Obesity Reviews, 12*(9), 709–723.

Beck, A. T., & Steer, R. A. (1990). *Beck Anxiety Inventory.* San Antonio, TX: Psychological Corp.

Beck, A. T., Steer, R. A., & Brown, G. K. (1996). *Beck Depression Inventory–II (BDI-II) manual.* San Antonio, TX: Harcourt Brace.

Bentley, T., & Widom, C. S. (2009). A 30-year follow-up of the effects of child abuse and neglect on obesity in adulthood. *Obesity, 17*(10), 1900–1905.

Berg, C., Lappas, G., Wolk, A., Strandhagen, E., Torén, K., Rosengren, A., et al. (2009). Eating patterns and portion size associated with obesity in a Swedish population. *Appetite, 52*(1), 21–26.

Bernstein, D. P., & Fink, L. (1998). *Childhood Trauma Questionnaire: A retrospective self-report—manual.* New York: Psychological Corp.

Bernstein, D. P., Stein, J. A., Newcomb, M. D., Walker, E., Pogge, D., Ahluvalia, T., et al. (2003). Development and validation of a brief screening version of the childhood trauma questionnaire. *Child Abuse and Neglect, 27*(2), 169–190.

Bhatti, J. A., Nathens, A. B., Thiruchelvam, D., Grantcharov, T., Goldstein, B. I., & Redelmeier, D. A. (2016). Self-harm emergencies after bariatric surgery: A population-based cohort study. *JAMA Surgery, 151*(3), 226–232.

Blaine, B. E., Rodman, J., & Newman, J. M. (2007). Weight loss treatment and psychological well-being: A review and meta-analysis. *Journal of Health Psychology, 12*(1), 66–82.

Block, G., Woods, M., Potosky, A., & Clifford, C. (1990). Validation of a self-administered diet history questionnaire using multiple diet records. *Journal of Clinical Epidemiology, 43*(12), 1327–1335.

Bouchard, C., Tremblay, A., Després, J., Nadeau, A., Lupien, P. J., Thériault, G., et al. (1990). The response to long-term overfeeding in identical twins. *New England Journal of Medicine, 322*(21), 1477–1482.

Burke, L. E., Ewing, L. J., Ye, L., Styn, M., Zheng, Y., Music, E., et al. (2015). The SELF trial: A self-efficacy-based behavioral intervention trial for weight loss maintenance: Self-efficacy weight loss maintenance intervention. *Obesity, 23*(11), 2175–2182.

Cardinal, T. M., Kaciroti, N., & Lumeng, J. C. (2006). The figure rating scale as an index of weight status of women on videotape. *Obesity, 14*(12), 2132–2135.

Carey, M., Small, H., Yoong, S. L., Boyes, A., Bisquera, A., & Sanson-Fisher, R. (2014). Prevalence of comorbid depression and obesity in general practice: A cross-sectional survey. *British Journal of General Practice, 64*(620), e122–e127.

Carroll, J. (2005). Gallup poll: Six in 10 Americans have attempted to lose weight. Retrieved from www.gallup.com/poll/17890/six-americans-attempted-lose-weight.aspx.

Casazza, K., Fontaine, K. R., Astrup, A., Birch, L. L., Brown, A. W., Bohan Brown, M. M., et al. (2013). Myths, presumptions, and facts about obesity. *New England Journal of Medicine, 368*(5), 446–454.

Chaput, J., Pérusse, L., Després, J., Tremblay, A., & Bouchard, C. (2014). Findings from the Quebec family study on the etiology of obesity: Genetics and environmental highlights. *Current Obesity Reports, 3*, 54.

Christakis, N. A., & Fowler, J. H. (2007). The spread of obesity in a large social network over 32 years. *New England Journal of Medicine, 357*(4), 370–379.

Cohen, S., Kamarck, T., & Mermelstein, R. (1983). A global measure of perceived stress. *Journal of Health and Social Behavior, 24*(4), 385–396.

Cox, T., Krukowski, R., Love, S. J., Eddings, K., DiCarlo, M., Chang, J. Y., et al. (2013). Stress management–augmented behavioral weight loss intervention for African American women: A pilot, randomized controlled trial. *Health Education and Behavior, 40*(1), 78–87.

Crerand, C. E., Wadden, T. A., Sarwer, D. B., Fabricatore, A. N., Kuehnel, R. H., Gibbons, L. M., et al. (2006). A comparison of weight histories in women with class III vs. class I–II obesity. *Obesity, 14*(3 Suppl.), 63S–69S.

Dawes, A. J., Maggard-Gibbons, M., Maher, A. R., Booth, M. J., Miake-Lye, I., Beroes, J. M., et al. (2016). Mental health conditions among patients seeking and undergoing bariatric surgery: A meta-analysis. *Journal of the American Medical Association, 315*(2), 150–163.

de Zwaan, M., Enderle, J., Wagner, S., Mühlhans, B., Ditzen, B., Gefeller, O., et al. (2011). Anxiety and depression in bariatric surgery patients: A prospective, follow-up study using structured clinical interviews. *Journal of Affective Disorders, 133*(1), 61–68.

Durso, L. E., & Latner, J. D. (2008). Understanding self-directed stigma: Development of the weight bias internalization scale. *Obesity, 16*(2, Suppl.), S80–S86.

Elder, C. R., Gullion, C. M., Funk, K. L., Debar, L. L., Lindberg, N. M., & Stevens, V. J. (2012). Impact of sleep, screen time, depression and stress on weight change in the intensive weight loss phase of the LIFE study. *International Journal of Obesity, 36*(1), 86–92.

Fabricatore, A. N., Crerand, C. E., Wadden, T. A., Sarwer, D. B., & Krasucki, J. L. (2006). How do mental health professionals evaluate candidates for bariatric surgery?: Survey results. *Obesity Surgery, 16*(5), 567–573.

Fabricatore, A. N., Wadden, T. A., Higginbotham, A. J., Faulconbridge, L. F., Nguyen, A. M., Heymsfield, S. B., et al. (2011). Intentional weight loss and changes in symptoms of depression: A systematic review and meta-analysis. *International Journal of Obesity, 35*(11), 1363–1376.

Fabricatore, A. N., Wadden, T. A., Womble, L. G.,

Sarwer, D. B., Berkowitz, R. I., Foster, G. D., et al. (2007). The role of patients' expectations and goals in the behavioral and pharmacological treatment of obesity. *International Journal of Obesity, 31*(11), 1739–1745.

Fairburn, C. G., & Beglin, S. (2008). Eating Disorder Examination Questionnaire. In C. G. Fairburn (Ed.), *Cognitive behavior therapy and eating disorders* (pp. 309–313). New York: Guilford Press.

Farooqi, I. S., & O'Rahilly, S. (2007). Genetic factors in human obesity. *Obesity Reviews, 8*(1), 37–40.

Felitti, V. J. (1993). Childhood sexual abuse, depression, and family dysfunction in adult obese patients: A case control study. *Southern Medical Journal, 86*(7), 732–736.

Folsom, A. R., Jacobs, D. R., Caspersen, C. J., Gomez-Marin, O., & Knudsen, J. (1986). Test–retest reliability of the Minnesota Leisure Time Physical Activity Questionnaire. *Journal of Chronic Diseases, 39*(7), 505–511.

Foster, G. D., Wadden, T. A., Vogt, R. A., & Brewer, G. (1997). What is a reasonable weight loss?: Patients' expectations and evaluations of obesity treatment outcomes. *Journal of Consulting and Clinical Psychology, 65*(1), 79.

Fuglestad, P. T., Jeffery, R. W., & Sherwood, N. E. (2012). Lifestyle patterns associated with diet, physical activity, body mass index and amount of recent weight loss in a sample of successful weight losers. *International Journal of Behavioral Nutrition and Physical Activity, 9*(1), 79–89.

Gallant, A. R., Lundgren, J., & Drapeau, V. (2012). The night-eating syndrome and obesity. *Obesity Reviews, 13*(6), 528–536.

Gibbons, L. M., Sarwer, D. B., Crerand, C. E., Fabricatore, A. N., Kuehnel, R. H., Lipschutz, P. E., et al. (2006). Previous weight loss experiences of bariatric surgery candidates: How much have patients dieted prior to surgery? *Obesity, 14*(3, Suppl.), 70S–76S.

Gloy, V. L., Briel, M., Bhatt, D. L., Kashyap, S. R., Schauer, P. R., Mingrone, G., et al. (2013). Bariatric surgery versus non-surgical treatment for obesity: A systematic review and meta-analysis of randomised controlled trials. *BMJ, 347*(7931), f5934.

Gordon-Larsen, P., Adair, L. S., & Suchindran, C. M. (2007). Maternal obesity is associated with younger age at obesity onset in U.S. adolescent offspring followed into adulthood. *Obesity, 15*(11), 2790–2796.

Gorin, A. A., Niemeier, H. M., Hogan, P., Coday, M., Davis, C., DiLillo, V. G., et al. (2008). Binge eating and weight loss outcomes in overweight and obese individuals with type 2 diabetes: Results from the look AHEAD trial. *Archives of General Psychiatry, 65*(12), 1447–1455.

Hamilton, M. (1959). The assessment of anxiety states by rating. *British Journal of Medical Psychology, 32*(1), 50–55.

Herring, L., Stevinson, C., Davies, M., Biddle, S., Sutton, C., Bowrey, D., & Carter, P. (2016). Changes in physical activity behaviour and physical function after bariatric surgery: A systematic review and meta-analysis. *Obesity Reviews, 17*(3), 250–261.

Hill, J. O., Wyatt, H. R., Reed, G. W., & Peters, J. C. (2003). Obesity and the environment: Where do we go from here? *Science, 299*(5608), 853–855.

Hutchesson, M. J., Rollo, M. E., Callister, R., & Collins, C. E. (2015). Self-monitoring of dietary intake by young women: Online food records completed on computer or smartphone are as accurate as paper-based food records but more acceptable. *Journal of the Academy of Nutrition and Dietetics, 115*(1), 87–94.

Jarry, J. L., & Ip, K. (2005). The effectiveness of stand-alone cognitive-behavioural therapy for body image: A meta-analysis. *Body Image, 2*(4), 317–331.

Jensen, M. D., Ryan, D. H., Apovian, C. M., Ard, J. D., Comuzzie, A. G., Donato, K. A., et al. (2014). 2013 AHA/ACC/TOS guideline for the management of overweight and obesity in adults: A report of the American College of Cardiology/American Heart Association Task Force on Practice Guidelines and The Obesity Society. *Journal of the American College of Cardiology, 63*(25, Pt. B), 2985.

Kase, C., Piers, A., Schaumberg, K., Forman, E., & Butryn, M. (2016). The relationship of alcohol use to weight loss in the context of behavioral weight loss treatment. *Appetite, 99*, 105–111.

King, T. K., Clark, M. M., & Pera, V. (1996). History of sexual abuse and obesity treatment outcome. *Addictive Behaviors, 21*(3), 283–290.

King, W. C., Chen, J., Mitchell, J. E., Kalarchian, M. A., Steffen, K. J., Engel, S. G., et al. (2012). Prevalence of alcohol use disorders before and after bariatric surgery. *Journal of the American Medical Association, 307*(23), 2516–2525.

Kolotkin, R. L., & Crosby, R. D. (2002). Psychometric evaluation of the Impact of Weight on Quality of Life–Lite questionnaire (IWQOL-lite) in a community sample. *Quality of Life Research, 11*(2), 157–171.

Kolotkin, R. L., Head, S., Hamilton, M., & Tse, C. K. (1995). Assessing impact of weight on quality of life. *Obesity Research, 3*(1), 49–56.

Kroenke, K., Spitzer, R. L., & Williams, J. B. W. (2001). The PHQ-9: Validity of a brief depression severity measure. *Journal of General Internal Medicine, 16*(9), 606–613.

LaRose, J. G., Leahey, T. M., Hill, J. O., & Wing, R. R. (2013). Differences in motivations and weight loss behaviors in young adults and older adults in the National Weight Control Registry. *Obesity (Silver Spring), 21*(3), 449–453.

Laurenius, A., Larsson, I., Bueter, M., Melanson, K. J., Bosaeus, I., Forslund, H. B., et al. (2012). Changes in eating behaviour and meal pattern following roux-en-Y gastric bypass. *International Journal of Obesity, 36*(3), 348–355.

Leahey, T. M., Larose, J. G., Fava, J. L., & Wing, R. R. (2011). Social influences are associated with BMI and weight loss intentions in young adults. *Obesity, 19*(6), 1157–1162.

Lent, M. R., Vander Veur, S. S., Peters, J. C., Herring, S. J., Wyatt, H. R., Tewksbury, C., et al. (2016). Initial weight loss goals—have they changed and do they matter?: Weight loss goals and outcomes. *Obesity Science and Practice, 2*(2), 154–161.

Levitsky, D. A., & Pacanowski, C. R. (2013). Effect of skipping breakfast on subsequent energy intake. *Physiology and Behavior, 119,* 9–16.

Lichtman, S. W., Pisarska, K., Berman, E. R., Pestone, M., Dowling, H., Offenbacher, E., et al. (1992). Discrepancy between self-reported and actual caloric intake and exercise in obese subjects. *New England Journal of Medicine, 327*(27), 1893–1898.

Livhits, M., Mercado, C., Yermilov, I., Parikh, J. A., Dutson, E., Mehran, A., et al. (2012). Preoperative predictors of weight loss following bariatric surgery: Systematic review. *Obesity Surgery, 22*(1), 70–89.

Lowe, M. R., Butryn, M. L., Didie, E. R., Annunziato, R. A., Thomas, J. G., Crerand, C. E., et al. (2009). The Power of Food Scale: A new measure of the psychological influence of the food environment. *Appetite, 53*(1), 114–118.

MacLean, P. S., Bergouignan, A., Cornier, M., & Jackman, M. R. (2011). Biology's response to dieting: The impetus for weight regain. *American Journal of Physiology: Regulatory Integrative, and Comparative Physiology, 301*(3), R581–R600.

Malik, V. S., Schulze, M. B., & Hu, F. B. (2006). Intake of sugar-sweetened beverages and weight gain: A systematic review. *American Journal of Clinical Nutrition, 84*(2), 274–288.

Mason, S., MacLehose, R., Katz-Wise, S., Austin, S., Neumark-Sztainer, D., Harlow, B., et al. (2015). Childhood abuse victimization, stress-related eating, and weight status in young women. *Annals of Epidemiology, 25*(10), 760–766.

Mechanick, J. I., Youdim, A., Jones, D. B., Garvey, W. T., Hurley, D. L., McMahon, M. M., et al. (2013). Clinical practice guidelines for the perioperative nutritional, metabolic, and nonsurgical support of the bariatric surgery patient—2013 update: Cosponsored by American Association of Clinical Endocrinologists, the Obesity Society, and American Society for Metabolic and Bariatric Surgery. *Obesity, 21*(1, Suppl.), S1–S27.

Mesas, A. E., Muñoz-Pareja, M., López-García, E., & Rodríguez-Artalejo, F. (2012). Selected eating behaviours and excess body weight: A systematic review. *Obesity Reviews, 13*(2), 106–135.

Mordes, J., Liu, C., & Xu, S. (2015). Medications for weight loss. *Current Opinion in Endocrinology Diabetes and Obesity, 22*(2), 91–97.

NIH Conference. (1991). Gastrointestinal surgery for severe obesity: Consensus development conference panel. *Annals of Internal Medicine, 115,* 956–961.

Pachucki, M. C., Lovenheim, M. F., & Harding, M. (2014). Within-family obesity associations: Evaluation of parent, child, and sibling relationships. *American Journal of Preventive Medicine, 47*(4), 382–391.

Paffenbarger, R. S., Wing, A. L., & Hyde, R. T. (1995). Physical activity as an index of heart attack risk in college alumni. *American Journal of Epidemiology, 142*(9), 889–903.

Pagoto, S., Schneider, K., Whited, M., Oleski, J., Merriam, P., Appelhans, B., et al. (2013). Randomized controlled trial of behavioral treatment for comorbid obesity and depression in women: The be active trial. *International Journal of Obesity, 37*(11), 1427–1434.

Paradis, A., Pérusse, L., Godin, G., & Vohl, M. (2008). Validity of a self-reported measure of familial history of obesity. *Nutrition Journal, 7*(1), 27.

Post, R. E., Mainous, A. G., Gregorie, S. H., Knoll, M. E., Diaz, V. A., & Saxena, S. K. (2011). The influence of physician acknowledgment of patients' weight status on patient perceptions of overweight and obesity in the United States. *Archives of Internal Medicine, 171*(4), 316–321.

Pournaras, D., & Le Roux, C. (2009). The effect of bariatric surgery on gut hormones that alter appetite. *Diabetes and Metabolism, 35*(6, Pt. 2), 508–512.

Puhl, R. M., Heuer, C., & Sarda, V. (2011). Framing messages about weight discrimination: Impact on public support for legislation. *International Journal of Obesity, 35*(6), 863–872.

Rogers, P. J. (1999). Eating habits and appetite control: A psychobiological perspective. *Proceedings of the Nutrition Society, 58*(1), 59–67.

Rooney, B. L., Mathiason, M. A., & Schauberger, C. W. (2011). Predictors of obesity in childhood, adolescence, and adulthood in a birth cohort. *Maternal and Child Health Journal, 15*(8), 1166–1175.

Rosenheck, R. (2008). Fast food consumption and increased caloric intake: A systematic review of a trajectory towards weight gain and obesity risk. *Obesity Reviews, 9*(6), 535–547.

Sarwer, D. B., Wadden, T. A., Moore, R. H., Baker, A. W., Gibbons, L. M., Raper, S. E., et al. (2008). Preoperative eating behavior, postoperative dietary adherence, and weight loss after gastric bypass surgery. *Surgery for Obesity and Related Diseases, 4*(5), 640–646.

Shephard, R. J. (2003). Limits to the measurement of habitual physical activity by questionnaires. *British Journal of Sports Medicine, 37*(3), 197–206.

Sherwood, N., Jeffery, R., & Wing, R. (1999). Binge status as a predictor of weight loss treatment outcome. *International Journal of Obesity, 23*(5), 485–493.

Shiroma, E., Sesso, H., Moorthy, M., Buring, J., & Lee, I. (2014). Do moderate-intensity and vigorous-intensity physical activities reduce mortality rates to the same extent? *Journal of the American Heart Association, 3*(5), e000802.

Sogg, S., Lauretti, J., & West-Smith, L. (2016). Recommendations for the presurgical psychosocial evaluation of bariatric surgery patients. *Surgery for Obesity and Related Diseases, 12*(4), 731–749.

Spalding, K. L., Arner, E., Westermark, P. O., Bernard, S., Buchholz, B. A., Bergmann, O., et al. (2008). Dynamics of fat cell turnover in humans. *Nature, 453*(7196), 783–787.

Spitzer, R. L., Kroenke, K., Williams, J. B. W., & Löwe, B. (2006). A brief measure for assessing generalized anxiety disorder: The GAD-7. *Archives of Internal Medicine, 166*(10), 1092–1097.

Steffen, K., Engel, S., Wonderlich, J., Pollert, G., & Sondag, C. (2015). Alcohol and other addictive disorders following bariatric surgery: Prevalence, risk factors and possible etiologies. *European Eating Disorders Review, 23*(6), 442–450.

Steinig, J., Wagner, B., Shang, E., Dölemeyer, R., & Kersting, A. (2012). Sexual abuse in bariatric surgery candidates—impact on weight loss after surgery: A systematic review. *Obesity Reviews, 13*(10), 892–901.

Stumbo, P. J. (2013). New technology in dietary assessment: A review of digital methods in improving food record accuracy. *Proceedings of the Nutrition Society, 72*(1), 70–76.

Stunkard, A. J. (1993). Talking with patients. In A. J. Stunkard & T. A. Wadden (Eds.), *Obesity: Theory and therapy* (2nd ed., pp. 355–363). New York: Raven Press.

Stunkard, A. J., & Messick, S. (1988). *Eating Inventory manual.* New York: Psychological Corp.

Svensson, P., Anveden, Å., Romeo, S., Peltonen, M., Ahlin, S., Burza, M. A., et al. (2013). Alcohol consumption and alcohol problems after bariatric surgery in the Swedish obese subjects study. *Obesity, 21*(12), 2444–2451.

Swift, D. L., Johannsen, N. M., Lavie, C. J., Earnest, C. P., & Church, T. S. (2014). The role of exercise and physical activity in weight loss and maintenance. *Progress in Cardiovascular Diseases, 56*(4), 441–447.

Swinburn, B. A., Sacks, G., Hall, K. D., McPherson, K., Finegood, D. T., Moodie, M. L., et al. (2011). Obesity 1: The global obesity pandemic—shaped by global drivers and local environments. *Lancet, 378*(9793), 804.

Thomas, J. G., Bond, D. S., Phelan, S., Hill, J. O., & Wing, R. R. (2014). Weight-loss maintenance for 10 years in the National Weight Control Registry. *American Journal of Preventive Medicine, 46*(1), 17–23.

Thorp, A. A., Healy, G. N., Owen, N., Salmon, J. O., Ball, K., Shaw, J. E., et al. (2010). Deleterious associations of sitting time and television viewing time with cardiometabolic risk biomarkers: Australian diabetes, obesity and lifestyle (AusDiab) study 2004–2005. *Diabetes Care, 33*(2), 327–334.

Tian, J., Venn, A., Otahal, P., & Gall, S. (2015). The association between quitting smoking and weight gain: A systemic review and meta-analysis of prospective cohort studies. *Obesity Reviews, 16*(10), 883–901.

Traversy, G., & Chaput, J. (2015). Alcohol consumption and obesity: An update. *Current Obesity Reports, 4*(1), 122.

Trief, P. M., Cibula, D., Delahanty, L. M., & Weinstock, R. S. (2014). Depression, stress, and weight loss in individuals with metabolic syndrome in SHINE: A DPP translation study. *Obesity, 22*(12), 2532–2538.

Tsai, A. G., Fabricatore, A. N., Wadden, T. A., Higginbotham, A. J., Anderson, A., Foreyt, J., et al. (2014). Readiness redefined: A behavioral task during screening predicted 1-year weight loss in the Look AHEAD study. *Obesity, 22*(4), 1016–1023.

Unick, J. L., Neiberg, R. H., Hogan, P. E., Cheskin, L. J., Dutton, G. R., Jeffery, R., et al. (2015). Weight change in the first 2 months of a lifestyle intervention predicts weight changes 8 years later. *Obesity, 23*(7), 1353–1356.

U.S. Department of Agriculture. (2017). Choose MyPlate. Retrieved from *www.choosemyplate.gov.*

U.S. Department of Health and Human Services & U.S. Department of Agriculture. (2015, December). 2015–2020 dietary guidelines for Americans (8th ed.). Available at *https://health.gov/dietaryguidelines/2015/guidelines.*

Wadden, T. A., Anderson, D. A., Foster, G. D., Bennett, A., Steinberg, C., & Sarwer, D. B. (2000). Obese women's perceptions of their physicians' weight management attitudes and practices. *Archives of Family Medicine, 9*(9), 854–860.

Wadden, T. A., Butryn, M. L., Sarwer, D. B., Fabricatore, A. N., Crerand, C. E., Lipschutz, P. E., et al. (2006). Comparison of psychosocial status in treatment-seeking women with class III vs. class I–II obesity. *Obesity, 14*(3, Suppl.), 90S–98S.

Wadden, T. A., & Foster, G. D. (2006). Weight and Lifestyle Inventory (WALI). *Obesity, 14*(3, Suppl.), 99S–118S.

Wadden, T. A., & Letizia, K. A. (1992). Predictors of attrition and weight loss in patients treated by moderate and severe caloric restriction. In T. A. Wadden & T. B. VanItallie (Eds.), *Treatment of the seriously obese patient* (pp. 383–410). New York: Guilford Press.

Wadden, T. A., & Sarwer, D. B. (2006). Behavioral assessment of candidates for bariatric surgery: A patient-oriented approach. *Obesity, 14*(3, Suppl.), 53S–62S.

Wahid, A., Manek, N., Nichols, M., Kelly, P., Foster, C., Webster, P., et al. (2016). Quantifying the association between physical activity and cardiovascular disease and diabetes: A systematic review and meta-analysis. *Journal of the American Heart Association, 5*(9), e002495.

Walley, A. J., Blakemore, A. I. F., & Froguel, P. (2006). Genetics of obesity and the prediction of risk for health. *Human Molecular Genetics, 15*(2), R124–R130.

Wansink, B. (2004). Environmental factors that increase the food intake and consumption volume of unknowing consumers. *Annual Review of Nutrition, 24*(1), 455–479.

Wansink, B. (2007). Portion size me: Downsizing our consumption norms. *Journal of the American Dietetic Association, 107*(7), 1103–1106.

Ware, J. E., Jr., & Sherbourne, C. D. (1992). The MOS 36-item short-form health survey (SF-36): I. Conceptual framework and item selection. *Medical Care, 30*(6), 473–483.

Warkentin, L. M., Majumdar, S. R., Johnson, J. A., Agborsangaya, C. B., Rueda-Clausen, C. F., Sharma, A. M., et al. (2014). Predictors of health-related quality of life in 500 severely obese patients: Health-related quality of life in severely obese. *Obesity, 22*(5), 1367–1372.

Wee, C., Mukamal, K., Huskey, K., Davis, R., Colten, M., Bolcic-Jankovic, D., et al. (2014). High-risk alcohol use after weight loss surgery. *Surgery for Obesity and Related Diseases, 10*(3), 508–513.

Whitaker, R. C., Wright, J. A., Pepe, M. S., Seidel, K. D., & Dietz, W. H. (1997). Predicting obesity in young adulthood from childhood and parental obesity. *New England Journal of Medicine, 337*(13), 869–873.

White, M. A., Whisenhunt, B. L., Williamson, D. A., Greenway, F. L., & Netemeyer, R. G. (2002). Development and validation of the Food-Craving Inventory. *Obesity Research, 10*(2), 107–114.

Wing, R. R., Lang, W., Wadden, T. A., Safford, M., Knowler, W. C., Bertoni, A. G., et al. (2011). Benefits of modest weight loss in improving cardiovascular risk factors in overweight and obese individuals with type 2 diabetes. *Diabetes Care, 34*(7), 1481–1486.

Yanovski, S. Z., Marcus, M. D., Wadden, T. A., & Walsh, B. T. (2015). The Questionnaire on Eating and Weight Patterns–5: An updated screening instrument for binge eating disorder. *International Journal of Eating Disorders, 48*(3), 259–261.

APPENDIX 16.1. Sample Letters Summarizing Presurgical Behavioral Assessment Findings and Recommendations

Mr. John Doe

May 1, 2017

James Smith, M.D.
Metabolic & Bariatric Surgery Program

RE: Mr. John Doe
DOB: 11/01/1966

Dear Dr. Smith:

I had the pleasure of meeting today with Mr. John Doe, whom you referred for a behavioral assessment of his appropriateness for bariatric surgery. Mr. Doe is a 50-year-old white male, with a height of 6'1" and weight of 339.4 lb., yielding a BMI of 44.8 kg/m^2. Mr. Doe is married and has three children, ages 11–19 years. He lives with his family and works as a security guard.

Biological Factors

Mr. Doe reported being overweight since age 15 years. He stated that his weight has increased gradually over time and that he is currently at his highest weight. Mr. Doe reported that his father, paternal grandparents, and sister are obese. He described his mother as overweight and his maternal grandmother and brother as normal weight.

Mr. Doe's adolescent onset and family history of obesity provide strong evidence for a biological predisposition to obesity.

Environmental Factors

Mr. Doe reported that problems with overeating at dinnertime, frequent snacking, and not feeling full after eating have contributed to his weight gain. He also reported frequently eating high-fat foods (e.g., fast food, cheesesteaks, pizza), which likely contributed. He reported no history of night eating, binge eating, or inappropriate compensatory behaviors.

Mr. Doe eats two to three meals per day with two to three snacks. He eats out approximately once per week. He is attending Medical Weight Management visits and has started to change his eating habits, including chewing his food thoroughly, separating his meals from drinks, and slowing his rate of eating. He has also increased his consumption of lean meats, fruits, and vegetables. He walks on 3–4 days per week for 20–40 minutes per bout. Of note, he has lost 8 lb. since beginning the bariatric surgery program.

Mr. Doe has engaged in previous behavioral weight loss attempts starting at age 35 years. These approaches have consisted of self-directed dieting (e.g., making healthier choices, reducing snacking), commercial programs (e.g., Weight Watchers), and increased exercise. He has also tried over-the-counter weight loss supplements. He lost up to 25 lb. with these attempts but was unable to maintain these losses.

In summary, Mr. Doe's history of frequently eating high-fat foods, overeating at dinnertime, frequent snacking, and not feeling full after eating have likely contributed to his weight gain. He has made adequate progress with behavior changes in preparation for the surgery.

Social/Psychological Factors

Mr. Doe reported no history of depression or anxiety. His Beck Depression Inventory–II score of 6 suggested minimal symptoms of depressed mood. He did not report any suicidal ideation. He reported no history of psychological treatment.

Mr. Doe reported no history of drug use or cigarette smoking. He rarely drinks alcohol (three or four times per year). During the interview, he was oriented to time, place, and person. He appears to be an appropriate candidate from a psychosocial perspective.

Timing

Mr. Doe has been considering bariatric surgery for the past 2 years. He reported that his family is supportive of his receiving bariatric surgery and that his wife is also preparing to have the surgery. He reported an average level of stress over the past 6 months. He indicated that he will be able to take time off from work to focus on his recovery following the surgery. Mr. Doe had an adequate understanding of the postoperative diet and is looking forward to surgery to improve his health, to reduce medication usage, to be more active with his children, and to extend life. Overall, the timing seems appropriate.

Summary

Mr. Doe appears to be an appropriate candidate for bariatric surgery from a behavioral perspective. I recommended that he continue to make healthier choices, eat his meals consistently throughout the day, chew his foods thoroughly, slow the pace of his eating, and separate his meals from drinks. I provided Mr. Doe with online resources to assist with nutrition education and to supplement his surgery support network.

These recommendations were discussed with him and presented in writing. Mr. Doe appeared to be in agreement with them. Please call me if you have any questions regarding the patient.

Diagnosis:
E66.01 Extreme obesity

Ms. Jane Doe

May 1, 2017

James Smith, M.D.
Metabolic & Bariatric Surgery Program

RE: Ms. Jane Doe
DOB: 02/01/1975

Dear Dr. Smith:

I had the pleasure of meeting today with Ms. Jane Doe, whom you referred for a behavioral assessment of her appropriateness for bariatric surgery. Ms. Doe is a 42-year-old, African American woman, with a height of 5'1" and weight of 238.0 lb., yielding a BMI of 45.0 kg/m^2. Ms. Doe is separated and has three children, aged 8, 14, and 17 years. She is not currently working and is seeking disability secondary to injuries sustained in a 2015 accident.

Biological Factors

Ms. Doe reported being overweight since age 25 years. She stated that her weight increased gradually over time, with larger gains following her third pregnancy. She indicated that she was recently at her highest weight of 247 lb. Ms. Doe reported that her father, paternal grandparents, maternal grandfather, and three siblings are obese. She indicated that one sister has had bariatric surgery. She described her mother, maternal grandmother, and two other siblings as normal weight.

Ms. Doe's family history provides strong evidence for a biological predisposition to obesity.

Environmental Factors

Ms. Doe reported that problems with frequent overeating, eating in response to cravings, and emotional eating have contributed to her weight gain. She reported no history of binge eating, inappropriate compensatory behaviors, or night eating.

Ms. Doe consumes two to three meals per day with one snack. She eats out approximately three times per week. She is attending Medical Weight Management and has started to chew her food thoroughly, separate her meals from drinks, and slow her rate of eating. Her physical activity is limited due to shoulder, neck, and back pain resulting from a 2015 injury. She currently engages in lifestyle activity.

Ms. Doe has engaged in previous behavioral weight loss attempts starting at age 35 years. These approaches have consisted of self-directed diets (e.g., reducing portion sizes) and exercise. She has also tried Weight Watchers, Jenny Craig, and weight loss supplements (e.g., Herbalife). She lost up to 25 lb. with these attempts but was unable to maintain these losses.

In summary, Ms. Doe's history of frequent overeating, eating in response to cravings, emotional eating, and limited physical activity have likely contributed to her weight gain. She has made adequate progress with behavior changes in preparation for the surgery.

Social/Psychological Factors

Ms. Doe reported financial stress over the past year as a result of being unable to work due to injuries sustained in a car accident. Currently, she is having difficulty paying her rent and buying food for herself and her children. She also reported stress related to problems with one of her children. As a result of these stressors, Ms. Doe is experiencing difficulty sleeping, worry, and depressed mood. Her Beck Depression Inventory–II score of 29 suggested moderate-to-severe symptoms of depressed mood. She did not report suicidal ideation or behavior. She reported that she and one of her children were seeing a therapist at the Mental Health Center; however, they stopped attending treatment 3 months ago due to the therapist's inattentive behavior.

Ms. Doe reported no history of drug abuse. She quit smoking cigarettes 15 years ago. She rarely drinks alcohol (two to three times per year).

Ms. Doe is experiencing stressors and symptoms of major depression. Her depression is not adequately treated at this time and could interfere with her adherence to postoperative recommendations. I recommended that she seek a psychiatric consultation, and I provided several referral options.

Timing

Ms. Doe reported that her children are supportive of her receiving bariatric surgery. She reported an above-average level of stress over the past 6 months, which she attributed to the stressors described above. She is not currently working, so she will be able to focus on her recovery following the surgery. Ms. Doe had an adequate understanding of the postoperative diet and is looking forward to surgery to improve her health, energy, and appearance. However, due to her current major depressive episode, I believe Ms. Doe should seek psychiatric care (or other mental health counseling) before undergoing bariatric surgery.

Summary

In many ways, Ms. Doe appears to be an appropriate candidate for bariatric surgery from a behavioral perspective. However, she currently appears to be experiencing a major depressive episode, as well as financial and family stressors that may affect her ability to adhere to the postoperative meal plan. I recommended that she seek psychiatric consultation and provided her with several options. I will follow up with Ms. Doe by phone in 2 weeks to discuss her progress with obtaining such care. I will also reevaluate Ms. Doe's mood and adjustment in a minimum of 3 months, following her final Medical Weight Management appointment.

In the meanwhile, I recommended that Ms. Doe continue to eat her meals consistently throughout the day, make healthier choices, chew her food thoroughly, slow the pace of her eating, and separate her meals from drinks. I provided Ms. Doe with online resources to assist with nutrition education and to supplement her surgery support network.

These recommendations were discussed with her and presented in writing. Ms. Doe appeared to be in agreement with them. Please call me if you have any questions regarding the patient.

Diagnoses:
F32.1 Major depressive episode
E66.01 Extreme obesity

PART V
Treatment of Obesity in Adults

CHAPTER 17

An Overview of the Treatment of Obesity in Adults

Thomas A. Wadden
Zayna M. Bakizada
Steven Z. Wadden
Naji Alamuddin

The first edition of this handbook appeared in 2002, 4 years after the publication of the Clinical Guidelines on the Identification, Evaluation, and Treatment of Overweight and Obesity in Adults: The Evidence Report (National Heart, Lung, and Blood Institute [NHLBI], 1998). This was a far-reaching report that provided practitioners with a broad summary of what was known about the etiology, consequences, assessment, and treatment of overweight and obesity. The treatment recommendations were based upon a thorough consideration of both the scientific literature and expert clinical opinion.

The second edition of this handbook appears 4 years after publication of the revised NHLBI guidelines, which were issued by a joint committee of the American Heart Association/American College of Cardiology/The Obesity Society (AHA/ACA/TOS; Jensen et al., 2014). In 2008, NHLBI leadership initiated the revision of the original guidelines and actively supported the review through 2012. However, the NHLBI ultimately opted for the update to be published and disseminated by the three professional societies identified. Titled "Guidelines for the Evaluation and Treatment of Overweight and Obesity in Adults," the revised document provided a systematic review of five critical questions and employed very stringent analytical methods. The resulting guidelines, as compared with those from 1998, yielded greater clarity and certainty about the five main areas reviewed—but, by design, omitted numerous topics, including pharmacotherapy and emerging weight loss devices for obesity.

This chapter provides an overview of options for the treatment of overweight and obesity, drawing upon the collective recommendations of the 1998 and 2014 NHLBI-related guidelines, as well as those from the Endocrine Society (Apovian et al., 2015), the National Institute for Health and Care Excellence (NICE; 2014), and the American Association of Clinical Endocrinologists/American College of Endocrinology (Garvey et al., 2016). Additional guidance is considered from the Canadian Clinical Practice Guidelines (Lau & Obesity Canada Clinical Practice Guidelines, 2007) and expert panels from the Department of Veterans Affairs/Department of Defense (VA/DoD, 2014) and professional societies, the latter charged with making recommendations for bariatric surgery (Mechanick et al., 2013; Rubino et al., 2016). Given the global scope of the obesity epidemic, numerous other countries and societies have issued weight management guidelines, including the World Health Organization (WHO, 1998). Despite the varied expert panels and resulting documents, there is remarkable agreement among the many guidelines in their recommendations for treating overweight and obesity.

Selecting Treatment

The decision to initiate weight loss should be based on an assessment of the individual's medical need to reduce, as described by Kumar and Aronne (Chapter 15, this volume), as well as the patient's desire for and behavioral appropriateness for weight reduction, as reviewed by Shaw Tronieri and Wadden (Chapter 16, this volume). These factors, together with the body mass index (BMI), provide initial guidance on which interventions are likely to be most appropriate for a given individual.

Treatment Algorithms

Kumar and Aronne (Chapter 15, this volume) have reviewed the obesity treatment algorithm developed by the AHA/ACC/TOS expert panel (Jensen et al., 2014). It is similar to one produced for the Canadian obesity guidelines, which calls for the calculation of the patient's BMI, measurement of waist circumference, and screening for cardiovascular disease (CVD) risk factors, including hypertension, hyperlipidemia, and type 2 diabetes (see Figure 17.1). Other obesity-related comorbidities, such as sleep apnea and degenerative joint disease, should also be assessed. Individuals with a BMI of 25–29.9 kg/m^2 and one or more CVD risk factors, who wish to lose weight, are encouraged to participate in an intensive lifestyle intervention, described in a later section of this chapter (Jensen et al., 2014). The goal is to lose 5–10% of initial weight, which is associated with improvements in CVD risk factors and quality of life (Jensen et al., 2014). Alternatively, prevention of further weight regain is recommended for persons who are not currently motivated to lose weight, as it is for individuals in the same BMI range but who are free of obesity-related comorbidities. The latter individuals have been referred to as "healthy, overweight/obese," for whom weight reduction is not required to improve health (Kramer, Zinman, & Retnakaran, 2013; Sharma & Kushner, 2009). Recent studies have shown that periodic encouragement from a primary care provider (e.g., quarterly visits) may be sufficient to prevent weight gain or induce modest weight loss (Wadden, Volger, et al., 2011).

As BMI increases, so generally do the health complications of obesity, the potential benefits of weight reduction, and the intensity of treatments available to patients. In the United States and Canada, persons with a BMI ≥ 30 kg/m^2 (or ≥ 27 kg/m^2 in the presence of a comorbid condition) are eligible to use weight loss medication as an adjunct to a reduced calorie diet and increased physical activity (see Bray & Ryan, Chapter 21, this volume). Bariatric surgery is an option for patients with a BMI ≥ 40 kg/m^2 who are unable to reduce successfully with lifestyle modification and/or pharmacotherapy, as it is for those with a BMI ≥ 35 kg/m^2 who have a significant weight-related comorbidity (see Hanipah, Aminian, & Schauer, Chapter 22, this volume).

Current treatment algorithms likely will expand in the next few years to incorporate a new generation of endoscopically placed devices, recently approved by the U.S. Food and Drug Administration (FDA), as well as new surgical procedures (e.g., transoral bypass). For example, endoscopically placed gastric balloons, which limit the amount of food that can be eaten, have been approved by the FDA for patients with a BMI of 30–40 kg/m^2, who are unable to reduce satisfactorily with intensive lifestyle intervention alone. These new approaches are reviewed in this volume by Soegaard Ballester, Halpern, Williams, and Dumon (Chapter 33).

Improving Health Outcomes

If improving CVD risk factors and other health conditions is the overriding goal of obesity treatment, then we believe that behavioral and pharmacological weight loss

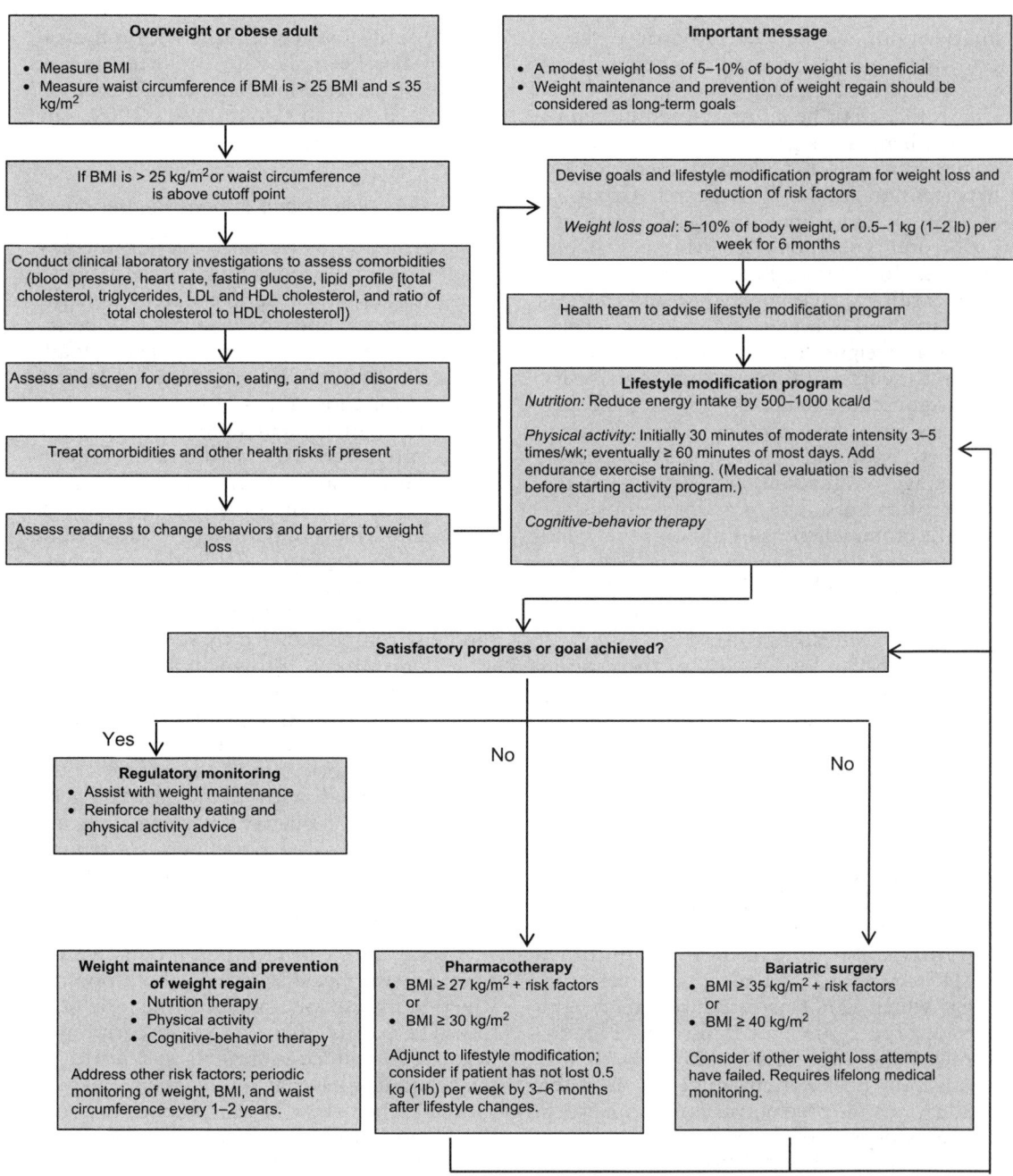

FIGURE 17.1. Algorithm for the assessment and stepwise management of the overweight or obese adult. LDL, low-density lipoprotein; HDL, high-density lipoprotein. BMI and waist circumference cut-off points are different for some ethnic groups. From Lau et al. (2007). Reprinted from the *Canadian Medical Association Journal* (ISSN: 0820-3946) 2007.

interventions, as well as bariatric surgery, generally should be used to complement well-established medical therapies for CVD risk, rather than being prescribed in lieu of them. There is far greater evidence, for example, that pharmacological therapies for hypertension (SPRINT Research Group et al., 2015), hyperlipidemia (Collins et al., 2016), and type 2 diabetes (Marso, Daniels, et al., 2016; Marso, Bain, et al., 2016) reduce cardiovascular morbidity and mortality than there is for behavioral or pharmacological weight loss interventions. Thus, when patients with overweight or obesity have significant CVD risk factors, prudence suggests providing pharmacological therapies first, as would be prescribed for person of average weight who presented with the same risk factors. This practice is consistent with recommendations of most of the existing guidelines (e.g., Jensen et al., 2014; Lau & Obesity Canada Clinical Practice Guidelines, 2007; National Institute for Health and Care Excellence, 2014).

If patients can lose 5–10% of their initial weight, practitioners may be able to reduce the amount of medication required, as observed in the Look AHEAD (Action for Health in Diabetes) Study (Look AHEAD Research Group, 2013). Similarly, losses of 20% or more of initial weight, achieved with bariatric surgery, frequently are associated with the remission of type 2 diabetes and the discontinuation of all diabetes medications (Schauer et al., 2012). Such patients, however, may still require medications for other CVD risk factors, such as hypercholesterolemia, which is not as responsive to weight loss as type 2 diabetes (Sjöström, Lissner, Wedel, & Sjöström, 1999). Similarly, weight loss usually does not eliminate the need for medications for psychiatric conditions, such as major depression or generalized anxiety disorder (Berkowitz & Fabricatore, 2011).

Weight reduction may be a more appropriate first intervention, prior to initiation of medical therapy, for individuals with overweight/obesity who have impaired glucose tolerance (i.e., pre-diabetes) or components of the metabolic syndrome. These individuals generally have a lower risk of CVD morbidity and mortality (compared with those with established cardiometabolic diseases), and weight loss combined with physical activity has been shown to reduce the risk of disease progression (Diabetes Prevention Program Research Group et al., 2002; Orchard et al., 2005).

Discussing Weight and Weight Reduction

Any discussion of weight reduction therapy should begin by considering the patient's thoughts about his or her weight and the potential desirability of weight loss. Obesity is a sensitive topic for many patients (Wadden & Didie, 2003; Volger et al., 2012), particularly for those not seeking treatment in a weight management clinic. This disease still is often portrayed as the result of simply overeating and underexercising, despite decades of research revealing the complex neuroendocrine regulation of body weight (Guyenet & Schwartz, 2012), the predisposing effects of genetics (van der Klaauw & Farooqi, 2015), and the ill effects of a toxic food environment fueled by economic interests (Pomeranz & Brownell, 2012). Negative social interactions leave many patients with obesity feeling stigmatized, including by health care practitioners (Foster et al., 2003). The emotionally laden nature of the topic, combined with many practitioners' perceptions that obesity treatments are not effective, probably contributes to reports that half of primary care practitioners do not discuss excess weight with their patients (Foster et al., 2003).

Several steps can facilitate productive patient–practitioner discussions about obesity. The first may involve avoiding the term *obesity*. The words *obesity* and *fat* carry such negative social connotations, as heard in jokes and insults, that some patients feel demeaned when their health practitioners use these descriptors. Patients prefer the use of the words *weight, weight problem,* or *problem BMI* in lieu of *obesity* (Volger et al., 2012; Wadden & Didie, 2003). Practitioners also may wish to broach the topic of obesity by asking, "Could we talk about your weight today?," followed by open-ended questions such as "How is your weight for you?" or "How does your weight affect your health or daily functioning?" The conversation should provide patients with an opportunity to discuss their likely concerns and frustrations with their weight (Wadden & Didie, 2003).

Practitioners should be prepared to accept that some patients do not wish to lose weight. This decision can be explored, using a motivational interviewing approach, but it should be respected (see Butryn, Schumacher, & Forman, Chapter 31, this volume). Treatment goals for such individuals can shift to ensuring optimal medical management of CVD risk factors, preventing further weight gain, and engaging in regular physical activity. With patients who wish to lose weight, a frequent challenge is offering new options and hope for weight management. This sometimes can be achieved by explaining that the loss of only 5–10% of initial weight can significantly improve health, without the need to achieve a statistically average body weight (Jensen et al., 2014). This conversation should include a review of the patient's previous weight loss efforts to determine which approaches the individual liked or did not like, and which interventions produced clinically meaningful weight loss (see Shaw Tronieri & Wadden, Chapter 16, this volume). Previously successful approaches are a good start with some individuals, whereas others may want a new approach. In either case, practitioners should applaud patients' previous weight losses efforts, noting that they contributed to improved health and well-being for the time they were undertaken, even if patients eventually regained the lost weight. A growing body of evidence suggests that prior weight loss, even with weight regain, may a have a beneficial legacy effect on some health complications, including type 2 diabetes (Wing et al., 2016). The safety and efficacy of treatment options should be discussed at length, as should the costs of treatment, particularly if out-of-pocket expenses are anticipated.

Developing a Treatment Plan

After reviewing treatment options, the patient and practitioner together should develop a plan that specifies the initial length of the intervention, the frequency and duration of visits, the mode of treatment delivery (e.g., individual vs. group care, in-person vs. remotely delivered sessions), the diet and physical activity regimens to be followed, and any additional considerations (e.g., pharmacotherapy, surgery). Patients benefit from having a written description of the treatment plan for at least the first few months, as well as clear expectations for weight loss, as described by Shaw Tronieri and Wadden (Chapter 16, this volume). The loss of approximately 5–10% of initial weight is a realistic expectation with an intensive lifestyle intervention, with potentially greater weight loss anticipated with the addition of portion-controlled diets or weight loss medications, as discussed later. Patients usually indicate that they wish to lose larger amounts, averaging approximately 20% of initial weight (Lent et al., 2016). They should not be discouraged from such goals, given that large weight loss goals do not adversely affect short- or long-term weight loss (Lent et al., 2016). However, bariatric surgery is currently the only intervention that reliably induces and maintains losses of 20% or more of initial weight.

Personalized Treatment

As discussed by Shaw Tronieri and Wadden (Chapter 16, this volume) and Astrup (Chapter 18, this volume), whenever possible, practitioners should select treatment components that are consistent with patients' preferences, such as in the selection of a reducing diet (e.g., low-fat vs, low-carbohydrate diet) or a program of physical activity. Similarly, treatments should be considered that address patients' complaints about their "always feeling hungry" or "never feeling full after eating" (i.e., impaired satiation). Garvey et al. (2016), for example, have discussed medications for chronic weight management that may help to control appetite or food cravings. The science and practice of personalized obesity treatment admittedly is in the early stages of development. However, practitioners should be mindful of the marked behavioral and biological heterogeneity among the patients whom they treat. Further research on the identification of behavioral phenotypes—and on the biology that underlies them—should ultimately facilitate more personalized treatment of patients with obesity.

Treatment Options: BMI < 30 kg/m² — A Comprehensive, High-Intensity Lifestyle Intervention

The AHA/ACC/TOS guidelines (Jensen et al., 2014) provide more detail and instruction concerning comprehensive lifestyle intervention than do other recently issued guidelines and are emphasized here. The AHA/ACC/TOS expert panel recommended that individuals who are overweight (BMI = 25.0–29.9 kg/m²) and would benefit from weight loss participate for ≥ 6 months in a comprehensive lifestyle program that would assist them in adhering to a lower-calorie diet and in increasing physical activity through the use of behavioral strategies. Face-to-face, high-intensity interventions are recommended that provide 14 or more individual or group sessions in 6 months, delivered by a trained interventionist (e.g., registered dietitian, exercise specialist) (Jensen et al., 2014). This approach, which produces an average loss of 5–8% of initial weight, is also recommended for patients with obesity (BMI ≥ 30 kg/m²) who have never had a course of intensive lifestyle intervention (which also is referred to as *intensive behavior therapy, behavioral weight control,* or *lifestyle modification*). Such an intervention also is indicated for patients who plan to take prescription weight loss medication, since the two approaches produce additive weight loss (Wadden et al., 2005). Behavioral weight control practices also may contribute to long-term success with bariatric surgery.

Table 17.1 summarizes the primary components and structure of a high-intensity intervention, as recommended by the AHA/ACC/TOS guidelines (Heymsfield & Wadden, 2017). Dietary modification seeks to induce an energy deficit of 500–750 kcal/day, usually achieved by prescribing 1,200–1,499 kcal/day for women and 1,500–1,800 kcal/day for men (with higher-calorie targets in the range for heavier individuals). Alternatively, calorie intake can be prescribed based on body weight, with 1,200–1,499 kcal/day for persons < 250 pounds (113.6 kg) and 1,500–1,800 kcal/day for those > 250 pounds (Look AHEAD Research Group, 2006). As described by Astrup (Chapter 18, this volume), a variety of diets, with differing macronutrient compositions—including low fat, low carbohydrate, low glycemic, high protein, or Mediterranean style—may be prescribed, provided they induce the desired energy deficit. Macronutrient composition may be more important for improving specific obesity-related comorbidities (e.g., type 2 diabetes) or for facilitating long-term weight control than it is for inducing weight loss (Jensen et al., 2014).

Patients are encouraged during the first 6 months to gradually increase their physical activity to 150–180 minutes/week, typically with brisk walking or others forms of moderately vigorous aerobic exercise (Jensen et al., 2014). Multiple short bouts of activity (e.g., 10 minutes), as well as increased lifestyle activity (e.g., using stairs rather than escalators, walking rather than riding) also facilitate weight control and improve cardiovascular health (see Jakicic et al., Chapter 19, this volume).

Behavior therapy provides patients with strategies and techniques for adopting diet and activity recommendations (see Gomez-Rubalcava, Stabbert, & Phelan, Chapter 20, this volume). Foremost among these strategies are regularly recording food intake, physical activity, and body weight—tasks facilitated by a new generation of smartphone applications (e.g., MyFitnessPal, Lose It!), activity counters (e.g., Fitbit, Jawbone), and cellular-connected scales (Webb & Wadden, 2017). Approximately weekly, patients review their progress with a trained interventionist, who provides encouragement and instruction in goal setting and problem solving. This feedback is critical to weight loss (Jensen et al., 2014).

Structured Lifestyle Intervention

A key to success with lifestyle intervention is ensuring that patients, during the first 6 months, receive a minimum of 14 individual or group counseling sessions. This is the definition of high-intensity counseling proposed by the AHA/ACC/TOS guidelines and one that is consistent with the recommendations of the Centers for Medicare and Medicaid Services (CMS; 2011) for the provision of intensive behavior therapy. Reviews of the literature by the AHA/ACC/TOS expert panel, as well as the U.S. Preventive Services Task Force (Moyer, 2012), found that less intensive (i.e., less frequent) counseling did

TABLE 17.1. Recommended Components of a High-Intensity Comprehensive Lifestyle Intervention to Achieve and Maintain a 5–10% Reduction in Body Weight

Component	Weight loss	Weight loss maintenance
Frequency and duration of treatment contact	• 14 or more in-person counseling sessions in 6 months with a trained interventionist (individual or group contact). • *Similarly structured, comprehensive web-based interventions, as well as evidence-based commercial programs may be recommended.*	• Monthly or more frequent in-person or telephone sessions for ≥ 1 year with a trained interventionist.
Diet	• Low-calorie diet (typically 1,200–1,500 kcal/day for women, 1,500–1,800 kcal/day for men), with macronutrient composition *based on patient's preferences and health status.*[a]	• Reduced-calorie diet, consistent with reduced body weight, with macronutrient composition based on patient's preferences and health status.
Physical activity[b]	• ≥ 150 minutes/week of aerobic physical activity (e.g., brisk walking).	• 200–300 minutes/week of aerobic activity (e.g., brisk walking).
Behavior therapy	• Daily monitoring of food intake and physical activity, facilitated by paper diaries or apps. • Weekly monitoring of weight. • Structured curriculum of behavior change (e.g., DPP), including goal setting, problem solving, and stimulus control. • Regular feedback and support from a trained interventionist.	• Occasional to frequent monitoring of food intake and physical activity, as needed. • Weekly to daily monitoring of weight. • Curriculum of behavior change, including problem solving, cognitive restructuring, and relapse prevention. • Regular feedback from trained interventionist.

Note. From Heymsfield & Wadden (2017). Mechanisms, pathophysiology, and management of obesity. *New England Journal of Medicine, 376*(3), 254–266. Copyright © 2017 Massachusetts Medical Society. Reprinted with permission from the Massachusetts Medical Society.

[a]The guidelines concluded that a variety of dietary approaches, which differ widely in macronutrient composition, can produce weight loss, provided they induce an adequate energy deficit. This includes ad libitum approaches in which a lower calorie intake is achieved by restriction or elimination of particular food groups or by the provision of prescribed foods. The guidelines recommended that practitioners, in selecting a reducing diet, consider its potential contribution to the management of obesity-related comorbidities (e.g., type 2 diabetes, hypertension).

[b]The guidelines did not address the possible benefits of strength training, in addition to aerobic activity.

not produce clinically meaningful weight loss. One year of monthly or less frequent treatment sessions produced a loss of only 1.7–4.0 kg (LeBlanc, O'Connor, Whitlock, Patnode, & Kapka, 2011). At the high end of the intensity (frequency) continuum, Perri et al. (2014) found that 24 counseling sessions delivered over 6 months (i.e., weekly visits) did not produce significantly greater weight loss than 16 sessions over the same period (losses of 10.9% and 9.3%, respectively). This finding questions the weight loss benefit, as well as cost effectiveness, of providing more than 16 sessions in 6 months to induce weight loss, although further dose–response studies of this type are needed to reach definitive conclusions.

Group versus Individual Care

The AHA/ACC/TOS guidelines recommend that patients attend traditional face-to-face counseling visits (Jensen et al., 2014). Treatment may be delivered in group or individual sessions. Group counseling usually includes 10–20 participants, lasts 60–90 min, and may induce somewhat larger (about 2 kg) weight loss than individual treatment (Renjilian et al., 2001; Paul-Ebhohimhen & Avenell, 2009). The greater losses likely are attributable to the increased social support and information sharing offered by group interactions, as well as to a healthy dose of competition among participants. Group care clearly is less expensive than individual counseling and can make treatment available to a greater number of patients in a clinical practice. Groups should be sufficiently small to allow all participants to report briefly each week on their success in adhering to their physical activity and food and calorie intake goals. Large groups (e.g., 30 participants), as compared with smaller ones (e.g., 12 members), may not provide adequate attention for each patient, potentially resulting in smaller weight losses, as found in a recent randomized controlled trial (losses of 3.2 and 6.5 kg, respectively, at 6 months; Dutton et al., 2014).

Structured lifestyle interventions are delivered following a curriculum of behavior change, in which one lesson typically builds on another, and participants are given weekly homework assignments to complete prior to the next session. The treatment manuals for the Diabetes Prevention Program and the Look AHEAD studies provide directions for interventionists to lead sessions, as well as homework assignments for participants. Both manuals are available to practitioners and researchers for nonprofit use (*https://dppos.bsc. gwu.edu/documents/1124073/1134992/ DPP_duringcore.pdf/a771d14f-fa3c-45b2-bd9f-5b17c0212892; www.lookaheadtrial. org/publicResources/interventionMaterial. cfm*). As described by Gomez-Rubalcava et al. (Chapter 20, this volume), treatment sessions typically begin with a weigh-in (in private) and then focus principally on patients' reporting on their completion of homework assignments (i.e., monitoring calorie intake and physical activity). Many patients report that counseling sessions provide not only important knowledge and support for behavior change but also much needed accountability to follow through on weekly goals and assignments.

Interventionist Training

Lifestyle interventionists typically include registered dietitians, exercise specialists, clinical psychologists, and related health counselors, as observed in the AHA/ACC/ TOS review of the literature (Jensen et al., 2014). However, trained laypersons who adhere to a structured treatment manual also have successfully served as interventionists (see West, Krukowski, & Larsen, Chapter 30, this volume). Further studies are needed to clarify the educational background and training required to provide intensive lifestyle intervention. Based on the current evidence, we believe that trained laypersons can deliver such counseling provided that patients do not have significant obesity-related comorbidities that may require additional nutritional or psychological expertise (e.g., type 2 diabetes, binge-eating disorder, significant depression). Such expertise potentially could be provided as an adjunct to lay-delivered counseling.

Examples of Intensive Lifestyle Interventions

The Diabetes Prevention Program (DPP) and Look AHEAD studies provide excellent examples of high-intensity lifestyle interventions that were delivered in multicenter trials, sponsored by the National Institutes of Health. (Look AHEAD is discussed in a later section of this chapter.) The DPP randomly assigned more than 3,200 patients with overweight/obesity and impaired glucose tolerance to placebo, metformin, or an intensive lifestyle intervention designed to induce and maintain a 7 kg reduction in initial weight (Diabetes Prevention Program Research Group et al., 2002). The study's primary outcome was the reduction in the incidence of type 2 diabetes. During the first 6 months, lifestyle participants attended 16 individual counseling sessions with a registered dietitian and then had one contact at least every other month for the remainder of the 4-year study. Patients were instructed to consume a low-fat, reduced-calorie diet (i.e., 1,200–2,000 kcal/day, based on body weight), comprised of conventional foods that they selected. The physical activity goal was 150 minutes/week, principally of brisk walking. The study was stopped after a mean of 2.8 years, at which time lifestyle participants had achieved a mean loss of 5.6 kg, compared with significantly smaller losses of 2.8 kg for metformin and 0.1 kg for placebo. The lifestyle intervention, compared with the placebo and metformin groups, reduced the risk of developing type 2 diabetes by 58% and 31%, respectively, leading to the study's early termination to provide lifestyle modification to the other two groups (Diabetes Prevention Program Research Group et al., 2002). A 10-year follow-up assessment found that, as compared with placebo, the lifestyle intervention group maintained a 34% reduction in the risk of developing type 2 diabetes, even though the latter patients had regained most of their lost weight (Diabetes Prevention Program Research Group, 2009).

Remotely Delivered Lifestyle Interventions

The AHA/ACC/TOS guidelines recommend the provision of traditional face-to-face counseling, primarily because this approach is supported by such a large evidence base (Jensen et al., 2014). Lifestyle interventions, however, are increasingly delivered by telephone, Internet, text messaging, social media, smartphones, and related approaches, which have the advantage of being more accessible, convenient, and affordable than traditional on-site interventions (Webb & Wadden, 2017). The AHA/ACC/TOS guidelines concluded that remotely delivered programs that include personalized feedback from a trained interventionist can be prescribed for weight loss but may result in smaller weight losses than face-to-face interventions. Tate, Nezami, and Valle reached similar conclusions in a thorough review of the literature for this volume (Chapter 28).

Telephone-Delivered Programs

The more that remotely delivered interventions resemble traditional face-to-face counseling, in terms of the frequency of contact with a trained interventionist, the greater the weight losses they produce. Telephone-delivered interventions, for example, have achieved approximately the same weight losses as face-to face programs, when matched for the number of treatment sessions (Appel et al., 2011; Donnelly et al., 2007, 2013; Rock et al., 2010). Figure 17.2 presents results of a randomized controlled trial by Appel et al. (2011), in which patients were randomly assigned to usual care (i.e., self-directed) or to a high-intensity lifestyle intervention delivered either by individual phone counseling (remotely delivered) or

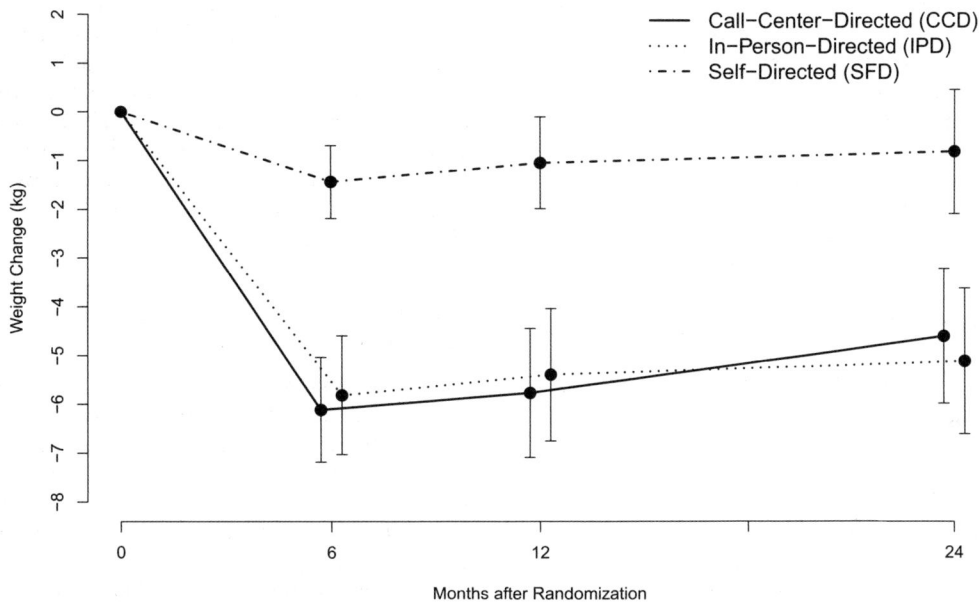

FIGURE 17.2. Mean weight change according to randomized group. From Appel, Clark, Yeh, Wang, Coughlin, Daumit, et al. (2011). Comparative effectiveness of weight-loss interventions in clinical practice. *New England Journal of Medicine, 365*(21), 1959–1968. Copyright © 2011 Massachusetts Medical Society. Reprinted with permission from Massachusetts Medical Society.

traditional in-person, group treatment with some individual sessions. Both lifestyle groups also were provided with a web-based program on which to record their food intake and physical activity. The remotely delivered and in-person interventions both produced mean weight losses of approximately 5 kg at both 6 and 24 months, with no significant differences between them, showing the benefits of telephone-delivered care. Both groups were superior to the self-directed group at all times.

Internet-Delivered Approaches

As reviewed by Tate and colleagues (Chapter 28, this volume), Internet-delivered programs have been most effective when they instructed participants to keep records (online) of their food intake, physical activity, and weight, which they reviewed regularly with a trained interventionist or received simulated feedback from a computer algorithm. However, weight losses produced by the most effective Internet-delivered programs have typically been one-third to one-half smaller than those resulting from traditional face-to-face treatment (Webb & Wadden, 2017). In the best designed and executed study of this topic to date, Harvey-Berino et al. (2010) provided adults with the same 24-session lifestyle intervention that was delivered in traditional face-to-face group meetings or by Internet sessions, which included having participants "meet" in a supervised chat room, with feedback from an interventionist. Participants in the Internet-delivered program lost 5.5 kg in 6 months, compared to a significantly greater 8.0 kg for those who received face-to-face treatment. A third "hybrid" group, which received a mix of Internet and face-to-face meetings, lost 6.0 kg.

Other Approaches

Smartphone-delivered programs and the dozens of weight loss applications (apps) that have been developed hold promise of simplifying the tasks of recording food intake, physical activity, body weight, and other outcomes (Webb & Wadden, 2017). A major challenge, however, is keeping patients engaged and accountable with these approaches in order to achieve clinically meaningful weight loss ($\geq 5\%$ of initial weight). Svetkey et al. (2015), for example, developed a smartphone-delivered intervention for young adults (ages 18–35) with overweight/obesity. Those who received a self-directed intervention, delivered by smartphone (and without interventionist feedback), lost only 0.9 kg in 6 months. Similarly modest weight losses were obtained in a randomized controlled trial of the currently popular MyFitnessPal app. Primary care patients who were randomly assigned to receive the app, along with usual medical care, lost no weight at the end of 6 months, compared with a gain of 0.6 pounds in those assigned to usual care alone (Laing et al., 2014). Most participants used the app for the first month, but few did at 6 months.

These findings underscore the need to identify methods to maintain accountability and motivation with self-directed apps and smartphone applications. The use of financial incentives provides a possibility, as discussed by Patel and Volpp (Chapter 32, this volume). In addition, some technologies and behavioral programs may be more reinforcing—and effective—than others, as illustrated by a promising study by Steinberg et al. (2013), which reported a 6.5% reduction in initial body weight at 6 months with the use of a cellular-connected smart scale. At present, however, practitioners and patients should know that the less structure and accountability that remotely delivered programs provide, the less weight patients will likely lose.

Commercial- and Community-Based Lifestyle Interventions

Many patients do not live near large medical centers that offer high-intensity lifestyle counseling. In such cases, commercial- and community-based programs may be considered. The AHA/ACC/TOS guidelines concluded that some commercial-based programs can be prescribed, provided there is peer-reviewed evidence of their safety and efficacy (Jensen et al., 2014). Gudzune and colleagues (2015) have summarized the safety and efficacy of leading commercial (non-medical) weight loss programs and concluded that Weight Watchers and Jenny

Craig have provided the strongest evidence of success (see Gudzune & Clark, Chapter 29, this volume). Weight Watchers offers behavioral counseling through either in-person group meetings or an online program. The in-person group program induces a mean loss of approximately 4–5% of initial weight in 6–12 months, with somewhat smaller losses for online programs (Heshka et al., 2003; Jebb et al., 2011). Randomized controlled trials of Jenny Craig have yielded larger weight losses—of approximately 7–8% of initial weight—most likely because of the program's provision of a diet of prepackaged, portion-controlled foods, which facilitates adherence to calorie goals (Rock et al., 2010, 2016). As discussed by Gudzune et al. (2015), the additional weight loss with Jenny Craig comes at a charge of about $100 per week, including the cost of the program's food, compared with $14 weekly for Weight Watchers. The latter costs do not include what participants spend on conventional foods.

As reviewed by West, Krukowski and Larsen (Chapter 30, this volume), local YMCAs may also provide high-intensity lifestyle group counseling as part of efforts to deliver the DPP intervention in community settings to persons with impaired glucose tolerance. Numerous controlled trials have shown that YMCA instructors, without prior weight management skills, were able to induce mean weight losses of 4–6% of initial weight in 6 months, using a modified version of the DPP protocol (Ali, Echouffo-Tcheugui, & Williamson, 2012). As important, the cost of providing weight management in the YMCA was estimated at $275–$325 per participant, compared to $1,400 for the original program delivered in academic medical centers (Ackermann & Marrero, 2007). These findings underscore that trained laypersons can play an important role in increasing the availability of high-intensity lifestyle interventions in community settings.

Lifestyle Interventions in Primary Care Practice

As summarized by Tsai and Wadden (Chapter 27, this volume), there have been few studies of primary care physicians, nurse practitioners, or physician assistants delivering high-intensity lifestyle counseling in primary care practice, as now prescribed and covered by the Centers for Medicare and Medicaid Services (CMS, 2011). CMS refers to such counseling as intensive behavior therapy (IBT) and reimburses weekly, brief (e.g., 15 minutes) visits the first month, followed by every-other-week visits in months 2–6, for a total of 14–15 visits. Patients who lose 3 kg are eligible for six additional monthly sessions, for a total of 20–21 visits in the year.

CMS's stipulation that counseling may be provided only by physicians and the other practitioners noted is surprising because these individuals generally have limited training in weight management and typically do not have the time or economic incentive to provide lifestyle counseling. (Registered dietitians apparently can deliver IBT if they work incident to a covered provider who is on the premises when counseling is delivered.) In addition, CMS has not provided a treatment protocol to guide practitioners' provision of IBT or assessed the efficacy of this approach. Wadden and colleagues currently are conducting a randomized controlled trial to evaluate 1-year changes in weight and CVD risk factors resulting from 21 brief counseling sessions, as prescribed by CMS. They have adapted the DPP protocol to include a 21-session guide for practitioners and patients (Wadden, Volger, et al., 2011). The entire protocol can be obtained at *www.med.upenn.edu/weight/wadden.html*.

Primary care practitioners play a critical role in the management of obesity by diagnosing this disease and providing medical therapies for the CVD risk factors and other weight-related health complications. They also can provide patients with critical guidance in selecting a weight reduction therapy, in prescribing chronic weight management medications, or in referring patients to bariatric surgery, as appropriate (Heymsfield & Wadden, 2017). We, however, do not believe that most primary care practitioners are well suited to deliver intensive lifestyle intervention (i.e., 14 sessions in 6 months), given the demands on their time and expertise. Other office personnel (e.g., dietitian, health counselor) potentially could provide such treatment, or patients could be referred to programs/providers in the community, as well as to remotely delivered interventions. These latter interventions have shown promise with patients encountered in primary care settings (Appel et al., 2011; Thomas, Leahey, & Wing, 2015).

A Structured Lifestyle Intervention for the Maintenance of Weight Loss

The maintenance of lost weight remains the Achilles' heel of intensive lifestyle interventions for obesity, as it is for other weight management approaches. Following weight loss and the end of counseling, patients typically regain one-third of lost weight in the year following treatment (Wadden, 1993), with continuing weight regain through year 5, when patients, on average, have returned to their baseline weight (Wadden, Sternberg, Letizia, Stunkard, & Foster, 1989). Reasons for weight regain are multiply determined and include (1) the termination of professional support and guidance with the end of lifestyle counseling; (2) the need for patients to continue to eat a low-calorie diet and engage in high levels of physical activity, in the face of returning to a toxic environment that thwarts such efforts; (3) an unfavorable work-to-reward ratio, in which patients' continued efforts are not rewarded with continued weight loss, which they still desire; (4) a loss of social support, as friends and family members stop applauding dieters when they stop losing weight; and (5) a host of compensatory biological changes, including reductions in resting and nonresting energy expenditures, as well as unfavorable changes in appetite-related hormones (e.g., ghrelin, leptin, neuropeptide Y-5), all of which serve to return body weight to baseline levels (Rosenbaum & Liebel, 2016; Sumithran et al., 2011; Webb & Wadden, 2017).

Continued Behavioral Counseling

As reviewed by Perri and Ariel-Donges (Chapter 23, this volume), continued behavioral counseling, following initial weight loss, facilitates the maintenance of lost weight. This also was the conclusion of the AHA/ACC/TOS guidelines, which recommend that overweight or obese individuals who have lost weight participate for 1 year or more in a comprehensive weight loss maintenance program, delivered in person or by telephone (Jensen et al., 2014). Monthly or more frequent visits are recommended with a trained interventionist who helps patients engage in high levels of physical activity (200–300 minutes/week), monitor body weight regularly (preferably daily), and consume a reduced-calorie diet that is needed to maintain the lower body weight. These are the same behaviors practiced by members of the National Weight Control Registry, all of whom have lost at least 30 pounds (13.6 kg) and maintained the loss for 1 year or more (Wing & Phelan, 2005).

The Look AHEAD Study

The Look AHEAD study provides the longest evaluation to date of the effectiveness of an intensive lifestyle intervention for inducing and maintaining weight loss. All study participants received at least 8 years of intervention. The trial enrolled participants with overweight/obesity and type 2 diabetes to determine whether the loss of 7% or more of initial weight, combined with 175 minutes/day of aerobic activity, would reduce the risk of CVD morbidity and mortality, as compared with a usual care group, referred to as *diabetes support and education* (DSE; Look AHEAD Research Group, 2013). (Gregg & Flores, Chapter 12, this volume, review the CVD findings.) During the first 6 months, lifestyle participants were provided with three face-to-face group counseling sessions and one individual meeting per month, which decreased to two group and one individual session from months 7–12. Details of the treatment protocol have been described previously and included the prescription of a 1,200–1,499 kcal/day diet for those who weighed ≤ 250 pounds (113.6 kg), with 1,500–1,800 for those >113.6 kg (Look AHEAD Research Group et al., 2006). During the first 4 months, these participants also were prescribed the use of liquid meal replacements (i.e., shakes) and meal bars (e.g., Glucerna, OPTIFAST, SlimFast, and Health Management Resources [HMR] products) to replace two meals and one snack per day to help them meet their calorie goals. Thereafter, they were offered one meal replacement daily to facilitate the maintenance of weight loss.

In years 2–4, lifestyle participants were provided with one individual face-to-face meeting per month and one monthly telephone or e-mail contact in which they reviewed their efforts to adhere to their diet and physical activity goals (increased to > 200 minutes/week) and maintain their weight loss (Look AHEAD Research Group et al., 2006). Individual monthly face-to-face meetings continued to be provided in years 5–8. In addition, throughout the maintenance period (years 2–8) participants were offered two to three group experiences per year, each typically 6–8 weeks in length, designed to help them lose additional weight or to reverse any weight regain. Throughout the study, DSE participants could attend one to three group sessions per year that provided information about aspects of healthy diet and physical activity but not instruction in how to change behavior.

Weight Loss in Look AHEAD

As shown in Figure 17.3, participants in the intensive lifestyle intervention (ILI) lost 8.6% of initial weight at year 1, compared with a significantly smaller 0.7% for those in the DSE. Fully 68% of lifestyle participants lost 5% or more of initial weight, and 37% lost 10% or more (Wadden et al., 2009). Despite the provision of weight loss maintenance therapy, lifestyle participants, on average, regained about 4% of their lost weight from years 2 to 5, after which their weight stabilized and then began to decline again. At year 8, these individuals achieved a mean loss from baseline of 4.7%, compared to 2.1% for the DSE participants; 50.3% of lifestyle participants maintained a loss of 5% or more of initial weight, compared with 35.7% for DSE (Look AHEAD Research Group, 2014). The Look AHEAD results represent the largest weight losses achieved with an intensive lifestyle intervention of 8 years or more.

The Biggest Losers in Look AHEAD

A great advantage of Look AHEAD was that its large sample of 2,500 lifestyle participants allowed the examination of subsets of individuals with different degrees of long-term weight loss success. Figure 17.4A presents findings for 787 participants who originally lost 10% or more of initial weight at year 1. Nearly 40% of these individuals maintained their full 10% weight loss at

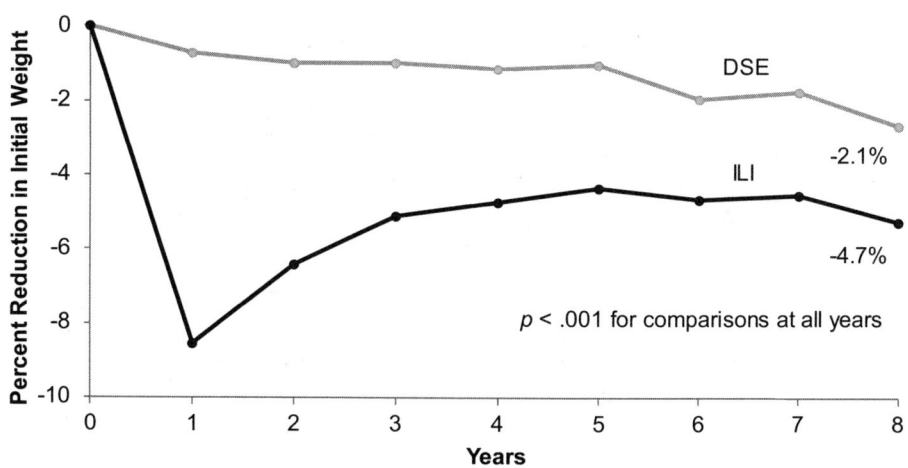

FIGURE 17.3. Mean (±SE) weight losses over 8 years for participants randomly assigned to an intensive lifestyle intervention (ILI) or diabetes support and education (DSE, usual care group). Differences between groups were significant (p < .001) at all years. From Look AHEAD Research Group (2014). Eight-year weight losses with an intensive lifestyle intervention: The Look AHEAD study. *Obesity*, *22*(1), 5–13. Copyright © 2014 Wiley. Reprinted by permission.

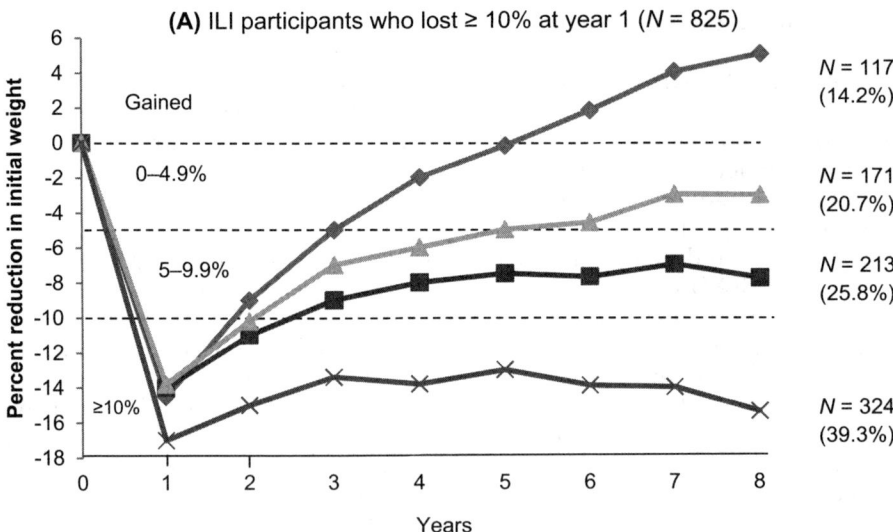

FIGURE 17.4A. Weight loss trajectories over 8 years in 825 participants in the intensive lifestyle intervention (ILI) who, at year 1, lost ≥ 10% of initial weight and, at year 8, provided a measured body weight. The figure shows the number of participants who, at year 8, maintained a loss of 10% or more of initial weight (N = 324), of 5–9.9% (N = 213), of 0–4.9% (N = 171), or who gained above their baseline weight (N = 117). The percentages shown in parentheses are based on the sample size for the subgroup. Thus, the 324 of 825 participants who maintained a ≥ 10% loss at year 8 comprised 39.3% of this subgroup of participants.

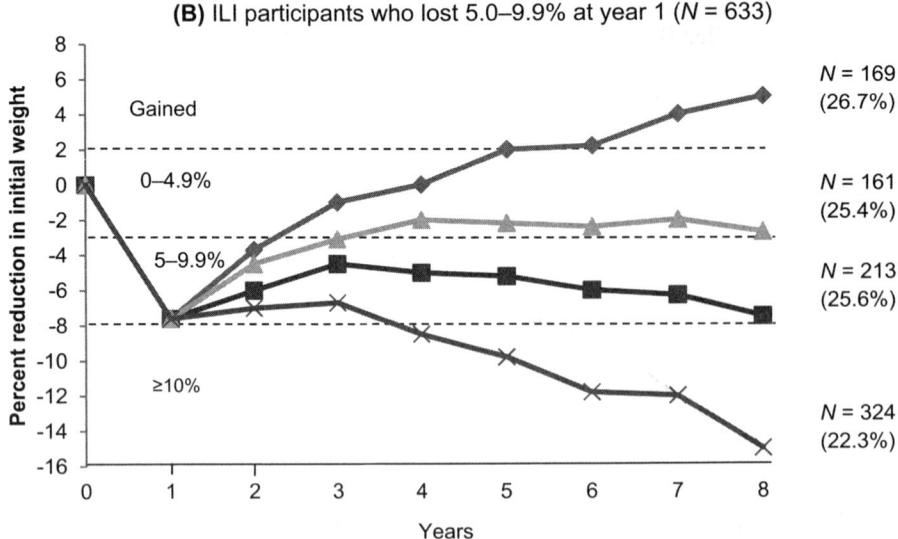

FIGURE 17.4B. Weight loss trajectories over 8 years in 633 ILI participants who, at year 1, lost 5–9.9% of initial weight and, at year 8, provided a measured body weight. The four categories of weight change that these participants achieved at year 8 are presented in the same manner as in Figure 17.4A.

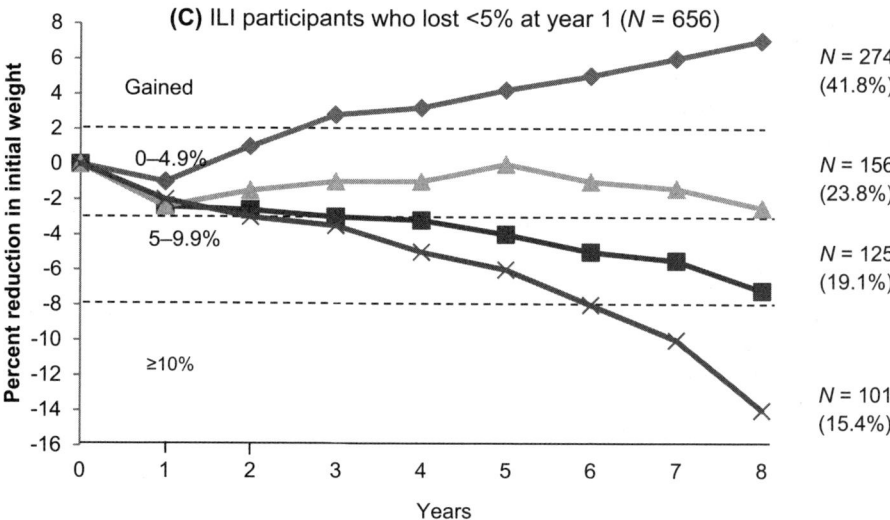

FIGURE 17.4C. Weight loss trajectories over 8 years in 656 ILI participants who, at year 1, lost < 5% of initial weight and, at year 8, provided a measured body weight. The four categories of weight change that these participants achieved at year 8 are presented in the same manner as in Figure 17.4A. From Look AHEAD Research Group (2014). Eight-year weight losses with an intensive lifestyle intervention: The Look AHEAD study. *Obesity, 22*(1), 5–13. Copyright © 2014 Wiley. Reprinted by permission.

year 8, suggesting the benefit of weight loss maintenance counseling when compared with the results of trials that provided minimal or no further treatment after weight loss (Look AHEAD Research Group, 2014). An additional, 25.8% of these participants who originally lost 10% of weight, maintained a loss at 8 years of 5.0% to 9.9% of initial weight, meeting the criterion for clinically meaningful weight loss. Only 14.2% of these successful 1-year participants regained all of their weight loss at year 8, substantially less than the 95%-regain figure frequently cited in media reports. Additional analyses showed that persons who maintained their full 10% weight loss at year 8 reported exercising more and expending significantly more calories at this time than those who regained their lost weight (1,472 vs. 800 kcal/week), a consistent finding among weight loss maintainers (see Jakicic et al., Chapter 19, this volume).

Treatment Nonresponders in Look AHEAD

The Look AHEAD data also reveal that what is frequently interpreted as a problem of weight regain in long-term weight loss trials partially reflects a problem of lack of initial weight loss. Figure 17.4C shows that 32% of lifestyle participants did not lose 5% of initial weight in the first year, and that 17% of ILI participants (430) did not lose this amount by the end of year 8. Results for such participants do not reflect upon the maintenance of weight reduction but instead upon the need to identify alternative treatments or rescue approaches to induce weight loss in persons who do not respond to intensive lifestyle intervention.

Treatment Options: BMI ≥ 30 kg/m²—Portion-Controlled Diets, Pharmacotherapy, and Weight Loss Devices

Intensive lifestyle intervention should be offered to all patients with a BMI ≥ 30 kg/m², given the safety, efficacy, and generally low cost of this approach. Individuals who are not successful with lifestyle intervention alone or who need to lose ≥ 10% of initial weight to better control obesity-related comorbidities are candidates for additional interventions, including portion-controlled diets, pharmacotherapy, and some newly approved weight loss devices. A question frequently asked is whether patients have to "fail" a course of lifestyle modification before being eligible to use weight loss medications or other approaches. We believe that a history of participating in structured lifestyle interventions should qualify patients for adjunctive care (e.g., pharmacotherapy), initiated from the outset of the new weight loss effort. For example, there is no need for another suboptimal outcome with lifestyle modification alone before adding pharmacotherapy. Adjunctive treatments, however, should be added to a robust program of lifestyle modification, rather than being used in lieu of it.

Low-Calorie, Portion-Controlled Diets

Individuals with overweight/obesity typically underestimate their calorie intake by 40–50% when instructed to consume a diet of 1,200–1,800 kcal/day of conventional foods (Lichtman et al., 1992). Persons of average weight similarly underestimate their energy intake by approximately 20%, as compared to energy requirements determined by doubly labeled water, the gold standard (Bandini, Schoeller, Cyr, & Dietz, 1990; Lichtman et al., 1992). In both cases, underestimation is thought to be attributable to difficulty in accurately determining the portion sizes and calories of the foods consumed, as well as simply forgetting to record all items. Patients' underestimation is not considered intentional but is one of the reasons that weight losses are often smaller than expected with the calorie levels prescribed.

Portion-controlled diets, including meal replacements, consist of liquid shakes, meal bars, and prepackaged or frozen servings of conventional foods (e.g., Lean Cuisine, Healthy Choice). These products provide dieters with a predetermined amount of food with a known calorie content, thereby removing much of the guesswork from counting calories (Tsai & Wadden, 2006). Using principles of stimulus control, portion-controlled servings reduce unwanted decision making about what to eat, as well as contact with potentially problem foods. This approach helps patients meet their calorie targets and achieve larger weight losses (Tsai & Wadden, 2006). Ditschuneit and colleagues reported that patients who met with a dietitian once a month and were prescribed a diet of 1,200–1,500 kcal/day, which included two servings a day of a liquid meal replacement (i.e., SlimFast), lost 7.1 kg in 3 months, compared with 1.3 kg for patients who were instructed to consume a self-selected diet of conventional foods with the same calorie target (Ditschuneit, Flechtner-Mors, Johnson, & Adler, 1999). In a meta-analysis of six studies, Heymsfield and colleagues found that portion-controlled diets produced a 2.5 kg greater weight loss at both 3 and 12 months than an equivalent calorie diet comprised of conventional foods (Heymsfield, van Mierlo, van der Knaap, Heo, & Friar, 2003).

In several trials, Wadden and colleagues prescribed 900–1,200 kcal/day portion-controlled diets that included four servings daily of a liquid diet (e.g., HMR 800, Boston, MA), combined with an evening meal of a frozen-food entrée, a cup of salad, and a fruit serving (Wadden, Vogt., et al., 1997; Wadden et al., 2004; Wadden, Faulconbridge, et al., 2011). This approach, as combined with intensive lifestyle intervention, reliably induced losses of 10–15% of initial weight in 12–16 weeks.

This mixed diet, combining a liquid diet with some conventional food, evolved from the use of very-low-calorie diets (VLCDs), providing 800 or fewer calories per day (Tsai & Wadden, 2006). Although some proprietary programs (e.g., OPTIFAST and HMR) still offer all-liquid VLCDs, in the form of five shakes per day with no other foods permitted, this aggressive regimen is now typically limited to patients with severe obesity immediately prior to their undergoing bariatric surgery (Gudzune et al., 2015; Jensen et al., 2014). As reviewed by Gudzune and Clark (Chapter 29, this volume), VLCDs produce mean weight losses as great as 15–20% of initial weight in 12–16 weeks, but weight regain is common even when patients are provided weekly weight loss maintenance sessions (Wadden, Foster, & Letizia, 1994). A minority of patients also complained of excessive fear of terminating the VLCD and of binge-eating once they did (Wadden &

Bartlett, 1992). Our research team found that these latter two problems were attenuated by providing patients with the higher calorie (900–1,200 kcal/day) mixed diet that included some conventional foods (Wadden et al., 2004). The problem of weight regain following the mixed diet remains but is less severe than with VLCDs (Wadden et al., 2004; Wadden, Falconbridge, et al., 2011).

Pharmacotherapy

Medications for chronic weight management are indicated for adults with a BMI ≥ 30 kg/m^2 or with a BMI ≥ 27 kg/m^2 who have at least one weight-related comorbidity (Apovian et al., 2015; Garvey et al., 2016). Pharmacotherapy is approved by the FDA as an adjunct to a reduced calorie diet and increased physical activity and appears to facilitate adherence to dietary recommendations by reducing hunger and/or increasing satiation (i.e., fullness) (Apovian et al., 2015; Wadden, Berkowitz, Sarwer, Prus-Wisniewski, & Steinberg, 2001). Some medications also may counteract compensatory hormonal changes precipitated by caloric restriction and weight loss (Ochner, Tsai, Kushner, & Wadden, 2015).

Bray and Ryan, in Chapter 21 of this volume, provide an excellent overview of (1) the five medications approved by the FDA for chronic weight management; (2) phentermine and other drugs approved for short-term use; and (3) medications frequently used off-label for weight management. As shown in Figure 17.5, the five medications approved for chronic use, as combined with low-to-moderate intensity lifestyle counseling (i.e., ≤1 counseling session per month, as provided in most industry-sponsored trials) are approximately equally effective as high intensity lifestyle intervention alone in helping patients lose ≥ 5% and ≥ 10% of initial weight (Heymsfield & Wadden, 2017). The sections that follow briefly discuss three issues relevant to the use of weight loss medications: (1) the importance of combining pharmacotherapy with intensive lifestyle intervention; (2) the benefit of chronic pharmacotherapy in facilitating the maintenance rather than induction of weight loss; and (3) the use of behavioral strategies to facilitate medication adherence.

Combining Lifestyle Modification and Medication

Intensive lifestyle modification helps patients consciously restrain their response to ubiquitous, high-calorie foods and opportunities to eat by using behavioral strategies such as cue control, self-monitoring, and slowing the rate of eating (see Gomez-Rubalcava et al., Chapter 20, this volume). Behavioral treatment helps patients cope with the external food environment. Pharmacotherapy, by contrast, facilitates weight loss by altering the internal environment—physiological factors, such as reducing hunger (i.e., the drive to initiate eating) and potentially food preoccupation (Wadden et al., 2001, Wadden, Foreyt, et al., 2011). In addition, some medications appear to help patients, once they have started eating, to feel full more quickly, thereby potentially correcting impaired satiation (Apovian et al., 2015; Garvey et al., 2016). From a clinical perspective, patients have reported that some medications stop them from thinking about specific foods or when they'll have their next meal (Wadden, Berkowitz, et al., 1997). Pharmacotherapy, at its best, appears to reduce vulnerability or responsiveness to the external food environment.

Given the complementary mechanisms by which lifestyle intervention and pharmacotherapy appear to induce weight loss, they could be expected to have additive effects. Such additive weight losses were demonstrated by Wadden et al. (2005) in a study of lifestyle modification combined with sibutramine, which was removed from the market in 2010 when found to increase the risk of cardiovascular morbidity and mortality (James et al., 2010). Nonetheless, the study illustrates the results likely to be obtained when currently approved FDA medications are combined with intensive lifestyle intervention. Patients who received sibutramine alone (10–15 mg/day) for 1 year, with eight brief medical visits but no lifestyle modification, lost 5 kg. Those provided with 30 group lifestyle modifications sessions, but no medication, lost 6.7 kg. Participants who received sibutramine (with eight medical visits) combined with the 30 group lifestyle modification sessions lost a significantly greater 12.1 kg, approximately the sum

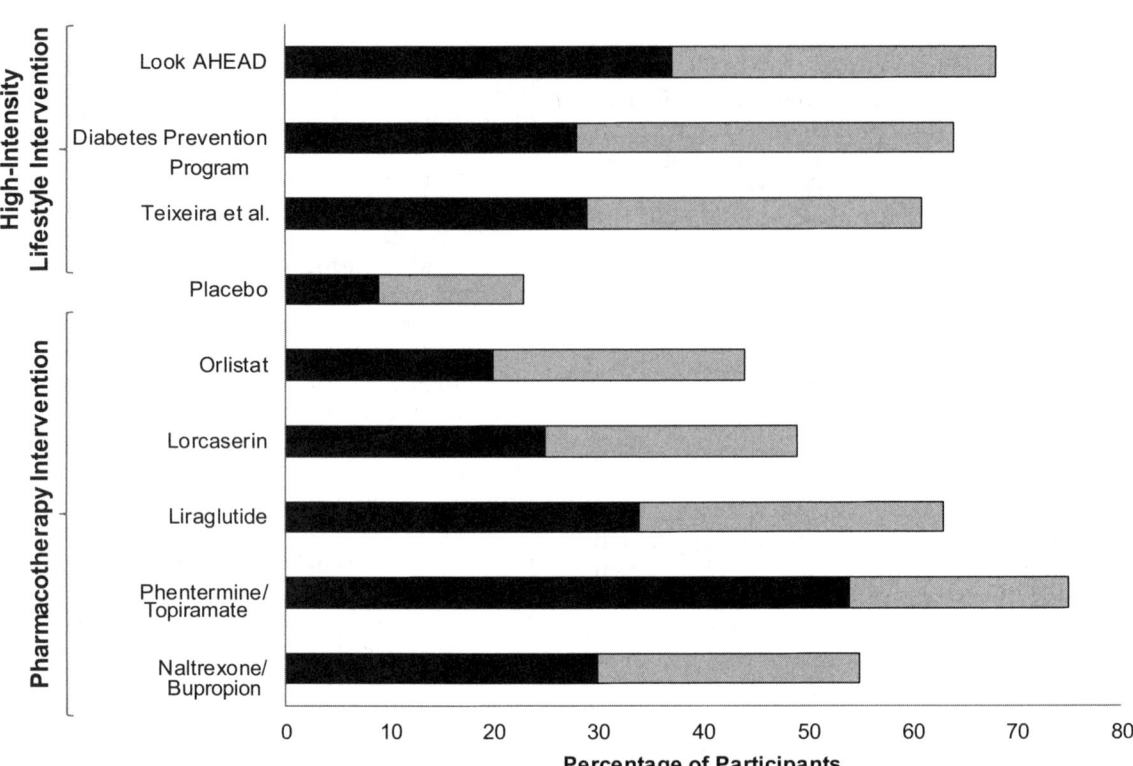

FIGURE 17.5. Weight loss at 1 year with high-intensity lifestyle interventions or pharmacotherapy combined with low- to moderate-intensity lifestyle counseling. This figure shows the percentages of participants in randomized controlled trials who lost ≥5% or ≥ 10% of their initial weight. Percentages shown are cumulative; the percentage of participants who lost ≥ 5% of initial weight includes the percentage who lost ≥ .0%. From Heymsfield and Wadden (2017). Mechanisms, pathophysiology, and management of obesity. *New England Journal of Medicine, 376*(3), 254–266. Copyright © 2017 Massachusetts Medical Society. Reprinted with permission from the Massachusetts Medical Society.

of the two separate treatments. Patients in a fourth group, who received sibutramine and eight brief visits of lifestyle modification, provided by a physician, lost 7.5 kg, suggesting the potential benefit of such counseling.

Other studies have shown that the addition of intensive lifestyle intervention to pharmacotherapy clearly increases weight loss, as compared to pharmacotherapy alone (Wadden et al., 2001). Similarly, the addition of pharmacotherapy to lifestyle modification alone significantly increases weight loss, as compared to the latter treatment alone (Wadden, Foreyt, et al., 2011). Such data should encourage physicians and other primary care practitioners to ensure that patients receive intensive lifestyle intervention when they are prescribed a medication for chronic weight management. Similarly, lifestyle interventionists should consider the benefits of adding medication to their high-intensity behavioral programs to increase weight loss (Wadden et al., 2005; Wadden, Foreyt, et al., 2011).

Chronic Pharmacotherapy for Weight Loss Maintenance

Pharmacotherapy was approved by the FDA for chronic weight management because of the recognition that patients may need to take obesity medications indefinitely, in the same manner as taking drugs daily for other chronic conditions, including hypertension, hyperlipidemia, and type 2 diabetes (Apovian et al., 2015; Garvey et al., 2016; Yanovski & Yanovski, 2014, 2015). Weight loss medications should not be expected to cure obesity in 6 months, any more than antihypertensive or antidiabetic agents should be expected to have lasting benefits if withdrawn after 6 months. Obesity, for most persons, is a chronic condition requiring long-term care.

Numerous randomized controlled trials have shown that the long-term ($\geq$ 1 year) use of weight loss medications significantly improves the maintenance of lost weight, as compared with placebo (Davidson et al., 1999; Smith et al., 2010; Torgerson, Hauptman, Boldrin, & Sjöström, 2004; Wadden et al., 2013). This finding holds true whether medication is used to induce weight loss and then is prescribed for weight loss maintenance (Smith et al., 2010) or whether initial weight loss is achieved with intensive lifestyle intervention alone and medication is then introduced to facilitate weight loss maintenance (Wadden et al., 2013).

Practitioners will need to prepare patients for the plateau in weight loss that typically occurs with pharmacotherapy between 6 and 9 months, after which most individuals stop losing weight, despite often remaining obese and still taking medication (Apovian et al., 2015). Patients should be informed that after the first 6 to 9 months the medication works to keep off the lost weight rather than inducing further weight loss (Wadden et al., 2001). Patients often are disappointed that they cannot lose more weight, and view this occurrence as evidence that the medication is not working. Discontinuing weight loss medication usually results in rapid regaining of lost weight (Wadden et al., 2013). This regain paradoxically illustrates how well the medication was working to facilitate weight maintenance.

Facilitating Medication Adherence

In addition to improving patients' eating and activity habits, behavioral principles may be used to facilitate adherence to weight loss medications. Practitioners may wish to review several issues with patients concerning medication adherence. These include:

1. Explaining the mechanisms by which the weight loss medication works. This includes describing what the medication will do (e.g., decrease hunger, increase satiation), as well as what the patient should do (e.g., decrease exposure to food triggers, record food intake).
2. Describing the medication's possible side effects and how the patient should respond to them. This includes having the patient call the practitioner before he or she stops taking the medication.
3. Inquiring whether the patient or the patient's family members have any health concerns about the use of medications or about their costs (which are not covered by most insurance plans).
4. Describing the course of treatment (at least for the first 6 months), outlining medication use and the frequency of office visits, and discussing behavioral goals of treatment.
5. Developing a medication schedule that identifies when and where patients will take their medication and what they should do in the event of missing a dose. The more concrete the schedule, the better patient adherence usually is.
6. Having patients keep a daily medication log, at least during the first few months. This log should be reviewed at subsequent office visits.
7. Reviewing how much weight patients can realistically expect to lose during the first 6 months of treatment and helping them define success in terms of non-weight-related outcomes. These might include improvements in health complications, increased fitness and mobility, or the ability to enjoy recreational or social activities that the individual has forgone because of excess weight (see Shaw Tronieri & Wadden, Chapter 16, this volume).

Weight Loss Devices

Since January 2015, the FDA's Center for Devices and Radiological Health has approved several nonsurgical weight management devices for patients with BMIs starting at 30, 35, and 40 kg/m^2 who have been unsuccessful with diet and exercise alone. These devices are viewed as an alternative to bariatric surgery for patients hesitant or unable to pursue this approach, or potentially as a bridge to surgery following device-induced weight loss. In some cases, initial device approval was based on randomized trials of only 171 participants, thereby limiting safety and efficacy data. The FDA has required additional postapproval studies of these devices.

In Chapter 33 of this volume, Soegaard Ballester et al. have provided a thorough review of both FDA-approved devices and those currently under review or in development. Three of the recently approved devices are space-occupying, intragastric silicone balloons, which are endoscopically placed and inflated with saline (Neylan, Dempsey, Tewksbury, Williams, & Dumon, 2016). Alternatively, some balloons can be swallowed in capsule form and then inflated with gas using a thin inflation catheter. Intragastric balloons are approved for individuals with a BMI of 30–40 kg/m² who have been unable to reduce successfully with lifestyle modification alone. They are approved for 6 months of use and produce mean weight losses of approximately 7–12% of initial weight, principally by limiting the amount of food consumed by occupying gastric space (Neylan et al., 2016). Single- and dual-balloon systems have been approved, each recommended with lifestyle counseling. Common complications include nausea, vomiting, and abdominal pain, with 5–15% of devices removed because of patient intolerance. Balloons must be removed after 6 months because of concerns about possible balloon deflation and attendant complications, including bowel obstruction. The current absence of long-term efficacy data combined with high costs (i.e., $5,000–$10,000) raise questions about the long-term benefits of this approach, particularly if not used as a bridge to bariatric surgery.

The FDA also recently approved a percutaneous endoscopic gastrostomy (PEG) tube, which is connected to a device that facilitates aspiration (evacuation) of about 30–40% of ingested calories when used 20–30 minutes after eating (Norén & Forssell, 2016). The device, combined with lifestyle counseling, produced a mean loss of 12.1% at 1 year, compared with 3.6% for counseling alone. Patient selection and monitoring are critical to ensuring that the device is not used by individuals with bulimia nervosa or related eating disorders and that such complications do not develop (Neylan et al., 2016). This device, as well as an FDA-approved vagus nerve stimulator, await further evaluation of their long-term safety and efficacy before they can be considered established weight reduction therapies (see Soegaard Ballester et al., Chapter 33, this volume).

Treatment Options: BMI ≥ 40 kg/m²—Bariatric Surgery

Multiple randomized controlled trials conducted in the past decade have shown definitively that bariatric surgery is the most effective long-term weight loss intervention for patients with a BMI > 40 kg/m², as well as for those with a BMI ≥ 35 kg/m² and one or more comorbid conditions (Dixon et al., 2008; Schauer et al., 2014; Ikramuddin et al., 2013). The two most frequently used procedures are Roux-en-Y gastric bypass (RYGB), considered the gold standard, and the newer vertical sleeve gastrectomy (VSG). These two operations accounted for 23.1% and 53.8%, respectively, of bariatric procedures performed in the United States in 2015 (American Society for Metabolic and Bariatric Surgery, 2016). Laparoscopic adjustable gastric banding (LAGB), which was widely used in the United States a decade ago, accounted for only 5.7% of procedures in 2015.

As described in detail by Nor Hanipah et al. (Chapter 22, this volume), RYGB is performed laparoscopically and involves dividing the stomach to create a small gastric pouch in the upper fundus. The pouch is anastomosed to a Roux limb of jejunum that bypasses 75–150 cm of small bowel, resulting in the bypass of the majority of the stomach, the entire duodenum, and most of the jejunum, thereby restricting food and limiting absorption. The procedure combines restrictive and malabsorptive mechanisms and produces a median loss of approximately 25–30% of initial weight at 3 years (Courcoulas et al., 2015). VSG, introduced in the United States in 2007, involves removing approximately 75% of the stomach, thus bypassing the gastric fundus and body (Schauer et al., 2017). In addition to its restrictive properties, VSG accelerates gastric emptying and dramatically reduces ghrelin levels, a hormone associated with hunger (Sumithran et al., 2011). VSG produces similar or slightly smaller weight losses as compared to RYGB. In a 5-year randomized controlled trial (RCT), Schauer et al. (2017) observed mean losses of 23% and 19% in patients who underwent RYGB vs. VSG, respectively. LAGB is the least invasive surgical procedure and involves placing an inflatable silicone band around the fundus of the stomach, creating a small pouch (Dixon et al., 2008). Saline can be added or removed through a subcutaneous port to adjust the diameter of the band. This is a restrictive procedure, with no changes in gut anatomy or hormones. LAGB results in median weight loss of approximately 15.9% of initial weight at 3 years (Courcoulas et al., 2015).

Comparative Treatment Trials

The most convincing evidence of the superiority of bariatric surgery has come from trials of patients with obesity and type 2 diabetes who were randomly assigned to medical therapy plus lifestyle intervention or medical therapy plus lifestyle intervention and bariatric surgery. Data from three RCTs found that approximately 55–60% of patients who received RYGB lost 25% or more of initial weight at 1 year, as did approximately 45% of those who underwent VSG; 85–95% of these patients, combined together, lost 15% or more of initial weight. With LAGB, 15% of patients lost ≥ 25% of weight, and 62% lost 15% or more, revealing why this therapy has been largely discontinued in the United States in favor of RYGB and VSG. In sharp contrast to surgical procedures, the most comprehensive lifestyle intervention, which used the treatment protocol from the Look AHEAD study, induced a loss ≥ 15% in only 12% of patients and a loss of 25% in only 4% of participants.

The primary outcome in these trials was remission of type 2 diabetes, not weight loss. Here again, bariatric surgery was superior to intensive lifestyle intervention. In the trial by Schauer et al. (2012), for example, the 1-year diabetes remission rates were 42% for RYGB, 37% for VSG, and 12% for medical therapy plus lifestyle modification. A similar difference was observed in the trial by Ikramuddin et al. (2013): 49% of RYGB-treated patients achieved diabetes remission, as compared with 19% for those who received medical care and intensive lifestyle intervention.

Weighing the Risks and Benefits of Bariatric Surgery

Bariatric surgery is associated with a substantially greater risk of serious adverse events, including death, during the first year of treatment than are intensive lifestyle intervention and pharmacotherapy (see Nor Hanipah et al., Chapter 22, this volume). It is also associated with substantially greater short-term costs than these other therapies, including those for rehospitalization and reoperation in a significant minority of patients. Thus, patient and practitioner must carefully review the potential risks of bariatric surgery against the expected benefits for the individual in question.

In 1991, after weighing the risks and benefits of surgery, the National Institutes of Health recommended that bariatric surgery be reserved for individuals with a BMI ≥ 40 kg/m^2 or a BMI ≥ 35 kg/m^2 in the presence of a significant comorbidity (National Institutes of Health, 1991). With the increased safety of surgery in the past decade, many bariatric surgeons and other health professionals believe that surgery should be considered for patients based on its capacity to ameliorate specific diseases, such as type 2 diabetes, with less concern for the patient's specific BMI. This is the case with type 2 diabetes, in particular, because RYGB and VSG are believed to ameliorate glucose metabolism by mechanisms independent of weight loss alone. The International Diabetes Federation has recently proposed that surgery be approved for individuals with this disease and a BMI as low as 30 kg/m^2, who are unable to achieve adequate glucose control with anti-diabetes medications and lifestyle intervention (Rubino et al., 2016). When pursued with caution and the collaboration of a multidisciplinary diabetes team, we believe that this is an appropriate use of bariatric surgery on an experimental basis. Additional safety and efficacy data are needed to confirm the benefits of surgery in this less obese and likely younger population.

Future Directions

The weight loss interventions described in this chapter clearly are of benefit in reducing excess weight and its associated health conditions. However, the treatments—ranging from intensive lifestyle intervention to bariatric surgery—will not be fully useful until they are universally covered by insurers and employers, as argued by Downey and Kyle (Chapter 25, this volume). Few insurers, for example, consistently cover high-intensity lifestyle modification, although it is mandated by the Affordable Care Act. Fewer still cover anti-obesity medications, requiring patients to pay out of pocket, which results in short-term use when chronic care is needed (Heymsfield & Wadden, 2017. Reimbursement of bariatric surgery, by both public and private insurers, has improved markedly over the past decade and serves as a model for expanding coverage for the other established weight reduction therapies.

Even if all of these weight loss therapies were well reimbursed, treatment alone clearly is not the answer to our nation's (or world's) epidemic of overweight and obesity. As discussed by Schwartz and Brownell (Chapter 42, this volume), far greater effort and resources must be directed to the prevention of obesity by addressing the environmental, financial, and socioeconomic factors that have driven the epidemic at a population level over the past 35 years. Bold public policy and legislative initiatives, combined with the sincere efforts of key industries (e.g., food, restaurant, leisure, and advertising) are needed to make healthier eating and physical activity habits the default (i.e., automatic) choice rather than the one that consumers must struggle to make. Individual responsibility for behavior change must be joined with social and institutional responsibility to prevent the development of overweight and obesity and thereby decrease the need for treatments discussed in this chapter.

References

Ackermann, R. T., & Marrero, D. G. (2007). Adapting the Diabetes Prevention Program lifestyle intervention for delivery in the community: The YMCA model. *The Diabetes Educator, 33*(1), 69, 74–75, 77–78.

Ali, M. K., Echouffo-Tcheugui, J., & Williamson, D. F. (2012). How effective were lifestyle interventions in real-world settings that were modeled on the Diabetes Prevention Program? *Health Affairs, 31*(1), 67–75.

American Society for Metabolic and Bariatric Surgery. (2016). *Estimate of bariatric surgery numbers, 2011–2015*. Retrieved February 20, 2017, from *https://asmbs.org/resources/estimate-of-bariatric-surgery-numbers*.

Apovian, C. M., Aronne, L. J., Bessessen, D. H., McDonnell, M. E., Murad, M. H., Pagotto, U., et al. (2015). Pharmacological management of obesity: An Endocrine Society clinical practice guideline. *Journal of Clinical Endocrinology and Metabolism, 100*(2), 342–362.

Appel, L. J., Clark, J. M., Yeh, H. C., Wang, N. Y., Coughlin, J. W., Daumit, G., et al. (2011). Comparative effectiveness of weight-loss interventions in clinical practice. *New England Journal of Medicine, 365*(21), 1959–1968.

Bandini, L. G., Schoeller, D. A., Cyr, H. N., & Dietz, W. H. (1990). Validity of reported energy intake in obese and nonobese adolescents. *American Journal of Clinical Nutrition, 52*(3), 421–425.

Berkowitz, R. I., & Fabricatore, A. N. (2011). Obesity, psychiatric status, and psychiatric medications. *Psychiatric Clinics of North America, 34*(4), 747–764.

Centers for Medicare and Medicaid Services. (2011). Decision memo for intensive behavioral therapy for obesity (CAG-00423N). Retrieved February 20, 2017, from *www.cms.gov/medicare-coverage-database/details/nca-decision-memo.aspx?&NcaName=Intensive%20Behavioral%20Therapy%20for%20Obesity&bc=ACAAAAAAIAAA&NCAId=253*.

Collins, R., Reith, C., Emberson, J., Armitage, J., Baignet, C., Blackwell, L., et al. (2016). Interpretation of the evidence for the efficacy and safety of statin therapy. *Lancet, 388*(10059), 2532–2561.

Courcoulas, A. P., Belle, S. H., Neiberg, R. H., Pierson, S. K., Eagleton, J. K., Kalarchian, M. A., et al. (2015). Three-year outcomes of bariatric surgery vs. lifestyle intervention for type 2 diabetes mellitus treatment: A randomized clinical trial. *JAMA Surgery, 150*(10), 931–940.

Department of Veterans Affairs, Department of Defense. (2014). *VA/DoD clinical practice guideline for screening and management of overweight and obesity*. Retrieved from *www.guideline.gov/summaries/summary/48461/vadod-clinical-practice-guideline-for-screening-and-management-of-overweight-and-obesity*.

Diabetes Prevention Program Research Group, Knowler, W. C., Barrett-Connor, E., Fowler, S. E., Hamman, R. F., Lachin, J. M., et al. (2002). Reduction in the incidence of type 2 diabetes with lifestyle intervention or metformin. *New England Journal of Medicine, 346*(6), 393–403.

Diabetes Prevention Program Research Group, Knowler, W. C., Fowler, S. E., Hamman, R. F., Christophi, C. A., Hoffman, H. J., et al. (2009). 10-year follow-up of diabetes incidence and weight loss in the Diabetes Prevention Program Outcomes Study. *Lancet, 374*(9702), 1677–1686.

Ditschuneit, H. H., Flechtner-Mors, M., Johnson, T. D., & Adler, G. (1999). Metabolic and weight-loss effects of a long-term dietary intervention in obese patients. *American Journal of Clinical Nutrition, 69*(2), 198–204.

Dixon, J. B., O'Brien, P. E., Playfair, J., Chapman, L., Schachter, L. M., Skinner, S., et al. (2008). Adjustable gastric banding and conventional therapy for type 2 diabetes: A randomized controlled trial. *Journal of the American Medical Association, 299*(3) 316–323.

Donnelly, J. E., Goetz, J., Gibson, C., Sullivan, D. K., Lee, R., Smith, B. K., et al. (2013). Equivalent weight loss for weight management programs delivered by phone and clinic. *Obesity, 21*(10), 1951–1959.

Donnelly, J. E., Smith, B. K., Dunn, L., Mayo, M. M., Jacobsen, D. J., Stewart, E. E., et al. (2007). Comparison of a phone vs clinic approach to achieve 10% weight loss. *International Journal of Obesity, 31*(8), 1270–1276.

Dutton, G. R., Nackers, L. M., Dubyak, P. J., Rushing, N. C., Huynh, T. V., Tan, F., et al. (2014). A randomized trial comparing weight loss treatment delivered in large versus small groups. *International Journal of Behavioral Nutrition and Physical Activity, 11*, 123.

Foster, G. D., Wadden, T. A., Makris, A. P., Davidson, D., Sanderson, R. S., Allison, D. B., et al. (2003). Primary care physicians' attitudes about obesity and its treatment. *Obesity Research, 11*(10), 1168–1177.

Garvey, W. T., Mechanick, J. I., Brett, E. M., Garber, A. J., Hurley, D. L., Jastreboff, A. M., et al. (2016). American Association of Clinical Endocrinologists and American College of Endocrinology clinical practice guidelines for comprehensive medical care of patients with obesity: Executive summary. *Endocrine Practice, 22*(Suppl. 3), 1–203.

Gudzune, K. A., Doshi, R. S., Mehta, A. K., Chaudhry, Z. W., Jacobs, D. K., Vakil, R. M., et al. (2015). Efficacy of commercial weight-loss programs: An updated systematic review. *Annals of Internal Medicine, 162*(7), 501–512.

Guyenet, S. J., & Schwartz, M. W. (2012). Clinical review: Regulation of food intake, energy balance, and body fat mass: Implications for the pathogenesis and treatment of obesity. *Journal of Clinical Endocrinology and Metabolism, 97*(3), 745–755.

Harvey-Berino, J., West, D., Krukowski, R., Prewitt, E., VanBiervliet, A., Ashikaga, T., et al. (2010). Internet delivered behavioral obesity treatment. *Preventive Medicine, 51*(2), 123–128.

Hauptman, J., DiGirolamo, M., Foreyt, J. P., Halsted, C. H., Heber, D., et al. (1999). Weight control and risk factor reduction in obese subjects treated for 2 years with orlistat: A randomized controlled trial. *Journal of the American Medical Association, 281*(3), 235–242.

Heshka, S., Anderson, J. W., Atkinson, R. L., Greenway, F. L., Hill, J. O., Phinney, S. D., et al. (2003). Weight loss with self-help compared with a structured commercial program: A randomized trial. *Journal of the American Medical Association, 289*(14), 1792–1798.

Heymsfield, S. B., van Mierlo, C. A., van der Knaap, H. C., Heo, M., & Frier, H. I. (2003). Weight management using a meal replacement strategy: Meta and pooling analysis from six studies. *International Journal of Obesity, 27*(5), 537–549.

Heymsfield, S. B., & Wadden, T. A. (2017). Mechanisms, pathophysiology, and management of obesity. *New England Journal of Medicine, 376*(3), 254–266.

Ikramuddin, S., Korner, J., Lee, W. J., Connett, J. E., Inabnet, W. B., Billington, C. J., et al. (2013). Roux-en-Y gastric bypass vs. intensive medical management for the control of type 2 diabetes, hypertension, and hyperlipidemia: The diabetes surgery study randomized clinical trial. *Journal of the American Medical Association, 309*(21), 2240–2249.

James, W. P., Caterson, I. D., Coutinho, W., Finer, N., Van Gaal, L. F., Maggioni, A. P., et al. (2010). Effect of sibutramine on cardiovascular outcomes in overweight and obese subjects. *New England Journal of Medicine, 363*(10), 905–917.

Jebb, S. A., Ahern, A. L., Olson, A. D., Aston, L. M., Holzapfel, C., Stoll, J., et al. (2011). Primary care referral to a commercial provider for weight loss treatment versus standard care: A randomized controlled trial. *Lancet, 378*(9801), 1485–1492.

Jensen, M. D., Ryan, D. H., Apovian, C. M., Ard, J. D., Comuzzie, A. G., Donato, K. A., et al. (2014). AHA/ACC/TOS guideline for the management of overweight and obesity in adults: A report of the American College of Cardiology/American Heart Association Task Force on Practice Guidelines and The Obesity Society. *Journal of the American College of Cardiology, 63*(25, Pt. B), 2985–3023.

Kramer, C. K., Zinman, B., & Retnakaran, R. (2013). Are metabolically healthy overweight and obesity benign conditions?: A systematic review and meta-analysis. *Annals of Internal Medicine, 159*(11), 758–769.

Laing, B. Y., Mangione, C. M., Tseng, C. H., Leng, M., Vaisberg, E., Mahida, M., et al. (2014). Effectiveness of a smartphone application for weight loss compared with usual care in overweight primary care patients: A randomized, controlled trial. *Annals of Internal Medicine, 161*(10, Suppl.), S5–S12.

Lau, D. C. W., & the Obesity Canada Clinical Practice Guidelines Steering Committee and Expert Panel. (2007). Synopsis of the 2006 Canadian clinical practice guidelines on the management and prevention of obesity in adults and children. *Canadian Medical Association Journal, 176*(8), 1103–1106.

LeBlanc, E., O'Connor, E., Whitlock, E. P., Patnode, C., & Kapka, T. (2011a). *Screening for and management of obesity and overweight in adults* (Evidence Report No 89; AHRQ Publication No. 11–05159-EF-1). Rockville, MD: Agency for Healthcare Research and Quality.

LeBlanc, E. S., O'Connor, E., Whitlock, E. P., Patnode, C. D., & Kapka, T. (2011b). Effectiveness of primary-core relevant treatments for obesity in adults: A systematic evidence review for the Preventive Services Task Force. *Annals of Internal Medicine, 155*(7), 434–447.

Lent, M. R., Vander Veur, S. S., Peters, J. C., Herring, S. J., Wyatt, H. R., Tewksbury, C., et al. (2016). Initial weight goals: Have they changed and do they matter? *Obesity Science and Practice, 2*(2), 154–161.

Lichtman, S. W., Pisarka, K., Berman, E. R., Pestone, M., Dowling, H., Offenbacher, E., et al. (1992). Discrepancy between self-reported and actual caloric intake and exercise in obese subjects. *New England Journal of Medicine, 327*(27), 1893–1898.

Look AHEAD Research Group. (2013). Cardiovascular effects of intensive lifestyle intervention in type 2 diabetes. *New England Journal of Medicine, 369*(2), 145–154.

Look AHEAD Research Group. (2014). Eight-year weight losses with an intensive lifestyle intervention: The Look AHEAD study. *Obesity, 22*(1), 5–13.

Look AHEAD Research Group, Wadden, T. A., West, D. S., Delahanty, L., Jakicic, J., Rejeski, J., et al. (2006). The Look AHEAD study: A description of the lifestyle intervention and the evidence supporting it. *Obesity, 14*(5), 737–752.

Marso, S. P., Bain, S. C., Consoli, A., Eliaschewitz, F. G., Jódar, E., Leiter, L. A., et al. (2016). Semaglutide and cardiovascular outcomes in patients with type 2 diabetes. *New England Journal of Medicine, 375*(19), 1834–1844.

Marso, S. P., Daniels, G. H., Brown-Frandsen, K., Kristensen, P., Mann, J. F., Nauck, M. A., et al. (2016). Liraglutide and cardiovascular outcomes in type 2 diabetes. *New England Journal of Medicine, 375*(4), 311–322.

Mechanick, J. I., Youdim, A., Jones, D. B., Timothy Garvey, W., Hurley, D. L., McMahon, M., et al. (2013). Clinical practice guidelines for the perioperative nutritional, metabolic, and nonsurgical support of the bariatric surgery patient—2013 update: Cosponsored by American Association of Clinical Endocrinologists, the Obesity Society, and American Society for Metabolic and Bariatric Surgery. *Surgery for Obesity and Related Diseases, 9*(2), 159–191.

Moyer, V. A., on behalf of the U.S. Preventive Services Task Force. (2012). Screening for and management of obesity in adults: U.S. Preventive Services Task Force recommendation statement. *Annals of Internal Medicine, 157*(5), 373–378.

National Heart, Lung, and Blood Institute. (1998). Clinical guidelines on the identification, evaluation, and treatment of overweight and obesity in adults: The evidence report. *Obesity Research, 6*(Suppl.), 51S–210S.

National Institute for Health and Care Excellence. (2014). Identification, assessment and management of overweight and obesity in children, young people and adults (NICE Clinical Guideline, No. 189). Retrieved from *www.nice.org.uk/guidance/cg189*.

National Institutes of Health. (1991). Gastrointestinal surgery for severe obesity. *NIH Consensus Statement, 9*(1), 1–20.

Neylan, C. J., Dempsey, D. T., Tewksbury, C. M., Williams, N. N., & Dumon, K. R. (2016). Endoscopic treatment of obesity: A comprehensive review. *Surgery for Obesity and Related Diseases, 12*(5), 1108–1115.

Norén, E., & Forssell, H. (2016). Aspiration therapy for obesity: A safe and effective treatment. *BMC Obesity, 3*, 56.

Ochner, C. N., Tsai, A. G., Kushner, R. F., & Wadden, T. A. (2015). Treating obesity seriously: When recommendations for lifestyle change confront biological adaptations. *Lancet Diabetes and Endocrinology, 3*(4), 232–234.

Orchard, T. J., Temprosa, M., Goldberg, R., Haffner, S., Ratner, R., Marcovina, S., et al. (2005). The effect of metformin and intensive lifestyle intervention on the metabolic syndrome: The Diabetes Prevention Program randomized trial. *Annals of Internal Medicine, 142*(8), 611–619.

Paul-Ebhohimhen, V., & Avenell, A. (2009). A systematic review of the effectiveness of group versus individual treatments for adult obesity. *Obesity Facts, 2*(1), 17–24.

Perri, M. G., Limacher, M. C., von Castel-Roberts, K., Daniel, M. J., Durning, P. E., Janicke, D. M., et al. (2014). Comparative effectiveness of three doses of weight-loss counseling: Two-year findings from the rural LITE trial. *Obesity, 22*(11), 2293–2300.

Pomeranz, J. L., & Brownell, K. D. (2012). Portion sizes and beyond: Government's legal authority to regulate food-industry practices. *New England Journal of Medicine, 367*(15), 1383–1385.

Renjilian, D. A., Perri, M. G., Nezu, A. M., McKelvey, W. F., Shermer, R. L., & Anton, S. D. (2001). Individual versus group therapy for obesity: Effects of matching participants to their treatment preferences. *Journal of Consulting and Clinical Psychology, 69*(4), 717–721.

Rock, C. L., Flatt, S. W., Pakiz, B., Barkai, H. S., Heath, D. D., & Krumhar, K. C. (2016). Randomized clinical trial of portion-controlled prepackaged foods to promote weight loss. *Obesity (Silver Spring), 24*(6), 1230–1237.

Rock, C. L., Flatt, S. W., Sherwood, N. E., Karanja, N., Pakiz, B., & Thomson, C. A. (2010). Effect of a free prepared meal and incentivized weight loss program on weight loss and weight loss maintenance in obese and overweight women: A randomized controlled trial. *Journal of the American Medical Association, 304*(16), 1803–1810.

Rosenbaum, M., & Leibel, R. L. (2016). Models of energy homeostasis in response to maintenance of reduced body weight. *Obesity (Silver Spring), 24*(8), 1620–1629.

Rubino, F., Nathan, D. M., Eckel, R. H., Schauer, P. R., Alberti, K. G., Zimmet, P. Z., et al. (2016). Metabolic surgery in the treatment algorithm for type 2 diabetes: A joint statement by international diabetes organizations. *Diabetes Care, 39*(6), 861–877.

Schauer, P. R., Bhatt, D. L., Kirwan, J. P., Wolski, K., Aminian, A., Brethauer, S. A., et al. (2017). Bariatric surgery versus intensive medical therapy for diabetes: 5-year outcomes. *New England Journal of Medicine, 376*(7), 641–651.

Schauer, P. R., Kashyap, S. R., Wolski, K., Brethauer,

S. A., Kirwan, J. P., Pothier, C. E., et al. (2012). Bariatric surgery versus intensive medical therapy in obese patients with diabetes. *New England Journal of Medicine, 366*(17), 1567–1576.

Sharma, A. M., & Kushner, R. F. (2009). A proposed clinical staging system for obesity. *International Journal of Obesity, 33,* 289–295.

Sjöström, C. D., Lissner, L., Wedel, H., & Sjöström, L. (1999). Reduction in incidence of diabetes, hypertension and lipid disturbances after intentional weight loss induced by bariatric surgery: The SOS intervention study. *Obesity Research, 7*(5), 477–484.

Smith, S. R., Weisman, N. J., Anderson, C. M., Sanchez, M., Chuang, E., Stubbe, S., et al (2010). *New England Journal of Medicine, 363*(3), 245–256.

SPRINT Research Group, Wright, J. T., Jr., Williamson, J. D., Whelton, P. K., Snyder, J. K., Sink, K. M., et al. (2015). A randomized trial of intensive versus standard blood-pressure control. *New England Journal of Medicine, 373*(22), 2103–2116.

Steinberg, D. M., Tate, D. F., Bennett, G. G., Ennett, S., Samuel-Hodge, C., & Ward, D. S. (2013). The efficacy of a daily self-weighing weight loss intervention using smart scales and e-mail. *Obesity, 21*(9), 1789–1797.

Sumithran, P., Prendergast, L. A., Delbridge, E., Purcell, K., Shulkes, A., Kriketos, A., et al. (2011). Long-term persistence of hormonal adaptations to weight loss. *New England Journal of Medicine, 365*(17), 1597–1604.

Svetkey, L. P., Batch, B. C., Lin, P. H., Intille, S. S., Corsino, L., Tyson, C. C., et al. (2015). *Obesity, 23*(11), 2133–2141.

Svetkey, L. P., Stevens, V. J., Brantley, P. J., Appel, L. J., Hollis, J. F., Loria, C. M., et al. (2008). Comparison of strategies for sustaining weight loss: The weight loss maintenance randomized controlled trial. *Journal of the American Medical Association, 299*(10), 1139–1148.

Thomas, J. G., Leahey, T. M., & Wing, R. R. (2015). An automated internet behavioral weight-loss program by physician referral: A randomized controlled trial. *Diabetes Care, 38*(1), 9–15.

Torgerson, J. S., Hauptman, J., Boldrin, M. N., & Sjöström, L. (2004). XENical in the prevention of diabetes in obese subjects (XENDOS) study: A randomized study of orlistat as an adjunct to lifestyle changes for the prevention of type 2 diabetes in obese patients. *Diabetes Care, 27*(1), 155–161.

Tsai, A. G., & Wadden, T. A. (2006). The evolution of very-low calorie diets: An update and meta-analysis. *Obesity, 14*(8), 1283–1293.

van der Klaauw, A. A., & Farooqi, I. S. (2015). The hunger genes: Pathways to obesity. *Cell 161*(1), 119–132.

Volger, S., Vetter, M. L., Dougherty, M., Panigrahi, E., Egner, R., Webb, V., et al. (2012). Patients' preferred terms for describing their excess weight: Discussing obesity in clinical practice. *Obesity, 20*(1), 147–150.

Wadden, T. A. (1993). Treatment of obesity by moderate and severe caloric restriction: Results of clinical research trials. *Annals of Internal Medicine, 119*(7, Pt. 2), 688–693.

Wadden, T. A., & Bartlett, S. J. (1992). Very low-calorie diets: An overview and appraisal. In T. A. Wadden & T. B. VanItallie (Eds.), *Treatment of the seriously obese patient* (pp. 44–79). New York: Guilford Press.

Wadden, T. A., Berkowitz, R. I., Sarwer, D. B., Prus-Wisniewski, R., & Steinberg, C. (2001). Benefits of lifestyle modification in the pharmacologic treatment of obesity: A randomized trial. *Archives of Internal Medicine, 161*(2), 218–227.

Wadden, T. A., Berkowitz, R. I., Vogt, R. A., Steen, S. N., Stunkard, A. J., & Foster, G. D. (1997). Lifestyle modification in the pharmacologic treatment of obesity: A pilot investigation of a potential primary care approach. *Obesity Research, 5*(3), 218–226.

Wadden, T. A., Berkowitz, R. I., Womble, L. G., Sarwer, D. B., Phelan, S., Cato, R. K., et al. (2005). Randomized trial of lifestyle modification and pharmacotherapy for obesity. *New England Journal of Medicine, 353*(20), 2111–2120.

Wadden, T. A., & Didie, E. (2003). What's in a name?: Patients' preferred terms for describing obesity. *Obesity Research, 11*(9), 1140–1146.

Wadden, T. A., Faulconbridge, L. F., Jones-Corneille, L. R., Sarwer, D. B., Fabricatore, A. N., Thomas, J. G., et al. (2011). Binge eating disorder and the outcome of bariatric surgery at one year: A prospective, observational study. *Obesity, 19*(6), 1220–1228.

Wadden, T. A., Foreyt, J. P., Foster, G. D., Hill, J. O., Klein, S., O'Neil, P. M., et al. (2011). Weight loss with naltrexone SR/bupropion SR combination therapy as an adjunct to behavior modification: The COR-BMOD trial. *Obesity, 19*(1), 110–120.

Wadden, T. A., Foster, G. D., & Letizia, K. A. (1994). One-year behavioral treatment of obesity: Comparison of moderate and severe caloric restriction and the effects of weight maintenance therapy. *Journal of Consulting and Clinical Psychology, 62*(1), 165–171.

Wadden, T. A., Foster, G. D., Sarwer, D. B., Anderson, D. A., Gladis, M., Sanderson, R. S., et al. (2004). Dieting and the development of eating disorders in obese women: Results of a randomized controlled trial. *American Journal of Clinical Nutrition, 80*(3), 560–568.

Wadden, T. A., Hollander, P., Klein, S., Niswender, K., Woo, V., Hale, P. M., et al. (2013). Weight maintenance and additional weight loss with liraglutide after low-calorie-diet-induced weight loss: The SCALE Maintenance randomized study. *International Journal of Obesity, 37*(11), 1443–1451.

Wadden, T. A., Sternberg, J. A., Letizia, K. A., Stunkard, A. J., & Foster, G. D. (1989). Treatment of obesity by very low calorie diet, behavior therapy, and their combination: A five-year perspective. *International Journal of Obesity, 13*(Suppl. 2), 39–46.

Wadden, T. A., Vogt, R. A., Andersen, R. E., Bartlett, S. J., Foster, G. D., Kuehnel, R. H., et al. (1997). Exercise in the treatment of obesity: Effects of four interventions on body composition, resting energy expenditure, appetite, and mood. *Journal of Consulting and Clinical Psychology, 65*(2), 269–277.

Wadden, T. A., Volger, S., Sarwer, D. B., Vetter, M. L., Tsai, A. G., Berkowitz, R. I., et al. (2011). A two-year randomized trial of obesity treatment in primary care practice. *New England Journal of Medicine, 365*(21), 1969–1979.

Wadden, T. A., West, D. S., Neiberg, R. H., Wing, R. R., Ryan, D. H., Johnson, K. C., et al. (2009). One-year weight losses in the Look AHEAD study: Factors associated with success. *Obesity, 17*(4), 713–722.

Webb, V. L., & Wadden, T. A. (2017). Intensive lifestyle intervention for obesity: Principles, practices, and results. *Gastroenterology, 152*(7), 1752–1764.

Wing, R. R., Espeland, M. A., Clark, J. M., Hazuda, H. P., Knowler, W. C., Pownall, H. J., et al. (2016). Association of weight loss maintenance and weight regain on 4-year changes in CVD risk factors: The Action for Health in Diabetes (Look AHEAD) clinical trial. *Diabetes Care, 39*(8), 1345–1355.

Wing, R. R., & Phelan, S. (2005). Long-term weight loss maintenance. *American Journal of Clinical Nutrition, 82*(1, Suppl.), 222S–225S.

World Health Organization. (1998). *Obesity: Preventing and managing the global epidemic.* Geneva, Switzerland: Author.

Yanovski, S. Z., & Yanovski, J. A. (2014). Long-term drug treatment for obesity: A systematic and clinical review. *Journal of the American Medical Association, 311*(1), 74–86.

Yanovski, S. Z., & Yanovski, J. A. (2015). Naltrexone extended-release plus bupropion extended-release for treatment of obesity. *Journal of the American Medical Association, 313*(12), 1213–1214.

CHAPTER 18

Dietary Treatment of Overweight and Obesity

Arne Astrup

The dietary goal for overweight and obese patients is to decrease energy intake while avoiding increased hunger between meals and maintaining the duration of the satiating effect of the diet. Moreover, the reduction in dietary energy intake should not compromise nutritional adequacy. Due to their enlarged body size, obese individuals have higher energy requirements for a given level of physical activity than their normal-weight counterparts. Reducing the obese patient's total energy intake to that of a normal-weight individual will inevitably cause weight loss, consisting of about 75% fat and 25% lean tissue, until weight normalization occurs at a new energy equilibrium. However, there is increasing evidence to suggest that reduced-obese individuals have lower energy expenditure than comparable never-obese individuals, and hence lower energy requirements than predicted by their body size and composition (Astrup et al., 1999; Knuth et al., 2014). This difference can be attributed to a physiological adaptation to reduced obesity involving suppressed sympathoadrenal activity, thyroid function, and lowered leptin levels. However, the energy requirements are only modestly reduced (i.e., by 5–10%).

The larger the daily deficit in energy balance, the more rapid the weight loss. A deficit of 300–500 kcal/day will produce a weight loss of 300–500 g/week, and a deficit of 500–1,000 kcal/day will produce a weight loss of 500–1,000 g/week (0.5–1.0 kg). Total energy expenditure declines and normalizes along with weight loss. Thus, total energy intake should gradually be reduced further to maintain the energy deficit. An alternative approach is to take advantage of the differences in the satiating power of the various dietary components in order to cause a spontaneous reduction in energy intake. This is the principle of the *ad libitum* higher-protein, low-glycemic-index (low-GI) or low-glycemic-load (low-GL) diets, as well as of the low-carbohydrate diets.

Choosing the Dietary Energy Deficit

The initial target of a weight loss program should be to decrease body weight by 10%. Once this is achieved, a new target can be set. However, patients with unrealistically high weight loss expectations should not be instructed to slow their weight loss rate and lower their goals, as these individuals tend to be more successful than those with more modest weight loss expectations (Casazza et al., 2013, 2015). Patients will generally want to lose more weight, and greater initial weight loss is associated with better long-term success. However, it should be remembered that even a 5–10% weight reduction improves risk factors and risk of comorbidities. Several factors should be taken into consideration, including the patient's degree of obesity, previous weight loss attempts, risk factors, comorbidities, and personal and social capacity to undertake the necessary lifestyle changes.

Theoretical Weight Loss versus Clinical Outcome

Translating the physiologically based considerations regarding energy balance and weight loss into clinical practice requires a high degree of compliance, which can be difficult to obtain. Adherence to the diet is the cornerstone of successful weight loss and the most complicated element of dietary management. In order to improve adherence, consideration should be given to the patient's food preferences, as well as to personal, educational, and social factors. Great efforts should be made to see the patient frequently and regularly.

Furthermore, long-term weight reduction is unlikely to succeed unless the patient actually changes eating and physical activity habits, and learns to cope with other obesity-promoting lifestyles, such as too little or impaired sleep, mental stress, and obesity-promoting medications.

Even with a high degree of compliance to the energy restriction, it can be difficult to predict weight loss trajectory and outcome in terms of effect size. The commonly used 7,000 kcal/kg weight loss rule (3,500 kcal/pound) is misleading and leads to overestimation of predicted weight loss in individuals and populations (Casazza et al., 2013). The most serious error of the 7,000-kcal rule is its failure to account for dynamic changes in energy balance that occur during loss and gain of weight. Moreover, it assumes that weight loss will continue without reaching a plateau. During weight loss, resting energy expenditure (REE) is reduced mainly due to the reduction in lean body mass, and the cost of movement and exercise is reduced due to the lower body weight. However, smaller adaptive reductions also occur.

A new, revised mathematical model, which takes the changes in energy requirements into consideration, predicts that every permanent 10-kcal change in caloric intake/day will lead to an eventual weight change of 0.45 kg (1 pound) when the body weight reaches a new steady state (~100 kJ/day/kg of weight change) (Sanghvi, Redman, Martin, Ravussin, & Hall, 2015). It will take nearly 1 year to achieve 50% and ~3 years to achieve 95% of the final steady-state weight loss. This model also eliminates the idea that small lifestyle changes producing small deficits in energy balance will lead to large weight losses over time. Older models suggested that an overweight or obese person should expend an additional daily 100 kcal by walking 1 mile a day, which would result in a weight loss of 23 kg (50 pounds) over 5 years. However, the resulting weight loss, as predicted by the new model, is only 4.5 kg (10 pounds) over 5 years. Moreover, even the revised model gives an optimistic assessment of weight change because it does not account for the potential active compensation in energy intake that occurs when physical activity is increased.

Options for Weight Loss Diets: Level of Energy Restriction

Therapeutic obesity diets distinguish between several recognized weight reduction regimens. Diets based on different levels of energy restriction are described in this section.

Very-Low-Energy Diets

Starvation (less than 200 kcal/day) is the ultimate dietary treatment of obesity, but it is no longer used because of the numerous and serious medical complications associated with prolonged starvation. Starvation has been replaced by very-low-energy diets (VLEDs, 200–800 kcal/day), which aim to supply very little energy while still providing all essential nutrients. The safety of these diets has been questioned, and today the 800 kcal/day VLED is the only version recognized as being both effective and safe. These diets are usually provided in the form of nutrition powders or in the form of protein, mineral, trace element, and vitamin enriched meals or drinks. VLEDs can induce very rapid weight loss over a 2- to 3-month period. The typical weight loss distribution after 8 weeks in obese individuals prescribed an 800–1,000 kcal/day diet, mainly based on meal replacements, is shown in Figure 18.1.

By themselves, VLEDs are not educational, nor do they facilitate the gradual modification of the patient's eating behavior, nutritional knowledge, and weight control skills, all of which seem to be required for long-term weight maintenance. However, after the initial weight loss achieved with a VLED, weight maintenance can be facilitated by using single-meal replacements (Casazza et al., 2015).

Low-Energy Diets

Low-energy diets (LEDs) usually provide 800–1,500 kcal/day and normally consist of natural, conventional foods, but may also include one to four meal replacement products per day. Although the macronutrient composition of the diet is of less importance for short-term weight loss, it is now usually modified to maximize the beneficial effect on cardiovascular risk factors and insulin resistance and to prevent cancers. This modification may also promote long-term weight maintenance. For practical reasons, LEDs are moderate-fat, higher-protein diets, with reduced refined carbohydrates (high GI) and a fixed energy allowance. A patient may choose an energy level of 1,000–1,200 kcal/day (for women) or 1,200–1,500 kcal/day (for men). LEDs produce a lower rate of weight loss than VLEDs, but randomized controlled trials (RCTs) demonstrate that the long-term (>1 year) weight loss is not different from that of the VLED (Tsai & Wadden, 2006). Furthermore, using LEDs for weight loss induction introduces healthy eating habits early in the weight reduction program, giving a longer period in which to familiarize the patient with the dietary changes that are a central element in a weight maintenance program.

Intermittent or Alternate-Day Fasting Diets

Intermittent fasting, which is also known as alternate-day fasting, is a relatively new and popular approach to weight management that involves interspersing normal daily caloric intake with a short period of severe calorie restriction. It has been claimed to be superior to conventional diets, both in terms of weight loss efficacy and in improvements in cardiometabolic risk factors (Harvie & Howell, 2017). Intermittent fasting involves the intermittent use of a VLED. There are still questions about the side effects of this approach, whether there is an optimal fasting pattern or calorie limit, and how sustainable this strategy is for long-term weight management.

Intermittent fasting has recently gained much popularity following significant media attention. One intermittent fasting approach is the "5:2 diet," which involves 5 days of habitual eating interchanged with 2 days of a VLED (maximum 500 kcal for women and 600 kcal for men). Other intermittent fasting patterns, such as alternate-day fasting, are also used. Despite the recent popularity of intermittent fasting and the much-publicized weight loss claims associated with this approach, the evidence base in humans remains small, and there is only one published systematic review examining the health benefits of this approach. The current evidence suggests that this option can be regarded as a safe alternative for obese patients who find the approach attractive and effective. However, the claim that it produces superior adherence to the energy restriction, as well as weight loss beyond what could be expected

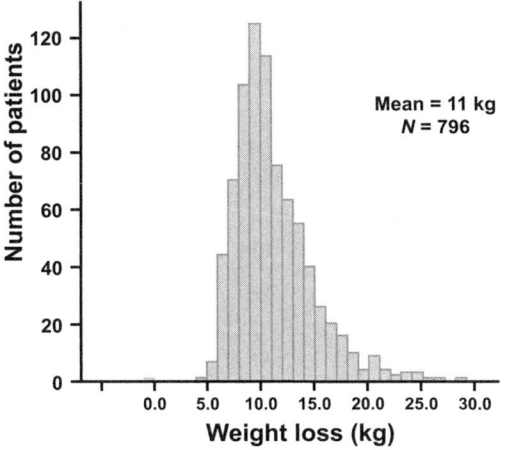

FIGURE 18.1. Weight loss achieved in 8 weeks in 796 obese patients who followed an 800–1,000 kcal/day very-low-energy diet using mainly meal replacements. Data from Larsen et al. (2010).

from the energy deficit, is unsubstantiated (Seimon et al., 2015).

Personalized Diets: One Diet Does Not Fit All

It is generally recognized that certain diets are more obesity promoting than others, and this is the basis for dietary recommendations aimed at preventing weight gain and obesity. There is no consensus about all elements, but most professionals would agree upon advice such as decreasing the intake of sugar-rich soft drinks and of energy-dense fast foods characterized by a high fat content and starchy carbohydrates with low fiber and whole-grain content. In addition, increasing the intake of nutrient-dense foods moderate in fat and higher in protein, fiber, and whole grains may lead to a spontaneous reduction in total energy intake and, thus, promote weight loss. The same principles are reflected in diets for weight loss. Changing diet composition can be a very effective tool for enhancing satiety and reducing spontaneous energy intake. However, there seems to be substantial variability in individual responsiveness to the different diets. So far, mapping of obesity genes has produced very limited advantages for the majority of obese patients. Carriers of the obesity promoting allele of the *FTO* gene are typically around 3 kg heavier than those without, but they do not have an impaired weight loss response to diet, exercise, obesity drugs, or bariatric surgery (Livingstone et al., 2016). Some promising genetic markers are listed in Table 18.1 (Heianza et al., 2016; Mattei, Qi, Hu, Sacks, & Qi, 2012; Stocks et al., 2013). Additional examples of the influence of various genes are shown in the review by Bray and Siri-Torino (2016).

Recent discoveries have identified pretreatment biomarkers that make it possible to select more effective diets for obese individuals based on simple fasting plasma glucose concentrations. The concept is based on the observation that normal insulin sensitivity and secretion is required for postprandial glucose uptake in the brain to produce satiety according to the glucostatic appetite control mechanism. It means that dietary carbohydrates exert a normal satiety signal in the normoglycemic obese individual, whereas increasing CNS insulin resistance limits glucose uptake and carbohydrate-induced satiety is gradually attenuated when moving from the normoglycemic to the prediabetic and further to the type 2 diabetic obese. Prediabetic and particularly type 2 diabetics are more likely prone to overeat on carbohydrate-rich diets, whereas diets with less carbohydrate and more protein and fat in these patients tend to rely on satiety signals such as the gastrointestinal satiety hormones (i.e., GLP-1 and PYY). This individualized diet therapy based on glucose metabolic status has proved effective in causing and maintaining weight loss in reanalyses of a number of clinical trials (Hjorth, Ritz, et al., 2017; Hjorth, Due, Larsen, & Astrup, 2017), and has contributed to understanding why low-fat diets may be more effective in some trials (predominantly normoglycemic obese), whereas low-carbohydrate diets are more effective in other trials (mainly type 2 diabetic obese subjects). For obese subjects with pre-diabetes, lower glycemic load diet with

TABLE 18.1. Examples of Potential Genetic Markers of Weight Loss Responsiveness on Diets with Different Macronutrient Composition

Genetic variant		Low fat/high carbohydrate	Low carbohydrate/ high fat	High protein	Low protein
TCFF7L2 (rs1225537)	TT	−9.5 [−5.0]	−4.8 [−2.0]		
TFAP2B (rs987237)	AA			−0.9	+1.5
	GG			+1.2	−1.4
FGF21 (rs838147)	C Carrier	−0.2 [−1.3]	+1.5 [+1.9]		

Note. Weight change (kg) and [fat loss].

high-fiber and whole-grain produce greater weight loss and maintenance.

Limitations of Randomized Dietary Intervention Trials

Evidence of the effects on body weight of diets with different macronutrient compositions, glycemic index, fiber and whole-grain contents stems mainly from mechanistic studies and RCTs, as it is difficult to get a true picture of these effects from longitudinal, observational studies. Results of numerous such RCTs are discussed in the next section. However, nutrition-related clinical trials also have major limitations arising from the difficulties in maintaining dietary adherence over the long term, the inherent complexity of diet change (in which changes in one dietary factor characteristically produce changes in others), variable background diet, and limited power to examine hard outcomes. Whereas pharmacological trials may require participants to do little more than take a drug or placebo, nutrition studies often demand alteration in food purchasing, food preparation, and eating behaviors. Unlike much industry-sponsored pharmacological research, diet studies rarely have multimillion-dollar annual budgets and the resources to properly support fundamental lifestyle changes. Indeed, most long-term behavioral diet studies suffer from poor treatment fidelity and differentiation between treatment groups, and consequently cannot provide a rigorous test of study hypotheses. One would not reject a promising treatment for Alzheimer's disease based on a null clinical trial if patients in the treatment group failed to take the drug as intended. Yet this leap is routinely made in the field of nutrition (Ludwig, Astrup, & Willett, 2015).

In contrast to behavioral diet trials, feeding studies aim to achieve better compliance within a sample of strongly motivated participants by providing meals prepared in a highly controlled setting. This study design can provide important insights into physiological mechanisms, but may lack generalizability to broad populations over the long term. Furthermore, the cost and logistical challenges of feeding studies usually limits duration to weeks or a few months, necessitating use of surrogate endpoints.

Diets with Different Macronutrient Distributions

Ad Libitum Lower-Fat Diets (25–30% Energy from Fat)

Data from animal and experimental research, observational studies, and RCTs have shown that a high dietary fat content plays some role in the development of obesity (Yu-Poth et al., 1999; Astrup, Ryan, et al., 2000) (Figures 18.2A and 18.2B). A high-fat diet has been shown to promote weight gain and obesity in many experimental studies, both in animals and in humans. The main mechanism seems to be passive overconsumption of energy, but it is difficult to disentangle the causal role of factors such as high-energy density, lower contents of fiber and whole grains, and other traits of fatty diets and foods. Lower-fat diets can be more satiating providing that the fat is replaced by protein and, to some extent, by more satiating carbohydrates—that is, low-GI carbohydrates, high-fiber foods, and whole grains. Low-fat diets in which fat is replaced by refined starch and simple carbohydrates will produce little or no weight loss and have adverse effects on cardiovascular risk factors. A meta-analysis of *ad libitum* low-fat interventions lasting >2 months found a weight loss difference of 3.3 kg (Astrup, Grunwald, Melanson, Saris, & Hill, 2000; Jéquier & Bray, 2002).

The lower-fat diet (25–30% of energy) is clinically relevant for obese patients who habitually consume a high-fat diet (35–50% of energy), but for the majority of the obese population, only a modest reduction in dietary fat content is possible. More emphasis should be put on nonfat dietary components—such as reduction of soft drinks and modification of protein, glycemic index, fiber, and whole grains—and on quality, in order to ensure the lowest cardiovascular risk profile.

Evidence supports that lower-fat diets are most effective among insulin-sensitive obese individuals with a low or impaired fat oxidation capacity. By contrast, these diets have little or no weight effect in more insulin-resistant individuals with obesity and impaired insulin-mediated glucose uptake (see the Personalized Diets section). Lower-fat diets may even have an adverse effect in such individuals.

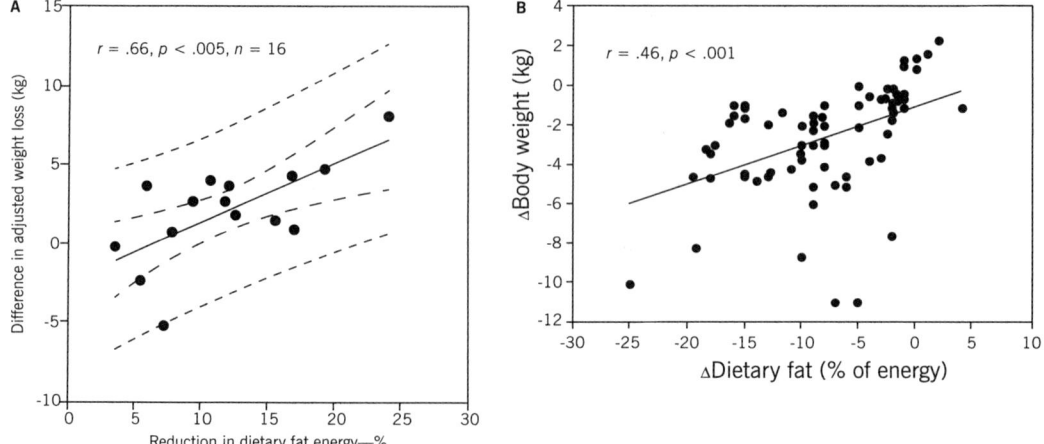

FIGURE 18.2. (A) The unweighted association between study means of difference in weight loss, adjusted for pretreatment body weight and change in percentage of dietary energy from fat. The weight loss and the change in percentage of dietary fat are calculated as the difference between mean changes in intervention and control groups. From Astrup et al. (2000). Reprinted by permission. (B) Correlation between changes (Δ) in body weight and changes in dietary total fat and energy intake and between changes in energy intake and dietary total fat. Pearson correlation coefficients (*r*) are significant for all correlations. From Yu-Poth, Zhao, Etherton, Naglak, Jonnalagadda, and Kris-Etherton (1999). Effects of the National Cholesterol Education Program's Step I and Step II dietary intervention programs on cardiovascular disease risk factors: A meta-analysis. *American Journal of Clinical Nutrition, 69*(4), 632–646. Reprinted by permission.

Ad Libitum Low-Carbohydrate Diets

Low-fat diets with higher protein have previously been recommended as the optimal weight loss diet. Numerous RCTs have been endeavored to assess their efficacy and safety. Many low-carbohydrate diets consist of an initial phase that restricts carbohydrate intake to < 50 g/day (~20% of energy), gradually increasing carbohydrate content to 30–40% as weight loss is achieved. The weight loss results in improvements in all cardiovascular and diabetes risk factors, but the major issue is whether the patient can adhere to a diet that dramatically reduces or almost eliminates all starchy and sugary carbohydrates over the long term. The low-carbohydrate intake depletes glycogen stores, and the patient develops "anorexia of starvation," also known from VLEDs. This is believed to be a partial mechanism behind the satiety effect and the spontaneous reduction in energy intake that results from this diet. There might be a slight thermogenic effect of this diet, but the effect size is too small to have clinical relevance (Hall et al., 2016). However, when starchy carbohydrates are restricted, meal plans typically increase the content of satiating high-protein foods and fiber-rich vegetables with low-energy density.

A number of meta-analyses of RCTs have compared low-fat with low-carbohydrate diets. They generally have found that low-carbohydrate diets are superior in producing weight loss in the short term, but the difference seems to diminish over time (Sackner-Bernstein, Kantner, & Kaul, 2015; Tobias et al., 2015; Mansoor, Vinknes, Veierød, & Retterstøl, 2016). One meta-analysis concluded that after 6 months, weight loss for participants on a low-carbohydrate diet was only 1.4 kg greater than on a low-fat diet. At 12 months the difference was only 0.8 kg.

Higher-Protein Diets

The normally recommended level of protein in the diet is determined by the minimum required to maintain nitrogen balance. However, there is some evidence that higher levels of dietary protein could help prevent and treat disorders such as obesity, metabolic syndrome, and type 2 diabetes. The literature on RCTs is inconsistent regarding the efficacy of higher-protein diets, rendering this topic contentious.

A higher-protein content is a feature of most lower-fat and lower-carbohydrate diets. Low-carbohydrate, high-fat diets are also much higher in protein, just as higher-protein diets are lower in carbohydrate, and in some cases, also lower in fat.

Short-term studies have illustrated the mechanisms by which higher-protein intake promotes negative fat balance and reduction of body fat stores. Protein generally exerts a greater satiety effect than other macronutrients, whether in drinks or in solid foods. There is accumulating evidence that this satiation is partly mediated by a synergistic effect of the satiety hormones glucagon-like peptide-1 (GLP-1) and peptide YY (PYY) released from the small intestine (Belza et al., 2013; see Figure 18.3). The thermic effect of protein is also greater than that of carbohydrate or fat (Mikkelsen, Toubro, & Astrup, 2000). During weight loss, higher-protein diets preserve lean body tissue, the major determinant of resting and 24-hour energy expenditure, curbing reduction in energy expenditure. This is particularly significant when higher-protein diets are combined with physical training.

A major study conducted in United States, the POUNDS Lost (Preventing Overweight Using Novel Dietary Strategies) trial, found similar weight loss after 6 months and 2 years among participants assigned to four diets that differed in their proportions of energy from the three major macronutrients (Sacks et al., 2009). The diets were low or high in total fat (20 or 40%) with normal or high protein (15 or 25%). Carbohydrate content ranged from 35 to 65% of calories. The diets all used the same calorie reduction goals and were low in saturated fat and high in dietary fiber. On average, participants lost 6–7 kg after 6 months and ~5 kg after 2 years. The results indicate that energy restriction is more important for induction of weight loss than macronutrient composition. The results provide clinicians with different options, allowing obese individuals to choose an approach that they are most likely to sustain and is most suited to their personal preferences and health needs.

Mediterranean Diet and Similar Regional Diets

A Mediterranean diet restricted to an energy intake of 1,500 kcal/day for women and 1,800 kcal/day for men, with a goal of no more than 35% of calories from fat, has been found to produce greater weight loss than a similarly energy-restricted low-fat diet in

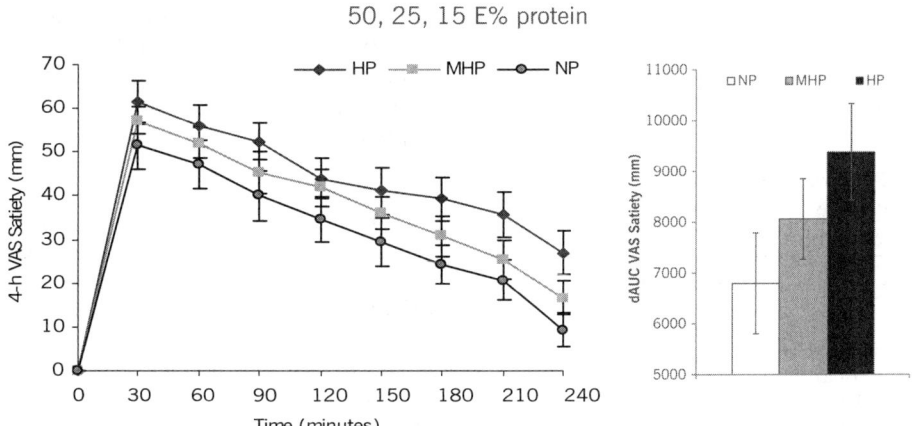

FIGURE 18.3. Replacement of carbohydrate for protein increases satiety in a dose-dependent manner. E%, energy percentage; VAS, visual analogue scale; HP, high protein; MHP, medium high protein; NP, normal protein. From Belza et al. (2013). Reprinted by permission.

some, but not all, studies (Shai et al., 2009; Astrup, 2008). In an RCT, the Mediterranean diet was found to be just as effective as an Atkins type of low-carbohydrate, *ad libitum* (non-calorie-restricted) diet aimed to provide 20 g of carbohydrates/day for the 2-month induction phase, with a gradual increase to a maximum of 120 g/day to maintain the weight loss (Shai et al., 2009).

After 2 years, the mean weight loss was 2.9 kg for the low-fat group, 4.4 kg for the Mediterranean-diet group, and 4.7 kg for the low-carbohydrate group (Shai et al., 2009). Similar results have been found with another regional diet based on very similar foods groups (see Table 18.2).

The new Nordic diet (NND) is a gastronomically driven regional, organic, and environmentally friendly diet. It was tested in a carefully controlled RCT, in a free-living setting, in individuals with abdominal obesity (Poulsen et al., 2014). The subjects were randomly assigned to receive either the NND (high in fruit, vegetables, whole grains, and fish) or an average Danish diet (ADD; a diet with fewer fruits, berries, and vegetables, and higher in meat and refined carbohydrates) for 6 months. Participants received cookbooks and all foods *ad libitum* and free of charge by using a shop model with no caloric restriction. The weight change was −4.7 kg for the NND and −1.5 kg for the ADD. The concept of using diets based on whole foods providing more fiber, whole grain, and less energy-dense content, without special emphasis, is gaining increasing attention and offers another option for weight loss and perhaps particularly for weight maintenance diets.

TABLE 18.2. Similarities and Differences between the New Nordic Diet and the Mediterranean Diet

Similarities	Differences
Both diets call for more vegetables, fruit, whole grains, fish, nonanimal proteins, moderate consumption of low-fat dairy, less meat and fewer sweets, and avoidance of processed food.	The Nordic diet uses rapeseed oil instead of olive oil, ramsons instead of garlic, buckthorn instead of lemon, etc.

GI and GL

An appreciable body of evidence supports the hypothesis that a reduced carbohydrate intake can enhance weight loss, though probably only in a subset of the obese subjects with insulin resistance (Chaput, Tremblay, Rimm, Bouchard & Ludwig, 2008; Ebbeling, Leidig, Feldman, Lovesky & Ludwig, 2007; Hron, Ebbeling, Feldman, & Ludwig, 2015). This does not mean that carbohydrates should be avoided in this group of patients. Carbohydrates that are present in different foods have distinct physiological effects, including differences in rate of digestion and absorption, thereby influencing appetite (hunger and satiety), fuel partitioning, metabolic rate, and postprandial glycaemia and insulinemia. The glycemic qualities of carbohydrates—defined by their GI and GL—are most relevant to insulin-resistant individuals who are overweight and at increased risk of diabetes. The GI is a food classification derived from the postprandial blood glucose response relative to a reference food, gram for gram of carbohydrate. The GL—the mathematical product of the GI and the amount of carbohydrate per serving—encapsulates both the quality and quantity of a carbohydrate, and is the single best predictor of postprandial glycaemia.

In overweight and insulin-resistant individuals, glycemic spikes and insulin demand are excessively increased. A meta-analysis of 24 prospective cohort studies with 7.5 million person-years of follow-up indicated that high dietary GL was positively associated with a 1.45-fold higher relative risk of type 2 diabetes per 100 g increment in GL. Meta-analyses of RCTs indicate that *ad libitum* low-GI and/or low-GL diets promote faster weight loss and greater loss of body fat than do conventional diets (Augustin et al., 2015). Whereas most diets exert their effect on energy balance via effects on appetite and rewarding systems, and hence work through effects on spontaneous energy intake, some diets may also affect energy expenditure and loss of energy by the stools.

Reduced energy expenditure following a period of weight loss is thought to contribute to weight regain. Studies have shown that the drop in REE is greatest for conventional low-fat diets (205 kcal/day, on average) and least for low-GI or low-GL diets (138–166 kcal/day) (Agus, Swain, Larson, Eckert, & Ludwig, 2000).

Individual Responsiveness to Weight Loss on Low-GI/GL Diets

Ebbeling et al. (2007) assigned 73 subjects to either a low-fat (55% carbohydrate and 20% fat) diet or a GL diet (40% carbohydrate and 35% fat), with no prescribed energy restriction (subjects could eat to satisfy appetite) (Ebbeling et al., 2007; Ludwig et al., 2015). The study found no difference in weight loss between the groups after 6 months of intervention or at the 18-month follow-up. However, there were differing responses in those with higher versus lower insulin concentrations—a marker of insulin resistance. Among the obese subjects with a high 30-minute insulin level following an oral glucose tolerance test, the low GL diet produced a much greater decrease in weight compared with the conventional low-fat diet. The diets produced similar results in those with low 30-minute insulin levels.

In another study, 21 overweight individuals were assigned to one of three diets with different levels of GL for 4 weeks each (Ebbeling et al., 2012). Again, those with high 30-minute insulin levels responded differently to those with low 30-minute insulin levels. Those with high insulin lost more fat tissue on the lower-GL diets. There were also differences in resting metabolic rate that favored the low-GL diets. These studies were relatively small, but the same phenomenon has also been observed in large observational studies. For example, in the Quebec Family Study 30-minute insulin levels were found to predict weight change over the subsequent 6-year observation period (Chaput et al., 2008). Subjects with the highest 30-minute insulin levels had the largest weight gain, and the effect was most pronounced among people consuming a high-GL diet. These studies support the concept that insulin-resistant individuals are more likely to lose weight on diets with reductions in carbohydrate content and GI than insulin-sensitive obese individuals.

Added Sugar and Sugar-Sweetened Beverages

A topic that continues to dominate the obesity debate is the role of sugar consumption in weight gain. The term *sugar* can refer to added or refined sugars, but scientifically it covers both naturally occurring and added sugars because the body is unable to distinguish between different sources. Theoretically, a diet that is high in sugar(s) may result in the suppression of fat oxidation, creating a metabolic environment likely to promote obesity. However, this is also true of a diet high in starch, particularly, high-GI starch. When added sugars are substituted with other carbohydrates (e.g., starch with the same calories), there is no effect on BMI, weight, or body fat. Although added sugars offer no nutritional benefits, their sweetness is an effective tool to increase enjoyment and consumption of nutrient-dense foods.

Meta-analyses of controlled feeding trials in which sugar-sweetened beverages (SSBs) were *added* to the diet showed a dose-dependent increase in weight, particularly among those with a high genetically determined obesity risk (Malik, Pan, Willett, & Hu, 2013; Kaiser, Shikany, Keating, & Allison, 2013). However, studies that attempted to *reduce* SSB intake show equivocal effects. When limited to overweight participants only, a small amount of weight loss or less weight gain is evident. Two large RCTs with children and adolescents, with a high degree of compliance, provided convincing data that reducing consumption of SSBs decreased weight gain and adiposity, although the effect size was small. There is evidence to support a special adverse effect of fructose (Bray, 2010), and future studies should distinguish between soft drinks that use high-fructose cornstarch (e.g., those produced in the United States) and those that use sucrose (e.g., the European Union) for soft drinks. One short-term randomized trial showed adverse effects on ectopic fat depositions and blood pressure by 1 liter/day of SSBs as compared to water or milk (Maersk et al., 2012).

Replacement of caloric sweeteners with lower or zero-calorie alternatives may be a useful dietary tool to improve compliance and facilitate weight loss and weight loss maintenance by helping to reduce energy intake. In systematic reviews low-calorie sweeteners modestly reduced BMI, fat mass, and waist circumference, but this reduction is not evident in prospective cohort studies. Indeed, the results of these studies indicate that low-calorie sweeteners are associated with a slightly higher BMI.

Fiber and Whole Grains

High intakes of fiber and whole grains are recommended for the population at large because of their high micronutrient density, bulk, and satiating qualities. In large prospective cohort studies, high intake of cereal fiber and whole-grain foods is strongly linked with decreased rates of weight gain, type 2 diabetes, ischemic heart disease, and hypertension. A recent meta-analysis of RCTs found a modest but potentially important effect on body fat (Pol et al., 2013). The positive effect of oat products may be ascribed to their slower digestion and absorption (low GI) rather than their fiber content. Thus, ascribing an equal health value to all types of whole-grain foods, without regard to the physical structure and type of cereal, may not be helpful. At present the evidence for recommending whole grains in place of refined grains for weight loss per se is weak.

Dietary Weight Maintenance Programs

In professional weight management programs, LEDs induce a ≥ 5% weight loss in more than 50% of the patients, and frequent clinical encounters during the initial 6 months of weight reduction appear to facilitate achievement of therapy goals. More ambitious success criteria (> 10% weight loss) can be met by 25–30% of patients if the treatment program also includes group therapy and behavior modification. A number of studies suggest that the use of information technology can further improve the cost–benefit of the programs. The real challenge is to maintain the reduced body weight and prevent subsequent relapse (Astrup, 2015; see Figure 18.4).

In a systematic review of long-term (> 3-year follow-up) efficacy of dietary treatment of obesity, success was defined as maintenance of all weight initially lost or maintenance of at least 9 kg of initial weight loss (Ayyad & Andersen, 2000; Anderson, Konz, Frederich, & Wood, 2001). Initial weight loss was 4–28 kg, 15% of the follow-up patients fulfilled one of the success criteria, and the success rate was stable for up to 14 years of observation. Diet combined with group therapy led to better long-term success rates (27%) than did diet alone (15%),

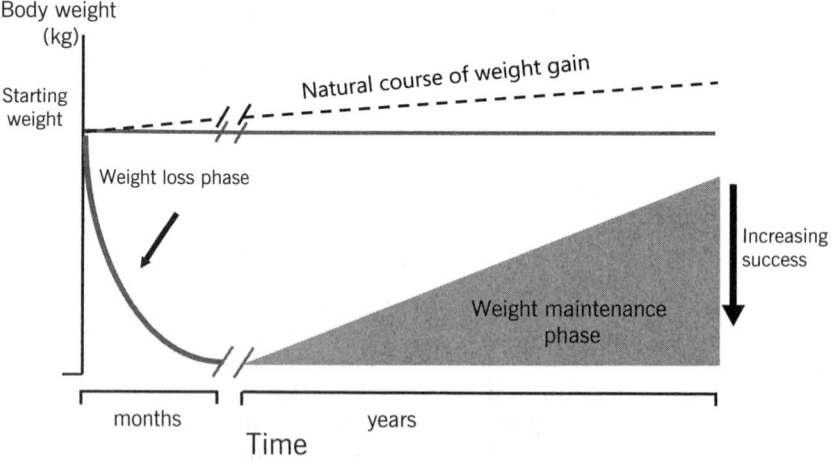

FIGURE 18.4. Maintenance of reduced body weight over time. From Astrup (2015). Treatment of obesity: Lifestyle and pharmacotherapy. In R. A. DeFronzo, E. Ferrannini, P. Zimmet, & K. G. M. M. Alberti (Eds.), *International textbook of diabetes mellitus* (4th ed., pp. 489–504). Chichester, UK: Wiley. Copyright © 2015 Wiley. Reprinted by permission.

or diet combined with behavior modification and active follow-up, although active follow-up produced better weight maintenance than passive follow-up (19% vs. 10%).

Diet Principles for Weight Loss Maintenance

Whereas energy restriction (LED) is successful for weight loss induction independent of dietary composition, the medium-fat, higher-protein/low GI diet seems to be more effective for long-term weight maintenance and prevention of weight regain. Weight maintenance diets need to be realistic, unrestrictive, and to fit into a food culture in order to be accepted over the long term and achieve compliance from the reduced-obese subjects.

In the diet, obesity, and genes (DioGenes) European multicenter trial, the impact of higher-protein and lower-GI diets for prevention of weight regain was studied in 800 obese families (Larsen et al., 2010). After an initial weight loss of 11 kg achieved by an 800 kcal/day diet over 8 weeks in the obese adults, they were randomized to five diets differing in protein content and GI. After 8 months, those randomized to higher protein and lower GI remained essentially weight stable, whereas those on diets with normal protein and higher GI regained weight. The effect of higher protein (23% of energy) and lower GI was additive. In this trial all diets were moderate in fat (25–30% of energy). In the normal-protein (NP) group, 10–15% of energy intake was comprised of protein. In the high-protein (HP) group, protein accounted for 22–24% of energy intake. Weight regain was ~1 kg less in the HP group than in the NP group, and ~1 kg less in the low GI (LGI) groups than in the high GI (HGI) groups. HP diets were more likely to produce an additional 5% weight loss after randomization than NP diets (odds ratio [OR], 1.92), and LGI diets were more likely to result in an additional 5% weight loss than were HGI diets (Handjieva-Darlenska et al., 2011). Thus a slight increase in dietary protein and corresponding reduction in carbohydrate, together with lowering GI by 5 units, exerted an additive effect on body weight maintenance after a LED-induced weight loss. After 14 months subjects on the HP diets had regained 2–3 kg less than those in the NP group, those on HP diets lost a total of 7.3 kg compared to 4.5 kg in the NP group. After 14 months the LGI diet was not found to have any effect.

This diet composition has also been shown to be effective in children (Papadaki et al., 2011) and to improve cardiometabolic risk. The HP–LGI diet produced a spontaneous 14.3% decline in the prevalence of overweight and obesity among the children ages 5–18 years who participated in the trial.

The challenge is to incorporate the weight maintenance diet into a food culture in order to achieve long-term adherence. It is important that weight maintenance diets are easily incorporated into normal food culture, and that availability, cost, and taste are not barriers for adopting the diet. Although meta-analyses suggest that there are long-term benefits on weight maintenance of higher protein diets, the effect size is small (Clifton, Condo, & Keogh, 2014).

Conclusions and Key Messages

This review has revealed that diet is a cornerstone of obesity management and that adherence to a reduced energy intake is a key challenge. The principal findings can be summarized as follows:

- LEDs and VLEDs using meal replacements effectively induce weight loss by ensuring a higher degree of adherence.
- A greater initial weight loss is associated with greater long-term retention and weight maintenance.
- Different diets take advantage of an enhanced satiety effect provided by higher protein content and lower content of fat, refined carbohydrates, and sugar-rich soft drinks.
- Higher-protein, low-carbohydrate diets are the most efficient and generally produce beneficial effects on all cardiometabolic risk factors. Long-term adherence may be a challenge.
- Greater weight loss can be achieved by using low-fat, high-carbohydrate diets in normoglycemic obese subjects, low glyce-

mic load diets with higher fiber and whole grain in the prediabetic obese, and lower carbohydrate, higher fat, and higher protein in type 2 diabetic obese subjects.

References

Agus, M. S., Swain J. F., Larson C. L., Eckert, E. A., & Ludwig D. S. (2000). Dietary composition and physiologic adaptations to energy restriction. *American Journal of Clinical Nutrition, 71*(4), 901–907.

Anderson, J. W., Konz, E. C., Frederich, R. C., & Wood, C. L. (2001). Long-term weight-loss maintenance: A meta-analysis of U.S. studies. *American Journal of Clinical Nutrition, 74*(5), 579–584.

Astrup, A. (2008). Weight loss with a low-carbohydrate, Mediterranean, or low-fat diet. *New England Journal of Medicine, 359*(20), 2169–2170.

Astrup, A. (2015). Treatment of obesity: Lifestyle and pharmacotherapy. In R. A. DeFronzo, E. Ferrannini, P. Zimmet, & K. G. M. M. Alberti (Eds.), *International textbook of diabetes mellitus* (4th ed., pp. 489–504). Chichester, UK: Wiley.

Astrup, A., Gøtzsche, P. C., van de Werken, K., Ranneries, C., Toubro, S., Raben, A., et al. (1999). Meta-analysis of resting metabolic rate in formerly obese subjects. *American Journal of Clinical Nutrition, 69*(6), 1117–1122.

Astrup, A., Grunwald, G. K., Melanson, E. L., Saris, W. H., & Hill, J. O. (2000). The role of low-fat diets in body weight control: A meta-analysis of ad libitum dietary intervention studies. *International Journal of Obesity, 24*(12), 1545–1552.

Astrup, A., Ryan, L., Grunwald, G. K., Storgaard, M., Saris, W., Melanson, E., et al. (2000). The role of dietary fat in body fatness: Evidence from a preliminary meta-analysis of ad libitum low fat dietary intervention studies. *British Journal of Nutrition, 83*(Suppl. 1), S25–S32.

Augustin, L. S., Kendall, C. W., Jenkins, D. J., Willett, W. C., Astrup, A., Barclay, A. W., et al. (2015). Glycemic index, glycemic load and glycemic response: An International Scientific Consensus Summit from the International Carbohydrate Quality Consortium (ICQC). *Nutrition, Metabolism and Cardiovascular Diseases, 25*(9), 795–815.

Ayyad, C., & Andersen, T. (2000). Long-term efficacy of dietary treatment of obesity: A systematic review of studies published between 1931 and 1999. *Obesity Reviews, 1*, 113–119.

Belza, A., Ritz, C., Sørensen, M. Q., Holst, J. J., Rehfeld, J. F., & Astrup, A. (2013). Contribution of gastroenteropancreatic appetite hormones to protein-induced satiety. *American Journal of Clinical Nutrition, 97*(5), 980–989.

Bray, G. A. (2010). Soft drink consumption and obesity: It is all about fructose. *Current Opinion in Lipidology, 21*(1), 51–57.

Bray, G. A., & Siri-Tarino, P. W. (2016). The role of macronutrient content in the diet for weight management. *Endocrinology Metabolism Clinics of North America, 45*, 581–604.

Casazza, K., Brown, A., Astrup, A., Bertz, F., Baum, C., Brown, M. B., et al. (2015). Weighing the evidence of common beliefs in obesity research. *Critical Reviews in Food Science and Nutrition, 55*(14), 2014–2053.

Casazza, K., Fontaine, K. R., Astrup, A., Birch, L. L., Brown, A. W., Brown, M. M. B., et al. (2013). Myths, presumptions, and facts about obesity. *New England Journal of Medicine, 368*(5), 446–454.

Chaput, J.-P., Tremblay, A., Rimm, E. B., Bouchard, C., & Ludwig, D. S. (2008). A novel interaction between dietary composition and insulin secretion: Effects on weight gain in the Quebec Family Study. *American Journal of Clinical Nutrition, 87*, 303–309.

Clifton, P. M., Condo, D., & Keogh, J. B. (2014). Long term weight maintenance after advice to consume low carbohydrate, higher protein diets: A systematic review and meta-analysis. *Nutrition, Metabolism and Cardiovascular Diseases, 24*, 224–235.

Ebbeling, C. B., Leidig, M. M., Feldman, H. A., Lovesky, M. M., & Ludwig, D. S. (2007). Effects of a low-glycemic load vs low-fat diet in obese young adults: A randomized trial. *Journal of the American Medical Association, 297*, 2092–2102.

Ebbeling, C. B., Swain, J. F., Feldman, H. A., Wong, W. W., Hachey, D. L., Garcia-Lago, E., & Ludwig, D. S. (2012). Effects of dietary composition on energy expenditure during weight loss maintenance. *Journal of the American Medical Association, 307*(24), 2627–2634.

Hall, K. D., Chen, K. Y., Guo, J., Lam, Y. Y., Leibel, R. L., Mayer, L. E., et al. (2016). Energy expenditure and body composition changes after an isocaloric ketogenic diet in overweight and obese men. *American Journal of Clinical Nutrition, 104*(2), 324–333.

Handjieva-Darlenska, T., Handjiev, S., Larsen, T. M., van Baak, M. A., Lindroos, A., Papadaki, A., et al., on behalf of DiOGenes. (2011). Predictors of weight loss maintenance and attrition during a 6-month dietary intervention period: Results from the DiOGenes study. *Clinical Obesity, 1*, 62–68.

Harvie, M., & Howell, A. (2017). Potential benefits and harms of intermittent energy restriction and intermittent fasting amongst obese, overweight and normal weight subjects: A narrative review of human and animal evidence. *Behavioral Sciences, 7*(1), 4.

Heianza, Y., Ma, W., Huang, T., Wang, T., Zheng, Y., Smith, S. R., et al. (2016). Macronutrient intake-associated FGF21 genotype modifies effects of weight-loss diets on 2-year changes of central adiposity and body composition: The POUNDS Lost Trial. *Diabetes Care, 39*(11), 1909–1914.

Hjorth, M. F., Due, A., Larsen, T. M., & Astrup, A. (2017). Pretreatment fasting plasma glucose modifies dietary weight loss maintenance success: Results from a stratified RCT. *Obesity, 25*, 2045–2048.

Hjorth, M. F., Ritz, C., Blaak, E. E., Saris, W. H., Langin, D., Paulsen, S. K., et al. (2017). Pretreatment fasting plasma glucose and insulin modify dietary weight loss success. Results from 3 randomized clinical trials. *American Journal of Clinical Nutrition, 106*, 479–505.

Hron, B. M., Ebbeling, C. B., Feldman, H. A., & Ludwig, D. S. (2015). Relationship of insulin dynamics to body composition and resting energy expenditure following weight loss. *Obesity, 23*, 2216–2222.

Jéquier, E., & Bray, G. A. (2002). Low-fat diets are preferred. *American Journal of Medicine, 113*(Suppl. 9B), 41S–46S.

Kaiser, K. A., Shikany, J. M., Keating, K. D., & Allison, D. B. (2013). Will reducing sugar-sweetened beverage consumption reduce obesity?: Evidence supporting conjecture is strong, but evidence when testing effect is weak. *Obesity Reviews, 14*(8), 620–633.

Knuth, N. D., Johannsen, D. L., Tamboli, R. A., Marks-Shulman, P. A., Huizenga, R., Chen, K. Y., et al. (2014). Metabolic adaptation following massive weight loss is related to the degree of energy imbalance and changes in circulating leptin. *Obesity, 22*(12), 2563–2569. (Erratum in *Obesity*, 2016, 24[10], 2248.)

Larsen, T. M., Dalskov, S.-M., van Baak, M., Jebb, S. A., Papadaki, A., Pfeiffer, A. F. H., et al., for the Diet, Obesity, and Genes (Diogenes) Project. (2010). Diets with high or low protein content and glycemic index for weight-loss maintenance. *New England Journal of Medicine, 363*(22), 2102–2113.

Ludwig, D. S., Astrup, A., & Willett, W. C. (2015). The glycemic index: Reports of its demise have been exaggerated. *Obesity, 23*(7), 1327–1328.

Maersk, M., Belza, A., Stødkilde-Jørgensen, H., Ringgaard, S., Chabanova, E., Thomsen, H., et al. (2012). Sucrose-sweetened beverages increase fat storage in the liver, muscle, and visceral fat depot: A 6-mo randomized intervention study. *American Journal of Clinical Nutrition, 95*(2), 283–289.

Malik, V. S., Pan, A., Willett, W. C., & Hu, F. B. (2013). Sugar-sweetened beverages and weight gain in children and adults: A systematic review and meta-analysis. *American Journal of Clinical Nutrition, 98*(4), 1084–1102.

Mansoor, N., Vinknes, K. J., Veierød, M. B., & Retterstøl, K. (2016). Effects of low-carbohydrate diets v. low-fat diets on body weight and cardiovascular risk factors: A meta-analysis of randomised controlled trials. *British Journal of Nutrition, 115*(3), 466–479.

Mattei, J., Qi, Q., Hu, F. B., Sacks, F. M., & Qi, L. (2012). TCF7L2 genetic variants modulate the effect of dietary fat intake on changes in body composition during a weight-loss intervention. *American Journal of Clinical Nutrition, 96*, 1129–1136.

Mikkelsen, P. B., Toubro, S., & Astrup, A. (2000). Effect of fat-reduced diets on 24-h energy expenditure: Comparisons between animal protein, vegetable protein, and carbohydrate. *American Journal of Clinical Nutrition, 72*(5), 1135–1141.

Papadaki, A., Linardakis, M., Larsen, T. M., van Baak, M. A., Lindroos, A. K., Pfeiffer, A. F. H., et al., on behalf of the DiOGenes Study Group. (2011). The effect of protein and glycemic index on children's body composition: The DiOGenes randomized study. *Pediatrics, 126*(5), e1143–e1152.

Pol, K., Christensen, R., Bartels, E. M., Raben, A., Tetens, I., & Kristensen, M. (2013). Whole grain and body weight changes in apparently healthy adults: A systematic review and meta-analysis of randomized controlled studies. *American Journal of Clinical Nutrition, 98*(4), 872–884.

Poulsen, S. K., Due, A., Jordy, A. B., Kiens, B., Stark, K. D., Stender, S., et al. (2014). Health effect of the New Nordic Diet in adults with increased waist circumference: A 6-mo randomized controlled trial. *American Journal of Clinical Nutrition, 99*(1), 35–45.

Sackner-Bernstein, J., Kanter, D., & Kaul, S. (2015). Dietary intervention for overweight and obese adults: Comparison of low-carbohydrate and low-fat diets—a meta-analysis. *PLOS ONE, 10*(10), e0139817.

Sacks, F. M., Bray, G. A., Carey, V. J., Smith, S. R., Ryan, D. H., Anton, S. D., et al. (2009). Comparison of weight-loss diets with different compositions of fat, protein, and carbohydrates. *New England Journal of Medicine, 360*(9), 859–873.

Sanghvi, A., Redman, L. M., Martin, C. K., Ravussin, E., & Hall, K. D. (2015). Validation of an inexpensive and accurate mathematical method to measure long-term changes in free-living energy intake. *American Journal of Clinical Nutrition, 102*(2), 353–358.

Seimon, R. V., Roekenes, J. A., Zibellini, J., Zhu, B., Gibson, A. A., Hills, A. P., et al. (2015). Do intermittent diets provide physiological benefits over continuous diets for weight loss?: A systematic review of clinical trials. *Molecular and Cellular Endocrinology, 418*(Pt. 2), 153–172.

Shai, I., Schwarzfuchs, D., Henkin, Y., Shahar, D. R., Witkow, S., Greenberg, I., et al., for the Dietary Intervention Randomized Controlled Trial (DIRECT) Group. (2009). Weight loss with a low-carbohydrate, Mediterranean, or low-fat diet. *New England Journal of Medicine, 359*(3), 229–241. (Erratum in *New England Journal of Medicine*, 2009, 361[27], 2681.)

Stocks, T., Angquist, L., Hager, J., Charon, C., Holst, C., Martinez, J. A., et al. (2013). TFAP2B-dietary protein and glycemic index interactions and weight maintenance after weight loss in the DiOGenes trial. *Human Heredity, 75*, 213–219.

Tobias, D. K., Chen, M., Manson, J. E., Ludwig, D. S., Willett, W., & Hu, F. B. (2015). Effect of low-fat diet interventions versus other diet interventions on long-term weight change in adults: A systematic review and meta-analysis. *Lancet Diabetes Endocrinology, 3*(12), 968–979.

Tsai, A. G., & Wadden, T. A. (2006). The evolution of very-low-calorie diets: An update and meta-analysis. *Obesity (Silver Spring), 14*(8), 1283–1293.

Yu-Poth, S., Zhao, G., Etherton, T., Naglak, M., Jonnalagadda, S., & Kris-Etherton, P. M. (1999). Effects of the National Cholesterol Education Program's Step I and Step II dietary intervention programs on cardiovascular disease risk factors: A meta-analysis. *American Journal of Clinical Nutrition, 69*(4), 632–646.

CHAPTER 19

Physical Activity and Weight Management

John M. Jakicic
Renee J. Rogers
Sally A. Sherman
Sara J. Kovacs

Given the prevalence of overweight and obesity in adults, there is a public health need to identify effective lifestyle factors that contribute to the prevention of additional weight gain. A growing literature supports physical activity as a key lifestyle factor that contributes to this important public health goal.

Data from population-based studies have shown an inverse association between measures of adiposity and physical activity, particularly moderate- to vigorous-intensity physical activity (MVPA). A study of more than 4,500 adults from the National Health and Nutrition Examination Survey (NHANES) showed that greater physical activity was associated with a lower body mass index (BMI) (Fan et al., 2013). However, of importance, only physical activity that was of moderate to vigorous intensity was inversely associated with BMI. This relationship did not hold with lower intensities of physical activity. These data suggest that there is a threshold of physical activity intensity necessary to affect body weight and prevent excessive weight gain. Cross-sectional baseline data from the Look AHEAD trial have also shown an inverse association between objectively measured physical activity and BMI (Jakicic et al., 2010). In this cohort of adults with type 2 diabetes who were also either overweight or obese, the data showed that MVPA was lower at higher categories of BMI. However, despite this evidence, these cross-sectional data alone are not sufficient to prove that engaging in physical activity will result in the prevention of excessive weight gain in adults.

There is compelling evidence from prospective cohort studies to support physical activity as a factor that contributes to the prevention of weight gain. Data from the NHANES I Epidemiologic Followup Study showed a higher odds of significant weight gain in adults who were at a low activity level at baseline and remained so at the 10-year follow-up period, compared to those who transitioned from low activity to high activity or those who remained highly active (Williamson et al., 1993). Moreover, a prospective cohort study of over 34,000 women showed that physical activity was inversely associated with weight gain over a mean follow-up period of approximately 3 years (Lee, Djousse, Sesso, Wang, & Buring, 2010). Approximately 60 minutes/day of MVPA were associated with prevention of weight gain or gaining less than 2.3 kg during the 3-year follow-up period. However, an important finding from this study was that this association was only observed in women who had an initial BMI of less than 25 kg/m^2; physical activity was not associated with prevention of weight gain in women with an initial BMI ≥ 25 kg/m^2. The threshold of 60 minutes/day of physical activity was also shown to be associated with prevention of weight gain over a 5-year period in older adult men in the Harvard Alumni Study (Shiroma, Sesso, & Lee, 2012).

Data from intervention trials also support the contribution of physical activity to the prevention of weight gain. However, close examination shows that many of these studies actually demonstrate that physical activity results in modest weight loss rather than solely preventing of weight gain. In a 12-month physical activity intervention, the mean difference in weight change between participants in the intervention and control groups was approximately 2.1 kg for women and 1.9 kg for men (McTiernan et al., 2007). For women, this was due to weight loss of 1.4 kg in the intervention and 0.7 kg weight gain in the control condition. In men, this was due to 1.8 kg weight loss in the intervention and 0.1 kg weight gain in the control condition. A similar pattern was shown in an 18-month study of 248 adults with an initial BMI of 25 to < 30 kg/m^2 in which 53.2% remained weight stable (within 3% of their baseline weight), 19.4% gained more than 3% of their baseline weight, and 27.4% lost more than 3% of their baseline weight (Jakicic et al., 2011). Participants who remained weight stable or gained weight over the 18-month period engaged in less than 80 minutes/week of MVPA, whereas those who lost weight engaged in more than 150 minutes/week of MVPA.

In summary, it appears that it may take 3–10 years to observe meaningful effects of physical activity on the prevention of weight gain, based on prospective cohort studies, and the dose of physical activity may need to approximate 60 minutes/day of MVPA. However, within the context of shorter interventions of 12–18 months, thresholds of MVPA that exceed 150 minutes/week may result in modest weight loss rather than prevention of weight gain. Regardless, physical activity should be considered an important lifestyle behavior that can prevent unhealthy weight gain. Progression of adults to a sustained level of 30–60 minutes/day of MVPA should be a public health target.

Physical Activity and Weight Loss

The public health need to prevent excessive weight gain is paralleled by a critical need for effective interventions to induce weight loss and prevent subsequent weight regain. As described in this chapter, substantial evidence supports physical activity as an important lifestyle behavior that significantly contributes to both short-term and long-term weight loss in adults.

Physical Activity in the Absence of Prescribed Dietary Restriction

One approach to weight loss is to prescribe physical activity in the absence of a diet focused on calorie restriction. Numerous studies have documented that the mean weight loss achieved with this approach is approximately 0.5–3.0 kg. Systematic reviews of these studies have concluded that physical activity alone induces modest weight loss (Wing, 1999; U.S. Department of Health and Human Services, 2008; Donnelly et al., 2009; Swift, Johannsen, Lavie, Earnest, & Church, 2014; Washburn et al., 2014).

Despite the limited average weight loss observed with physical activity alone, the dose of physical activity may make a difference (Donnelly et al., 2009). Although physical activity of approximately 150 minutes/week produces a loss of up to only 3 kg, weight loss of 5 kg or more can be achieved when physical activity is increased to 225 or more minutes/week. Thus, to achieve greater weight loss without caloric restriction, a higher dose of physical activity appears necessary. There also is considerable variability in weight change in response to a similar dose of physical activity without caloric restriction. An example of this variability comes from the Midwest Exercise Trial in which men and women were prescribed the same duration and intensity of physical activity across a 16-month period (Donnelly et al., 2003). On average, men reduced weight by 5.2 kg compared to nonexercise controls, whereas women had 2.3 kg less weight gain compared to nonexercise controls. However, given differences in weight and lean body mass between men and women, it is likely that the same duration and intensity of physical activity resulted in greater energy expenditure in men versus women, which may have contributed to the differential effects on body weight change. Thus, in a follow-up study in which the prescribed dose of physical activity for men and women was matched for energy expenditure, there was no significant difference in weight loss between the sexes. Moreover, regardless of sex, a dose–response relationship was observed with 400 kcal of activity/session, producing a mean loss of 3.9 kg and 600 kcal/session, resulting in a mean weight loss of 5.2 kg at the end of the 10-month intervention. These findings suggest that although there may be differences between men and women in weight loss achieved with physical activity, when they engage in a similar dose of physical activity, based on energy expenditure, the weight loss is comparable. In addition, as energy expenditure from physical activity increases, more weight is lost.

Physical Activity Combined with Prescribed Dietary Restriction

A more commonly recommended clinical approach to weight loss is to combine physical activity with a diet designed to induce calorie restriction, along with behavior change strategies (Jensen et al., 2014). Calorie restriction combined with physical activity appears to produce greater weight loss than calorie restriction alone. In a systematic review of studies of at least 12 months in duration, the combination of a calorie-restricted diet plus physical activity resulted in a median weight loss of 8.8% of initial body weight, compared to 6.9% for a calorie-restricted diet alone (Washburn et al., 2014). Moreover, even in adults with class 2 obesity or greater (defined as a BMI of ≥ 35 kg/m²), the combination of physical activity and a calorie-restricted diet resulted in 2.7 kg more weight loss than diet alone in a 6-month intervention (Goodpaster et al., 2010). Thus, it appears that the addition of physical activity to a calorie-restricted diet enhances the weight loss achieved in a 6- to 12-month period of time.

Physical Activity and Long-Term Weight Loss

Physical activity, particularly MVPA, also appears to be an important predictor of improved long-term weight loss (Donnelly et al., 2009), and MVPA may have been one of the strongest correlates of the ability to achieve ≥ 10% weight loss within a comprehensive weight loss intervention that included calorie restriction and behavior change strategies (Unick, Jakicic, & Marcus, 2010). However, a relatively high amount of physical activity may be necessary to enhance weight loss at 12 months and beyond. For example, data from the Look AHEAD Study showed that a mean of 287 minutes/week of MVPA was associated with a 1-year weight loss of 11.9%, and physical activity was a strong correlate of weight loss at this time (Wadden et al., 2009). Moreover, our research team has consistently found that ≥ 250 minutes/week of MVPA (~2,000–2,500 kcal/week) is associated with the greatest weight loss and prevention of weight regain in lifestyle interventions of at least 12 months in duration (Jakicic, Winters, Lang, & Wing, 1999; Jakicic, Marcus, Gallagher, Napolitano, & Lang, 2003; Jakicic, Marcus, Lang, & Janney, 2008) (see Figures 19.1 and 19.2). This finding is consistent with the findings of others based on secondary data analysis from clinical trials (Tate, Jeffery, Sherwood, & Wing, 2007) and from the National Weight Control Registry (Klem, Wing, McGuire, Seagle, & Hill, 1997; Catenacci et al., 2008, 2011).

Many of the studies that have found that a relatively high dose of physical activity is important for enhancing long-term weight loss have relied on self-reported physical activity. However, we recently obtained similar findings when physical activity was measured objectively using a wearable activity monitor (Jakicic et al., 2014). The findings from this study also support that MVPA of approximately 250 minutes/week should be performed in bouts of at least 10 minutes, as this was associated with the greatest magni-

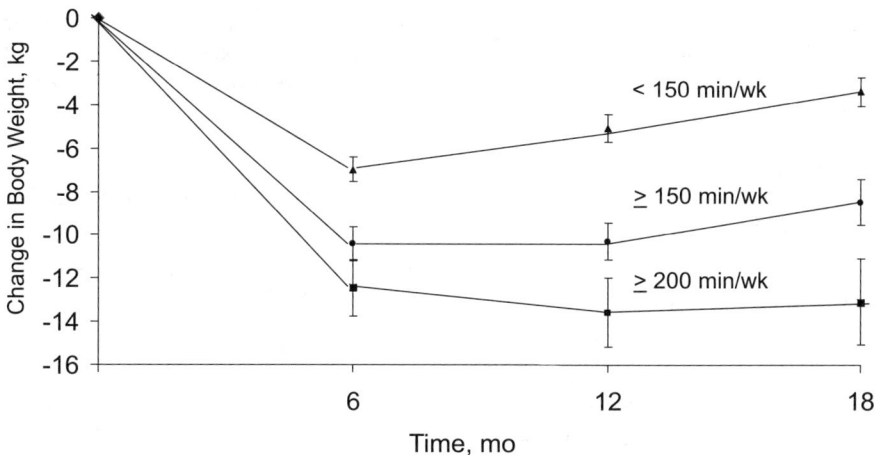

FIGURE 19.1. Dose response of exercise on weight loss. Reprinted with permission from Jakicic, Winters, Lang, and Wing (1999). Effects of intermittent exercise and use of home exercise equipment on adherence, weight loss, and fitness in overweight women: A randomized trial. *Journal of the American Medical Association, 282*(16), 1554–1560. Copyright © 1999 the American Medical Association. All rights reserved.

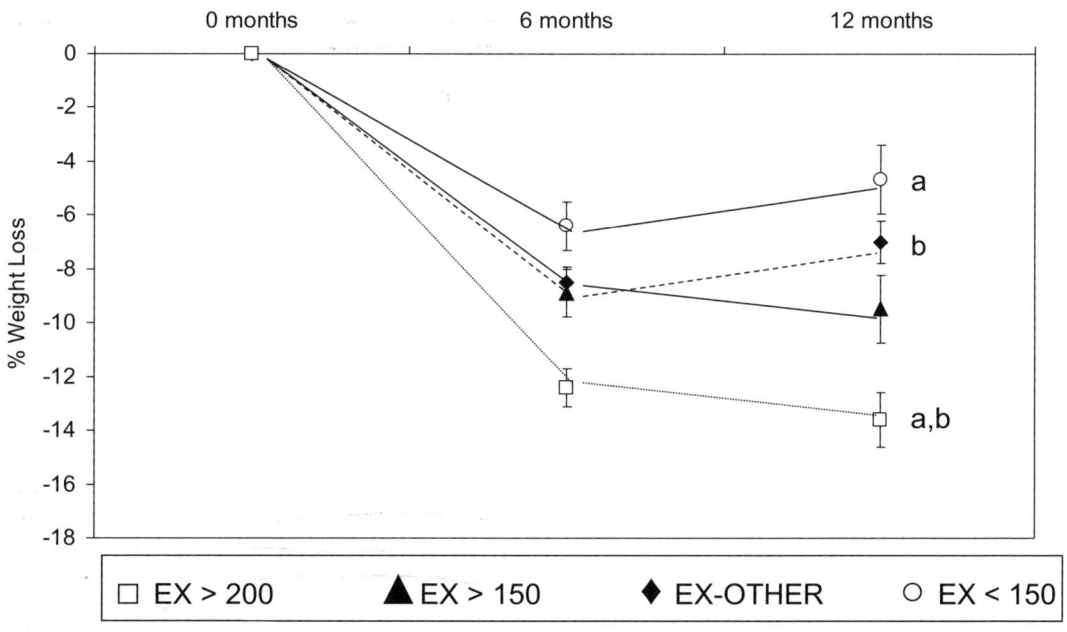

FIGURE 19.2. Percent change (+ standard error) in weight loss based on exercise participation ($N = 196$). Groups with the same letters are significantly different at 12 months, based on Bonferroni adjustment ($p < .05$). Adapted with permission from Jakicic, Marcus, Gallagher, Napolitano, and Lang (2003). Effect of exercise duration and intensity on weight loss in overweight, sedentary women: A randomized trial. *Journal of the American Medical Association, 290*(10), 1323–1330. Copyright © 2003 the American Medical Association. All rights reserved.

tude of weight loss following an 18-month intervention. Thus, lifestyle interventions for weight loss that include a calorie-restricted diet should also include a sufficient dose of physical activity to further enhance short-term weight loss (≤ 6 months) and to maximize weight loss achieved and maintained at 12 months and beyond.

Physical Activity Combined with Bariatric Surgery

Bariatric surgery has become a more common intervention for patients with severe obesity and is highly effective in inducing weight loss and improvements in obesity-related comorbidities. However, physical activity appears to be an important lifestyle behavior that needs to be included within the bariatric surgery approach. For example, observational studies have shown that engagement in physical activity is associated with improved weight loss following bariatric surgery (Bond et al., 2004, 2009; Evans et al., 2007; Josbeno, Kalarchian, Sparto, Otto, & Jakicic, 2011; King et al., 2012, 2015). However, following bariatric surgery, most patients remain insufficiently active (Josbeno et al., 2011; King et al., 2012, 2015).

Interventions are needed to increase physical activity in patients undergoing bariatric surgery (King & Bond, 2013). In one of the few randomized studies of this issue, patients were assigned to supervised exercise or a health education control for 6 months (Coen et al., 2015). The supervised exercise consisted of progressing to 120 minutes/week of moderate-intensity physical activity. Results showed that adherence to this dose of physical activity resulted in greater improvements in insulin sensitivity, glucose effectiveness, and cardiorespiratory fitness. However, this dose of physical activity did not enhance weight loss, reductions in body fatness, or retention of lean body mass during this 6-month period. Thus, these data suggest that within the initial 6 months following bariatric surgery, engagement in physical activity is not associated with improved weight loss or favorable body composition changes but may be associated with other important health-related outcomes. Moreover, the benefits of physical activity on weight loss during the postbariatric surgery period may become more apparent with longer periods of follow-up at 12 months or beyond.

Intervention Considerations to Enhance Physical Activity

Self-Directed versus Center-Based Physical Activity

In the physical activity literature, particularly that pertinent to obesity treatment, there is variability in the settings in which physical activity is promoted. Numerous studies have evaluated the effects of center-based (i.e., in-person) physical activity training that allows for supervision and direct observation of the prescribed dose of physical activity (Ross et al., 2000, 2004; Donnelly et al., 2003; Slentz et al., 2004; Church, Earnest, Skinner, & Blair, 2007). Many studies also have examined the effect of self-directed physical activity that allows for the activity to be performed at home or other settings outside of a supervised center (Jakicic, Wing, Butler, & Robertson, 1995; Wing, Venditti, Jakicic, Polley, & Lang, 1998; Jeffery, Wing, Sherwood, & Tate, 2003; Jakicic et al., 2003, 2008, 2011, 2012; Jakicic, King, et al., 2015; Jakicic, Rickman, et al., 2015). Both center-based and self-directed approaches to increase physical activity have been shown to be effective.

Additional studies have directly compared self-directed and center-based physical activity interventions to determine if there are differences in weight-related outcomes. When combined with a calorie-reduced diet and behavior change strategies, self-directed physical activity programs appear to induce greater weight loss and may result in continued engagement in physical activity, compared to programs that require center-based physical activity (Perri, Martin, Leermakers, Sears, & Notelovitz, 1997; Andersen et al., 1999). A more recent study that directly compared self-directed and center-based physical activity programs for adults who were overweight or obese showed similar improvements in physical activity, reductions in weight, and increases in cardiorespiratory fitness (Creasy, Rogers, Byard, Kowalsky, & Jakicic, 2016). Thus, in situations

Prescribing Short Bouts of Physical Activity

Common barriers to engaging in physical activity include a lack of time and low self-efficacy for physical activity. One strategy that has been shown to be effective, at least for a period of 5–6 months, is to encourage multiple short bouts of activity per day rather than one long session per day, as is customary.

A 20-week behavioral weight loss study found that prescribing physical activity in multiple 10-minute bouts/day, as compared with one 40-minute bout, resulted in more minutes of activity per week and a trend toward greater weight loss at the end of treatment (see Figure 19.3) (Jakicic et al., 1995). These results were replicated across the initial 6 months of an additional trial (Jakicic, Winters, Lang, & Wing, 1999). However, at 18 months, the short-bout strategy was no longer superior to prescribing physical activity in one long bout. Thus, this strategy of prescribing multiple short bouts of physical activity may be most effective at increasing initial engagement and adoption of physical activity in adults who are overweight or obese. The short-bout approach should be considered by health care providers and health–fitness professionals for this patient population.

Encouraging Increased Steps per Day of Physical Activity

Guidelines commonly recommend that adults increase their movement in the form of increased steps per day to improve health, with a goal of accumulating approximately 10,000 steps/day. Typical daily physical activity results in approximately 6,000–7,000 steps/day, with some adults, including those with obesity, potentially taking fewer steps (Tudor-Locke & Bassett, 2004).

A systematic review of the literature showed that an increase in 2,100 steps/day, equivalent to approximately 1 mile of walking/day, was associated with a modest yet significant decrease in BMI (Donnelly et al., 2009). Moreover, an intervention that increased steps by 3,000/day across a 12-week period showed a positive association between steps walked and reduction in waist circumference (Chan, Ryan, & Tudor-Locke, 2004). Another 12-week weight loss intervention, which included a calorie-reduced diet and behavioral strategies, also evaluated a physical activity intervention focused on steps per day (Creasy et al., 2016). At the end of the intervention, there was a significant mean increase of 2,595 steps/day, with 1,584 of these steps taken at a moderate to vigorous intensity and in bouts

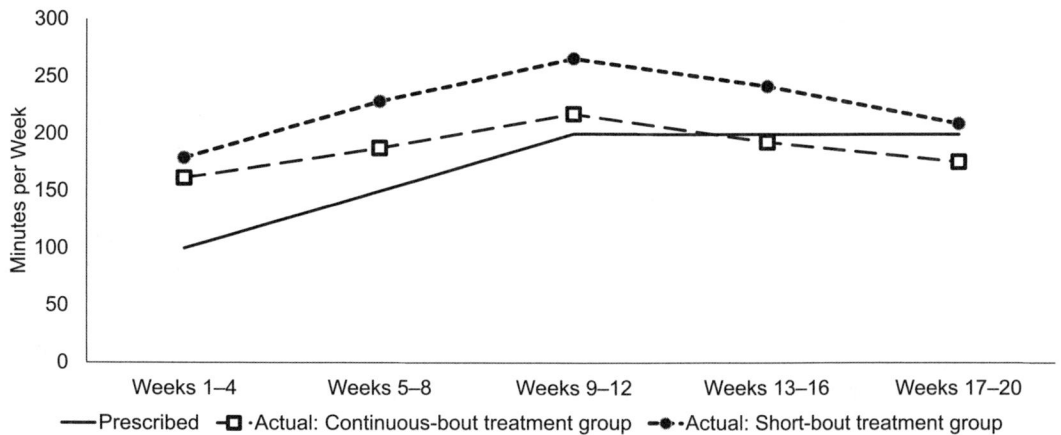

FIGURE 19.3. Physical activity engagement when prescribed in one continuous bout or in multiple short bouts. Data from Jakicic et al. (1995).

of at least 10 minutes in duration. This resulted in an increase in total steps/day to a mean of 10,323 by the end of the 12 weeks. Moreover, the weight loss achieved in this step-based intervention (–5.3 kg) was similar to that achieved when physical activity involved center-based sessions (–3.8 kg) or was self-directed and prescribed as minutes/day (–5.1 kg).

These data suggest that movement accumulated in steps/day is associated with improved weight regulation. Moreover, interventions that focus on increasing steps can be effective at increasing total physical activity in adults who are overweight or obese. This approach appears to be an effective strategy for increasing physical activity to both prevent and treat overweight and obesity.

Wearable Physical Activity Monitors

Numerous wearable devices are available that focus on measuring and encouraging physical activity. However, there is variability in the success of these devices in promoting activity and weight loss in adults with overweight/obesity. Initial research in this area showed that the addition of wearable physical activity technology to an individual or group-based weight loss intervention produced modest improvements in weight loss in studies of 3–9 months' duration (Polzien, Jakicic, Tate, & Otto, 2007; Shugar et al., 2011). However, when these devices were paired with a less intensive intervention that involved only one brief telephone contact with a health coach, weight loss and physical activity were comparable to what was achieved with a more intensive program that involved regular in-person contact with a weight loss interventionist (Pellegrini et al., 2012; Rogers et al., 2016). As shown in Figure 19.4, a more recent large-scale randomized trial that added wearable technology following the initial 6 months of weight loss treatment actually showed significantly less weight loss across 24 months and no improvement in physical activity, when compared to a weight loss treatment that received no wearable technology (Jakicic et al., 2016).

Thus, there appears to be variability in the effectiveness of including wearable technology that tracks and provides feedback on physical activity within the context of weight loss interventions. Studies consistently indicate that simply providing the wearable technology results in little impact on physical activity engagement, and that there is a significant decrease in the use of the technology after approximately 6 months (Finkelstein et al., 2016). More research is needed to better understand how to best apply these technologies to improve health behaviors, weight, and related health outcomes (Piwek, Ellis, Andrews, & Joinson, 2016).

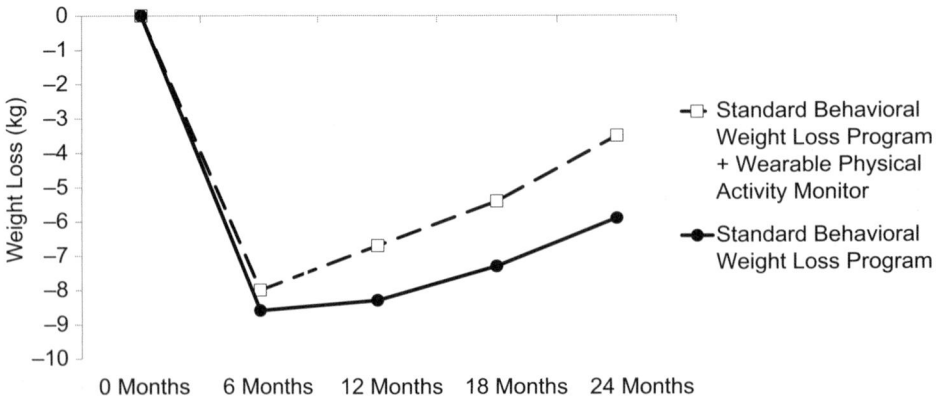

FIGURE 19.4. Weight loss with and without the addition of a wearable physical activity monitor. Data from Jakicic et al. (2016).

Additional Physical Activity Considerations

The majority of the studies that demonstrated the importance of physical activity for preventing weight gain or inducing weight loss included primarily aerobic or endurance modes of physical activity, such as walking or cycling. However, other popular forms of physical activity should be considered for their potential influence on obesity management.

Resistance Exercise

Resistance exercise, primarily in the form of weight lifting, is a common form of physical activity that may be recommended for adults who are overweight or obese. However, the vast majority of data suggests that resistance exercise may result in only modest reductions in weight or body fatness, as summarized in systematic reviews of the literature (Donnelly et al., 2004, 2009; U.S. Department of Health and Human Services, 2008; Swift et al., 2014). This lack of a substantial influence on body weight or body fatness may reflect the less than optimal energy expenditure resulting from resistance exercise in these studies. Resistance exercise typically was prescribed only 2–3 days/week, and most studies of this topic have typically been less than 6 months in duration.

There may be barriers to resistance exercise that are not present with other forms of physical activity, which may affect participant engagement and compliance. For example, when walking is prescribed, there is great flexibility with where an individual can engage in this physical activity (e.g., outdoors, indoors, on a treadmill). However, in most circumstances, resistance exercise has typically required specific equipment and supervision that may only be available at a health–fitness facility, which may limit participant access and feasibility. Thus, alternative home-based approaches to resistance exercise may be necessary to enhance engagement. This may require home exercise equipment or home-based approaches that do not require equipment and that are tailored specifically to adults who are overweight or obese. Given that resistance exercise may contribute to improved strength, function, and metabolic factors, such as reduced insulin resistance, it may also be important for clinicians and health–fitness professionals to encourage this approach with interested patients.

Yoga

Yoga also may be considered for weight management. *Yoga* is a broad term used to describe mental, physical, and spiritual disciplines that originated in ancient India and which now have been translated into different styles and interpretations.

A key consideration of whether yoga may contribute to body weight regulation is its ability to increase energy expenditure through the *asanas* (poses) that comprise a practice. Yoga that includes mostly poses for relaxation and the holding of postures has been shown to elicit a mean energy expenditure of 3.2 ± 1.1 kcal/minute, equivalent to 2.5 ± 0.8 metabolic equivalents (METs) (Hagins, Moore, & Rundle, 2007). This type of yoga reflects a light-intensity form of physical activity, as defined by the commonly accepted threshold of 1.5 to < 3.0 METs, which would be equivalent to walking at a speed of approximately 2.0 miles per hour (mph). Our research team recently evaluated the energy expenditure of a vinyasa style of yoga, which is often referenced as being a type of "power yoga" due to its continuous patterns that flow through a dynamic series of movements, rather than the static holding of poses. Results showed that the energy cost of vinyasa yoga was 4.1 ± 0.6 METs, which meets the lower criterion of MVPA (i.e., ≥ 3 METs) (Sherman, 2016). Moreover, energy expenditure during vinyasa yoga in participants who were overweight or obese was 4.0 METs, which was not significantly different than the energy expenditure in nonoverweight and nonobese individuals (4.2 METs). Thus, vinyasa yoga elicits an energy expenditure typical of other forms of MVPA (e.g., brisk walking) that are recommended within behavioral weight control interventions.

In addition to the asanas (poses), which is the physical component, yoga may also be beneficial in other ways for treating obesity.

As described in a recent review (Sherman, 2016), yoga may contribute to body weight regulation through its potential to decrease stress (Michalsen et al., 2005; Li & Goldsmith, 2012), mitigate pain (Sherman, Cherkin, & Wellman, 2011), enhance mood and diminish depression (Woolery, Myers, Sternlieb, & Zelter, 2004; Uebelacker et al., 2010), enhance sleep (Khalsa, 2004; Mustian et al., 2013), and increase energy expenditure (Carroll, Blansit, Otto, & Wygand, 2003; Hagins et al., 2007). Traditional forms of yoga also include mindfulness meditation, which focuses on heightening awareness to make conscious decisions. The mindfulness mediation component of yoga may also contribute to regulation of body weight through improved psychological functioning and flexibility (Lillis, Hayes, Bunting, & Masuda, 2009; Forman & Butryn, 2015), awareness (Sears & Kraus, 2009; Brown, Goodman, & Inzlicht, 2013), and self-regulation (Kristeller & Wolever, 2011; Forman & Butryn, 2015). The mindfulness component of yoga may also contribute to decreased emotional reactivity, rumination (Baer, 2009), and stress (Kabat-Zinn, 1991; Goyal et al., 2014). These factors may improve eating and physical activity behaviors, which may contribute to enhanced body weight regulation.

Despite the potential for yoga to influence body weight, few studies have examined the effect of including yoga in a weight loss intervention. Unpublished data from our laboratory illustrate the potential of yoga to enhance weight loss when added to a comprehensive intervention that included a calorie-restricted diet, physical activity, and behavior change strategies. This pilot study found that the addition of yoga to a comprehensive intervention produced an additional 2.5-kg weight loss in 6 months of treatment. This study also showed that adults who were overweight or obese could engage in yoga as a form of physical activity. The inclusion of yoga into a comprehensive behavioral weight loss approach may be a promising strategy in the treatment of overweight and obesity, although further research clearly is needed

Sedentary Behavior

There is growing interest in the influence of sedentary behavior on a variety of health-related outcomes, including the influence on overweight and obesity. Investigators have suggested that increasing energy expenditure by 100 kcal/day, while maintaining a consistent energy intake, could potentially prevent population weight gain (Hill, Wyatt, Reed, & Peters, 2003). Moreover, occupational-related energy expenditure has declined by approximately 140 kcal/day since 1960 in the United States, which could account for the population-based weight gain during that same period (Church et al., 2011). Thus, modest reductions in sedentary behavior that result in modest increases in energy expenditure may be important to counter weight gain and may contribute to the successful treatment of overweight and obesity.

Much of the early literature in this area focused on the association between sedentary behavior and risk of obesity, with sedentary behavior typically defined as television viewing. These data typically show positive associations between sedentary behavior and risk of obesity (Foster, Gore, & West, 2006). For example, television viewing has been shown to be positively associated with the risk of gaining weight or with the development of obesity (Ball, Brown, & Crawford, 2002; Hu, Li, Colditz, Willett, & Manson, 2003). Thus, reducing sedentary behavior, such as television viewing, has the potential to prevent or attenuate weight gain.

A potential pathway that may explain the association between sedentary behavior and weight gain is that sedentary behavior replaces physical activity and therefore reduces total daily energy expenditure. Studies have shown that there is greater energy expenditure when standing compared to sitting, and these differences range from approximately 9 to 50 kcal/hour (Levine, Schleusner, & Jensen, 2000; Levine & Miller, 2007; McAlpine, Manohar, McCrady, Hensrud, & Levine, 2007; Beers, Roemmich, Epstein, & Horvath, 2008; Reiff, Marlatt, & Dengel, 2012; Buckley, Mellor, Morris, & Joseph, 2014). A recent study confirmed that standing versus sitting will elicit approximately an additional 9 kcal/hour, and that there is greater energy expenditure when transitioning from sitting to walking, compared to sitting to standing (Creasy, 2016). Thus, encouraging standing versus sitting may elicit a modest increase in energy expenditure, whereas encouraging breaks in sitting that are replaced with periods of walking elicits greater energy expenditure that may be important for body weight regulation.

Within the context of an intervention to treat overweight or obesity, few studies have specifically isolated the contribution of sedentary behavior on weight loss success. However, data from a 6-month behavioral weight loss intervention of young adults (ages 18–35), which included a calorie-reduced diet, physical activity, and behavioral strategies, showed that change in sedentary behavior was not associated with weight loss (Jakicic, King, et al., 2015). Rather, increased MVPA, performed in bouts of at least 10 minutes in duration, and increased light-intensity physical activity were predictive of weight loss in this study. Thus, for weight loss, focusing the intervention on increasing light- and moderate-intensity physical activity may result in greater weight loss than simply encouraging reduced sedentary behavior in adults.

Clinical Application with Patients with Obesity

The majority of the evidence suggests that promoting higher levels of physical activity in patients who are overweight or obese will enhance weight loss and potentially improvements in obesity-related health outcomes. Physicians, other health care providers, and health–fitness professionals should encourage patients to increase their physical activity, while considering the following points.

1. Engagement in physical activity has been shown to be relatively safe when appropriate screening and risk stratification are considered. Updated guidelines of the American College of Sports Medicine provide information on when more extensive medical evaluation is required prior to participating in a program of regular physical activity (Magal & Riebe, 2016). A summary of these updated recommendations is provided in Table 19.1.

2. For adults who are overweight or obese, gradual progression of physical activity to at least 150 minutes/week of moderate-intensity physical activity (e.g., brisk walking or activities of similar intensity) should be encouraged. In some circumstances, a higher threshold of physical activity may be needed to enhance and sustain long-term weight loss.

3. Engaging in sufficient levels of physical activity can benefit patients who undergo bariatric surgery by potentially enhancing long-term weight loss success and improving other health-related outcomes beyond what can be achieved with bariatric surgery alone.

TABLE 19.1. Determining the Need for Medical Clearance to Engage in Structured Physical Activity

Current activity level	No known cardiovascular, metabolic, or renal disease		Known cardiovascular, metabolic, or renal disease	
	Asymptomatic	Symptomatic	Asymptomatic	Symptomatic
Active[a]	Medical clearance not required to continue physical activity program	Medical clearance recommended before continuing with physical activity	Medical clearance not required provided that prior medical clearance obtained within the previous 12 months	Medical clearance recommended before continuing with physical activity
Inactive	Medical clearance not required to engage in light-intensity to moderate-intensity physical activity	Medical clearance recommended prior to initiating physical activity program	Medical clearance recommended prior to initiating physical activity program	Medical clearance recommended prior to initiating physical activity program

[a]Defined as performing planned structured physical activity for at least 30 minutes at moderate intensity on at least 3 days/week for at least the last 3 months.

4. Self-directed physical activity approaches that do not require attendance at center-based sessions can be effective in increasing physical activity and inducing weight loss. Within the context of self-directed physical activity approaches, encouraging initial engagement in multiple short bouts of activity that are at least 10 minutes in duration may be a particularly effective strategy within the first 6 months of treatment. However, the evidence is mixed with regard to the effectiveness of wearable physical activity monitors to facilitate engagement in physical activity and weight loss.

5. Alternative physical activities such as yoga and resistance training may be considered for weight management. Certain styles of yoga may reach low levels of MVPA and potentially contribute to weight loss. Although increased physical strength and functional improvements may be realized with resistance exercise, there is little evidence that this form of physical activity improves weight loss outcomes beyond what can be achieved with activity such as brisk walking.

6. Based on the current evidence, encouraging patients to reduce sedentary behavior may have limited impact on weight unless coupled with a prescription to also increase participation in moderate-intensity physical activity.

Conclusion

In summary, increased physical activity can play a critical role in the prevention of weight gain and in the treatment of overweight and obesity. Effective methods are needed to encourage individuals to both adopt and maintain greater daily physical activity.

References

Andersen, R. E., Wadden, T. A., Bartlett, S. J., Zemel, B., Verde, T. J., & Franckowiak, S. C. (1999). Effects of lifestyle activity vs. structured aerobic exercise in obese women: A randomized trial. *Journal of the American Medical Association, 281*(4), 335–340.

Baer, R. A. (2009). Self-focused attention and mechanisms of change in mindfulness-based treatment. *Cognitive Behaviour Therapy, 38*(Suppl. 1), 15–20.

Ball, K., Brown, W., & Crawford, D. (2002). Who does not gain weight?: Prevalence and predictors of weight maintenance in young women. *International Journal of Obesity, 26*(12), 1570–1578.

Beers, E. A., Roemmich, J. N., Epstein, L. H., & Horvath, P. J. (2008). Increasing passive energy expenditure during clerical work. *European Journal of Applied Physiology, 103*(3), 353–360.

Bond, D. S., Evans, R. K., Wolfe, L. G., Meador, J. G., Sugerman, H. J., Kellum, J. M., et al. (2004). Impact of self-reported physical activity participation on proportion of excess weight loss and BMI among gastric bypass surgery patients. *The American Surgeon, 70*(9), 811–814.

Bond, D. S., Phelan, S., Wolfe, L. G., Meador, J. G., Kellum, J. M., Maher, J. W., et al. (2009). Becoming physically active after bariatric surgery is associated with improved weight loss and health-related quality of life. *Obesity, 17*(1), 78–83.

Brown, K. W., Goodman, R. J., & Inzlicht, M. (2013). Dispositional mindfulness and the attenuation of neural responses to emotional stimuli. *Social Cognitive and Affective Neuroscience, 8*(1), 93–99.

Buckley, J. P., Mellor, D. D., Morris, M., & Joseph, F. (2014). Standing-based office work shows encouraging signs of attenuating post-prandial glycaemic excursion. *Occupational and Environmental Medicine, 71*(2), 109–111.

Carroll, J., Blansit, A., Otto, R. M., & Wygand, J. W. (2003). The metabolic requirements of Vinyasa yoga. *Medicine and Science in Sports and Exercise, 35*(5), S155.

Catenacci, V. A., Grunwald, G. K., Ingebrigtsen, J. P., Jakicic, J. M., McDermott, M. D., Phelan, S., et al. (2011). Physical activity patterns using accelerometry in the National Weight Control Registry. *Obesity, 19*(6), 1163–1170.

Catenacci, V. A., Ogden, L. G., Stuht, J., Phelan, S., Wing, R. R., Hill, J. O., et al. (2008). Physical activity patterns in the National Weight Control Registry. *Obesity, 16*(1), 153–161.

Chan, C. B., Ryan, D. A., & Tudor-Locke, C. (2004). Health benefits of a pedometer-based physical activity intervention in sedentary workers. *Preventive Medicine, 39*(6), 1215–1222.

Church, T. S., Earnest, C. P., Skinner, J. S., & Blair, S. N. (2007). Effects of different doses of physical activity on cardiorespiratory fitness among sedentary, overweight, or obese postmenopausal women with elevated blood pressure. *Journal of the American Medical Association, 297*(19), 2081–2091.

Church, T. S., Thomas, D. M., Tudor-Locke, C., Katzmarzyk, P. T., Earnest, C. P., Rodarte, R. Q., et al. (2011). Trends over 5 decates in U.S. occupation-related physical activity and their associations with obesity. *PLOS ONE, 6*(5), e19657.

Coen, P. M., Tanner, C. J., Helbling, N. L., Dubis, G. S., Hames, K. M., Hui, X., et al. (2015). Clinical trial demonstrates exercise following bariatric surgery improves insulin sensitivity. *Journal of Clinical Investigation, 125*(1), 248–257.

Creasy, S. A. (2016). *Comparison of supervised and unsupervised physical activity programs during a* standard behavioral weight loss intervention for adults who are overweight or obese. Unpublished doctoral dissertation, University of Pittsburgh, Pittsburgh, PA.

Creasy, S. A., Rogers, R. J., Byard, T. D., Kowalsky, R. J., & Jakicic, J. M. (2016). Energy expenditure during acute periods of sitting, standing, and walking. *Journal of Physical Activity and Health, 13*(6), 573–578.

Donnelly, J. E., Blair, S. N., Jakicic, J. M., Manore, M. M., Rankin, J. W., & Smith, B. K. (2009). ACSM position stand on appropriate intervention strategies for weight loss and prevention of weight regain for adults. *Medicine and Science in Sports and Exercise, 42*(2), 459–471.

Donnelly, J. E., Hill, J. O., Jacobsen, D. J., Potteiger, J., Sullivan, D. K., Johnson, S. L., et al. (2003). Effects of a 16-month randomized controlled exercise trial on body weight and composition in young, overweight men and women: The Midwest Exercise Trial. *Archives of Internal Medicine, 163*(11), 1343–1350.

Donnelly, J. E., Jakicic, J. M., Pronk, N. P., Smith, B. K., Kirk, E. P., Jacobsen, D. J., et al. (2004). Is resistance exercise effective for weight management? *Evidence-Based Preventive Medicine, 1*(1), 21–29.

Evans, R. K., Bond, D. S., Wolfe, L. G., Meador, J. G., Herrick, J. E., Kellum, J. M., et al. (2007). Participation in 150 minutes/week of moderate or higher intensity physical activity yields greater weight loss following gastric bypass surgery. *Surgery for Obesity and Related Disorders, 3*(5), 526–530.

Fan, J. X., Brown, B. B., Hanson, H., Kowaleski-Jones, L., Smith, K. R., & Zick, C. D. (2013). Moderate to vigorous physical activity and weight outcomes: Does every minute count? *American Journal of Preventive Medicine, 28*(1), 41–49.

Finkelstein, E. A., Haaland, B. A., Bilger, M., Sahasranaman, A., Sloan, R. A., Nang, E. E. K., et al. (2016). Effectiveness of activity trackers with and without incentives to increase physical activity (TRIPPA): A randomised controlled trial. *Lancet Diabetes and Endocrinology, 4*(12), 983–995.

Forman, E. M., & Butryn, M. L. (2015). A new look at the science of weight control: How acceptance and commitment strategies can address the challenge of self-regulation. *Appetite, 84*, 171–180.

Foster, J. A., Gore, S. A., & West, D. S. (2006). Altering TV viewing habits: An unexplored strategy for adult obesity intervention? *American Journal of Health Behavior, 30*(1), 3–14.

Goodpaster, B. H., DeLany, J. P., Otto, A. D., Kuller, L. H., Vockley, J., South-Paul, J. E., et al. (2010). Effects of diet and physical actvity interventions on weight loss and cardiometabolic risk factors in severely obese adults: A randomized trial. *Journal of the American Medical Association, 304*(16), 1795–1802.

Goyal, M., Singh, S., Sibinga, E. M., Gould, N. F., Rowland-Seymour, A., Sharma, R., et al. (2014). Meditation programs for psychological stress and well-being: A systematic review and meta-analysis. *JAMA Internal Medicine, 174*(3), 357–368.

Hagins, M., Moore, W., & Rundle, A. (2007). Does practicing hatha yoga satisfy recommendations for intensity of physical activity which improves and maintains health and cardiovascular fitness? *BMC Complementary and Alternative Medicine, 7*, 40.

Hill, J. O., Wyatt, H. R., Reed, G. W., & Peters, J. C. (2003). Obesity and the environment: Where do we go from here? *Science, 7*(299), 853–855.

Hu, F. B., Li, T. Y., Colditz, G. A., Willett, W. C., & Manson, J. E. (2003). Television watching and other sedentary behaviors in relation to risk of obesity and type 2 diabetes mellitus in women. *Journal of the American Medical Association, 289*(14), 1785–1791.

Jakicic, J. M., Davis, K. K., Rogers, R. J., King, W. C., Marcus, M. D., Helsel, D., et al. (2016). Effect of wearable technology combined with a lifestyle intervention on long-term weight loss: The IDEA randomized clinical trial. *Journal of the American Medical Association, 316*(11), 1161–1171.

Jakicic, J. M., Gregg, E., Knowler, W., Kelley, D. E, Lang, W., Miller, G. D., et al. (2010). Physical activity patterns of overweight and obese individuals with type 2 diabetes in the Look AHEAD Study. *Medicine and Science in Sports and Exercise, 42*(11), 1995–2005.

Jakicic, J. M., King, W. C., Marcus, M. D., Davis, K. K., Helsel, D., Rickman, A. D., et al. (2015). Short-term weight loss with diet and physical activity in young adults: The IDEA Study. *Obesity, 23*(12), 2385–2397.

Jakicic, J. M., Marcus, B. H., Gallagher, K. I., Napolitano, M., & Lang, W. (2003). Effect of exercise duration and intensity on weight loss in overweight, sedentary women: A randomized trial. *Journal of the American Medical Association, 290*(10), 1323–1330.

Jakicic, J. M., Marcus, B. H., Lang, W., & Janney, C. (2008). Effect of exercise on 24-month weight loss in overweight women. *Archives of Internal Medicine, 168*(14), 1550–1559.

Jakicic, J. M., Otto, A. D., Semler, L., Polzien, K., Lang, W., & Mohr, K. (2011). Effect of physical activity on 18-month weight change in overweight adults. *Obesity, 19*(1), 100–109.

Jakicic, J. M., Rickman, A. D., Lang, W., Davis, K. K., Barone Gibbs, B., Neiberg, R. H., et al. (2015). Time-based physical activity interventions for weight loss: A randomized trial. *Medicine and Science in Sports and Exercise, 47*(5), 1061–1069.

Jakicic, J. M., Tate, D., Davis, K. K., Polzien, K., Rickman, A. D., Erickson, K., et al. (2012). Effect of a stepped-care intervention approach on weight loss in adults: The Step-Up Study Randomized Trial. *Journal of the American Medical Association, 307*(24), 2617–2626.

Jakicic, J. M., Tate, D. F., Lang, W., Davis, K. K., Polzien, K., Neiberg, R., et al. (2014). Objective physical activity and weight loss in adults: The Step-Up randomized clinical trial. *Obesity, 22*(11), 2284–2292.

Jakicic, J. M., Wing, R. R., Butler, B. A., & Robertson, R. J. (1995). Prescribing exercise in multiple short bouts versus one continuous bout: Effects on adherence, cardiorespiratory fitness, and weight loss in overweight women. *International Journal of Obesity, 19*(12), 893–901.

Jakicic, J. M., Winters, C., Lang, W., & Wing, R. R. (1999). Effects of intermittent exercise and use of home exercise equipment on adherence, weight loss, and fitness in overweight women: A randomized trial. *Journal of the American Medical Association, 282*(16), 1554–1560.

Jeffery, R. W., Wing, R. R., Sherwood, N. E., & Tate, D. F. (2003). Physical activity and weight loss: Does prescribing higher physical activity goals improve outcome? *American Journal of Clinical Nutrition, 78*(4), 684–689.

Jensen, M. D., Ryan, D. H., Apovian, C. M., Ard, J. D., Comuzzie, A. G., Donato, K. A., et al. (2014). 2013 AHA/ACC/TOS guideline for the management of overweight and obesity in adults: A report of the American College of Cardiology/American Heart Association Task Force on Practice Guidelines and The Obesity Society. *Journal of the American College of Cardiology, 63*(25), 2985–3023.

Josbeno, D. A., Kalarchian, M., Sparto, P. J., Otto, A. D., & Jakicic, J. M. (2011). Physical activity and physical function in individuals post-bariatric surgery. *Obesity Surgery, 21*(8), 1243–1249.

Kabat-Zinn, J. (1991). *Full catastrophe living: Using the wisdom of your body and mind to face stress, pain, and illness.* New York: Dell.

Khalsa, S. B. S. (2004). Treatment of chronic insomnia with yoga: A preliminary study with sleep–wake diaries. *Applied Psychophysiology and Biofeedback, 29*(4), 269–278.

King, W. C., & Bond, D. S. (2013). The importance of pre and postoperative physical activity counseling in bariatric surgery. *Exercise and Sport Sciences Review, 41*(6), 26–35.

King, W. C., Chen, C. Y., Bond, D. S., Belle, S. H., Courcoulas, A. P., Patterson, E. J., et al. (2015). Objective assessment of changes in physical activity and sedentary behavior: Pre- through 3 years post-bariatric surgery. *Obesity, 23*(6), 1143–1150.

King, W. C., Hsu, J. Y., Belle, S. H., Courcoulas, A. P., Eid, G. M., Flum, D. R., et al. (2012). Pre- to postoperative changes in physical activity: Report from the Longitudinal Assessment of Bariatric Surgery-2 (LABS-2). *Surgery for Obesity and Related Diseases, 8*(5), 522–532.

Klem, M. L., Wing, R. R., McGuire, M. T., Seagle, H. M., & Hill, J. O. (1997). A descriptive study of individuals successful at long-term maintenance of substantial weight loss. *American Journal of Clinical Nutrition, 66*(2), 239–246.

Kristeller, J. L., & Wolever, R. Q. (2011). Mindfulness-based eating awareness training for treating binge eating disorder: The conceptual foundation. *Eating Disorders, 19*(1), 49–61.

Lee, I., Djousse, M. L., Sesso, H. D., Wang, L., & Buring, J. E. (2010). Physical activity and weight gain prevention. *Journal of the American Medical Association, 303*(12), 1173–1179.

Levine, J. A., & Miller, J. M. (2007). The energy expenditure of using a "walk-and-work" desk for office workers with obesity. *British Journal of Sports Medicine, 41*(9), 558–561.

Levine, J. A., Schleusner, S. J., & Jensen, M. D. (2000). Energy expenditure of nonexercise activity. *American Journal of Clinical Nutrition, 72*(6), 1451–1454.

Li, A. W., & Goldsmith, C. A. (2012). The effects of yoga on anxiety and stress. *Alternative Medicine Review, 17*(1), 21–35.

Lillis, J., Hayes, S. C., Bunting, K., & Masuda, A. (2009). Teaching acceptance and mindfulness to improve the lives of the obese: A preliminary test of a theoretical model. *Annals of Behavioral Medicine, 37*(1), 58–69.

Magal, M., & Riebe, D. (2016). New preparticipation health screening recommendations: What exercise professionals need to know. *ACSM Health and Fitness Journal, 20*(3), 22–27.

McAlpine, D. A., Manohar, C. U., McCrady, S. K., Hensrud, D., & Levine, J. A. (2007). An office-place stepping device to promote workplace physical activity. *British Journal of Sports Medicine, 41*(12), 903–907.

McTiernan, A., Sorensen, B., Irwin, M. L., Morgan, A., Yasui, Y., Rudolph, R. E., et al. (2007). Exercise effect on weight and body fat in men and women. *Obesity, 15*(6), 1496–1512.

Michalsen, A., Grossmon, P., Acil, A., Langhorst, J., Ludtke, R., Esch, T., et al. (2005). Rapid stress reduction and anxiolysis among distressed women as a consequence of a three-month intensive yoga program. *Medical Science Monitor, 11*(12), 555–561.

Mustian, M., Sproad, L. K., Janelsins, M., Peppone, L. J., Palesh, O. G., Chandwani, K., et al. (2013). Multicenter, randomized controlled trial of yoga for sleep quality among cancer survivors. *Journal of Clinical Oncology, 10*(31), 3233–3241.

Pellegrini, C. A., Verba, S. D., Otto, A. D., Helsel, D. L., Davis, K. K., & Jakicic, J. M. (2012). The comparison of a technology-based system and an in-person behavioral weight loss intervention. *Obesity, 20*(2), 356–363.

Perri, M. G., Martin, A. D., Leermakers, E. A., Sears, S. F., & Notelovitz, M. (1997). Effects of group- versus home-based exercise in the treatment of obesity. *Journal of Consulting and Clinical Psychology, 65*(2), 278–285.

Piwek, L., Ellis, D. A., Andrews, S., & Joinson, A. (2016). The rise of consumer health wearables: Promises and barriers. *PLOS Medicine, 13*(2), e1001953.

Polzien, K. M., Jakicic, J. M., Tate, D. F., & Otto, A. D. (2007). The efficacy of a technology-based system in a short-term behavioral weight loss intervention. *Obesity, 15*(4), 825–830.

Reiff, C., Marlatt, K., & Dengel, D. R. (2012). Difference in caloric expenditure in sitting versus standing desks. *Journal of Physical Activity and Health, 9*(7), 1009–1011.

Rogers, R. J., Lang, W., Gibbs, B. B., Davis, K. K., Burke, L. E., Kovacs, S. I., et al. (2016). Comparison of a technology-based system and in-person behavioral weight loss intervention in adults with severe obesity. *Obesity Science and Practice, 2*(1), 3–12.

Ross, R., Dagnone, D., Jones, P. J. H., Smith, H., Paddags, A., Hudson, R., et al. (2000). Reduction in obesity and related comorbid conditions after diet-induced weight loss or exercise-induced weight loss in men. *Annals of Internal Medicine, 133*(2), 92–103.

Ross, R., Janssen, I., Dawson, J., Kungl, A. M., Kuk, J. L., Wong, S. L., et al. (2004). Exercise-induced reduction in obesity and insulin resistance in women: A randomized controlled trial. *Obesity Research, 12*(5), 789–798.

Sears, S., & Kraus, S. (2009). I think therefore I om: Cognitive distortions and coping style as mediators for the effects of mindfulness meditation on anxiety, positive and negative affect, and hope. *Journal of Clinical Psychology, 65*(6), 561–573.

Sherman, K. J., Cherkin, D. C., & Wellman, R. D. (2011). A randomized trial comparing yoga, stretch, and a self-care book for chronic low back pain. *Archives of Internal Medicine, 171*(22), 2019–2026.

Sherman, S. A. (2016). *Energy expenditure in yoga versus other forms of physical activity.* Unpublished doctoral dissertation, University of Pittsburgh, Pittsburgh, PA.

Shiroma, E. J., Sesso, H. D., & Lee, I. M. (2012). Physical activity and weight gain prevention in older men. *International Journal of Obesity (London), 36*(9), 1165–1169.

Shugar, S. L., Barry, V. W., Sui, X., McClain, A., Hand, G. A., Wilcox, S., et al. (2011). Electronic feedback in a diet- and physical activity-based lifestyle intervention for weight loss: A randomized controlled trial. *International Journal of Behavioral Nutrition and Physical Activity, 8*, 41–49.

Slentz, C. A., Duscha, M. S., Johnson, J. L., Ketchum, K., Aiken, L. B., Samsa, G. P., et al. (2004). Effects of the amount of exercise on body weight, body composition, and measures of central obesity: STRIDDE—a randomized controlled study. *Archives of Internal Medicine, 164*(1), 31–39.

Swift, D. L., Johannsen, N. M., Lavie, C. J., Earnest, C. P., & Church, T. S. (2014). The role of exercise and physical activity in weight loss and maintenance. *Progress in Cardiovascular Diseases, 56*(4), 441–447.

Tate, D. F., Jeffery, R. W., Sherwood, N. E., & Wing, R. R. (2007). Long-term weight losses associated with prescription of higher physical activity goals: Are higher levels of physical activity protective against weight regain? *American Journal of Clinical Nutrition, 85*(4), 954–959.

Tudor-Locke, C., & Bassett, D. R. (2004). How many steps/day are enough?: Preliminary pedometer indices for public health. *Sports Medicine, 34*(1), 1–8.

Uebelacker, L. A., Epstein-Lubow, G., Guadiano, B. A., Tremont, G., Battle, C. L., & Miller, I. W. (2010). Hatha yoga for depression: Critical review of the evidence for efficacy, plausible mechanisms of action, and directions for future research. *Journal of Psychiatric Practice, 16*(1), 22–23.

Unick, J. L., Jakicic, J. M., & Marcus, B. H. (2010). Contribution of behavior intervention components to 24 month weight loss. *Medicine and Science in Sports and Exercise, 42*(4), 745–753.

U.S. Department of Health and Human Services. (2008). Physical activity guidelines advisory committee report 2008. Retrieved January 19, 2009, from *www.health.gov/paguidelines/report/pdf/ CommitteeReport.pdf.*

Wadden, T. A., West, D. S., Neiberg, R. H., Wing, R. R., Ryan, D. H., Johnson, K. C., et al. (2009). One-year weight losses in the Look AHEAD Study: Factors associated with success. *Obesity, 17*(4), 713–722.

Washburn, R. A., Szabo, A. N., Lambourne, K., Willis, E. A., Ptomey, L. T., Honas, J. J., et al., (2014). Does the method of weight loss effect the long-term changes in weight, body composition or chronic disease risk factors in overweight or obese adults?: A systematic review. *PLOS ONE, 9*(10), e109849.

Williamson, D. F., Madans, J., Anda, R. F., Kleinman, J. C., Kahn, H. S., & Byers, T. (1993). Recreational physical activity and ten-year weight change in a US national cohort. *International Journal of Obesity, 17*(5), 279–286.

Wing, R. R. (1999). Physical activity in the treatment of adulthood overweight and obesity: Current evidence and research issues. *Medicine and Science in Sports and Exercise, 31*(11, Suppl. 1), S547–S552.

Wing, R. R., Venditti, E. M., Jakicic, J. M., Polley, B. A., & Lang, W. (1998). Lifestyle intervention in overweight individuals with a family history of diabetes. *Diabetes Care, 21*(3), 350–359.

Woolery, A., Myers, H., Sternlieb, B., & Zelter, L. (2004). Yoga intervention for young adults with depression. *Alternative Therapies in Health and Medicine, 10*(2), 60–63.

CHAPTER 20

Behavioral Treatment of Obesity

Stephanie Gomez-Rubalcava
Kaitlin Stabbert
Suzanne Phelan

Behavioral treatment of obesity is a theory-based approach for fostering long-term weight control. The treatment applies principles from learning theories, including classical conditioning, operant conditioning, and social learning, to help patients learn skills to modify eating and activity behaviors. The approach recognizes that genetic and metabolic factors may predispose individuals to obesity, but emphasizes the interplay between the individual and the environment in shaping behavior. Behavioral treatment is arguably the most thoroughly evaluated weight control approach. When combined with diet and exercise strategies, behavioral treatment produces clinically significant weight loss and improves patients' health status. Behavioral treatment has been delivered through many modalities (Tsai & Wadden, Chapter 27, this volume), applied to many populations (Downey & Kyle, Chapter 25, and Lawman, Wojtanowski, & Foster, Chapter 38, this volume), and integrated with other treatment approaches (West, Krukowski, & Larsen, Chapter 30, this volume). This chapter reviews the key components of typical behavioral treatment programs for adults, describes the results of current behavioral interventions, and discusses future directions.

Theoretical Foundation

Behavioral treatment is largely derived from classical conditioning, operant conditioning, and social learning theories. Classical conditioning is based on associative learning and posits that when two stimuli are repeatedly paired, they become linked, and eventually one stimulus will automatically trigger the other. As applied to eating, a person who repeatedly eats while watching television or driving in the car might experience an urge to eat whenever watching television or driving. Several studies provide evidence of the powerful role that environmental factors play in influencing eating and activity behaviors (Cohen, 2008). Proximity and visibility of food are especially strong environmental eating cues. Behavior therapy aims to identify and uncouple learned associations that promote overeating and inactivity. Patients are encouraged to eat only in one place instead of multiple rooms and to do nothing else while eating in order to break apart the many associations that build between eating and other activities (Butryn, Webb, & Wadden, 2011; Stuart, 1967). Behavioral treatment also strives to build new associations that promote healthy eating and activity. For example, a patient might be encouraged to leave a pair of walking sneakers repeatedly by the bed to serve as a prompt for a morning walk. A fruit bowl might be left on the kitchen table to prompt healthy eating.

Behavioral treatment is also derived from operant conditioning principles. Operant conditioning holds that behaviors that are rewarded (reinforcement) tend to be repeated more frequently over time, whereas behaviors that produce negative consequences (punishment) tend to be repeated less frequently over time (Skinner, 1953). New behavior is established most quickly when it is rewarded immediately and often. As applied to weight control, patients are taught to closely monitor the outcomes of their eating and activity behaviors. Positive rewards are planned for achieving desired goals. Rewards might include feeling confident, receiving praise from an interventionist, or buying a new book after a behavioral success (Alamuddin & Wadden, 2016; Chapman & Jeffrey, 1978). Treatment also aims to lessen potential negative consequences associated with increasing activity and eating less (Butryn, Clark, & Coletta, 2012). For example, a gradual increase in activity is encouraged to prevent fatigue, and the selection of enjoyable activities is promoted to reduce boredom. Eating small meals throughout the day and choosing foods that enhance feelings of fullness are also recommended to reduce feelings of hunger during treatment.

Using principles of both classical and operant conditioning, behavioral treatment incorporates functional analysis to help patients identify the cues and consequences of eating and activity behaviors. Functional analysis helps patients identify the events (e.g., items, places, people, feelings) associated with unhealthy eating and physical activity patterns and the consequences of each behavioral choice (Sturmey, 2007). Creating a behavioral chain is helpful in identifying opportunities for intervention (Brownell, 1998; Haynes & O'Brien, 1990; Wadden, Crerand, & Brock, 2005). Figure 20.1 shows an example of a behavioral chain. In this example, the patient might be encouraged to plan to get additional sleep, to eat before shopping, and/or to shop from a list in order to break links in the chain that lead to overeating.

Behavioral treatment also draws, in large part, from social cognitive theory (Bandura, 1977). Social cognitive theory emphasizes self-efficacy as a crucial determinant of behavior. *Self-efficacy* is defined as an individual's perceived ability to successfully engage in the behaviors needed to reach desired

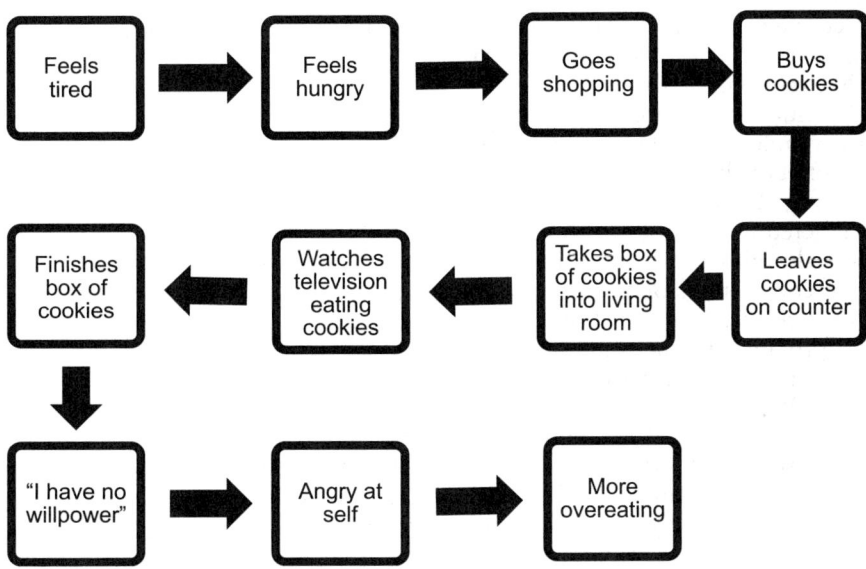

FIGURE 20.1. Behavioral chain used for a functional analysis of a patient's overeating episode. Links in the chain can be broken and seen as opportunities for intervention.

goals. In the behavioral treatment of obesity, patients with high self-efficacy believe that they can and will successfully meet their eating, physical activity, and other treatment goals. They are confident that their efforts will result in benefits. Behavioral interventionists may target improvements in self-efficacy by setting achievable weekly goals, reinforcing the positive consequences of achieving goals, and providing ongoing positive feedback for every behavioral success (Wadden et al., 2005). Higher self-efficacy has been consistently related to weight loss. A recent clinical trial (Burke et al., 2015) found that a behavioral intervention that emphasized self-efficacy improved 18-month weight loss outcomes compared with a standard behavioral treatment approach (8% vs. 6% loss of initial body weight, respectively), underscoring the importance of bolstering self-efficacy in behavioral treatment.

Format of Behavioral Treatment

Behavioral treatment typically consists of a structured series of lessons (Table 20.1). Treatment often takes place over weekly patient–provider visits for the first 6 months, followed by every-other-week meetings for 6 months, and monthly meetings thereafter (Butryn et al., 2011; Wadden et al., 2005). Continued contact appears to be critical to lasting success (Perri et al., 2001). Behavioral treatment is commonly led by interventionists trained in nutrition, exercise physiology, or clinical psychology, but lay interventionists may also effectively administer treatment (Leahey & Wing, 2013). Treatment meetings may be conducted in person, in groups, one on one, over the phone, over the Internet, or as part of commercial or hospital-based weight loss programs. Some level of face-to-face patient–provider interaction appears to be critical to maximizing long-term success (Svetkey et al., 2015). If delivered in a group format, meetings typically last 1 hour; one-on-one visits may last 30 minutes.

In a typical visit, treatment begins with the interventionist privately measuring the patient's weight. The interventionist informs the patient as to the amount of weight lost since the last visit and the total loss since the beginning of treatment (Alamuddin & Wadden, 2016; Wadden et al., 2005). Positive reinforcement is provided for successful weight loss and support and encouragement are offered to patients who are unhappy with their weight change. During the weigh-in, the interventionist reinforces the connection between the patient's specific weekly behaviors and the resulting weight loss. After the weigh-in, the interventionist reviews the patient's successes and barriers in completing any assigned homework since the last visit. New materials or topics are discussed (Table 20.1). Finally, time is reserved at the end of each session to review goals and assign new homework for the next visit.

TABLE 20.1. Sample List of Lessons Covered during the First 6 Months of a Behavioral Treatment Program for Obesity

1. Behavioral approach to weight control
2. Goal setting
3. Daily self-monitoring
4. Increasing your physical activity: Programmed exercise
5. Healthy food choices
6. Cues in your physical environment for eating and exercise
7. Increasing lifestyle exercise
8. Eating in social situations
9. Eating patterns
10. Barriers to exercise
11. Problem solving
12. Simple ways to reduce calories
13. Eating out in restaurants
14. Building social support
15. Thoughts and weight control
16. Exercising for aerobic fitness
17. Mediterranean eating
18. Reducing sedentary time
19. Recipe modification
20. High-risk situations
21. Assertion and eating
22. Motivation
23. Getting back on track: Lapses
24. Stress and eating
25. Mindfulness
26. Maintaining long-term weight control

Behavioral Skills

Behavioral treatment is delivered as a "package" comprised of multiple components designed to teach patients the skills needed to modify their eating and activity behaviors. The intervention can differ widely in the extent to which emphasis is placed on different behavior change strategies. Moreover, the independent contribution to weight loss of each strategy within a package is difficult to isolate. Even though millions of possible variations exist, behavioral treatment's key components most commonly include goal setting, self-monitoring, stimulus control, positive reinforcement, problem solving, and cognitive restructuring (Wadden, Butryn, & Wilson, 2007).

Goal Setting

Behavioral treatment encourages patients to set specific goals for weight, eating, and physical activity, which are identified and defined in behavioral terms early in care. The interventionist guides the selection of these goals, and the patient is actively involved in the process. Long-term and short-term weight, eating, and activity goals are made explicit and then operationalized, using functional analysis to describe how, when, and where specific actions will be performed to meet desired goals (Pearson, 2012).

For weight loss, the overall target goal is typically equivalent to a 10% loss of initial body weight. Although health improvements occur with as little as a 3–5% weight loss (Jensen et al., 2014), overall weight loss goals that are more challenging are associated with greater weight loss success (Jeffery, Wing, & Mayer, 1998). Long-term weight-loss goals are then subdivided into achievable goals of a 1- to 2-pound weight loss per week (0.45–0.9 kg). Caloric restriction is emphasized rather than macronutrient composition, as diets may differ markedly in macronutrient composition yet still promote weight loss (Sacks et al., 2009). Moderate calorie restriction is typically recommended; patients weighing ≥ 113.5 kg (250 pounds) are advised to consume 1,500–1,800 kcal/day, and those weighing less than 113.5 kg to eat 1,200–1,500 kcal/day. Given variations in caloric needs based on a patient's height, weight, sex, age, activity level, and other factors, calorie goals may be modified depending on weekly progress (Smith & Wing, 2000).

A gradual increase in structured physical activity is advised, with the long-term goal of 180–200 minutes or more of activity each week. At the outset of treatment, an initial activity goal might be to walk at least 10 minutes per day for 4 days. Then, each week, the physical activity goal might be increased by approximately 10 minutes to an eventual goal of 200 minutes of activity per week. A gradual increase in lifestyle activity is also targeted, with the eventual goal of walking at least 10,000 steps per day (Butryn et al., 2012). Steps are typically monitored using a pedometer. However, the inclusion of wearable technology devices that monitor physical activity during treatment may not improve long-term weight loss outcomes (Jakicic et al., 2016).

Self-Weighing

Patients are instructed to weigh themselves at home and track progress using weight graphs. Daily, as opposed to less frequent self-weighing, appears to promote the best weight control (Linde, Jeffery, French, Pronk, & Boyle, 2005). Frequent self-weighing helps patients learn the link between their behaviors and weight changes. Literature reviews on the topic have concluded that self-weighing is a significant and independent predictor of greater weight loss (Vanwormer, French, Pereira, & Welsh, 2008; Zheng et al., 2015). Regular self-weighing has also been shown to promote greater long-term weight loss maintenance (Zheng et al., 2016) and to prevent weight gain (Wing et al., 2016) in adults. Frequent self-weighing is not associated with adverse psychological outcomes, such as depressive symptoms, eating disorders, or binge eating (Wing et al., 2007; Zheng et al., 2015).

Self-Monitoring of Behaviors

The systematic recording of behaviors has long been considered the cornerstone of behavioral treatment. Self-monitoring increases awareness of target behaviors and provides feedback on progress (Burke, Wang, &

Sevick, 2011; Turk et al., 2013). Patients are taught to write down everything they eat, to estimate or count calories in foods using a calorie counting book, and to keep a running total of their intake to ensure they stay within their calorie goal. Since individuals may underestimate their food intake (Lichtman et al., 1992), treatment provides training in reading food labels and using measuring cups and spoons. Patients are also encouraged to record the type and the total minutes of physical activity completed each day and to use a pedometer to objectively track their daily number of steps (Butryn et al., 2012). Typically, record keeping is increased over time to include information about times, places, thoughts, and feelings associated with eating and activity.

A number of clinical trials (Baker & Kirschenbaum, 1993; Fabricatore et al., 2009; Jeffery et al., 1993) and reviews of the literature (Burke, Conroy, et al., 2011) have found self-monitoring of eating and activity to be significantly correlated with short- and long-term weight loss outcomes. A new generation of online trackers and applications (apps) has greatly simplified the tracking of eating and activity behaviors. A variety of apps to monitor dietary intake are available from major smartphone platforms such as iPhone, Android, Nokia, and BlackBerry, but relatively few have been tested in research studies to determine their effectiveness in promoting weight loss (Coughlin et al., 2015). New technologies to monitor physical activity (e.g., Fitbit) have also emerged and may hold promise for enhancing long-term adherence (Turner-McGrievy et al., 2013). However, a randomized trial found that the inclusion of wearable technology devices to monitor physical activity during behavioral treatment did not improve 24-month weight loss outcomes during behavioral treatment (Jakicic et al., 2016).

Stimulus Control

Behavioral treatment also teaches stimulus control techniques to reduce the cues for overeating and inactivity and to strengthen the cues for desired behaviors (Alamuddin & Wadden, 2016; Butryn et al., 2011). In order to limit exposure to cues that prompt overeating, patients are taught to store foods out of sight, to limit the places that they eat to only one or two rooms, and to refrain from engaging in other activities while eating (e.g., watching television). Stimulus control strategies are also used to create positive cues for healthy behaviors (Alamuddin & Wadden, 2016; Butryn et al., 2011). A patient might move a treadmill from the basement to a more visible location in the house to prompt exercise.

Randomized clinical trials have found that behavioral treatment programs that emphasize restructuring cues in the home environment tend to improve long-term weight loss success. Jakicic and colleagues found that access to exercise equipment in the home facilitated the maintenance of short bouts of physical activity (Jakicic, Wing, Butler, & Jeffery, 1997; Jakicic, Winters, Lang, & Wing, 1999). Gorin et al. (2008) found that behavioral treatment that emphasized restructuring the physical and social home environment was effective in enhancing weight loss for women but not men. Use of meal plans, prepackaged foods, and liquid meal replacements offers another stimulus control strategy. Meal plans and prepackaged foods may serve to enhance positive food cues and reduce the number of high-calorie food options in the home. Several studies have suggested that meal plans and meal replacements improve dietary adherence and produce greater weight loss than diets comprised of conventional foods (Flechtner-Mors, Ditschuneit, Johnson, Suchard, & Adler, 2000; Heymsfield, 2010; Wadden et al., 2009).

Positive Reinforcement and Feedback

An integral part of treatment is the provision of positive consequences for engaging in weight control behaviors. At each visit, interventionists review food and activity records and provide supportive feedback for the patient. Weight loss is perhaps the strongest positive consequence that patients experience after successfully adhering to behavioral and environmental change goals (Alamuddin & Wadden, 2016; Chapman & Jeffrey, 1978). During maintenance, additional positive reinforcers are especially important and may include interpersonal (e.g., self-praise, praise from interventionist) and tangible (e.g., family bike ride) rewards. Financial reinforcers or deposit contracts can also be effective reinforcers for promoting desired behavior changes (Jeffery, 2012; Volpp et al., 2008).

Problem Solving

Behavioral programs teach patients to anticipate and plan for lapses and to prevent them from escalating to relapse (Marlatt & Gordon, 1979, 1985). To this end, problem solving is used, especially during later weeks of a behavioral program. Patients are taught to (1) identify the problem situation and describe it in detail using a behavioral chain; (2) brainstorm solutions to the problem, considering the pros and cons of each possible solution; and (3) choose, implement, and evaluate the effectiveness of one solution. If the problem is not successfully solved, the process is repeated. Increasing problem-solving skills has been associated with improved weight loss and weight loss maintenance (Murawski et al., 2009; Perri et al., 2001).

Cognitive Restructuring

Cognitive theory posits that a person's thoughts determine emotional and behavioral responses to events (Beck, 1976). For example, a person may overeat and think "I've totally blown it, I should just give up." This irrational thinking may lead to feelings of despair and to continued overeating and relapse. In treatment, cognitive strategies are aimed at identifying and modifying aversive thinking patterns and mood states that may interfere with successful weight control. Patients are taught to monitor their thoughts and feelings and to replace cognitive distortions with rational responses (Cooper, Fairburn, & Hawker, 2003). Thus, a patient might be taught to replace the thought of "totally blowing it" with the thought "I know that was not the best choice, but I am going to stick with my eating plan for the rest of the day." A meta-analysis (Shaw, O'Rourke, Del Mar, & Kenardy, 2005) found that cognitive therapy, when combined with diet and exercise interventions, produced greater weight losses than diet and exercise treatment alone. However, a 3-year study that focused strongly on cognitive modification showed no greater weight loss with this approach than with traditional behavioral treatment (Cooper et al., 2010).

Long-Term Efficacy

Behavioral treatment combined with diet and exercise intervention consistently produces greater weight losses than diet and exercise intervention alone (Shaw et al., 2005). Clinical trials testing the efficacy of comprehensive behavioral treatment packages have found weight losses averaging about 8–10% of initial body weight over 20–30 weeks. After initial weight loss, gradual weight regain is observed, resulting in a 4–5% weight loss maintained for up to 8 years (Butryn et al., 2011; Look AHEAD Research Group, 2014; Look AHEAD Research Group & Wing, 2010). These long-term results are modest, yet meet the criteria for success (i.e., 5–10% weight loss) endorsed by the World Health Organization (1998), the Dietary Guidelines for Americans (U.S. Department of Health and Human Services, 2010), and the Guidelines for the Management of Overweight and Obesity in Adults, published by the American Heart Association, the American College of Cardiology, and the Obesity Society (Jensen et al., 2014). Even with weight regain, improvements in long-term health are observed with comprehensive behavioral treatment programs (Knowler et al., 2002).

Findings from the three largest and longest studies of behavioral treatment provide perhaps the strongest evidence that this approach can promote sustained, modest weight losses that translate into significant health benefit (Table 20.2). The Diabetes Prevention Program (DPP) Research Group conducted a large, randomized clinical trial involving U.S. adults (> 25 years) who had a body mass index (BMI) ≥ 24 kg/m^2 and elevated glucose concentrations, making them at high risk for the development of type 2 diabetes mellitus. The DPP comprehensive behavioral treatment program produced a 5.6 kg weight loss at an average of 2.8 years and reduced the risk of developing diabetes by 58%. The intervention also reduced high blood pressure and metabolic syndrome

TABLE 20.2. Large-Scale (> 1,000) and Long-Term (> 2 Year) Randomized Controlled Trials of Behavioral Weight Loss Interventions in Adults

Reference	n	Pretreatment Patient characteristics	Pretreatment Randomized groups	Long-term outcome Duration	Long-term outcome Weight loss	Long-term outcome Duration	Long-term outcome Weight loss
Diabetes Prevention Program Research Group et al. (2009); Florez et al. (2006)	3,234	Males + females with pre-diabetes	Placebo	2.8 y	0.1 kg	10 y	1.0 kg
			Lifestyle intervention		5.6 kg		2.0 kg
Look AHEAD Research Group (2007, 2010, 2014)	5,145	Males + females with Type 2 diabetes	Support and education	1 y	0.7%	8 y	2.1%
			Behavioral treatment		8.6%		4.7%
Weight Loss Maintenance Trial (Svetkey et al., 2008)	1,032	Males + females who had achieved ≥ 4-kg weight loss in phase 1	Monthly contact control	2.5 y	2.9 kg		
			Self-directed behavioral tx		4.2 kg		
			Web-based behavioral tx		3.3 kg		

Note. Tx, treatment; y, year. Participants in the lifestyle arm of the Diabetes Prevention Program received standard behavioral treatment for 2.8 years. Thereafter, semiannual group lifestyle intervention was offered to both the lifestyle intervention and placebo groups. Participants in the Look AHEAD trial received standard behavioral treatment for the first 2 years followed by less intensive intervention (one or two contacts/month) thereafter.

(Diabetes Prevention Program Research et al., 2009; Florez et al., 2006; Knowler et al., 2002). The Finnish DPP produced similar results (Lindstrom et al., 2003).

In the Look AHEAD study of patients with type 2 diabetes, the intensive lifestyle behavioral intervention produced an 8.6% weight loss at 1 year and maintained nearly a 5% weight loss at 8 years (Look AHEAD Research Group, 2014; Look AHEAD Research Group et al., 2007; Look AHEAD Research Group & Wing, 2010). The intervention did not reduce cardiovascular events, such as heart attack and stroke (Look AHEAD Research Group et al., 2013), but was associated with improved diabetes control and a reduction in cardiovascular disease risk factors and medication use (Pi-Sunyer et al., 2007; Wing, 2010).

The Weight Loss Maintenance (WLM) trial compared three different behavioral treatments to promote weight loss maintenance among 1,032 individuals with overweight or obesity and high blood pressure and/or high cholesterol. Patients who had lost an average of 8.5 kg during an initial 6-month weight loss phase were randomly assigned to one of three programs for weight loss maintenance: monthly behavioral treatment delivered primarily over the phone, monthly web-delivered behavioral intervention, or a self-directed control group (Svetkey et al., 2008). At the end of 2.5 years, participants who received brief behavioral counseling retained an average weight loss of 4.2 kg, compared to an average 3.3-kg loss for those who used the web-based intervention, and 2.9 kg for those in the self-directed group. Thus monthly, brief behavioral counseling, delivered by phone, produced the best long-term weight loss outcomes.

Predictors of Weight Loss

Extensive research has examined whether certain individuals respond better than others to behavioral weight loss treatment. For the most part, treatment induces weight loss regardless of demographic background. Thus, the outcomes of treatment generally do not differ by gender (French, Jeffery, & Wing, 1994; Hoie & Bruusgaard, 1999), age (Hoie & Bruusgaard, 1999; Wing et al., 2016), age of onset of obesity (Rupp, Taverno Ross, Lang, & Jakicic, 2016), dieting history (Hoie & Bruusgaard, 1999; Pekkarinen, Takala, & Mustajoki, 1996), marital status (Pekkarinen et al., 1996), education, or employment (Neumark-Sztainer, Kaufmann, & Berry, 1995). Similarly, most research suggests that treatment is beneficial regardless of pretreatment levels of depression and anxiety (Karlsson et al., 1994; Pekkarinen et al., 1996; Wadden, Foster, & Letizia, 1992), binge eating (Sherwood, Jeffery, & Wing, 1999), and personality variables (Poston et al., 1999). Findings are mixed regarding the role of race/ethnicity. Some weight loss trials have shown that minorities, particularly African American women, lose less weight than European American participants at 6–12 months (Hollis et al., 2008; Kumanyika, Obarzanek, Stevens, Hebert, & Whelton, 1991; Sutton, Magwood, Jenkins, & Nemeth, 2016). However, other studies have shown that African American and Hispanic participants achieve long-term (> 1 year) weight losses that are comparable to those achieved by European American participants (Wadden et al., 2011; Wing, 2004).

Future Directions

Behavioral treatment can promote sustained, modest weight losses that translate into significant health benefits. However, the average 5–10% reduction in body weight masks heterogeneity in treatment effects. There are several avenues for future investigation.

First Responders

Most participants in behavioral treatment trials are highly motivated and often must undergo a behavioral "run-in" before enrollment to ensure treatment adherence. For example, the Look AHEAD trial required participants to record their food intake for 1–2 weeks before becoming eligible for study participation. Participants in the study who kept more detailed food records during this run-in lost more weight after 1 year than individuals who kept sparser records (Tsai et al., 2014). As a corollary, magnitude of initial weight loss early in treatment has been consistently and positively correlated with long-term weight loss success. In the Look AHEAD trial, larger 1- and 2-month weight losses were associated with larger 8-year losses (Unick et al., 2015). The factors that lead some individuals to respond and others to fail early in treatment merit further investigation.

Minimizing Burden

Behavioral treatment requires that patients complete homework assignments, attend ongoing visits, and self-monitor every day. Treatment is intensive and time-consuming, as well as somewhat reliant on literacy, language, motivation, and time management skills. Some individuals may not have the immediate resources—perceived or actual—to engage in standard treatment regimens. New technologies hold promise for lessening the burden of some behavioral tasks, such as self-monitoring. However, other innovations are needed to reduce treatment demands on time, attention, and effort, while maintaining treatment efficacy.

Adaptive Interventions

Adaptive interventions that are tailored to fit individual patient needs throughout the treatment process may prove beneficial (Sherwood et al., 2016). Adaptive interventions provide a sequential, individualized approach to treatment that is adapted and readapted over time in response to specific patient needs. For example, a patient who did not initially respond to five sessions of standard behavioral treatment could have treatment augmented to include meal replacements (Sherwood et al., 2016). A patient with a history of emotional eating could have treatment augmented with acceptance and commitment therapy (West, Krukowski, & Larsen, Chapter 30, this volume). Adaptive interventions provide one way to integrate and optimize behavioral treatment strategies, leading to individualized sequences of treatment that may prove beneficial (Lei, Nahum-Shani, Lynch, Oslin, & Murphy, 2012).

Mechanisms

The specific cognitive and behavioral mechanisms through which behavioral weight loss interventions work are still poorly understood. Behavioral pathways toward weight loss include greater physical activity, more frequent attendance at treatment sessions, greater consumption of meal replacements, and more frequent weight and diet monitoring (Wadden et al., 2009, 2011). However, the optimal intensity, sequence, and synergy of behavioral strategies remain unclear. Researchers are only beginning to explore relevant cognitive mediators (Crane, Ward, Lutes, Bowling, & Tate, 2016; Nezami et al., 2016). Teixeira et al. (2010) examined cognitive and psychosocial mechanisms underlying a 2-year behavioral weight loss program in women, and found different determinants of success depending on treatment phase. During the first year of treatment, improvements in cognitive restraint, emotional eating, and eating self-efficacy were important. During maintenance, treatment worked mostly through improvements in exercise self-efficacy, reductions in perceived barriers, and increases in exercise motivation (Teixeira et al., 2010). Burke et al. (2015) found that a behavioral treatment approach that emphasized self-efficacy had greater weight loss maintenance than standard behavioral treatment. Understanding the cognitive and behavioral mechanisms through which treatment works can lead to more targeted and efficacious interventions and inform which behavioral treatment components should be emphasized at different stages of treatment.

Timing Interventions

Behavioral treatment may be particularly effective if timed to occur during certain life transitions when individuals are naturally motivated to adopt healthy eating and activity behaviors (Phelan, 2010). For example, ongoing research in pregnancy is studying the efficacy of behavioral interventions to prevent excessive gestational weight gain—an independent risk factor for long-term weight gain, obesity, and related comorbidities in women (Clifton et al., 2016). Unlike results in nonpregnant populations, behavioral interventions during pregnancy appear to have enduring effects on maternal postpartum behaviors, even after treatment termination (Phelan et al., 2014). Moreover, behavioral interventions during pregnancy have the added potential benefit of reducing risk of obesity in the offspring (Haire-Joshu & Tabak, 2016; Mourtakos et al., 2015; Oken, Rifas-Shiman, Field, Frazier, & Gillman, 2008), signaling a potential avenue for primary prevention.

Ripple Effects

Although the direct effects of standard behavioral weight loss interventions have been extensively documented, the potential "indirect" benefits are often overlooked. Standard behavioral weight loss interventions have been shown to have positive "ripple" effects on weight of untreated partners in the home (Gorin et al., 2008; Hagobian et al., 2016). Future work should examine the ways in which behavioral treatment might impact untreated family members, their home environment, and social modeling behaviors.

Conclusions

Research on the behavioral treatment of obesity over the past 30 years has shown that eating and physical activity habits can be changed to promote successful weight control. A comprehensive behavioral treatment program produces an average 8–10% reduction in initial body weight and a long-term 4–5% weight loss that can be maintained for up to 8 years. This weight loss is associated with clinically meaningful improvements in several cardiovascular disease risk factors, including the prevention of type 2 diabetes. As reviewed in other chapters, innovative approaches to improving behavioral treatment are on the horizon. Potential treatment targets include strengthening motivation, self-efficacy, mindfulness/acceptance, self-regulation, and weight stability skills. Although behavioral treatment is an individual-level intervention, ultimately, behaviorists must work within all layers of society to foster change. Industries, the government, and community organizations must work in conjunction to (1) reduce the number of environmental prompts for overeating and inactivity; (2) increase positive visual cues and provide rewards for healthy eating and activity behaviors; and (3) promote rational cognitions surrounding eating, activity, and weight regulation. Engagement from various segments of society will maximize behavioral treatment's success in fostering long-term weight loss and positive health outcomes.

References

Alamuddin, N., & Wadden, T. A. (2016). Behavioral treatment of the patient with obesity. *Endocrinology Metabolism Clinics of North America, 45*(3), 565–580.

Baker, R. C., & Kirschenbaum, D. S. (1993). Self-monitoring may be necessary for successful weight control. *Behavior Therapy, 24*(3), 377–394.

Bandura, A. (1977). *Social learning theory*. Englewood Cliffs, NJ: Prentice-Hall.

Beck, A. T. (1976). *Cognitive therapy and the emotional disorders*. New York: International Universities Press.

Brownell, K. D. (1998). *The LEARN Program for weight control* (7th ed.). Dallas, TX: American Health.

Burke, L. E., Conroy, M. B., Sereika, S. M., Elci, O. U., Styn, M. A., Acharya, S. D., et al. (2011). The effect of electronic self-monitoring on weight loss and dietary intake: A randomized behavioral weight loss trial. *Obesity (Silver Spring), 19*(2), 338–344.

Burke, L. E., Ewing, L. J., Ye, L., Styn, M., Zheng, Y., Music, E., et al. (2015). The SELF trial: A self-efficacy-based behavioral intervention trial for weight loss maintenance. *Obesity (Silver Spring), 23*(11), 2175–2182.

Burke, L. E., Wang, J., & Sevick, M. A. (2011). Self-monitoring in weight loss: A systematic review of the literature. *Journal of the American Dietetic Association, 111*(1), 92–102.

Butryn, M., Clark, V. L., & Coletta, M. C. (2012). Behavioral approaches. In S. R. Akabas, S. A. Lederman, & B. J. Moore (Eds.), *Textbook of obesity: Biological, psychological, and cultural influences* (pp. 253–272). Chichester, UK: Wiley-Blackwell.

Butryn, M. L., Webb, V., & Wadden, T. A. (2011). Behavioral treatment of obesity. *Psychiatric Clinics of North America, 34*(4), 841–859.

Chapman, S. L., & Jeffrey, D. B. (1978). Situational management, standard setting, and self-reward in a behavior modification weight loss program. *Journal of Consulting and Clinicl Psychology, 46*(6), 1588–1589.

Clifton, R. G., Evans, M., Cahill, A. G., Franks, P. W., Gallagher, D., Phelan, S., et al. (2016). Design of lifestyle intervention trials to prevent excessive gestational weight gain in women with overweight or obesity. *Obesity (Silver Spring), 24*(2), 305–313.

Cohen, D. A. (2008). Obesity and the built environment: Changes in environmental cues cause energy imbalances. *International Journal of Obesity, 32*(Suppl. 7), S137–S142.

Cooper, Z., Doll, H. A., Hawker, D. M., Byrne, S., Bonner, G., Eeley, E., et al. (2010). Testing a new cognitive behavioural treatment for obesity: A randomized controlled trial with three-year follow-up. *Behavior Research and Therapy, 48*(8), 706–713.

Cooper, Z., Fairburn, C. G., & Hawker, D. M. (2003). *Cognitive-behavioral treatment of obesity: A clinician's guide*. New York: Guilford Press.

Coughlin, S. S., Whitehead, M., Sheats, J. Q., Mastromonico, J., Hardy, D., & Smith, S. A. (2015). Smartphone applications for promoting healthy diet and nutrition: A literature review. *Jacobs Journal of Food and Nutrition, 2*(3), 021.

Crane, M. M., Ward, D. S., Lutes, L. D., Bowling, J. M., & Tate, D. F. (2016). Theoretical and behavioral mediators of a weight loss intervention for men. *Annals of Behavioral Medicine, 50*(3), 460–470.

Diabetes Prevention Program Research, Knowler, W. C., Fowler, S. E., Hamman, R. F., Christophi, C. A., Hoffman, H. J., et al. (2009). 10-year follow-up of diabetes incidence and weight loss in the Diabetes Prevention Program Outcomes Study. *Lancet, 374*(9702), 1677–1686.

Fabricatore, A. N., Wadden, T. A., Moore, R. H., Butryn, M. L., Heymsfield, S. B., & Nguyen, A. M. (2009). Predictors of attrition and weight loss success: Results from a randomized controlled trial. *Behavioral Research and Therapy, 47*(8), 685–691.

Flechtner-Mors, M., Ditschuneit, H. H., Johnson, T. D., Suchard, M. A., & Adler, G. (2000). Metabolic and weight loss effects of long-term dietary intervention in obese patients: Four-year results. *Obesity Research, 8*(5), 399–402.

Florez, J. C., Jablonski, K. A., Bayley, N., Pollin, T. I., de Bakker, P. I., Shuldiner, A. R., et al. (2006). TCF7L2 polymorphisms and progression to diabetes in the Diabetes Prevention Program. *New England Journal of Medicine, 355*(3), 241–250.

French, S., Jeffery, R. W., & Wing, R. R. (1994). Food intake and physical activity: A comparison of three measures of dieting. *Addictive Behaviors, 19*(4), 401–409.

Gorin, A. A., Wing, R. R., Fava, J. L., Jakicic, J. M., Jeffery, R., West, D. S., et al. (2008). Weight loss treatment influences untreated spouses and the home environment: Evidence of a ripple effect. *International Journal of Obesity (London), 32*(11), 1678–1684.

Hagobian, T. A., Phelan, S., Gorin, A. A., Phipps, M. G., Abrams, B., & Wing, R. R. (2016). Effects of maternal lifestyle intervention during pregnancy on untreated partner weight: Results from the Fit for Delivery study. *Obesity (Silver Spring), 24*(1), 23–25.

Haire-Joshu, D., & Tabak, R. (2016). Preventing obesity across generations: Evidence for early life intervention. *Annual Reviews of Public Health, 37*, 253–271.

Haynes, S. N., & O'Brien, W. H. (1990). Functional analysis in behavior therapy. *Clinical Psychology Review, 10*, 649–668.

Heymsfield, S. B. (2010). Meal replacements and energy balance. *Physiology of Behavior, 100*(1), 90–94.

Hoie, L. H., & Bruusgaard, D. (1999). Predictors of long-term weight reduction in obese patients after initial very-low-calorie diet. *Advances in Therapy, 16*(6), 285–289.

Hollis, J. F., Gullion, C. M., Stevens, V. J., Brantley, P. J., Appel, L. J., Ard, J. D., et al. (2008). Weight loss during the intensive intervention phase of the weight-loss maintenance trial. *American Journal of Health Promotion, 35*(2), 118–126.

Jakicic, J. M., Davis, K. K., Rogers, R. J., King, W. C., Marcus, M. D., Helsel, D., et al. (2016). Effect of wearable technology combined with a lifestyle intervention on long-term weight loss: The IDEA randomized clinical trial. *Journal of the American Medical Association, 316*(11), 1161–1171.

Jakicic, J. M., Wing, R. R., Butler, B. A., & Jeffery, R. W. (1997). The relationship between presence of exercise equipment in the home and physical activity level. *American Journal of Health Promotion, 11*(5), 363–365.

Jakicic, J. M., Winters, C., Lang, W., & Wing, R. R. (1999). Effects of intermittent exercise and use of home exercise equipment on adherence, weight loss, and fitness in overweight women: A randomized trial. *Journal of the American Medical Association, 282*(16), 1554–1560.

Jeffery, R. W. (2012). Financial incentives and weight control. *Preventive Medicine, 55*(Suppl. 1), S61–S67.

Jeffery, R. W., Wing, R. R., & Mayer, R. R. (1998). Are smaller weight losses or more achievable weight loss goals better in the long term for obese patients? *Journal of Consulting and Clinical Psychology, 66*(4), 641–645.

Jeffery, R. W., Wing, R. R., Thornson, C., Burton, L. R., Raether, C., Harvey, J., et al. (1993). Strengthening behavioral interventions for weight loss: A randomized trial of food provision and monetary incentives. *Journal of Consulting and Clinical Psychology, 61*(6), 1038–1045.

Jensen, M. D., Ryan, D. H., Apovian, C. M., Ard, J. D., Comuzzie, A. G., Donato, K. A., et al. (2014). 2013 AHA/ACC/TOS guidelines for the management of overweight and obesity in adults: A report of the American College of Cardiology/American Heart Association Task Force on Practice Guidelines and The Obesity Society. *Circulation, 129*(25, Suppl. 2), S102–S138.

Karlsson, J., Hallgren, P., Kral, J. G., Lindross, A. K., Sjostrom, L., & Sullivan, M. (1994). Predictors and effects of long-term dieting on mental well-being and weight loss in obese women. *Appetite, 23*(1), 15–26.

Knowler, W. C., Barrett-Connor, E., Fowler, S. E., Hamman, R. F., Lachin, J. M., Walker, E. A., et al. (2002). Reduction in the incidence of type 2 diabetes with lifestyle intervention or metformin. *New England Journal of Medicine, 346*(6), 393–403.

Kumanyika, S. K., Obarzanek, E., Stevens, V. J., Hebert, P. R., & Whelton, P. K. (1991). Weight-loss experience of black and white participants in NHLBI-sponsored clinical trials. *American Journal of Clinical Nutrition, 53*(6, Suppl.), 1631S–1638S.

Leahey, T. M., & Wing, R. R. (2013). A randomized controlled pilot study testing three types of health coaches for obesity treatment: Professional, peer, and mentor. *Obesity (Silver Spring), 21*(5), 928–934.

Lei, H., Nahum-Shani, I., Lynch, K., Oslin, D., & Murphy, S. A. (2012). A "SMART" design for building individualized treatment sequences. *Annual Review of Clinical Psychology, 8*, 21–48.

Lichtman, S. W., Pisarska, K., Berman, E. R., Pestone, M., Dowling, H., Offenbacher, E., et al. (1992). Discrepancy between self-reported and actual caloric intake and exercise in obese subjects. *New England Journal of Medicine, 327*(27), 1893–1898.

Linde, J. A., Jeffery, R. W., French, S. A., Pronk, N. P., & Boyle, R. G. (2005). Self-weighing in weight gain prevention and weight loss trials. *Annals of Behavioral Medicine, 30*(3), 210–216.

Lindstrom, J., Louheranta, A., Mannelin, M., Rastas, M., Salminen, V., Eriksson, J., et al. (2003). The Finnish Diabetes Prevention Study (DPS): Lifestyle intervention and 3-year results on diet and physical activity. *Diabetes Care, 26*(12), 3230–3236.

Look AHEAD Research Group. (2014). Eight-year weight losses with an intensive lifestyle intervention: The look AHEAD study. *Obesity (Silver Spring), 22*(1), 5–13.

Look AHEAD Research Group, Pi-Sunyer, X., Blackburn, G., Brancati, F. L., Bray, G. A., Bright, R., et al. (2007). Reduction in weight and cardiovascular disease risk factors in individuals with type 2 diabetes: One-year results of the Look AHEAD trial. *Diabetes Care, 30*(7), 1374–1383.

Look AHEAD Research Group, & Wing, R. R. (2010). Long-term effects of a lifestyle intervention on weight and cardiovascular risk factors in individuals with type 2 diabetes mellitus: Four-year results of the Look AHEAD trial. *Archives of Internal Medicine, 170*(17), 1566–1575.

Look AHEAD Research Group, Wing, R. R., Bolin, P., Brancati, F. L., Bray, G. A., Clark, J. M., et al. (2013). Cardiovascular effects of intensive lifestyle intervention in type 2 diabetes. *New England Journal of Medicine, 369*(2), 145–154.

Marlatt, G. A., & Gordon, J. R. (1979). Determinants of relapse: Implications for the maintenance of behavior change. In P. O. Davidson & S. M. Davidson (Eds.), *Behavioral medicine: Changing health lifestyles* (pp. 410–452). New York: Brunner/Mazel.

Marlatt, G. A., & Gordon, J. R. (1985). *Relapse prevention: Maintenance strategies in addictive behavior change.* New York: Guilford Press.

Mourtakos, S. P., Tambalis, K. D., Panagiotakos, D. B., Antonogeorgos, G., Arnaoutis, G., Karteroliotis, K., et al. (2015). Maternal lifestyle characteristics during pregnancy, and the risk of obesity in the offspring: A study of 5,125 children. *BMC Pregnancy Childbirth, 15*, 66.

Murawski, M. E., Milsom, V. A., Ross, K. M., Rickel, K. A., DeBraganza, N., Gibbons, L. M., et al. (2009). Problem solving, treatment adherence, and weight-loss outcome among women participating in lifestyle treatment for obesity. *Eating Behavior, 10*(3), 146–151.

Neumark-Sztainer, D., Kaufmann, N. A., & Berry, E. M. (1995). Physical activity within a community-based weight control program: Program evaluation and predictors of success. *Public Health Reviews, 23*(3), 237–251.

Nezami, B. T., Lang, W., Jakicic, J. M., Davis, K. K., Polzien, K., Rickman, A. D., et al. (2016). The effect of self-efficacy on behavior and weight in a behavioral weight-loss intervention. *Health Psychology, 35*(7), 714–722.

Oken, E., Rifas-Shiman, S. L., Field, A. E., Frazier, A. L., & Gillman, M. W. (2008). Maternal gestational weight gain and offspring weight in adolescence. *Obstetrics and Gynecology, 112*(5), 999–1006.

Pearson, E. S. (2012). Goal setting as a health behavior change strategy in overweight and obese adults: A systematic literature review examining intervention components. *Patient Education and Counselling, 87*(1), 32–42.

Pekkarinen, T., Takala, I., & Mustajoki, P. (1996). Two year maintenance of weight loss after a VLCD and behavioural therapy for obesity: Correlation to the scores of questionnaires measuring eating behaviour. *International Journal of Obesity and Related Metabolic Disorders, 20*(4), 332–337.

Perri, M. G., Nezu, A. M., McKelvey, W. F., Shermer, R. L., Renjilian, D. A., & Viegener, B. J. (2001). Relapse prevention training and problem-solving therapy in the long-term management of obesity. *Journal of Consulting and Clinical Psychology, 69*(4), 722–726.

Phelan, S. (2010). Pregnancy: A "teachable moment" for weight control and obesity prevention. *American Journal of Obstetrics and Gynecology, 202*(2), 135. e1–135.e8.

Phelan, S., Phipps, M. G., Abrams, B., Darroch, F., Grantham, K., Schaffner, A., et al. (2014). Does behavioral intervention in pregnancy reduce postpartum weight retention?: Twelve-month outcomes of the Fit for Delivery randomized trial. *American Journal of Clinical Nutrition, 99*(2), 302–311.

Pi-Sunyer, X., Blackburn, G., Brancati, F. L., Bray, G. A., Bright, R., Clark, J. M., et al. (2007). Reduction in weight and cardiovascular disease risk factors in individuals with type 2 diabetes: One-year results of the Look AHEAD trial. *Diabetes Care, 30*(6), 1374–1383.

Poston, W. S., II, Ericsson, M., Linder, J., Nilsson, T., Goodrick, G. K., & Foreyt, J. P. (1999). Personality and the prediction of weight loss and relapse in the treatment of obesity. *International Journal of Eating Disorders, 25*(3), 301–309.

Rupp, K., Taverno Ross, S. E., Lang, W., & Jakicic, J. M. (2016). Response to a standard behavioral weight loss intervention by age of onset of obesity. *Obesity Science and Practice, 2*(3), 248–255.

Sacks, F. M., Bray, G. A., Carey, V. J., Smith, S. R., Ryan, D. H., Anton, S. D., et al. (2009). Comparison of weight-loss diets with different compositions of fat, protein, and carbohydrates. *New England Journal of Medicine, 360*(9), 859–873.

Shaw, K., O'Rourke, P., Del Mar, C., & Kenardy, J. (2005). Psychological interventions for overweight or obesity. *Cochrane Database Systematic Reviews,* (2), CD003818.

Sherwood, N. E., Butryn, M. L., Forman, E. M., Almirall, D., Seburg, E. M., Lauren Crain, A., et al. (2016). The BestFIT trial: A SMART approach to developing individualized weight loss treatments. *Contemporary Clinical Trials, 47,* 209–216.

Sherwood, N. E., Jeffery, R. W., & Wing, R. R. (1999). Binge status as a predictor of weight loss treatment outcome. *International Journal of Obesity and Related Metabolic Disorders, 23*(5), 485–493.

Skinner, B. F. (1953). *Science and human behavior.* New York: Macmillan.

Smith, C. F., & Wing, R. R. (2000). New directions in behavioral weight-loss programs. *Diabetes Spectrum, 13*(3), 142–148.

Stuart, R. B. (1967). Behavioral control of overeating. *Behavior Research and Therapy, 5,* 357–365.

Sturmey, P. (2007). *Functional analysis in clinical treatment.* Boston: Academic Press.

Sutton, S. M., Magwood, G. S., Jenkins, C. H., & Nemeth, L. S. (2016). A scoping review of behavioral weight management interventions in overweight/obese African American females. *Western Journal of Nursing Research, 38*(8), 1035–1066.

Svetkey, L. P., Batch, B. C., Lin, P. H., Intille, S. S., Corsino, L., Tyson, C. C., et al. (2015). Cell phone intervention for you (CITY): A randomized, controlled trial of behavioral weight loss intervention for young adults using mobile technology. *Obesity (Silver Spring), 23*(11), 2133–2141.

Svetkey, L. P., Stevens, V. J., Brantley, P. J., Appel, L. J., Hollis, J. F., Loria, C. M., et al. (2008). Comparison of strategies for sustaining weight loss: The weight loss maintenance randomized controlled trial. *Journal of the American Medical Association, 299*(10), 1139–1148.

Teixeira, P. J., Silva, M. N., Coutinho, S. R., Palmeira, A. L., Mata, J., Vieira, P. N., et al. (2010). Mediators of weight loss and weight loss maintenance in middle-aged women. *Obesity (Silver Spring), 18*(4), 725–735.

Tsai, A. G., Fabricatore, A. N., Wadden, T. A., Higginbotham, A. J., Anderson, A., Foreyt, J., et al. (2014). Readiness redefined: A behavioral task during screening predicted 1-year weight loss in the Look AHEAD study. *Obesity (Silver Spring), 22*(4), 1016–1023.

Turk, M. W., Elci, O. U., Wang, J., Sereika, S. M., Ewing, L. J., Acharya, S. D., et al. (2013). Self-monitoring as a mediator of weight loss in the SMART randomized clinical trial. *International Journal of Behavioral Medicine, 20*(4), 556–561.

Turner-McGrievy, G. M., Beets, M. W., Moore, J. B., Kaczynski, A. T., Barr-Anderson, D. J., & Tate, D. F. (2013). Comparison of traditional versus mobile app self-monitoring of physical activity and dietary intake among overweight adults participating in an mHealth weight loss program. *Journal of the American Medical Informatics Association, 20*(3), 513–518.

Unick, J. L., Neiberg, R. H., Hogan, P. E., Cheskin, L. J., Dutton, G. R., Jeffery, R., et al. (2015). Weight change in the first 2 months of a lifestyle intervention predicts weight changes 8 years later. *Obesity (Silver Spring), 23*(7), 1353–1356.

U.S. Department of Health and Human Services. (2010). *Dietary guidelines for Americans, 2010* (7th ed.). Washington, DC: U.S. Government Printing Office.

Vanwormer, J. J., French, S. A., Pereira, M. A., & Welsh, E. M. (2008). The impact of regular self-weighing on weight management: A systematic literature review. *International Journal of Behavioral Nutrition and Physical Activity, 5*, 54.

Volpp, K. G., John, L. K., Troxel, A. B., Norton, L., Fassbender, J., & Loewenstein, G. (2008). Financial incentive-based approaches for weight loss: A randomized trial. *Journal of the American Medical Association, 300*(22), 2631–2637.

Wadden, T. A., Butryn, M. L., & Wilson, C. (2007). Lifestyle modification for the management of obesity. *Gastroenterology, 132*(6), 2226–2238.

Wadden, T. A., Crerand, C. E., & Brock, J. (2005). Behavioral treatment of obesity. *Psychiatric Clinics of North America, 28*(1), 151–170.

Wadden, T. A., Foster, G. D., & Letizia, K. A. (1992). Response of obese binge eaters to treatment by behavior therapy combined with very low calorie diet. *Journal of Consulting and Clinical Psychology, 60*(5), 808–811.

Wadden, T. A., Volger, S., Sarwer, D. B., Vetter, M. L., Tsai, A. G., Berkowitz, R. I., et al. (2011). A two-year randomized trial of obesity treatment in primary care practice. *New England Journal Medicine, 365*(21), 1969–1979.

Wadden, T. A., West, D. S., Neiberg, R. H., Wing, R. R., Ryan, D. H., Johnson, K. C., et al. (2009). One-year weight losses in the Look AHEAD study: Factors associated with success. *Obesity (Silver Spring), 17*(4), 713–722.

Wing, R. R. (2004). Behavioral approaches to the treatment of obesity. In G. A. Bray & C. Bouchard (Eds.), *Handbook of obesity: Clinical applications* (pp. 147–168). New York: Marcel Dekker.

Wing, R. R. (2010). Long-term effects of a lifestyle intervention on weight and cardiovascular risk factors in individuals with type 2 diabetes mellitus: Four-year results of the Look AHEAD trial. *Archives of Internal Medicine, 170*(17), 1566–1575.

Wing, R. R., Tate, D. F., Espeland, M. A., Lewis, C. E., LaRose, J. G., Gorin, A. A., et al. (2016). Innovative self-regulation strategies to reduce weight gain in young adults: The Study of Novel Approaches to Weight Gain Prevention (SNAP) randomized clinical trial. *Journal of the American Medical Association, 176*(6), 755–762.

Wing, R. R., Tate, D. F., Gorin, A. A., Raynor, H. A., Fava, J. L., & Machan, J. (2007). STOP regain: Are there negative effects of daily weighing? *Journal of Consulting and Clinical Psychology, 75*(4), 652–656.

World Health Organization. (1998). *Obesity: Preventing and managing the global epidemic*. Geneva, Switzerland: World Health Organization.

Zheng, Y., Burke, L. E., Danford, C. A., Ewing, L. J., Terry, M. A., & Sereika, S. M. (2016). Patterns of self-weighing behavior and weight change in a weight loss trial. *International Journal of Obesity (London), 40*(9), 1392–1396.

Zheng, Y., Klem, M. L., Sereika, S. M., Danford, C. A., Ewing, L. J., & Burke, L. E. (2015). Self-weighing in weight management: A systematic literature review. *Obesity (Silver Spring), 23*(2), 256–265.

CHAPTER 21

The Role of Medications in Weight Management

George A. Bray
Donna H. Ryan

The impact of obesity on well-being, health, and economic costs is well known (Apovian, Aronne, & Powell, 2015; Bray, Frühbeck, Ryan, & Wilding, 2016; Bray, 2011; Bray & Bouchard, 2014; Jensen et al., 2014). Even if the percentage of Americans who is overweight does not rise any further, the fact that 40% of U.S. adults are obese is unacceptable (Ogden, Carroll, Kit, & Flegal, 2014). Although prevention is desirable, there will always be some people who are susceptible to weight gain and need management of their obesity. This handbook deals with the breadth of options to manage overweight and obesity. This chapter focuses on the use of medications as an adjunct to lifestyle intervention to produce and sustain weight loss. We discuss the use of U.S. Food and Drug Administration (FDA)-approved medications indicated for chronic weight management in patients with obesity (Apovian, Aronne, & Powell, 2015). Our discussion also encompasses the use of medications that affect body weight in patients with and without obesity but which are not explicitly approved by the FDA to manage obesity.

When evaluating a patient with obesity, a good first step is to identify the medications he or she is taking, noting the drugs that might affect body weight. This step gathers the "low-hanging fruit." If medications that drive weight gain can be eliminated or replaced with those that also promote weight loss, the primary care physician has the opportunity to help patients reduce body weight.

Body mass index (BMI) is widely used for screening for the presence of obesity and its overall risks (Jensen et al., 2014). Using a matrix of BMI and other health risk factors, the NIH Review in 1998 and the AHA/ACC/TOS Guidelines, which updated evidence on risk assessment, provide recommendations on the selection among various treatments for management of weight, including the use of medications (see Figure 21.1). The latest guidelines, based on systematic evidence reviews (Jensen et al., 2014; Apovian, Aronne, & Powell, 2015), endorse initiating use of medications as an adjunct to lifestyle intervention for patients with a BMI > 27 kg/m2 (in the presence of diabetes, hypertension, dyslipidemia, or other weight-related comorbidity) or with a BMI ≥ 30 kg/m² if patients without comorbid conditions have been unable to achieve

Treatment	BMI Category				
	25–26.9	27–29.9	30–34.9	35–39.9	≥40
Diet, physical activity, and behavior therapy	with comorbidities	with comorbidities	+	+	+
Pharmacotherapy		with comorbidities	+	+	+
Surgery				with comorbidities	+

- Prevention of weight gain with lifestyle therapy is indicated for any patient with a BMI ≥ 25 kg/m², even without comorbidities, whereas weight loss is not necessarily recommended for those with a BMI of 25–29.9 kg/m² or a high waist circumference, unless they have two or more comorbidities.
- Combined therapy with a low-calorie diet, increased physical activity, and behavior therapy provides the most successful intervention for weight loss and weight maintenance.
- Consider pharmacotherapy only if a patient has not lost 1 pound/week after 6 months of combined lifestyle therapy.

FIGURE 21.1. Using BMI to select treatment for chronic weight management. This framework reflects a BMI-centric and complications-centric approach to selecting medications for weight management (Jensen et al., 2014; Apovian, Aronne, & Powell, 2015).

or sustain weight loss with behavioral intervention alone.

FDA-Approved Medications for Weight Management in Patients with Obesity

Two groups of medications are approved by the FDA to treat obesity (Apovian, Aronne, & Powell, 2015; Bray et al., 2016). The first are the agents approved for "chronic weight management" and include orlistat, lorcaserin, liraglutide, the combination of phentermine and topiramate as an extended-release (ER) formulation, and the combination of naltrexone and bupropion, both in sustained-release (SR) forms. The second are the medications approved by the FDA for short-term use, which is usually considered to be less than 12 weeks. These drugs are shown in Table 21.1.

Orlistat (Marketed as Xenical Worldwide)

Orlistat (tetrahydrolipstatin) is approved by the FDA for long-term treatment of obesity. Orlistat, as a potent and selective inhibitor of pancreatic lipase, reduces intestinal absorption of fat. It is available as a prescription drug (120 mg three times a day before meals).

Clinical Efficacy

A number of long-term clinical trials with orlistat in patients with uncomplicated obesity and in those with obesity and diabetes have been published (Sjöström et al., 1998; Torgerson, Hauptman, Boldrin, & Sjöström, 2004; Chanoine, Hampl, Jensen, Boldrin, & Hauptman, 2005; LeBlanc, O'Connor, Whitlock, Patnode, & Kapka, 2011). The pooled 2-year data from pivotal randomized clinical trials are summarized in Figure 21.2 (Bray, 2011). The figure compares the placebo-treated group, which initially lost weight and then began to regain, against groups treated with 60 or 120 mg of orlistat three times a day. A dose–response relationship is clear, showing greater weight loss efficacy with 120 mg three times daily, intermediate efficacy with 60 mg, and the lowest efficacy with placebo, all in conjunction with lifestyle intervention. In a meta-analysis of trials with orlistat, the weighted mean weight loss in the placebo group was 2.4 kg and the weight loss in those treated with orlistat was 5.7 kg, for a net effect of –2.9 kg (LeBlanc et al., 2011).

TABLE 21.1. Drugs That Have Been Approved by the FDA for Treatment of Obesity

Drug and mechanism of action (year approved)	Trade names	Dosage	Comments
Pancreatic lipase inhibitor approved for long-term use orally			
Orlistat (not scheduled) (1999)	Xenical	120 mg tid before meals	GI side effects from bloating and diarrhea are principal drawbacks; should be taken with a multivitamin.
Serotonin receptor agonist approved for long-term use orally			
Lorcaserin DEA Schedule IV (2012)	BELVIQ	110 mg twice daily	Headache, dizziness, nausea, dry mouth, and constipation are generally mild. Do not use with other serotonin-active drugs.
Glucagon-like receptor-1 agonist approved for long-term use by injection			
Liraglutide (not scheduled) (2014)	Saxenda	3.0 mg/day by injection; dose escalation over 5 weeks from 0.6 mg/day to 3.0 mg/day	Nausea with some vomiting are principal side effects; acute pancreatitis or gall bladder disease can occur; hypoglycemia with some anti-diabetic drugs; do not prescribe in patients with personal or family history of medullary thyroid cancer or MEN 2.
Combination of two drugs approved for long-term use orally			
Phentermine/topiramate ER DEA Schedule IV (2012)	Qsymia	3.75 mg/23 mg, first week; 7.5 mg/46 mg thereafter; can increase to 15 mg/92 mg for inadequate response	Paresthesias and change in taste (dysgeusia); metabolic acidosis and glaucoma are rare; do not use within 14 days of an MAOI antidepressant; obtain negative pregnancy test before prescribing and avoid during pregnancy.
Naltrexone SR/bupropion SR (not scheduled) (2014)	CONTRAVE	8 mg/90 mg tabs; take 2 twice daily after dose escalation.	Nausea, constipation, headache; avoid in patients receiving opioids, MAOI, antidepressants, and with history of seizure disorder.
Noradrenergic drugs approved for short-term use orally			
Diethylpropion DEA Schedule IV (1959)	Tenuate Tepanil	25 mg tid	Dizziness, dry mouth, insomnia, constipation, irritability, and cardiostimulatory side effects.
	Tenuate Dospan	75 mg q A.M.	
Phentermine DEA Schedule IV (1959)	Adipex Fastin	15–37.5 mg/day	Dizziness, dry mouth, insomnia, constipation, irritability, and cardiostimulatory side effects.
	Oby-Cap Ionamin slow release	15–30 mg/day	
Benzphetamine DEA Schedule III (1960)	Didrex	25–50 mg tid	Dizziness, dry mouth, insomnia, constipation, irritability, and cardiostimulatory side effects.
Phendimetrazine DEA Schedule III (1959)	Bontril Plegine Prelu-2 X-Trozine	17.5–70 mg tid 105 mg daily	Dizziness, dry-mouth, insomnia, constipation, irritability, and cardiostimulatory side effects.

Note. Data from McEvoy, Miller, and Litvak (2005). MAOI, monoamine oxidase inhibitors; MEN2, multiple endocrine neoplasia type 2

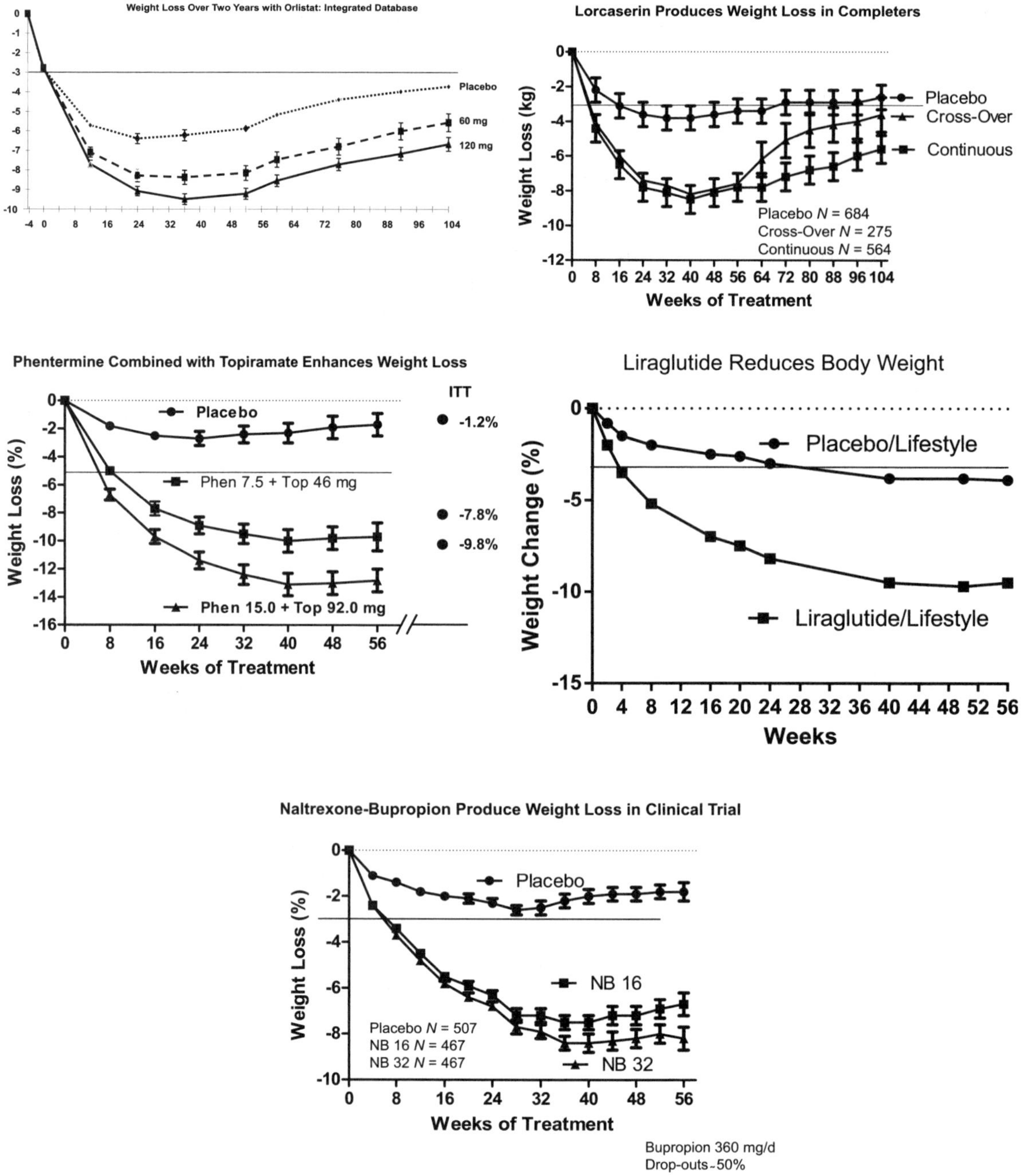

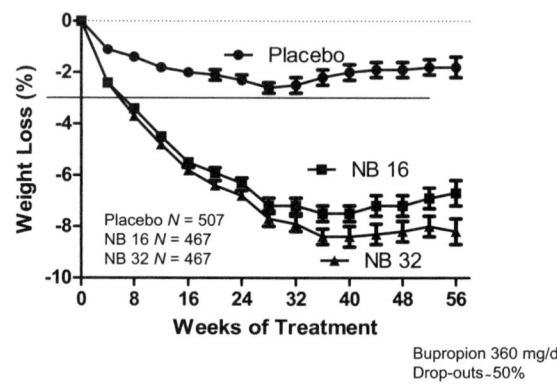

FIGURE 21.2. Weight loss for five FDA-approved medications for chronic weight management. Medication and placebo groups each received a background of lifestyle intervention. The transverse line represents the 5% weight loss line for comparison across the five medications. Orlistat was given at 60 mg or 120 mg three times daily and compared to placebo in the pooled 2-year trials of orlistat (Bray, 2011); data for lorcaserin 10 mg twice daily from Smith et al. (2010); data for liraglutide 3.0 mg/day from Pi-Sunyer et al. (2015); data on phentermine/topiramate SR at 7.5 mg/46 mg/day or 15 mg/92 mg/day from Garvey et al. (2012); data for naltrexone/bupropion ER 16 mg/360 mg/day and 32 mg/360 mg/day from Greenway et al. (2010).

A 4-year double-blind, randomized, placebo-controlled trial with orlistat in 3,304 overweight patients, 21% of whom had impaired glucose tolerance (Torgerson et al., 2004), observed a mean loss during the first year of more than 11% of baseline weight in the lifestyle + orlistat-treated group, compared to 6% in the lifestyle + placebo-treated group. Over the remaining 3 years of the trial, there was a small regain in mean body weight, with the orlistat-treated patients remaining 6.9% below baseline, compared with 4.1% for those receiving placebo. In this study, there was a 37% reduction in the conversion of patients from impaired glucose tolerance to diabetes with the use of orlistat 120 mg three times daily plus lifestyle counseling as compared with placebo.

Orlistat has also been studied in 539 adolescents who received lifestyle intervention with either 120 mg of orlistat three times per day or placebo (Chanoine et al., 2005). BMI decreased on average by 0.6 kg/m² in the drug-treated group compared to a mean increase of 0.3 kg/m² in the placebo group. Orlistat has an FDA-approved indication in adolescents.

Safety Profile

Orlistat is not absorbed through the gastrointestinal (GI) track to any significant degree, and its side effects are thus related mainly to the blockade of triglyceride digestion in the intestine (Bray, 2011). Oily stools, flatus with discharge, and related GI symptoms are common initially, but they subside as patients learn not to eat high-fat meals or snacks when they take the drug. Orlistat can cause small but significant decreases in fat-soluble vitamins. Levels usually remain within the normal range, but a few patients may need vitamin supplementation. Because it is clinically challenging to tell which patients need vitamins, it is wise to provide a multivitamin routinely with instructions to take it before bedtime. Orlistat does not seem to affect the absorption of other drugs, except acyclovir. Rare cases of severe liver injury have been reported with the use of orlistat; at a time when an estimated 40 million people took orlistat, only one case of severe liver injury occurred in the United States, and 13 elsewhere. A causal relationship has not been established, but patients who take orlistat should contact their health care provider if itching, jaundice, pale-color stools, or anorexia develop.

Lorcaserin (Marketed as BELVIQ in the United States)

Lorcaserin is approved by the FDA for chronic weight management. Fenfluramine and dexfenfluramine, two previously approved serotonergic drugs for weight loss, were removed from the market because of damage to the heart valves, and lorcaserin was carefully evaluated for this potential concern (Rothman & Baumann, 2009). Lorcaserin selectively targets the serotonin 2C ($5\text{-}HT_{2C}$) receptor, and not the 2B receptors that were involved in the heart damage. When the $5\text{-}HT_{2C}$ receptor is activated in the hypothalamus, food intake is reduced (Halford, Harrold, Boyland, Lawton, & Blundell, 2007). Lorcaserin is prescribed at 10 mg twice daily (see BELVIQ prescribing information).

Clinical Efficacy

Three clinical studies provided evidence for approval of lorcaserin at a dose of 10 mg twice daily (Smith et al., 2010; Fidler et al., 2011; O'Neil et al., 2012). The data from one trial are summarized in Figure 21.2, which shows the weight loss over 2 years and allows comparison with a subgroup of treated patients who were switched to placebo after 52 weeks on lorcaserin and subsequently returned to placebo-treated weight loss levels (Smith et al., 2010). Two of these studies—BLOOM (Behavioral Modification and Lorcaserin for Overweight and Obesity Management; Smith et al., 2010) and BLOSSOM (Behavioral Modification and Lorcaserin Second Study for Obesity; Fidler et al., 2011)—enrolled volunteers who were obese or had a BMI ≥ 27 kg/m² with one comorbidity. The third study—BLOOM-DM (BLOOM—Diabetes Millitus) O'Neill et al., 2012)—enrolled patients with type 2 diabetes and hemoglobin A1C (HbA1C) of 7–10% and a BMI of 27–45 kg/m². In these studies all patients (including the placebo group) received counseling in diet and physical activity. There were improvements in cardiovascular risk factors in these studies, particularly when the patient population had abnormal risk factors at baseline. In the BLOOM-DM study, mean HbA1C decreased by 0.9 with lorcaserin twice daily, compared to a 0.4 decrease with placebo ($p < .001$), and mean fasting glucose decreased 27.4 ± mg/dL compared to a decrease of 11.9 mg/dL for placebo ($p < .001$) (O'Neil et al., 2012). Weight maintenance was demonstrated in the BLOOM-DM study with a small amount of regain in the second year. Energy intake was significantly reduced with lorcaserin by 286 kcal/day compared to a decrease of 147 kcal/day in the placebo group. Hunger ratings were also reduced by lorcaserin treatment (Martin et al., 2011).

Safety Profile

Lorcaserin was scrutinized for potential effects on heart valves during Phase III studies in which echocardiograms were done on more than 5,200 subjects. There was no statistically significant increase in FDA-defined valvulopathy with drug treatment as compared to placebo. In the FDA briefing report, using combined data on all patients who were exposed to lorcaserin or to placebo in the three studies, the relative risk of FDA-defined valvulopathy in lorcaserin-treated participants, as compared with those who received placebo, was reported as 1.16 (95% confidence interval [CI], 0.81 to 1.67), which is not statistically significant. However, since lorcaserin has much greater selectivity for the $5-HT_{2C}$ receptor than the $5-HT_{2B}$ receptor, it is very unlikely that lorcaserin will increase the risk of valvulopathy in humans. The FDA has not recommended routine echocardiography for prescription of the medication.

Another issue with lorcaserin arose in preclinical studies, in which an increased number of brain and mammary tumors were found in rats in long-term toxicology studies. These were reanalyzed, and there were fewer malignant tumors than first thought (Food and Drug Administration, 2012a). Additionally, the drug does not achieve high levels in the central nervous system of humans, whereas it does in rats (Food and Drug Administration, 2012a).

Lorcaserin is well tolerated. The most common adverse events in clinical trials were headache, nausea, dizziness, fatigue, dry mouth, and constipation. These were mild and resolved quickly. However, a primary concern is that the drug should not be used with selective serotonin reuptake inhibitors (SSRIs) or with monoamine oxidase inhibitors (MAOIs) because of the risk of serotonin syndrome.

Liraglutide (Marketed as Saxenda in the United States)

Liraglutide is a glucagon-like peptide-1 (GLP-1) agonist that has a 97% homology to GLP-1. The molecular change extends the circulating half-life from 1–2 minutes to 13 hours. Liraglutide reduces body weight in animals and human beings. This drug is indicated as an adjunct to a reduced-calorie diet and increased physical activity for chronic weight management in adult patients with an initial BMI of > 30 kg/m² or > 27 kg/m² if diabetes, hypertension, or dyslipidemia are present.

Clinical Efficacy

In a 20-week multicenter European trial, extended to 2 years, Astrup et al. (2009, 2012) reported that on a background of lifestyle intervention, daily injections of liraglutide at 1.2, 1.8, 2.4, or 3.0 mg produced mean weight losses of 4.8, 5.5, 6.3 and 7.2 kg respectively, compared to a loss of 2.8 kg in the placebo-treated group and 4.1 kg in the orlistat-treated comparator group. In the group treated with 3.0 mg/day, 76% achieved a ≥ 5% weight loss compared to 30% in the placebo group. In a much larger multi-center trial, 3,731 patients without diabetes were instructed to adhere to a 500 kcal/day deficit diet and lifestyle recommendations and were treated in a ratio of 2:1 with liraglutide 3.0 mg/day (after dose titration) or with placebo + lifestyle. Mean baseline weight was 106.3 kg, and mean BMI was 38.3 kg/m². Liraglutide reduced body weight at 56 weeks by 8.4 kg on average compared to 2.8 kg on average in the placebo + placebo-treated group (Pi-Sunyer et al., 2015). Weight loss of ≥ 5% was achieved by 62.3% of those receiving liraglutide but only 34.4% in those with placebo. The corresponding numbers losing ≥ 10% were 33.9% for those on liraglutide and 15.4% for those assigned to placebo. In another trial, weight loss was induced with a low-calorie diet before patients were randomized to lifestyle counseling and either placebo or 3.0 mg/day (after titration) liraglutide (Wadden et al., 2013). The mean weight was 99.6 kg, slightly less than in the previous trial. Weight loss before randomization was approximately 6% on average, and after randomization those receiving liraglutide lost an additional 6.8 kg (completers; 4.9 kg by intention to treat) compared to no additional loss in the placebo group at 56 weeks (and a small gain in the intention-to-treat analysis). The percentage of participants losing ≥ 5% and 10% of body weight was more than twice as high in the liraglutide-treated patients, compared to placebo.

Safety Profile

Liraglutide is contraindicated in people with a family history of medullary thyroid carcinoma or multiple endocrine neoplasia syndrome type 2 (MEN2). It also is contraindicated in pregnancy. Liraglutide should not be used in patients with a history of pancreatitis and should be discontinued if pancreatitis develops. Its safety, when combined with other drugs for weight management, has not been established. This drug is given by injection, and nausea was one of its most troublesome side effects, occurring in 39.3% of those on liraglutide compared to 13.8% in the placebo-treated group. Diarrhea, constipation, vomiting, dyspepsia and abdominal pain also occurred in more than 5% of those treated with liraglutide. Mean serum calcitonin was significantly higher in the liraglutide group but did not require further follow-up. Hypoglycemia was only a problem in patients also taking sulfonylureas. Blood pressure was significantly reduced, but pulse rate increased by > 10 beats/minute in 34% of the liraglutide-treated group, compared with 19% in the placebo-treated group. There were no changes in serum lipids. Liraglutide should be used with caution in patients with renal impairment. Liraglutide has been approved by both the European Medicines Agency and the FDA for the treatment of obesity in a dose of 3.0 mg/day. If weight loss does not exceed 4% by 16 weeks, the drug should be discontinued. Liraglutide has been approved at a lower dose of 1.8 mg/day for the treatment of diabetes and has a different retail name (Victoza). The indications for these two doses are distinct—if patients with and without diabetes are undertaking a weight loss effort, liraglutide 3.0 mg may be indicated. However, if the primary goal is management of glycemia in patients with diabetes, then liraglutide 1.8 mg is indicated.

Phentermine/Topiramate Combination (Marketed as Qsymia in the United States)

The combination of phentermine and topiramate (PHEN/TPM) as an ER medication is marketed as Qsymia and was the first new drug combination approved for chronic weight management in overweight and obese persons in more than a decade. The combination uses lower doses of phentermine (i.e., 3.75 mg in the starting dose, 7.5 mg in the recommended dose, and 15 mg in the dose that may be used if patients do not achieve success at the recommended dose) than are usually prescribed when phentermine is used as a single agent. The topiramate is an ER formulation, not available other than in this combination. The dose of topiramate in the combination (i.e., 23 mg in the starting dose, 46 mg in the recommended dose, and 92 mg in the full dose) is also lower than that when topiramate is used for migraine prophylaxis or to control seizures. In terms of mechanism of action, phentermine acts to reduce appetite through increasing norepinephrine in the hypothalamus. The appetite-reducing mechanism of topiramate is not thoroughly understood, although it may be through its effect on gamma-aminobutyric acid (GABA) receptors.

Clinical Efficacy

Two clinical studies provided efficacy and safety data that formed the basis for FDA (Food and Drug Administration, 2010b) approval of the medication (Allison et al., 2012; Gadde et al., 2011). The first, EQUIP, enrolled subjects ≤ 70 years of age with BMI ≥ 35 kg/m^2 (no upper limit) and required blood pressure to be controlled (≤ 140/90 mmHg using 0–2 antihypertensive medications), fasting blood glucose ≤ 110 mg/dL, and triglycerides ≤ 200 mg/dL using 0 or 1 lipid-lowering medication (Allison et al., 2012). The other study, CONQUER, enrolled adults ≤ 70 years of age with BMI ≥ 27 and ≤ 45 kg/m^2, but for patients with type 2 diabetes, no lower BMI limit was required (Gadde et al., 2011). The CONQUER study also required patients to have two or more of the following comorbidities: hypertension, hypertriglyceridemia, dysglycemia (impaired fasting glucose, impaired glucose tolerance, or type 2 diabetes), or an elevated waist circumference (≥ 40 inches for men or ≥ 35 inches for women). Thus, the patient population in these two studies represents those with higher-risk profiles from the consequences of excess weight. A titration period of 2 weeks is recommended for PHEN/TPM ER, starting at the combination dose of 3.75 mg phentermine/23 mg topiramate, although in these studies it was shorter. All subjects in these studies received a lifestyle modification program based on the LEARN manual (Brownell, 2000). This combination medication has produced the largest mean weight losses observed in clinical trials of obesity medications, approaching 10% on average.

The CONQUER study was extended for a second year of observation with 78% of patients continuing in their treatment assignment; this was called the SEQUEL study (Garvey et al., 2012). At the end of the second year of treatment, patients who completed the trial taking the recommended dose (7.5 mg/46 mg) maintained a mean weight loss of 9.3% below baseline, and those on the top dose maintained a 10.7% mean weight loss from baseline. The 2-year weight loss for this trial is shown in Figure 21.2.

The weight loss with PHEN/TPM ER is accompanied by improvements in most risk factors. In the CONQUER study, there were clinically and statistically significant improvements in blood pressure, glycemic measures, HDL cholesterol, and triglycerides with both the recommended and the top doses of the medication (Gadde et al., 2011). In the EQUIP, CONQUER, and SEQUEL studies, improvements in risk factors were related to the amount of weight loss, with greater benefit being observed with greater weight loss (Allison et al., 2012; Gadde et al., 2011; Garvey et al., 2012). Further, a population with abnormal risk factors is more likely to demonstrate improvement in those risk factors. PHEN/TPM ER has also been studied in patients with sleep apnea and shown to reduce the severity of symptoms from sleep apnea (Garvey et al., 2012).

Safety Profile

The most commonly observed side effects in the clinical trials of PHEN/TPM ER were paraesthesia, dizziness, dysgeusia (altered taste), insomnia, constipation, and dry mouth (Vivus, Inc., 2012). These side effects are related to the constituents of PHEN/TPM ER or, in the case of constipation, to weight loss per se. Phentermine, as a sympathomimetic agent, causes insomnia and dry mouth, usually early in treatment, which then resolves. Topiramate is a carbonic anhydrase inhibitor that is associated with altered taste for carbonated beverages and tingling in fingers, toes and perioral areas and may lead to mild metabolic acidosis.

Safety concerns with PHEN/TPM ER are also associated with the two components. Weight loss is contraindicated in pregnancy, as are all weight loss medications. Topiramate is associated with oral clefts if used during early pregnancy, and PHEN/TPM ER is pregnancy Category X (see Vivus, Inc., 2012, for Qsymia prescribing information). A rare side effect of topiramate is acute glaucoma, and the drug is contraindicated in glaucoma. PHEN/TPM ER is also contraindicated in hyperthyroidism and within 14 days of treatment with MAOIs. It is also contraindicated in patients with hypersensitivity to any of the ingredients in the medication. Because of the risk of oral clefts, a negative pregnancy test before treatment (and monthly thereafter) and use of effective contraception are required. If a patient becomes pregnant while taking PHEN/TPM ER, treatment should be terminated immediately. Other potential issues, though rare, include risk of kidney stones (associated with topiramate) and increased heart rate in patients susceptible to sympathomimetic drugs (associated with phentermine).

Naltrexone/Bupropion Combination (Marketed as CONTRAVE in the United States)

Bupropion reduces food intake by acting on adrenergic and dopaminergic receptors in the hypothalamus. Naltrexone is an opioid receptor antagonist with minimal effect on weight loss on its own. The rationale for combining bupropion with naltrexone is that naltrexone might block inhibitory influences of opioid receptors activated by the beta-endorphin that is released in the hypothalamus and stimulates feeding, while allowing alpha-melanocyte-stimulating hormone to inhibit food intake (Greenway, Whitehouse, et al., 2009). The combination of bupropion and naltrexone (called CONTRAVE) was favorably reviewed by an FDA Advisory Panel in 2012 (Food and Drug Administration, 2012a, 2012c).

Clinical Efficacy

Four clinical trials, encompassing over 4,000 patients, have demonstrated the clinical effectiveness of this combination for chronic management of weight (Apovian et al., 2013; Greenway et al., 2010). Mean weight loss with the naltrexone/bupropion SR combination (32 mg naltrexone, 360 mg bupropion) plus lifestyle at 56 weeks was 6.1% below baseline ($N = 471$) compared to 1.6% in the placebo + lifestyle group ($N = 511$). In a second trial mean weight loss was 6.4% ($N = 825$) in the drug + lifestyle group versus 1.2% ($N = 456$) in the placebo + lifestyle group (Greenway et al., 2010). In both trials the proportion achieving weight loss ≥ 5% was more than twice as large in the combination-treated group as in the placebo-treated group. In both cases, too, the mean placebo-subtracted weight loss was intermediate to that of PHEN/TPM ER and lorcaserin. Naltrexone/bupropion (SR) produced significantly greater weight loss when combined with intensive rather than minimal lifestyle counseling (Wadden et al., 2011) and also was effective in inducing weight loss in patients with diabetes (Hollander et al., 2013). Significant improvements were seen in HDL cholesterol and triglycerides in all four trials. Mean diastolic blood pressure fell by 2–3 mmHg in the placebo-treated groups, but blood pressure increased slightly from baseline in the bupropion/naltrexone-treated group at 4 and 8 weeks; blood pressure was similar to baseline at 12 weeks and only decreased by about 1 mmHg at the end of 24–56 weeks. Systolic blood pressure and pulse rate were also higher in the drug-treated patients compared to the placebo-treated groups. Because of these cardiovascular effects, patients receiving this combination should be monitored for undesirable increases in heart rate or blood pressure.

Safety Profile

This combination is contraindicated in individuals with uncontrolled hypertension, seizure disorders, anorexia nervosa, or those undergoing the abrupt withdrawal of alcohol, benzodiazepines, barbiturates, or antiepileptic drugs. Since it contains an opioid antagonist, it is contraindicated in people using opioids chronically. It should not be used within 14 days of taking an MAOI. Finally, it is contraindicated in pregnancy. Care should be taken in patients with a history of suicidal thoughts and behaviors, since bupropion used for treatment of depression has been associated with suicidal risk. Naltrexone and bupropion are metabolized by several different hepatic enzymes, and care needs to be taken to check for potential drug–drug interactions. Bupropion may produce dilation of the pupils, which poses a risk for individuals with angle-closure glaucoma. A history of bipolar disorder should raise concern when thinking of this drug combination because bupropion may exacerbate mania. Weight loss in patients with diabetes may increase the risk of hypoglycemia, particularly in patients taking insulin or insulin secretogogues.

FDA-Approved Drugs for Short-Term Use in Weight Management of Patients with Obesity

The sympathomimetic drugs—benzphetamine, diethylpropion, phendimetrazine, and phentermine—are grouped together because they act like norepinephrine and were tested before 1975. Phentermine and diethylpropion are classified by the U.S. Drug Enforcement Agency as Schedule IV drugs; benzphetamine and phendimetrazine are Schedule III drugs. This regulatory classification indicates the government's belief that these drugs have the potential for abuse, although this potential appears to be very low. Phentermine and diethylpropion are approved for only a "few weeks," which usually is interpreted as up to 12 weeks. Most of the data on these drugs come from short-term trials.

Phentermine

Phentermine, as a single agent, remains the most frequently prescribed drug for weight loss in the United States. Because phentermine was approved in 1959 for short-term use for weight loss, there are few current data to evaluate its long-term efficacy. In 2011, the FDA (2011) approved a new formulation of the drug, Suprenza, marketed by Akrimax Pharmaceuticals, LLC. Since the FDA only approved the new, orally dissolving formulation, no clinical weight loss data were submitted with the New Drug Application (NDA; Food and Drug Administration, 2011). However, several studies are worthy of note because they provide recent data on the safety and efficacy of phentermine as a single agent.

A 6-month study that was presented to the FDA in the briefing document for the PHEN/TPM combination had four treatment arms and 200 subjects, with 158 subjects completing 6 months (Ryan et al., 2010). For the phentermine 15 mg daily treatment group, mean weight loss at 6 months was 4.6%, compared to a mean loss of 2.1% for placebo. Another phentermine study that is relatively current was presented as a poster at the European Congress on Obesity in 2009 (Aronne et al., 2013; Ryan et al., 2010). This study also explored the PHEN/TPM combination and overall had seven treatment arms among 756 subjects. Thus, it is one of the largest studies of phentermine alone at two doses (> 100 subjects per dose) with over 6 months of observation. In that study, at 28 weeks, completion rates were 65%. Mean weight loss at 28 weeks for the placebo group was 1.7% from baseline, compared with 5.5% for phentermine 7.5 mg/day and 6.1% for phentermine 15 mg/day. Finally, a report from Korea evaluated a diffuse, controlled-release form of phentermine at 30 mg (n = 37) versus placebo (n = 37) (Kim, Cho, Kang, Youn, & Lee, 2006). At 12 weeks, mean weight loss was 8.1 ±3.9 kg for drug-treated patients versus 1.7 ± 2.9 kg for placebo patients. These trials suggest that the degree of weight loss with phentermine is dose-related.

Safety Profile

The sympathomimetic drugs produce central excitation, manifested clinically as insomnia and in some individuals as nervousness. This effect is most obvious shortly after the drug is started and wanes substantially with continued use. Dry mouth is among the most common side effects. To a variable extent, these drugs may also increase heart rate and blood pressure. The prescribing information usually recommends that the drugs not be given to individuals with a history of cardiovascular disease. There is little evidence of quantitative effects on blood pressure and pulse, especially after 6 months of treatment. A short-term study, which evaluated phentermine and taranabant (an experimental cannabinoid receptor antagonist), administered singly or together for up to 28 days, revealed no significant differences in mean blood pressure and heart rate as compared with placebo (Kang, Park, Kang, Park, & Park, 2010). In a 12-week study from Korea, 68 obese individuals were randomized to either phentermine HCl 37.5 mg/day or placebo (Kim et al., 2006). There were no significant differences in mean blood pressure changes between groups at 12 weeks, although the phentermine group lost significantly more weight, on average (7.2 kg vs. 1.9 kg, p < .001). In the previously described Korean study of a new formulation of phentermine (i.e., diffuse, controlled release; not marketed in the United States), there were no significant differences between the phentermine and placebo groups in systolic or diastolic blood pressure. However, despite clinically significant weight loss in the phentermine group (8.1 kg) at 12 weeks, expected decreases in blood pressure were not observed. Furthermore, the phentermine group had a mean increase in heart rate of

2.7 beats/minute, compared to a decrease of 4.3 in the placebo-treated subjects (Addy et al., 2009).

Lacking good quantitative measures of the effects of phentermine diethylpropion, phendimetrazine, and benzphetamine on heart rate and pulse, we recommend caution in prescribing these drugs. They should not be prescribed to persons with a history of cardiovascular disease. The blood pressure and pulse should be monitored while taking sympathomimetics. Even though there is no convincing evidence of mean blood pressure increases, the lack of the expected reductions in blood pressure with weight loss is an indication that the drugs do have some stimulatory effect on blood pressure. Should these drugs have come before the FDA today for approval for long-term use, the FDA would undoubtedly have required a cardiovascular outcome study.

In one survey of bariatric physicians, use of sympathomimetic amines was more frequent than use of sibutramine (a drug that was withdrawn by the FDA, based on results of a cardiovascular outcome trial) or orlistat, and the medications were often used for longer than approved by the FDA (Hendricks, Rothman, & Greenway, 2009). Prescribers should be aware of the local and federal regulations governing prescribing limits and the lack of long-term clinical trial data for phentermine.

Treatment of Patients with Overweight/Obesity and Comorbid Diabetes, Depression, Migraine, or Epilepsy

Weight gain, or weight loss, are side effects of many drugs used by physicians to treat their patient's diseases. When selecting medications for managing chronic disease, if there is a reasonable choice that will produce weight loss for the patient with obesity, good clinical practice would recommend that choice.

Treatment of Patients with Obesity and Diabetes

Many would say that the epidemic of diabetes is following on the heels of the obesity epidemic. The rate of developing diabetes can clearly be slowed by weight loss, which is the first line of treatment (Diabetes Prevention Program Research Group, 2002, 2009; Tuomilehto et al., 2001). There is growing interest in the ability of weight loss to "reverse" diabetes, and this has been demonstrated in association with various surgical procedures (Buchwald et al., 2004; Sjöström et al., 2014) and even with a lifestyle intervention (Gregg et al., 2012). Table 21.2 lists the drugs that are available to treat diabetes. Insulin produces a weight gain that ranges from 1.8 to 6.6 kg (Leslie, Hankey, & Lean, 2007). Two widely used sulfonylurea drugs (i.e., glipizide and glibenclamide) also produce weight change, which in most studies ranges from −0.3 to 4.0 kg (Leslie et al., 2007), and this is also true for the thiazolidinediones (e.g., rosiglitazone and pioglitazone), which lead to weight gains of 0.2–1.5 kg or more (Smith et al., 2005). Other drugs are weight neutral or can cause weight loss (Bray & Ryan, 2012).

Metformin

Metformin is a biguanide that is approved by the FDA for the treatment of diabetes mellitus and has a good safety profile. This drug reduces hepatic glucose production, decreases intestinal glucose absorption from

TABLE 21.2. Categorization of Anti-Diabetic Drugs by Their Effects on Body Weight

Produce weight loss	Are weight neutral	Produce weight gain
Metformin	Dipeptidyl peptidase-4 inhibitors (DPP-4)	Insulin
Pramlintide	Acarbose	Sulfonylureas[a]
Exenatide	Miglitol	Glitinides
Liraglutide	Bromocriptine	Thiazolidinediones[b]
		Gliflazones

[a]Glipizide, glimepride, glibenclamide, chlorpropamide.
[b]Pioglitazone, rosiglitazone.

the gastrointestinal tract, and enhances insulin sensitivity. One mechanism for the reduction in hepatic glucose production by metformin may depend on the phosphorylation of a nuclear binding protein, cyclic AMP-responsive element-binding (CREB) protein (CBP) at Ser436 AMPK. This mechanism disrupts a number of other signals, including a master transcription factor, peroxisome profliferator-activated receptor gamma coactivator 1A (PPARGC1A), which in turn leads to the suppression of hepatic glucose output (He et al., 2009).

The longest and best study of metformin on body weight comes from the Diabetes Prevention Program Research Group (2012). During the first 2.8 years of the double-blind, placebo-controlled trial, the metformin-treated group lost an average of 2.1 kg versus a loss of only 0.1 kg in the placebo group ($p < .001$). The degree of weight loss was related to the adherence to metformin. Those who were the most adherent lost, on average, 3.5 kg at 2 years, compared with a small weight gain of 0.5 kg in those who were assigned to, but never took, metformin. This differential mean weight loss persisted throughout the 8 years of follow-up, with highly adherent patients remaining 3–4 kg below baseline and those who were not adherent being no different from placebo.

Metformin has been evaluated in people treated with antipsychotic drugs. In a systematic review, Bushe, Bradley, Doshi, and Karagianis (2009) found that metformin may have some value in reducing or preventing weight gain and adverse changes in metabolic parameters during treatment with antipsychotic medications.

Pramlintide

Pramlintide is a modified form of amylin, a peptide secreted from the beta cells of the pancreas along with insulin. Pramlintide has been approved by the FDA for treatment of diabetes and in clinical trials produced weight loss. A meta-analysis of pramlintide's effect on weight, when used in the treatment of diabetes, demonstrated a mean weight loss of 2.6 kg for those taking pramlintide versus the control groups (Singh-Franco, Perez, & Harrington, 2011).

GLP-1 Receptor Agonists

GLP-1 is a naturally occurring peptide released by the GI tract in response to food. It is a known suppressor of food intake. Because of their favorable weight loss profile, GLP-1 agonists may be of value in treating patients with diabetes.

Several GLP-1 receptor agonists are available in the United States (i.e., albiglutide, dulaglutide, exenatide, and liraglutide) and one agonist in Europe (i.e., lixisenatide). As a class, GLP-1 receptor agonists are associated with weight loss at dosage levels approved for the treatment of diabetes. Only liraglutide (Astrup et al., 2009) and exenatide (Rosenstock et al., 2006; Dushay et al., 2012; Kelly et al., 2013) have been systematically studied in the setting of lifestyle intervention to produce weight loss. As discussed previously, liraglutide 3.0 mg is approved for chronic weight management, but liraglutide 1.8 mg is the maximum dose indicated for the management of diabetes.

Liraglutide (once daily) and exenatide (twice daily) are short-acting compounds approved for treatment of type 2 diabetes. A systematic evidence review that evaluated effects on weight of exenatide and liraglutide, at doses approved for the management of diabetes, concluded that there was no difference in the weight loss effects of exenatide given weekly or daily versus daily liraglutide (Potts et al., 2015). That study showed a weight loss effect of 1.3–2.4 kg for the various doses of the two medications.

Long-acting GLP-1 receptor agonists have more recently been marketed for the management of type 2 diabetes. Exenatide long-acting release (LAR), albiglutide, and dulaglutide are all administered weekly and are associated with weight loss (Amori, Lau, & Pittas, 2007). However, no head-to-head comparisons of weight loss efficacy have been published.

As a class, GLP-1 receptor agonists have a side-effect profile of headache, nausea, and vomiting that is lessened by a gradual dose escalation (Apovian et al., 2010). This class of drugs is associated with pancreatitis, and because of rodent findings of C cell tumors, the drugs are contraindicated in patients with a personal or family history of med-

Gliflozins

Familial renal glucosuria results from a deficiency in the sodium–glucose cotransporter-2 (SGLT-2) and serves as a model for the effects of drugs that inhibit this pathway and might be useful to treat diabetics. Glucose is removed from the urinary filtrate by the action of two SGLTs. SGLT-2 is located primarily in the proximal tubule, where 90% of the glucose is reabsorbed, in contrast to SGLT-1, which is located more distally in the nephron. Several drugs have been developed in this class and marketed in the United States for management of type 2 diabetes: dapaglifozin, canaglifozin, and empaglifozin (Clar, Gill, Court, & Waugh, 2012; Cefalu et al., 2013; Kim & Babu, 2012). These are all selective, orally active, once-daily SGLT-2 inhibitors. All are associated with weight loss. In a randomized, placebo-controlled study of 182 patients, dapaglifozin was associated with a 2.1-kg placebo-subtracted weight loss at 24 weeks (Bolinder et al., 2012). Canaglifozin at doses of 100 and 300 mg per day, in a pooled analysis of four studies ($N = 2,250$), was shown to produce weight loss compared to placebo (Cefalu et al., 2015). In a meta-analysis of 10 trials of empaglifozin 10 mg and 25 mg used for diabetes management, weight loss was 1.9 and 1.8 kg for each dose, respectively (Liakos et al., 2014). There are no head-to-head comparisons of the SGLT-2 inhibitors, but the weight loss efficacy of the drugs in this class seems to be similar. Side effects with this class of drugs include urinary tract infections, hypoglycemia, reduction in blood pressure, postural hypotension, dehydration, renal dysfunction, and metabolic acidosis.

Treatment of Patients with Obesity and Comorbid Neuropsychiatric Disorders Such as Depression, Epilepsy, and Migraine

This category of patients includes those with obesity who are depressed, those with migraine symptoms, and those needing antipsychotic drugs. Some of the approved drugs for managing neuropsychiatric conditions produce weight gain, and others are associated with weight loss (see Table 21.3). One option for the health provider is to change to an effective medication that produces weight loss from one that produces weight gain. The magnitude of mean weight gain for the drugs in the weight gain column ranges from 1.2 to 5.8 kg for valproate, from 4.0 kg to 5.3 kg for lithium, from 2.1 to 2.3 kg for risperidone, from 2.8 to 7.1 kg for olanzapine, and from 4.2 to 9.9 kg for clozapine (Leslie et al., 2007). This degree of weight gain can make continuation of treatment more difficult, and using weight neutral drugs or the alternatives that produce weight loss is good clinical practice.

TABLE 21.3. Categorization of Neurobehavioral Drugs by Their Effects on Body Weight

Produce weight loss	Are weight neutral	Produce weight gain
Bupropion	Haloperidol	Tricyclic antidepressants[a]
Venlafaxine	Aripiprazole	Monoaine oxidase inhibitors
Desvenlafaxine		Paroxetine
Topiramate		Escitalopram
Zonisamide		Lithium
Lamotrigine		Olanzapine
Ziprasidone		Clozapine
		Risperidone
		Carbamazepine
		Valproate
		Divalproex
		Mirtazapine

[a]Nortriptyline, amitriptyline, doxepin.

Bupropion

Bupropion is FDA approved for the treatment of depression and as an aid in helping patients stop smoking. It reduces food intake by acting on adrenergic and dopaminergic receptors in the hypothalamus. These neurotransmitters are involved in the regulation of food intake.

In a study with uncomplicated and nondepressed people with obesity, 327 subjects were randomized in equal proportions to bupropion 300 mg/day, bupropion 400 mg/day, or placebo (Anderson et al., 2002). All patients were prescribed a hypocaloric diet that included the use of liquid meal replacements. At 24 weeks, 69% of those randomized remained in the study, and body weight was reduced, on average, by 5.0%, 7.2%, and 10.1% for the placebo, bupropion 300-mg, and bupropion 400-mg groups, respectively ($p < .0001$). The placebo group was randomized to the 300-mg or 400-mg group at 24 weeks, and the trial was extended to week 48. By the end of the trial, the dropout rate was 41%, and the mean weight losses in the bupropion 300-mg and bupropion 400-mg groups were 6.2% and 7.2% of initial body weight, respectively (Anderson et al., 2002). For patients with obesity and depression, this drug would be a good option.

Topiramate

Topiramate is FDA approved for the use in certain types of epilepsy and for the prophylaxis of migraine headache. It was found to induce weight loss in clinical trials for epilepsy treatment, with losses of 3.9% of initial weight at 3 months and 7.3% at 1 year. In a 6-month, placebo-controlled, dose-ranging study, 385 subjects were randomized to five groups: topiramate at 64 mg/day, 96 mg/day, 192 mg/day, 384 mg/day, or placebo (Bray et al., 2003). These doses were gradually increased over 12 weeks and were tapered off in a similar manner at the end of the trial. Mean weight losses from baseline to 24 weeks were 5.0%, 4.8%, 6.3%, 6.3%, and 2.6%, in the five groups, respectively. The most frequent adverse events were paresthesias (tingling or prickly feelings in skin), somnolence, and difficulty with concentration, memory, and attention.

Other Medications That Can Affect Weight

A systematic evidence review conducted by the Endocrine Society (Apovian, Aronne, Bessesen, et al., 2015) discusses additional medications that can affect body weight. Of particular concern are the newer atypical antipsychotics, which may cause weight gain in susceptible individuals. That review identified ziprasidone and aripiprazole as most likely to be weight neutral. Similarly, the anticonvulsants carbamazepine, gabapentin, and valproate were found to be associated with weight gain, whereas topiramate (discussed above) and zonisamide with weight loss (Apovian, Aronne, Bessesen, et al., 2015). Other medications associated with gain included progestational steroids used for contraception or for treatment of endometriosis (Apovian, Aronne, Bessesen, et al., 2015).

Conclusions

It is important that physicians who manage patients with health problems related to obesity prescribe medications appropriately. This includes prescribing medications as adjuncts to comprehensive lifestyle intervention and choosing medications wisely for management of chronic diseases. Figure 21.1 provides a framework for selecting treatments for chronic weight management in patients who are overweight or obese. This framework was provided in the guidelines of the National Heart, Lung, and Blood Institute in 1998 and basically was reconfirmed in the 2013 guidelines (Jensen et al., 2014). It uses BMI as the major factor in making treatment selections, but this singular focus needs to be tempered with clinical judgment based on cultural considerations and the presence of risk factors for the metabolic syndrome. Medications as adjuncts to comprehensive lifestyle intervention are indicated in chronic weight management for patients with a BMI > 30 kg/m^2 or with a comorbidity and BMI > 27 kg/m^2.

Medications are useful in the management of patients with obesity because they can reinforce behavioral intentions that lead to lifestyle changes. Five medications are now approved by the FDA for chronic weight management. Since treating a patient with obesity with one of these agents may improve the management of weight-related comorbidities and prevent others from developing, these medications should be considered for patients in which lifestyle modification does not produce the desired weight loss. As noted above, no patient responds to all treatments and, thus, rules for discontinuing medications are needed. As a generalization, the label recommendations for these medications advocate assessing weight loss response at 12 weeks and stopping the medication if weight loss is not at least 4–5% below the starting weight. After discontinuing the medication, alternative approaches need to be considered. Other ways of personalizing the response to therapy with genetic markers may become available, but none is currently of important predictive value. Physicians could help their patients who struggle with overweight or obesity by avoiding the prescription of medications that promote weight gain, and, when possible, selecting medications that promote weight loss when treating diabetes, depression, migraine, or epilepsy. Obesity is a chronic disease and its management is a long-term proposition. With good medication management, patients who struggle with obesity and its complications can achieve healthier weights and improvement in obesity risks and complications.

References

Addy, C., Jumes, P., Rosko, K., Li, S., Li, H., Maes, A., et al. (2009). Pharmacokinetics, safety, and tolerability of phentermine in healthy participants receiving taranabant, a novel cannabinoid-1 receptor (CB1R) inverse agonist. *Journal of Clinical Pharmacology, 49*(10), 1228–1238.

Allison, D. B., Gadde, K. M., Garvey, W. T., Peterson, C. A., Schwiers, M. L., Najarian, T., et al. (2012). Controlled-release phentermine/topiramate in severely obese adults: A randomized controlled trial (EQUIP). *Obesity, 20*(2), 330–342.

Amori, R. E., Lau, J., & Pittas, A. G. (2007). Efficacy and safety of incretin therapy in type 2 diabetes: Systematic review and meta-analysis. *Journal of the American Medical Association, 298*(2), 194–206.

Anderson, J. W., Greenway, F. L., Fujioka, K., Gadde, K. M., McKenney, J., & O'Neil, P. M. (2002). Bupropion SR enhances weight loss: A 48-week double-blind, placebo- controlled trial. *Obesity Research, 10*(7), 633–641.

Apovian, C. M., Aronne, L. J., Bessesen, D. H., McDonnell, M. E., Murad, M. H., Pagotto, U., et al. (2015). Pharmacologic management of obesity: An Endocrine Society clinical practice guideline. *Journal of Clinical Endocrinology and Metabolism, 100*(2), 342–362.

Apovian, C. M., Aronne, L., & Powell, A. G. (2015). *Clinical management of obesity*. West Islip, NY: Professional Communcations.

Apovian, C. M., Aronne, L., Rubino, D., Still, C., Wyatt, H., Burns, C., et al. (2013). A randomized, phase 3 trial of naltrexone SR/bupropion SR on weight and obesity-related risk factors (COR-II). *Obesity (Silver Spring), 21*(5), 935–943.

Apovian, C. M., Bergenstal, R. M., Cuddihy, R. M., Qu, Y., Lenox, S., & Lewis, M. S., et al. (2010). Effects of exenatide combined with lifestyle modification in patients with type 2 diabetes. *American Journal of Medicine, 123*(5), 468.e9–468.e17.

Aronne, L. J., Wadden, T. A., Peterson, C., Winslow, D., Odeh, S., & Gadde, K. M. (2013). Evaluation of phentermine and topiramate versus phentermine/topiramate extended-release in obese adults. *Obesity (Silver Spring), 21*(11), 2163–2171.

Astrup, A., Carraro, R., Finer, N., Harper, A., Kunesova, M., Lean, M. E., et al. (2012). Safety, tolerability and sustained weight loss over 2 years with the once-daily human GLP-1 analog, liraglutide. *International Journal Obesity (London), 36*(6), 843–854.

Astrup, A., Rössner, S., Van Gaal, L., Rissanen, A., Niskanen, L., Al Hakim, M., et al. (2009). Effects of liraglutide in the treatment of obesity: A randomised, double-blind, placebo-controlled study. *Lancet, 374*(9701), 1606–1616.

Bolinder, J., Ljunggren, Ö., Kullberg, J., Johansson, L., Wilding, J., Langkilde, A. M., et al. (2012). Effects of dapagliflozin on body weight, total fat mass, and regional adipose tissue distribution in patients with type 2 diabetes mellitus with inadequate glycemic control on metformin. *Journal of Clinical Endocrinology and Metabolism, 97*(3), 1020–1031.

Bray, G. A. (2011). *A guide to obesity and the metabolic syndrome*. Boca Raton, FL: CRC Press.

Bray, G. A., & Bouchard, C. (Eds.). (2014). *Handbook of obesity: Clinical applications* (Vol. 2, 4th ed.). Boca Raton, FL: CRC Press.

Bray, G. A., Frühbeck, G., Ryan D. H., & Wilding J. P. (2016). Management of obesity. *Lancet, 387*(10031), 1947–1956.

Bray, G. A., Hollander, P., Klein, S., Kushner, R., Levy, B., Fitchet, M., et al. (2003). A 6-month randomized, placebo-controlled, dose-ranging trial of topiramate for weight loss in obesity. *Obesity Research, 11*(6), 722–733.

Bray, G. A., & Ryan, D. H. (2012). Medical therapy for the patient with obesity. *Circulation, 125,* 1695–1703.

Brownell, K. D. (2000). *The LEARN manual for weight management*. Dallas, TX: American Health.

Buchwald, H., Avidor, Y., Braunwald, E., Jensen, M. D., Pories, W., Fahrbach, K., et al. (2004). Bariatric surgery: A systematic review and meta-analysis. *Journal of the American Medical Association, 292*(14), 1724–1737.

Bushe, C. J., Bradley, A. J., Doshi, S., & Karagianis, J. (2009). Changes in weight and metabolic parameters during treatment with antipsychotics and metformin: Do the data inform as to potential guideline development?: A systematic review of clinical studies. *International Journal of Clinical Practice, 63*(12), 1743–1761.

Cefalu, W. T., Leiter, L. A., Yoon, K. H., Arias, P., Niskanen, L., Xie, J., et al. (2013). Efficacy and safety of canagliflozin versus glimepiride in patients with type 2 diabetes inadequately controlled with metformin (CANTATA-SU): 52 week results from a randomised, double-blind, phase 3 non-inferiority trial. *Lancet, 382*(9896), 941–950.

Cefalu, W. T., Stenlöf, K., Leiter, L. A., Wilding, J. P., Blonde, L., Polidori, D., et al. (2015). Effects of canagliflozin on body weight and relationship to HbA1c and blood pressure changes in patients with type 2 diabetes. *Diabetologia, 58*(6), 1183–1187.

Chanoine, J. P., Hampl, S., Jensen, C., Boldrin, M., & Hauptman, J. (2005). Effect of orlistat on weight and body composition in obese adolescents: A randomized controlled trial. *Journal of the American Medical Association, 293*(23), 2873–2883.

Clar, C., Gill J. A., Court, R., & Waugh, N. (2012). Systematic review of SGLT2 receptor inhibitors in dual or triple therapy in type 2 diabetes. *BMJ Open, 2*(5), e001007.

Diabetes Prevention Program Research Group. (2002). Reduction in the incidence of type 2 diabetes with lifestyle intervention or metformin. *New England Journal of Medicine, 346*, 393–403.

Diabetes Prevention Program Research Group. (2009). 10-year followup of diabetes incidence and weight loss in the Diabetes Prevention Program Outcomes Study. *Lancet, 374*, 1677–1686.

Diabetes Prevention Program Research Group. (2012). Long term safety, tolerability and weight loss associated with metformin in the Diabetes Prevention Program Outcomes Study. *Diabetes Care, 35*(4), 731–737.

Dushay, J., Gao, C., Gopalakrishnan, G. S., Crawley, M., Mitten, E. K., Wilker, E., et al. (2012). Short-term exenatide treatment leads to significant weight loss in a subset of obese women without diabetes. *Diabetes Care, 35*(1), 4–11.

Fidler, M. C., Sanchez, M., Raether, B., Weissman, N. J., Smith, S. R., Shanahan, W. R., et al. (2011). A one-year randomized trial of lorcaserin for weight loss in obese and overweight adults: The BLOSSOM trial was significantly greater than with placebo. *Journal of Clinical Endocrinology and Metabolism, 96*(10), 3067–3077.

Food and Drug Administration. (2010a). *CONTRAVE (naltrexone SR/bupropion SR combination) Advisory Committee briefing document* (NDA 200063). Silver Spring, MD: Endocrinologic and Metabolic Drugs Advisory Committee.

Food and Drug Administration. (2010b). *VI-0521 (QNEXA®) Advisory Committee briefing document* (NDA 022580). Silver Spring, MD: Endocrinologic and Metabolic Drugs Advisory Committee.

Food and Drug Administration. (2011). Drug approval package. Retrieved from *www.accessdata.fda.gov. drugsatfda_docs/nda/2011/201088_suprenza_toc. cfm.*

Food and Drug Administration. (2012a). *Lorcaserin hydrochloride tablets, 10 mg briefing document* (NDA 22529). Silver Spring, MD: Endocrinologic and Metabolic Drugs Advisory Committee.

Gadde, K. M., Allison, D. B., Ryan, D. H., Peterson, C. A., Troupin, B., Schwiers, M. L., et al. (2011). Effects of low-dose, controlled-release, phentermine plus topiramate combination on weight and associated comorbidities in overweight and obese adults (CONQUER): A randomised, placebo-controlled, phase 3 trial. *Lancet, 377*(9774), 1341–1352.

Garvey, W. T., Ryan, D. H., Look, M., Gadde, K. M., Allison, D. B., Peterson, C. A., et al. (2012). Two-year sustained weight loss and metabolic benefits with controlled-release phentermine/topiramate in obese and overweight adults (SEQUEL): A randomized, placebo-controlled, phase 3 extension study. *American Journal of Clinical Nutrition, 95*(2), 297–308.

Greenway, F. L., Dunayevich, E., Tollefson, G., Erickson, J., Guttadauria, M., Fujioka, K., et al. (2009). Comparison of combined bupropion and naltrexone therapy for obesity with monotherapy and placebo. *Journal of Clinical Endocrinology and Metabolism, 94*(12), 4898–4906.

Greenway, F. L., Fujioka, K., Plodkowski, R. A., Mudaliar, S., Guttadauria, M., Erickson, J., et al. (2010). Effect of naltrexone plus bupropion on weight loss in overweight and obese adults (COR-I): A multicenter, randomised, double-blind, placebo-controlled, phase 3 trial. *Lancet, 376*(9741), 595–605.

Greenway, F. L., Whitehouse, M. J., Guttadauria, M., Anderson, J. W., Atkinson, R. L., Fujioka, K., et al. (2009). Rational design of a combination medication for the treatment of obesity. *Obesity (Silver Spring), 17*(1), 30–39.

Gregg, E. W., Chen, H., Wagenknecht, L. E., Clark, J. M., Delahanty, L. M., Bantle, J., et al. (2012). Association of an intensive lifestyle intervention with remission of type 2 diabetes. *Journal of the American Medical Association, 308*(23), 2489–2496.

Halford, J. C., Harrold, J. A., Boyland, E. J., Lawton, C. L., & Blundell, J. E. (2007). Serotonergic drugs: Effects on appetite expression and use for the treatment of obesity. *Drugs, 67*(1), 27–55.

He, L., Sabet, A., Djedjos, S., Miller, R., Sun, X., Hussain, M. A., et al. (2009). Metformin and insulin suppress hepatic gluconeogenesis through phosphorylation of CREB binding protein. *Cell, 137*(4), 635–646.

Hendricks, E. J., Rothman, R. B., & Greenway, F. L. (2009). How physician obesity specialists use drugs to treat obesity. *Obesity (Silver Spring), 17*(9), 1730–1735.

Hollander, P., Gupta, A. K., Plodkowski, R., Greenway, F., Bays, H., Burns, C., et al. (2013). Effects of naltrexone sustained-release/bupropion sustained-release combination therapy on body weight and glycaemic parameters in overweight and obese patients with type 2 diabetes. *Diabetes Care, 36*(12), 4022–4029.

Jensen, M. D., Ryan, D. H., Donato, K. A., Apovian, C. M., Ard, J. D., Comuzzie, A. G., et al. (2014). Guidelines (2013) for managing overweight and obesity in adults. *Obesity (Silver Spring), 22*(Suppl. 2), S1–S410.

Kang, J. G., Park, C. Y., Kang, J. H., Park, Y. W., & Park S. W. (2010). Randomized controlled trial to investigate the effects of a newly developed formulation of phentermine diffuse-controlled release for obesity. *Diabetes, Obesity, and Metabolism, 12,* 876–882.

Kelly, A. S., Rudser, K. D., Nathan, B. M., Fox, C. K., Metzig, A. M., Coombes, B. J., et al. (2013). The effect of glucagon-like peptide-1 receptor agonist therapy on body mass index in adolescents with severe obesity: A randomized, placebo-controlled, clinical trial. *Journal of the American Medical Association Pediatrics, 167*(4), 355–360.

Kim, K. K., Cho, H. J., Kang, J. C., Youn, B. B., & Lee, K. R. (2006). Effects on weight reduction and safety of short-term phentermine administration in Korean obese people. *Yonsei Medical Journal, 47*(5), 614–625.

Kim, Y., & Babu, A. R. (2012). Clinical potential of sodium–glucose cotransporter 2 inhibitors in the management of type 2 diabetes. *Diabetes, Metabolic Syndrome, and Obesity: Targets and Therapy, 5,* 313–327.

LeBlanc, E. S., O'Connor, E., Whitlock, E. P., Patnode, C. D., & Kapka, T. (2011). Effectiveness of primary care—relevant treatments for obesity in adults: A systematic review of evidence for the U.S. Preventive Task Force. *Annals of Internal Medicine, 155*(7), 434–447.

Leslie, W. S., Hankey, C. R., & Lean, M. E. (2007). Weight gain as an adverse effect of some commonly prescribed drugs: A systematic review. *Quarterly Journal of Medicine, 100*(7), 395–404.

Liakos, A., Karagiannis, T., Athanasiadou, E., Sarigianni, M., Mainou, M., Papatheodorou, K., et al. (2014). Efficacy and safety of empagliflozin for type 2 diabetes: A systematic review and metaanalysis. *Diabetes, Obesity and Metabolism, 16*(10), 984–993.

Martin, C. K., Redman, L. M., Zhang, J., Sanchez, M., Anderson, C. M., Smith, S. R., et al. (2011). Lorcaserin, a 5-HT(2C) receptor agonist, reduces body weight by decreasing energy intake without influencing energy expenditure. *Journal of Clinical Endocrinology and Metabolism, 96*(3), 837–845.

McEvoy, G. K., Miller, J., & Litvak, K. (Eds.). (2005). *AHFS drug information.* Bethesda, MD: American Society of Health-System Pharmacists.

National Heart, Lung, and Blood Institute (NHLBI). (1998). Clinical guidelines on the identification, evaluation, and treatment of overweight and obesity in adults: The evidence report. *Obesity Research, 6*(Suppl.), 51S–210S.

Ogden, C. L., Carroll, M. D., Kit, B. K., & Flegal, K. M. (2014). Prevalence of childhood and adult obesity in the United States, 2011–2012. *Journal of the American Medical Association, 311*(8), 806–814.

O'Neil, P. M., Smith, S. R., Weissman, N. J., Fidler, M. C., Sanchez, M., Zhang, J., et al. (2012). Randomized placebo-controlled clinical trial of lorcaserin for weight loss in type 2 diabetes mellitus: The BLOOM-DM study. *Obesity (Silver Spring), 20*(7), 1426–1436.

Pi-Sunyer, F. X., Astrup, A., Fujioka, K., Greenway, F., Halpern, A., Krempf, M., et al. (2015). A randomized, controlled trial of 3.0 mg of liraglutide in weight management. *New England Journal of Medicine, 373*(1), 11–22.

Potts, J. E., Gray, L. J., Brady, E. M., Khunti, K., Davies, M. J., & Bodicoat, D. H. (2015). The effect of glucagon-like peptide 1 receptor agonists on weight loss in type 2 diabetes: A systematic review and mixed treatment comparison meta-analysis. *PLOS ONE, 10*(6), e0126769.

Rosenstock, J., Klaff, L. J., Schwartz, S., Northrup, J., Holcombe, J. H., Wilhelm, K., et al. (2006). Effects of exenatide and lifestyle modification on body weight and glucose tolerance in obese subjects with and without pre-diabetes. *Diabetes Care, 33*(6), 1173–1175.

Rothman, R. B., & Baumann, M. H. (2009). Serotonergic drugs and valvular heart disease. *Expert Opinion on Drug Safety, 8*(3), 317–329.

Ryan, D., Peterson, C., Troupin, B., Najarian, T., Tam, P., & Day, W. (2010). Weight loss at 6 months with VI-0521 (PHEN/TPM combination) treatment. *Obesity Facts, 3,* 139–146.

Singh-Franco, D., Perez, A., & Harrington, C. (2011). The effect of pramlintide acetate on glycemic control and weight in patients with type 2 diabetes mellitus and in patients without diabetes: A systematic review and meta-analysis. *Diabetes, Obesity and Metabolism, 13*(2), 169–180.

Sjöström, L., Peltonen, M., Jacobson, P., Ahlin, S., Andersson-Assarsson, J., Anveden, Å., et al. (2014). Association of bariatric surgery with long-term remission of type 2 diabetes and with microvascular and macrovascular complications. *Journal of the American Medical Association, 311*(22), 2297–2304.

Sjöström, L., Rissanen, A., Andersen, T., Boldrin, M., Golay, A., Koppeschaar, H. P., et al. (1998). Randomised placebo-controlled trial of orlistat for weight loss and prevention of weight regain in obese patients: European Multicentre Orlistat Study Group. *Lancet, 352*(9123), 167–172.

Smith, S. R., De Jonge, L., Volaufova, J., Li, Y., Xie, H., & Bray, G. A. (2005). Effect of pioglitazone on body composition and energy expenditure: A randomized controlled trial. *Metabolism, 54,* 24–32.

Smith, S. R., Weissman, N. J., Anderson, C. M., Sanchez, M., Chuang, E., Stubbe, S., et al. (2010). Multicenter, placebo-controlled trial of lorcaserin for weight management. *New England Journal of Medicine, 363*(3), 245–256.

Torgerson, J. S., Hauptman, J., Boldrin, M. N., & Sjöström, L. (2004). Xenical in the prevention of diabetes in obese subjects (XENDOS) study: A randomized study of orlistat as an adjunct to lifestyle changes for the prevention of type 2 diabetes in obese patients. *Diabetes Care, 27*(1), 155–161.

Tuomilehto, J., Lindström, J., Eriksson, J. G., Valle, T. T., Hämäläinen, H., Ilanne-Parikka, P., et al. (2001). Prevention of type 2 diabetes mellitus by changes in lifestyle among subjects with impaired glucose tolerance. *New England Journal of Medicine, 344*(18), 1343–1350.

Vivus, Inc. (2012). Qsymia: Full prescribing information. Retrieved from *https://qsymia.com/patient/include/media/pdf/prescribing-information.pdf*.

Wadden, T. A., Foreyt, J. P., Foster, G. D., Hill, J. O., Klein, S., O'Neil, P. M., et al. (2011). Weight loss with naltrexone SR/bupropion SR combination therapy as an adjunct to behavior modification: The COR-BMOD trial. *Obesity (Silver Spring), 19*(1), 110–120.

Wadden, T. A., Hollander, P., Klein, S., Niswender, K., Woo, V., Hale, P. M., et al. (2013). Weight maintenance and additional weight loss with liraglutide after low-calorie-diet-induced weight loss: The SCALE Maintenance randomized study. *International Journal of Obesity (London), 37*(11), 1443–1451.

CHAPTER 22

Surgical Treatment of Obesity

Zubaidah Nor Hanipah
Ali Aminian
Philip R. Schauer

Lifestyle modification, drug therapy, and bariatric–metabolic surgery are the three modalities for the treatment of obesity. Intensive lifestyle intervention (ILI) and drug therapy are relatively low risk, but their weight loss efficacy is modest, especially in patients with severe obesity (Heymsfield & Wadden, 2017). Although surgery involves greater risk, it produces a greater magnitude and durability of weight loss and corresponding improvement in comorbidity and long-term survival. This chapter provides a comprehensive review of the surgical treatment of obesity.

The surgical treatment of severe obesity, historically referred to as *bariatric surgery* (derived from the Greek word *barrios,* for *weight*), originated in the 1950s with jejunoileal bypass (JIB) procedures that have become obsolete due to severe long-term metabolic and nutritional complications (Hocking, Duerson, O'Leary, & Woodward, 1983). Many other gastrointestinal (GI) weight loss operations have evolved since that time (with varying degrees of success), leading to the emergence of the commonly performed procedures of today (see Figure 22.1). Fundamental advances in bariatric–metabolic surgery occurred in the last two decades with the introduction of new, less invasive laparoscopic procedures, along with outcome studies demonstrating reliable, long-term weight loss and comorbidity improvement.

Classification of Bariatric–Metabolic Surgery

Bariatric and metabolic procedures have traditionally been classified as restrictive, malabsorptive, or both (Table 22.1), based on presumed mechanisms of weight loss. This classification system, though commonly used, may be an oversimplification of weight loss mechanisms based on recent studies pointing to neurohormonal mechanisms. Nevertheless, restrictive procedures reduce the gastric luminal diameter, and malabsorptive procedures divert nutrient flow and reduce the absorptive surface of the GI tract. These GI procedures have resulted in the resolution of obesity-related comorbidities through weight loss, neuroendocrine, or hormonal mechanisms. Thus, the term *bariatric surgery* is now frequently replaced with *metabolic surgery*. The mechanisms of bariatric–metabolic surgery are yet to be determined. Alteration of the GI tract by reducing stomach capacity and absorption in

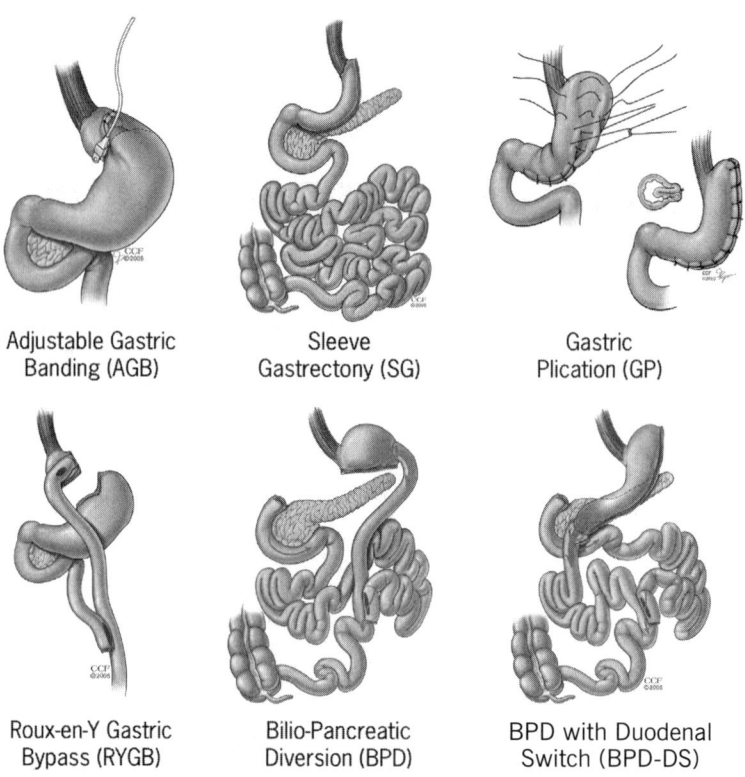

FIGURE 22.1. Bariatric operation performed in clinical practice. Reprinted with permission, Cleveland Clinic Center for Medical Art & Photography. Copyright © 2005–2017. All rights reserved.

the small intestine appears to alter satiety, calorie absorption, neuroendocrine pathways, and the gut microbiome, leading to weight loss and resolution of type 2 diabetes (T2D) and other comorbidities (Batterham & Cummings, 2016).

As noted, Figure 22.1 shows the common operations currently performed. Some procedures have been modified over time, and others have become obsolete. Single-anastomosis modifications of the Roux-en-Y gastric bypass (RYGB) (not shown), sometimes referred to as the *loop gastric bypass* or *mini-gastric bypass,* are popular in some regions (Quan et al., 2015). Similarly, single-anastomosis modifications of the duodenal switch (DS) have emerged, but have shown limited long-term outcomes (Sánchez-Pernaute et al., 2015). Gastric plication (GP) has emerged as a new restrictive procedure in recent years, but its long-term results have yet to be verified (Talebpour, Motamedi, Talebpour, & Vahidi, 2012; Brethauer, Harris, Kroh, & Schauer, 2011). JIB and vertical banded gastroplasty (VBG) have fallen out of favor because of significant long-term complications and suboptimal long-term results (Schirmer & Schauer, 2010).

While pure restrictive procedures are virtually all performed through the minimally invasive approach, either the laparoscopic or the open approach may be used for more complex diversionary procedures, including RYGB and biliopancreatic diversion (BPD). It has been shown that the laparoscopic approach is associated with fewer postoperative complications than the open approach, most notably the risk of wound infection and incisional hernia (Schirmer & Schauer, 2010; Reoch et al., 2011). The open approach is generally reserved for revisional operations or whenever laparoscopic surgery cannot be performed for technical reasons. Today, more than 95% of all primary bariatric operations are performed laparoscopically.

TABLE 22.1. Classification of Bariatric–Metabolic Procedures

Restrictive (satiety enhancing)
  Adjustable gastric banding (AGB)
  Sleeve gastrectomy (SG)
  Gastric plication (GP)
  Vertical banded gastroplasty (VBG)[a]

Malabsorptive
  Biliopancreatic diversion (BPD)[b]
  Jejunoileal bypass (JIB)[a]

Combined restrictive and malabsorptive
  Roux-en-Y gastric bypass (RYGB)[b]
  BPD with duodenal switch (BPD-DS)[b]

Experimental metabolic operations[c]
  Duodenal–jejunal bypass (DJB)
  Ileal interposition (II)

Note. From Aminian and Schauer (2014). Surgical procedures in the treatment of obesity and its comorbidities. In G. A. Bray & C. Bouchard (Ed.), *Handbook of obesity: Vol. 2. Clinical applications* (4th ed., pp. 365–383). Boca Raton, FL: CRC Press. Reprinted with permission from Taylor & Francis.

[a]Now offered infrequently and of historic interest only.

[b]Diversionary procedures that are performed through laparoscopic or open approach.

[c]Produce metabolic effects without significant weight loss; for use in experimental setting only at this time.

Several novel procedures (e.g., duodenal–jejunal bypass [DJB] and ileal interposition [II]), aimed to treat T2D and not necessarily to reduce weight, have been developed in recent years (see Figure 22.2). Although experimental and clinical studies show promising weight-independent antidiabetic results, their clinical use should still be considered investigational (Rubino et al., 2010).

A remarkable increase in the utilization of bariatric–metabolic surgery (> 135%) has occurred in the last two decades, with the realization of the relative ineffectiveness of conventional weight loss therapies with severely obese individuals (Eldar, Heneghan, Brethauer, & Schauer, 2011b). In the United States, an estimated total of 196,000 bariatric procedures were performed in 2015. Sleeve gastrectomy (SG) has recently become the most common procedure (53.8%), followed by RYGB (23.1%), adjustable gastric banding (AGB; 5.7%), BPD with or without duodenal switch (BPD-DS; 0.6%), and surgical revision or other procedures (16.8%) (Ponce et al., 2016). SG and RYGB together are the most popular procedures (77%), whereas AGB has declined in use due to poor long-term results. BPD is the least frequently performed procedure, most likely due to the significant risk of severe nutritional deficiencies (3–18%; Scopinaro, 2012; Sethi et al., 2016). In some countries, SG is even more common (> 70%); the estimated worldwide utilization of bariatric–

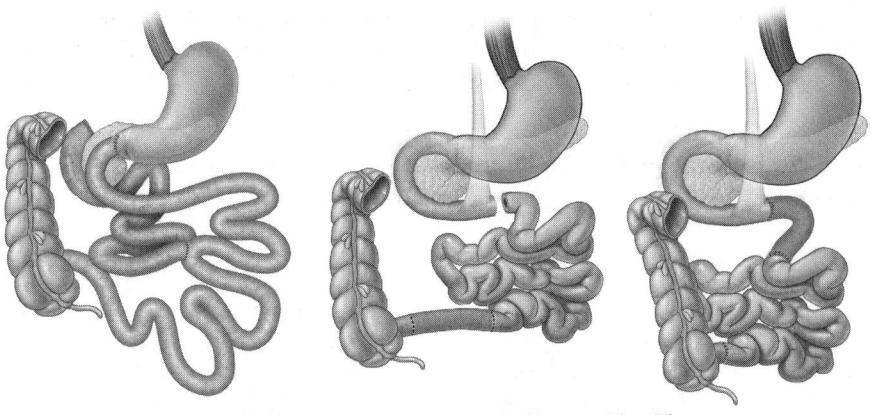

Duodenal-Jejunal Bypass (DJB) Ileal Interposition (II)

FIGURE 22.2. Novel experimental metabolic procedures. Reprinted with permission, Cleveland Clinic Center for Medical Art & Photography. Copyright © 2005–2017. All rights reserved.

metabolic surgery was 468,609 procedures performed in 2013 (Angrisani et al., 2015). Despite this growth, fewer than 2% of eligible patients are estimated to undergo surgical treatment for severe obesity.

Anatomic Description of Surgical Procedures

AGB

AGB uses a restrictive mechanism for weight loss by placing an inflatable silicone band just below the gastroesophageal junction, creating a small gastric pouch and a narrow stoma (Figure 22.1). The band is attached to a subcutaneous port that allows adjustment of the band's tightness. Saline is injected into the port usually beginning 1 month after surgery. Frequent follow-up is essential after the AGB operation to achieve the optimal band tightness for each patient.

SG

Sleeve gastrectomy (SG) was originally intended to be the initial procedure for very high-risk, super-obese patients who ultimately would have BPD-DS or RYGB surgery. The intent of this first stage was to perform a relatively safe and simple procedure in patients who could not tolerate a complex procedure due to comorbidities or anatomic limitations. After very good weight loss results were reported with SG, it rapidly gained popularity as a stand-alone bariatric operation. Currently, SG is recognized as a standard weight loss operation. In this procedure, a linear cutting stapler is used to make a narrow gastric tube along the lesser curvature of the stomach (Figure 22.1). The remaining 75–80% of the gastric body and fundus are removed.

GP

GP is a newer procedure in the treatment of morbid obesity. It appears to produce results that are similar to those of SG with potentially fewer complications. Without gastric resection, the greater curve of the stomach is invaginated with suturing to create a tubular stomach. In GP, the stomach is not cut or crushed by staplers, no anastomoses are made, and no foreign body is used. Similar weight loss compared to other restrictive procedures, lower chance of GI leak and bleeding due to elimination of stapling and resection, reversibility, and lower cost are among the potential advantages of GP. The true role of GP as a weight loss procedure awaits clarification with long-term data (Talebpour et al., 2012; Brethauer, Harris, et al., 2011).

RYGB

RYGB was the most widely performed bariatric surgery in the United States until recently being overtaken by SG. In laparoscopic RYGB, which is the most common approach, the jejunum is divided approximately 50 cm from the ligament of Treitz, and the proximal end of the jejunum is anastomosed to the distal part of the jejunum at 150 cm below the site of transection (jejunojejunostomy). The resultant 150-cm Roux limb of proximal jejunum is brought up and anastomosed to the small proximal gastric pouch (15–30 ml).

BPD and BPD-DS

In BPD, a horizontal partial gastrectomy (resection of the distal half to two-thirds of the stomach) is performed. Then the terminal ileum is divided 250 cm proximal to the ileocecal valve. The distal end of that divided ileum (alimentary Roux limb) is anastomosed to the stomach (gastroileostomy). The proximal end of the ileum (biliopancreatic limb) is then anastomosed to the terminal ileum approximately 50–100 cm proximal to the ileocecal valve to create a small common channel. Prophylactic cholecystectomy is performed due to the high incidence of gallstone formation following the malabsorption of bile salts. High incidence of marginal ulcers at gastroileal anastomosis after BPD led to a modification of the original technique. The modified procedure, BPD-DS, differs from BPD only in the gastric portion of the operation. In the BPD-DS variant, instead of horizontal gastrectomy, a narrow sleeve gastrectomy is performed and the pylorus is preserved. After division of the duodenum, the Roux alimentary limb is anastomosed to the first portion of the duodenum after the pylorus (duodenoileostomy), and the distal duodenal end is closed. A short common channel is created by connecting the biliopancreatic limb to the alimentary limb 50–100 cm from the ileocecal valve.

Indications for Bariatric–Metabolic Surgery

Historically, indications for bariatric–metabolic surgery have been based on the National Institutes of Health (NIH; 1991) Consensus Conference, which developed guidelines based strictly on BMI and the presence or absence of comorbidity. According to the NIH guidelines, patients are eligible for bariatric–metabolic surgery if they have a BMI ≥ 40 kg/m^2, or if their BMI is ≥ 35 kg/m^2 with comorbidity, and they do not have medical or psychological contraindications (Table 22.2). More recent evidence-based guidelines (2013) endorsed by the American Heart Association, the American College of Cardiology, and the Obesity Society, advocate very similar criteria for surgery (Jensen et al., 2014). The Edmonton obesity staging system (stages 0–4) proposed by Sharma and Kushner (2009) has gained international recognition as an obesity staging system that emphasizes disease severity and deemphasizes BMI, which is often a poor indicator of disease burden. Some countries and third-party payers have adopted the Edmonton approach and reserve bariatric–metabolic surgery for advanced stages of obesity (stages 2–4) regardless of BMI (Gill, Karmali, & Sharma, 2011). Until recently, guidelines for bariatric–metabolic surgery have generally excluded patients with BMI < 35 kg/m^2 due to inadequate evidence for the efficacy of surgery in these patients. However, the Second Diabetes Surgery Summit (DSS-II) guidelines, endorsed by more than 50 international medical societies, including the American Diabetes Association and the International Diabetes Federation, recommend that bariatric–metabolic surgery be considered for patients with T2D and a BMI of 30–34 kg/m^2 (BMI of 27.5 kg/m^2 for people of Asian ancestry) who are not well controlled with lifestyle modification and/or drug therapy (Rubino et al., 2016). Age per se is not a limiting factor. Carefully selected elderly and adolescent patients can benefit significantly from bariatric–metabolic surgery (Buchwald & Consensus Conference Panel, 2005; Brethauer, Chand, & Schauer, 2006).

TABLE 22.2. Indications and Contraindications of Bariatric–Metabolic Surgery

Indications	• BMI ≥ 40 kg/m^2 with or without comorbid medical conditions associated with obesity. • BMI 35–39 kg/m^2 with comorbid medical conditions. • Patients must be psychiatrically stable.
Bariatric–metabolic surgery recommended	• Patients with T2D and patients with class 3 obesity (BMI ≥ 40 kg/m^2), regardless of glycemic control or complexity of glucose lowering regimes. • Patients with T2D and patients with class 2 obesity (BMI 35–39.9 kg/m^2) with inadequate glycemic control, despite lifestyle and optimal medical treatment (either oral or injectable medications, including insulin).
Bariatric–metabolic surgery should be considered	• Patients with T2D and patients with class 1 obesity (BMI 30–34.9 kg/m^2) with inadequate glycemic control, despite optimal medical treatment (either oral or injectable medications, including insulin).
Relative contraindication for bariatric–metabolic surgery	• Incompetent mentally to understand procedure. • Inability or unwillingness to change lifestyle postoperatively. • Uncontrolled substance abuse. • Psychologically unstable.

Perioperative Management

A multidisciplinary approach to preoperative and postoperative management has been broadly adopted in order to optimize outcomes. The multidisciplinary team consists of the bariatric surgeon, obesity medicine specialist, psychologist, and dietitian. Obesity medicine has recently emerged as a board certified specialty (see Kushner & Kahan, Chapter 24, this volume). Other specialists, who may include the endocrinologist, cardiologist, anesthetist, pulmonologist, and sleep physician, play an important role in patient care, as do the family and social supports.

The perioperative management for bariatric patients is outlined in Tables 22.3, 22.4, and 22.5, based on the updated clinical practice guidelines in perioperative nutritional, metabolic, and nonsurgical support of bariatric surgery patients by the American Association of Clinical Endocrinologists (AACE), The Obesity Society (TOS), and the American Society for Metabolic and Bariatric Surgery (ASMBS; Mechanick et al., 2013).

Although success with diet and exercise alone is very limited for severely obese individuals, all patients are encouraged to attempt this safest method of weight loss prior to undertaking any surgical intervention. In this way, patients with severe obesity practice the lifestyle changes that are the key to long-term success after any bariatric operation. Moreover, some surgeons instruct patients to follow a low-calorie diet in the immediate preoperative period (e.g., 800–1,200 calories/day for 2 weeks prior to surgery) to reduce liver volume and improve operative exposure. In addition, some data indicate that preoperative weight loss may be associated with better outcomes (Schirmer & Schauer, 2010). Weeks and sometimes months are needed for a careful preoperative evaluation and optimization of bariatric surgical candidates (Table 22.3). A multidisciplinary team approach is essential for both preoperative and postoperative care of these patients.

Careful nutritional, medical, and psychological assessments are essential steps in the preparation of patients for surgery. Cardiac evaluation for patients over age 50 or for those with known cardiovascular disease is necessary. Pulmonary evaluation is indicated for patients with asthma, hypoventilation syndrome, or pulmonary hypertension. In patients with symptoms suggestive of obstructive sleep apnea (OSA), including a history of loud snoring, tiredness, and falling asleep easily, a sleep study is indicated prior to surgery for diagnosis. Initiation of treatment with continuous positive airway pressure (CPAP) is recommended for patients with OSA to reduce postoperative complications such as severe hypoxia and dysrhythmia. A preoperative screening upper gastrointestinal (UGI) endoscopy is indicated in patients with a history of UGI diseases, including gastroesophageal reflux disease (GERD), to rule out internal pathologies such as Barrett's esophagus. This evaluation is especially important for patients planning to undergo RYGB, with which the distal stomach and duodenum will not be easily accessible after operation. Baseline routine blood tests; renal, liver, and thyroid function tests; and arterial blood gas analysis are indicated, as shown in Table 22.3. Before surgery, a preoperative visit from the anesthesiologist for assessment of airway issues and comorbid medical problems is also advised for all patients undergoing bariatric surgery (Schirmer & Schauer, 2010; Eldar et al., 2011b).

Early postoperative care emphasizes prevention and management of complications commonly occurring in the first month after surgery (Table 22.4). Nausea, vomiting, and dehydration are the most common early side effects and are usually self-limited but can lead to serious conditions that may require hospitalization for rehydration or treatment of deficiencies. Acute thiamine deficiency (Wernicke encephalopathy) caused by vomiting is the most feared deficiency. It may result in permanent neurological deficit unless promptly treated with thiamine. Patients should begin vitamin supplementation within a week of surgery and start an exercise program when recovered from surgery. Long-term follow-up care is outlined in Table 22.5. Prophylactic ursodiol taken daily in divided doses of at least 300 mg for the first 6 months after surgery has been shown to decrease the incidence of gallstone formation (Mechanick et al., 2013). Pro-

Surgical Treatment of Obesity

TABLE 22.3. Perioperative Care

Complete history and physical examination	• Causes for obesity, related comorbidities and their treatment, diet history, weight loss history and commitment to lose weight, weight, height, and BMI.
Blood investigations	• Fasting blood glucose and lipid panel, renal function, liver profile, lipid profile, prothrombin time/international normalized ratio (INR), blood type, complete blood count.
Nutritional assessment	• Appropriate clinical nutritional evaluation, nutrient screening with iron studies, B12, and folic acid and 25-vitamin D levels. • Optional screening: red blood cell (RBC) folate, homocysteine, methylmalonic acid, vitamins A and E. • Consider more extensive testing in patients undergoing malabsorptive procedures based on ASMBS guidelines.
Cardiopulmonary assessment	• Chest X-ray (CXR), electrocardiogram (ECG), sleep apnea screening (± confirmatory polysomnography). • In patients with cardiac disease or pulmonary hypertension: echocardiogram. • In patients with intrinsic lung disease or disordered sleep patterns: arterial blood gas (ABG), formal pulmonary evaluation. • In patients with risk of venous thromboembolism (VTE): deep vein thrombosis (DVT) evaluation.
Endocrine assessment	• Prediabetic or diabetic: HbA1C level; optimization of glycemic control (including HbA1C ≤ 7%, fasting blood sugar ≤ 110 mg/dL, 2-hour postprandial blood glucose of ≤ 140 mg/dL). • In long-standing diabetic patients: HbA1C 7–8%. • Thyroid disease: thyroid-stimulating hormone (TSH) test. • Patients with suspected polycystic ovary syndrome (PCOS): total or bioavailable testosterone, dehydroepiandrosterone sulfate (DHEAS), D4-androstenedione. • Screening for Cushing's syndrome: 1 mg overnight dexamethasone test, 24-hour urinary-free cortisol, 11 P.M. salivary cortisol.
GI assessment (test: optional or if indicated)	• Ultrasound abdomen (to rule out gallstones, liver assessment). • Upper endoscopy for history of upper gastrointestinal (UGI) disease. • *H. pylori* screening in high-prevalence areas.
Psychosocial–behavioral assessment	• Evaluation of environmental, familial, and behavioral factors. • In patients with suspected psychiatric illness or substance abuse: formal mental health evaluation.
Informed consent for surgery	• Written documentation of patient education and understanding of risks and benefits of surgery.
Preoperative weight loss (desirable but not mandatory)	• Rationale: reduce intraoperative and postoperative complications. Goal: 5–10% weight loss.
Counseling	• Childbearing women: pregnancy and contraception. • Smokers: stop smoking at least 6 weeks prior to surgery. • Long-term dietary and vitamin adherence and monitoring.
Cancer screening	• Verified by primary care physician. • Screening for breast, colorectal, endometrium, cervical, and prostate cancers.

TABLE 22.4. Early Postoperative Care

Cardiopulmonary care	• High risk of myocardial infarction (MI): at least 24-hour telemetry monitoring. • Pulmonary toilet, incentive spirometry. • Early CPAP if required. • DVT prophylaxis; encourage ambulation. • If unstable: consider leak or pulmonary embolism (PE).
Hydration	• Maintain adequate hydration (usually 1.5 liter/day, oral administration).
Healthy eating education	• Protocol-derived stage meal progression by registered dietitian.
Monitoring	• Bleeding, leak, severe nausea, vomiting, dehydration, stricture, bowel obstruction, DVT/PE, hypoglycemia, hyperglycemia, wound infection, pneumonia, acute thiamine deficiency (Wernike's encephalopathy).
Pressure sore prevention	• Early ambulation. • Adequate padding at pressure points. • For suspected rhabdomyolysis: check for creatine kinase level.
Supplemental vitamins and nutrients	• One or two adult multivitamin–mineral supplements containing iron, 1,200–1,500 mg/day of calcium, and a vitamin B-complex preparation. • Protein 60–80 g/day.

Note. Adapted from Hanipah and Schauer (2017). Surgical treatment of obesity and diabetes. *Gastrointestinal Endoscopy Clinics of North America, 27*(2), 191–211. Copyright © 2017 Elsevier. Adapted with permission.

TABLE 22.5. Follow-Up Care

Follow-up visit	• 1, 3, 6, and 12 months, then annually. • Patients with gastric banding require more frequent visits for band adjustments.
Monitoring	• Weight loss trend. • Nutritional assessment. • Psychological assessment (if support group needed). • Evidence of postoperative complications. • Physical activity (average 150 minutes of aerobic activity/week).
Evaluation and medication adjustment	• Need for antihypertensive, anti-diabetic, and lipid medications.
Substances/habits to avoid	• Nonsteroidal anti-inflammatory drugs. • Smoking.
Prophylactic medication	• Gout as needed. • Gallstones: ursodial 600 mg/day for 6 months. • Marginal ulcers: antisecretory agent for 6 months.
Investigations to be monitored	• Complete blood count (CBC)/platelet, serum chemistry, and lipid profile every 6–12 months. • Thiamine evaluation for signs of thiamine deficiency. • 24-hour urinary calcium excretion at 6 months and then annually. • B12 (annually; then 3–6 months if supplemented). • Bone density scan at 2 years. • In malabsorptive surgery: folic acid, iron studies, 25-vitamin D, iPTH, vitamin A (initially and 6–12 months thereafter), copper, zinc, and selenium evaluation with specific findings.

phylatic use of an antisecretory agent for 6 months may prevent marginal ulceration after gastric bypass.

Complications

The morbidity and mortality rates associated with bariatric–metabolic surgery are generally comparable to morbidity and mortality rates for other major abdominal operations such as cholecystectomy, appendectomy, and hysterectomy. Surgical complications are dependent on several factors: (1) the skill and the stage in the learning curve of the bariatric surgeon; (2) the type of surgical approach (open vs. laparoscopic) and procedure performed (lower risk for restrictive procedures); and (3) the presence of significant comorbidities, such as systemic hypertension, OSA, pulmonary hypertension, ischemic heart disease, or history of deep vein thrombosis (DVT). Certainly, the best preventive measure is good operative technique and wise perioperative selection. When complications do occur, the best outcomes result from early diagnosis and prompt treatment.

The complications after bariatric–metabolic surgery can be divided into procedure-independent complications (Table 22.6), which can occur after any type of weight loss surgery, or procedure-specific complications (Table 22.7; Moustarah, Brethauer, & Schauer, 2010; Brethauer et al., 2006). Four main complications that need emergent assessment and management are described in the following sections. Keys to the recognition and management of other complications are outlined in Table 22.8 (Moustarah et al., 2010; Al Harakeh, 2011).

Bariatric–Metabolic Surgery Emergencies

Recognition and diagnosis of emergencies after bariatric–metabolic surgery can be challenging. Severely obese patients may not present with typical signs and symptoms, so a high index of suspicion is warranted. In addition, these patients usually do not have enough physiological reserve to adequately tolerate complications, intensifying the necessity of rapid emergency care. It is generally recommended that patients or caretakers contact a bariatric surgeon, preferably the one who performed the operation, to handle bariatric–metabolic surgical emergencies. If the bariatric surgeon is not available, a general surgeon should be involved in the emergent care of bariatric patients.

TABLE 22.6. Procedure-Independent Complications of Bariatric Surgery

Early complications	Late complications
• Surgical site infection (superficial, deep). • Bleeding (GI, intraperitoneal). • Pulmonary complications (airway obstruction, atelectasis, pneumonia, pneumothorax, respiratory failure). • DVT and pulmonary embolism. • Nausea and vomiting, food intolerance, dehydration. • Prolonged ileus. • Intestinal obstruction (due to intraluminal clot, adhesion, abdominal wall hernia). • Cardiac arrhythmia (induced by hypoxia). • Myocardial infarction. • Dehiscence and evisceration (open surgery only). • Rhabdomyolysis (due to pressure necrosis of the gluteal muscles), acute tubular necrosis. • Pancreatitis. • Sepsis and multiple organ failure.	• Intractable nausea and vomiting, food intolerance, dehydration. • Intestinal obstruction (due to adhesion, abdominal wall hernia). • Incisional hernia. • Weight loss failure. • Weight regain. • Nutritional deficiencies. • Hypoglycemia.

Note. From Aminian and Schauer (2014). Surgical procedures in the treatment of obesity and its comorbidities. In G. A. Bray & C. Bouchard (Ed.), *Handbook of obesity: Vol. 2. Clinical applications* (4th ed., pp. 365–383). Boca Raton, FL: CRC Press. Reprinted with permission from Taylor & Francis.

Bleeding

Postoperative bleeding is classified as GI bleeding and intraperitoneal bleeding. Signs and symptoms of acute bleeding include hematemesis, rectal bleeding, melena, blood in drains, tachycardia, hypotension, pallor, fainting, and drowsiness. Hemoperitoneum usually occurs in the initial 48 hours after surgery. The possible sources of intraperitoneal bleeding include staple lines, iatrogenic injury (e.g., spleen), and trocar sites (Bal, Koch, Finelli, & Sar, 2010). Hematemasis often suggests bleeding from the gastrojejunal anastomosis. Lower GI bleeding potentially indicates bleeding from the staple line of the gastric remnant, gastrojejunostomy, or jejunojejunostomy. Marginal ulceration at the gastrojejunostomy can also cause GI bleeding, usually within 48 hours of surgery. These ulcers are consequent to exposure of

TABLE 22.7. Procedure-Specific Complications of Bariatric Surgery

Procedure	Early complications	Late complications
AGB	• Gastroesophageal reflux. • Band misplacement. • Band slippage. • GI leak (generalized peritonitis, abscess, fistula formation).	• Gastroesophageal reflux. • Pouch enlargement, esophageal dilation. • Gastric prolapse. • Band slippage. • Mechanical port and tubing complications. • Band erosion into the stomach. • Necessity for multiple adjustments. • Gallstones.
SG, GP	• GI leak (generalized peritonitis, abscess, fistula formation). • Gastric obstruction. • Gastroesophageal reflux.	• Gastroesophageal reflux. • Gastric dilation. • Gallstones. • Nutritional deficiencies (calcium, vitamins D and B12). • Iron deficiency anemia.
RYGB	• GI leak (generalized peritonitis, abscess, fistula formation). • Acute distal gastric dilatation and rupture. • Roux limb obstruction.	• Stomal stenosis (at gastrojejunostomy). • Marginal ulcer (at gastrojejunostomy). • Dumping syndrome. • Internal hernia. • Staple line disruption and gastrogastric fistula. • Stomal dilation. • Gallstones. • Nutritional deficiencies (calcium, iron, vitamins D and B12). • Iron deficiency anemia.
BPD, BPD-DS	• GI leak (generalized peritonitis, abscess, fistula formation). • Roux limb obstruction.	• Diarrhea and flatulence. • Marginal ulcer (after BPD). • Dumping syndrome (after BPD). • Internal hernia. • Electrolyte abnormalities. • Liver failure. • Gallstones. • Renal stone. • Nutritional deficiencies (calcium, iron, vitamins D and B12). • Iron deficiency anemia. • Protein-calorie malnutrition. • Hypocalcemia, osteoporosis. • Night blindness—vitamin A deficiency.

Note. From Aminian and Schauer (2014). Surgical procedures in the treatment of obesity and its comorbidities. In G. A. Bray & C. Bouchard (Ed.), *Handbook of obesity: Vol. 2. Clinical applications* (4th ed., pp. 365–383). Boca Raton, FL: CRC Press. Reprinted with permission from Taylor & Francis. AGB, adjustable gastric banding; SG, sleeve gastrectomy; GP, gastric plication; RYGB, Roux-en-Y gastric bypass; BPD, biliopancreatic diversion; BPD-DS, with duodenal switch.

TABLE 22.8. Postoperative Complications of Bariatric Surgery and in the Management.

Complication	Incidence	Presentation	Diagnostic tool	Management
Wound infection	2% after laparoscopic vs. 7% after open approach	Wound swelling, erythema, discharge, pain, and fever	Wound examination	Drainage ± antibiotics
Acute gastric remnant dilatation	≤ 1% after RYGB	Hiccups, abdominal bloating	Abdominal X-ray Abdominal CT	Needle decompression, surgical decompression
Dumping syndrome	50–75% after RYGB and BPD	GI symptoms (nausea, abdominal cramps, bloating, diarrhea) and vasomotor symptoms (facial flushing, lightheadedness, palpitations) after the consumption of carbohydrate-rich meals	Clinical history	*Dietary modification*: consumption of foods high in fiber and protein instead of simple carbohydrates *Medications*: octreotide, acarbose
Marginal ulceration	About 1–5% after RYGB and BPD	Epigastric pain (no relation to food), nausea, vomiting, bleeding	UGI endoscopy	*Medical* (90% effective): proton pump inhibitors, sucralfate, *H. pylori* eradication (if present), no NSAIDs/smoking/alcohol. *Indications for surgery*: development of gastrogastric fistula, severe stenosis, nonhealing ulcers
Stomal stenosis	3–10% after RYGB (at gastrojejunal anastomosis)	Vomiting, dysphagia, pain, mostly 6–12 weeks postoperatively	UGI endoscopy UGI contrast study	Endoscopic balloon dilation (one to two sessions); revisional surgery (< 10% of cases)
Gallstones	About 10–25% after RYGB	Nausea, vomiting, abdominal pain, tenderness, fever	Ultrasound	Ursodiol for 6 months after bariatric surgery to reduce the incidence of gallstone formation to < 5%; cholecystectomy for symptomatic patients
Weight regain	10–25% between 2–5 years after surgery	> 15% regain of lost weight, recurrence of comorbidities	Rule out anatomic abnormalities (gastric pouch dilation, wide gastrojejunal anastomosis, gastrogastric fistula): UGI endoscopy, small-bowel series, or diagnostic laparoscopy	Dietary modification and exercise; weight loss medications; endoscopic or endoluminal therapies; if unsuccessful, surgical revision

Note. From Aminian and Schauer (2014). Surgical procedures in the treatment of obesity and its comorbidities. In G. A. Bray & C. Bouchard (Ed.), *Handbook of obesity: Vol. 2. Clinical applications* (4th ed., pp. 365–383). Boca Raton, FL: CRC Press. Reprinted with permission from Taylor & Francis. CT, computed tomography; NSAID, nonsteroidal anti-inflammatory drug; RYGB, Roux-en-Y gastric bypass; BPD, bilipoancreatic diversion.

the unprotected jejunal mucosa to gastric acidity (Bal et al., 2010).

Resuscitation with intravenous fluid (normal saline or Ringer's lactate) and then blood products, as necessary, are first-line therapy. Close monitoring of vital signs, urine output, and hemoglobin level is critical. Individuals who are unresponsive to blood transfusion (i.e., persistent tachycardia, hypotension, or drop in hemoglobin levels) need surgical intervention. UGI endoscopy may facilitate detection and local treatment of upper GI bleeding in stable patients (Bal et al., 2010; Heneghan et al., 2012).

GI Leak

Anastomotic and staple line leaks have been reported to occur in 0.5–5% of bariatric cases and continue to be a major cause of surgical mortality. In the case of RYGB, leaks occur most frequently at the gastrojejunal anastomosis, but can also occur from the staple line of the gastric pouch or bypassed remnant, the jejunojejunostomy, or an unrecognized iatrogenic bowel injury. Leakage can occur at the gastric staple line in the case of SG or at the anastomotic sites in BPD (Brethauer et al., 2006; Moustarah et al., 2010).

Leaks can occur early after surgery or present up to 2–3 weeks postoperatively. The diagnosis of a leak in severely obese patients is challenging. Although fever, tachycardia, tachypnea, and abdominal pain are common, often the only presenting sign is tachycardia in the absence of classical peritoneal signs of guarding and rebound tenderness. Careful vigilance and a high index of suspicion are necessary for early diagnosis. Unexplained persistent and progressive tachycardia (>120 beats per minute for more than 4 hours) should alert the surgeon or physician to the possibility of a leak, even if other findings are not present. Abdominal CT scan with oral contrast and UGI radiography with gastrografin are the most useful diagnostic tools, but negative results do not definitively rule out a leak. In many cases, the presentation of a leak is similar to that of a pulmonary embolism (tachycardia, tachypnea, hypoxia). Once pulmonary embolism is ruled out with a helical computed tomography (CT) scan of the chest, immediate surgical exploration may be warranted even in the presence of normal abdominal imaging studies (Schirmer & Schauer, 2010; Brethauer et al., 2006; Moustarah et al., 2010; Al Harakeh, 2011).

GI leakage can be contained (i.e., an abscess) or result in diffuse peritonitis. In selected stable patients, contained leaks can be managed nonoperatively with adequate radiologic drainage, bowel rest, and antibiotics (Thodiyil et al., 2008). If the patient is not stable or the leak is not contained, surgical reexploration involving copious irrigation, oversewing and repair of the leak as feasible, wide drainage, and creation of access for enteral feeding are advised (Schirmer & Schauer, 2010; Bal et al., 2010; Al Harakeh, 2011).

Pulmonary Embolism

Because all obese surgical candidates have an increased risk for thromboembolic complications, mechanical and pharmacological prophylactic measures for DVT are commonly practiced to reduce this risk (Brethauer et al., 2006). Nonetheless, postoperative pulmonary embolism remains a leading cause of mortality after bariatric–metabolic surgery and can occur after discharge from hospital. The condition can be difficult to diagnose, as the patients may become tachycardic and/or hypotensive with clinical findings similar to those indicating leak and sepsis. In such patients, the diagnosis of a pulmonary embolism and intra-abdominal complications (e.g., leak or strangulated obstruction) should be concurrently considered. Chest and abdominal CT scans should be performed without delay. When large body size precludes diagnostic CT imaging, surgical exploration of the abdomen may be warranted. If no intra-abdominal source is found, empiric anticoagulant therapy should be considered (Moustarah et al., 2010; Bal et al., 2010).

Small-Bowel Obstruction

Patients may present with colicky abdominal pain, vomiting, abdominal distention, obstipation, constipation, tachycardia, hypotension, and dehydration. The most common causes of small-bowel obstruction after bariatric–metabolic surgery include adhesive bands, internal hernia due to inadequate closure or nonclosure of the mesenteric defects by the surgeon at the time of operation (specific for RYGB and BPD), narrowing at the anastomosis (e.g., narrowing or kinking of jejunojejunal anastomosis after RYGB), incarcerated abdominal wall hernia, and intraluminal blood clot (in early postoperative period; Moustarah et al., 2010; Al Harakeh, 2011; Hwang, Swartz, & Felix, 2004). Adequate hydration by intravenous resuscitation is mandatory. Blind placement of a nasogastric tube should generally be avoided, or performed with caution, due to risk of perforation. In stable patients, examination with abdominal CT, UGI series, or both may be helpful in the diagnosis. If a patient presents with severe abdominal pain, surgical abdomen, or unstable vital signs, he or she should be taken directly to the operating room without any further delay (Rogula, Yenumula, & Schauer, 2007).

In the setting of RYGB or BPD, a small-bowel obstruction must be managed differently from obstruction after general surgical procedures, which is usually caused by adhesions and often will resolve with conservative, nonoperative management. Bowel obstruction after RYGB or BPD may be due to an internal hernia, which may rapidly progress to bowel strangulation and infarction, leading to high morbidity and mortality (Rogula et al., 2007; Shimizu, Maia, Kroh, Schauer, & Brethauer, 2013).

Perioperative Mortality

An analysis of a national database on 13,871 bariatric procedures reported a total 60-day mortality rate of 0.25% (Morino et al., 2007). The type of surgical procedure significantly influenced mortality risk: 0.1% with AGB, 0.15% with VBG, 0.54% for RYGB, and 0.8% with BPD. Pulmonary embolism represented the most common cause of death (38.2%), followed by cardiac failure (17.6%) and intestinal leak (17.6%). Open surgery and caseload per center were among the major risk factors of mortality (Morino et al., 2007). In a more recent prospective multicenter study (Longitudinal Assessment of Bariatric Surgery [LABS] Consortium et al., 2009), the overall 30-day mortality was 0.3% (Flum et al., 2009). Mortality rates following open and laparoscopic RYGB (LRYGB) were 2.1% and 0.2%, respectively. Aminian et al. (2015) showed that the 30-day morbidity rate after LRYGB (n = 16,509) was 3.4%, which was comparable to the morbidity rates for laparoscopic cholecystectomy (n = 15,306) and laparoscopic hysterectomy (n = 2,309) with 3.7% and 3.5%, respectively. The 30-day mortality was 0.3% in the LRYGB group, which was similar to the mortality in the total knee arthroplasty group (n = 9,184).

Outcome of Bariatric–Metabolic Surgery

Weight Loss

Percentages of excess weight and BMI loss are used most commonly in the surgical literature (Deitel & Greenstein, 2003). Percentage of excess weight loss (% EWL) is defined as [(operative weight–follow-up weight)/(operative weight–ideal weight)] × 100, and percentage of excess BMI loss (% EBMIL) is defined as 100–[(follow-up BMI–25/operative BMI–25) × 100]. At this time, bariatric surgery is the most well-established and successful method of facilitating durable weight loss in severely obese patients. Relative weight loss is shown in Table 22.9 (Moustarah et al., 2010; Smith, Schauer, & Nguyen, 2011; Chikunguwo, Brethauer, & Schauer, 2008). Malabsorptive procedures produce greater and more durable weight loss results compared to purely restrictive procedures, although these results come at the expense of higher morbidity and nutritional complications (Eldar et al., 2011a; Moustarah et al., 2010).

On average, at long-term follow-up, purely restrictive procedures are associated with a 45–50% EWL, RYGB with 60–65% EWL, and BPD with 70–75% EWL (i.e., BPD > RYGB > SG = GP > AGB; Brethauer et al., 2006). Weight reduction after AGB is more gradual than that after other procedures, such that maximal weight loss is achieved between 2 and 3 years after AGB versus 1 to 1.5 years after other procedures (Dixon, le Roux, Rubino, & Zimmet, 2012; Eldar et al., 2011a; Smith et al., 2011). Overall, approximately 1 in 10 bariatric patients experiences failure to achieve significant weight loss (defined as % EWL < 25% at 2 years after surgery) or regains lost weight (defined as > 15% weight regain after 2

TABLE 22.9. Weight-Reducing Effects of Commonly Performed Bariatric Procedures

	Restrictive procedures (AGB, SG, GP)	RYGB	BPD, BPD-DS
Mean weight loss (%) at long term	20–30	25–35	30–40
Excess weight loss (%) at long term	45–50	60–65	70–75
Pattern of weight loss	Gradual, maximum 2–3 years	Rapid, maximum at 1–1.5 years	Rapid, maximum at 1–1.5 years
Relative chance of weight regain and need for revision	Moderate	Low	Very low

Note. From Aminian and Schauer (2014). Surgical procedures in the treatment of obesity and its comorbidities. In G. A. Bray & C. Bouchard (Ed.), *Handbook of obesity: Vol. 2. Clinical applications* (4th ed., pp. 365–383). Boca Raton, FL: CRC Press. Reprinted with permission from Taylor & Francis. AGB, adjustable gastric banding; SG, sleeve gastrectomy; GP, gastric plication; RYGB, Roux-en-Y gastric bypass; BPD, biliopancreatic diversion; BPD-DS, with duodenal switch.

years). The etiology of failed bariatric surgery and weight regain is complex and most likely multifactorial. Contributing factors include anatomical failure and poor compliance with postoperative regimens. In these situations, dietary modification and assessment of GI anatomy are imperative. Some types of anatomical failures are amenable to endoscopic corrections. Conversion to RYGB is the most commonly practiced intervention after failed restrictive procedures and has been documented to achieve good salvage rates (Brolin & Cody, 2008; Spyropoulos, Kehagias, Panagiotopoulos, Mead, & Kalfarentzos, 2010; Kellogg, 2011).

Resolution or Improvement of Metabolic Comorbidities

In addition to significant weight loss effects, bariatric–metabolic surgical procedures are associated with other favorable metabolic outcomes, including resolution or improvement of T2D, hypertension, dyslipidemia, metabolic syndrome, and overall survival. These improvements may be the result of weight loss or weight-loss-independent factors (Schauer et al., 2016).

T2D

Obesity is considered a major contributing factor in the pathogenesis of T2D, such that more than 80% of diabetic patients are overweight or obese. Although medical interventions, including lifestyle modifications and pharmacotherapy, are the cornerstone of treatment for obesity and T2D, adequate glycemic control is not achieved in many obese patients with T2D. By contrast, bariatric procedures cause amelioration, and even complete remission, of T2D in a substantial number of severely obese patients. No other intervention that is currently available has been shown to achieve complete remission of this progressive disease (Schauer et al., 2016; Rubino et al., 2016). Observational studies have shown remarkable improvements in glycemic control after surgery, as measured by HbA1C, with remission rates as high as 70% (Panunzi, De Gaetano, Carnicelli, & Mingrone, 2015; Buchwald et al., 2009). Duration of diabetes and severity of diabetes based on insulin use appear to be the key predictors of diabetes improvement and remission after surgery (Schauer et al., 2003). The prospective, nonrandomized Swedish Obese Subjects (SOS) trial has shown a decrease in all-cause mortality, cardiovascular disease mortality, and microvascular complications (retinopathy and nephropathy) in patients with T2D and obesity who had bariatric surgery, compared to nonoperated controls (Sjöström et al., 2012).

A recent review of 11 randomized controlled trials (RCTs; $n = 794$) that compared bariatric–metabolic surgery with medical treatment showed that superior glycemic control was achieved after surgery compared to medical therapy, with no mortality and a perioperative morbidity of 5% (Schauer et al., 2016; Courcoulas et al., 2015; Courcoulas et al., 2014; Cummings et al., 2016; Ding et al., 2015; Dixon et al., 2008; Halperin et al., 2014; Ikramuddin et al., 2015; Ikramuddin et al., 2013; Liang et al., 2013; Mingrone et al., 2015; Mingrone et al., 2012; Parikh et al., 2014; Schauer et al., 2017; Schauer et al., 2014; Wentworth et al., 2014). Surgery resulted in an absolute decrease in HbA1C of 2–3.5% compared to a 1–1.5% decrease after medications only. Most of these studies showed the superiority of surgery in achieving secondary endpoints such as weight loss, remission of metabolic syndrome, reduction in diabetes and cardiovascular medications, and improvement in triglycerides, high-density lipoprotein (HDL), and quality of life. Results were mixed in terms of improvements in blood pressure and low-density lipoprotein (LDL) cholesterol after surgery compared with medical treatment, but many studies did show a corresponding reduction in medication usage. Two long-term (i.e., 5 years) RCTs showed superior and durable weight loss and glycemic control (remission) with RYGB, SG, and BPD compared with medical therapy (Mingrone et al., 2015; Schauer et al., 2017). In the RCTs, the most common predictors of diabetes remission included duration of diabetes, weight loss, requirement for insulin, and disease status (HbA1C). None of these 11 RCTs were powered sufficiently to detect differences in macrovascular or microvascular events, especially at the relatively short follow-up. Longer follow-up or larger studies will be required to determine whether the reductions in mortality and microvascular events demonstrated in the SOS study can be validated (Sjöström et al., 2012).

Strong evidence now supports bariatric–metabolic surgery even for patients with class 1 obesity (BMI of 30–34 kg/m²). In a meta-analysis (N = 94,579) of patients undergoing bariatric–metabolic surgery, the diabetes remission rate was nearly equal for patients with BMI < 35 vs. patients with BMI > 35 kg/m² (72 vs. 71% respectively). Diabetes remission in BPD, RYGB, AGB, and SG was 89%, 77%, 62%, and 60%, respectively (Panunzi et al., 2015). Waist circumference was the only predictor of diabetes remission in this study, suggesting that the arbitrary exclusion of patients with BMI < 35 kg/m² is not scientifically valid. The Surgical Treatment and Medications Potentially Eradicate Diabetes Efficiently (STAMPEDE) RCT study showed similar improvements in HbA1C among patients with a BMI of 27–34 kg/m2 compared to patients with a BMI > 35 kg/m² (Schauer et al., 2017). Furthermore, most of the 11 RCTs comparing bariatric–metabolic surgery to medical treatment for T2D included patients with BMI < 35 kg/m² (Schauer et al., 2016). Collectively, these studies confirmed that patients with class 1 obesity (BMI 30–34 kg/m²) received benefits from bariatric–metabolic surgery comparable to those of patients with severe obesity (BMI ≥ 35 kg/m²), and there appeared to be no increased risk of excessive weight loss or nutritional complications in this lower BMI group.

Based on this level-1 evidence, guidelines from international diabetes organizations, including the American Diabetes Association, recommend bariatric–metabolic surgery as an important treatment for patients with T2D and obesity (Rubino et al., 2016; Marathe, Gao, & Close, 2017). Specifically, surgery is recommended for patients with T2D and BMI ≥ 40 kg/m² regardless of glycemic control on medications. For patients with a BMI of 35–39 kg/m² and T2D, surgery is recommended for those who are not in adequate glycemic control with medications. Surgery should be considered for patients with a BMI of 30–34 kg/m² and T2D if they are not in adequate glycemic control with medications. This BMI threshold is lowered to 27.5 kg/m² for patients of certain ethnic origins such as Asia (India, China) who are particularly prone to complications of T2D.

Hyperlipidemia

Many studies have shown consistent improvement of dyslipidemia following bariatric–metabolic surgery. The 1990 report of the Program on the Surgical Control of the Hyperlipidemias (POSCH) described reductions in the levels of total cholesterol (23%) and LDL cholesterol (38%), in association with an increase in HDL cholesterol (4%), after a surgical distal ileal malabsorptive procedure (Buchwald et al., 1990). In two meta-analyses, hyperlipidemia improved in 79% and 65% of patients, respectively (Buchwald et al., 2004; Vest, Heneghan, Agarwal, Schauer, & Young, 2012). However, relapse of dyslipidemia by as much as 25% over 10 years may occur, as reported in the SOS study (Vest et al., 2012). In terms of the effects of various bariatric procedures on lipoproteins, RCTs reported an average of 20–30 mg/dL greater reduction in LDL levels after BPD and BPD-DS, as compared with RYGB. However, RYGB was the most effective in raising HDL levels (Schauer et al., 2014; Mingrone et al., 2015).

Hypertension

Bariatric–metabolic surgery has been shown to improve systolic and diastolic blood pressure. In a study by Adams et al. (2012), remission rates of hypertension at year 6 remained significantly improved in the RYGB group compared with nonsurgical, severely obese control groups (42% vs. 18% and 9%). Two meta-analyses showed 62% improvement or resolution of hypertension (Buchwald et al., 2004; Vest et al., 2012). The SOS trial showed that RYGB was associated with a sustained blood pressure reduction at a median follow-up of 10 years (Hallersund et al., 2012). As stated previously, more recent RCTs in patients with T2D have been inconsistent in showing relative improvements in blood pressure after surgery compared to medical treatment, but surgery consistently reduces antihypertensive medication requirements.

Cardiovascular Disease

Beneficial effects of bariatric–metabolic surgery on T2D, dyslipidemia, and hypertension translate into a lower risk of coronary artery disease in the surgical group (Heneghan et al., 2012; Brethauer, Heneghan, et al., 2011). One meta-analysis has shown a 10-year coronary heart disease Framingham Risk Score reduction from 5.9 to 3.3% following bariatric surgery (Vest et al., 2012). Multiple retrospective cohort studies have suggested that bariatric surgery is associated with reduced incidence of cardiovascular events (MacDonald et al., 1997; Christou et al., 2004; Adams et al., 2007; Arterburn et al., 2015). The SOS study showed that for both diabetic and nondiabetic patients, bariatric–metabolic surgery was associated with a reduced number of cardiovascular deaths (1.3 vs. 2.4%; adjusted hazard ratio = 0.47). The number of total first-time (fatal or nonfatal) cardiovascular events (myocardial infarction or stroke) was also lower in the surgical group (9.9%) than in the control group (11.5%, adjusted hazard ratio = 0.67; Sjöström et al., 2012).

The hemodynamic, neurohumoral, and metabolic abnormalities characteristic of obesity are associated with alterations in the structure of the myocardium and the arterial wall (i.e. remodeling), which may lead to ventricular dysfunction and susceptibility to heart failure. Restoration of insulin sensitivity and blood pressure to normal range after bariatric–metabolic surgery has been related to favorable changes in cardiac metabolism, structure, and function (Algahim, Sen, & Taegtmeyer, 2012; Poirier et al., 2011). Clinically significant improvements in left ventricular function in severely obese adults (Garza et al., 2010; Valezi & Machado, 2011) and in obese patients with severe cardiomyopathy (McCloskey et al., 2007; Ristow, Rabkin, & Haeusslein, 2008; Vest et al., 2016) after bariatric surgery have been reported. One meta-analysis demonstrated regression of left ventricular hypertrophy and improved diastolic function following weight loss surgery (Vest et al., 2012).

Nonalcoholic Fatty Liver Disease

Nonalcoholic fatty liver disease (NAFLD) is associated with metabolic risk factors such as obesity, T2D, and dyslipidemia. The spectrum of NAFLD histologically ranges from hepatic steatosis to the more severe nonalcoholic steatohepatitis (NASH) and fibrosis that can progress to cirrhosis, end-stage liver disease, and hepatocellular carcinoma. Twenty percent of patients with NASH will progress to cirrhosis, and no medical treatment, thus far, has been shown to reduce progression. The prevalence of NAFLD and NASH in patients with severe obesity is estimated to be as high as 90% and 33%, respectively (Chalasani et al., 2012; Mummadi, Kasturie, Chennareddygari, & Sood, 2008). Due to the high incidence of this disease, some experts have advocated routine liver biopsy at the time of bariatric–metabolic surgery (Schirmer & Schauer, 2010).

One study that prospectively correlated clinical data with liver histology before and after bariatric surgery in 381 adult patients showed a significant improvement in the prevalence and severity of steatosis and NASH at 1 and 5 years following bariatric surgery (Mathurin et al., 2009). Most histological benefits were evident at 1 year, with no differences in liver histology between 1 and 5 years after surgery. A meta-analysis of 15 available studies (766 paired liver biopsies) reported improvement or remission after bariatric surgery in steatosis (92%), NASH (81.3%), and fibrosis (65.5%). Taken together, bariatric surgery resulted in an improvement of histopathologic features of NAFLD in more than three-fourths of patients (Mummadi et al., 2008). Recognizing that treatment of NASH with lifestyle intervention or medical therapy thus far has been very limited in effect, bariatric surgery appears to be the only treatment to improve or reverse NASH. However, due to the lack of RCTs, bariatric surgery has not been widely endorsed as a treatment for NASH (Chalasani et al., 2012).

Resolution or Improvement of Obesity-Related Comorbidities

Bariatric–metabolic surgery is able to resolve or at least improve many, if not all, of the comorbidities associated with obesity (Figure 22.3).

OSA

Obesity is a major risk factor for OSA, and weight loss is recommended as part of the overall management of it in obese patients. The presence of OSA is associated with significant morbidity and mortality. In the meta-analysis by Buchwald et al. (2004), over 80% of patients experienced improvement in OSA after bariatric surgery. An RCT comparing conventional weight loss therapy versus AGB for OSA showed significant improvement in symptoms and polysomnographic indices after both interventions (Dixon, Schachter, et al., 2012). Another RCT showed that patients with severe obesity who underwent bariatric–metabolic surgery had significant reductions in neck and waist circumference and increases in maximum ventilatory pressures at 3 months postsurgery as compared to the control group. These improvements enhance sleep architecture and reduce OSA (Aguiar et al., 2014). The effect of weight loss on OSA indicated in various studies suggests that weight loss should be a key arm of OSA treatment (Greenburg, Lettieri, & Eliasson, 2009; Dixon, Schachter, et al., 2012).

GERD

Since the prevalence of GERD is markedly higher in obese populations as compared to those with normal BMI, GERD is now recognized as one of the obesity-related comorbidities. The outcomes of anti-reflux surgery (e.g., fundoplication) in severely obese patients are not as good as the outcomes in patients who are not obese. Gastric bypass is approximately 90% effective in eliminating GERD, which is thought to be related to the relatively low acid production by the small-volume gastric pouch, reduction of esophageal bile reflux by use of a roux limb, and weight loss (Madalosso et al., 2016; El-Hadi, Birch, Gill, & Karmali, 2014). Higher rate of GERD resolution after RYGB as compared with BPD-DS, despite the greater weight loss produced by the latter procedure, indicates the importance of the small gastric pouch. Patients generally show no improvement or worsening in GERD following AGB, SG, and GP, so these procedures are not recommended in patients with severe GERD (El-Hadi et al., 2014). Therefore, when surgical treatment of GERD is indicated in a severely obese patient, RYGB (rather than a fundoplication) should be strongly considered (Prachand & Alverdy, 2010; Schauer, Hamad, & Ikramuddin, 2001).

Other Comorbidities

Salutary effects have been reported of bariatric surgery on a long list of comorbid conditions, including asthma, stress urinary incontinence, polycystic ovarian syndrome, infertility, musculoskeletal problems (especially degenerative joint disease and low-back pain), varicose veins, lymphedema, migraine headaches, pseudotumor cerebri, and depression (Schirmer & Schauer, 2010; Brethauer et al., 2006). The overall out-

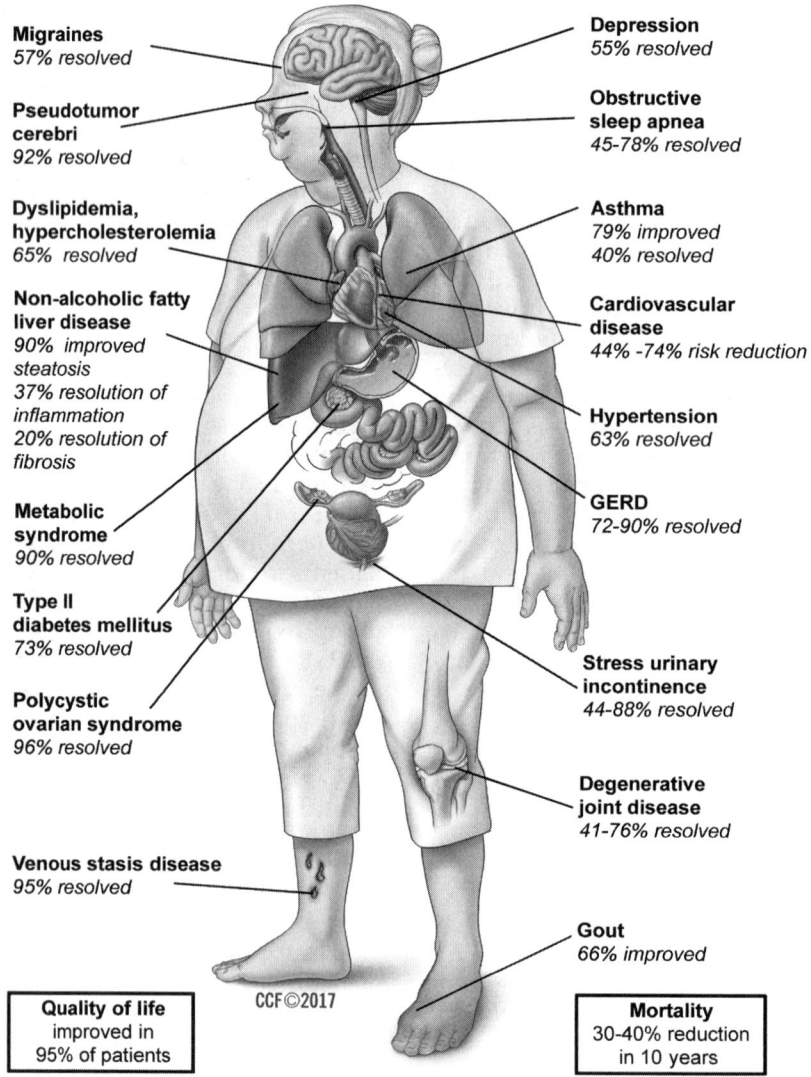

FIGURE 22.3. Impact of bariatric surgery on obesity-related comorbidities. Reprinted with permission, Cleveland Clinic Center for Medical Art & Photography. Copyright © 2005–2017. All rights reserved.

comes of bariatric-metabolic surgery are summarized in Figure 22.3.

From Treatment to Prevention of Comorbidities

In addition to effects in reversing or improving comorbidities, bariatric surgery can be reasonably presumed to prevent the development of the conditions explained earlier. Specifically, the protective effects of bariatric surgery on T2D, cancer, and mortality have been well studied and are discussed in the following sections.

T2D

Bariatric–metabolic surgery is not only an effective therapeutic intervention for T2D, but it also prevents the development of diabetes in the severely obese. A report from the

SOS study compared the incidence of T2D in 1,658 patients who underwent bariatric surgery and in 1,771 obese matched controls, none of whom had T2D at baseline. During the follow-up period of 15 years, bariatric surgery, as compared with standard medical care, reduced the incidence of T2D by 78%; diabetes did not develop in approximately 10 of 13 obese patients who underwent bariatric surgery (Carlsson et al., 2012). Similarly, in the study by Adams et al. (2012), T2D incidence during a 6-year period was significantly lower in the RYGB surgery group than in the two nonsurgical severely obese control groups (2% vs. 17% and 15%). In addition, the incidence of hypertension and dyslipidemia was also lower in the surgical group. Although lifestyle modification and/or pharmacotherapy have also been shown to prevent T2D, bariatric surgery generally appears to result in a greater reduction in T2D incidence, especially in severely obese patients (Knowler et al., 2005; Sjöström, 2013).

Cancer

Obesity is an established risk factor for the development of a long list of cancers, including, but not limited to, endometrial cancer, postmenopausal female breast cancer, colorectal cancer, renal cell carcinoma, and esophageal adenocarcinoma. Metabolic and endocrine changes are involved in the increased cancer risk with obesity. Chronic inflammation and associated oxidative stress, increased sex-steroid hormones (estrogens and testosterone), and hyperinsulinemia have been implicated in cancer development (Ashrafian et al., 2011).

Bariatric surgical patients have lower rates of cancer incidence and mortality than obese patients who have not undergone surgery (Ashrafian et al., 2011). Christou and colleagues reported an 82% decrease in breast cancer incidence and a 76% decrease in cancer incidence overall at a maximum follow-up of 5 years (Christou, Lieberman, Sampalis, & Sampalis, 2008). During a mean follow-up of 7.1 years after RYGB, Adams and colleagues showed that, whereas all-cause mortality was reduced by 40% in the surgical group compared with severely obese controls, the reduction in cancer-related deaths was 60% for the surgical group compared with the control group (Adams et al., 2007; Adams & Hunt, 2009). In their next report, when the follow-up was increased to a mean of 12.5 years, the cancer mortality was 46% lower in the RYGB group, and was accompanied by a 24% decrease in overall cancer incidence. Of the specific cancers, the incidence of uterine cancer was significantly lower among surgical patients than severely obese control subjects (Adams et al., 2009). These findings are in line with the results of the SOS trial, which reported a 30% reduction in cancer incidence after bariatric surgery, mostly for women (Sjöström et al., 2009). Studies have shown that the cancer-protective role of bariatric surgery is strongest for female obesity-related tumors (i.e., breast and endometrial cancer; Ashrafian et al., 2011).

Long-Term Mortality

Observational studies evaluating long-term mortality after bariatric surgery consistently show a survival benefit for surgery patients when compared with nonsurgical obese controls. Patients treated by bariatric surgery, as compared with nonoperated cohorts, have experienced significantly greater reductions in long-term mortality, although the magnitude of the reduction has varied among studies (Ashrafian et al., 2011). In their cohort study, Christou et al. (2004) found that the 5-year mortality rate in the bariatric surgical group was 0.68% compared with 6.17% in the medically managed patients, which translates to an 89% relative risk reduction. Flum and Dellinger (2004) evaluated survival after RYGB in a retrospective cohort study and found a 27.6% lower mortality rate in severely obese patients who underwent RYGB, as compared with those who did not. After the surgical patients reached the first postoperative year, the long-term survival advantage increased to 33%. Adams et al. (2009) reported that during a mean follow-up of 7.1 years, adjusted long-term mortality from any cause in the RYGB group decreased by 40%, as compared with that in the control group. Cause-specific mortality in the RYGB group decreased by 56% for coronary artery disease, by 92% for T2D, and by 60% for cancer. The SOS study also showed a 30% decrease in mortality rates after 10 years of follow-up, with cancer and myocardial infarction being the leading causes of death (Sjöström et al., 2007). A meta-analysis involving 44,022 participants from eight clinical trials with a mean follow-up of 7.5 years indicated that, compared with controls, bariatric surgery was associated with a reduced risk of all-cause mortality (odds ratio = 0.55) and cardiovascular mortality (odds ratio = 0.58; Pontiroli & Morabito, 2011). More recently, in a study involving older, mostly male veterans, Arterburn et al. (2015) demonstrated a 42% reduction in mortality after bariatric surgery compared to matched controls. At present, there have been no prospective RCTs with sufficient sample size or follow-up duration to determine a mortality benefit of bariatric surgery.

Comparison of Standard Bariatric Procedures

The GI configuration in each bariatric procedure results in unique risks, merits, and limitations (Eldar et al., 2011a). The general consensus, based on the results of comparative studies and meta-analyses, suggests the presence of an efficacy gradient among standard bariatric operations for the resolution of excess weight and cardiovascular risk factors (i.e., BPD > RYGB > SG > AGB). More extensive diversionary procedures are generally associated with greater weight loss (Table 22.9) and more profound metabolic benefits in the long term, but at the cost of more surgical complications, especially ones related to nutritional deficiencies.

Choice of Bariatric–Metabolic Surgical Procedures

The choice of bariatric surgery requires assessment of risk versus benefit for each procedure and must be individualized for each surgical candidate. Factors to be considered when choosing a weight loss surgical procedure include the following:

- Expertise and experience of the surgical team.
- Patient's preference after being fully informed about the risks and benefits of each procedure.
- Patient's BMI.
- Presence of metabolic comorbidities, especially pre-diabetes and T2D.
- Patient's risk factors associated with high perioperative morbidity and mortality.
- Follow-up regimen for the procedure and the patient's commitment to adhere to it.

AGB

With no resection and anastomosis, the relative operative risk of AGB is lower than that of most other bariatric operations. However, long-term results indicate a relatively high revision rate for complications or poor weight loss. For this reason, the popularity of AGB has decreased dramatically over the past 5 years across the globe, such that relatively few (5–8%) new patients receive this procedure. Patients who are extremely motivated and will participate in frequent assessments for band adjustments are most suitable for this procedure. In general, this procedure should be avoided in patients with high BMI (> 50 kg/m^2), severe GERD, or advanced T2D.

SG

SG is the most common bariatric procedure worldwide. Appropriate indications for SG include the first component of a two-stage approach for high-risk super obese patients (i.e., BMI > 50 kg/m^2) who are considering BPD-DS or RYGB as an eventual completion operation. SG also is indicated as a stand-alone procedure in the following conditions (Brethauer, Hammel, & Schauer, 2009; Rosenthal et al., 2012):

- Patient's preference to have a relatively simple restrictive operation without use of a foreign body.
- In patients considered high risk.
- In the presence of gastric lesions that require monitoring (e.g., adenomatous polyps).
- In endemic area for gastric cancer.
- In patients with inflammatory bowel disease, for whom the integrity of an intestinal anastomosis is a concern.
- In liver and kidney transplant candidates.
- In the presence of liver cirrhosis.

GP

Along with other restrictive procedures, GP can be an appropriate option in high-risk surgical patients. The cost of surgery is lower than that of other bariatric procedures, which makes it an affordable choice for patients in places with limited resources. Patients may choose it as a simple and potentially reversible procedure without any opening of the GI tract (i.e., reduced risk of leakage) or use of a foreign body (Brethauer, Harris, et al., 2011; Talebpour et al., 2012; Abdelbaki et al., 2012). However, long-term follow-up data for GP are limited.

RYGB

As a procedure that has been consistently used for decades, RYGB is an appropriate consideration for most patients who are eligible for bariatric surgery. RYGB carries more perioperative risk than AGB, SG, and GP, but it is more effective in controlling weight and comorbidities. RYGB is the preferred option in patients with severe GERD. In appropriate risk patients with pre-diabetes or established T2D, RYGB is probably the best overall option (in our opinion). Relative contraindications to RYGB include severe iron deficiency anemia, extensive prior abdominal surgery, severe dysplasia of distal esophagus (which may require resectioning of the esophagus and reconstruction with the stomach in the future), and distal gastric or duodenal lesions that require future endoscopic surveillance (Schauer & 2004; ABS Consensus Conference, 2005; Schirmer & Schauer, 2010; Smith et al., 2011).

BPD and BPD-DS

BPD and BPD-DS appear to be the most effective weight loss and antidiabetic procedures but carry a higher operative risk and lifelong risk of malnutrition. Therefore, they are reasonable options for super obese patients (BMI > 50 kg/m^2) with low to moderate surgical risk who are expected to be highly compliant with follow-up regimen and monitoring. Contraindications to the procedure include high-risk patients; presence of obstacles for follow-up (e.g., geographic distance from the surgeon, lack of financial means to afford lifelong supplements); and preexisting calcium, iron, or other vitamin deficiencies (Schirmer & Schauer, 2010; Smith et al., 2011).

Body Contouring Following Massive Weight Loss

Body contouring after bariatric surgery is not a luxury; rather, it is often necessary to achieve not only reasonable cosmetic results but also appropriate health care. Large skin folds can lead to back strain, maceration under folds, fungal intertriginous dermatitis, and body image dissatisfaction. Excess skin folds can also be a limiting factor in exercise and sexual activity. Plastic surgery procedures following massive weight loss range from simple panniculectomies to upper-, lower-, and total-body lifts. Total-body lift may include a circumferential abdominoplasty, lower-body lift, medial thighplasty, upper-body lift, and breast reshaping. The procedure can involve up to 10 hours in the operating room (Shermak, 2012; Buckley, 2007).

Conclusions

The growing epidemic of obesity, along with unsatisfactory results of conventional weight reduction programs, has led to a remarkable rise in the number of bariatric surgeries performed in the last decade; yet, fewer than 2% of eligible patients choose to undergo surgery. In addition to achieving significant and durable weight loss, bariatric surgery is associated with favorable metabolic effects and a survival benefit far beyond those obtained by behavioral and pharmacological therapies. Outcomes of bariatric–metabolic surgery have steadily improved over the last half-century, especially after the advent of minimally invasive laparoscopic techniques. Early perioperative morbidity (4–5%) and mortality (0.3%) are relatively low following bariatric surgery, as compared to other abdominal procedures such as cholecystectomy. Surgical interventions with a very good risk–benefit ratio are available now, and surgical and nonsurgical innovations will, most certainly, revolutionize management of severe obesity in the near future. Whatever the next decade holds for the treatment of severe obesity is uncertain. However, scientific evidence indicates that bariatric–metabolic surgery, thus far, is the only weight loss therapy that consistently results in clinically significant long-term weight loss for severely obese patients. Moreover, bariatric–metabolic surgery for T2D has shown significant improvement in glycemic control as compared to medical therapy alone. Patients with class 1 obesity (BMI of 30–34 kg/m^2) may also benefit from bariatric–metabolic surgery, especially if their T2D is poorly controlled with optimal medical therapy. Bariatric–metabolic surgery will likely play a more prominent role in the management of obesity and diabetes in the near future.

References

Abdelbaki, T. N., Huang, C. K., Ramos, A., Neto, M. G., Talebpour, M., & Saber, A. A. (2012). Gastric plication for morbid obesity: A systematic review. *Obesity Surgery, 22*(10), 1633–1639.

Adams, T. D., Davidson, L. E., Litwin, S. E., Kolotkin, R. L., LaMonte, M. J., Pendleton, R. C., et al. (2012). Health benefits of gastric bypass surgery after 6 years. *Journal of the American Medical Association, 308*(11), 1122–1131.

Adams, T. D., Gress, R. E., Smith, S. C., Halverson, R. C., Simper, S. C., Rosamond, W. D., et al. (2007). Long-term mortality following gastric bypass surgery. *New England Journal of Medicine, 357*(8), 753–761.

Adams, T. D., & Hunt, S. C. (2009). Cancer and obesity: Effect of bariatric surgery. *World Journal of Surgery, 33*(10), 2028–2033.

Adams, T. D., Stroup, A. M., Gress, R. E., Adams, K. F., Calle, E. E., Smith, S. C., et al. (2009). Cancer incidence and mortality after gastric bypass surgery. *Obesity (Silver Spring), 17*(4), 796–802.

Aguiar, I. C., Freitas, W. R., Santos, I. R., Apostolico, N., Nacif, S. R., Urbano, J. J., et al. (2014). Obstructive sleep apnea and pulmonary function in patients with severe obesity before and after bariatric surgery: A randomized clinical trial. *Multidisciplinary Respiratory Medicine, 9*(1), 43.

Al Harakeh, A. B. (2011). Complications of laparoscopic Roux-en-Y gastric bypass. *Surgical Clinics of North America, 91*(6), 1225–1237.

Algahim, M. F., Sen, S., & Taegtmeyer, H. (2012). Bariatric surgery to unload the stressed heart: A metabolic hypothesis. *American Journal of Physiology: Heart and Circulatory Physiology, 302*(8), H1539–H1545.

Aminian, A., Brethauer, S. A., Kirwan J. P., Kashyap, S. R., Burguera, B., & Schauer, P. R. (2015). How safe is metabolic/diabetes surgery? *Diabetes, Obesity and Metabolism, 17*(2), 198–201.

Aminian, A., & Schauer, P. R. (2014). Surgical procedures in the treatment of obesity and its comorbidities. In G. A. Bray & C. Bouchard (Ed.), *Handbook of obesity: Vol. 2. Clinical applications* (4th ed., pp. 365–383). Boca Raton, FL: CRC Press.

Angrisani, L., Santonicola, A., Iovino, P., Formisano, G., Buchwald, H., & Scopinaro, N. (2015). Bariatric surgery worldwide 2013. *Obesity Surgery, 25*(10), 1822–1832.

Arterburn, D. E., Olsen, M. K., Smith, V. A., Livingston, E. H., Van Scoyoc, L., Yancy, W. S., et al. (2015). Association between bariatric surgery and long-term survival. *Journal of the American Medical Association, 313*(1), 62–70.

Ashrafian, H., Ahmed, K., Rowland, S. P., Patel, V. M., Gooderham, N. J., Holmes, E., et al. (2011). Metabolic surgery and cancer: Protective effects of bariatric procedures. *Cancer, 117*(9), 1788–1799.

Bal, B., Koch, T. R., Finelli, F. C., & Sarr, M. G. (2010). Managing medical and surgical disorders after divided Roux-en-Y gastric bypass surgery. *Gastroenterology and Hepatology, 7*(6), 320–334.

Batterham, R. L., & Cummings, D. E. (2016). Mechanisms of diabetes improvement following bariatric/metabolic surgery. *Diabetes Care, 39*(6), 893–901.

Brethauer, S. A., Chand, B., & Schauer, P. R. (2006). Risks and benefits of bariatric surgery: Current evidence. *Cleveland Clinical Journal of Medicine, 73*(11), 993–1007.

Brethauer, S. A., Hammel, J. P., & Schauer, P. R. (2009). Systematic review of sleeve gastrectomy as staging and primary bariatric procedure. *Surgery for Obesity and Related Diseases, 5*(4), 469–475.

Brethauer, S. A., Harris, J. L., Kroh, M., & Schauer, P. R. (2011). Laparoscopic gastric plication for treatment of severe obesity. *Surgery for Obesity and Related Disorders, 7*(1), 15–22.

Brethauer, S. A., Heneghan, H. M., Eldar, S., Gatmaitan, P., Huang, H., Kashyap, S., et al. (2011). Early effects of gastric bypass on endothelial function, inflammation, and cardiovascular risk in obese patients. *Surgical Endoscopy, 25*(8), 2650–2659.

Brolin, R. E., & Cody, R. P. (2008). Weight loss outcome of revisional bariatric operations varies according to the primary procedure. *Annals of Surgery, 248*(2), 227–232.

Buchwald, H., Avidor, Y., Braunwald, E., Jensen, M. D., Pories, W., Fahrbach, K., et al. (2004). Bariatric surgery: A systematic review and meta-analysis. *Journal of the American Medical Association, 292*(14), 1724–1737.

Buchwald, H., & Consensus Conference Panel. (2005). Bariatric surgery for morbid obesity: Health implications for patients, health professionals, and third-party payers. *Journal of the American College of Surgery, 200*(4), 593–604.

Buchwald, H., Estok, R., Fahrbach, K., Banel, D., Jensen, M. D., Pories, W. J., et al. (2009). Weight and type 2 diabetes after bariatric surgery: Systematic review and meta-analysis. *American Journal of Medicine, 122*(3), 248–256.

Buchwald, H., Varco, R. L., Matts, J. P., Long, J. M., Fitch, L. L., Campbell, G. S., et al. (1990). Effect of partial ileal bypass surgery on mortality and morbidity from coronary heart disease in patients with hypercholesterolemia: Report of the Program on the Surgical Control of the Hyperlipidemias (POSCH). *New England Journal of Medicine, 323*(14), 946–955.

Buckley, M. C. (2007). Body contouring after massive weight loss. In H. Buchwald, W. Pories, & G. M. Cowan (Eds.), *Surgical management of obesity* (pp. 325–333). Philadelphia: Elsevier.

Carlsson, L. M., Peltonen, M., Ahlin, S., Anveden, A., Bouchard, C., Carlsson, B., et al. (2012). Bariatric surgery and prevention of type 2 diabetes in Swedish obese subjects. *New England Journal of Medicine, 367*(8), 695–704.

Chalasani, N., Younossi, Z., Lavine, J. E., Diehl, A. M., Brunt, E. M., Cusi, K., et al. (2012). The diagnosis and management of non-alcoholic fatty liver disease: Practice guideline by the American Gastroenterological Association, American Association for the Study of Liver Diseases, and American College of Gastroenterology. *Gastroenterology, 142*(7), 1592–1609.

Chikunguwo, S., Brethauer, S. A., & Schauer, P. R. (2008). Bariatric surgery. In K. I. Bland, M. G. Sarr, & M. W. Buchler (Eds.), *General surgery: Principles and international practice* (2nd ed., pp. 557–566). London: Springer.

Christou, N. V., Lieberman, M., Sampalis, F., & Sampalis, J. S. (2008). Bariatric surgery reduces cancer risk in morbidly obese patients. *Surgery for Obesity and Related Disorders, 4*(6), 691–695.

Christou, N. V., Sampalis, J. S., Liberman, M., Look, D., Auger, S., McLean, A. P. H., et al. (2004). Surgery decreases long-term mortality, morbidity, and health care use in morbidly obese patients. *Annals of Surgery, 240*(3), 416–424.

Courcoulas, A. P., Belle, S. H., Neiberg, R. H., Pierson, S. K., Eagleton, J. K., Kalarchian, M. A., et al. (2015). Three-year outcomes of bariatric surgery vs. lifestyle intervention for type 2 diabetes mellitus treatment: A randomized clinical trial. *JAMA Surgery, 150*(10), 931–940.

Courcoulas, A. P., Goodpaster, B. H., Eagleton, J. K., Belle, S. H., Kalarchian, M. A., Lang, W., et al. (2014). Surgical vs. medical treatments for type 2 diabetes mellitus: A randomized clinical trial. *JAMA Surgery, 149*(7), 707–715.

Cummings, D. E., Arterburn, D. E., Westbrook, E. O., Kuzma, J. N., Stewart, S. D., Chan, C. P., et al. (2016). Gastric bypass surgery vs. intensive lifestyle and medical intervention for type 2 diabetes: The CROSSROADS randomised controlled trial. *Diabetologia, 59*(5), 945–953.

Deitel, M., & Greenstein, R. J. (2003). Recommendations for reporting weight loss. *Obesity Surgery, 13*(2), 159–160.

Ding, S. A., Simonson, D. C., Wewalka, M., Halperin, F., Foster, K., Goebel-Fabbri, A., et al. (2015). Adjustable gastric band surgery or medical management in patients with type 2 diabetes: A randomized clinical trial. *Journal of Clinical Endocrinology and Metabolism, 100*(7), 2546–2556.

Dixon, J. B., le Roux, C. W., Rubino, F., & Zimmet, P. (2012). Bariatric surgery for type 2 diabetes. *Lancet, 379*(9833), 2300–2311.

Dixon, J. B., O'Brien, P. E., Playfair, J., Chapman, L., Schachter, L. M., Skinner, S., et al. (2008). Adjustable gastric banding and conventional therapy for type 2 diabetes: A randomized controlled trial. *Journal of the American Medical Association, 299*(3), 316–323.

Dixon, J. B., Schachter, L. M., O'Brien, P. E., Jones, K., Grima, M., Lambert, G., et al. (2012). Surgical vs. conventional therapy for weight loss treatment of obstructive sleep apnea: A randomized controlled trial. *Journal of the American Medical Association, 308*(11), 1142–1149.

Eldar, S., Heneghan, H. M., Brethauer, S. A., & Schauer, P. R. (2011a). Bariatric surgery for treatment of obesity. *International Journal of Obesity, 35*(Suppl. 3), S16–S21.

Eldar, S., Heneghan, H. M., Brethauer, S., & Schauer, P. R. (2011b). A focus on surgical preoperative evaluation of the bariatric patient: The Cleveland Clinic protocol and review of the literature. *Surgeon, 9*(5), 273–277.

El-Hadi, M., Birch, D. W., Gill, R. S., & Karmali, S. (2014). The effect of bariatric surgery on gastroesophageal reflux disease. *Canadian Journal of Surgery, 57*(2), 139–144.

Flum, D. R., Belle, S. H., King, W. C., Wahed, A. S., Berk, P., Chapman, W., et al. (2009). Perioperative safety in the longitudinal assessment of bariatric surgery. *New England Journal of Medicine, 361*(5), 445–454.

Flum, D. R., & Dellinger, E. P. (2004). Impact of gastric bypass operation on survival: A population-based analysis. *Journal of the American College of Surgeons, 199*(4), 543–551.

Garza, C. A., Pellikka, P. A., Somers, V. K., Sarr, M. G., Collazo-Clavell, M. L., Korenfeld, Y., et al. (2010). Structural and functional changes in left and right ventricles after major weight loss following bariatric surgery for morbid obesity. *American Journal of Cardiology, 105*(4), 550–556.

Gill, R. S., Karmali, S., & Sharma, A. M. (2011). The potential role of the Edmonton obesity staging system in determining indications for bariatric surgery. *Obesity Surgery, 21*(12), 1947–1949.

Greenburg, D. L., Lettieri, C. J., & Eliasson, A. H. (2009). Effects of surgical weight loss on measures of obstructive sleep apnea: A meta-analysis. *American Journal of Medicine 122*(6), 535–542.

Hallersund, P., Sjöström, L., Olbers, T., Lönroth, H., Jacobson, P., Wallenius, V., et al. (2012). Gastric bypass surgery is followed by lowered blood pressure and increased diuresis: Long-term results from the Swedish Obese Subjects (SOS) study. *PLOS ONE, 7*(11), e49696.

Halperin, F., Ding, S. A., Simonson, D. C., Panosian, J., Goebel-Fabbri, A., Wewalka, M., et al. (2014). Roux-en-Y gastric bypass surgery or lifestyle with intensive medical management in patients with type 2 diabetes: Feasibility and 1-year results of a randomized clinical trial. *JAMA Surgery, 149*(7), 716–726.

Hanipah, Z. N., & Schauer, P. R. (2017). Surgical treatment of obesity and diabetes. *Gastrointestinal Endoscopy Clinics of North America, 27*(2), 191–211.

Heneghan, H. M., Meron-Eldar, S., Brethauer, S. A., Schauer, P. R., & Young, J. B. (2011). Effect of bariatric surgery on cardiovascular risk profile. *American Journal of Cardiology, 108*(10), 1499–1507.

Heneghan, H. M., Meron-Eldar, S., Yenumula, P., Rogula, T., Brethauer, S. A., & Schauer, P. R. (2012). Incidence and management of bleeding complications after gastric bypass surgery in the morbidly obese. *Surgery for Obesity and Related Diseases, 8*(6), 729–735.

Heymsfield, S. B., & Wadden, T. A. (2017). Mechanisms, pathophysiology, and management of obesity. *New England Journal of Medicine, 376*(3), 254–266.

Hocking, M. P., Duerson, M. C., O'Leary, J. P., & Woodward, E. R. (1983). Jejunoileal bypass for morbid obesity: Late follow-up in 100 cases. *New England Journal of Medicine, 308*(17), 995–999.

Hwang, R. F., Swartz, D. E., & Felix, E. L. (2004). Causes of small bowel obstruction after laparoscopic gastric bypass. *Surgical Endoscopy, 18*(11), 1631–1635.

Ikramuddin, S., Billington, C. J., Lee, W. J., Bantle, J. P., Thomas, A. J., Connett, J. E., et al. (2015). Roux-en-Y gastric bypass for diabetes (the Diabetes Surgery Study): 2-year outcomes of a 5-year, randomised, controlled trial. *Lancet Diabetes and Endocrinology, 3*(6), 413–422.

Ikramuddin, S., Korner, J., Lee, W. J., Connett, J. E., Inabnet, W. B., Billington, C. J., et al. (2013). Roux-en-Y gastric bypass vs. intensive medical management for the control of type 2 diabetes, hypertension, and hyperlipidemia: The Diabetes Surgery Study randomized clinical trial. *Journal of the American Medical Association, 309*(21), 2240–2249.

Jensen, M. D., Ryan, D. H., Apovian, C. M., Ard, J. D., Comuzzie, A. G., Donato, K. A., et al. (2014). 2013 AHA/ACC/TOS guideline for the management of overweight and obesity in adults: A report of the American College of Cardiology/American Heart Association Task Force on Practice Guidelines and the Obesity Society. *Circulation, 129*(25, Suppl. 2), S102–S138.

Kellogg, T. A. (2011). Revisional bariatric surgery. *Surgical Clinics of North America, 91*(6), 1353–1371.

Knowler, W. C., Hamman, R. F., Edelstein, S. L., Barrett-Connor, E., Ehrmann, D. A., Walker, E. A., et al. (2005). Prevention of type 2 diabetes with troglitazone in the diabetes prevention program. *Diabetes, 54*(4), 1150–1156.

Liang, Z., Wu, Q., Chen, B., Yu, P., Zhao, H., & Ouyang, X. (2013). Effect of laparoscopic Roux-en-Y gastric bypass surgery on type 2 diabetes mellitus with hypertension: A randomized controlled trial. *Diabetes Research and Clinical Practice, 101*(1), 50–56.

Longitudinal Assessment of Bariatric Surgery (LABS) Consortium (2009). Perioperative safety in the longitudinal assessment of bariatric surgery. *New England Journal of Medicine, 361*(5), 445–454.

MacDonald, K. G., Long, S. D., Swanson, M. S., Brown, B. M., Morris, P., Dohm, G. L., et al. (1997). The gastric bypass operation reduces the progression and mortality of non-insulin-dependent diabetes mellitus. *Journal of Gastrointestinal Surgery, 1*(3), 213–220.

Madalosso, C. A., Gurski, R. R., Callegari-Jacques, S. M., Navarini, D., Mazzini, G., Pereira Mda, S., et al. (2016). The impact of gastric bypass on gastroesophageal reflux disease in morbidly obese patients. *Annals of Surgery, 263*(1), 110–116.

Marathe, P. H., Gao, H. X., & Close, K. L. (2017). American Diabetes Association standards of medical care in diabetes 2017. *Journal of Diabetes* [Epub ahead of print].

Mathurin, P., Hollebecque, A., Arnalsteen, L., Buob, D., Leteurtre, E., Caiazzo, R., et al. (2009). Prospective study of the long-term effects of bariatric surgery on liver injury in patients without advanced disease. *Gastroenterology, 137*(2), 532–540.

McCloskey, C. A., Ramani, G. V., Mathier, M. A., Schauer, P. R., Eid, G. M., Mattar, S. G., et al. (2007). Bariatric surgery improves cardiac function in morbidly obese patients with severe cardiomyopathy. *Surgery for Obesity and Related Disorders, 3*(5), 503–507.

Mechanick, J. I., Youdim, A., Jones, D. B., Garvey, W. T., Hurley, D. L., McMahon, M., et al. (2013). Clinical practice guidelines for the perioperative nutritional, metabolic, and nonsurgical support of the bariatric surgery patient—2013 update: Cosponsored by American Association of Clinical Endocrinologists, The Obesity Society, and American Society for Metabolic and Bariatric Surgery. *Obesity, 21*(Suppl. 1), S1–S27.

Mingrone, G., Panunzi, S., De Gaetano, A., Guidone, C., Iaconelli, A., Leccesi, L., et al. (2012). Bariatric surgery versus conventional medical therapy for type 2 diabetes. *New England Journal of Medicine, 366*(17), 1577–1585.

Mingrone, G., Panunzi, S., De Gaetano, A., Guidone, C., Iaconelli, A., Nanni, G., et al. (2015). Bariatric–metabolic surgery versus conventional medical treatment in obese patients with type 2 diabetes: 5 year follow-up of an open-label, single centre, randomised controlled trial. *Lancet, 386*(9997), 964–973.

Morino, M., Toppino, M., Forestieri, P., Angrisani, L., Allaix, M. E., & Scopinaro, N. (2007). Mortality after bariatric surgery: Analysis of 13,871 morbidly obese patients from a national registry. *Annals of Surgery, 246*(6), 1002–1007.

Moustarah, F., Brethauer, S. A., & Schauer, P. R. (2010). Laparoscopic surgery for severe obesity. In J. L. Cameron & A. M. Cameron (Eds.), *Current* surgical therapy (10th ed., pp. 1304–1316). Philadelphia: Elsevier.

Mummadi, R. R., Kasturi, K. S., Chennareddygari, S., & Sood, G. K. (2008). Effect of bariatric surgery on nonalcoholic fatty liver disease: Systematic review and meta-analysis. *Clinical Gastroenterology and Hepatology, 6*(12), 1396–1402.

National Institutes of Health. (1991). Gastrointestinal surgery for severe obesity: National Institutes of Health Consensus Development Conference Panel. *Annals of Internal Medicine, 115*(12), 956–961.

Panunzi, S., De Gaetano, A., Carnicelli, A., & Mingrone, G. (2015). Predictors of remission of diabetes mellitus in severely obese individuals undergoing bariatric surgery: Do BMI or procedure choice matter?—a meta-analysis. *Annals of Surgery, 261*(3), 459–467.

Parikh, M., Chung, M., Sheth, S., McMacken, M., Zahra, T., Saunders, J. K., et al. (2014). Randomized pilot trial of bariatric surgery versus intensive medical weight management on diabetes remission in type 2 diabetic patients who do not meet NIH criteria for surgery and the role of soluble RAGE as a novel biomarker of success. *Annals of Surgery, 260*(4), 617–622; discussion 622–624.

Poirier, P., Cornier, M. A., Mazzone, T., Stiles, S., Cummings, S., Klein, S., et al. (2011). Bariatric surgery and cardiovascular risk factors: A scientific statement from the American Heart Association. *Circulation, 123*(15), 1683–1701.

Ponce, J., DeMaria, E. J., Nguyen, N. T., Hutter, M., Sudan, R., & Morton, J. M. (2016). American Society for Metabolic and Bariatric Surgery estimation of bariatric surgery procedures in 2015 and surgeon workforce in the United States. *Surgery for Obesity and Related Diseases, 12*(9), 1637–1639.

Pontiroli, A. E., & Morabito, A. (2011). Long-term prevention of mortality in morbid obesity through bariatric surgery: A systematic review and meta-analysis of trials performed with gastric banding and gastric bypass. *Annals of Surgery, 253*(3), 484–487.

Prachand, V. N., & Alverdy, J. C. (2010). Gastroesophageal reflux disease and severe obesity: Fundoplication or bariatric surgery? *World Journal of Gastroenterology, 16*(30), 3757–3761.

Quan, Y., Huang, A., Ye, M., Xu, M., Zhuang, B., Zhang, P., et al. (2015). Efficacy of laparoscopic mini gastric bypass for obesity and type 2 diabetes mellitus: A systematic review and meta-analysis. *Gastroenterology Research and Practice, 2015*, 152852.

Reoch, J., Mottillo, S., Shimony, A., Fillion, K. B., Christou, N. V., Joseph, L., et al. (2011). Safety of laparoscopic vs. open bariatric surgery: A systematic review and meta-analysis. *Archives of Surgery, 146*(11), 1314–1322.

Ristow, B., Rabkin, J., & Haeusslein, E. (2008). Improvement in dilated cardiomyopathy after bariatric surgery. *Journal of Cardiac Failure, 14*(3), 198–202.

Rogula, T., Yenumula, P. R., & Schauer, P. R. (2007). A complication of Roux-en-Y gastric bypass: Intestinal obstruction. *Surgical Endoscopy, 21*(11), 1914–1918.

Rosenthal, R. J., International Sleeve Gastrectomy Expert Panel, Diaz, A. A., Arvidsson, D., Baker, R. S., Basso, N., et al. (2012). International Sleeve Gastrectomy Expert Panel consensus statement: Best practice guidelines based on experience of > 12,000 cases. *Surgery for Obesity and Related Diseases, 8*(1), 8–19.

Rubino, F., Nathan, D. M., Eckel, R. H., Schauer, P. R., Alberti, K. G., Zimmet, P. Z., et al. (2016). Metabolic surgery in the treatment algorithm for type 2 diabetes: A joint statement by international diabetes organizations. *Diabetes Care, 39*(6), 861–877.

Rubino, F., R'bibo, S. L., del Genio, F., Mazumdar, M., & McGraw, T. E. (2010). Metabolic surgery: The role of the gastrointestinal tract in diabetes mellitus. *Nature Reviews Endocrinology, 6*(2), 102–109.

Sánchez-Pernaute, A., Rubio, M. Á., Conde, M., Arrue, E., Pérez-Aguirre, E., & Torres, A. (2015). Single-anastomosis duodenoileal bypass as a second step after sleeve gastrectomy. *Surgery for Obesity and Related Diseases, 11*(2), 351–325.

Schauer, P. R., & 2004 ABS Consensus Conference. (2005). Gastric bypass for severe obesity: Approaches and outcomes. *Surgery for Obesity and Related Diseases, 1*(3), 297–300.

Schauer, P. R., Bhatt, D. L., Kirwan, J. P., Wolski, K., Aminian, A., Brethauer, S. A., et al. (2017). Bariatric surgery vs. intensive medical therapy for diabetes: 5-year outcomes. *New England Journal of Medicine, 376*(7), 641–651.

Schauer, P. R., Bhatt, D. L., Kirwan, J. P., Wolski, K., Brethauer, S. A., Navaneethan, S. D., et al. (2014). Bariatric surgery versus intensive medical therapy for diabetes: 3-year outcomes. *New England Journal of Medicine, 370*(21), 2002–2013.

Schauer, P. R., Burguera, B., Ikramuddin, S., Cottam, D., Gourash, W., Hamad, G., et al. (2003). Effect of laparoscopic Roux-en Y gastric bypass on type 2 diabetes mellitus. *Annals of Surgery, 238*(4), 467–485.

Schauer, P. R., Hamad, G., & Ikramuddin, S. (2001). Surgical management of gastroesophageal reflux disease in obese patients. *Seminars in Laparoscopic Surgery, 8*(4), 256–264.

Schauer, P. R., Mingrone, G., Ikramuddin, S., & Wolfe, B. (2016). Clinical outcomes of metabolic surgery: Efficacy of glycemic control, weight loss, and remission of diabetes. *Diabetes Care, 39*(6), 902–911.

Schirmer, B., & Schauer, P. R. (2010). The surgical management of obesity. In F. C. Brunicardi, D. K. Andersen, & T. R. Billiar (Eds.), *Schwartz's principles of surgery* (9th ed., pp. 949–978). New York: McGraw-Hill.

Scopinaro, N. (2012). Thirty-five years of biliopancreatic diversion: Notes on gastrointestinal physiology to complete the published information useful for a better understanding and clinical use of the operation. *Obesity Surgery, 22*(3), 427–432.

Sethi, M., Chau, E., Youn, A., Jiang, Y., Fielding, G., & Ren-Fielding, C. (2016). Long-term outcomes after biliopancreatic diversion with and without duodenal switch: 2-, 5-, and 10-year data. *Surgery for Obesity and Related Diseases, 12*(9), 1697–1705.

Sharma, A. M., & Kushner, R. F. (2009). A proposed clinical staging system for obesity. *International Journal of Obesity, 33*(3), 289–295.

Shermak, M. A. (2012). Pearls and perils of caring for the post-bariatric body contouring patient. *Plastic and Reconstructive Surgery, 130*(4), 585e–596e.

Shimizu, H., Maia, M., Kroh, M., Schauer, P. R., & Brethauer, S. A. (2013). Surgical management of early small bowel obstruction after laparoscopic Roux-en-Y gastric bypass. *Surgery for Obesity and Related Diseases, 9*(5), 718–724.

Sjöström, L. (2013). Review of the key results from the Swedish Obese Subjects (SOS) trial: A prospective controlled intervention study of bariatric surgery. *Journal of Internal Medicine, 273*(3), 219–234.

Sjöström, L., Gummesson, A., Sjöström, C. D., Narbro, K., Peltonen, M., Wedel, H., et al. (2009). Effects of bariatric surgery on cancer incidence in obese patients in Sweden (Swedish Obese Subjects study): A prospective, controlled intervention trial. *Lancet Oncology, 10*(7), 653–662.

Sjöström, L., Narbro, K., Sjöström, C. D., Karason, K., Larsson, B., Wedel, H., et al. (2007). Effects of bariatric surgery on mortality in Swedish obese subjects. *New England Journal of Medicine, 357*(8), 741–752.

Sjöström, L., Peltonen, M., Jacobson, P., Sjöström, C. D., Karason, K., Wedel, H., et al. (2012). Bariatric surgery and long-term cardiovascular events. *Journal of the American Medical Association, 307*(1), 56–65.

Smith, B. R., Schauer, P., & Nguyen, N. T. (2011). Surgical approaches to the treatment of obesity: Bariatric surgery. *Endocrinology Metabolism Clinics of North America, 37*(4), 943–964.

Spyropoulos, C., Kehagias, I., Panagiotopoulos, S., Mead, N., & Kalfarentzos, F. (2010). Revisional bariatric surgery: 13-year experience from a tertiary institution. *Archives of Surgery, 145*(2), 173–177.

Talebpour, M., Motamedi, S. M. K., Talebpour, A., & Vahidi, H. (2012). Twelve year experience of laparoscopic gastric plication in morbid obesity: Development of the technique and patient outcomes. *Annals of Surgical Innovation and Research, 6*(1), 7.

Thodiyil, P. A., Yenumula, P., Rogula, T., Gorecki, P., Fahoum, B., Goursash, W., et al. (2008). Selective nonoperative management of leaks after gastric bypass: Lessons learned from 2,675 consecutive patients. *Annals of Surgery, 248*(5), 782–792.

Valezi, A. C., & Machado, V. H. (2011). Morphofunctional evaluation of the heart of obese patients before and after bariatric surgery. *Obesity Surgery, 21*(11), 1693–1697.

Vest, A. R., Heneghan, H. M., Agarwal, S., Schauer, P. R., & Young, J. B. (2012). Bariatric surgery and cardiovascular outcomes: A systematic review. *Heart, 98*(24), 1763–1777.

Vest, A. R., Patel, P., Schauer, P. R., Satava, M. E., Cavalcante, J. L., Brethauer, S., et al. (2016). Clinical and echocardiographic outcomes after bariatric surgery in obese patients with left ventricular systolic dysfunction. *Circulation: Heart Failure, 9*(3), e002260.

Wentworth, J. M., Playfair, J., Laurie, C., Ritchie, M. E., Brown, W. A., Burton, P., et al. (2014). Multidisciplinary diabetes care with and without bariatric surgery in overweight people: A randomised controlled trial. *Lancet Diabetes and Endocrinology, 2*(7), 545–552.

CHAPTER 23

Maintenance of Weight Lost in Behavioral Treatment of Obesity

Michael G. Perri
Aviva H. Ariel-Donges

Behavioral treatment for obesity, also commonly referred to as *comprehensive lifestyle treatment,* employs principles from learning and social–cognitive theories (Bandura, 1991; Ferster, Nurnberger, & Levitt, 1996; Kanfer, 1970) to help individuals lose weight by achieving a negative energy balance via reduced caloric consumption and increased physical activity. Behavioral treatment reliably results in body weight reductions of 8–10% (Butryn, Webb, & Wadden, 2011). Weight losses of this magnitude typically produce improvements in cardiovascular risk factors and obesity-related medical conditions (Diabetes Prevention Program Research Group, 2002; Look AHEAD Research Group, 2010; Jensen et al., 2014). Despite the notable benefits of behavioral treatment, the regaining of weight that commonly follows initial weight loss remains a pressing problem—one that has even led some to question the ethics of psychological treatments for obesity (Cooper et al., 2010).

For more than three decades, obesity researchers have struggled to understand the factors associated with posttreatment weight regain (MacLean et al., 2015). Poor maintenance appears to have multiple interactive determinants, including biological, environmental, and psychological factors. Following diet-induced weight loss, biological influences such as the persistence of adaptive thermogenesis (Rosenbaum, Hirsch, Gallagher, & Leibel, 2008) and environmental contributors such as continuous exposure to stimuli that promote the consumption of appetizing, low-cost, energy-dense foods (Drewnowski & Rolls, 2005) prime the individual for regaining weight. Psychological factors then come into play to potentiate the predisposition to relapse (Fuglestad, Rothman, & Jeffery, 2008).

Indeed, the most rewarding aspect of obesity treatment from the participant's perspective is weight loss. However, after several months of caloric restriction, the rate of weight loss slows or stops—often at a point that is far from the participant's desired weight—leaving unfulfilled expectations for personal and social benefits of weight loss. The individual is confronted with the need to continue substantial behavioral efforts to avoid weight gain, creating a perception that the behavioral costs exceed the personal benefits of the weight management endeavor (Hsu & Blanford, 2014). The drop in reinforcement (i.e., absence of further weight loss) can trigger a decrease in the diet and exercise behaviors required for further weight loss or the maintenance of lost weight. Furthermore, a decrease in behavioral adherence, coupled with the unfavorable influences of biological and environmental factors, often leads to weight regain. Attributions of personal ineffectiveness commonly follow, which can trigger negative emotions, a sense of hopelessness, and ultimately abandonment of the weight control effort (Andersson & Rossner, 1997; Jeffery, French, & Schmid, 1990; Ratcliffe & Ellison, 2015).

To overcome this sobering set of challenges, researchers have tested an array of strategies designed to enhance the maintenance of lost weight. In this chapter, we examine the progress made (since the publication of the prior edition of this handbook) toward solving the "maintenance problem." Accordingly, we conducted a review of randomized trials of behavioral treatment for obesity in an effort to document the effects of various treatment strategies on long-term weight change. We were particularly interested in determining whether the incorporation of particular intervention methods either *during* or *following* the weight loss phase of behavioral treatment produces meaningful improvements in maintenance.

A number of studies entail modifications that are implemented during the *initial* "weight loss" phase of behavioral treatment, with the expectation that the inclusion of new components will have a direct or indirect impact on long-term weight change or the maintenance of weight lost. For example, the inclusion of training in weight maintenance skills during initial treatment is an example of an approach expected to have a *direct* impact on the maintenance of lost weight. Alternatively, modifying the home environment during initial treatment to support weight change behaviors represents an approach that would be expected to boost initial weight loss *and* have a beneficial although *indirect* impact on the maintenance of lost weight. We include both of these approaches, along with a review of studies that entail interventions delivered following the initial weight loss phase that are specifically designed to improve the maintenance of lost weight.

The inclusion criteria for our review entailed the following elements: (1) publication between 2001 and 2015; (2) the use of behavioral treatment procedures (i.e., defined operationally as the inclusion of daily self-monitoring of food consumption); (3) the implementation of a randomized design to test methods intended to improve the effectiveness or efficiency of behavioral treatment; (4) a study sample consisting of adults with body mass indices (BMIs) ≥ 25 kg/m^2; (5) an initial weight loss intervention phase conducted over a period of 3 months or longer; and (6) a follow-up evaluation completed 12 or more months after the initiation of treatment. Studies were excluded if they involved the use of medications, surgical procedures, inpatient care, very-low-calorie diets (< 800 kcal/day), or meal replacements as the *primary* means of achieving weight loss. Studies were also excluded if they contained a methodological flaw that threatened the validity of findings.

We identified 31 studies that met the inclusion and exclusion criteria and sorted them into two groups: (1) investigations that tested modifications or additions to the initial (weight loss) phase of behavioral treatment; and (2) studies that examined the effects of an extended-care (i.e., "maintenance") program after the initial phase of treatment. We summarize the findings from these studies and discuss implications for future research and clinical care.

Modifications of the Initial Phase of Behavioral Treatment

A number of studies have investigated the effects of intervention components delivered *during* the initial (weight loss) phase of behavioral treatment that were expected to have a long-term impact on weight loss success. Table 23.1 contains key information about the study samples, treatment conditions, and data regarding long-term retention rates and weight changes.

Size of Treatment Groups

Behavioral treatment of obesity is typically conducted in a group treatment format, with group size varying widely across studies. Does size matter? Dutton et al. (2014) tested the delivery of behavioral treatment

TABLE 23.1. Studies with Modifications to the Initial Phase of Behavioral Treatment

Study			Intervention content and outcomes				
Author (year)	Sample N	Baseline M BMI (kg/m²)	Treatment conditions	Posttreatment (mos. from baseline)	M weight change from baseline to posttreatment (kg)	Follow-up (mos. from baseline)	Follow-up retention (%)	M weight change from baseline to follow-up (kg)
Appel et al. (2011)	415	36.8	BT + online BT/e-mail/phone	6	−5.8 (SE = 0.6)[a]	24	96	−5.1 (SE = 0.8)[a]
		36.0	Online BT + e-mail/phone		−6.1 (SE = 0.5)[a]		94	−4.6 (SE = 0.7)[a]
		36.8	Self-directed control		−1.4 (SE = 0.4)[b]		93	−0.8 (SE = 0.6)[b]
Carels et al. (2005)	53	37.2	BT			12	~74	~−7.6
		38.0	BT + glycemic index education					~−7.6
Cooper et al. (2010)	150	34.8	BT	11	−11.6 (SD = 12.9)	23	88	−7.0 (SD = 12.8)
		33.9	Reformulated CBT		−8.2 (SD = 10.0)		96	−3.3 (SD = 10.2)
		35.4	Guided self-help		−5.2 (SD = 10.4)		98	−2.3 (SD = 10.1)
Donnelly et al. (2013)	395	34.9	BT	6	−13.5 (SD = 7.3)	18	74	−8.4 (SD = 9.1)
		34.6	Group phone BT		−12.6 (SD = 8.1)		72	−7.5 (SD = 8.1)
Dutton et al. (2014)	66	36.9	BT with large groups	6	−0.2 (SE = 1.1)[a]	12	88	−1.7 (SE = 1.2)[a]
		36.1	BT with small groups		~−6.5 (SE = 1.3)[b]		91	~−7.0 (SE = 1.5)[b]
Foster et al. (2010)	307	36.1	BT + low-fat diet	6	−11.3 (CI: −12.4, −10.3)	24	68	−7.4 (CI: −9.1, −5.6)
		36.1	BT + low-carbohydrate diet		−12.1 (CI: −13.1, −11.2)		58	−6.3 (CI: −8.1, −4.6)
Foster-Schubert et al. (2012)	439	31.0	BT with diet + exercise			12	92	−10.8[a]
		31.1	BT with diet only				89	−8.5[a]
		30.7	Exercise only				91	−2.4[b]
		30.7	Control				92	−0.8[c]
Micco et al. (2007)	23	32.3	Online BT	6	−6.8 (SD = 7.8)	12	~63	−5.1 (SD = 7.1)
		31.0	Online BT + FtF groups		−5.1 (SD = 4.8)			−3.5 (SD = 5.1)

(continued)

TABLE 23.1. (continued)

Study			Intervention content and outcomes				
Author (year)	Sample N	Baseline M BMI (kg/m²)	Treatment conditions	Posttreatment (mos. from baseline)	M weight change from baseline to posttreatment (kg)	Follow-up (mos. from baseline)	Follow-up retention (%)	M weight change from baseline to follow-up (kg)
Goodpaster et al. (2010)	130	43.5	BT with exercise	6	−10.9 (CI: −9.1, −12.7)[a]	12	73	−12.1 (CI: −10.0, −12.7)
		43.7	BT with delayed exercise		−8.2 (CI: −6.4, −9.9)[b]		83	−9.9 (CI: −8.0, −11.7)
Gorin et al. (2013)	201	36.1	BT + FtF ExtCare	6	−6.8 (SE = 2.2)[a]	18	87	−5.5 (SE = 1.0)
		36.7	BT + home changes + FtF ExtCare		−9.1 (SE = 0.7)[b]		97	−7.3 (SE = 1.0)
Jakicic et al. (2008)	201	32.7	BT + vigorous-intensity/high-duration exercise	6	−9.5 (SD = 11.1)	24	90	−5.8 (SD = 11.9)
		32.7	BT + vigorous-intensity/moderate-duration exercise		−7.5 (SD = 14.6)		88	−2.9 (SD = 15.0)
		32.4	BT + moderate-intensity/high-duration exercise		−8.2 (SD = 15.1)		82	−4.7 (SD = 16.4)
		32.8	BT + moderate-intensity/moderate-duration exercise		−7.3 (SD = 12.9)		78	−3.5 (SD = 14.1)
Jeffery et al. (2003)	202	~31.7	BT + 1,000 kcal/week EE	6	−8.1 (SD = 7.4)	18	90	−4.1 (SD = 8.3)[a]
		~31.7	BT + 2,500 kcal/week EE		−9.0 (SD = 7.1)		94	−6.7 (SD = 8.1)[b]
Tate et al. (2007)		~31.7	BT + 1,000 kcal/week EE			30	79	−0.9 (SD = 8.9)
		~31.7	BT + 2,500 kcal/week EE				77	−2.9 (SD = 8.6)
Kalarchian et al. (2011)	203	34.3	BT	6	−6.0 (SE = 1.7)[a]	18	56	−3.3 (SE = 1.3)
		34.1	Appearance-focused BT		−8.7 (SE = 0.8)[b]		53	−6.3 (SE = 1.4)
		33.9	Health-focused BT		−7.1 (SE = 0.7)[a,b]		64	−5.9 (SE = 1.2)
		34.3	Appearance and health-focused BT		−8.9 (SE = 0.7)[b]		57	−6.4 (SE = 1.2)
Kiernan et al. (2013)	267	32.1	Maintenance training prior to BT	6	−7.3 (SD = 5.0)	18	94	~−5.9 (SD = 4.9)[a]
		32.1	Maintenance training following BT		−7.7 (SD = 6.1)		93	~−4.4 (SD = 5.3)[b]

Study	N	BMI	Intervention	mos	%	Posttreatment	Follow-up
Leahey et al. (2015)	268	32.9	Online BT + website	3	87	~−3.9^a	~−1.1^a
		33.5	Online BT + website + incentives		94	~−5.9^b	~−2.9^b
		34.3	Online BT + website + FtF groups		93	~−5.4^{a,b}	~−4.2^b
Nackers et al. (2013)	125	38.1	BT with 1,000 kcal/day goal	6	88	−10 (SE = 0.92)^a	−8.52 (SE = 1.17)^a
		37.6	BT with 1,500 kcal/day goal		90	−6.2 (SE = 0.94)^b	−5.84 (SE = 1.11)^b
Perri et al. (2014)	612	36.7	High-dose BT and ExtCare	6	78	~−11.1 (CI: 9.8, 11.9)^a	~−6.9 (CI: 5.5, 8.1)^a
		36.2	Moderate-dose BT and ExtCare		84	~−9.2 (CI: 8.2, 10.3)^a	~−6.6 (CI: 5.3, 7.9)^a
		36.1	Low-dose BT and ExtCare		76	~−7.2 (CI: 6.1, 8.3)^b	~−3.6 (CI: 2.0, 4.8)^b
		36.3	Education control		84	~−4.1 (CI: 3.1, 5.1)^c	~−2.9 (CI: 1.7, 4.3)^b
Raynor et al. (2012)	202	35.3	BT	6	95	~−10.9 (SD = 5.8)	−9.6 (SD = 9.2)
		34.5	BT with limited energy dense foods		93	~−10.9 (SD = 5.8)	−9.9 (SD = 7.6)
Rejeski et al. (2002)	316	34.2	BT with diet + exercise	18	76		~−4.1^a
		34.7	BT with diet only		80		~−5.4^a
		34.6	Exercise only		82		~−2.4^b
		34.8	Education control		78		~−1.3^b
Villareal et al. (2011)	107	37.2	BT with diet + exercise	12	89	−7.7 (SD = 4.2)^a	−8.6 (SD = 3.8)^a
		37.2	BT with diet only		88	−9.0 (SD = 5.4)^a	−9.7 (SD = 5.4)^a
		36.9	Exercise only		85	−0.3 (SD = 2.3)^b	−0.5 (SD = 3.6)^b
		37.3	No intervention control		85	+0.9 (SD = 2.8)^b	−0.1 (SD = 3.5)^b
Sacks et al. (2009)	811	33.0	BT with low-fat/average-protein diet	24	~80	~−5.8	~−2.8
		33.0	BT with low-fat/high-protein diet			~−6.1	~−3.8
		32.0	BT with high-fat/average-protein diet			~−5.7	~−3.0
		33.0	BT with high-fat/high-protein diet			~−6.0	~−3.4

Note. Differing letters next to means represent significant between-group differences at posttreatment or follow-up ($p < .05$). *M*, mean; BMI, body mass index; EE, energy expenditure; mos, months; BT, standard behavioral treatment for obesity; Maint., maintenance program; *SD*, standard deviation; FtF, face-to-face treatment; *SE*, standard error; CI, 95% confidence interval; RPT, relapse prevention training; PST, problem-solving training; ExtCare, extended-care treatment.

^{a}Significant between-group differences compared to groups with superscript b or c, $p < .05$.
^{b}Significant between-group differences compared to groups with superscript a or c, $p < .05$.
^{c}Significant between-group differences compared to groups with superscript a or b, $p < .05$.

in small versus large groups (~12 vs. ~30 participants). The investigators found that participants in the small-group condition reported better treatment engagement, completed more self-monitoring records, and achieved greater *maintenance* of lost weight than those in the large-group intervention. One year after the start of treatment, the small-group condition showed a mean net weight loss of 7.0 kg versus 1.7 kg for the large-group condition. Moreover, the frequency of self-monitoring mediated the relation between group size and weight loss. Compared with those in the small groups, the decreased individual attention received by the large-group participants may have contributed to poorer adherence and smaller weight changes. What remains to be determined is the group size with which treatment efficiency is maximized without diminishing treatment effectiveness. More specifically, is there a group size larger than 12 but smaller than 30 that increases treatment efficiency without decreasing treatment effectiveness?

Dose of Treatment

Similarly, it is important to understand the relation between the dose (i.e., number of treatment sessions) of behavioral treatment and the magnitude of weight loss. Perri et al. (2014) examined the effects of small, moderate, and large doses of behavioral treatment on both short- and long-term changes in body weight. The small-, moderate-, and high-dose conditions involved 8, 16, and 24 sessions of treatment, respectively, during both the initial 6 months and subsequent 12 months of the program. At 24 months, participants in the moderate- and high-dose conditions had equivalent weight reductions (6.7% and 6.8%, respectively), and both had weight losses superior to those achieved by the low-dose participants (3.5%). An additional analysis showed that moderate dose treatment was more cost-effective than the low- and high-dose conditions. Thus, it appears that bigger is not necessarily better when it comes to dose of treatment. A longer initial phase of treatment with a greater number of sessions (i.e., higher treatment dose) generally increases mean weight loss (Perri, Nezu, Patti, & McCann, 1989). However, very high doses of treatment often result in higher group means due to larger losses achieved by a few high performers rather than uniformly higher weight losses for all participants. Identifying the dose of treatment associated with long-term success has an indirect, as well as a direct, impact on improving the maintenance of lost weight. In the clinical arena, cost-effectiveness is critical to policymakers who determine whether third-party payers will cover treatments. Treatments with long-term cost-effectiveness, as well as long-term weight loss effectiveness, are more likely to be disseminated and implemented and thereby produce the intended benefits of improving the health of people with obesity in the general population.

Telephone Counseling

The mode of treatment delivery has the potential to influence long-term weight loss. Appel et al. (2011) compared the effectiveness of treatment provided to primary care patients through (1) telephone counseling, (2) face-to-face sessions, or (3) a control group with instructions for self-directed weight management. Participants in telephone and face-to-face interventions also had access to a website with weight management tools, and they received encouragement for weight loss from their primary care providers. At 24 months, telephone and face-to-face counseling showed equivalent mean reductions (M's = 4.6 and 5.1 kg, respectively) that were significantly larger than the mean loss in the control condition (0.8 kg). In a similar vein, Donnelly et al. (2013) conducted an equivalence trial to test whether telephone counseling conducted via conference calls with groups of participants would produce weight losses equivalent to those produced by face-to-face group counseling. At 18 months, the net reduction in initial body weight was the same in both conditions (6.6%), but the calculated cost of treatment (to the participant) was $790 less for the conference call intervention compared with face-to-face clinic sessions. The findings from Appel et al. (2011) and Donnelly et al. (2013) show that telephone delivery can provide a level of effectiveness equivalent to the gold standard of face-to-face sessions, not only in the short run, but also at long-term follow-ups of 18 and 24 months. Moreover, the findings from Donnelly et al. (2013) suggest that telephone-delivered treatments have the potential to yield substantial savings in costs versus clinic-based treatments.

Internet Delivery

With its ubiquity and continuous availability, Internet delivery of behavioral treatment could be a boon to the long-term management of weight. Early research by Tate, Wing, and Winett (2001) that focused on initial weight loss showed that behavioral treatment delivered via the Internet produced significantly larger 6-month losses than diet education via the Internet (M's = 4.1 and 1.6 kg, respectively). In an effort to improve the *long-term* effects of behavioral counseling via the Internet, Micco et al. (2007) randomized participants to a 12-month behavioral weight loss program delivered via the Internet alone or to an identical Internet program supplemented with *monthly* in-person support meetings led by trained interventionists. An intention-to-treat analysis indicated no significant between-group differences in weight loss at 12 months, with 5.1 versus 3.5 kg for Internet alone versus Internet plus in-person support conditions, respectively. However, in the context of a statewide weight loss campaign, Leahey et al. (2015) tested whether the long-term effectiveness of behavioral counseling via the Internet might be improved by adding (1) optional in-person group meetings (maximum of 12 weekly sessions conducted at the start of treatment and led by dietitians or exercise physiologists); or (2) small financial incentives for good adherence (maximum of $45 in total). A 12-month assessment showed significantly larger mean percent reductions in body weight for the treatment conditions with group support (4.5%) or financial incentives (3.1%) compared with behavioral counseling alone (1.2%). The study also found that the incentive program was the most cost-effective approach to improving the long-term effects of behavioral counseling via the Internet.

The findings from Micco et al. (2007) and Leahey et al. (2015) showed mixed results for supplementing Internet interventions with face-to-face contacts. The timing of personal support may be critical to its impact on short- and long-term weight change. Providing frequent support early in the intervention phase (weekly for 3 months) appears to be more effective than less frequent contact distributed over the course of a year (monthly for 12 months). Historically, the use of financial incentives has yielded mixed findings (Jeffery et al., 1993). However, in the context of an Internet-based program, the addition of small incentives might be a cost-effective approach to enhancing the long-term effectiveness of behavioral treatment (Leahey et al., 2015). Demonstrations that weight losses achieved via the Internet, even if modest in size, can be maintained over the long run would represent an important public health accomplishment.

Modifying the Home Environment

The influence of environmental factors on behavior change has long been an area of interest to behavioral psychologists. Gorin et al. (2013) examined the short- and long-term effects of modifying the home environment to support weight reduction as an adjunct to standard behavioral treatment. Modifications to the home environment included the provision of exercise equipment, a full-length mirror, a scale, fitness magazines, and portion plates, coupled with the inclusion of a home partner in treatment sessions. The home environment program improved weight losses at 6 months compared to standard behavioral treatment, but the impact of the environmental enhancements did not persist over time. There were no significant between-group differences in weight or weight regain at the 18-month follow-up. Modifying the home environment to support weight loss, though promising with respect to initial weight reduction, does not seem to provide a long-term impact on weight change.

Motivation-Focused Treatment

The two most important reasons that people seek to lose weight are to improve their health and/or their physical appearance. Kalarchian et al. (2011) examined whether highlighting treatment-induced changes that were in alignment with different motivations for weight loss might improve treatment effectiveness. The researchers randomly assigned participants to one of four conditions: standard behavioral treatment, appearance-focused behavioral treatment, health-focused behavioral treatment, or a combination of both appearance- and health-focused behavioral treatment. The appearance-focused and the combined appearance- and health-focused interventions showed greater weight reductions at 6 months compared with standard behavioral treatment, but the superior outcomes for these conditions were not maintained at 18 months. Thus, motivation-focused treatment does not appear to enhance long-term weight loss.

Reformulated Cognitive-Behavioral Treatment

Concerned about the problem of poor maintenance of weight lost via standard behavioral treatment, Cooper and Fairburn (2001) proposed a reformulated cognitive-behavioral therapy (CBT) intervention for obesity. They designed their intervention to address the key factors that they believed were responsible for relapse following standard behavioral treatment for obesity (i.e., unrealistic expectations about the personal benefits of weight loss and a failure to acquire the skills needed to maintain a stable body weight). Cooper et al. (2010) subsequently reported findings from a trial that tested the new CBT versus standard behavioral treatment and a guided self-help (GSH) control condition. An individual therapy format was used to deliver behavioral treatment and CBT over the course of 44 weeks, while GSH was completed in 24 weeks. At week 44, behavioral treatment and CBT groups had weight reductions that did not differ significantly (12.7% and 8.9%, respectively), but only behavioral treatment showed a significantly greater reduction than GSH (5.4%). Over the course of 3 years of follow-up with no posttreatment contact, participants in all three conditions on average regained virtually 100% of their initial losses, and no significant between-group differences were observed among any of the conditions.

Cooper and Fairburn's (2001) debut of a new CBT treatment for obesity was published without data supporting the superiority of their intervention versus standard behavioral treatment. However, findings from their trial of CBT versus behavioral treatment showed no advantage for CBT, and both the behavioral treatment and CBT conditions demonstrated poorer long-term maintenance than is typically accomplished with standard behavioral treatment (Cooper et al., 2010). Cooper et al. (2010) argued that the failure of their CBT intervention was evidence that relapse following obesity treatment is likely controlled by (unspecified) nonpsychological factors, and they concluded that it is "ethically questionable to claim that psychological treatments for obesity work in the absence of data on their longer-term outcome" (p. 712). However, others investigators (Perri, Sears, & Clark, 1993), as well as scientific and professional associations (American College of Cardiology, American Heart Association, and The Obesity Society; see Jensen et al., 2014), have recognized that obesity should be viewed as a complex, chronic condition requiring a continuous-care approach to treatment. Indeed, the Look AHEAD Study (Look AHEAD Research Group, 2010, 2014), which achieved successful behavioral management of obesity over the course of more than 8 years, provides compelling evidence that psychological interventions "work" when they are based on a model that appreciates the multiple biobehavioral contributors to relapse and when they employ a continuous-care approach to long-term treatment.

Maintenance Training Prior to Weight Loss

In a novel approach to the maintenance problem, Kiernan et al. (2013) tested the effectiveness of providing participants with maintenance training *prior* to initiating weight reductions rather than *after* weight loss. Participants in the "stability first" condition had 2 months of training in how to maintain a stable body weight before beginning the weight loss phase of treatment. Those in the "weight loss first" condition received training in maintenance strategies after the weight loss phase was completed. The mean losses accomplished in the initial phase of treatment were equivalent (~7.5 kg). However, consistent with the researchers' hypothesis, training participants in how to maintain a stable weight before embarking on a weight loss intervention resulted in significantly greater maintenance of lost weight compared with the traditional approach of addressing maintenance after an initial period of weight loss (i.e., 81 vs. 57% of initial weight loss maintained). Thus, training participants in body weight stability skills prior to the initiation of weight loss seems to improve long-term outcomes. Indeed, if replicated, the findings from the innovative study by Kiernan et al. (2013) have the potential to change how we approach the development of maintenance skills. The timing and methods used to train participants in body weight stability skills represent a fertile avenue for future study.

Manipulations of Diet and/or Exercise

Behavioral treatment of obesity commonly includes prescriptions for a balanced deficit diet of 1,200–1,500 kcal/day and for the addition of 30 minutes/day of moderate-intensity physical activity, typically brisk walking, 5–7 days per week. A number of studies have examined the effects of different variations in energy intake, diet education, diet composition, exercise, and combinations of diet and exercise on the short- and long-term effects of behavioral treatment. The specific characteristics of the exercise and diet regimens have varied from study to study, as have the target populations (e.g., older adults, people with specific medical conditions). The findings from such studies have been remarkably consistent. The inclusion of diet or diet plus exercise produces superior weight reductions compared with exercise alone (Rejeski et al., 2002; Villareal et al., 2011; Foster-Schubert et al., 2012). Indeed, a systematic review and meta-analysis of studies that included diet or exercise or their combination in behavioral weight loss treatment led to the conclusion that the addition of diet to exercise increases weight loss, but the addition of exercise to diet does not (Johns, Hartmann-Boyce, Jebb, & Aveyard, 2014). These findings are not surprising, given that caloric consumption has the potential to contribute to larger changes in energy balance than does energy expenditure (e.g., it takes more than 2 hours of brisk walking to expend the > 700 kcal contained in one Cinnabon Classic Cinnamon Roll). Thus, the contribution of exercise to initial weight loss is typically small (Goodpaster et al., 2010), and its effects are often difficult to detect due to variability in participant adherence to exercise prescriptions (Jakicic, Marcus, Lang, & Janney, 2008). Nonetheless, exercise provides many benefits in addition to caloric expenditure (e.g., increased metabolic rate, muscle preservation, mood enhancement), and exercise engagement is associated with *long-term* success in weight management (American College of Sports Medicine, 2009).

Exercise Variations

Jakicic et al. (2008) examined the effects of four different exercise regimens based on *energy expenditure* (1,000 vs. 2,000 kcal/week) and *exercise intensity* ("moderate" vs. "vigorous"), combined with standard behavioral treatment using a low-calorie diet. There were no significant weight loss differences between any of the regimens over the short or long run. However, post-hoc analyses indicated that those participants who maintained weight reductions ≥ 10% at 24 months reported that they engaged in higher levels of exercise than those maintaining losses of < 10%. Jeffery and colleagues examined the short- and long-term effects of prescribing 2,500 versus 1,000 kcal/week of physical activity and found no between-group difference in weight loss at posttreatment, but observed a greater weight loss at 18 months for participants in the high- versus low-exercise conditions (M's = 6.7 vs. 4.1 kg, respectively; Jeffery, Wing, Sherwood, & Tate, 2003; Tate, Jeffery, Sherwood, & Wing, 2007). However, a 30-month follow-up showed equivalent weight changes, and, similar to the findings from Jakicic et al. (2008), participants who reported higher levels of exercise maintained greater amounts of weight loss.

The largely unsuccessful efforts to boost short- and long-term weight losses by increasing the frequency, duration, intensity, or type of exercise is likely due to the highly variable response of participants to exercise prescriptions (American College of Sports Medicine, 2009). Nonetheless, participants who exercise more show better *long-term* weight loss outcomes. The larger weight losses of successful participants may be due to their higher levels of physical activity. Alternatively, the greater losses could also be due to other factors commonly observed in people who are highly successful in weight management, such as better adherence to all components of treatment. Future research in this area might benefit from the use of adaptive clinical trial designs (Chow, 2014). For example, after a fixed period of time with randomized assignment to a particular exercise prescription, a participant's adherence would be assessed and the results of that evaluation would determine whether the participant continues on that particular exercise regimen or is assigned to a prespecified alternative prescription. Such an approach might allow investigators to more quickly identify which exercise prescriptions work best for different subsets of their sample.

Caloric Intake Levels

Low-calorie regimens ($\geq$ 800 kcal/day but less than the amount required for a balanced energy equation) are standard components of behavioral treatment, but the specific level of prescribed energy intake varies widely across studies. Nackers et al. (2013) tested the effect of prescribing 1,000 versus 1,500 kcal/day to women who weighed 91–136 kg (i.e., 200–300 pounds). Participants in the 1,000 kcal/day program achieved significantly larger weight losses at 6 months than those prescribed 1,500 kcal/day (M's = 10.0 vs. 6.2 kg, respectively), but the 1,000 kcal/day participants experienced greater weight regain during months 7–12 than those in the 1,500 kcal/day condition (M net losses from baseline = 8.5 vs. 5.8 kg, respectively, p = .32). However, a significantly greater percentage of participants prescribed 1,000 versus 1,500 kcal/day achieved losses $\geq$ 5% of initial body weight at 12 months (62 vs. 42%, respectively), suggesting that there may be some longer-term benefits associated with the use of a lower-calorie prescription.

The findings from Nackers et al. (2013) showed that a prescription for lower-caloric intake boosts initial weight reduction but does not increase long-term weight loss. Nonetheless, lower-calorie targets may increase the percentage of participants who achieve body weight reductions $\geq$ 5%. This finding runs counter to the "small changes" approach to weight management (Lutes et al., 2013), which posits that smaller caloric restrictions ultimately lead to larger long-term reductions and better maintenance of weight loss than more restrictive caloric prescriptions. Larger losses are more rewarding to participants than smaller ones, yet they are harder to maintain. Future research might examine the use of various schedules of caloric intake in which, after a prespecified period of time or weight reduction, participants are moved from a lower- to a higher-caloric level that is easier to maintain over the long run.

Dietary Variety

Dietary *variety* influences food consumption, with greater variety leading to greater consumption. Raynor and colleagues tested the effects of lifestyle treatment (i.e., behavioral treatment) with or without limited food variety (Raynor, Looney, Steeves, Spence, & Gorin, 2012). The lifestyle plus limited variety intervention included a prescription to limit energy-dense, low-nutritional-value foods (e.g., baked goods, snack bars, candy, chips) to two servings per day. Although the limited variety manipulation resulted in decreased dietary diversity and lower energy consumption compared with standard treatment, there were no significant between-group differences in percent weight loss from baseline to 18 months. Thus, reducing dietary variety appears to have a beneficial effect on food selections, but it does not appear to produce a large enough impact on caloric intake to improve long-term weight loss.

Glycemic Index Education

The role of carbohydrates in weight reduction is often a topic of heated debate. In recent years, various "low-carb" approaches to weight loss have been popular. The glycemic index (GI) measures how foods containing carbohydrates influence blood glucose levels. A low-GI diet may enhance weight loss by decreasing insulin levels, hunger, and caloric intake. Accordingly, Carels and colleagues examined the addition of GI education to standard behavioral treatment and found that participants in the education condition demonstrated improved knowledge at posttreatment related to the GI rating of foods compared to those in standard behavioral treatment (Carels, Darby, Douglass, Cacciapaglia, & Rydin, 2005). However, there were no significant between-group differences with respect to weight loss at either posttreatment or at a 12-month follow-up. Thus, education regarding the GI of foods enhances knowledge, but that knowledge does not translate into sufficient changes in eating patterns to influence weight change.

Macronutrient Composition

Sacks et al. (2009) compared the effects of different dietary compositions of fat, protein, and carbohydrates on 2-year changes in body weight. The experimental design entailed a 2 × 2 factorial comparison of low-fat (20% of total caloric intake) versus high-fat (40% of total caloric intake) and average-protein (15% of total caloric intake) versus high-protein (25% of total caloric intake) regimens, all against a background of comprehensive behavioral treatment. The mean weight losses across all participants were ~6 kg at 6 months and ~4 kg at 24 months, and no significant between-group effects were observed at either assessment. The authors concluded, "reduced-calorie diets result in clinically meaningful weight loss regardless of which macronutrients they emphasize" (p. 859). Similarly, Foster et al. (2010) compared comprehensive behavioral treatment coupled with either a low-carbohydrate or a low-fat diet. The low-carbohydrate regimen prescribed 20 g/day of carbohydrates during the first 3 months without restrictions on protein or fat consumption, followed by monthly increases of 5 g/day of carbohydrates until a stable weight was achieved. The low-fat diet prescribed 1,200–1,800 kcal/day with < 30% of energy from fats. Over the course of the study, the two interventions produced similar patterns of weight change, with mean 1-year losses of approximately 11 kg in both groups. Two-year findings revealed equivalent mean losses for the low-fat and low-carbohydrate conditions (7.4 and 6.3 kg, respectively), indicating that both dietary regimens produce good long-term reductions when coupled with behavioral treatment. However, neither diet substantially improved the maintenance of lost weight.

The macronutrient composition of diet may not play an important role in the amount of weight loss induced or maintained in behavioral treatment. Collectively, the results from Sacks et al. (2009) and Foster et al. (2010) indicate that similar long-term weight changes can be achieved with the combination of behavioral treatment plus either a low-fat or a low-carbohydrate diet. These findings are consistent with a recent meta-analysis that compared the effects of various popular diets and found equivalent weight losses regardless of diet composition (Johnston et al., 2014). Thus, clinicians should feel free to counsel patients to select a dietary approach (e.g., low-fat or low-carb) based on their personal preferences and expectations of likely adherence.

Extended-Care Maintenance Programs

The most common approach to enhancing the maintenance of lost weight has been to provide participants with additional sessions *after* an initial phase of weight loss treatment has ended. The sessions commonly focus on different ways to improve participants' *skills* for coping with the challenges associated with maintaining lost weight. In a series of studies conducted in the 1980s, Perri and colleagues examined the effects of providing every-other-week, face-to-face sessions, 90 minutes in length, that included a weigh-in, a review of participant progress, group problem solving, and goal setting. These early studies demonstrated that delivering extended care during the year following initial treatment successfully enhanced the maintenance of lost weight compared to behavior therapy without posttreatment care (Perri et al., 1987; Perri, McAdoo, McAllister, Lauer, & Yancey, 1986; Perri, McAdoo, Spevak, & Newlin, 1984; Perri et al., 1988; Perri, Shapiro, Ludwig, Twentyman, & McAdoo, 1984).

Although extended care improves the maintenance of weight loss, weight regain of 25–40% of initial weight loss is common at

18-month evaluations, even with extended care (Perri & Corsica, 2002). Longer-term changes in weight are difficult to characterize due to the limited number of studies that follow participants beyond 2 years. Nonetheless, findings from large trials such as the Diabetes Prevention Program and the Look AHEAD Study indicate that weight regain levels off, and that participants maintain on average 50% of their initial weight loss for 3 or more years with continuous care (Diabetes Prevention Program Research Group, 2002; Look AHEAD Research Group, 2014). Table 23.2 contains key information and data for studies published from 2001 through 2015 that tested extended-care regimens following an initial weight loss phase of behavioral treatment.

Relapse Prevention and Problem Solving

Does the *content* of extended-care sessions matter? Perri et al. (2001) examined the effects of extended-care programs consisting of instruction in relapse prevention training (RPT) strategies versus the application of problem-solving therapy (PST) in comparison with a control condition that received standard behavioral treatment without follow-up care. All groups had equivalent initial losses of approximately 8.7 kg after 5 months of weekly sessions. At 17 months, the mean losses from baseline were 10.8, 5.9, and 4.1 kg for the PST, RPT, and control conditions, respectively. Only the difference between PST and the behavioral control treatment was statistically significant at 17 months. These findings suggest extended care utilizing the application of PST (but not RPT) may enhance the long-term effects of behavioral treatment, compared to initial behavioral treatment without extended care. The focus of PST on developing solutions for the immediate challenges facing participants may enhance its salience and effectiveness. An advantage of PST is that it allows the interventionist to assist participants in developing ways to deal with problems in all spheres of their lives, including family stresses, coping with other illnesses, dealing with depression, and interacting with treatment providers, as well as issues that represent impediments to weight loss progress (Perri, Nezu, & Viegener, 1992).

Motivation-Focused Extended Care

West et al. (2011) examined the effectiveness of a motivation-focused extended-care program in comparison with skill-based extended care group and a no-treatment control group. Participants in the two active conditions completed 6 months of standard behavioral treatment before beginning 12 months of extended care. The skill-based program focused on PST and RPT, whereas the motivation-focused intervention incorporated strategies designed to strengthen participants' satisfaction with weight loss and to cultivate an identity as a successful weight loser. At an 18-month follow-up, equivalent mean reductions from baseline were observed for the motivation-focused and skill-based conditions (M's = 5.3 and 5.2 kg, respectively), and both were significantly larger than the reduction for the control condition (M = 1.4 kg). Most extended-care programs focus on teaching participants the skills needed to cope with weight-related challenges that arise after the initial weight loss phase of treatment. However, the findings of West et al. (2011) demonstrate that motivation-focused maintenance programs may produce benefits equivalent to skill-based extended-care regimens, thereby providing options in the approach to extended care.

Maintenance-Tailored Treatment

Jeffery and colleagues compared the effects of manipulating both the *schedule* and *content* of treatment sessions to standard behavioral treatment in an effort to enhance maintenance of lost weight (Jeffery et al., 2009; Levy et al., 2010). In *maintenance-tailored treatment* (MTT), the investigators delivered the intervention in six units, each of which was 8 weeks long and devoted to a specific theme (e.g., caloric intake goals, exercise, diet composition). This alternative schedule was designed to alleviate the potential monotony associated with the schedule of 24 weekly sessions followed by 12 every-other-week and then 6 monthly sessions typically used in standard behavioral treatment. To further enhance variety, MTT participants were prescribed alternating 2-week periods with and without caloric restriction (e.g.,

TABLE 23.2. Studies of Behavioral Treatment with Extended Care or Maintenance Programs

Study Author (year)	Sample N	Baseline M BMI (kg/m²)	Intervention content and outcomes				
			Treatment conditions	Posttreatment (mos. from baseline)	M weight change from baseline to posttreatment (kg)	Follow-up (mos. from baseline)	Retention at follow-up (%)	M weight change from baseline to follow-up (kg)

Study Author (year)	Sample N	Baseline M BMI (kg/m²)	Treatment conditions	Posttreatment (mos. from baseline)	M weight change from baseline to posttreatment (kg)	Follow-up (mos. from baseline)	Retention at follow-up (%)	M weight change from baseline to follow-up (kg)
Cussler et al. (2008)	13	31.0	BT + Internet behavioral maint.	4	−5.3 (SD = 3.6)	16	79	~ −4.9 (SD = 4.3)
	5	30.4	BT + no posttreatment contact		−5.2 (SD = 3.8)		86	~ −4.6 (SD = 3.9)
Harvey-Berino et al. (2002)	12	31.5	BT + frequent FtF maint.	6	−9.8 (SD = 5.9)	18	~76	−10.4 (SD = 6.3)[a]
	2	32.8	BT + minimal FtF maint.		−11.0 (SD = 6.5)			−10.4 (SD = 9.3)[a]
		32.2	BT + Internet maint.		−8.0 (SD = 5.0)			−5.7 (SD = 5.9)[b]
Harvey-Berino et al. (2004)	23	28.9	BT + frequent FtF maint.	6	−7.6 (SD = 5.0)	18	79	−3.9 (SD = 5.9)
	2	29.0	BT + minimal FtF maint.		−7.6 (SD = 4.9)		80	−4.2 (SD = 7.9)
		29.3	BT + Internet maint.		−8.4 (SD = 6.1)		67	−4.7 (SD = 6.9)
Jeffery et al. (2009)	213	35.2	BT	6	−7.4 (SD = 3.9)[a]	18	74	−9.3 (SD = 8.8)
		34.6	Maint.-tailored BT		−5.7 (SD = 5.0)[b]		75	−8.3 (SD = 8.9)
Levy et al. (2010)			BT			30	74	~ −5.8
			Maint.-tailored BT				71	~ −5.8
Perri et al. (2001)	80	35.0	BT + RPT	5	−9.1 (SD = 5.0)	17	68	−5.9 (SD = 6.4)[a, b]
		36.1	BT + PST		−8.4 (SD = 4.7)		71	−10.8 (SD = 8.7)[b]
		36.4	BT + no posttreatment contact		−8.9 (SD = 4.8)		83	−4.1 (SD = 4.9)[a]
Perri et al. (2008)	234	36.9	BT + phone ExtCare	6	−9.4 (SE = 0.6)	18	97	−8.2 (SE = 0.7)[a]
		37.1	BT + FtF ExtCare		−10.1 (SE = 0.6)		90	−8.9 (SE = 0.6)[a]
		36.2	BT + mail ExtCare		−10.5 (SE = 0.6)		95	−6.8 (SE = 0.7)[b]
Svetkey et al. (2008)	1032	34.2	BT + interactive technology maint.	12	~ −5.5	36	93	−3.3 (SE = 0.4)[a]
		34.2	BT + FtF maint.		~ −7.5		94	−4.2 (SE = 0.4)[b]
		34.0	BT + self-directed control maint.		~ −7.5		94	−2.9 (SE = 0.4)[a]
West et al. (2011)	338	~36.0	BT + FtF motivation-based ExtCare	6	−7.8 (CI: −9.1, −6.6)[a]	18	91	−5.3 (CI: −7.0, −3.7)[a]
		~36.0	BT + FtF skilled-based ExtCare		−7.6 (CI: −9.3, −6.0)[a]		87	−5.2 (CI: −7.2, −3.2)[a]
		~36.0	Education control		−1.5 (CI: −2.6, −0.4)[b]		79	−1.4 (CI: −3.1, 0.3)[b]

Note. Differing letters next to means represent significant between-group differences at posttreatment or follow-up, $p < .05$. M, mean; BMI, body mass index; mos, months; BT, standard behavioral treatment for obesity; Maint., maintenance program; SD, standard deviation; FtF, face-to-face treatment; SE, standard error; CI, 95 confidence interval; RPT, relapse prevention training; PST, problem-solving training; ExtCare, extended-care treatment.

[a]Significant between-group differences compared to groups with superscript b, $p < .05$.
[b]Significant between-group differences compared to groups with superscript a, $p < .05$.

1,000–2,300 kcal/day). Mean weight reductions were equivalent across treatment conditions at the 6-, 12-, and 18-month assessments. However, the MTT group showed a trend toward smaller weight regain than the standard behavioral treatment group between 18 and 30 months (M's = 2.8 vs. 4.4 kg regained, respectively, p = .078). MTT may make extended-care programs more interesting and attractive to many participants, which may improve treatment satisfaction and *potentially* improve weight loss outcomes.

Extended Care via Telephone Counseling

Perri et al. (2008) examined the effects of extended care delivered via individual telephone contacts or face-to-face group sessions versus a comparison group that received advice on weight maintenance via newsletters delivered by mail. All three treatment groups completed an initial 6-month standard behavioral treatment program before being randomly assigned to a 12-month extended-care program delivered by phone, face-to-face, or mail. The mean 6-month loss across all participants completing initial behavioral treatment was ~10 kg, with no differences between groups prior to the extended-care phase. At the 18-month assessment, both the face-to-face intervention and the telephone program showed significantly better maintenance of weight loss than the program delivered by mail. On average, participants in the telephone extended-care program achieved a level of maintenance that was virtually identical to the face-to-face condition (87 vs. 88% of initial loss maintained, respectively) and significantly greater than the newsletter comparison group (65% of initial loss maintained). Furthermore, the costs of extended care delivered via telephone were significantly lower than the costs for face-to-face sessions.

Extended Care via the Internet

Easy access and continuous availability make the Internet a potentially valuable medium for long-term weight control programs. Harvey-Berino et al. (2002) randomized participants who received an identical 24 weeks of in-person behavioral treatment (and achieved mean reductions of 9.5 kg) to one of three 12-month maintenance programs: Internet support (26 every-other-week chat sessions), in-person support (26 every-other-week sessions), or minimal in-person support (6 in-person monthly sessions followed by no further contact). Both in-person groups sustained losses of 10.4 kg, which were significantly larger than the Internet support group's loss of 5.7 kg. However, in a subsequent study with a similar experimental design, Harvey-Berino and colleagues failed to replicate these findings (Harvey-Berino, Pintauro, Buzzell, & Gold, 2004). Similarly, after 4 months of behavioral treatment that produced mean reductions of approximately 5 kg, Cussler et al. (2008) randomized participants to either an Internet-based maintenance program or a self-directed control group. Over the course of a 12-month follow-up period, study completers in the Internet and control conditions experienced minimal regains (0.4 and 0.6 kg, respectively), and the between-group difference was not significant.

In the largest trial (N = 1,032) of weight loss maintenance programs, Svetkey et al. (2008) compared the effects of (1) unlimited access to an interactive Internet-based program for weight management, (2) monthly personal contacts (primarily 10- to 15-minute phone calls with an interventionist), and (3) a self-directed control condition. Eligibility for randomization required achievement of a weight loss of 4 kg or more during a 6-month weight loss phase that preceded the 30-month maintenance phase of the trial. The mean initial weight loss of the randomized participants was 8.5 kg. All groups regained weight over the 30 months of the study. The means for percentages of initial weight loss maintained were 35%, 39%, and 53% for the self-directed, Internet, and personal contact conditions, respectively. The personal contact condition demonstrated significantly better maintenance than both the Internet and self-directed conditions, and the Internet program failed to show a weight loss maintenance benefit compared to the control condition. The findings from Svetkey et al. (2008) highlight the unfulfilled promise of Internet technology as a means of fostering successful maintenance of weight loss. However, as noted earlier, supplementing the initial weeks of Internet programs with face-to-face support or providing small monetary incentives may be fruitful additions to help realize the potential of web-based interventions (Leahey et al., 2015).

Conclusions

Have we made progress over the past 15 years in the long-term behavioral management of obesity? The answer is a qualified "yes." Decades of research on the development of an intervention model and behavioral treatment strategies, tested in smaller studies, contributed to the comprehensive lifestyle treatment that produced good long-term outcomes in the Look AHEAD Study (Look AHEAD Research Group, 2006). Indeed, the intensive lifestyle program in Look AHEAD was light years ahead of the first and second generations of behavioral treatment for obesity. In addition to core behavioral procedures of goal setting, self-monitoring, and stimulus control, the Look AHEAD intervention included cognitive-behavioral techniques, motivational strategies, problem solving, group competitions, a strong exercise component, partial meal replacements, and a "toolbox" of assorted techniques to enhance maintenance. Perhaps most importantly, the intervention adopted a *continuous care* model of treatment (Perri et al., 1993) with ongoing contacts conducted throughout the entire study. Look AHEAD achieved good long-term maintenance of weight loss. After 1 year, participants had lost a mean of 8.6% of their initial body weight and, over the course of 8 years, they succeeded in maintaining on average 55% of their initial losses (Look AHEAD Research Group, 2014).

Over the past 15 years, we have also learned much about strategies that do and do not work. Among the approaches that seemed promising but have not (yet) come to fruition are modification to the home environment (Gorin et al., 2013) and limitations on the variety of foods consumed (Raynor et al., 2012). Minor accomplishments include findings that suggest that smaller groups may produce bigger weight losses than larger groups (Dutton et al., 2014) and that moderate doses of treatment may produce outcomes comparable to higher doses of behavioral treatment (Perri et al., 2014). We have learned that exercise often does not improve initial weight loss but is routinely associated with better long-term outcomes (Jakicic et al., 2008; Tate et al., 2007). We have found that more restrictive caloric intake goals may not lead to greater losses in the long run but may help more people achieve clinically meaningful reductions (Nackers et al., 2013). We have learned that diets consisting of different macronutrient contents produce similar long-term reductions (Foster et al., 2010; Sacks et al., 2009). We have seen that therapies based on alternative cognitive-behavioral treatments delivered *outside* the context of continuous care do not improve long-term weight losses (Cooper et al., 2010), and we have learned that the promise of the Internet as an effective means of long-term weight management remains largely unfulfilled (Svetkey et al., 2008).

Nonetheless, we have also identified several promising avenues for future research. We have seen intriguing results suggesting that training in maintenance skills before, rather than after, initial weight loss may boost long-term success (Kiernan et al., 2013). Moreover, we have seen clear indications that behavioral treatment can be successfully administered via telephone counseling for both the induction and maintenance of weight loss (Appel et al., 2011; Perri et al., 2008), and that telephone counseling can be accomplished in a more cost-effective manner than face-to-face sessions (Donnelly et al., 2013).

All in all, although there has been no single breakthrough to solve the maintenance problem, we have witnessed substantial *incremental* progress. What we have learned over the past 15 years has increased our understanding of strategies and tactics that decrease the risk of weight regain. Equipped with this knowledge, we are better prepared to approach the next 15 years with new insights and promising leads toward improving the long-term management of obesity.

References

American College of Sports Medicine. (2009). American College of Sports Medicine Position Stand: Appropriate physical activity intervention strategies for weight loss and prevention of weight regain for adults. *Medicine and Science in Sports and Exercise, 41*(2), 459–471.

Andersson, I., & Rossner, S. (1997). Weight development, drop-out pattern and changes in obesity-related risk factors after two years treatment of obese men. *International Journal of Obesity and Related Metabolic Disorders, 21*(3), 211–216.

Appel, L. J., Clark, J. M., Yeh, H. C., Wang, N. Y., Coughlin, J. W., Daumit, G., et al. (2011). Comparative effectiveness of weight loss interventions in clinical practice. *New England Journal of Medicine, 365*(21), 1959–1968.

Bandura, A. (1991). Social cognitive theory of self-regulation. *Organizational Behavior and Human Decision Processes, 50*(2), 248–287.

Butryn, M. L., Webb, V., & Wadden, T. A. (2011). Behavioral treatment of obesity. *Psychiatric Clinics of North America, 34*(4), 841–859.

Carels, R. A., Darby, L. A., Douglass, O. M., Cacciapaglia, H. M., & Rydin, S. (2005). Education on the glycemic index of foods fails to improve treatment outcomes in a behavioral weight loss program. *Eating Behaviors, 6*(2), 145–150.

Chow, S. C. (2014). Adaptive clinical trial design. *Annual Review of Medicine, 65*(1), 405–415.

Cooper, Z., Doll, H. A., Hawker, D. M., Byrne, S., Bonner, G., Eeley, E., et al. (2010). Testing a new cognitive behavioural treatment for obesity: A randomized controlled trial with three-year follow-up. *Behaviour Research and Therapy, 48*(8), 706–713.

Cooper, Z., & Fairburn, C. G. (2001). A new cognitive behavioural approach to the treatment of obesity. *Behaviour Research and Therapy, 39*(5), 499–511.

Cussler, E. C., Teixeira, P. J., Going, S. B., Houtkooper, L. B., Metcalfe, L. L., Blew, R. M., et al. (2008). Maintenance of weight loss in overweight middle-aged women through the Internet. *Obesity, 16*(5), 1052–1060.

Diabetes Prevention Program Research Group. (2002). The Diabetes Prevention Program (DPP) description of lifestyle intervention. *Diabetes Care, 25*(12), 2165–2171.

Donnelly, J. E., Goetz, J., Gibson, C., Sullivan, D. K., Lee, R., Smith, B. K., et al. (2013). Equivalent weight loss for weight management programs delivered by phone and clinic. *Obesity, 21*(10), 1951–1959.

Drewnowski, A., & Rolls, B. J. (2005). How to modify the food environment. *Journal of Nutrition, 135*(4), 898–899.

Dutton, G. R., Nackers, L. M., Dubyak, P. J., Rushing, N. C., Huynh, T. V. T., Tan, F., et al. (2014). A randomized trial comparing weight loss treatment delivered in large versus small groups. *International Journal of Behavioral Nutrition and Physical Activity, 11*, 123–133.

Ferster, C. B., Nurnberger, J. I., & Levitt, E. B. (1996). The control of eating: 1962. *Obesity Research, 4*(4), 401–410.

Foster, G. D., Wyatt, H. R., Hill, J. O., Makris, A. P., Rosenbaum, D. L., Brill, C., et al. (2010). Weight and metabolic outcomes after 2 years on a low-carbohydrate versus low-fat diet: A randomized trial. *Annals of Internal Medicine, 153*(3), 147–157.

Foster-Schubert, K. E., Alfano, C. M., Duggan, C. R., Xiao, L., Campbell, K. L., Kong, A., et al. (2012). Effect of diet and exercise, alone or combined, on weight and body composition in overweight-to-obese postmenopausal women. *Obesity, 20*(8), 1628–1638.

Fuglestad, P. T., Rothman, A. J., & Jeffery, R. W. (2008). Getting there and hanging on: The effect of regulatory focus on performance in smoking and weight loss interventions. *Health Psychology, 27*(3S), S260–S270.

Goodpaster, B. H., DeLany, J. P., Otto, A. D., Kuller, L., Vockley, J., South-Paul, J. E., et al. (2010). Effects of diet and physical activity interventions on weight loss and cardiometabolic risk factors in severely obese adults: A randomized trial. *Journal of the American Medical Association, 304*(16), 1795–1802.

Gorin, A. A., Raynor, H. A., Fava, J., Maguire, K., Robichaud, E., Trautvetter, J., et al. (2013). Randomized controlled trial of a comprehensive home environment-focused weight loss program for adults. *Health Psychology, 32*(2), 128–137.

Harvey-Berino, J., Pintauro, S., Buzzell, P., DiGiulio, M., Gold, B. C., Moldovan, C., et al. (2002). Does using the Internet facilitate the maintenance of weight loss? *International Journal of Obesity and Related Metabolic Disorders, 26*(9), 1254–1261.

Harvey-Berino, J., Pintauro, S., Buzzell, P., & Gold, E. C. (2004). Effect of Internet support on the long-term maintenance of weight loss. *Obesity Research, 12*(2), 320–329.

Hsu, A., & Blandford, A. (2014). Designing for psychological change: Individuals' reward and cost valuations in weight management. *Journal of Medical Internet Research, 16*(6), e138.

Jakicic, J. M., Marcus, B. H., Lang, W., & Janney, C. (2008). Effect of exercise on 24-month weight loss maintenance in overweight women. *Archives of Internal Medicine, 168*(14), 1550–1559.

Jeffery, R. W., French, S. A., & Schmid, T. L. (1990). Attributions for dietary failures: Problems reported by participants in the Hypertension Prevention Trial. *Health Psychology, 9*(3), 315–329.

Jeffery, R. W., Levy, R. L., Langer, S. L., Welsh, E. M., Flood, A. P., Jaeb, M. A., et al. (2009). A comparison of maintenance-tailored therapy (MTT) and standard behavior therapy (SBT) for the treatment of obesity. *Preventive Medicine, 49*(5), 384–389.

Jeffery, R. W., Wing, R. R., Sherwood, N. E., & Tate, D. F. (2003). Physical activity and weight loss: Does prescribing higher physical activity goals improve outcome? *American Journal of Clinical Nutrition, 78*(4), 684–689.

Jeffery, R. W., Wing, R. R., Thorsen, C., Burton, L. R., Raether, C., Harvey, J., et al. (1993). Strengthening behavioral interventions for weight loss: A randomized trial for food provision and monetary incentives. *Journal of Consulting and Clinical Psychology, 61*(6), 1038–1045.

Jensen, M. D., Ryan, D. H., Apovian, C. M., Ard, J. D., Comuzzie, A. G., Donato, K. A., et al. (2014). 2013 AHA/ACC/TOS guidelines for the management of overweight and obesity in adults: A report of the American College of Cardiology/American Heart Association Task Force on Practice Guidelines and The Obesity Society. *Circulation, 129*(25, Suppl. 2), S102–S138.

Johns, D. J., Hartmann-Boyce, J., Jebb, S. A., & Aveyard, P. (2014). Diet or exercise interventions vs. combined behavioral weight management programs: A systematic review and meta-analysis of direct comparisons. *Journal of the Academy of Nutrition and Dietetics, 114*(10), 1557–1568.

Johnston, B. C., Kanters, S., Bandayrel, K., Wu, P., Naji, F., Siemieniuk, R. A., et al. (2014). Comparison of weight loss among named diet programs in overweight and obese adults: A meta-analysis. *Journal of the American Medical Association, 312*(9), 923–933.

Kalarchian, M. A., Levine, M. D., Klem, M. L., Burke, L. E., Soulakova, J. N., & Marcus, M. D. (2011). Impact of addressing reasons for weight loss on behavioral weight control outcome. *American Journal of Preventive Medicine, 40*(1), 18–24.

Kanfer, F. H. (1970). Self-regulation: Research, issues, and speculations. In C. Neuringer & J. L. Michael (Eds.), *Behavior modification in clinical psychology* (pp. 178–220). New York: Appleton-Century-Crofts.

Kiernan, M., Brown, S. D., Schoffman, D. E., Lee, K., King, A. C., Taylor, C. B., et al. (2013). Promoting healthy weight with "stability skills first": A randomized trial. *Journal of Consulting and Clinical Psychology, 81*(2), 336–346.

Leahey, T. M., Subak, L. L., Fava, J., Schembri, M., Thomas, G., Xu, X., et al. (2015). Benefits of adding small financial incentives or optional group meetings to a web-based statewide obesity initiative. *Obesity, 23*(1), 70–76.

Levy, R. L., Jeffery, R. W., Langer, S. L., Graham, D. J., Welsh, E. M., Flood, A. P., et al. (2010). Maintenance-tailored therapy vs. standard behavior therapy for 30-month maintenance of weight loss. *Preventive Medicine, 51*(6), 457–459.

Look AHEAD Research Group. (2006). The Look AHEAD study: A description of the lifestyle intervention and the evidence supporting it. *Obesity, 14*(5), 737–752.

Look AHEAD Research Group. (2010). Long-term effects of a lifestyle intervention on weight and cardiovascular risk factors in individuals with type 2 diabetes mellitus: Four-year results of the Look AHEAD trial. *Archives of Internal Medicine, 170*(17), 1566–1575.

Look AHEAD Research Group. (2014). Eight-year weight losses with an intensive lifestyle intervention: The Look AHEAD study. *Obesity, 22*(1), 5–13.

Lutes, L. D., DiNatale, E., Goodrich, D. E., Ronis, D. L., Gillon, L., Kirsh, S., et al. (2013). A randomized trial of a small changes approach for weight loss in veterans: Design, rationale, and baseline characteristics of the ASPIRE-VA trial. *Contemporary Clinical Trials, 34*(1), 161–172.

MacLean, P. S., Wing, R. R., Davidson, T., Epstein, L., Goodpaster, B., Hall, K. D., et al. (2015). NIH working group report: Innovative research to improve maintenance of weight loss. *Obesity, 23*(1), 7–15.

Micco, N., Gold, B. C., Buzzell, P., Leonard, H., Burke, S., Pintauro, S., et al. (2007). Minimal in-person support as an adjunct to Internet obesity treatment. *Annals of Behavioral Medicine, 33*(1), 49–56.

Nackers, L. M., Middleton, K. R., Dubyak, P. J., Daniels, M. J., Anton, S. D., & Perri, M. G. (2013). Effects of prescribing 1,000 versus 1,500 kilocalories per day in the behavioral treatment of obesity: A randomized trial. *Obesity, 21*(12), 2481–2487.

Perri, M. G., & Corsica, J. A. (2002). Improving the maintenance of weight lost in behavioral treatment of obesity. In T. A. Wadden & A. J. Stunkard (Eds.), *Handbook of obesity treatment* (pp. 357–379). New York: Guilford Press.

Perri, M. G., Limacher, M. C., Castel-Roberts, K., Daniels, M. J., Durning, P. E., Janicke, D. M., et al. (2014). Comparative effectiveness of three doses of weight loss counseling: Two-year findings from the Rural LITE trial. *Obesity, 22*(11), 2293–2300.

Perri, M. G., Limacher, M. C., Durning, P. E., Janicke, D. M., Lutes, L. D., Bobroff, L. B., et al. (2008). Extended-care programs for weight management in rural communities: The treatment of obesity in underserved rural settings (TOURS) randomized trial. *Archives of Internal Medicine, 168*(21), 2347–2354.

Perri, M. G., McAdoo, W. G., McAllister, D. A., Lauer, J. B., Jordan, R. C., Yancey, D. Z., et al. (1987). Effects of peer support and therapist contact on long-term weight loss. *Journal of Consulting and Clinical Psychology, 55*(4), 615–617.

Perri, M. G., McAdoo, W. G., McAllister, D. A., Lauer, J. B., & Yancey, D. Z. (1986). Enhancing the efficacy of behavior therapy for obesity: Effects of aerobic exercise and a multicomponent maintenance program. *Journal of Consulting and Clinical Psychology, 54*(4), 670–675.

Perri, M. G., McAdoo, W. G., Spevak, P. A., & Newlin, D. B. (1984). Effect of a multicomponent maintenance program on long-term weight loss. *Journal of Consulting and Clinical Psychology, 52*(3), 480–481.

Perri, M. G., McAllister, D. A., Gange, J. J., Jordan, R. C., McAdoo, W. G., & Nezu, A. M. (1988). Effects of four maintenance programs on the long-term management of obesity. *Journal of Consulting and Clinical Psychology, 56*(4), 529–534.

Perri, M. G., Nezu, A. M., McKelvey, W. F., Shermer, R. L., Renjilian, D. A., & Viegener, B. J. (2001). Relapse prevention training and problem-solving therapy in the long-term management of obesity. *Journal of Consulting and Clinical Psychology, 69*(4), 722–726.

Perri, M. G., Nezu, A. M., Patti, E. T., & McCann,

K. L. (1989). Effect of length of treatment on weight loss. *Journal of Consulting and Clinical Psychology, 57*(3), 450–452.

Perri, M. G., Nezu, A. M., & Viegener, B. J. (1992). *Improving the long-term management of obesity: Theory, research, and clinical guidelines.* New York: Wiley.

Perri, M. G., Sears, S. F., & Clark, J. E. (1993). Strategies for improving maintenance of weight loss: Toward a continuous care model of obesity management. *Diabetes Care, 16*(1), 200–209.

Perri, M. G., Shapiro, R. M., Ludwig, W. W., Twentyman, C. T., & McAdoo, W. G. (1984). Maintenance strategies for the treatment of obesity: An evaluation of relapse prevention training and posttreatment contact by mail and telephone. *Journal of Consulting and Clinical Psychology, 52*(3), 404–413.

Ratcliffe, D., & Ellison, N. (2015). Obesity and internalized weight stigma: A formulation model for an emerging psychological problem. *Behavioural and Cognitive Psychotherapy, 43*(2), 239–252.

Raynor, H. A., Looney, S. M., Steeves, E. A., Spence, M., & Gorin, A. A. (2012). The effects of an energy density prescription on diet quality and weight loss: A pilot randomized controlled trial. *Journal of the Academy of Nutrition and Dietetics, 112*(9), 1397–1402.

Rejeski, W. J., Focht, B. C., Messier, S. P., Morgan, T., Pahor, M., & Penninx, B. (2002). Obese, older adults with knee osteoarthritis: Weight loss, exercise, and quality of life. *Health Psychology, 21*(5), 419–426.

Rosenbaum, M., Hirsch, J., Gallagher, D. A., & Leibel, R. L. (2008). Long-term persistence of adaptive thermogenesis in subjects who have maintained a reduced body weight. *American Journal of Clinical Nutrition, 88*(4), 906–912.

Sacks, F. M., Bray, G. A., Carey, V. J., Smith, S. R., Ryan, D. H., Anton, S. D., et al. (2009). Comparison of weight loss diets with different compositions of fat, protein, and carbohydrates. *New England Journal of Medicine, 360*(9), 859–873.

Svetkey, L. P., Stevens, V. J., Brantley, P. J., Appel, L. J., Hollis, J. F., Loria, C. M., et al. (2008). Comparison of strategies for sustaining weight loss: The Weight Loss Maintenance randomized controlled trial. *Journal of the American Medical Association, 299*(10), 1139–1148.

Tate, D. F., Jeffery, R. W., Sherwood, N. E., & Wing, R. R. (2007). Long-term weight losses associated with prescription of higher physical activity goals: Are higher levels of physical activity protective against weight regain? *American Journal of Clinical Nutrition, 85*(4), 954–959.

Tate, D. F., Wing, R. R., & Winett, R. A. (2001). Using Internet technology to deliver a behavioral weight loss program. *Journal of the American Medical Association, 285*(9), 1172–1177.

Villareal, D. T., Chode, S., Parimi, N., Sinacore, D. R., Hilton, T., Armamento-Villareal, R., et al. (2011). Weight loss, exercise, or both and physical function in obese older adults. *New England Journal of Medicine, 364*(13), 1218–1229.

West, D. S., Gorin, A. A., Subak, L. L., Foster, G., Bragg, C., Hecht, J., et al. (2011). A motivation-focused weight loss maintenance program is an effective alternative to a skill-based approach. *International Journal of Obesity, 35*(2), 259–269.

PART VI
Additional Approaches to and Resources for the Treatment of Obesity

CHAPTER 24

The Emerging Field of Obesity Medicine

Robert F. Kushner
Scott Kahan

Obesity medicine is an emerging field in health care. Previously called *bariatrics,* a shift in nomenclature to *obesity medicine* has occurred to coincide with other newly recognized disciplines, such as addiction medicine and exercise medicine. Furthermore, the term *bariatrics* was often associated with practitioners who dispensed non-evidence-based or unregulated treatments. In contrast, the surgeons who perform weight loss surgery have embraced the name *metabolic and bariatric surgery* and continue to be identified as bariatric surgeons.

The deluge of knowledge and new science in obesity over the past 20 years has helped to propel this field forward. With the recognition of obesity as a chronic medical condition like diabetes or coronary heart disease, this new field of medicine is gaining wider acceptance. Yet despite the publication of multiple guidelines and recommendations regarding assessment and treatment, few physicians feel that they are successful in helping patients with obesity lose weight (Bleich, Bennett, Gudzune, & Cooper, 2012). Multiple barriers exist that present challenges to the provision of obesity care; one is the perceived need for improved medical education related to obesity. Although the entire medical community would benefit from achieving an increased competency in care for persons with obesity, a pathway has been established to recognize physicians who have chosen to become more educated in obesity and to focus their practice on the treatment of patients with obesity. They can become Diplomates of the American Board of Obesity Medicine. In this chapter, we briefly review the recommendations and guidelines for the screening and treatment of obesity, the current provision of obesity care, the barriers to practice among primary care providers, and the creation of the obesity medicine specialist.

Recommendations and Guidelines for Screening and Treatment

There has been an emergence of clinical guidance for adult obesity treatment, both in the form of evidence-based clinical guidelines and in practical consensus recommendations (Table 24.1). Clear, science-based guidelines are particularly important in the field of obesity management, where confusion, dogmatic beliefs, and dueling practices are common.

The first obesity management guidelines, published by the National Heart, Lung, and

TABLE 24.1. Guidelines and Recommendations for the Assessment and Management of Obesity

	AHA/ACC/TOS	Endo	AACE	OMA	USPSTF	Dietary Guidelines for Americans	Physical Activity Guidelines for Americans
Primary target audience	Primary care providers	Primary care providers and specialists	Endocrinologists	Obesity medicine practitioners	Primary care providers	Public	Public
Process	Systematic review, primarily RCTs	Systematic review and expert consensus	Systematic review and expert consensus	Expert and member consensus	Systematic review	Systematic review and expert consensus	Systematic review and expert consensus
Focus	Obesity assessment and treatment	Obesity pharmacotherapy	Obesity assessment and treatment	Obesity assessment and treatment	Obesity screening and counseling	Dietary intake	Physical activity

Note. AHA/ACC/TOS, American Heart Association/American College of Cardiology/The Obesity Society; Endo, Endocrine Society; AACE, American Association of Clinical Endocrinology; OMA, Obesity Medical Association; USPSTF, U.S. Preventive Services Task Force; RCTs, randomized controlled trials.

Blood Institute (NHLBI) in 1998, filled a critical void for obesity medicine and established many of the best-practice recommendations that continue to be used today (Pi-Sunyer et al., 1998). However, these guidelines were limited, did not adhere to evidence-based guideline development, and were not kept updated. In recent years, several guidelines and recommendations have been published to extend the initial NHLBI guidelines. Most notably, updated, evidence-based guidelines published by the American Heart Association (AHA), American College of Cardiology (ACC), and The Obesity Society (TOS; Jensen et al., 2014), and those published by the Endocrine Society (Apovian et al., 2016) and the American Association of Clinical Endocrinologists (AACE; Garvey et al., 2016) offer authoritative recommendations for clinical obesity practice.

Published 15 years after the initial NHLBI guidelines, the 2013 AHA/ACC/TOS *Guideline for the Management of Overweight and Obesity in Adults,* originally launched by NHLBI and disseminated by the three societies, provides in-depth guidance on five key areas of weight management and obesity treatment (Jensen et al., 2014). The guidelines were developed based on high-level systematic literature reviews, guided by strict criteria for acceptability of studies, with a primary focus on (1) randomized controlled trials; (2) graded recommendations; and (3) specific, a priori-defined outcomes, inclusion and exclusion criteria, populations, and subgroups. They adhere to the Institute of Medicine's (IOM) criteria for the development of guidelines (Graham, Mancher, Miller Wolman, Greenfield, & Steinberg, 2011). The central findings and recommendations include:

- Use body mass index (BMI) as a first-line screening tool for weight status classification.
- Initial goal of treatment is a moderate weight loss of 5–10% of initial body weight, with evidence that as little as 3–5% weight loss leads to improvements in risk factors.
- Caloric reduction should be the primary objective of all diets, with dietary composition based on personal preference and potential for comorbidity improvement; no single diet is clearly superior.
- Intensive, multicomponent lifestyle counseling should be offered to patients, including access to at least 14 sessions over the initial 6 months and long-term follow-up for at least a year.
- Bariatric surgery should be considered in appropriate patient candidates with severe obesity.

Though scientifically rigorous and in-depth, a clear limitation of the AHA/ACC/TOS guideline is its limited scope. It focuses on just five key questions out of 23 initially proposed, due to the expense, time, and difficulty that covering additional topics would require. Moreover, the guideline focuses on the highest threshold of evidence for the recommendations, primarily randomized controlled trials of relatively long duration (> 6 months) and high subject retention. For this reason, much of the published literature is excluded, including most observational research and studies of self-reported outcomes. Notably absent are recommendations on pharmacotherapy, behavioral medicine, and physical activity.

To expand on these recommendations, several other guidelines have been created. In 2015, the Endocrine Society published clinical practice guidelines focused on obesity pharmacotherapy to fill a key gap in the AHA/ACC/TOS guidelines. The *Pharmacological Management of Obesity* guidelines focus on systematic reviews of evidence for pharmacotherapy options and prescribing practices, but also include broader suggestions on best clinical practices based on expert consensus (Apovian et al., 2016). "Recommendations" in the guidelines are based on high-quality evidence, whereas clinical "suggestions" are based on consensus opinion. Core recommendations include the following:

- Prescribe pharmacotherapy for obesity as an adjunct to diet, exercise, and behavior modification for individuals with BMI > 30 kg/m^2 or > 27 kg/m^2 with at least one comorbidity; for individuals who are unable to lose or successfully maintain weight loss; and for individuals who meet label indications.
- Continue pharmacotherapy if the patient has lost at least 5% of initial body weight

within 3 months of use; if not, discontinue and seek alternative approaches.
- In patients with uncontrolled hypertension and/or history of cardiovascular disease (CVD), do not use sympathomimetic agents.
- Use weight-losing and weight-neutral medications as first- and second-line therapies and discuss potential weight gain effects of medications with patients.
- Use a shared decision-making process in selecting medications, providing patients with estimates of the weight loss effects of each possible medication.

Additional clinical consensus recommendations from AACE and the Obesity Medicine Association (OMA) add to these evidence-based guidelines. The AACE obesity management algorithm was developed primarily for clinical endocrinology practice as part of a broader set of diabetes prevention and treatment guidelines (Garvey et al., 2014). The AACE process accepted a broader range of evidence, including observational data and expert opinion, and did not explicitly grade the strength of recommendations. An updated iteration focuses explicitly on obesity, independent of diabetes prevention, and includes evidence grading (Garvey et al., 2016). A notable difference of the AACE guidelines is the explicit recommendation for complication-centric assessment. The presence of obesity comorbidities, in addition to anthropometric measures such as BMI, guides treatment indication, intensification, and goals, with the intent of targeting the most aggressive treatments to those who might derive the highest benefit. The OMA obesity algorithm, essentially a "toolkit" for obesity-focused and primary care clinicians, is the most inclusive of the recently published guidelines (Seger et al., 2016). This algorithm is not intended as an objective evidence review, but rather as a broad, practical, expert-opinion-based overview of obesity medicine concepts. In contrast to the other guidelines, it is descriptive (i.e., "Here are the options") rather than prescriptive (i.e., "Do this"). For example, it lists benefits and weaknesses of several body weight classifications (e.g., BMI, waist circumference, body composition) but does not offer authoritative recommendations or hierarchical grading of evidence for their use.

In addition to these clinical guidelines, the U.S. Preventive Services Task Force (USPSTF) has offered its own recommendations for treatment of obesity. The USPSTF is an independent panel appointed by the Department of Health and Human Services' Agency for Healthcare Research and Quality (AHRQ) to provide recommendations for preventive services in primary care based on robust systematic reviews. It published strong recommendations to screen all adults for obesity and offer intensive, multicomponent, behavioral intervention for those individuals (Moyer et al., 2012). Coverage of USPSTF recommended services is required by the Affordable Care Act. Further, broad, science-based recommendations on dietary intake, via the 2015 Dietary Guidelines for Americans (U.S. Department of Health and Human Services & U.S. Department of Agriculture, 2015), and physical activity, via the "2008 Physical Activity Guidelines for Americans" (U.S. Department of Health and Human Services, 2008), offer additional guidance for practitioners and patients on behavioral goals relevant to obesity management.

Although there are some differences between the published guidelines, these are dwarfed by overwhelming agreement. Several general concepts are consistent among the guidelines:

- Obesity is a chronic disease requiring long-term management.
- Patients should be appropriately screened for obesity.
- Practitioners should understand and be prepared to address obesity using a collaborative, shared decision-making approach.
- Use of appropriate treatment modalities should be considered, as indicated.
- Multicomponent interventions are preferred over individual treatments.

Current Provision of Obesity Care

Current practice and provision of obesity-related care, including screening, counseling, treatment, and documentation, are largely inconsistent with the published guidelines. Despite clear and uniform recommendations to measure weight status and screen for obesity, few patients receive these basic practices. For example, a 2013 analysis of electronic medical record (EMR) data from 25 primary care practices found that one-third of patients did not have BMI information recorded (Baer, Karson, Soukup, Williams, & Bates, 2013). Among those whose BMIs were recorded, only 17% of patients with a BMI > 25 kg/m² received a formal diagnosis of overweight, and just 30% of patients with BMI > 30 kg/m² had a formal obesity diagnosis documented in the EMR. Among 9,827 patients in a Mayo Clinic primary care data base, just 5% of all patients received a diagnosis of obesity, despite 26% having recorded BMIs greater than 30 kg/m² (Bardia, Holtan, Slezak, & Thompson, 2007). A 2011 NHANES analysis of 7,090 individuals showed that only 45% of patients with BMI > 25 kg/m² were told by a physician that they were overweight, and just 66% of patients with BMI > 30 kg/m² received a diagnosis of obesity (Post et al., 2011). Even those with severe and extreme obesity are frequently undiagnosed. A 2010 analysis of more than 6 million EMR records showed that fewer than 23% of individuals with BMI of 35–40 kg/m² received a formal obesity diagnosis, and 43% of patients with BMI > 50 kg/m² had no diagnosis (Crawford et al., 2010). Lastly, in a 2014 study of 33,718 patients receiving bariatric surgery, fewer than 40% had a documented *International Classification of Diseases*–9 (ICD-9) diagnosis of severe obesity (278.01) prior to surgery (Hatoum et al., 2016).

Similarly, provision of basic counseling for individuals with obesity is limited. In a study assessing 16 outpatient clinics, only 2% of patient discussions included mention of BMI, and only 1% mentioned waist circumference (Antognoli et al., 2014). Among 1,002 male firefighters surveyed, 69% of subjects overall and 48% of subjects with obesity reported never having received weight loss advice from their health care provider (Wilkinson et al., 2014). Although the likelihood of receiving weight loss advice increased with age and severity of obesity, just 67% of persons with BMI > 35 kg/m² received weight loss advice from their health care provider. Moreover, data from the National Ambulatory Medical Care Survey suggest that obesity counseling may be declining: Among 32,519 adult primary care visits, obesity counseling was provided in 7.8% of visits in 1995–1996 and in 6.2% of visits in 2007–2008 (Kraschnewski, Sciamanna, Pollak, Stuckey, & Sherwood, 2013). In 2012, just 4.9 visits per 100 persons, ages 20 and over, were for obesity, amounting to 2% of all visits by nonpregnant, nonpostpartum adults (Talwalkar & McCarty, 2016). Although obesity counseling is recommended in primary care and covered for Medicare beneficiaries, fewer than 10% of 1,000 primary care providers surveyed reported using the Current Procedural Terminology (CPT) code for obesity counseling (G0447; Petrin, Kahan, Turner, Gallagher, & Dietz, 2016).

One study that assessed content of obesity counseling discussions found that only 35% of weight-related conversations offered assessment and treatment recommendations consistent with those recommended by the initial NHLBI guidelines (Antognoli et al., 2014). A 2013 systematic review found that most physicians only prescribe one or two interventions to their patients, rather than offering counseling on the range of treatment options, and rarely refer to dietitians or obesity specialists (van Dillen, van Binsbergen, Koelene, & Hiddinka, 2013). The review found that current weight counseling fixates on general education, such as informing patients of the risks of obesity or the benefits of weight loss, rather than specific behavioral guidance. Counseling also tends to be overly confrontational, with little opportunity for collaboration or realistic goal setting, and is unlikely to promote actual lifestyle changes. Although nine medications are approved for obesity treatment, fewer than 2% of eligible patients with obesity receive pharmacotherapy for obesity as part of their management plan (Xian, Kelton, Guo, Bian, & Heaton, 2015; Zhang, Manne, Lin, & Yang, 2016). Most recently, a review of weight loss programs in a large metropolitan area found that 91% had low adherence to the AHA/ACC/TOS guidelines (Block, DeSalvo, & Fisher, 2016).

Barriers to Obesity Care

Numerous barriers to care underlie the disparities between guidelines and practice. Physicians primarily cite time limitations, insufficient reimbursement, and lack of training as barriers. A focus group of internal medicine, family medicine, obstetrics and gynecology (OB-GYN), pediatrics, and nurse practitioner providers cited payment as the top barrier to treatment for obesity. Other treatment barriers included time constraints, legal issues, perceived inconsistency between guidelines and available resources, and concern that discussions regarding weight might be offensive or be perceived as "lecturing" (Ayres & Griffith, 2007). Another focus group of general practitioners, nurse practitioners, and patients echoed these findings, particularly the difficulty of educating patients within a constrained time frame and a cumbersome referral process. Several physicians viewed obesity as a nonmedical issue that did not fall under the responsibility of the physician (Gunther, Guo, Sinfield, Rogers, & Baker, 2012). In a survey of 1,000 primary care providers, including family practitioners, internists, OB-GYN physicians, and nurse practitioners, the three greatest reported barriers to improved obesity counseling were time constraints, lack of training in obesity management, and limited reimbursement (Kahan & Zvenyach, 2016).

Among the barriers cited, lack of training in obesity management and related skills, including nutrition and physical activity counseling and behavioral medicine techniques, is one that requires particular attention. Fewer than 30% of medical schools meet the minimum National Academy of Sciences (NAS) recommended hours of education devoted to nutrition and physical activity. The time devoted to nutrition and physical activity education in medical schools has decreased from an average of 22.3 hours in 2004 to 19.6 hours in 2009 (Adams, Kohlmeier & Zeisel, 2010). A review of obesity coverage on medical licensing examinations showed that few obesity-specific test questions were included, and the vast majority of obesity-related questions were focused on obesity comorbidities rather than obesity science or management itself (Kushner et al., 2015). A survey of 290 primary care physicians conducted by the Strategies to Overcome and Prevent (STOP) Obesity Alliance found that 72% of those polled said that neither they nor anyone in their practice had any training in obesity diagnosis or management (STOP Obesity Alliance, 2010). Among 87 internal medicine residents, 60% did not know the basic BMI cutoff for diagnosing obesity; 69% did not recognize waist circumference as a reasonable measure of overweight/obesity; 39% incorrectly reported their own BMI; only 44% felt qualified to treat obesity; and 31% felt that obesity treatment was futile (Block et al., 2003). A survey of 315 academic faculty physicians and residents showed similar results, with 48% of practicing physicians being unable to adequately counsel patients about common obesity treatments (Jay et al., 2008). Among 500 primary care physicians polled in 2012, 48% felt that dietitians were more qualified to help patients with obesity, 41% believed that physicians were the most qualified to help, and 44% reported success in helping their patients with obesity lose weight (Bleich et al., 2012).

Concerns about time limitations and insufficient reimbursement are consistent with similar concerns related to provision of preventive services. A 2003 study estimated that it would take 7.4 hours per day to satisfy USPSTF recommended services in primary care (Yarnall, Pollak, Ostbye, Krause, & Michener, 2003). However, in the past few years, several policies have been introduced to increase the feasibility of primary care screening and management of obesity. In 2011, the Centers for Medicare and Medicaid Services issued a national determination memo to cover intensive obesity counseling in primary care settings, consistent with USPSTF guidelines and without cost-sharing (Centers for Medicare and Medicaid Services, 2011). The Affordable Care Act mandates coverage for obesity preventive services, including screening and counseling for obesity, though most plans do not cover obesity treatments such as weight loss programs, pharmacotherapy, and bariatric surgery (Kahan & Zvenyach, 2016). EMR incentive programs also support documentation of BMI and follow-up care for patients with obesity (Centers for Medicare and Medicaid Services, 2009). In 2013, the American Medical Association issued an official policy recognizing "obesity as a disease requiring a range of medical interventions to advance obesity treatment and prevention" (American Medical Association, 2013). In 2014, an official letter by the U.S. Office of Personnel Management, which is responsible for health insurance coverage for nearly 9 million Americans and serves as an important benchmark for private health plan coverage determinations, explicitly stated that obesity exclusions are no longer permissible in health plans (Office of Personnel Management, 2014). Unless overturned by Congress, these and other policy developments should improve access to and reimbursement for obesity counseling and other services, and also contribute to improved provision of care.

Creation of Obesity Medicine Specialists

Rationale

It is clear from the previous discussion that more needs to be done to increase the competency of physicians to provide obesity care. One integral aspect of increasing competency is improving the inadequate training that medical students, residents, and physicians receive during undergraduate, graduate, and postgraduate education, respectively. In 2007, the Association of American Medical Colleges (AAMC) published a Contemporary Issues in Medicine Report VIII statement, "The Prevention and Treatment of Overweight and Obesity" (Association of American Medical Colleges, 2007). The report concluded by stating:

> Medical education must assume that future physicians will be better prepared to provide respectful, effective care of overweight and obese patients and to appropriately participate in overweight/obesity prevention efforts. Education on assessing, preventing and treating overweight and obesity should be included in basic science, clinical experiences, and population health sciences.

Others have voiced similar recommendations, including a call for improved residency training (Colbert & Jangi, 2013). The American Academy of Pediatrics and the American Academy of Family Medicine have responded to the needs of their members and trainees with grant funding to residency programs to develop residency curricula for obesity (American Academy of Family Physicians, 2010). Additionally, obesity-related topics are increasingly included in many continuing medical education (CME) live conferences and specialty seminars, and provided as online durable materials (Obesity CE, 2016). However, despite the need to develop greater competency in obesity care and provision of evidence-based treatment modalities, implementation in the practice setting has been slow.

Development of the Obesity Medicine Specialty

Although a broad-based intervention is needed to adequately train current and future health care providers in the prevention and treatment of obesity, initiatives have begun to immediately meet this increased need. The rationale for developing certification in obesity medicine includes the following arguments:

- The increased prevalence and burden of overweight and obesity among U.S. adults and children present an important public health challenge that requires an expanded and dedicated physician work force (Flegal, Kruszon-Moran, Carroll, Fryar, & Ogden, 2016; Ogden et al., 2016).
- Obesity has recently been recognized as a chronic disease by several health care organizations including the American Medical Association (2013).
- Steep increases in severe, complicated, and recalcitrant obesity demand specialist referral options for intensive care.
- Certification would bring increased recognition and competency to the obesity field and may lay the foundation for improved reimbursement for obesity care.
- Offering a certification examination would increase the number of physicians choosing to train in obesity and/or seek obesity-related CME activities.
- Over the next decade, anticipated advances in pharmacotherapy and surgical procedures and devices for obesity care will require specialty training and expertise.
- There is an insufficient number of physicians to provide perioperative care for the increasing number of patients undergoing bariatric surgery and placement of intraluminal devices.
- Certified physicians can serve as clinical

and educational champions at local and national levels.

One of the first initiatives to create obesity specialization is the SCOPE (Specialist Certification in Obesity Professional Education) certification program, launched by the World Obesity Organization in 2003 and designed for all health professionals. According to its website, SCOPE's mission is to develop a coherent approach to obesity management through education and recognition of professional expertise in obesity and its management (World Obesity, 2016). SCOPE equips health professionals with up-to-date, evidence-based obesity management resources through e-learning online modules and live training courses. Certification is granted to those health professionals who demonstrate evidence of 6 months of practical experience related to obesity management within a medical or allied health care professional setting, and who earn 12 points of credit through e-learning and accredited courses.

Specialization efforts in the United States began with creation of the American Board of Bariatric Medicine (ABBM), established by the American Society of Bariatric Physicians (ASBP) in 1997. Over the course of 10 years, nearly 400 physicians were certified as ABBM diplomates. However, in 2007, The Obesity Society (TOS) felt that a broader approach was needed to further advance the field. Thus, TOS, along with 13 other professional societies and organizational partners, formed a Certified Obesity Medicine Physician (COMP) steering committee with the goal of establishing a new certification process. Involvement of multiple societies and organizations on the steering committee was instrumental for providing legitimacy to the process as well as a broad representation of the field of medicine. Under the direction of the Professional Examination Service (PES) as the vendor to guide the examination development process, a Practice Analysis Task Force created the first-draft description of the specialized body of knowledge required by physicians of obesity medicine. Subsequently, 238 physicians from internal medicine, family practice, and pediatrics completed an Internet-based validation survey to assess importance and time spent for each item. The item-writing phase of the initiative was conducted from October, 2009 through September, 2010.

The American Board of Obesity Medicine

Instead of creating two competing certification pathways, the ABBM and the COMP steering committee cooperated to establish the American Board of Obesity Medicine (ABOM). After coordinating administrative and operational issues, the ABOM was incorporated as a nonprofit 501 c (6) corporation in Denver, Colorado in 2011. Whereas the content rubric and domains from COMP were used for the new examination structure, examination items were initially taken from both the ABBM and COMP as appropriate. Furthermore, a 12-member board of directors was formed in order to merge the two organizations and give representation to primary specialty boards from internal medicine, family practice, OB-GYN, pediatrics, and surgery. The established mission of the ABOM is to serve the public and the field of obesity medicine by maintaining standards for assessment and credentialing of obesity medicine physicians. Certification as an ABOM diplomate signifies specialized knowledge in the practice of obesity medicine and distinguishes a physician as having achieved competency in obesity care. The board describes an obesity medicine physician as follows:

- A physician with expertise in the field of obesity medicine. This field requires competency in and a thorough understanding of the treatment of obesity and the genetic, biological, environmental, social, and behavioral factors that contribute to obesity.
- The obesity medicine physician employs therapeutic interventions that include diet, physical activity, behavioral change, and pharmacotherapy.
- The obesity medicine physician utilizes a comprehensive approach and may collaborate with other specialists such as nutritionists, exercise physiologists, psychologists, and bariatric surgeons, as indicated to achieve optimal results.
- Additionally, the obesity medicine physician maintains competency in providing pre-, peri-, and postsurgical care of bariatric surgery patients, promotes the pre-

The Examination and Certification Process

In order to maintain the highest standards of professional integrity, the ABOM partnered with the National Board of Medical Examiners (NBME), the same premier organization that administers the three-step United States Medical Licensing Examination (USMLE) required for medical licensure in this country. The NBME serves two valuable functions for the examination process: annual administration to candidates and quality improvement of the examination itself. By providing item-writing workshops, mentoring, and item editorial review, the ABOM Board and item-writing committee have been able to develop a unique skill set and high level of competency in item-writing construction. In turn, this expertise improves the quality and robustness of the examination to assess the candidates' knowledge and practice application.

The current examination rubric contains 4 domains and 107 subdomains (Table 24.2). The rubric was developed by a job task analysis conducted among primary care physicians in 2009 to identify core competency topics in obesity medicine. Overall, 65%, 20%, and 15% of the examination items are allocated to content relevant to the entire life cycle, adults, and children/adolescents, respectively.

In lieu of the paucity of fellowships available in obesity medicine, candidates for the ABOM examination are expected to gain knowledge about obesity through CME activities and self-directed practice experience. ABOM certification qualifications include the following:

- An active U.S. medical license
- Completion of U.S. or Canadian medical residency
- Active board certification in an American Board of Medical Specialties (ABMS) member board or osteopathic medicine equivalent
- At least 60 credit hours of CME on obesity topics recognized by the American Medical Association Physician Recognition Award (AMA PRA) Category 1 credit hours *or* successful completion of a clinical fellowship that included at least 500 hours of training in obesity or obesity-related conditions

ABOM diplomates have time-limited board certification for 10 years. To recertify, diplomates must maintain an active medical license, complete a minimum of 120 credit hours of CME on the topic of obesity, and successfully pass the examination.

ABOM Diplomates

Since provision of the first certifying examination in 2012, the number of candidates enrolling in the examination has steadily increased (see Figure 24.1). As of the 2016 examination, there were 2,068 ABOM diplomats, of which 52.8% were women. As an indication of a new specialty, 63.9% of diplomates have spent less than 5 years in the practice of obesity medicine. It is also interesting to note that the time spent devoted to obesity medicine varies among the diplomates: 38% spend less than a quarter of their time focused on obesity care; 31.2% allocate 25–50% of their time; and 19.4% dedicate more than 75% of their time exclusively to obesity medicine. The first group is represented by family medicine or internal medicine primary care physicians who designate the equivalent of 1 day a week to obesity care. In contrast, the group that devotes more than three-quarters of its time to obesity is primarily represented by physicians who practice in a specialty care setting. Overall, 57.4% of diplomates help care for patients who have received bariatric surgery.

TABLE 24.2. ABOM Examination Rubric Domains, Subdomains, and Percentage Contribution

Domain	Percent of examination	Number of subdomains
Basic concepts	25	21
Diagnosis and evaluation	30	23
Treatment	40	37
Practice management	5	12

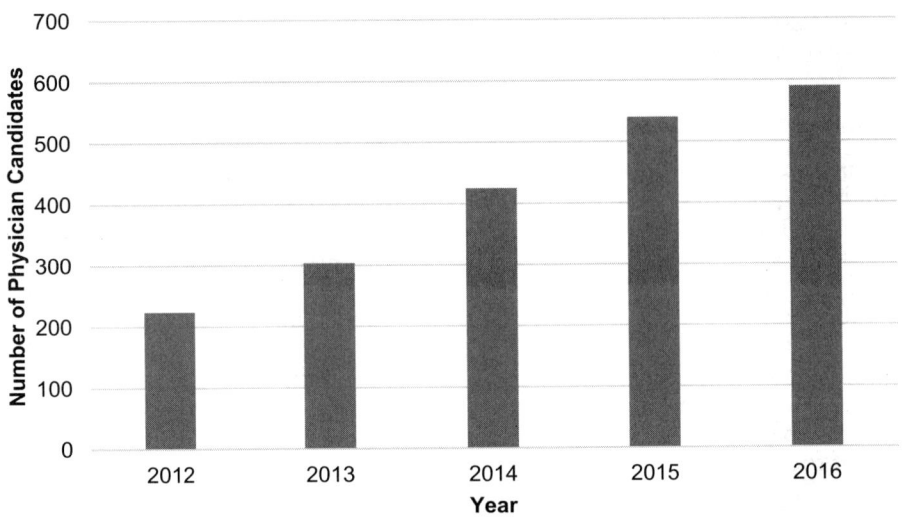

FIGURE 24.1. Number of candidates taking the ABOM examination by year of administration.

What Is the Future of the ABOM?

The ABOM Board of Directors is carefully monitoring the changing climate of board certification and maintenance of certification as guided by the ABMS and its member boards. The discipline of obesity medicine potentially meets several of the criteria for recognition as a subspecialty (e.g., it has a unique body of knowledge that cannot be fully incorporated into an existing discipline, has clinical applicability, contributes to the scholarly generation of new information, advances research in the field, and has an important social need). However, there is one essential stumbling block that precludes further movement in this direction (American Board of Internal Medicine, 2006). With the exception of a few fellowships, there is no formal, generalized training that provides supervision and direct observation for at least 12 months to demonstrate the competence needed for certification. All existing ABMS specialties and subspecialties meet this criterion. If it is officially adopted by the ABMS and member boards, focused practice and maintenance of certification recognition will be a potentially viable alternative pathway for subspecialization. As of this time, the ABOM is proceeding as a stand-alone board. Under the direction of the NBME, the ABOM recently completed an updated practice analysis study to assess the knowledge, skills, and ability of physicians so that the examination content and rubric remain relevant and up-to-date.

Conclusions

A number of obesity guidelines and recommendations have recently been published to assist clinicians in the assessment and management of patients with obesity. However, provision of comprehensive obesity care in the primary and specialty care settings remains challenging due to multiple practice-, system-, and patient-based factors. These barriers will not be easy to overcome. A multifaceted approach is required in order to assure that obesity is routinely addressed in these settings. Although creation of a new specialty of obesity medicine will not be sufficient to address the obesity crisis, Diplomates of the American Board of Obesity Medicine can serve as referral resources, as well as local and national champions.

References

Adams, K. M., Kohlmeier, M., & Zeisel, S. H. (2010). Nutrition education in U.S. medical schools: Latest update of a national survey. *Academic Medicine*, 85(9), 1537–1542.

American Academy of Family Physicians (2010). Residencies seek to boost training in obesity management, lifestyle issues. Retrieved from *www.aafp.org/news/obesity/20100517residencies.html*.

American Board of Internal Medicine. (2006). Final report of the committee on recognizing new and emerging disciplines in internal medicine (NEDIM)-2. Retrieved July 31, 2016, from *www.abim.org/~/media/ABIM%20Public/Files/pdf/report/nedim-2-report.pdf*.

American Medical Association House of Delegates. (2013). Recognition of obesity as a disease: Resolution 420 (A-13).

Antognoli, E. L., Smith, K. J., Mason, M. J., Milliner, B. R., Davis, E. M., Harris-Haywood, S., et al. (2014). Direct observation of weight counselling in primary care: Alignment with clinical guidelines. *Clinical Obesity, 4*(2), 69–76.

Apovian, C. M., Aronne, L. J., Bessessen, D. H., McDonnell, M. E., Murad, M. H., Pagotto, U., et al. (2016). Pharmacological management of obesity: An Endocrine Society clinical practice guideline. *Journal of Clinical Endocrinology and Metabolism, 100*(2), 342–362.

Association of American Medical Colleges. (2007). Report VIII: Contemporary issues in medicine—the prevention and treatment of overweight and obesity. Retrieved from *https://members.aamc.org/eweb/upload/Contemporary%20Issues%20in%20Med%20The%20Prevention%20and%20Treatment%20Report%20VIII.pdf*.

Ayres, C. G., & Griffith, H. M. (2007). Perceived barriers to and facilitators of the implementation of priority clinical preventive services guidelines. *American Journal of Managed Care, 13*(3), 150–155.

Baer, H. J., Karson, A. S., Soukup, J. R., Williams, D. H., & Bates, D. W. (2013). Documentation and diagnosis of overweight and obesity in electronic health records of adult primary care patients. *JAMA Internal Medicine, 173*(17), 1648–1652.

Bardia, A., Holtan, S. G., Slezak, J. M., & Thompson, W. G. (2007). Diagnosis of obesity by primary care physicians and impact on obesity management. *Mayo Clinic Proceedings, 82*(8), 927–932.

Bleich, S. N., Bennett, W. L., Gudzune, K. A., & Cooper, L. A. (2012). National survey of US primary care physicians' perspectives about causes of obesity and solutions to improve care. *BMJ Open, 2*(6), e001871.

Block, J. P., DeSalvo, K. B., & Fisher, W. P. (2003). Are physicians equipped to address the obesity epidemic?: Knowledge and attitudes of internal medicine residents. *Preventive Medicine, 36*(6), 669–675.

Centers for Medicare and Medicaid Services. (2009). Electronic health records (HER) incentive programs. Retrieved August 8, 2016, from *www.cms.gov/Regulations-and-Guidance/Legislation/EHRIncentivePrograms/index.html*.

Centers for Medicare and Medicaid Services. (2011). National coverage determination for intensive behavioral therapy for obesity. Retrieved August 8, 2016, from *www.cms.gov/medicare-coverage-database/details/ncd-details*.

Colbert, J. A., & Jangi, S. (2013). Training physicians to manage obesity—back to the drawing board. *New England Journal of Medicine, 369*(25), 1389–1391.

Crawford, A. G., Cote, C., Couto, J., Daskiran, M., Gunnarsson, C., Haas, K., et al. (2010). Prevalence of obesity, type II diabetes mellitus, hyperlipidemia, and hypertension in the United States: Findings from the GE Centricity Electronic Medical Record database. *Population Health Management, 13*(3), 151–161.

Flegal, K. M., Kruszon-Moran, D., Carroll, M. D., Fryar, C. D., & Ogden, C. L. (2016). Trends in obesity among adults in the United States, 2005 to 2014. *Journal of the American Medical Association, 315*(21), 2284–2291.

Garvey, W. T., Garber, A. J., Mechanick, J. I., Bray, G. A., Dagogo-Jack, S., Einhorn, D., et al. (2014). American Association of Clinical Endocrinologists and American College of Endocrinology position statement on the 2014 advanced framework for a new diagnosis of obesity as a chronic disease. *Endocrine Practice, 20*(9), 977–989.

Garvey, W. T., Mechanick, J. I., Brett, E. M., Garber, A. J., Hurley, D. L., Jastreboff, A. M., et al. (2016). American Association of Clinical Endocrinologists and American College of Endocrinology comprehensive clinical practice guidelines for medical care of patients with obesity. *Endocrine Practice, 22*(Suppl. 3), 1–202.

Graham, R., Mancher, M., Miller Wolman, D., Greenfield, S., & Steinberg, E. (2011). *Clinical practice guidelines we can trust*. Washington, DC: National Academies Press.

Gunther, S., Guo, F., Sinfield, P., Rogers, S., & Baker, R. (2012). Barriers and enablers to managing obesity in general practice: A practical approach for use in implementation activities. *Quality in Primary Care, 20*(2), 93–103.

Hatoum, I. J., Blackstone, R., Hunter, T. D., Francis, D. M., Steinbuch, M., Harris, L., et al. (2016). Clinical factors associated with remission of obesity-related comorbidities after bariatric surgery. *JAMA Surgery, 151*(2), 130–137.

Jay, M., Gillespie, C., Ark, T., Richter, R., McMacken, M., Zabar, S., et al. (2008). Do internists, pediatricians, and psychiatrists feel competent in obesity care?: Using a needs assessment to drive curriculum design. *Journal of General Internal Medicine, 23*(7), 1066–1070.

Jensen, M. D., Ryan, D. H., Apovian, C. M., Ard, J. D., Comuzzie, A. G., Donato, K. A., et al. (2014). 2013 AHA/ACC/TOS guideline for the management of overweight and obesity in adults: A report of the American College of Cardiology/American Heart Association Task Force on Practice Guidelines and The Obesity Society. *Circulation, 129*(25, Suppl. 2), S102–S138.

Kahan, S., & Zvenyach, T. (2016). Obesity as a disease: Current policies and implications for the future. *Current Obesity Reports, 5*(2), 291–297.

Kraschnewski, J. L., Sciamanna, C. N., Pollak, K. I., Stuckey, H. L., & Sherwood, N. E. (2013). The epidemiology of weight counseling for adults in the United States: A case of positive deviance. *International Journal of Obesity, 37*(5), 751–753.

Kushner, R. F., Brittan, D., Cleek, J., Hes, D., English, W., Kahan, S. et al. (2017). The American Board of Obesity Medicine: Five year report. *Obesity, 25*(6), 982–983.

Moyer, V. A., LeFevre, M. L., Siu, A. L., Baumann, L. C., Bibbins-Domingo, K., Curry, S. J., et al. (2012). Screening for and management of obesity in adults: U.S. Preventive Services Task Force recommendation statement. *Annals of Internal Medicine, 157*(5), 373–378.

Obesity Hyperguide. (2016). Retrieved July 30, 2016, from *https://cme.healio.com/obesityce*.

Office of Personnel Management. (2014). FEHB program carrier letter. Retrieved August 8, 2016, from *www.opm.gov/healthcare-insurance/healthcare/carriers/2014/2014-04.pdf*.

Ogden, C. L., Carroll, M. D., Lawman, H. G., Fryar, C. D., Kruszon-Morgan, D., & Flegal, K. M. (2016). Trends in obesity prevalence among children and adolescents in the United States, 1988–1994 through 2013–2014. *Journal of the American Medical Association, 315*(21), 2292–2299.

Petrin, C., Kahan, S., Turner, M., Gallagher, C., & Dietz, W. H. (2016). Current practices of obesity pharmacotherapy, bariatric surgery referral and coding for counselling by healthcare professionals. *Obesity Science and Practice, 2*(3), 266–271.

Pi-Sunyer, F. X., Becker, D. M., Bouchard, C., Carleton, R. A., Colditz, G. A., Dietz, W. H., et al. (1998). *Clinical guidelines on the identification, evaluation, and treatment of overweight and obesity in adults* (NIH Publication No. 98-4083). Bethesda, MD: National Heart, Lung, and Blood Institute, National Institutes of Health.

Post, R. E., Mainous, A. G., III, Gregorie, S. H., Knoll, M. E., Diaz, V. A., & Saxena, S. K. (2011). The influence of physician acknowledgment of patients' weight status on patient perceptions of overweight and obesity in the United States. *Archives of Internal Medicine, 171*(4), 316–321.

Seger, J. C., Horn, D. B., Westman, E. C., Primack, C., Long, J., Clark, T., et al. (2016). Obesity algorithm: Clinical guidelines for obesity treatment. Retrieved September 24, 2016, from *www.obesityalgorithm.org*.

STOP Obesity Alliance. (2010). New survey from the STOP Obesity Alliance shows primary care doctors and patients see shared role in weight loss, but ask, now what? Retrieved August 8, 2016, from *http://stopobesityalliance.org/newsroom/press-releases/new-surveys-from-stop-obesity-alliance-show-primary-care-doctors-and-patients-see-shared-role-in-weight-loss-but-ask-now-what*.

Talwalkar, A., & McCarty, F. (2016). *Characteristics of physician office visits for obesity by adults aged 20 and over: United States, 2012* (NCHS Data Brief, No. 237). Hyattsville, MD: National Center for Health Statistics.

U.S. Department of Health and Human Services, Office of Disease Prevention and Health Promotion. (2008). 2008 physical activity guidelines for Americans (ODPHP Publication No. U0036). Retrieved from *https://health.gov/PAGuidelines/guidelines*.

U.S. Department of Health and Human Services & U.S. Department of Agriculture. (2015). 2015–2020 dietary guidelines for Americans (8th ed.). Retrieved from *http://health.gov/dietaryguidelines/2015/guidelines*.

van Dillen, S. M. E., van Binsbergen, J. J., Koelenc, M. A., & Hiddinka, G. J. (2013). Nutrition and physical activity guidance practices in general practice: A critical review. *Patient Education and Counseling, 90*(2), 155–169.

Wilkinson, M. L., Brown, A. L., Poston, W. S., Haddock C. K., Jahnke, S. A., & Day, R. S. (2014). Physician weight recommendations for overweight and obese firefighters, United States, 2011–2012. *Preventing Chronic Disease, 11*, E116.

World Obesity. (2016). SCOPE program. Retrieved July 30, 2016, from *www.worldobesity.org/scope*.

Xian, Y., Kelton, C. M., Guo, J. J., Bian, B., & Heaton, P. C. (2015). Treatment of obesity: Pharmacotherapy trends in the United States from 1999 to 2010. *Obesity, 23*(8), 1721–1728.

Yarnall, K. S., Pollak, K. I., Ostbye, T., Krause, K. M., & Michener, J. L. (2003). Primary care: Is there enough time for prevention? *American Journal of Public Health, 93*(4), 635–641.

Zhang, S., Manne, S., Lin, J., & Yang, J. (2016). Characteristics of patients potentially eligible for pharmacotherapy for weight loss in primary care practice in the United States. *Obesity Science and Practice, 2*(2), 104–114.

CHAPTER 25

Coverage of Obesity Treatment
Costs and Benefits

Morgan Downey
Theodore K. Kyle

Third-party reimbursement for obesity treatment is a complex subject. Relevant to the discussion is the evolution of framing obesity as a disease that should be treated medically. Governmental and nongovernmental programs present a mix of coverages and limitations. Successful advocacy for expanding reimbursement of obesity treatment requires knowledge of evolving scientific research and medical developments, as well as awareness of changes in health policy and the health care delivery system. In spite of numerous studies showing the deleterious effects of obesity on health and the benefits of evidence-based treatments, coverage for obesity treatments is lagging. This is an indicator of continuing stigmatization and failure by physicians to treat obesity like other chronic diseases. Expanding coverage is essential to addressing the lack of access to care for low-income patients, including members of minority groups, and incentivizing the development of more effective treatments and research on comparative effectiveness. The movement away from fee-for-service methods of payment to value-based systems may make the utilization of obesity treatments more attractive.

This review principally considers reimbursement programs in Medicare, Medicaid, and managed care. It also covers changes brought about by the Affordable Care Act (ACA) in Medicaid, private insurance, and employer wellness programs (The Affordable Care Act is undergoing continuing legislative, regulatory, and market changes. Therefore, its provisions may change over time.) It does not include population-specific programs, such as the military's health insurance program, the Veterans Administration health services, the Indian Health Service, state employees, or coverage for institutionalized persons in long-term care facilities and prisons.

The high level of obesity in the United States imposes well-documented costs on the health care system, both directly, through medical expenses, and indirectly through, for example, lost productivity. Obesity ranks third, behind smoking and armed violence (including war and terrorism), in its global social burden: about $2 trillion or 2.8% of global gross domestic product (GDP), approximately equal to the GDP of Russia or Italy. Lost productivity may be responsible for 70% of total costs.

According to the World Health Organization Global Burden of Disease data base, "In the United States, armed conflict (and especially spending on the military) has the highest social and economic impact, and obesity is second; obesity generated an impact in the United States of $664 billion a year in 2012, or 4.1% of GDP" (Dobbs et al., 2014). High costs attributed to obesity indicate the many critical comorbid conditions that lead to great human suffering. Yet the public policy response across the globe has been poor, inconsistent, and of limited effectiveness.

This inadequate response by policymakers reflects the misunderstanding of obesity and the stigmatization of persons with obesity, as well as the lack of direct and effective solutions. One glaring omission in public policy response is the lack of comprehensive, adequate third-party reimbursement for evidence-based obesity care. This omission reflects many inconsistencies endemic to any discussion of obesity. Should limited resources be committed to prevention or treatment? Are treatments effective in the long term? Is obesity the result of personality weakness in resisting temptations and establishing a healthy lifestyle? Would reimbursing obesity treatments create a "moral hazard," in which poor behavior is encouraged by a safety net to limit the damage? How much would coverage cost, and should persons with obesity be required to pay more for coverage?

Several studies and the experience of clinicians persuaded the obesity community leadership in the late 1990s that greater third-party access would address the glaring inequalities regarding those who receive treatment and those who do not (Lewis, Edwards-Hampton, & Ard, 2016). Because most patients pay for treatment out of pocket, it is usually the more financially secure patients who can afford treatment. It is safe to assume that expansion of third-party reimbursement would facilitate the provision of treatment, especially for those with a financial obstacle to receiving treatment. Excess mortality has been found among candidates for bariatric surgery who were subjected to extensive prior authorization processes (Flanagan, Ghaderi, Overby, & Farrell, 2016). A survey by Arterburn et al. (2008) showed that expanding insurance coverage of weight management programs may encourage more men and women to enroll in such programs.

Historical Perspective on Obesity as a Disease

In the 1990s, advocates for greater third-party reimbursement adopted a strategy to change the categorization of obesity to a medical disease, as opposed to merely a lack of personal willpower, as a prerequisite for improving reimbursement. The idea of changing both policymakers' and the public's perception of obesity was consistent with major scientific breakthroughs in the understanding of obesity, especially the discovery of leptin and other neuroendocrine mediators that affect perceptions of hunger and satiety and contribute to body weight regulation. A consensus among obesity clinicians emerged that mere exhortations for reductions in food consumption and increased levels of energy expenditure were unlikely to change the trends in obesity prevalence.

With the creation of a Washington, DC-based advocacy organization, the American Obesity Association (AOA), a strategy evolved to have federal health care agencies recognize obesity as a disease. (Morgan Downey served as executive director of AOA from 1997 to 2006 and of The Obesity Society from 2006 to 2008.) AOA's position that Medicare should recognize obesity as a disease was delivered in testimony on March 1, 2000, before a Medicare Coverage Executive Committee (2000).

A paper published in 2001 was among the first to directly address reframing obesity as a disease rather than as a personal character flaw (Downey, 2001). In 2001, the Social Security Administration removed obesity from a listing of impairments that facilitated determinations of disability. Following a petition from the AOA, the Social Security Administration reopened the rule-making process. In its final determination, the Social Security Administration (2002) stated that "Obesity is a complex, chronic disease characterized by excessive accumulation of body fat."

In 2002, the AOA petitioned the Internal Revenue Service (IRS) to allow the costs of weight loss treatment to be included as a medical deduction on individual tax returns. The IRS responded by requesting documentation that obesity is a disease. The AOA response argued that obesity met existing definitions of "disease" (e.g., an impairment of the normal functioning of the body, characteristic signs and symptoms, and affecting mortality and morbidity). Following AOA's response, the IRS reversed an earlier revenue ruling and accepted obesity as a disease, making physician-prescribed treatments eligible for the medical deduction (U.S. Department of the Treasury, Internal Revenue Service, 2016). As the federal government moved to recognize obesity as a disease, so did professional societies. The Obesity Society (formerly the North American Association for the Study of Obesity) adopted a policy that recommended describing obesity as a disease (Allison et al., 2008). The American College of Clinical Endocrinology did so in 2012, and the American Medical Association recognized obesity as a disease in 2013.

In 2014, the Office of Personnel Management, which oversees the Federal Employee Health Benefit program, advised participating insurance companies that they could no longer exclude drugs and surgery for weight management on the basis that these were "lifestyle" conditions. The letter, after noting the applicability of the United States Preventive Services Task Force (USPSTF) recommendations, stated:

> Given the impact of obesity on individual and population health, we also encourage issuers to provide enrollees with access to a full range of weight reduction treatment interventions. Issuers that specifically exclude coverage for weight reduction and/or management interventions should review the clinical rationales for those exclusions and document how enrollees will receive appropriate care to achieve and sustain a healthy weight. (O'Brien, 2014)

Categorizing obesity as a disease was only the first step toward improving reimbursement for obesity treatments. Acceptance by payers in both the public sector (e.g., Medicare and Medicaid) and the private sector (e.g., group health insurance) has lacked comprehensiveness and flexibility. Where there is coverage, it is frequently inadequate. Some payers cover bariatric surgery but not pharmacology. Where behavioral counseling or drugs are covered, limitations on the amount, duration, and frequency are inconsistent with the general rules for treating a long-term, chronic disease.

Public Sector Coverage

Medicare

The Medicare program is the country's largest health care reimbursement program, covering most persons age 65 years and older, as well as persons with disabilities covered by the Social Security Disability Insurance program. Medicare and Medicaid are administered by the Centers for Medicare and Medicaid Services.

Up until 2004, the Centers for Medicare and Medicaid Services policy on obesity stated that "obesity itself cannot be considered an illness." Therefore, no claims for treating obesity could be paid. After requests from the AOA and The Obesity Society, Centers for Medicare and Medicaid Services eliminated this language. It is important to note that Centers for Medicare and Medicaid Services did not actively recognize obesity as a disease, instead adopting a neutral position on the issue of classification. However, this reprieve created the opportunity for a more detailed Centers for Medicare and Medicaid Services review of specific obesity treatments (Glassman, 2004).

In 2006, Centers for Medicare and Medicaid Services reviewed bariatric surgery amid national concerns over the safety of the procedure. A Centers for Medicare and Medicaid Services Advisory Committee review resulted in a significant turnaround, with a recommendation to expand coverage of bariatric surgery for patients with a body mass index (BMI) ≥ 35 kg/m^2 and at least one comorbid condition (Centers for Medicare and Medicaid Services, 2013).

In 2003, the USPSTF recommended that "clinicians screen adult patients for obesity and offer intensive counseling and behavioral interventions to promote sustained weight loss for obese adults." Centers for Medicare and Medicaid Services incorporated this recommendation as a covered service for Medicare beneficiaries in 2011 (Centers for Medicare and Medicaid Services, 2011). Despite this progress, the Centers for Medicare and Medicaid Services policy has drawn criticism for several reasons. First, it requires patients to lose 3 kg or more after 6 months for intervention to continue, a policy that some regard as unreasonable, especially for members of high-risk groups. Second, the amount that can be charged to Medicare is quite low compared to other interventions. Third, the policy does not include nonphysician providers, notably registered dietitians and psychologists (Bennett, Steinberg, & Pogoto, 2015). Coverage of pharmacology for the treatment of obesity was explicitly excluded from Medicare by Congressional action in the enactment of Part D of Medicare (Medicare Prescription Drug, Improvement, and Modernization Act of 2003). However, Medicare Advantage plans are allowed to exceed the scope of the defined Part D benefit, so some beneficiaries may have coverage (Baum et al., 2015). Efforts to amend Part D's exclusion have been unsuccessful to date.

Medicaid

The Medicaid program is a joint federal–state health program serving low-income families with dependent children and persons who are disabled. Medicaid and the Children's Health Insurance Program provide acute and long-term health coverage for approximately 40 million children and adults. The ACA has expanded the population covered by Medicaid in states that choose to participate in the expansion. It has been estimated that new enrollees in Medicaid would be approximately 14.7 million if each eligible individual chose to enroll. One out of three were expected to be obese (Decker, Kostova, Kenney, & Long, 2013).

All Medicaid programs cover at least one obesity treatment modality. Montana and Mississippi explicitly exclude drugs and surgery for weight loss (Petrin, 2016). State Medicaid programs may request a waiver from the Department of Health and Human Services to cover obesity drugs, but few have taken advantage of this option (Lee, Sheer, Lopez, & Rosenbaum, 2010).

The ACA contains two provisions that provide a platform for advocacy to expand coverage of obesity treatments in the Medicaid program. These provisions apply to the contracts that states enter into with managed care organizations. Approximately 70% of Medicaid recipients receive services in managed care organizations. The first provision, §1557, bans discrimination "based on health status or the need for health services or on race, color, national origin, sex, sexual orientation, gender identity, or disability." The nondiscrimination clause extends to both de facto as well as intentional discrimination. Clearly, obesity is both a "health status" as well as (in some cases) a "disability."

The second provision allows for the provision of substitute services "in lieu" of covered services. This allows states to be innovative in developing evidence-based alternatives (Rosenbaum, 2016). The systematic exclusion of services (other than intensive behavioral counseling) can be challenged as illegal discrimination, as substitute services "in lieu" of covered services, such as bariatric surgery and pharmacology, could be available for patients with obesity.

The ACA

In March 2010, Congress enacted the signature legislative accomplishment of President Barack Obama, the Patient Protection and Affordable Care Act (ACA). The primary goal of the ACA is to expand access to health insurance for persons who do not have coverage due either to health or economic factors. The secondary goal is to control health care costs by including younger, healthier individuals in the health insurance pool and making structural changes to the health care delivery system.

In addition to expanding Medicaid, the ACA expands access to health insurance for uninsured individuals by creating state health marketplaces (formerly called *exchanges*). The marketplaces come in three varieties: state-administered, joint federal–state run, and federally administered. They have been described as an "Expedia" of health insurance, where one can enter one's age, gender, smoking status, and income to receive information about four potential coverage plans (bronze, silver, gold, and platinum). Individuals can then pick the plan that gives them the best coverage at an affordable cost. The cheapest plans (i.e., bronze) have high out-of-pocket costs and are designed for those who do not expect to have high medical expenses. The most costly plans (i.e., platinum) have high premiums but lower out-of-pocket requirements. Federal subsidies are available for low-income purchasers.

What are the health status characteristics of the population expected to enroll in state exchanges/marketplaces? A study undertaken by the Urban Institute investigated the population of individuals who were uninsured and without group insurance, and whose income was too high to qualify for Medicaid (approximately 16.1 million Americans). Interestingly, these individuals are significantly less likely than insured individuals to be obese (23.7 compared to 27.2%), but are more likely to smoke (16.8 vs. 13.7%). Even so, under this model, 3.8 million adults with a BMI $\geq$ 30 kg/m^2 between the ages of 19 to 64 years would be expected to join the health exchanges (Blumberg & Holahan, 2013).

Under the ACA, there are 10 minimum "essential health benefits" that each plan listed on the federal or state exchanges must provide: ambulatory care, emergency services, hospitalizations, maternity and newborn care, mental health treatment, prescription drugs, rehabilitative and habilitative services and devices, laboratory services, preventive and wellness services, and pediatric services. Centers for Medicare and Medicaid Services has established a "benchmark plan" for each state as a model for other plans to use. Unfortunately, this approach only institutionalized the lack of adequate coverage in the private sector. The Obesity Care Continuum has provided a very helpful analysis of each state's benchmark plan and obesity treatment modalities (Gallagher, 2012). The coverage of bariatric surgery is highly variable in these marketplaces (Yang & Pomeranz, 2015). The ACA bans the imposition of annual or lifetime limits, but only on essential health benefits, and excludes many plans that were in existence when the law was enacted. Therefore, limits can still be applied to bariatric surgery (U.S. Department of Health and Human Services, 2014).

Coverage of approved pharmaceutical products for the treatment of obesity is problematic. The final regulations require coverage of either one or more drugs from each class (as listed in the U.S. Pharmacopeia Model Guidelines), or the "benchmark" plan the state has selected as its model plan. Most benchmark plans do not include drugs approved by the U.S. Food and Drug Administration (FDA) for weight loss. The U.S. Pharmacopeia Model Guidelines do not have a category of drugs for weight loss or appetite suppressants, even though the FDA (U.S. Food and Drug Administration, 2016) includes a "weight loss" category.

The regulations stress that an issuer "does not provide essential health benefits if its benefit design, or the implementation of its benefit design, discriminates based on an individual's age, expected length of life, or present or predicted disability, degree of medical dependency, quality of life or other health conditions" (CCI Center for Consumer Information, 2015). The Department of Health and Human Services has undertaken investigations into whether some plans violate the discriminatory benefit design standard in regard to mental health, autism, and Alzheimer's disease coverages (Millman, 2015). Appeals of adverse decisions may be required to obtain the necessary coverage.

Private Insurance

The private health insurance market has historically provided little coverage of weight loss treatments (Cook, 2002). Nevertheless, companies such as Blue Cross and Blue Shield of North Carolina (2004) have started to lead the way, setting an example for other insurance providers (BCBSNC, 2004. Managed care organizations (e.g., health maintenance organizations, preferred provider organizations, accountable care organizations, and state health care exchanges) are major providers of care through commercial insurance plans, Medicare, and Medicaid. To allow comparisons among programs, quality care standards are established and monitored by the National Committee on Quality Assessment (NCQA; 2015a).

The NCQA established standards for children and adolescents (ages 3–17) with obesity in 2008, after several years of development and testing. The standards require evaluation of the child's BMI percentile, as well as nutritional and physical activity counseling. The assessment rate for BMI percentile assessment in 2014 was 61% for commercial health maintenance organizations (HMOs) and 64% for Medicaid HMOs. Counseling for nutrition and physical activity in both categories ranged from 53 to 60%. Adult obesity assessment involves measuring the percentage of adults (ages 18–74) who had an outpatient visit and whose BMI was documented in the past 2 years. Assessment rates in 2014 ranged between 75% for commercial HMOs and 92% for Medicare HMOs (NCQA, 2015b).

In the private insurance market, the ACA makes three major changes of interest for persons with obesity. First, it prohibits the denial of coverage based on "pre-existing conditions." Many persons, especially those with a high BMI, can be unable to obtain any health insurance at all. In one study, lack of insurance coverage was the predominant reason why patients were not accepted for bariatric surgery (Tsuda, Barros, Schneider, & Jones, 2009). Another study indicated a rise in the number of patients forgoing bariatric surgery because of insurance denials or unattainable coverage prerequisites (Sadhasivam, Larson, Lambert, Mathiason, & Kothari, 2007). Yet another study indicated that lack of health insurance was the probable reason for the racial disparities in the receipt of bariatric surgery (Mainous, Johnson, Saxena, & Wright, 2013). Another group of persons with obesity may have health insurance but not have coverage for treatment of obesity. Changes to one's health care coverage under the ACA depends, in large part, on which market or program a specific individual is in (e.g., has insurance through an employer or pays for an individual plan, is on Medicaid, or is uninsured and not eligible for Medicaid).

The ACA requires that newer private insurance plans include free preventive services, including the USPSTF recommendation (see above) for intensive adult behavioral counseling at no charge to patients. The ACA also requires a robust and independent appeals process in §1001. It is often necessary for persons with obesity to appeal denials of claims. Formerly, these appeals were reviewed by the insurance company itself. Important and overlooked changes in the ACA are the new federal regulations for internal and external appeal processes. These new procedures may be especially helpful in cases of denial of bariatric surgery. Under the ACA, all consumers have the right to appeal coverage decisions made by a health insurance company to an outside, independent decision panel.

Plans must have an internal claims appeal process in effect and provide notice to enrollees of the available internal and external appeals process and the availability of consumer assistance. Plans must allow enrollees to review their files, present evidence and testimony, and receive continued coverage pending the outcome of their appeal (Internal Revenue Service, Employee Benefits, 2011). The three federal departments involved in implementing the ACA decided what types of adverse benefit determinations involved "medical judgments" and therefore could be appealed. Among those included were (1) "A plan's general exclusion of an item or service (such as speech therapy), if the plan covers the item or service in certain circumstances (such as, to aid in the restoration of speech loss or impairment or speech resulting from a medical condition)"; (2) "Whether a participant or beneficiary is entitled to a reasonable alternative standard for a reward under the plan's wellness program"; and (3) "The frequency, method, treatment, or setting for a recommended preventive service, to the extent not specified, in the recommendation or guideline of the U.S. Preventive Services Task Force, etc." All three of these areas are applicable to obesity treatments.

The ACA also expands employer wellness programs. A full discussion of employer wellness programs is beyond the scope of this chapter. Nevertheless, health professionals should be aware that the ACA regulations require employers who mandate employees to participate in a wellness program to provide employees with the opportunity to have their own physicians provide alternative programs, and that the company must pay for these programs (Downey, 2014a).

There are several systemic changes to the health insurance marketplace, which, although not mandating coverage, may provide employers, payers, and policymakers with a data-driven platform on which to make future coverage decisions. For example, the ACA provides financial incentives for improved care and preventive health measures, including the prevention of obesity. Affordable Care Organizations (ACOs) and the Medicare Shared Savings Program (MSSP) encourage individual and organizational providers to assume financial risk for defined populations of elderly and disabled citizens. Among MSSP and ACOs' quality measures are BMI screening and follow-up, which are expected to benefit millions of Medicare beneficiaries. The same measures are incorporated in the Healthcare Effectiveness Data and Information Set program of the NCQA.

Future Challenges

The evolution of third-party reimbursement for obesity treatment has often involved long discussions with policymakers, employers, and insurance companies. Throughout these discussions, several themes keep emerging. These include fears of high, added costs if treatments are covered; doubts about the effectiveness and safety of treatments; and the issue of individual responsibility. Preparation to engage these themes is essential for effective advocacy.

The Cost Issue

Many people look at the very high prevalence of obesity and raise concerns over how overweight or obese persons will utilize a new or expanded benefit. They could also argue that their wellness program and/or implementation of the intensive behavioral counseling preventive care benefit address the issue at low cost compared to an insured product, such as bariatric surgery. In response, it may be helpful to point to several studies that report lower than expected utilization of bariatric surgery and pharmacology. For example, only 1.3–4.2% of weight loss medication users continued for over 1 year (Hampp, Kang, & Borders-Hemphill, 2013). Another study of 1.85 million patients found that the use of weight loss drugs was "rare," at 0.6%. Many more patients used antihypertensive drugs (17.9%), antidepressants (14.2%), lipid-lowering drugs (17.9%), nonsteroidal anti-inflammatory drugs (NSAIDs; 12.1%) and antidiabetic drugs (7.8%; Zhang, Manne, Lin, & Yang, 2016). Less than 1% of the clinically eligible population has bariatric–metabolic surgery (Dixon, 2015). It is also important to stress that education programs and encouragement to eat more healthfully and to exercise more have been in place for decades, with little observable impact on the rates of obesity. In the best cases, individual efforts for behavioral change produce small changes that are largely insufficient to achieve significant weight loss and affect the expression of comorbid conditions.

It is useful to look at the lack of coverage of obesity treatments in the context of stigma and discrimination in the workplace. Not only has stigma been documented in the hiring and promotion of employees who are obese, but other more subtle expressions of discrimination are evident. For example, there is a well-documented pattern of people with obesity, especially white women, receiving lower compensation in companies that provide health insurance compared to their peers in companies that do not provide such benefits (Han, Norton, & Stearns, 2009). Lower compensation puts an additional burden on the discretionary income available to employees with obesity. Personal expenditures for people with obesity are higher than similar expenditures for people without obesity, as documented in a study carried out by George Washington University School of Public Health and Health Policy (Dor, Ferguson, Langwith, & Tan, 2010). These additional expenditures range between $6,518 for men and $8,365 for women. Another possible cost of being obese is the penalty imposed in employer wellness plans for those who fail to meet specific weight loss metrics. Such penalties can be as high as 30% of the health insurance premium paid by the employer and employee for a single-person plan, about $5,000 in the current economic environment (Downey, 2014b). The accumulation of lower compensation and higher costs can mean that employees with obesity have fewer resources for lifestyle changes and/or medical or surgical treatments for obesity.

Finally, there is the matter of equity. Employees who have a normal weight or have obesity will pay the same amount for health insurance coverage and have similar deductibles and copayments. However, nonobese employees enjoy insurance coverage for their diseases; not so for employees with obesity, whose health insurance program excludes obesity treatments. Thus, the employees with obesity are actually subsidizing the health care of nonobese employees.

The absence of covered treatments for obesity allows for the progression of greater complications. Payers can look at nonsurgical treatments for obesity and conclude that many of the comorbid conditions related to obesity take years to develop. By that time, the thinking goes, the employee will have moved on to a different employer. So why pay now when the benefit may not be evident? In this environment, the ill effects of obesity continue to mature, becoming even more resistant to treatment.

Weight loss in persons with obesity can have a significant impact on health care costs. Cawley and colleagues showed that health care plans could expect savings from a 5% reduction in initial weight in people whose BMI exceed 40 kg/m^2. In the elderly population alone, Medicare could save a considerable amount if seniors with a BMI of 30 kg/m^2 or greater lost 10–15% of their weight, using weight loss drugs (Cawley, Meyerhoefer, Biener, Hammer, & Wintfield, 2015). Even modest weight loss in a low-income population may yield significant effects. The Tennessee Medicaid Program (TennCare) partnered with the commercial program Weight Watchers to offer recipients participation in the Weight Watchers program. The mean weight loss for all participants was 1.9 kg (i.e., 1.8% of initial weight). (The average American adult gains 0.9 kg a year.) However, 20% of participants lost 5% or more of their initial body weight. After the program concluded, TennCare maintained the arrangement for all of its low-income population (Mitchell, Ellison, Hill, & Tsai, 2013).

Different payers will have different perceptions of the cost of expanding coverage. For example, Medicare has an interest in seeing incoming beneficiaries have as low a weight as possible, because this may postpone the development of obesity-related conditions later in life. Lower weights would also be expected to reduce complications after surgery, decrease length of stay in hospitals, and delay admission to rehabilitation facilities. Medicaid would also be interested in strategies to delay institutionalization in long-term care facilities for as long as possible. For example, one study estimates that obesity and related chronic diseases lead to a higher probability of entering a long-term care facility at a younger age, more long-term care days before death, and higher lifetime long-term care costs paid by Medicaid. The authors project that, at the population level, overweight and obesity will induce 1.3 billion or more long-term care patient days and $68 billion or more in Medicaid costs among Baby Boomers (Yang & Zhang, 2014). Another study estimated that severe obesity costs state Medicaid programs almost $8 billion a year (Wang et al., 2015).

Employers and commercial payers may have more concern over what their competition is doing. However, they may be more interested in reducing absenteeism and costs of disability or worker's compensation insurance. They may also be concerned about their future employees—that is, overweight or obese children in their catchment area.

Effectiveness of Interventions

Approximately 45 million Americans attempt weight loss each year, and many are successful in the short term. However, up to 50% of the lost weight is typically regained in the first year and the rest thereafter. It is well accepted in the public and among clinicians that weight regain after weight loss is a common phenomenon. Too often, this regain is seen as indicating poor self-control or lack of willpower. However, research has identified the biological mechanism at work, called metabolic or adaptive *thermogenesis*. This mechanism reinforces the validity of categorizing obesity as a disease (Ochner, Barrios, Lee, & Pi-Sunyer, 2013). In fact, the metabolic changes favoring weight regain persist after weight loss for up to 1 year, possibly longer. According to the authors of one study, "One year after initial weight reduction, levels of the circulation mediators of appetite that encourage weight regain after diet-induced weight loss do not revert to the levels recorded before weight loss" (Sumithran et al., 2011). Unfortunately, the obesity epidemic is of relatively recent origin, so many, if not most, treatments and preventive strategies were developed recently and have weak to poor success rates. But this disappointing outcome is not unique to obesity. Many diseases that are well covered by insurance products, such as type 2 diabetes, hypertension, heart disease, and cancer, are still difficult to treat effectively, even with many more covered treatment options. Obesity, like other long-term chronic diseases, is complicated, and treatment setbacks or recurrences are common. Poor third-party reimbursement is felt to be a disincentive in the development of new drugs, devices, and surgical approaches to finding more effective treatments.

Personal Responsibility

No conversation about providing help or resources goes on for very long without someone imploring, "What about personal responsibility?" On the surface, this question is simply an attempt to direct the conversation away from a greater sense of social responsibility and turn the topic back to stigmatized views of persons with obesity. To be generous, such a statement may only reflect the marketing of numerous products and services for weight loss, as well as statements from official health agencies asserting that weight regulation is up to individual. This is somewhat akin to saying that global economic problems can be cured by individuals balancing their checkbooks. The response is "Yes, but. . . . " Most diseases are, according to our current understanding, a mix of genetic (or epigenetic) factors, the environment, and personal behavior. There are numerous diseases that we can look to for comparison. Two of the diseases most amenable to behavioral influence are melanoma and sexually transmitted diseases (e.g., HIV/AIDS). Regarding melanoma, influences include genetic susceptibility (e.g., fair skin complexion), environmental exposure to sunlight, and failure to take personal protective measures. Nevertheless, treatments for melanoma, which can be very expensive, are well covered by insurance. No insurer says, "We are not covering your cancer because you could have worn long-sleeve shirts and a hat." Likewise, most sexually transmitted diseases can be prevented by simple, inexpensive, and widely available protection (e.g., condoms). Nevertheless, no insurer says, "We are not covering the costs of HIV/AIDS treatments because you did not use a condom when you should have." Yet this is precisely the type of reasoning that occurs in discussions of obesity. No one tells a person with type 2 diabetes or hypertension, "You did it to yourself—we are not going to help you," or "You have to control your blood glucose by diet and exercise alone, without drugs." With most diseases, personal responsibility or "self-management" is part of the discussion; with obesity, it is all too often the end of the conversation.

Implicit in these discussions is a view that persons with obesity have a personality defect that impedes their ability to limit food intake and/or sustain a regimen of physical activity. Rather than ignore such views, it is helpful to see how research on personality and obesity provides us with enhanced understanding. A series of papers by Angela Sutin and colleagues offer some helpful insights. A study from 2011 found that the most disciplined consumers had lower rates of obesity, whereas large weight gains were found among consumers scoring high on measures of impulsiveness, low conscientiousness, and willingness to take risks (Sutin, Ferrucci, Zonderman, & Terraciano, 2011). In another study, Sutin, Zonderman, et al. (2013) found that persons who rated high on impulsiveness, low on conscientiousness, or lacked discipline had high circulating levels of leptin, which pays a critical role in weight regulation, even after controlling for BMI, waist circumference, or inflammatory markers. A third paper asked whether weight gain or loss of 10% or more led to personality changes, specifically changes in impulsiveness and deliberation. The researchers found that compared to participants who remained weight stable, those who gained weight became more impulsive. Those who did not gain weight showed a predicted decrease in impulsiveness. But contrary to their hypothesis, weight gain was also associated with increases in deliberation. In other words, subjects who were gaining weight became more thoughtful before acting. The authors opined that as participants gained weight, they bought into the American stereotypes about persons with obesity. So they saw themselves as more impulsive even as they were increasing in deliberativeness. There was no observable change in self-discipline (Sutin, Costa, et al., 2013).

Conclusions

Third-party reimbursement for obesity treatment stands at the crossroads of science, stigma, health policy, and the dynamics of changes in the health care delivery system. The move from fee-for-service reimbursement to value-based reimbursement may create positive incentives for addressing treatments for obesity. Third-party reimbursement is essential to make treatments for obesity accessible to low-income (often minority) populations, and to create incentives for the development of new drugs and devices. The accumulation of more data about patients and their weight-related conditions may demonstrate the usefulness of reimbursing for obesity treatments.

To date, efforts to expand third-party reimbursement have depended on the efforts, usually uncoordinated, of professional societies, corporations, and advocacy groups. They have lacked a necessary focus on developing a strategy to expand coverage across a range of interventions and assisting the most at-risk populations: those with severe obesity and low-income individuals and minorities. There also has been a lack of attention to the evolution of the health care delivery system, which may hold promise for greater attention to persons with obesity. This is an unmet structural defect in the obesity field that must be fixed in order to facilitate continued progress in obesity treatments.

References

Allison, D. B., Downey, M., Atkinson, R. L., Billington, C. J., Bray, G. A., Eckel, R. H., et al. (2008). Obesity as a disease: A white paper on evidence and arguments commissioned by the Council of The Obesity Society. *Obesity, 16*(6), 1161–1177.

Arterburn, D., Westbrook, E. O., Wiese, C. J., Ludman, E. J., Grossman, D. C., Fishman, P. A., et al. (2008). Insurance coverage and incentives for weight loss among adults with metabolic syndrome. *Obesity, 16*(1), 70–76.

Baum, C., Andiono, K., Wittbrodt, E., Stewart, S., Szymanski, K., & Turpin, R. (2015). The challenges and opportunities associated with reimbursement for obesity pharmacology in the USA. *Pharmacoeconomics, 33*(7), 643–653.

Bennett, G. G., Steinberg, D. M., & Pogoto, S. L. (2015). Will obesity treatment reimbursement benefit those at highest risk? *American Journal of Medicine, 128*(7), 670–671.

Blue Cross and Blue Shield of North Carolina. (2004, October). Blue Cross and Blue Shield of North Carolina expands coverage to treat obesity. Retrieved from *http://mediacenter.bcbsnc.com/news/59743*.

Blumberg, L. J., & Holahan, J. (2013). Health status of exchange enrollees: Putting rate shock in perspective. Retrieved from *www.urban.org/UploadedPDF/412859-Health-Status-of-Exchange-Enrollees-Putting-Rate-Shock-in-Perspective.pdf*.

Cawley, J., Meyerhoefer, C., Biener, A., Hammer, M., & Wintfeld, N. (2015). Savings in medical expenditures associated with reductions in body mass index among U.S. adults with obesity, by diabetes status. *Pharmacoeconomics, 33*(7), 707–722.

CCI Consumer Information and Insurance Oversight & Centers for Medicare and Medicaid Services. (2015). Final 2016 letter to issuers in the federally-facilitated marketplaces. Retrieved from *www.cms.gov/CCIIO/Resources/Regulations-and-Guidance/Downloads/2016-Letter-to-Issuers-2-20-2015-R.pdf*.

Centers for Medicare and Medicaid Services. (2011). Decision memo for intensive behavioral therapy for obesity, CAG-00423N. Retrieved from *www.cms.gov/medicare-coverage-database/details/nca-decision-memo.aspx?&NcaName=Intensive%20Behavioral%20Therapy%20for%20Obesity&bc=ACAAAAAAIAAA&NCAId=253*.

Centers for Medicare and Medicaid Services. (2013). Decision memo for bariatric surgery for the treatment of morbid obesity—facility certification requirement, CAG-00250R3. Retrieved from *www.cms.gov/medicare-coverage-database/details/nca-decision-memo.aspx?NCAId=266*.

Cook, D. (2002). Coverage of obesity problematic for most health plans. Retrieved from *www.managedcaremag.com/archives/2002/7/coverage-obesity-problematic-most-health-plans*.

Decker, S. L., Kostova, D., Kenney, G. M., & Long, S. K. (2013). Health status, risk factors, and medical conditions among persons enrolled in Medicaid vs. uninsured low-income adults potentially eligible for Medicaid under the Affordable Care Act. *Journal of the American Medical Association, 309*(24), 2579–2586.

Dixon, J. B. (2015). Regional differences in the coverage and uptake of bariatric–metabolic surgery: A focus on type 2 diabetes. *Surgery for Obesity and Related Diseases, 12*(6), 1171–1177.

Dobbs, R., Sawers, C., Thompson, F., Manyika, J., Woetzel, J., Child, P., et al. (2014). Overcoming obesity: An initial economic analysis. Retrieved from *www.mckinsey.com/mgi/overview*.

Dor, A., Ferguson, C., Langwith, C., & Tan, E. (2010). A heavy burden: The individual cost of being overweight and obese in the United States. Retrieved June 15, 2016, from *http://stopobesityalliance. org/wp-content/themes/stopobesityalliance/pdfs/ Heavy_Burden_Report.pdf*.

Downey, M. (2001). Results of expert meetings: Obesity and cardiovascular disease—obesity as a disease entity. *American Heart Journal, 142*(6), 1091–1094.

Downey, M. (2014a). The doctor is in charge: How the ACA puts the employee's physician in charge of the wellness program. *Journal of Policy Analysis and Management, 33*(3), 820–826.

Downey, M. (2014b). Response to Dr. Cawley. *Journal of Policy Analysis and Management, 33*(3), 820–826.

Flanagan, E., Ghaderi, I., Overby, D. W., & Farrell, T. M. (2016). Reduced survival in bariatric surgery candidates delayed or denied by lack of insurance approval. *American Journal of Surgery, 82*(2), 166–170.

Gallagher, C. (2012). Summary of obesity treatment state benchmark plan coverage. Retrieved from *www.obesityaction.org/wp-content/uploads/1212-OCC-Summary-of-Obesity-Treatment-State-Benchmark-Plan-Coverage.pdf*.

Glassman, M. (2004). A deletion opens Medicare to coverage for obesity. Retrieved July 16, 2004, from *www.nytimes.com*.

Hampp, C., Kang, E. M., & Borders-Hemphill, V. (2013). Use of prescription anti-obesity drugs in the United States. *Pharmacotherapy, 33*(12), 1299–1307.

Han, E., Norton, E. C., & Stearns, S. C. (2009). Weight and wages: Fat versus lean paychecks. *Health Economics, 18*(5), 535–548.

Internal Revenue Service, Employee Benefits Security Administration, & Health and Human Services Department. (2011). Group health plans and health insurance issuers: Rules relating to internal claims and appeals and external review processes. Retrieved from *www.federalregister.gov/ articles/2011/06/24/2011-15890/group-health-plans-and-health-insurance-issuers-rules-relating-to-internal-claims-and-appeals-and-external-review-processes*.

Lee, J. S., Sheer, J. L., Lopez, N., & Rosenbaum, S. (2010). Coverage of obesity treatment: A state-by-state analysis of Medicaid and state insurance laws. *Public Health Reports, 125*(4), 596–604.

Lewis, K. H., Edwards-Hampton, S. A., & Ard, J. D. (2016). Disparities in treatment uptake and outcomes of patients with obesity in the USA. *Current Obesity Reports, 5*(2), 282–290.

Mainous, A. G., Johnson, S. P., Saxena, S. K., & Wright, R. U. (2013). Inpatient bariatric surgery among eligible black and white men and women in the United States, 1999–2010. *American Journal of Gastroenterology, 108*(8), 1218–1223.

Medicare Coverage Executive Committee. (2000). Transcript for March 1, 2000 meeting: Health Care Financing Administration, Baltimore, MD. Retrieved from *http://lobby.la.psu.edu/014_Medical_ Devices/Agency_Activities/HCFA/HCFA_Transcript_of_MCAC_EC_Meeting_030100.htm*.

Medicare Prescription Drug, Improvement, and Modernization Act of 2003, Pub.L.108-173. 149 U.S.C. §§ 2066–2480.

Millman, J. (2015). Health insurers may be finding new ways to discriminate against patients. Retrieved January 28, 2015, from *www.washingtonpost.com/ news/wonk/wp/2015/01/28/health-insurers-may-be-finding-new-ways-to-discriminate-against-patients*.

Mitchell, N. S., Ellison, M. C., Hill, J. O., & Tsai, A. G. (2013). Evaluation of the effectiveness of making Weight Watchers available to Tennessee Medicaid (TennCare) recipients. *Journal of General Internal Medicine, 28*(1), 12–17.

NCQA. (2015a). Adult BMI assessment. Retrieved from *www.ncqa.org/report-cards/health-plans/ state-of-health-care-quality/2015-table-of-contents/adult-bmi*.

NCQA. (2015b). Weight assessment and counseling for nutrition and physical activity for children/adolescents. Retrieved from *www.ncqa.org/report-cards/ health-plans/state-of-health-care-quality/2015-table-of-contents/weight-assessment*.

O'Brien, J. (2014). Supplemental guidance: Management of obesity in adults (Letter No. 2014-04). Retrieved from *www.opm.gov/healthcare-insurance/ healthcare/carriers/2014/2014-04.pdf*.

Ochner, C. N., Barrios, D. M., Lee, C. D., & Pi-Sunyer, F. X. (2013). Biological mechanisms that promote weight regain following weight loss in obese humans. *Physiology and Behavior, 120*, 106–113.

Patient Protection and Affordable Care Act of 2010, Pub. L. 111-148. 124 U.S.C. §§ 119-1024.

Petrin, C. (2016). Medicaid fee-for-service treatment of obesity interventions. Retrieved June 15, 2016, from *http://stopobesityalliance.org/wp-content/ assets/2016/04/Medicaid%20FFS%20Treatment%20of%20Obesity.%202016%20(4)%20(1). pdf*.

Rosenbaum, S. (2016). Twenty-first century Medicaid: The final managed care rule. Retrieved May 6, 2017, from *http://healthaffairs.org/blog/2016/05/05/ twenty-first-century-medicaid-the-final-managed-care-rule*.

Sadhasivam, S., Larson, C. J., Lambert, P. J., Mathiason, M. A., & Kothari, S. N. (2007). Refusals, denials, and patient choice: Reasons prospective patients do not undergo bariatric surgery. *Surgery for Obesity and Related Diseases, 3*(5), 531–535.

Social Security Administration. (2002). Policy interpretation ruling Titles II and XVI: Evaluation of obesity. Retrieved from *www.ssa.gov/OP_Home/ rulings/di/01/SSR2000-03-di-01.html*.

Sumithran, P., Prendergast, L. A., Delbridge, E., Purcell, K., Shulkes, A., Kriketos, A., et al. (2011). Long-term persistence of hormonal adaptions to weight loss. *New England Journal of Medicine, 365*, 1597–1604.

Sutin, A. R., Costa, P. T., Jr., Chan, W., Milaneschi, Y., Eaton, W. W., Zonderman, A. B., et al. (2013).

I know not to, but I can't help it: Weight gain and changes in impulsivity-related personality traits. *Pyschological Science, 24*(7), 1323–1328.

Sutin, A. R., Ferrucci, L., Zonderman, A. B., & Terracciano, A. (2011). Personality and obesity across the adult life span. *Journal of Personality and Social Psychology, 101*(3), 579–592.

Sutin, A. R., Zonderman, A. B., Uda, M., Deiana, B., Taub, D. D., Longo, D. L., et al. (2013). Personality traits and leptin. *Psychosomatic Medicine, 75*(5), 505–509.

Tsuda, S., Barrios, L., Schneider, B., & Jones, D. B. (2009). Factors affecting rejection of bariatric patients from an academic weight loss program. *Surgery for Obesity and Related Diseases, 5*(2), 199–202.

U.S. Department of Health and Human Services. (2014). Lifetime and annual limits. Retrieved from *www.hhs.gov/healthcare/about-the-law/benefit-limits/index.html*.

U.S. Department of the Treasury, Internal Revenue Service. (2016). Medical and dental expenses (including the Health Coverage Tax Credit) (Publication No. 502). Retrieved from *www.irs.gov/pub/irs-pdf/p502.pdf*.

U.S. Food and Drug Administration. (2016). Information by drug class. Retrieved from *www.fda.gov/Drugs/DrugSafety/InformationbyDrugClass*.

Wang, Y. C., Pamplin, J., Long, M. W., Ward, Z. J., Gortmaker, S. L., & Andreyeva, T. (2015). Severe obesity in adults cost state Medicaid programs nearly $8 billion in 2013. *Health Affairs, 34*(11), 1923–1931.

Yang, Y. T., & Pomeranz, J. L. (2015). States variations in the provision of bariatric surgery under the Affordable Care Act exchanges. *Surgery for Obesity and Related Diseases, 11*(3), 715–720. See also, the American Society for Metabolic and Bariatric Surgery coverage of bariatric surgery in state exchanges available at *https://asmbs.org/wp/uploads/2014/06/State-Exchange-and-Bariatric-Coverage-Stories-for-Selected-States.pdf*.

Yang, Z., & Zhang, N. (2014). The burden of overweight and obesity on long-term care and Medicaid financing. *Medical Care, 52*(7), 658–663.

Zhang, S., Manne, S., Lin, J., & Yang, J. (2016). Characteristics of patients potentially eligible for pharmacotherapy for weight loss in primary care practice in the United States. *Obesity Science and Practice, 2*(2), 104–114.

CHAPTER 26

Obesity Treatment Perspectives in U.S. Racial/Ethnic Minority Populations

Shiriki K. Kumanyika

The importance of giving special consideration to racial/ethnic minority populations for addressing obesity as a public health and clinical challenge in the United States is a well-established principle. It addresses the changing demographics of the U.S. population, as well as the above-average prevalence of obesity in some minority populations. The most recent obesity treatment guidelines acknowledge the need for a better understanding of racial/ethnic differences in obesity-related health risks, especially in relation to African American and Hispanic/Latino populations (Jensen et al., 2014). These guidelines also call for further research to identify appropriate approaches to behavioral as well as surgical treatments of obesity in different racial/ethnic groups. The additional recommendation for studies to evaluate approaches for translating treatments to community settings has special relevance to minority populations. There are substantial racial/ethnic differences within the sociocultural, physical, and economic environments that influence obesity.

This chapter highlights evidence supporting the applicability of currently recommended treatment approaches to racial/ethnic minority populations and considers theoretical and empirical evidence related to translating these approaches for effectiveness with these populations. The review draws primarily on evidence from studies of African Americans, who are the most well-studied minority population. The scope is limited to obesity treatment with lifestyle modification approaches, which are the major foci of clinical guidelines and important as supportive approaches to both pharmacological and surgical treatments. The scope of the chapter is limited to adults—and adults influence children's environments and behaviors. Effective treatment of obesity in adults in minority populations can, therefore, be expected to also contribute to addressing the higher-than-average rates of obesity among children and adolescents in these populations (U.S. Department of Health and Human Services, Centers for Disease Control and Prevention, National Center for Health Statistics, 2015). Balantekin, Wilfley, and Epstein (Chapter 39, this volume) discuss obesity treatment in children and adolescents.

Background

Minority Populations

The U.S. Census Bureau minority population categories and selected demographic data for these population groups are shown in Table 26.1; data for non-Hispanic whites are included for reference. The main Census Bureau minority populations are "black or African American," "Hispanic or Latino American," "American Indian or Alaska Native," "Native Hawaiian or other Pacific Islander," or "Asian American" (Humes, Nicholas, & Ramirez, 2011). However, each of these categories as well as non-Hispanic whites are very heterogeneous and have limited specificity with respect to ethno–cultural–regional variation. More than a third of the U.S population is in a minority racial/ethnic category—that is, identifies in a category other than "white" and does not indicate Hispanic or Latino ethnicity. Hispanic or Latino Americans are the largest minority population (17%) overall; Hispanic and Asian Americans comprise the majority of the foreign-born population (Colby & Ortman, 2015). The overall U.S. population is expected to become "majority" minority within the next three decades (Colby & Ortman, 2015). The term *"majority–minority"* is currently used to describe jurisdictions where minority populations constitute more than 50% of the population—for example, California; Washington, DC, Hawaii; New Mexico; and Texas (Humes et al., 2011).

Low socioeconomic status (SES) is relatively more common among minority populations compared to whites, although this varies among subgroups, especially among Asian Americans (Macartney, Bishaw, & Fontenot, 2013; Ryan & Bauman, 2016; U.S. Department of Health and Human Services, Office of Minority Health, 2016). Up to one-quarter of individuals live below the poverty line in some U.S. ethnic groups, and substantial proportions of minority populations have no regular source of health care (Table 26.1) (U.S. Department of Health and Human Services, Centers for Disease Control and Prevention, National Center for Health Statistics, 2015).

Prevalence of Obesity and Related Health Risks

Self-reported data on the percent of people with obesity, diabetes, and/or hypertension in each racial/ethnic group are also shown in Table 26.1 (Blackwell, Lucas, & Clarke, 2014; U.S. Department of Health and Human Services, Centers for Disease Control and Prevention, National Center for Health Statistics, 2016a, 2016b). Self-reported data may underestimate prevalence but provide a picture of the group differences across the racial/ethnic categories. Except for Asian Americans, obesity prevalence is higher in minority than in white populations. As a caveat, a BMI cutoff of 25 or 30 kg/m^2 might seriously underestimate fatness-related metabolic risks in populations of Asian descent (World Health Organization Consultation, 2004). For example, diabetes prevalence is higher in Asian Americans than in whites—higher than would be expected based on the low prevalence of obesity at the BMI cutoff of 30 kg/m^2 (Table 26.1). Non-Hispanic black and Native Hawaiian/Pacific populations are more likely than non-Hispanic white or the other minority populations to have hypertension.

Figure 26.1 shows the distribution of BMI ≥ 25 kg/m^2 by gender for the three largest racial/ethnic groups, for whom height and weight measurements are available from the National Health and Nutrition Examination Survey (NHANES; U.S. Department of Health and Human Services, Centers for Disease Control and Prevention, National Center for Health Statistics, 2015). Hispanic and non-Hispanic white men have similar levels of overweight, but more Hispanic men have obesity (39 vs. 34%, respectively). A smaller percent of black men are overweight, but the percent with obesity is similar to that in Hispanic men (38%). Among men with obesity, more black men have class 2 (BMI = 35.0–39.9 kg/m^2) or class 3 (BMI $\geq$ 40 kg/m^2) obesity. In women, the percent with obesity is higher in both black and Hispanic women compared to white women—highest in black women, among whom 32% have class 2 or class 3 obesity. This high prevalence at the upper end of the BMI distribution reflects baseline BMI levels that were al-

TABLE 26.1. Characteristics of U.S. Racial/Ethnic Subgroups

Variable	Non-Hispanic white	Non-Hispanic black	Hispanic/Latino	Asian	American Indian or Alaska Native	Native Hawaiian/ Pacific Islander
Basis for racial/ethnic classification[a]	Origins in any of the original peoples of Europe, the Middle East, or North Africa	Origins in any of the black racial groups of Africa	Origins in Cuba, Mexico, Puerto Rico, South or Central America, or other Spanish culture or origin regardless of race	Origins in any of the original peoples of the Far East, Southeast Asia, or the Indian subcontinent	Origins in any of the original peoples of North and Central or South America and maintaining tribal affiliation or community attachment	Original peoples of Hawaii, Guam, Samoa, or other Pacific Islands
Percent distribution of U.S. population[b]	62.2	13.3	17.4	5.4	1.2	0.2
Percent distribution of foreign-born population[b]	18.8	8.1	45.8	25.8	0.1	0.3
Percent with at least high school education[c]	93.3	87.0	66.7	89.1	82	87.4
Percent with a bachelor's degree or more[c]	36.2	22.5	15.5	53.9	17.0	21.5
Percent below poverty[d]	9.9	25.8	16.2–26.3	5.8–15.0	27.0	17.6
No usual source of health care[e]	15.0	19.6	28.9	18.1	23.4	Not reported
Percent with BMI ≥ 30[f]	28.5	39.5	31.8	11.0	43.7	34.6
Percent with type 2 diabetes[g]	7.6	13.0	12.2	9.0	20.9	11.7
Percent with hypertension[b]	23.4	33.2	20.9	21.2	24.8	36.5

[a]Humes et al. (2011); people who indicate Hispanic ethnicity may be of any race, although most check either "white" race or "other" race.
[b]Colby and Ortman (2015); population distribution percentages are approximate due to overlap between Hispanic and Latino ethnicity with the race categories. Data for race do not include the 2.5% of census respondents who identify more than one race.
[c]Ryan and Bauman (2016); The two italicized numbers were taken from data in profiles from the following source: U.S. Department of Health and Human Services, Office of Minority Health (2016).
[d]Macartney et al. (2013).
[e]U.S. Department of Health and Human Services, Centers for Disease Control and Prevention, National Center for Health Statistics (2015).
[f]U.S. Department of Health and Human Services, Centers for Disease Control and Prevention, National Center for Health Statistics (2016a).
[g]U.S. Department of Health and Human Services, Centers for Disease Control and Prevention, National Center for Health Statistics (2016b).
[h]Blackwell, Lucas, and Clarke (2014).

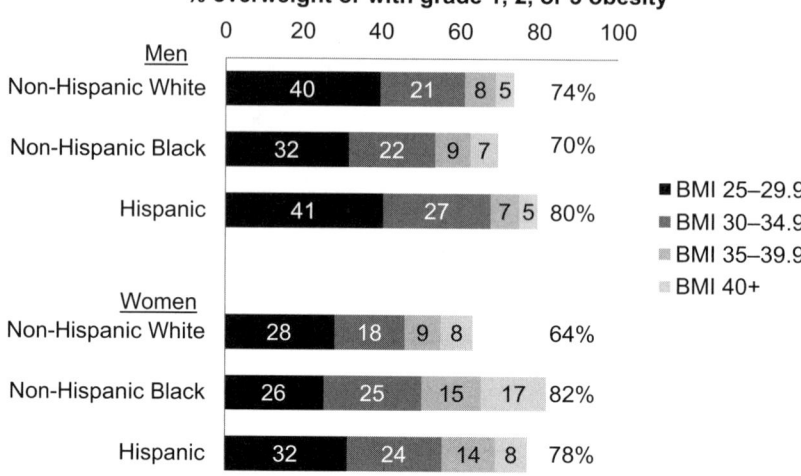

FIGURE 26.1. Combined prevalence and distribution of overweight and obesity in adults ages 20 years and over, age-adjusted and rounded to whole numbers, by race/ethnicity/gender; based on height and weight measurements in the National Health and Nutrition Examination Survey, 2011–2014. Data from U.S. Department of Health and Human Services, Centers for Disease Control and Prevention, National Center for Health Statistics (2015).

ready higher than average when the upward BMI shift began in the U.S. population as a whole.

Race and Ethnicity as Obesity Treatment Variables

Special attention to race and ethnicity in considering approaches to obesity treatment is justified on theoretical grounds and is supported by empirical data. Potential pathways of interest are shown in Figure 26.2. Pretreatment variables that may alter obesity treatment outcomes include biological or psychosocial and behavioral predispositions, as well as environmental contextual factors, which influence participation in and adherence to treatment. The behavioral and psychosocial factors operate at the individual level but are conditioned, in part, by the sociocultural and environmental factors. The pathways shown are interdependent. Documented racial/ethnic differences occur in the direction of predisposing to excess weight gain or limiting treatment motivations or effectiveness.

Biological Predispositions

An example of a supposed biological difference is a "thrifty genotype" that predisposes to efficiency in caloric utilization and fat storage, and that might have conferred an evolutionary survival advantage for some ethnic groups in times of famine (Neel, 1999). Efforts, however, to pinpoint such a gene have been unsuccessful. Among American Indians with a very high prevalence of obesity (for whom a genetic predisposition might be presumed responsible), obesity prevalence is much lower among people of the same heritage who live a traditional lifestyle (Ravussin, Valencia, Esparza, Bennett, & Schulz, 1994). This finding suggests the influence of environmental factors. A large cross-national study showing a gradient of increase in obesity prevalence from Africa through the Caribbean to the United States also suggests that environmental exposures have a much larger role than genetic predisposition among people of African descent (Luke, Cooper, Prewitt, Adeyemo, & Forrester, 2001).

Whether or not genetically mediated, a lower resting energy expenditure in some racial/ethnic groups has been examined as a possible contributor to excess weight gain or to difficulty in losing weight (Allison, Nezin, & Clay-Williams, 1997; Foster, Wadden, Swain, Anderson, & Vogt, 1999; Goran & Weinsier, 2000; Weyer, Snitker, Bogardus, & Ravussin, 1999). For example, lower resting energy expenditure, which may be a function of ethnic differences in body composition, has been proposed as an explanation for smaller weight losses observed in black versus white women. However, data to support this hypothesis have been contradictory (Goran & Weinsier, 2000). Racial/ethnic differences in regional fat distribution may influence obesity treatment effects on clinical outcomes as well—for example, differences in the proportion of visceral fat at a given level of BMI or waist circumference (Camhi et al., 2011).

Psychosocial and Behavioral Predispositions

Weight loss motivations differ by race/ethnicity and tend to be lower in racial/ethnic minorities that have a high prevalence of obesity. These differences are usually attributed to cultural factors: that is, to differences in body image, particularly among women (Brown & Konner, 1987; Craig, 2009). Although combined overweight and obesity affect more than half of the populations in all of the ethnic categories, the perception that obesity is normative, if not physiologically normal, is likely to be more common in minority populations where prevalence is high. In addition, the common association of extreme thinness or what appears to be too much weight loss with wasting illnesses such as cancer, tuberculosis, HIV/AIDS or substance abuse may foster the belief that being heavy is healthier than being thin. This belief may, in turn, affect body image, standards of personal attractiveness, perceptions of whether a heavier or thinner body size is "healthier," and motivations for seeking or continuing with weight loss treatment—particularly among those with obesity but no diagnosed comorbidities.

Standards of attractiveness vary across cultures, and it is now recognized that the preoccupation with thinness among women in the U.S. mainstream culture is not of the same intensity in some ethnic minority populations. As described by Ritenbaugh (1982), obesity is a "culture-bound" syndrome—that is, understandable only within a specific culture and with an etiology that "summarizes and symbolizes core meanings and behavioral norms of that culture" (p. 351). In an account of the evolution of fat storage, distribution, and related attitudes, Craig (2009) refers to the survival advantages associated with excess fat storage as a protec-

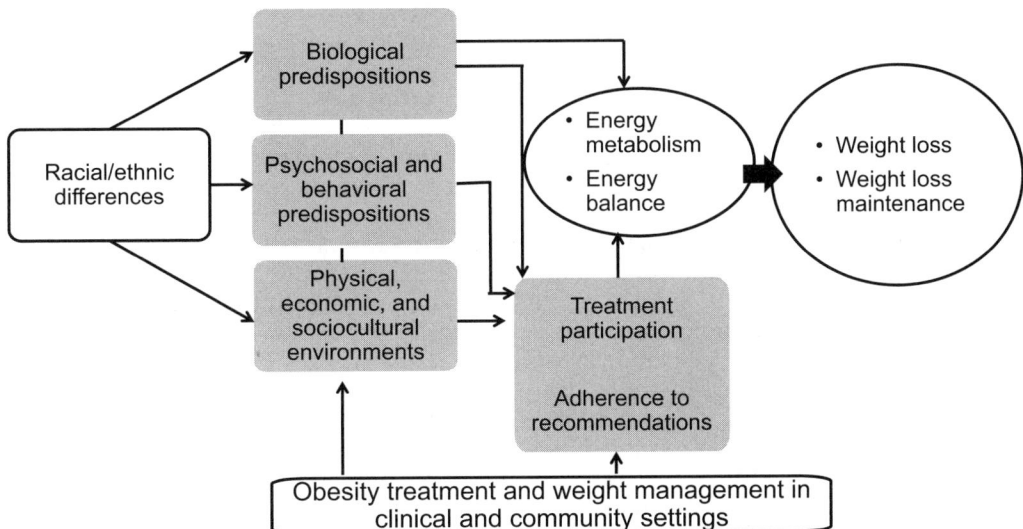

FIGURE 26.2. Pathways of racial/ethnic differences on obesity treatment outcomes.

tion against famine, noting that "Plumpness in women, particularly as lower body fat, evolved to ensure survival of the human race and thus became a rational cultural preference supporting a biologic norm" (Craig, 2009, p. 42). Very overweight individuals in almost all ethnic groups may aspire to weigh less. However, the cosmetic goal of achieving a slender body image may be much less common than expected on the basis of data in non-Hispanic white populations (Flynn & Fitzgibbon, 1998; Striegel-Moore, 1996). In addition, body image in African American women is strongly influenced by considerations of shape and robustness as well as weight, and body size is not necessarily central to the perception of oneself as attractive (Allan, Mayo, & Michel, 1993; Faith, Manibay, Kravitz, Griffith, & Allison, 1998). This less negative experience of obesity may also apply to Hispanic/Latino and other minority populations (Fiery, Martz, Webb, & Curtin, 2016).

Acceptance of a heavier body size may persist despite knowledge and medical advice indicating that obesity is associated with increased risks of diabetes and other chronic diseases, and in spite of exposure to mass media images and fashions that promote weight loss and smaller body sizes. Some cultural differences may fall along a continuum across populations, whereas others reflect qualitative differences in the way certain issues are viewed. At any given point in time, people will tend to judge their weight in reference to their peers or people in their social networks. Winston and colleagues demonstrated the direct association of social norms about obesity with the prevalence of obesity in the social networks of black and Hispanic adults (Winston et al., 2015). Langellier and colleagues, based on an analysis of NHANES data within and across two time periods (1988–1994 and 1999–2000), found several indications that, compared to whites, weight perceptions of black and Mexican Americans were less likely to align with clinical definitions of overweight or obesity and that weight loss motivations were lower and, in some cases, had declined more over time (Langellier, Glik, Ortega, & Prelip, 2015). Self-perceptions as overweight generally did not change in spite of increases in obesity prevalence and in mean BMI among those who were overweight, except that self-perceptions as overweight decreased among white and black women. Consistent with this finding, the percent who reported weight loss efforts in the past year declined by 10 percentage points in both female populations: from 67 to 57% ($p < .001$) in white women and from 63 to 52% ($p < .001$) in black women.

Eating and activity patterns are also rooted in cultural traditions and attitudes—for example, food preferences and preparation practices that add fat to foods or a pattern of sedentary forms of entertainment and low levels of physical activity—which influence receptivity to behavioral change advice. Many Americans are insufficiently active according to national guidelines. The percent, however, of adults classified as "sufficiently active" in the 2012 National Health Interview Survey was lower than whites in all racial/ethnic minority populations (54% for non-Hispanic whites and 41%, 43%, 46%, and 49%, respectively, in non-Hispanic blacks, Hispanics, American Indians/Alaska Natives, and Asian Americans), except for Native Hawaiians/Pacific Islanders, among whom 70% were sufficiently active. However, apart from and sometimes despite cultural preferences, eating and activity behaviors are strongly anchored in and influenced by contextual factors, such as where a person lives, his or her daily routines, and obligations at work and at home (Institute of Medicine, 2012; Kumanyika et al., 2008). These behaviors are also influenced by socioeconomic factors such as education, discretionary income, exposure to financial and other socioecological stressors, and a person's ability to cope, as well as by health variables such as mobility limitations due to osteoarthritis. Some examples of environmental influences that are particularly relevant to racial/ethnic minority populations with a high prevalence of obesity are presented in Table 26.2 (Grier & Kumanyika, 2008; Institute of Medicine, 2013; Kumanyika, Whitt-Glover, & Haire-Joshu, 2014; Lovasi, Hutson, Guerra, & Neckerman, 2009; Yancey, Ory, & Davis, 2006). Not all of the implied constraints can be overcome by the individual, even by one who is well motivated and has been counseled extensively.

TABLE 26.2. Aspects of Environmental Contexts That May Increase Risks of Developing Obesity and Decrease Responsiveness to Interventions

Food-related aspects	Physical-activity-related aspects
Physical environment	
• Limited access to full-service supermarkets • Numerous fast-food outlets • Prominent advertisements for high-sugar, high-fat foods inside of stores and outdoors • Limited availability of fresh fruits and vegetables • Provision of high-fat, high-sugar foods in schools, workplaces, and other community settings • Lack of public transportation	• Heavy traffic • Poor air quality • Lack of pedestrian and cycling pathways • Concern about crime • Limited access to high-quality parks and recreation centers • Lack of safe and appealing school playgrounds
Economic environment	
• Unemployment or unstable employment • Low incomes • Costs of healthier foods and promotion of less healthy foods at low cost • Limited funds available for school meals • Prominence of fast-food and soft-drink companies as employers or funders of scholarships and community events and projects • Cost of supervised preschool and afterschool child care	• Costs of private gyms • Marketing of digital devices and other sedentary forms of entertainment • Limited local investment in parks and recreational facilities • Lack of funds to hire trained physical education teachers in schools • Cost of supervised preschool and after-school child care
Sociocultural environment	
• High-fat, high-sugar foods in traditional cuisine • Awareness of or experiences with food insecurity • Child care and food related responsibilities of women • Body image and perceptions that relatively large body size is the cultural norm • High exposure to television commercials for food	• Cultural attitudes about physical activity and importance of rest • Lack of social support or role models for active living • Fears about safety or for child safety • Gender norms about appropriate physical activity • Reliance on TV and digital devices for entertainment

Note. From Kumanyika, Whitt-Glover, and Haire-Joshu (2014). What works for obesity prevention and treatment in black Americans?: Research directions. *Obesity Review, 15*(Suppl., 4), 204–212. Copyright © 2014 Wiley. Reprinted by permission.

Evidence from Randomized Trials

African Americans

Findings that lifestyle modification interventions for weight loss were less effective with black than white Americans raise questions as to whether this is a consistent pattern and, if so, why. For example, one study compared weight loss in black and white adults from two multicenter high blood pressure prevention trials: the Hypertension Prevention Trial (HPT) and the Trials of Hypertension Prevention, Phase 1 (TOHP I) (Kumanyika, Obarzanek, Stevens, Hebert, & Whelton, 1991). These trials recruited otherwise healthy adults with high-normal blood pressure and included treatment arms with weight loss alone or in combination with sodium reduction, each with a follow-up of 36 and 18 months, respectively. Findings indicated smaller initial weight losses in blacks than whites, particularly among women, but relatively similar trajectories of weight regain. No explanatory data for this pattern were available, although the authors discussed possible explanations based on differences in education, weight loss skills, social norms, or exercise.

Wing and Anglin (1996) compared weight loss outcomes of black and white participants randomized to receive a low-calorie diet or intermittent use of a very-low-calorie diet over 1 year of treatment for type 2 diabetes. They found smaller weight losses in blacks overall, regardless of intervention arm, with a steeper trajectory of weight regain during months 6–12. The authors cited differences in baseline dietary intake and dietary changes during treatment, as well as poorer attendance during months 6–12, as possible reasons for their findings. Clinical outcomes for diabetes control were not significantly different.

More recent studies that have compared weight loss outcomes for black and white participants include five multicenter trials of hypertension or of diabetes prevention or management: Phase II of the Trials of Hypertension Prevention (TOHP II) with 36 months of follow-up (Hebert et al., 1995; Stevens et al., 2001); the Trial of Nonpharmacologic Interventions in the Elderly (TONE), with a median follow-up of 29 months (Kumanyika et al., 2002; Whelton et al., 1998); the PREMIER study (Funk et al., 2008; Svetkey et al., 2005) with 18 months of follow-up; the Diabetes Prevention Program (DPP) with an average of ~30 months of follow-up (Knowler et al., 2002; West, Prewitt, Bursac, & Felix, 2008); and the Action for Health in Diabetes (Look AHEAD) study, which has reported long-term follow-up at 4 and 8 years (Look Ahead Research Group, 2014; Pi-Sunyer, 2014; Wadden et al., 2011). The most recent trials have included special provisions to recruit black participants and, in some cases, other minority populations in diverse geographic areas, and have well-documented and executed interventions and excellent retention for follow-up.

Results of these several multicenter trials (i.e., HPT, TOHP I and the above-cited additional five trials) were included in a systematic review by Wingo, Carson, and Ard (2014). The trials were somewhat comparable in that the weight loss interventions all involved an intensive (i.e., weekly) period of group or individual counseling, or both, which focused on restricting calorie intake and increasing physical activity, with varying levels of continued counseling support during the follow-up period. Age groups and study populations varied and included young to middle-age adults with overweight or moderate level of obesity and at relatively high risk of developing hypertension requiring pharmacological treatment (HPT, TOHP I, TOHP II); older adults already taking medications for high blood pressure but sufficiently well controlled to be potentially managed by lifestyle interventions without medications (TONE); adults with overweight or obesity and at high risk of developing type 2 diabetes (DPP); and middle-age and older adults with overweight/obesity being treated for type 2 diabetes (Look AHEAD).

Smaller weight losses in black than white participants, in both men and women or women at 6 months (i.e., after the initial, most intensive phase of counseling), were a consistent finding of the systematic review (Wingo et al., 2014). Blacks lost approximately 2–6 kg, compared to 5–8 kg in whites. The statistical significance of these initial weight losses, net of control, and of the black–white differences varied, but the same pattern was observed in six of the seven studies. The review did not include 6-month data from Look AHEAD but reported data for the period between 6 months and 1 year, which showed the largest weight loss for both blacks (6.8% of body weight) and whites (9.6% of body weight), although still smaller in blacks, a difference that was statistically significant. Smaller weight losses for black than white participants were also observed in the other studies with a 6-month to < 1-year time period, except for men in the DPP (Wingo et al., 2014).

Concerns raised by the finding of a relatively consistent pattern of less initial weight loss in blacks than whites, under the theoretically ideal circumstances of multicenter efficacy trials, are mitigated by two additional findings from these studies. One is that the black–white differences in initial weight loss were attenuated over 1.5–3 years of follow-up, apparently associated with better maintenance of lost weight in blacks than whites (Wingo et al., 2014). This impression is strongly supported in the 8-year results from Look AHEAD (Look Ahead Research Group, 2014). The mean percent weight loss in Look AHEAD at 1, 4, and 8 years was 6.4, 3.8, and 5.0%, respectively, among black participants and 9.4, 4.6, and 4.7%, respectively, among white participants. Only the 1-year black–white difference in weight loss of 3 percentage points was statistically significant; the percent weight loss at 8 years was essentially the same. Although not included in the Wingo et al. (2014) review, this impression of comparable weight maintenance in black and white participants after smaller initial weight losses was also observed in the Weight Loss Maintenance trial, which randomized participants who achieved a requisite level of initial weight loss to one of three maintenance conditions (Svetkey et al., 2012).

The other mitigating finding is that, despite the smaller initial weight losses, the black participants obtained long-term improvements in blood pressure and diabetes status comparable to those observed for whites in the same study. Wingo et al. (2014) identified only one study in which this was not observed; weight loss among black women in the PREMIER study did not result in a significant change in blood pressure (Svetkey et al., 2005).

Hispanics/Latinos and other Racial/Ethnic Groups

Both the DPP and Look AHEAD trials included and reported subgroup analyses for Hispanic/Latino participants (Look Ahead Research Group, 2014; West et al., 2008). Look AHEAD also included American Indians, Asians, and Pacific Islanders, but the numbers of Asians and Pacific Islanders were too small to support separate statistical analyses. Weight losses and other outcomes for Hispanics in the DPP were comparable to those in the white participants over the course of the 3 years of follow-up. In Look AHEAD, weight losses in Hispanics and American Indians followed a similar pattern as those reported for black participants, i.e., significantly lower weight loss at 1 year but better maintenance than in whites, with no significant difference at the 8-year follow up).

Effectiveness of Lifestyle Interventions in Clinical and Community Settings

The longer-term findings from Look AHEAD, in particular, suggest that lifestyle modification interventions can be effective in diverse ethnic minority populations, particularly when strategies that support weight loss maintenance are available. Although no such efficacy data were identified for adults in Asian or Pacific Islander Americans, it is reasonable to assume that these strategies would also apply to these populations. Thus, the question of how to translate these findings for effectiveness in clinical and community settings becomes critical. The highly selected participants and "best-case scenario" aspects of efficacy trials constitute artificial conditions that presumably are not replicable in day-to-day clinical settings or community programs generally, and perhaps especially not in black and many other minority communities. Evidence on the efficacy-to-effectiveness continuum suggests that effects seen in efficacy trials are diluted when adapted and implemented in clinical and community settings (Glasgow, McKay, Piette, & Reynolds, 2001). Thus, the smaller weight losses that can be expected outside of specialized obesity treatment programs may become problematic where clinically significant weight losses are less common even in efficacy trials. Evidence from weight loss trials in racial/ethnic minority populations in clinical and community settings is still very limited. Summaries of evidence in African Americans are highlighted below.

DPP Translations

A systematic review of short-term weight loss outcomes of DPP translational studies with African Americans confirmed the expectation of notably smaller weight losses. Samuel-Hodge and colleagues identified 17 DPP translation studies, of which 7 involved all African American samples and 10 involved mixed samples and reported subgroup data for African Americans (Samuel-Hodge, Johnson, Braxton, & Lackey, 2014). The mean weight loss and estimated rate of weight loss on a monthly basis for African Americans in the studies for which these could be calculated were compared with results for African Americans in the DPP (Figure 26.3). Compared with the 1.1 or 0.8 kg weight loss in African American men and women, respectively, in the DPP, mean loss in the translational studies was 0.5–0.7 kg per month. Samuel-Hodge et al. (2014) noted several differences between these studies

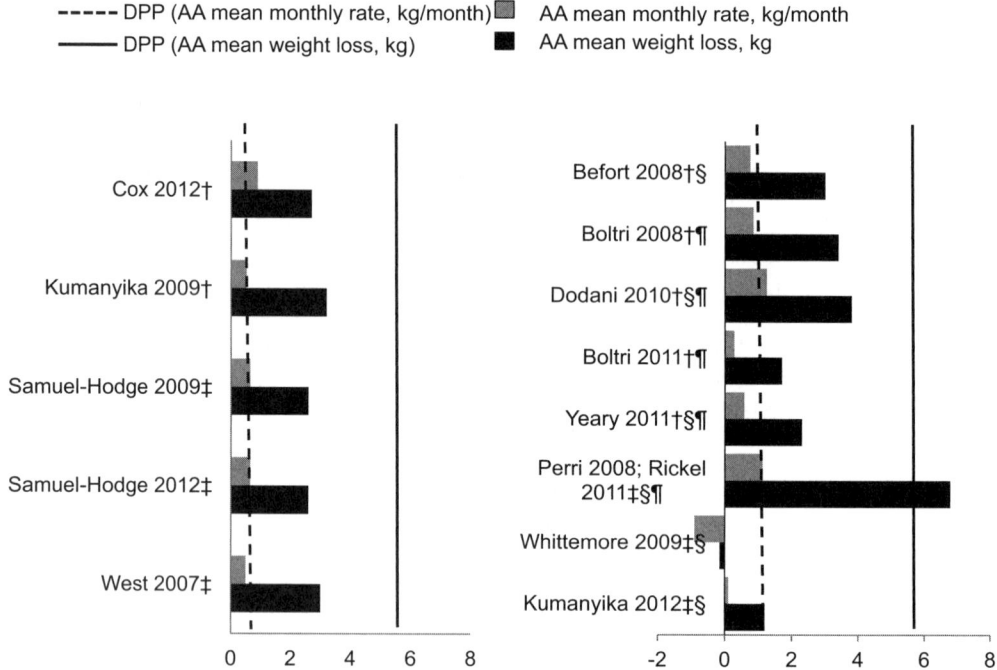

FIGURE 26.3. Comparisons of weight loss among African Americans (AA) in the DPP with that of African Americans in DPP translation studies. *Higher quality studies (left panel) were defined by the following three criteria: (1) randomized, controlled trial during the weight loss phase; (2) sample size > 30; and (3) intention-to-treat analysis or attrition < 20%. Studies not meeting this definition are in the right panel. †AA-only sample; ‡mixed sample; §nonrandomized controlled trials (during the weight loss phase); ¶completers-only outcome analysis. Adapted from Samuel-Hodge, Johnson, Braxton, and Lackey, M. (2014). Effectiveness of Diabetes Prevention Program translations among African Americans. *Obesity Reviews, 15*(Suppl. 4), 107–124. Copyright © 2014 Wiley. Adapted by permission.

and the DPP, such as the higher proportion of women in the translational studies (68% in the DPP compared with 70–100% in the translational studies), the fact that only six of these studies included people with prediabetes or diabetes, and higher attrition rates (7% in the DPP vs. 18–22% on average and as high as 41% in the translational studies). Although the evidence from these heterogeneous studies was difficult to summarize, the authors concluded that specific enhancements to the DPP, related to social support, stress reduction, as well as more staff training, might improve effectiveness.

Faith-Based Programs

Faith organizations have also been used for several community-based weight loss programs with African Americans because of their central role as community institutions. A systematic review of faith-based interventions that targeted diet, physical activity, or weight loss identified 27 studies; randomized controlled trials (RCTs), quasi-experiments, and single-group designs were included (Lancaster, Carter-Edwards, Grilo, Shen, & Schoenthaler, 2014). Statistically significant changes in weight and other outcomes were reported by two-thirds of the studies that targeted weight loss, but this outcome applied to only two of the five RCTs assessed. Significant findings for behavior change were reported by 7 of the 11 RCTs that reported such measurements. This review was valuable for describing the different approaches used and their potential implications for further research, emphasizing that these approaches should be evaluated in more RCTs or quasi-experiments using theory-based approaches. Research needs identified by the authors included evaluation of the potential value of intervening at multiple levels of relevant social contexts (intra- and interpersonal, organizational, and neighborhood/community level), as well as issues associated with incorporation of spiritual content and the involvement of church members as lay intervention providers.

Culturally Adapted Interventions

Kong and colleagues conducted a systematic review of 28 interventions (20 RCTs and 8 quasi-experiments) with data for African American women, of which 17 reported statistically significant net improvements in weight or dietary change (Kong, Tussing-Humphreys, Odoms-Young, Stolley, & Fitzgibbon, 2014). All except four of the studies had solely African American participants, and most were conducted in churches, community centers, or health clinics. The authors coded the interventions according to Kreuter's classification of types of cultural adaptation strategies as (1) *peripheral* (modifying characteristics of materials or other elements to be recognized as culturally relevant; (2) *evidential* (using ethnically based health information to contextualize the salience of the intervention for the population; (3) *linguistic* (using language that increases accessibility of the information to the audience, including the use of languages other than English, entirely or in a bilingual format; (4) *constituent-involving* (using experiences or input from the population of interest to inform the study design or procedures); and (5) *sociocultural* (incorporating content that aligns with the underlying beliefs, values, and group norms) (Kreuter, Lukwago, Bucholtz, Clark, & Sanders-Thompson, 2003). Kong et al. also assessed the use of "tailoring," an additional concept from Kreuter's framework defined as adapting aspects of the intervention for individual characteristics. Tailoring can be contrasted with "targeting," which usually refers to studies that focus on recruiting members of a particular group, but without necessarily tailoring to individuals within the group.

Key findings of this review with respect to cultural adaptations included the following: Peripheral strategies were used by about half of the studies (15 of 28), primarily during participant recruitment. Constituent-involving and sociocultural strategies were each used by 23 of the 28 studies. Various forms of constituent involvement were used, and at various study phases. Sociocultural strategies included faith-based content, cultural foods, aspects of body image, and social support. Three studies mentioned health risks (evidential), and one adapted program materials for literacy appropriateness (linguistic). Because most studies used at least two of the five types of cultural adaptations, there was not a clear distinction in the categories of cultural adaptations that were associated with significant weight loss. In addition, the types of approaches within these categories differed. Kong et al. (2014) also recommended a more systematic basis for designing and reporting cultural adaptations. Their impression was that the use of culturally adapted strategies was probably a positive factor in the number of studies that did show significant behavioral change, and that constituent involvement and individual tailoring were important approaches to include (Kong et al., 2014). A separate systematic review from the same group that focused on weight loss maintenance in African American women suggested that cultural adaptations were associated with preventing weight regain during the maintenance phase (Tussing-Humphreys, Fitzgibbon, Kong, & Odoms-Young, 2013)

Men in general and men in racial/ethnic minority populations are underrepresented in weight loss intervention trials (Pagoto et al., 2012). Authors of a systematic review of weight loss studies in African American men reported that there was insufficient evidence to draw meaningful conclusions about effectiveness in community settings (Newton, Griffith, Kearney, & Bennett, 2014). This is a critical area for future research in African American communities, given that African American men have above-average risks of obesity-related diseases and rising obesity prevalence (U.S. Department of Health and Human Services, Centers for Disease Control and Prevention, National Center for Health Statistics, 2015). The efficacy and effectiveness of e-health interventions in minority populations has also not been well studied to date but will become an increasingly important approach to consider, given that these interventions can be delivered through mobile devices (Bennett et al., 2014). Survey data indicate that 70% percent of black Americans and 71% of Hispanic Americans own a smartphone, compared to 61% of whites (Smith, 2015).

The evidence in other minority populations includes promising reports about successful approaches, for example: the Lawrence Latino Diabetes Prevention Project (LLDPP) in Massachusetts (Merriam et al., 2009; Ockene et al., 2012); the De Por Vida pilot study with Mexican American women in Portland, Oregon (Lindberg et al., 2012); the PILI 'Ohana study with Native Hawaiians and Pacific Islanders (Kaholokula et al., 2013, 2014); and strategies within American Indian communities described by Teufel-Shone (2006). However, there appear to be few systematic reviews. Those identified found relatively few studies, often of poor quality (Bender, Choi, Won, & Fukuoka, 2014; Corona, Flores, & Arab, 2016; Lindberg & Stevens, 2007).

The underlying issues for translational studies identified in the systematic reviews of data for African Americans may be applicable to other minority populations. However, generalized approaches, even when based on certain principles, cannot meet the needs of diverse minority populations and subpopulations (National Heart, Lung, and Blood Institute, 1998). A program of well-designed and conducted studies is needed within each population or in mixed studies with adequate subgroup sizes.

Conclusions and Implications

Despite the limitations of the evidence base on obesity treatment in minority populations, multicenter efficacy trials of obesity treatment that have well-designed and executed interventions can result in clinically significant and sustainable outcomes in diverse racial/ethnic groups. Some trials suggest that black women may face greater challenges in this respect, perhaps due to greater severity of obesity (see Figure 26.1). For example, in the DPP, the proportion of black women with BMI ≥ 35 kg/m^2 was greater than in the other race/ethnicity-gender groups, and black women also comprised the group with the smallest weight loss and least favorable trajectory compared to the other groups (West et al., 2008).

The Look AHEAD group reported that at least modest initial weight loss was a key factor in successful long-term weight outcomes (Look AHEAD Research Group, 2014). This study also reported that a 4-year lifestyle program achieved significant weight losses and clinical outcomes results among those with class 3 obesity that were comparable to those with less severe obesity (Unick et al., 2011). Thus, finding accessible, affordable, effective, and scalable weight loss approaches emerges as a particularly pressing priority for black women within the overall priority for all ethnic minority populations with above-average obesity prevalence. According to a meta-analysis of 14 studies by Admiraal et al. (2012), black women and men receiving bariatric surgery appear to benefit in terms of diabetes remission in spite of the significantly lower percent (by about 8 percentage points) of excess weight loss in blacks than whites postsurgery. However, bariatric surgery is often an infeasible option for most people with severe obesity, and those who do have surgery will still need effective, culturally appropriate, lifestyle modification counseling after surgery.

Whether the problem of limited effectiveness of obesity treatment outside of efficacy trials is solvable through current approaches has been questioned. Available data indicate that cultural adaptations may help, particularly if designed and applied in more rigorous study designs than has been the case to date. High attrition rates and low session attendance are other areas needing attention. Although the available data do not lend themselves to systematic analyses of the impact of these participation issues on outcomes, good retention and attendance in efficacy trials are closely linked to success in these trials. Selectivity of treatment populations for community and clinical programs—although not a major focus of reviews cited here—may be worth considering as a contributing factor. Unlike efficacy trials, community- and clinically based programs may be open to "all comers," leading to heterogeneity in treatment groups on variables such as health status, motivation, and a range of contextual factors. Stratifying treatment populations, or the use of adaptive designs or individual tailoring to accommodate differences in predispositions, are possible approaches. Finally, Mitchell and colleagues have suggested that community-based weight loss programs, including commercial programs, could meet the need for an infrastructure to support effectiveness studies with the potential to reach populations at large, including medically underserved populations (Mitchell, Nassel, & Thomas, 2015; Mitchell, Prochazka, & Glasgow, 2016). They mentioned four possible programs: The National Diabetes Prevention Program, which is based on the DPP; Jenny Craig; Weight Watchers; and TOPS (Take Off Pounds Sensibly). This line of reasoning merits further consideration.

The findings about cultural adaptations potentially influence all types of interventions, approaches, and settings. The theoretical importance of such adaptations is meaningless unless they are conceptualized, operationalized, assessed, and found to make a difference in outcomes. Information about how and when these adaptations matter during the recruitment, enrollment, intervention, and follow-up process would also be needed. Interventions should strive to leverage social and cultural assets of minority communities to foster healthy eating and active living rather than only view cultural influences as "barriers" to be removed. Approaches based in faith organizations may be particularly promising in this respect, and strategies that partner with other types of well-established community organizations that offer access and resources should also be explored.

References

Admiraal, W. M., Celik, F., Gerdes, V. E., Dallal, R. M., Hoekstra, J. B., & Holleman, F. (2012). Ethnic differences in weight loss and diabetes remission after bariatric surgery: A meta-analysis. *Diabetes Care, 35*(9), 1951–1958.

Allan, J. D., Mayo, K., & Michel, Y. (1993). Body size values of white and black women. *Research in Nursing and Health, 16*(5), 323–333.

Allison, D. B., Nezin, L. E., & Clay-Williams, G. (1997). Obesity among African American women: Prevalence, consequences, causes, and developing research. *Women's Health Research, 2*(3–4), 243–274.

Bender, M. S., Choi, J., Won, G. Y., & Fukuoka, Y. (2014). Randomized controlled trial lifestyle interventions for Asian Americans: A systematic review. *Preventative Medicine, 67,* 171–181.

Bennett, G. G., Steinberg, D. M., Stoute, C., Lanpher, M., Lane, I., Askew, S., et al. (2014). Electronic health (eHealth) interventions for weight management among racial/ethnic minority adults: A systematic review. *Obesity Reviews, 15*(4, Suppl.), 146–158.

Blackwell, D. L., Lucas, J. W., & Clarke, T. C. (2014). Summary health statistics for U.S. adults: National Health Interview Survey, 2012. *Vital and Health Statistics Series, 10*(260), 1–161.

Brown, P. J., & Konner, M. (1987). An anthropological perspective on obesity. *Annals of New York Academy of the Sciences, 499,* 29–46.

Camhi, S. M., Bray, G. A., Bouchard, C., Greenway, F. L., Johnson, W. D., Newton, R. L., et al. (2011). The relationship of waist circumference and BMI to visceral, subcutaneous, and total body fat: Sex and race differences. *Obesity (Silver Spring), 19*(2), 402–408.

Colby, S. L., & Ortman, J. M. (2015, March). *Projections of the size and composition of the U.S. population: 2014 to 2060. Population estmates and projections.* Current Population Reports (Report No. P25-1143). Washington, DC: U.S. Census Bureau.

Corona, E., Flores, Y. N., & Arab, L. (2016). Trends in evidence-based lifestyle interventions directed at obese and overweight adult Latinos in the US: A systematic review of the literature. *Journal of Community Health, 41*(3), 667–673.

Craig, P. (2009). Obesity and culture. In P. G. Kopelman, I. D. Caterson, & W. H. Dietz (Eds.), *Clinical obesity in adults and children* (3rd ed., pp. 41–57). New Jersey: Wiley-Blackwell.

Faith, M. S., Manibay, E., Kravitz, M., Griffith, J., & Allison, D. B. (1998). Relative body weight and self-esteem among African Americans in four nationally representative samples. *Obesity Research, 6*(6), 430–437.

Fiery, M. F., Martz, D. M., Webb, R. M., & Curtin, L. (2016). A preliminary investigation of racial differences in body talk in age-diverse U.S. adults. *Eating Behaviors, 21,* 232–235.

Flynn, K. J., & Fitzgibbon, M. (1998). Body images and obesity risk among black females: A review of the literature. *Annals of Behavioal Medicine, 20*(1), 13–24.

Foster, G. D., Wadden, T. A., Swain, R. M., Anderson, D. A., & Vogt, R. A. (1999). Changes in resting energy expenditure after weight loss in obese African American and white women. *American Journal of Clinical Nutrition, 69*(1), 13–17.

Funk, K. L., Elmer, P. J., Stevens, V. J., Harsha, D. W., Craddick, S. R., Lin, P. H., et al. (2008). PREMIER: A trial of lifestyle interventions for blood pressure control—intervention design and rationale. *Health Promotion Practice, 9*(3), 271–280.

Glasgow, R. E., McKay, H. G., Piette, J. D., & Reynolds, K. D. (2001). The RE-AIM framework for evaluating interventions: What can it tell us about approaches to chronic illness management? *Patient Education Counseling, 44*(2), 119–127.

Goran, M. I., & Weinsier, R. L. (2000). Role of environmental vs. metabolic factors in the etiology of obesity: Time to focus on the environment. *Obesity Research, 8*(5), 407–409.

Grier, S. A., & Kumanyika, S. K. (2008). The context for choice: Health implications of targeted food and beverage marketing to African Americans. *American Journal of Public Health, 98*(9), 1616–1629.

Hebert, P. R., Bolt, R. J., Borhani, N. O., Cook, N. R., Cohen, J. D., Cutler, J. A., et al. (1995). Design of a multicenter trial to evaluate long-term lifestyle intervention in adults with high-normal blood pressure levels. *Annals of Epidemiology, 5*(2), 130–139.

Humes, K. R. J., Nicholas A., & Ramirez, R. R. (2011). Overview of race and Hispanic origins, 2010. *2010 Census Briefs*. Washington, DC: U.S. Census Bureau.

Institute of Medicine. (2012). *Accelerating progress in obesity prevention: Solving the weight of the nation*. Washington, DC: National Academies Press.

Institute of Medicine. (2013). *Creating equal opportunities for a healthy weight: Workshop summary*. Washington, DC: National Academy of Sciences.

Jensen, M. D., Ryan, D. H., Apovian, C. M., Ard, J. D., Comuzzie, A. G., Donato, K. A., et al. (2014). 2013 AHA/ACC/TOS guideline for the management of overweight and obesity in adults: A report of the American College of Cardiology/American Heart Association Task Force on Practice Guidelines and The Obesity Society. *Circulation, 129*(25, Suppl. 2), S102–S138.

Kaholokula, J. K., Kekauoha, P., Dillard, A., Yoshimura, S., Palakiko, D. M., Hughes, C., et al. (2014). The PILI 'Ohana Project: A community–academic partnership to achieve metabolic health equity in Hawai'i. *Hawaii Journal of Medicine Public Health, 73*(12, Suppl. 3), 29–33.

Kaholokula, J. K., Townsend, C. K., Ige, A., Sinclair, K., Mau, M. K., Leake, A., et al. (2013). Sociodemographic, behavioral, and biological variables related to weight loss in Native Hawaiians and other Pacific Islanders. *Obesity (Silver Spring), 21*(3), E196–E203.

Knowler, W. C., Barrett-Connor, E., Fowler, S. E., Hamman, R. F., Lachin, J. M., Walker, E. A., et al. (2002). Reduction in the incidence of type 2 diabetes with lifestyle intervention or metformin. *New England Journal of Medicine, 346*(6), 393–403.

Kong, A., Tussing-Humphreys, L. M., Odoms-Young, A. M., Stolley, M. R., & Fitzgibbon, M. L. (2014). Systematic review of behavioural interventions with culturally adapted strategies to improve diet and weight outcomes in African American women. *Obesity Review, 15*(Suppl. 4), 62–92.

Kreuter, M. W., Lukwago, S. N., Bucholtz, D. C., Clark, E. M., & Sanders-Thompson, V. (2003). Achieving cultural appropriateness in health promotion programs: Targeted and tailored approaches. *Health Education and Behavior, 30*(2), 133–146.

Kumanyika, S. K., Espeland, M. A., Bahnson, J. L., Bottom, J. B., Charleston, J. B., Folmar, S., et al. (2002). Ethnic comparison of weight loss in the Trial of Nonpharmacologic Interventions in the Elderly. *Obesity Research, 10*(2), 96–106.

Kumanyika, S. K., Obarzanek, E., Stettler, N., Bell, R., Field, A. E., Fortmann, S. P., et al. (2008). Population-based prevention of obesity: The need for comprehensive promotion of healthful eating, physical activity, and energy balance—a scientific statement from American Heart Association Council on Epidemiology and Prevention, Interdisciplinary Committee for Prevention (formerly the expert panel on population and prevention science). *Circulation, 118*(4), 428–464.

Kumanyika, S. K., Obarzanek, E., Stevens, V. J., Hebert, P. R., & Whelton, P. K. (1991). Weight-loss experience of black and white participants in NHLBI-sponsored clinical trials. *American Journal of Clinical Nutrition, 53*(6, Suppl.), 1631S–1638S.

Kumanyika, S. K., Whitt-Glover, M. C., & Haire-Joshu, D. (2014). What works for obesity prevention and treatment in black Americans?: Research directions. *Obesity Review, 15*(Suppl. 4), 204–212.

Lancaster, K. J., Carter-Edwards, L., Grilo, S., Shen, C., & Schoenthaler, A. M. (2014). Obesity interventions in African American faith-based organizations: A systematic review. *Obesity Review, 15*(Suppl. 4), 159–176.

Langellier, B. A., Glik, D., Ortega, A. N., & Prelip, M. L. (2015). Trends in racial/ethnic disparities in overweight self-perception among US adults, 1988–1994 and 1999–2008. *Public Health Nutrition, 18*(12), 2115–2125.

Lindberg, N. M., & Stevens, V. J. (2007). Review: Weight-loss interventions with Hispanic populations. *Ethnicity and Disease, 17*(2), 397–402.

Lindberg, N. M., Stevens, V. J., Vega-Lopez, S., Kauffman, T. L., Calderon, M. R., & Cervantes, M. A. (2012). A weight-loss intervention program designed for Mexican-American women: Cultural adaptations and results. *Journal of Immigrant and Minority Health, 14*(6), 1030–1039.

Look Ahead Research Group. (2014). Eight-year weight losses with an intensive lifestyle intervention: The Look AHEAD study. *Obesity (Silver Spring), 22*(1), 5–13.

Lovasi, G. S., Hutson, M. A., Guerra, M., & Neckerman, K. M. (2009). Built environments and obesity in disadvantaged populations. *Epidemiologic Reviews, 31*, 7–20.

Luke, A., Cooper, R. S., Prewitt, T. E., Adeyemo, A. A., & Forrester, T. E. (2001). Nutritional consequences of the African diaspora. *Annual Review of Nutrition, 21*, 47–71.

Macartney, S., Bishaw, A., & Fontenot, K. (2013). *Poverty Rates for Selected Detailed Race and Hispanic Groups by State and Place: 2007–2011* (ACSBR/11-17). Washington, DC: U.S. Census Bureau.

Merriam, P. A., Tellez, T. L., Rosal, M. C., Olendzki, B. C., Ma, Y., Pagoto, S. L., et al. (2009). Methodology of a diabetes prevention translational research

Mitchell, N. S., Nassel, A. F., & Thomas, D. (2015). Reach of effective, nationally-available, low-cost, nonprofit weight loss program in medically underserved areas (MUAs). *Journal of Community Health, 40*(6), 1201–1206.

Mitchell, N. S., Prochazka, A. V., & Glasgow, R. E. (2016). Time to RE-AIM: Why community weight loss programs should be included in academic obesity research. *Preventing Chronic Disease, 13*, E37.

National Heart, Lung, and Blood Institute. (1998). Clinical guidelines on the identification, evaluation, and treatment of overweight and obesity in adults—the evidence report. *Obesity Research, 6*(Suppl. 2), 51S–209S.

Neel, J. V. (1999). Diabetes mellitus: A "thrifty" genotype rendered detrimental by "progress"? *Bulletin of the World Health Organization, 77*(8), 694–703; discussion 692–693.

Newton, R. L., Jr., Griffith, D. M., Kearney, W. B., & Bennett, G. G. (2014). A systematic review of weight loss, physical activity and dietary interventions involving African American men. *Obesity Review, 15*(Suppl. 4), 93–106.

Ockene, I. S., Tellez, T. L., Rosal, M. C., Reed, G. W., Mordes, J., Merriam, P. A., et al. (2012). Outcomes of a Latino community-based intervention for the prevention of diabetes: The Lawrence Latino Diabetes Prevention Project. *American Journal of Public Health, 102*(2), 336–342.

Pagoto, S. L., Schneider, K. L., Oleski, J. L., Luciani, J. M., Bodenlos, J. S., & Whited, M. C. (2012). Male inclusion in randomized controlled trials of lifestyle weight loss interventions. *Obesity (Silver Spring), 20*(6), 1234–1239.

Pi-Sunyer, X. (2014). The Look AHEAD trial: A review and discussion of its outcomes. *Current Nutrition Reports, 3*(4), 387–391.

Ravussin, E., Valencia, M. E., Esparza, J., Bennett, P. H., & Schulz, L. O. (1994). Effects of a traditional lifestyle on obesity in Pima Indians. *Diabetes Care, 17*(9), 1067–1074.

Ritenbaugh, C. (1982). Obesity as a culture-bound syndrome. *Culture, Medicine, and Psychiatry, 6*(4), 347–364.

Ryan, C. L., & Bauman, K. (2016). Educational attainment in the United States: 2015 population characteristics. *Current Population Reports* (pp. 20–578). Washington, DC: U.S. Census Bureau.

Samuel-Hodge, C. D., Johnson, C. M., Braxton, D. F., & Lackey, M. (2014). Effectiveness of Diabetes Prevention Program translations among African Americans. *Obesity Review, 15*(Suppl. 4), 107–124.

Smith, A. (2015). U.S. smartphone use in 2015. Retrieved from *www.pewinternet.org/2015/04/01/us-smartphone-use-in-2015*.

Stevens, V. J., Obarzanek, E., Cook, N. R., Lee, I. M., Appel, L. J., Smith West, D., et al. (2001). Long-term weight loss and changes in blood pressure: Results of the Trials of Hypertension Prevention, phase II. *Annals of Internal Medicine, 134*(1), 1–11.

Striegel-Moore, R. H. (1996). Weight-related attitudes and behaviors of women who diet to lose weight: A comparison of black dieters and white dieters. *Obesity Research, 4*, 109–116.

Svetkey, L. P., Ard, J. D., Stevens, V. J., Loria, C. M., Young, D. Y., Hollis, J. F., et al. (2012). Predictors of long-term weight loss in adults with modest initial weight loss, by sex and race. *Obesity (Silver Spring), 20*(9), 1820–1828.

Svetkey, L. P., Erlinger, T. P., Vollmer, W. M., Feldstein, A., Cooper, L. S., Appel, L. J., et al. (2005). Effect of lifestyle modifications on blood pressure by race, sex, hypertension status, and age. *Journal of Human Hypertension, 19*(1), 21–31.

Teufel-Shone, N. I. (2006). Promising strategies for obesity prevention and treatment within American Indian communities. *Journal of Transcultural Nursing, 17*(3), 224–229.

Tussing-Humphreys, L. M., Fitzgibbon, M. L., Kong, A., & Odoms-Young, A. (2013). Weight loss maintenance in African American women: A systematic review of the behavioral lifestyle intervention literature. *Journal of Obesity, 2013*, 437369.

Unick, J. L., Beavers, D., Jakicic, J. M., Kitabchi, A. E., Knowler, W. C., Wadden, T. A., et al. (2011). Effectiveness of lifestyle interventions for individuals with severe obesity and type 2 diabetes: Results from the Look AHEAD trial. *Diabetes Care, 34*(10), 2152–2157.

U.S. Department of Health and Human Services, Centers for Disease Control and Prevention, National Center for Health Statistics. (2015). *Health, United States, 2014: With special feature on adults aged 55–64*. Washington, DC: U.S. Government Printing Office.

U.S. Department of Health and Human Services, Centers for Disease Control and Prevention, National Center for Health Statistics. (2016a). Age-adjusted percent distribution (with standard errors) of body mass index among adults aged 18 years and over, by selected characteristics, United States, 2015. Retrieved from *http://ftp.cdc.gov/pub/Health_Statistics/NCHS/NHIS/SHS/2015_SHS_Table_A-15.pdf*.

U.S. Department of Health and Human Services, Centers for Disease Control and Prevention, National Center for Health Statistics. (2016b). Age-adjusted percent distribution (with standard errors) of selected diseases and conditions among adults aged 18 years and over, by selected characteristics: United States, 2015. Retrieved from *http://ftp.cdc.gov/pub/Health_Statistics/NCHS/NHIS/SHS/2015_SHS_Table_A-4.pdf*.

U.S. Department of Health and Human Services, Office of Minority Health. (2016). Minority population profiles. Retrieved March 6, 2017, from *www.minorityhealth.hhs.gov/omh/browse.aspx?lvl=2&lvlid=26*.

Wadden, T. A., Neiberg, R. H., Wing, R. R., Clark, J. M., Delahanty, L. M., Hill, J. O., et al. (2011).

Four-year weight losses in the Look AHEAD study: Factors associated with long-term success. *Obesity (Silver Spring), 19*(10), 1987–1998.

West, D. S., Prewitt, T. E., Bursac, Z., & Felix, H. C. (2008). Weight loss of black, white, and Hispanic men and women in the Diabetes Prevention Program. *Obesity (Silver Spring), 16*(6), 1413–1420. Erratum in *Obesity (Silver Spring)* 2009, *17*(11), 2119–2120.

Weyer, C., Snitker, S., Bogardus, C., & Ravussin, E. (1999). Energy metabolism in African Americans: Potential risk factors for obesity. *American Journal of Clinical Nutrition, 70*(1), 13–20.

Whelton, P. K., Appel, L. J., Espeland, M. A., Applegate, W. B., Ettinger, W. H., Jr., Kostis, J. B., et al. (1998). Sodium reduction and weight loss in the treatment of hypertension in older persons: A randomized controlled Trial of Nonpharmacologic Interventions in the Elderly (TONE). *Journal of the American Medical Association, 279*(11), 839–846.

Wing, R. R., & Anglin, K. (1996). Effectiveness of a behavioral weight control program for blacks and whites with NIDDM. *Diabetes Care, 19*(5), 409–413.

Wingo, B., Carson, T., & Ard, J. (2014). Differences in weight loss and health outcomes among African Americans and whites in multicentre trials. *Obesity Reviews, 15*(Suppl. 4), 46–61.

Winston, G., Phillips, E., Wethington, E., Wells, M., Devine, C. M., Peterson, J., et al. (2015). The relationship between social network body size and the body size norms of black and Hispanic adults. *Preventive Medicine Reports, 2*, 941–945.

World Health Organization Consultation. (2004). Appropriate body-mass index for Asian populations and its implications for policy and intervention strategies. *Lancet, 363*(9403), 157–163.

Yancey, A. K., Ory, M. G., & Davis, S. M. (2006). Dissemination of physical activity promotion interventions in underserved populations. *American Journal of Preventive Medicine, 31*(4, Suppl.), S82–S91.

# CHAPTER 27

Treatment of Obesity in Primary Care

Adam G. Tsai
Thomas A. Wadden

Obesity continues to be the most important chronic health problem facing the United States. The prevalence of obesity is not decreasing, and among women, appears still to be rising (Flegal, Kruszon-Moran, Carroll, Fryar, & Ogden, 2016). With the decreasing prevalence of tobacco use, obesity is now likely to represent the most important risk factor for other chronic diseases treated in primary care. These diseases include diabetes, hypertension, obstructive sleep apnea, various forms of cardiovascular disease, arthritis of weight-bearing joints, and depression. Thus, better control of obesity has the potential to dramatically reduce the burden of chronic disease being treated by primary care physicians and other providers.

The medical profession seems to be coming around to the idea that obesity is not simply a risk factor for chronic disease, but is also a chronic disease in its own right, and one that requires long-term management. This view is supported by several developments in health care over the past 7 years. First, in 2010, the Patient Protection and Affordable Care Act (ACA) was passed. The ACA, in addition to expanding health insurance for millions of Americans, also mandated that any service receiving an "A" or a "B" grade recommendation from the U.S. Preventive Services Task Force be covered without patient copayments (United States Congress, 2010). High-intensity weight loss counseling received a "B" grade from the Task Force in 2003 and again in 2012 (U.S. Preventive Services Task Force, 2003; Moyer, U.S. Preventive Services Task Force, 2012). (A "B" grade means that there is high certainty that the net benefit of providing a service is moderate, or a moderate certainty that the net benefit of providing a service is moderate to substantial.) Following this, in 2011 the Centers for Medicare and Medicaid Services created a new benefit for the treatment of obesity in the primary care setting, allowing for up to 20 15-minute visits over 1 year. Additionally, in 2013, the American Medical Association recognized obesity as a chronic disease in its own right (American Medical Association, 2013). A separate development was the publication of updated obesity treatment guidelines. Guidelines covering the behavioral and surgical treatment of obesity were published in 2014 by the American Heart Association, the American College of Cardiology, and The Obesity Society (Jensen et al., 2014), and in 2015, U.S. guidelines on the use of medications to treat obesity were published by the Endocrine Society (including four new medications approved by the U.S. Food and Drug Administration [FDA] since 2012 for the long-term management of obesity) (Apovian et al., 2015). Other professional societies and organizations recently have provided guidelines on weight management (Garvey et al., 2016; Brauer et al., 2015)

Together, these developments have helped physicians to understand the importance of treating obesity on a chronic basis. An increasing number of physicians are pursuing the board certification offered by the American Board of Obesity Medicine (ABOM; 2016). In 2015, the number of internal medicine physicians who pursued this board exam was greater than the numbers for several traditional internal medical subspecialties, such as endocrinology and infectious diseases (American Board of Internal Medicine, 2016). The majority of applicants for the obesity medicine board certification are from primary care specialties—internal medicine, family medicine, and pediatrics.

At the same time that treatment of obesity is receiving increased attention from physicians and from health care regulatory organizations and insurance payers, the practice of primary care medicine is not thriving. The percentage of graduates of U.S. medical schools and residency programs going into adult primary care has increased slightly from its nadir but remains close to an all-time low. Burnout rates among practicing primary care physicians are high (Roberts, Shanafelt, Dyrbye, & West, 2014). There is a perception in the medical community and among the public that primary care medicine is not prestigious.

In this context, what can primary care physicians (PCPs) do to manage obesity? This chapter reviews the literature on interventions to treat obesity that have been tested in primary care populations. We also discuss the role of the PCP in evaluating and treating obesity and suggest a few key messages that PCPs can deliver to help engage patients in therapy. We conclude with recommendations for how PCPs can make the best use of office visits to manage obesity along with their patients' other health concerns.

Behavioral Treatment of Obesity

The 2013 obesity treatment guidelines (American Heart Association [AHA]/American College of Cardiology [ACC]/The Obesity Society [TOS]) gave a strong recommendation for high-intensity treatment of obesity (Jensen, 2014). The standard for high intensity is at least 14 visits, provided over a period of 6 months, which offer personalized counseling and feedback from a trained interventionist. An evidence review of "primary care relevant" studies, supported by the U.S. Preventive Services Task Force (USPSTF) and serving as the basis for the updated 2012 recommendation from the Task Force, similarly concluded that high-intensity behavioral programs (providing 12–26 visits in the first year) were more likely to produce clinically significant weight loss, compared to programs that provided fewer than 12 visits (Leblanc, O'Connor, Whitlock, Patnode, & Kapka, 2011). We focus our attention primarily on describing studies that met the 2003 USPSTF standard for high-intensity treatment (i.e., greater than monthly visits for at least 6 months). In a 2014 systematic review of obesity treatment provided in primary care, weight losses were more closely associated with the intensity of treatment than with the modality used to deliver treatment (in-person vs. telephone) (Wadden, Butryn, Hong, & Tsai, 2014). The review of studies that follows is not a systematic review of the literature, but rather a highlighting of relevant studies that tested different types of interventions and with varying intensities of treatment.

Low- to Moderate-Intensity Counseling in Primary Care

A number of studies have offered low- to moderate-intensity counseling (i.e., ≤ one session/month; see Table 27.1 for additional study details). Davis and colleagues randomly assigned primary care patients to standard care or to monthly counseling visits with their PCPs. Weight loss was significantly greater in the treatment arm than in the control group after 12 months (–1.4 kg vs. 0.3 kg; $p = .01$), but not at 18 months (–0.5 kg vs. + 0.1 kg; $p = .39$) (Davis et al., 2006; Davis-Martin, 2008). Christian and

TABLE 27.1. Studies of Low- to Moderate-Intensity Treatment

Study	Demographics	Duration	Weight change	p value
Davis (2006); Davis-Martin (2008)	N = 144 BMI = 38.9 kg/m² Age = 41.8 years 100% female	18 months	Treatment: −0.5 kg Control: +0.1 kg	.39
Christian (2008)	N = 310 BMI = 35.1 kg/m² Age = 53.2 years 66% female	12 months	Treatment: −0.1 kg Control: +0.6 kg	.23
Christian (2011)	N = 279 BMI = 34.3 kg/m²[a] Age = 49.6 years[a] 68.4% female	12 months	Treatment: −1.5 kg Control: +0.2 kg	.002
Whittemore (2009)	N = 58 BMI = 38.9 kg/m²[a] Age = 45.9 years[a] 89.7% female	6 months	Treatment: −1.6%[b] Control: −0.3%[b]	.08
ter Bogt (2011)	N = 457 BMI = 29.6 kg/m² Age = 56.1 years 52% female	12 months	Treatment: −1.9% Control: −0.9%	< .05
Kumanyika (2012)	N = 261 BMI = 37.2 kg/m² Age = 47.2 years 84% female	12 months	Treatment: −1.6 kg Control: −0.6 kg	.15
Tsai (2010)	N = 50 BMI = 36.5 kg/m² Age = 49.4 years 88% female	12 months	Treatment: −2.3 kg Control: −1.1 kg	.31

[a]Estimated from table in published paper.
[b]Estimated from figure in published paper.

colleagues conducted two randomized trials in primary care practices, both also using PCPs to deliver counseling to study participants (Christian et al., 2008, 2011). Both studies employed low-intensity counseling, with visits conducted quarterly in one trial and twice per year in the second trial. In both trials, the active intervention arm included a computer-based assessment that gave patients an individualized assessment of their weight and weight loss history and provided personalized recommendations. These recommendations were printed for the patients to review with their PCPs during counseling visits. In the first trial, control group participants gained 0.6 kg at 1 year, compared to a weight loss of 0.1 kg in the intervention group ($p = 0.23$ for difference) (Christian et al., 2008). In the second study, the intervention group lost 1.5 kg at 1 year, whereas the control group gained 0.2 kg ($p = .002$) (Christian et al., 2011).

Two trials used midlevel providers (nurse practitioners) instead of physicians as counselors. A study by Whittemore et al. (2009) adapted the Diabetes Prevention Program (DPP) for use in a primary care office and reduced the number of sessions from 16 to 6, providing a phone visit between monthly in-person visits over a 6-month period. Weight losses after 6 months (estimated from a figure in the study) were 0.3% and 1.6% of initial body weight in the control and intervention groups, respectively ($p = .08$). In a study by ter Bogt et al. (2011), nurse practitioners provided quarterly counseling visits, using a computerized treatment protocol developed by the study investigators. Weight losses were 0.9% and 1.9% of initial body weight after 12 months in the control and intervention groups, respectively (ter Bogt et al., 2011). Kumanyika et al. (2012) randomized primary care patients to low-intensity counseling, defined as visits every 4 months with their PCP or provider, or to moderate-intensity counseling, defined as monthly weight loss counseling visits with a medical assistant in the practice. Weight losses at 12 months were 0.6 kg in the low-intensity group and 1.6 kg in the moderate-intensity group ($p = .15$) (Kumanyika et al., 2012).

Taken together, these studies show very similar outcomes. Specifically, low- to moderate-intensity counseling, whether delivered by primary care physicians themselves or by other primary care team members (midlevel providers or medical assistants), produces modest weight loss among participants (approximately 1–2 kg greater than standard care). Thus, for the majority of patients, these interventions have limited clinical benefit with regard to reducing the burden of comorbid medical illness or improving health. Although a minority of patients may benefit from having monthly or less frequent counseling visits with a dietitian, a physician, or another team member from the primary care office, PCPs do not have a reliable method to determine which individuals would benefit from a low- to moderate-intensity intervention. Thus, although the likelihood of harm from such interventions is small, the likelihood of benefit is also small. PCPs should counsel their patients that such interventions are unlikely to produce clinically significant weight loss.

High-Intensity Weight Loss Counseling

A limited number of trials have been able to deliver high-intensity weight loss counseling to patients recruited from primary care settings. The small number of trials that have achieved this goal is likely a consequence of the logistical and financial barriers to delivering such treatment in the physical settings of the primary care office and the conflicting demands and high workload of a primary care medical practice.

In a study by Tsai et al. (2010), primary care patients were randomized to quarterly counseling visits with their PCPs or to a series of eight lifestyle counseling visits over 6 months with a medical assistant in the practice, using a shortened version of the DPP curriculum. Weight loss at 6 months was significantly greater in the treatment than control arm (4.4 kg vs. 0.9 kg; $p < .001$), but at 12 months the difference was no longer significant (2.3 kg vs. 1.1 kg; $p = .31$).

Appel et al. (2011) recruited participants from primary care offices affiliated with a large academic medical center. Participants were randomly assigned to usual care, telephone-delivered counseling, or in-person counseling. The latter two groups had access to a web-based program to record food intake and physical activity. Those in the phone group were provided with 12 initial weekly phone sessions, followed by monthly calls through year 2. Participants in the in-person group were offered a combination of group and individual treatment, up to 57 visits over the 2 years. Weight losses at 2 years were 0.8, 4.6, and 5.1 kg, respectively ($p < .001$ for both intensive groups vs. control arm).

In a 2-year randomized controlled trial, Wadden, Volger, et al. (2011) assigned individuals with at least two out of five criteria for the metabolic syndrome to usual care; brief lifestyle counseling (25 10- to 15-minute visits over 2 years with a trained medical assistant from the primary care practice); or "enhanced" brief lifestyle counseling (the same 25 counseling visits, combined with the patient's choice of meal replacements, orlistat, or sibutramine). At year 2, weight losses in the three groups were 1.7, 2.9, and 4.6 kg, respectively ($p = .08$ for brief counseling vs. usual care; $p = .003$ for enhanced brief lifestyle counseling vs. usual care).

In a study by Ma et al. (2013), primary care patients who had either pre-diabetes or metabolic syndrome were randomly assigned to usual care; an in-person group version of the DPP; or to the DPP curriculum, delivered via a self-directed DVD. Participants assigned to the in-person intervention received weekly sessions for 12 weeks, followed by monthly sessions for the remainder of the 2-year trial. At year 2, weight losses in the usual care, in-person, and self-directed groups were 2.4, 5.4, and 4.5 kg, respectively ($p = .001$ for in-person vs. control; $p = .03$ for self-directed vs. control) (Ma et al., 2013; Xiao, Yank, Wilson, Lavori, & Ma, 2013).

In a 1-year randomized controlled trial, Ashley et al. (2001) randomly assigned participants to dietitian-led groups; dietitian-led groups plus the use of a partial meal replacement diet (replacement of two meals/day); or individual counseling visits with a PCP, combined with the use of meal replacements. (This study was conducted in a primary care practice, but participants were not patients from the practice; instead, they were recruited from the local community.) Dietitian-led groups lasted for 1 hour, whereas PCP visits lasted 10–15 minutes. All participants received 26 every-other-week visits. Weight losses at 1 year were 3.4, 7.7, and 3.5 kg, respectively ($p < .001$ for dietitian plus meal replacement group compared to the other two groups).

In a trial by Tsai and colleagues, 106 individuals recruited from primary care offices were provided with 12 in-person counseling visits during the first 6 months of treatment and were given access to a subsidized program of portion-controlled foods (Nutrisystem®) (Tsai, Felton, Wadden, Hosokawa, & Hill, 2015). Of these 106 participants, 84 persons completed the first 6 months and were randomly assigned to a maintenance condition. Participants randomized to the "intensive" maintenance condition, involving one in-person and one individualized phone or e-mail contact per month, retained a loss of 6.1 kg at month 18, compared to 2.2 kg in the "standard" maintenance arm ($p < .001$).

Ryan et al. (2010) randomly assigned state employees in Louisiana to usual care or a multimodality intervention. The treatment program started with a 3-month, 900 kcal/day, medically supervised diet using meal replacements (HealthOne Formula). It then continued for an additional 4 months with high-intensity group weight loss counseling, with a partial meal replacement diet and optional weight loss medication, followed by continued use of medication and monthly group sessions for the final 17 months (with the option for intermittent short-term use of full meal replacement). Mean weight loss at month 24 was 4.9% of initial weight in the intervention group and 0.2% in control participants ($p < .001$). Attrition in the trial was nearly 50%; weight loss in the 51% of participants in the intervention who completed the study was 8.3% of initial weight.

In a study by Weinstock and colleagues, primary care patients with metabolic syndrome were randomly assigned to receive the DPP curriculum, delivered in either group conference calls or individual phone calls (Weinstock, Trief, Cibula, Morin, & Delahanty, 2013). The first five calls were delivered weekly; calls were then delivered monthly for the remainder of the first year. All participants were offered monthly maintenance calls during a second year. At year 2, mean weight loss with group conference calls was 6.2 kg, compared with 2.2 kg in the individual call group ($p < .001$). (Only 52.5% of participants, however, completed the 2-year assessment.)

Taken together, the majority of the studies just described found that high-intensity counseling, using different modalities (e.g., in-person or phone visits), produced clinically meaningful weight loss. This conclusion is tempered by high attrition in two of the trials (Ryan et al., 2010; Weinstock et al., 2013), as well as by the fact that in one trial, participants were not primary care patients, but instead were recruited from the local community (Ashley et al., 2001). However, this group of studies also demonstrates that a number of different treatment modalities, if delivered with adequate intensity, can be effective. These range from telephone-delivered interventions to in-person individual or group counseling sessions, counseling supplemented with meal replacements or medication, or in one case, a multimodality intervention that varied the type of treatment offered over time.

Studies Using Alternative Methods of Behavioral Counseling in Primary Care

As mentioned, a systematic review of obesity management in primary care (Wadden et al., 2014) found that high-intensity treatment leads to greater weight loss than low- or moderate-intensity counseling. The other major finding of this review was that "traditional" behavioral interventions produced larger weight losses than interventions that used "alternative" methods of counseling. Traditional methods of behavioral counseling were defined as those that included a prescription for a reduced calorie diet, a specific target for physical activity, and the use of behavioral strategies (e.g., goal setting, self-monitoring) to improve adherence to diet and physical activity plans. In this review, alternative methods of behavioral counseling were defined as interventions that used primarily motivational interviewing (Miller & Rollnick, 2002) or stages of change (Prochaska, Redding, & Evers, 1997) without including specific targets for calorie intake or physical activity.

Summary of Behavioral Treatment in Primary Care

The studies reviewed previously demonstrate that (1) low- to moderate-intensity counseling alone does not lead to clinically significant weight loss; (2) high-intensity weight loss counseling, provided by a variety of health care professionals, produces a weight loss of approximately 5–10% of initial weight; (3) the modality of providing counseling (in-person vs. telephone, individual vs. group treatment) is less important than the intensity of treatment; and (4) traditional methods of behavioral counseling produce greater weight loss than alternative methods, such as motivational interviewing.

Referring Primary Care Patients to Commercial Weight Loss Programs

In its recommendations on obesity, the USPSTF advised that PCPs should "offer or refer patients with a body mass index of 30kg/m^2 or higher to intensive, multicomponent behavioral interventions" (p. 373; Moyer & U.S. Preventive Services Task Force, 2012). In this context, PCPs who work in settings where high-intensity treatment is not offered can refer patients to weight loss services in the community, such as commercial weight loss programs. The 2013 AHA/ACC/TOS guidelines indicate that commercial programs can be considered as an option for high-intensity treatment, provided that the programs have published evidence of their safety and efficacy in peer-reviewed medical literature.

Since the publication of a review article in 2005 (Tsai & Wadden, 2005), several commercial weight loss programs have conducted randomized trials to evaluate the effectiveness of their interventions. An updated review published by Gudzune et al. (2015), as well as a separate chapter in this book (Gudzune & Clark, Chapter 29), review in detail the studies conducted by these programs, as well as the relative costs and benefits of the different interventions. Weight Watchers, Jenny Craig, Nutrisystem, Health Management Resources, Medifast, and Optifast are among the structured commercial and meal replacement programs reviewed by Gudzune et al. (2015). Self-directed meal plans with published evidence of safety and efficacy include Atkins and Slim-Fast. PCPs who work in low-resource settings and who do not have access to intensive behavioral interventions may also consider referring their patients to low-cost programs such as Take Off Pounds Sensibly (TOPS; Mitchell, Dickinson, Kempe, & Tsai, 2011). TOPS is not supported by randomized trial evidence, but we believe that it is a reasonable option for providing high-intensity behavioral treatment when participation in other programs is not feasible.

Medical and Surgical Options for PCPs to Consider

Adding Medications to Behavioral Treatment

Bray and Ryan (Chapter 21, this volume) review the use of FDA-approved medications to treat obesity. None of the pivotal Phase-3 trials of these medications were conducted in primary care settings per se. However, the behavioral interventions provided in these studies, with the exception of the Contrave Obesity Research—Behavior Modification (COR-BMOD) trial (Wadden, Foreyt, et al., 2011), were of low to moderate intensity. Thus, the weight losses achieved in these trials are likely to be similar to weight losses expected among primary care patients who are prescribed these medicines with minimal lifestyle counseling.

Three randomized trials have studied the effectiveness of medications when added to weight loss counseling provided in primary care settings. Hauptman and colleagues randomly assigned 796 individuals from 17 primary care offices to placebo, orlistat 60 mg 3x/day, or orlistat 120 mg 3x/day (Hauptman, Lucas, Boldrin, Collins, & Segal, 2000). All participants were given videos on weight management every 3 months in year 1, and were given written materials on weight management every 3 months in year 2. After 2 years, weight losses in the three groups were 1.7, 4.5, and 5.0 kg, respectively ($p = .001$ for both treatment groups vs. control). Wadden et al. (2005) tested the effect of sibutramine in a randomized trial, with or without a series of eight brief 10- to 15-minute lifestyle counseling visits delivered by a physician or nurse practitioner. At 1 year, mean weight loss in the medication-alone group was 5.0 kg and in the combined group was 7.5 kg ($p > .05$). (Sibutramine was removed from European and U.S. markets in 2011 after the SCOUT trial reported an increased risk of major cardiovascular events among patients taking the drug [James et al., 2010].) Poston et al. (2006) randomly assigned 250 individuals to monthly weight loss counseling, orlistat (120 mg 3x/day), or the combination of counseling plus orlistat. At 1 year, participants in the orlistat alone and combination therapy group both lost 1.7 kg, whereas those in the counseling only group gained 1.7 kg ($p < .001$ for both orlistat groups compared to counseling alone). Two of these trials suggest that medication, when added to low- to moderate-intensity lifestyle counseling provided in primary care settings, increases weight loss compared to counseling alone. Conversely, multiple trials have demonstrated that when high-intensity counseling is added to medication, it nearly doubles the weight loss achieved with medication alone (Stunkard, Craighead, & O'Brien, 1980; Wadden et al., 2001, 2005; Digenio, Mancuso, Gerber, & Dvorak, 2009). This consistent finding in the literature again highlights the importance of high-intensity behavioral treatment of obesity. The additive effect of weight management medications and high-intensity behavioral counseling is a key message for PCPs, particularly those who prescribe medications. PCPs should explain that weight management medications help patients reduce their food and calorie intake, and as such, serve as a tool to facilitate lifestyle modification. Thus, the more structured the behavioral program undertaken by the patient, the greater the weight loss achieved with adjunctive weight management medication.

Surgical Treatment of Obesity

The safety and effectiveness of bariatric surgery are covered in detail by Hanipah, Aminian, and Schauer (Chapter 22, this volume). PCPs should be aware that bariatric surgery is dramatically safer now than when it was first developed (Longitudinal Assessment of Bariatric Surgery [LABS] Consortium, 2009). It also is by far the most effective intervention for severe obesity, producing long-term (i.e., 3- to 15-year) reductions in initial weight of 20–25%. PCPs also should know that when they refer a patient for weight loss surgery, the patient may or may not turn out to be a good candidate. All patients referred for bariatric surgery undergo a structured medical and behavioral evaluation before they are approved for a procedure. Referral for evaluation for bariatric surgery is indicated when desired weight loss outcomes or improvements in health cannot be achieved by high-intensity lifestyle counseling alone or in combination with pharmacotherapy.

Figure 27.1 provides an algorithm to help providers select an appropriate weight management intervention. The first goal is to determine if weight loss is medically indicated. If so, the PCP should offer or refer the patient to high-intensity behavioral treatment. If the patient accepts this recommendation, then success is defined as a loss of 5–10% of initial body weight that is maintained for at least 1 year from the end of treatment. If treatment intensification is needed, then partial or full meal replacement plans may be considered, as well as weight loss medication. If a combination of these therapies is not effective in producing a weight loss of 5–10% of initial body weight, consideration of bariatric surgery is appropriate.

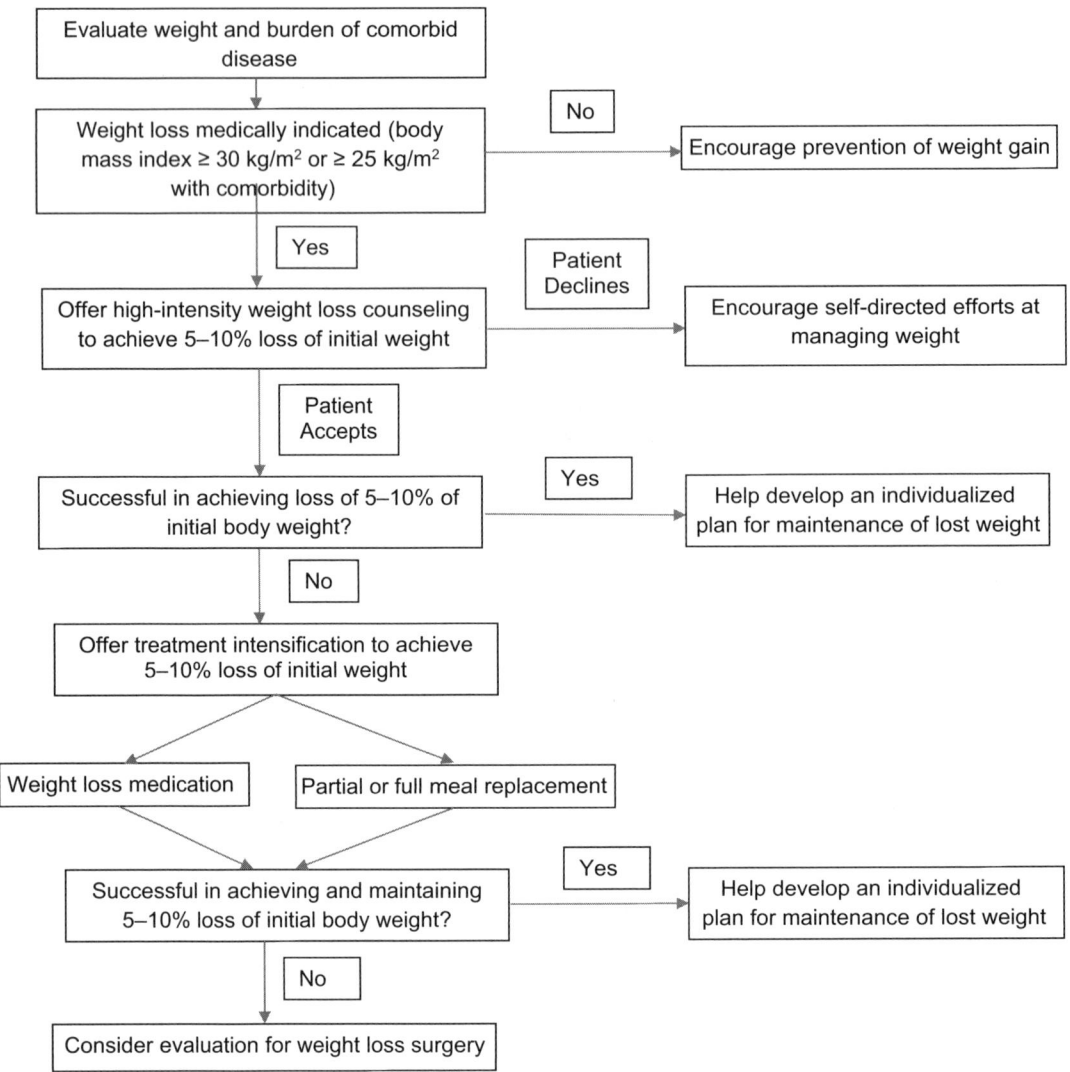

FIGURE 27.1. A stepped-care algorithm to help providers identify appropriate weight loss interventions for individuals with overweight or obesity.

Key Messages for PCPs Concerning Obesity

Physicians and policymakers alike are paying increased attention to obesity. However, this is occurring within the context of an ongoing "crisis" in primary care, with a shortage of physicians and a perception that specialty medical practice is more desirable. Many of the intensive behavioral interventions described in this chapter are simply not realistic in most primary care practices. PCPs can use medications to help their patients lose weight, but medication alone, without a structured behavioral program, is only modestly effective and usually does not come close to achieving the weight loss goals desired by patients and their physicians (Foster, Wadden, Vogt, & Brewer, 1997; Wadden et al., 2003). PCPs can recommend that their patients with severe obesity undergo an evaluation for bariatric surgery, but this evaluation takes place largely outside of the primary care office. In the following material we suggest several key messages that PCPs can deliver to their patients. Some of these were discussed by Rutledge, Groesz, Linke, Woods, and Herbst (2011). Delivery of these messages by PCPs has not been tested in a clinical trial. However, all of the underlying principles are supported by strong evidence.

The first message that PCPs should deliver is the *value of engaging in high-intensity behavioral treatment*. As reviewed above, low- to moderate-intensity behavioral interventions do not benefit most patients. Thus, patients who are interested in engaging in structured treatment should be encouraged to participate in high-intensity programs, whether inside or outside of the health care system in which they are being treated. Admittedly, this is a hard sell for physicians, given the time commitment required for treatment and some patients' beliefs that they do not need a class or a counselor to teach them how to eat healthy foods. For patients willing to engage in high-intensity interventions, however, the studies reviewed in this chapter show that treatment delivered by phone can produce clinically meaningful weight loss (Appel et al., 2011; Weinstock et al., 2013) Thus, high-intensity treatment delivered by phone (or potentially by Internet) has the potential to increase the reach of this effective therapy. A nonrandomized study suggested that a live "webinar" using the DPP curriculum also produced clinically meaningful weight loss among program completers (Sepah, Jiang, & Peters, 2015). The key goal for patient and clinician is engagement in the intervention and the presence of a live counselor providing feedback, whether that is in-person, by phone, or by Internet (Jensen et al., 2014).

A second message that PCPs can deliver concerns the *benefits of moderate weight loss*. Patients have been shown to have unrealistic weight loss goals (Foster et al., 1997; Wadden et al., 2003), and many PCPs likely share these unrealistic expectations. Numerous studies have demonstrated the value of a 5–10% loss of initial body weight (Goldstein, 1992; Jensen et al., 2014; Wing et al., 2011). Patients may ask their PCP, "What should I weigh?" An appropriate answer is not necessarily the weight that gives them a body mass index of less than 25 kg/m^2, but rather a weight that reduces medication use for comorbid conditions such as diabetes or hypertension, reduces the severity of other comorbid conditions (obstructive sleep apnea, osteoarthritis of weight-bearing joints), and improves functional status. Of note, in elderly patients with obesity, increased physical activity appears to be at least as effective for improving functional status as weight loss alone (Villareal et al., 2011).

A third message that PCPs can deliver invokes the *challenge of weight loss maintenance*. Although researchers have known about metabolic adaptations to weight loss for over 20 years (Leibel, Rosenbaum, & Hirsch, 1995), recently this issue has become better publicized, specifically with the publication of results from participants on *The Biggest Loser* television show (Fothergill et al., 2016). Most patients work hard for several months (restricting their calorie intake and increasing their physical activity) and then hit a "plateau" after losing 5–10% of initial body weight. Many patients, frustrated by the inability to lose more weight, give up their efforts, resulting in weight regain. The PCP can help the patient to understand that the hard work begins when the scale stops moving. Although this is a sobering message, if patients understand the changes in diet and physical activity that are required for long-term success, it can help them work harder to maintain their 5–10% loss of initial weight.

A fourth message that PCPs can deliver involves the *use of "biological" therapies to treat obesity (i.e., medications and bariatric surgery)*. Patients may be hesitant to try medication or surgery because they feel that doing so is taking the "easy way out," or they may not want to take a medication for years to maintain their weight loss. In the context of metabolic adaptations to weight loss, patients with severe obesity are likely to be challenged in maintaining long-term weight loss. PCPs can explain that no viable medical treatments currently exist to raise metabolic rate when patients are weight-reduced. PCPs can also explain that medications and surgery can help to maintain weight loss by reducing hunger and the sensitivity of the brain to food cues (Wang et al., 2014; Faulconbridge et al., 2016). Stated another way, PCPs can help their patients understand the chronic nature of obesity and make it feel more acceptable to use these biological therapies.

A fifth message that PCPs can deliver concerns the *importance of adequate sleep in maintaining a healthy body weight*. This issue was reviewed in detail by Rutledge et al. (2011). Only 65% of Americans report a healthy sleep duration, defined as greater than 7 hours per night (Liu et al., 2016). Strong data from both epidemiological and intervention studies indicate that most individuals need 7–9 hours of sleep per night to maintain optimal health (Nedeltcheva, Kilkus, Imperial, Schoeller, & Penev, 2010; Ogilvie et al., 2016). Whether due to untreated sleep apnea or insomnia, PCPs can help patients improve their sleep as a means of better managing their weight.

Summary

Primary care physicians have been urged to routinely treat obesity in their practices. Although it is clinically appropriate for them to do so, the call for them to manage obesity comes at a time when primary care practices generally are in a poor position to take on additional work with no new resources. The literature on primary-care-based treatment of obesity shows that high-intensity interventions are the most likely to produce clinically meaningful weight loss. However, such intervention cannot be provided in most practices. Instead, PCPs should refer patients with obesity to high-intensity interventions that are available in their health care institution or in the greater community. PCPs should keep in mind that high-intensity treatments are effective, regardless of the delivery modality used, provided that the intervention offers personalized counseling and feedback from a trained interventionist (Jensen et al., 2014). PCPs can also help their patients by delivering a few key messages regarding weight loss goals, the challenge of long-term weight loss maintenance, and the potential benefits of adjunctive weight management medications. With patients who have made repeated efforts to lose weight with lifestyle modification but have not been successful, PCPs should not hesitate to refer such individuals for an evaluation for bariatric surgery.

Regardless of the degree to which PCPs choose to engage in treating obesity in their patients, it is important to be respectful and empathic in discussing weight—a sensitive subject for many patients. Respectful treatment includes the use of appropriate language (e.g., *weight* rather than *obesity*; Wadden & Didie, 2003; Volger et al., 2012), as well as acknowledging the challenge of successful long-term weight management, given the behavioral and biological barriers for patients. Many patients will not reach their weight loss goals; with these individuals, the clinician's role is to provide encouragement, refocus the conversation on health status rather than the number on the scale, and continue to treat the medical comorbidities of excess weight. PCPs who want to manage obesity in their practice will need to employ a combination of scientific knowledge, behavioral counseling, and sensitivity to produce the best possible outcomes.

References

American Board of Internal Medicine. (2016). Number of candidates certified annually by the American Board of Internal Medicine, 2011–2015. Retrieved July 25, 2016, from *www.abim.org/~/media/ABIM%20Public/Files/pdf/statistics-data/candidates-certiified-annually.pdf*.

American Board of Obesity Medicine. (2016). Statistics and data: ABOM exam pass rate. Retrieved July 25, 2016, from *www.abom.org/stats*.

American Medical Association. (2013). Business of the American Medical Association host of delegates 2013 annual meeting. Retrieved July 15, 2014, from *www.ama-assn.org/ama/pub/news/news/2013/2013-06-18-new-ama-policies-annual-meeting.page*.

Apovian, C. M., Aronne, L. J., Bessesen, D. H., McDonnell, M. E., Murad, M. H., Pagotto, U., et al. (2015). Pharmacological management of obesity: An Endocrine Society clinical practice guideline. *Journal of Clinical Endocrinology and Metabolism, 100*(2), 342–362.

Appel, L. J., Clark, J. M., Yeh, H. C., Wang, N. Y., Coughlin, J. W., Daumit, G., et al. (2011). Comparative effectiveness of weight-loss interventions in clinical practice. *New England Journal of Medicine, 365*(21), 1959–1968.

Ashley, J. M., St. Jeor, S. T., Schrage, J. P., Perumean-Chaney, S. E., Gilbertson, M. C., McCall, N. L., et al. (2001). Weight control in the physician's office. *Archives of Internal Medicine*, 161(13), 1599–1604.

Brauer, P., Conner Gorber, S., Shaw, E., Singh, H., Bell, N., Shane, A. R., et al. (2015). Recommendations for prevention of weight gain and use of behavioural and pharmacologic interventions to manage overweight and obesity in adults in primary care. *Canadian Medical Association Journal*, 187(3), 184–195.

Centers for Medicare and Medicaid Services (2011). Decision memo for intensive behavioral therapy for obesity (CAG-00423N). Retrieved December 14, 2013, from *www.cms.gov/medicare-coverage-database/details/nca-decisionmemo.aspx?&NcaName=Intensive%20Behavioral%20Therapy%20forObesity&bc=ACAAAAAAIAAA&NCAId=253&*.

Christian, J. G., Bessesen, D. H., Byers, T. E., Christian, K. K., Goldstein, M. G., & Bock, B. C. (2008). Clinic-based support to help overweight patients with type 2 diabetes increase physical activity and lose weight. *Archives of Internal Medicine*, 168(2), 141–146.

Christian, J. G., Byers, T. E., Christian, K. K., Goldstein, M. G., Bock, B. C., Prioreschi, B., et al. (2011). A computer support program that helps clinicians provide patients with metabolic syndrome tailored counseling to promote weight loss. *Journal of the American Dietetic Association*, 111(1), 75–83.

Davis, P., Rhode, P. C., Dutton, G. R., Redmann, S. M., Ryan, D. H., & Brantley, P. J. (2006). A primary care weight management intervention for low-income African-American women. *Obesity*, 14(8), 1412–1420.

Davis-Martin, P. D., Dutton, G. R., Rhode, P. C., Horswell, R. L., Ryan, D. H., & Brantley, P. J. (2008). Weight loss maintenance following a primary care intervention for low-income minority women. *Obesity*, 16(11), 2462–2467.

Digenio, A. G., Mancuso, J. P., Gerber, R. A., & Dvorak, R. V. (2009). Comparison of methods for delivering a lifestyle modification program for obese patients: A randomized trial. *Annals of Internal Medicine*, 150(4), 255–262.

Faulconbridge, L. F., Ruparel, K., Loughead J., Allison, K. C., Hesson, L. A., Fabricatore, A. N., et al. (2016). Changes in neural responsivity to highly palatable foods following Roux-en-Y gastric bypass, sleeve gastrectomy, or weight stability: An fMRI study. *Obesity*, 24(5), 1054–1060.

Flegal, K. M., Kruszon-Moran, D., Carroll, M. D., Fryar, C. D., & Ogden, C. L. (2016). Trends in obesity among adults in the United States, 2005 to 2014. *Journal of the American Medical Association*, 315(21), 2284–2291.

Foster, G. D., Wadden, T. A., Vogt, R. A., & Brewer, G. (1997). What is a reasonable weight loss?: Patients' expectations and evaluations of obesity treatment outcomes. *Journal of Consulting and Clinical Psychology*, 65(1), 79–85.

Fothergill, E., Guo, J., Howard, L., Kerns, J. C., Knuth, N. D., Brychta, R., et al. (2016). Persistent metabolic adaptation 6 years after "The Biggest Loser" competition. *Obesity*, 24(8), 1612–1619.

Garvey, W. T., Mechanick, J. I., Brett, E. M., Garber, A. J., Hurley, D. L., Jastreboff, A. M., et al. (2016). American Association of Clinical Endocrinologists and American College of Endocrinology comprehensive clinical practice guidelines for medical care of patients with obesity executive summary. *Endocrine Practice*, 22(7), 842–884.

Goldstein, D. J. (1992). Beneficial health effects of modest weight loss. *International Journal of Obesity and Related Metabolic Disorders*, 16(6), 397–415.

Gudzune, K. A., Doshi, R. S., Mehta, A. K., Chaudhry, Z. W., Jacobs, D. K., Vakil, R. M., et al. (2015). Efficacy of commercial weight-loss programs: An updated systematic review. *Annals of Internal Medicine*, 162(7), 501–512.

Hauptman, J., Lucas, C., Boldrin, M. N., Collins, H., & Segal, K. R. (2000). Orlistat in the long-term treatment of obesity in primary care settings. *Archives of Family Medicine*, 9(2), 160–167.

James, W. P. T., Caterson, I. D., Coutinho, W., Finer, N., Van Gaal, L. F., Maggioni, A. P., et al. (2010). Effect of sibutramine on cardiovascular outcomes in overweight and obese subjects. *New England Journal of Medicine*, 363(10), 905–917.

Jensen, M. D., Ryan, D. H., Apovian, C. M., Ard, J. D., Comuzzie, A. G., Donato, K. A., et al (2014). 2013 AHA/ACC/TOS guideline for the management of overweight and obesity in adults: A report of the American College of Cardiology/American Heart Association Task Force on Practice Guidelines and The Obesity Society. *Circulation*, 129(25, Suppl. 2), S102–S138.

Kumanyika, S. K., Fassbender, J. E., Sarwer, D. B., Phipps, E., Allison, K. C., Localio, R., et al. (2012). One-year results of the Think Health! study of weight management in primary care practices. *Obesity*, 20(6), 1249–1257.

Leblanc, E. S., O'Connor, E., Whitlock, E. P., Patnode, C. D., & Kapka, T. (2011). Effectiveness of primary care-relevant treatments for obesity in adults: A systematic evidence review for the U.S. Preventive Services Task Force. *Annals of Internal Medicine*, 155(7), 434–447.

Leibel, R. L., Rosenbaum, M., & Hirsch, J. (1995). Changes in energy expenditure resulting from altered body weight. *New England Journal of Medicine*, 332(10), 621–628.

Liu, Y., Wheaton, A. G., Chapman, D. P., Cunningham, T. J., Lu, H., & Croft, J. B. (2016). Prevalence of healthy sleep duration among adults—United States, 2014. *Morbidity and Mortality Weekly Report*, 65(6), 137–141.

Longitudinal Assessment of Bariatric Surgery (LABS) Consortium. (2009). Perioperative safety in the longitudinal assessment of bariatric surgery. *New England Journal of Medicine*, 361(5), 445–454.

Ma, J., Yank, V., Xiao, L., Lavori, P. W., Wilson, S.

R., Rosas, L. G., et al. (2013). Translating the Diabetes Prevention Program Lifestyle Intervention for weight loss into primary care: A randomized trial. *Journal of the American Medical Association Internal Medicine, 173*(2), 113–121.

Miller, W. R., & Rollnick, S. (2002). *Motivational interviewing: Preparing people for change* (2nd ed.). New York: Guilford Press.

Mitchell, N. S., Dickinson, L. M., Kempe, A., & Tsai, A. G. (2011). Determining the effectiveness of Take Off Pounds Sensibly (TOPS), a nationally available nonprofit weight loss program. *Obesity, 19*(3), 568–573.

Moyer, V. A., & U.S. Preventive Services Task Force. (2012). Screening for and management of obesity in adults: U.S. Preventive Services Task Force recommendation statement. *Annals of Internal Medicine, 157*(5), 373–378.

Nedeltcheva, A. V., Kilkus, J. M., Imperial, J., Schoeller, D. A., & Penev, P. D. (2010). Insufficient sleep undermines dietary efforts to reduce adiposity. *Annals of Internal Medicine, 153*(7), 435–441.

Ogilvie, R. P., Redline, S., Bertoni, A. G., Chen, X., Ouyang, P., Szklo, M., et al. (2016). Actigraphy measured sleep indices and adiposity: The Multi-Ethnic Study of Atherosclerosis (MESA). *Sleep, 39*(9), 1701–1708.

Poston, W. S., Haddock, C. K., Pinkston, M. M., Pace, P., Reeves, R. S., Karakoc, N., et al. (2006). Evaluation of a primary care-oriented brief counseling intervention for obesity with and without orlistat. *Journal of Internal Medicine, 260*(4), 388–398.

Prochaska, J. O., Redding, C. A., & Evers, K. E. (1997). The transtheoretical model and stage of change. In K. Glanz, F. M. Lewis, & B. K. Rimer (Eds.), *Health behavior and health education: Theory, research, and practice* (pp. 60–84). San Francisco: Jossey-Bass.

Roberts, D. L., Shanafelt, T. D., Dyrbye, L. N., & West, C. P. (2014). A national comparison of burnout and work–life balance among internal medicine hospitalists and outpatient general internists. *Journal of Hospital Medicine, 9*(3), 176–181.

Rutledge, T., Groesz, L. M., Linke, S. E., Woods, G., & Herbst, K. L. (2011). Behavioural weight management for the primary care provider. *Obesity Reviews, 12*(5), e290–e297.

Ryan, D. H., Johnson, W. D., Myers, V. H., Prather, T. L., McGlone, M. M., Rood, J., et al. (2010). Nonsurgical weight loss for extreme obesity in primary care settings: Results of the Louisiana Obese Subjects Study. *Archives of Internal Medicine, 170*(2), 146–154.

Sepah, S. C., Jiang, L., & Peters, A. L. (2015). Long-term outcomes of a web-based diabetes prevention program: 2-year results of a single-arm longitudinal study. *Journal of Medical Internet Research, 17*(4), e92.

Stunkard, A. J., Craighead, L. W., & O'Brien, R. (1980). Controlled trial of behaviour therapy, pharmacotherapy, and their combination in the treatment of obesity. *Lancet, 2*(8203), 1045–1047.

ter Bogt, N. C., Bemelmans, W. J., Beltman, F. W., Broer, J., Smit, A. J., & van der Meer, K. (2011). Preventing weight gain by lifestyle intervention in a general practice setting: Three-year results of a randomized controlled trial. *Archives of Internal Medicine, 171*(4), 306–313.

Tsai, A. G., Felton, S., Wadden, T. A., Hosokawa, P. W., & Hill, J. O. (2015). A randomized clinical trial of a weight loss maintenance intervention in a primary care population. *Obesity, 23*(10), 2015–2021.

Tsai, A. G., & Wadden, T. A. (2005). Systematic review: An evaluation of major commercial weight loss programs in the United States. *Annals of Internal Medicine, 142*(1), 56–66.

Tsai, A. G., Wadden, T. A., Rogers, M. A., Day, S. C., Moore, R. H., & Islam, B. J. (2010). A primary care intervention for weight loss: Results of a randomized controlled pilot study. *Obesity, 18*(8), 1614–1618.

United States Congress. (2010). Patient Protection and Affordable Care Act (PPACA), section 2713. Retrieved April 6, 2016, from *www.gpo.gov/fdsys/pkg/PLAW-111publ148/pdf/PLAW-111publ148.pdf.*

U.S. Preventive Services Task Force. (2003). Screening for obesity in adults: Recommendations and rationale. *Annals of Internal Medicine, 139*(11), 930–932.

Villareal, D. T., Chode, S., Parimi, N., Sinacore, D. R., Hilton, T., Armamento-Villareal, R., et al. (2011). Weight loss, exercise, or both and physical function in obese older adults. *New England Journal of Medicine, 364*(13), 1218–1229.

Volger, S., Vetter, M. L., Dougherty, M., Panigrahi, E., Egner, R., Webb, V., et al. (2012). Patients' preferred terms for describing their excess weight: Discussing obesity in clinical practice. *Obesity, 20*(1), 147–150.

Wadden, T. A., Berkowitz, R. I., Sarwer, D. B., Prus-Wisniewski, R., & Steinberg, C. (2001). Benefits of lifestyle modification in the pharmacologic treatment of obesity: A randomized trial. *Archives of Internal Medicine, 161*(2), 218–227.

Wadden, T. A., Berkowitz, R. I., Womble, L. G., Sarwer, D. B., Phelan, S., Cato, R. K., et al. (2005). Randomized trial of lifestyle modification and pharmacotherapy for obesity. *New England Journal of Medicine, 353*(20), 2111–2120.

Wadden, T. A., Butryn, M. L., Hong, P. S., & Tsai, A. G. (2014). Behavioral treatment of obesity in patients encountered in primary care settings: A systematic review. *Journal of the American Medical Association, 312*(17), 1779–1791.

Wadden, T. A., & Didie, E. (2003) What's in a name?: Patients' preferred terms for describing obesity. *Obesity Research, 11*(9), 1140–1146.

Wadden, T. A., Foreyt, J. P., Foster, G. D., Hill, J. O., Klein, S., O'Neil, P. M., et al. (2011). Weight loss with naltrexone SR/bupropion SR combination therapy as an adjunct to behavior modification: The COR-BMOD trial. *Obesity, 19*(1), 110–120.

Wadden, T. A., Volger, S., Sarwer, D. B., Vetter, M. L., Tsai, A. G., Berkowitz, R. I., et al. (2011). A two-year randomized trial of obesity treatment in primary care practice. *New England Journal of Medicine, 365*(21), 1969–1979.

Wadden, T. A., Womble, L. G., Sarwer, D. B., Berkowitz, R. I., Clark, V. L., & Foster, G. D. (2003). Great expectations: "I'm losing 25% of my weight no matter what you say." *Journal of Consulting and Clinical Psychology, 71*(6), 1084–1089.

Wang, G. J., Tomasi, D., Volkow, N. D., Wang, R., Telang, F., Caparelli, E. C., et al. (2014). Effect of combined naltrexone and bupropion therapy on the brain's reactivity to food cues. *International Journal of Obesity, 38*(5), 682–688.

Weinstock, R. S., Trief, P. M., Cibula, D., Morin, P. C., & Delahanty, L. M. (2013). Weight loss success in metabolic syndrome by telephone interventions: Results from the SHINE Study. *Journal of General Internal Medicine, 28*(12), 1620–1628.

Whittemore, R., Melkus, G., Wagner, J., Dziura, J., Northrup, V., & Grey, M. (2009). Translating the diabetes prevention program to primary care: A pilot study. *Nursing Research, 58*(1), 2–12.

Wing, R. R., Lang, W., Wadden, T. A., Safford, M., Knowler, W. C., Bertoni, A. G., et al. (2011). Benefits of modest weight loss in improving cardiovascular risk factors in overweight and obese individuals with type 2 diabetes. *Diabetes Care, 34*(7), 1481–1486.

Xiao, L., Yank, V., Wilson, S. R., Lavori, P. W., & Ma, J. (2013). Two-year weight-loss maintenance in primary care-based Diabetes Prevention Program lifestyle interventions. *Nutrition and Diabetes, 3*, e76.

CHAPTER 28

Remotely Delivered Interventions for Obesity

Deborah F. Tate
Brooke T. Nezami
Carmina G. Valle

Obesity is a pressing public health problem, with 37.9% of adults currently obese in the United States (Flegal, Kruszon-Moran, Carroll, Fryar, & Ogden, 2016). Because obesity is associated with a greater risk of hypertension, heart disease, type 2 diabetes, stroke, and several cancers (National Institutes of Health, 1998), treatment options are needed that are effective and keep participants engaged. The current nonmedical gold-standard treatment for obesity is a structured behavioral weight loss program that supports reduced dietary intake and increased energy expenditure (Knowler et al., 2002; Wadden, Butryn, & Byrne, 2004). The core pieces of lifestyle weight management programs include the provision of counseling support, goal setting, self-monitoring, and individualized feedback from a trained interventionist (Alamuddin, Bakizada, & Wadden, 2016).

Behavioral weight loss programs have traditionally been delivered in a face-to-face format with weekly group sessions that last 60–90 minutes, but often decrease in frequency to biweekly or monthly following the first 3–6 months of the program. These face-to-face interventions produce clinically significant weight losses of 5–10% by 6 months, which are known to reduce the risk of weight-related chronic diseases (National Institutes of Health, 1998; Alamuddin et al., 2016). Unfortunately, there are several barriers to in-person session attendance, including lack of transportation, travel costs, scheduling conflicts, the time burden of travel and attendance, and child care. In order to increase the accessibility and effectiveness of behavioral weight loss programs for individuals who may have barriers to in-person treatment, there is a great need to improve the access and convenience of treatments, and potentially reducing the cost as well.

Evolution of Remotely Delivered Interventions

Historically, remote counseling methods were used to provide additional intervention strategies during the later months of treatment, when the frequency of face-to-face visits reduced from weekly to biweekly or monthly (e.g., 6–18 months). Print materials with psychoeducational content sent via postal mail and telephone calls facilitated continued contact with study participants and served to cue continued efforts, maintain accountability, facilitate goal setting, reinforce positive behaviors, and promote problem solving to overcome barriers (Jakicic, Marcus, Gallagher, Napolitano, & Lang, 2003). As interest grew in reaching wider populations, studies began to examine remote delivery of entire weight loss treatments, replacing all or most clinic visits with mail or telephone counseling contacts.

With the advancement of computer and mobile technologies in the last several decades, the methods for and interest in providing counseling support and feedback remotely have continued to increase. Figure 28.1 displays the steadily increasing number of interventions that have been delivered using remote methods since 2000. The ability to communicate using email, the Internet, text messaging, smartphones, and social networking platforms has enabled researchers to incorporate remote methods that increasingly mimic many of the successful features of face-to-face delivery. Recent practice guidelines for managing overweight and obesity in adults indicated moderate evidence supporting the use of remotely delivered weight loss programs that include tailored feedback from trained interventionists (Jensen et al., 2014). Several systematic reviews have concluded that remotely delivered interventions are more efficacious than control groups or minimal treatments for weight loss (Saperstein, Atkinson, & Gold, 2007; Wieland et al., 2012).

The goal of this chapter is to highlight the emergence and effectiveness of the various types of remotely delivered behavioral weight loss interventions for adults that have been conducted to date. Rather than providing a systematic review of the literature, we have limited the examples to intervention studies that delivered a comprehensive behavioral program, including some form of remote counseling support, and specified weight loss as the primary outcome. We have also excluded studies with a focus on weight maintenance, those that used remote contact methods after in-person weight loss treatment, studies in children or adolescents, and trials with a primary goal of improving dietary behaviors or increasing physical activity. To summarize the efficacy of these interventions, we have prioritized studies that have compared remotely delivered interventions to either standard face-to-face interventions or control groups. Details of the studies included in this chapter can be found in Table 28.1.

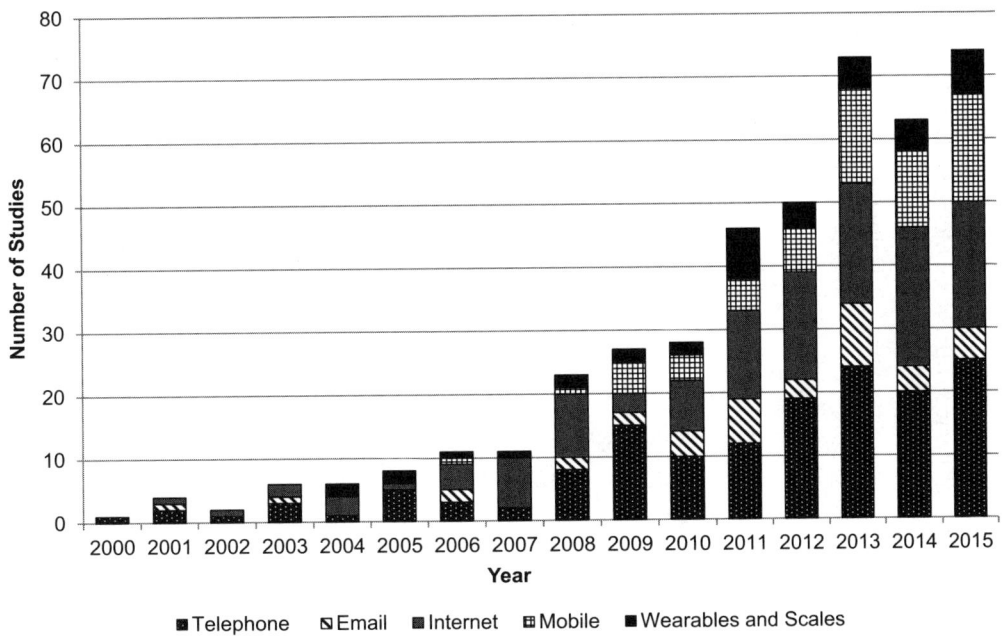

FIGURE 28.1. The number of publications focused on remote treatment of obesity over time.

TABLE 28.1. Types of Remotely Delivered Methods Used, Utilization Rates, and Initial Weight Losses in Remotely Delivered Interventions

	Remote modalities used	Utilization	Initial weight losses
Jeffery et al. (2003)	Mail[a] Telephone[b]	Not available	6 months: Mail = 1.9 kg;[d, e] Telephone = −2.4 kg;[d] Usual Care = −1.5 kg[e]
Sherwood et al. (2010)	Phone	10-session group: median 10 telephone contacts 20-session group: median 19 telephone contacts	6 months: 10 phone sessions = −3.2 kg;[d] 20 phone sessions = −4.9 kg;[d] Self-directed = −2.3 kg[d]
Digenio et al. (2009)	Telephone[a] Email[b]	Telephone contacts: 76% Email contacts: 80%	6 months: Telephone = −7.7%;[d] Email = −5.9%;[e] Self-directed = −5.2%;[e] High-frequency FTF = −8.9%;[d] Low-frequency FTF = −6.4%[e]
Appel et al. (2011)	Telephone Website Email	Median 14 (out of 15) telephone contacts, median 23 (out of 26) weekly website logins	6 months: Remote = −6.1 kg;[d] Remote + FTF = −5.8 kg;[d] Control = −1.4 kg[e]
Bennett et al. (2010)	Telephone Website	80% call completion Week 1 website logins (mean) = 5.5 Week 12 website logins (mean) = 2.7	12 weeks: Intervention = −2.6 kg;[d] Control = +0.3 kg[e]
Donnelly et al. (2013)	Telephone Email	73% telephone contacts completed	6 months: Phone = −12.3 ± 7.0%;[d] FTF = −13.4 ± 6.7%[d]
Rock et al. (2010)	Telephone Email	Months 0–6: Not available Months 18–24: 39% completed weekly calls, 24% completed no calls	12 months: FTF = −10.1 kg;[d] Telephone = −8.5 kg;[d] Usual care = −2.4 kg[e]
Gold et al. (2007)	Website Email	Months 0–6: median 21 out of 26 online group chats	6 months: VTrim = −8.3 kg;[d] eDiets.com = −4.1 kg[e]
Micco et al. (2007)	Website Email	Months 0–6: 77% attendance in online group chats Months 7–12: 56% attendance in online group chats	6 months: Internet = −6.8 kg;[d] Internet + FTF = −5.1 kg[d]
Harvey-Berino et al. (2010)	Website	76% attendance in online group chats	6 months: Internet = −5.5 kg;[d] FTF = −8.0 kg;[e] Hybrid = −6.0 kg[d]
Tate et al. (2003)	Website Email	Logins greater in internet + email counseling group vs. internet group	12 months: Internet + Email counseling = −4.4 kg;[d] Internet = −2.0 kg[e]

Study	Modality	Engagement	Outcomes
Tate et al. (2006)	Website, Email	Internet + Human Email Counseling = 32.5 logins; Internet + Automated Counseling = 20 logins; No Counseling = 34 logins	6 months: Internet + Human email counseling = −7.3 kg;[d] Internet + Automated email counseling = −4.9 kg;[e] No counseling = −2.6 kg
Thomas et al. (2015)	Website	Interactive Internet: Mean of 10 out of 12 weeks with 1+ login; Education-Only Internet: Mean of 9.5 out of 12 weeks with 1+ login	3 months: Interactive internet = Education-only internet = −5.5 kg;[d] −1.3 kg
Steinberg et al. (2013)	Website, Email	Not available	6 months: Intervention = −6.6%;[d] Control = −0.4%[e]
Crane et al. (2015)	Website, Email	Mean of 11.2 out of 13 online contacts	6 months: Intervention = −5.3 kg;[d] Control = −0.6 kg
Patrick et al. (2009)	Telephone, Text messages	Week 1: Mean of 3/3 text message replies; Week 16: Mean of 2/3 text message replies	4 months: Intervention = −2.9 kg;[d] Control = −0.9 kg
Shapiro et al. (2012)	Text messages, Website	SMS response rate ranged from 60–69%	6 months: Intervention = −1.7 kg;[d] Control = −0.7 kg[d]
Haapala et al. (2009)	Text messages, Website	Months 1–3: Mean of 8.2 text and website contacts per week; Months 10–12: Mean of 3.1 text and website contacts per week	12 months: Intervention = −5.4%;[d] Control = −1.3%[e]
Martin et al. (2015)	Email, Text messages, Telephone	Email contacts (mean): 11.5; Text message contacts (mean): 6.8; Telephone contacts (mean): 8.8	12 weeks: Intervention = −7.8 kg;[d] Control = −0.6 kg[e]
Svetkey et al. (2015)	Smartphone Application	Months 0–6: Interaction with smartphone app mean of 4.6 times/day	6 months: Smartphone = −0.9 kg;[d] In-Person + Telephone = −3.1 kg;[e] Control = −1.1 kg[d]
Turner-McGrievy & Tate (2011)	Social media (Twitter), Podcasts	Podcast + Twitter: Mean of 25.4 out of 48 podcasts downloaded; Podcast-Only: Mean of 22.7 out of 48 podcasts downloaded	6 months: Podcast + Twitter = −2.6 kg;[d] Podcast-only = −2.6 kg
Napolitano et al. (2013)	Social media (Facebook), Text messages	Facebook: 24% "liked" at least 1 post, 41% commented at least once; Facebook + Texts: 22% "liked" at least one post, 78% commented at least once	8 weeks: Facebook = −0.5 kg;[d] Facebook + Texts = −1.7 kg;[e] Control = 0.3 kg[d]

Note. FTF, face-to-face.

[a,b,c] Indicates modalities compared by different treatment groups, rather than used together in the same treatment group.

[d,e] Means with unshared superscripts indicate significant weight loss differences.

Types of Remotely Delivered Interventions

Telephone

Weigh-to-Be was the largest of several trials conducted by Jeffery and colleagues (2003) that studied the use of telephone-delivered weight loss treatment. The study compared a mail-based intervention to phone-based or usual care among 1,801 managed-care patients over 1- and 2-year follow-up periods. In both intervention groups, a series of 10 lessons were mailed to participants. Each lesson included a rationale for and introduction of a new behavioral skill, as well as related homework assignments. In the mail intervention, participants returned a report of progress to the counselor each week via mail and received written feedback and a new lesson the following week. The phone group reported their progress and received feedback from counselors through 20-minute phone calls that corresponded to each of the 10 lessons. At 6 months, only the phone intervention resulted in significantly greater weight loss than usual care; however, no between-group differences were observed in mean weight losses at 1 year (–2.3 kg mail, –2.3 kg phone, and –1.9 kg usual care) or at 2 years (–0.7 kg mail, –1.0 kg phone, and –0.6 kg usual care). The results of this study suggested that regular interactive discussions with a counselor could be more effective for weight loss during the first 6 months of treatment compared to passively receiving written feedback through the mail.

A follow-up study by this research team evaluated the intervention dose that might be required for efficacy in telephone-delivered weight loss programs. The DIAL (Drop It At Last) study compared a self-directed program to two interventions that differed in dose of telephone counseling delivered (10 vs. 20 calls) in a sample of 63 adults (Sherwood, Jeffery, Welsh, VanWormer, & Hotop, 2010). The 6-month weight losses were 2.3 kg, 3.2 kg, and 4.9 kg in the self-directed, 10-call, and 20-call groups, respectively. Although these differences did not reach statistical significance, the effect size for the 20-call treatment compared to the self-directed group was $d = 0.49$. Twice as many participants achieved a 5% weight loss in the 20-call condition compared to the self-directed condition, suggesting that the dose required to produce clinically significant weight losses in the absence of face-to-face visits is perhaps more similar to the 16- to 24-session dose delivered over the first 6 months of successful face-to-face weight loss interventions (DPP Research Group, 2002; Look AHEAD Research Group, 2007). A 6-month pharmacotherapy study by Digenio and colleagues added to the evidence that high-frequency (i.e., 19 contacts over 6 months) in-person or telephone counseling yield similar weight losses (–8.9% in person and –7.7% telephone) that are superior to the losses yielded by lower-frequency (6 contacts over 6 months) in-person or high-frequency email methods (6.4 and 5.9%, respectively) (Digenio, Mancuso, Gerber, & Dvorak, 2009).

Several studies have used telephone counseling to deliver weight loss treatment remotely in primary care settings. One of the largest and longest studies, conducted by Appel et al. (2011), randomized 415 adults to a remote-only intervention, an in-person intervention, or a usual-care control group, all with long-term follow-up at 24 months. The remote-only group received web-based learning modules, self-monitoring, email reminders, and progress summaries, plus weekly telephone coaching for the first 3 months, followed by monthly coaching calls through 24 months. The in-person group also received the web and email remote contacts, but coaching was provided face-to-face in either group or individual sessions: weekly for the first 3 months, three visits per month during months 3–6, and two visits per month thereafter. Weight losses at 24 months were significantly greater in both the remote-only and in-person treatment arms than in usual care (–4.6, –5.1, and –0.8 kg, respectively). The weight losses achieved at 2 years in the remote-only group are notable. This intervention provides an example of a potentially sustainable remote care model that is a hybrid of human and automated contacts.

Similar to Appel et al. (2011), Bennett et al. (2010) studied the efficacy of an intervention that used a website and telephone calls to reduce the burden on primary care patients. They randomly assigned 101 patients to a 12-week intervention, primarily delivered through a website, supplemented with two in-person sessions and two individual telephone sessions, or to a usual-care control group. Participants in the intervention group lost 2.3 kg at 3 months compared to a gain of 0.3 kg among participants in usual care. A greater number of website logins was associated with greater weight loss.

Most studies of telephone counseling to date have used individual or one-on-one telephone counseling to replace a clinic visit that involves group counseling support. Donnelly et al. (2013) studied the delivery of behavioral weight loss treatment using weekly group telephone conference calls compared with standard group-based clinical care in an equivalency design with 285 adults. After 6 months, weight losses were sizable and not different between groups, averaging 12% and 13% reductions in initial weight in the conference-call and clinic groups, respectively. Use of liquid meal replacements was required as the primary method for calorie control in both groups and likely contributed to the magnitude of weight loss. Another large study (N = 442) of a commercial meal replacement program compared weekly telephone counseling coupled with web and email follow-up against in-person support to facilitate weight loss, along with provision of free portion-controlled foods (Rock et al., 2010). Both remote and in-person support programs produced greater weight losses than a usual-care group. At 1 year, phone and in-person groups had lost 9.2 and 10.9% of initial body weight, respectively, though the study was not designed to compare these differences. The effects of phone and in-person support cannot be separated from the effects of portion-controlled meals.

Online Chats

Consistent with delivery of face-to-face standard behavioral weight loss using a group treatment model, Harvey-Berino and colleagues have conducted a series of studies examining provision of remote weight loss support via online therapist-led group meetings (i.e., chats). In a 2007 study, 124 participants received a web-based program that included lessons in an online workbook-style self-monitoring diary, a peer discussion board, weekly email feedback from a counselor on self-monitoring data, and weekly group meetings led by the counselor in an online chat room. The intervention lasted for 6 months, followed by 6 months of biweekly chat support (Gold, Burke, Piuntaro, Buzzell, & Harvey-Berino, 2007). Weight losses at 12 months were significantly greater for the intervention (−5.5% of initial weight) than for a web-based commercial comparison group (i.e., eDiets, −2.8%). Micco et al. (2007) compared the same remote Internet program with online chat group support to a program with online chat group support plus in-person counseling. The Internet plus in-person group participated in three online chats and one in-person group meeting per month. Surprisingly, the Internet plus in-person group did not lose more weight than the group receiving only remote Internet support at 6 months (−5.1 vs. −7.8 kg) or 12 months (−3.5 vs. −5.1 kg). Attendance at weekly online chat groups was significantly lower in the group that received the hybrid in-person plus remote support treatment.

In a larger study (N = 481) Harvey-Berino et al. (2010) conducted a randomized comparative effectiveness trial of a 24-session program that was delivered weekly for 6 months. Participants were randomly assigned to receive the program provided in one of three ways: (1) the Internet group chat approach, (2) the standard in-person group treatment, or (3) the hybrid online group with once-per-month in-person group meetings described previously. At 6 months, weight losses were significantly greater for the in-person group treatment (−7.9% of initial weight), compared with the Internet-only (−5.7%) or hybrid approach (−6.0%). Collectively, these studies demonstrate that counselor-led, online group behavioral support produces clinically meaningful weight loss, though weight losses are about 1–2 kg less than those produced by in-person group behavioral treatment. Further, substituting an online group meeting with one in-person group session once per month does not appear to add to the efficacy of a comprehensive remote online group support intervention.

Email

In standard face-to-face behavioral programs, attendance at clinic visits and call completion rates decline over time (Donnelly et al., 2013), perhaps due to declining motivation or because continued attendance at meetings becomes a barrier to busy adults. Researchers have speculated that using asynchronous forms of communication such as email might overcome this barrier, and that email would also be superior to postal mail, another form of asynchronous communication, because exchanges between participants and counselors could occur more quickly and at lower cost. In addition, email use is becoming increasingly common, with 92% of adults using email and 61% using it every day (Purcell, 2011).

Email counseling has been studied as an individual form of remote behavioral treatment support with one-on-one email feedback or messaging. A series of early studies examined remote behavioral interventions using a website or email to deliver behavioral lesson content, web-based self-monitoring, online peer support message boards, and email as the main form of counseling support. Email counseling provided prompting, accountability, feedback, review of goals, limited problem solving, and reinforcement (Tate, Jackvony, & Wing, 2003, 2006; Tate, Wing, & Winett, 2001). A study by Tate et al. (2003) of 92 adults used an additive, randomized design to compare provision of web-based content, self-monitoring, and peer support to a program that included the same features plus weekly email counseling exchange with participants. At 12 months, weight losses were greater in participants who received weekly email counseling (−4.8 vs. −2.2% reduction in initial weight), though weight losses were not of the magnitude achieved with intensive face-to-face behavioral programs. A subsequent study compared fully automated, weekly, computer-generated messages to weekly human email counseling and to web content with no counseling (Tate et al., 2006). Weight losses in both the computer-generated and email counseling groups were significantly greater than no counseling at 3 months (−5.8%, −6.8%, and −3.2% of initial weight, respectively) and did not differ significantly from each other. However, at 6 months, only the human email counseling group was superior to control (−5.3% for automated counseling, −8.1% for human counseling, and −2.8%

for no counseling). A more recent study by Thomas, Leahey, and Wing (2015) demonstrated that a program that used fully automated weekly feedback, coupled with a website that included interactive lesson content, videos, quizzes, and goal setting, produced significantly greater weight losses at 3 months (5.5 kg) than a control condition (1.3 kg) in primary care patients.

Remotely delivered programs that include computer-generated, fully automated feedback and recommendations based on participant progress are appealing due to the potential for reach and low cost. However, engagement has been a concern in programs that do not use some human support as part of remote treatment delivery. Advances in machine learning may enable the creation of more engaging and appropriate messages that consider complex behavior patterns and contexts in ways that more closely mimic human counseling support.

Semiautomated feedback involves creating feedback messages that apply to groups of individuals based on their weekly data, but sending the grouped messages from a study staff person rather than from a generic study email address. There are advantages to this approach over individualized email counseling in terms of reduced study staff time and increased intervention fidelity, and over fully automated systems in terms of heightened level of participant accountability, since study staff emails may be familiar. Steinberg et al. (2013) remotely delivered an intervention with semiautomated weekly email feedback and behavioral lessons compared to a wait-list control group. Following one group session, participants received weekly emails and used cellular-connected wireless scales to transmit daily weights. The primary behavioral strategy encouraged by the program was daily weighing, which was used as a self-monitoring strategy to gauge progress without detailed monitoring of calories and exercise. Weekly feedback focused on adherence to daily weighing and weight loss progress; participants were grouped based on these factors and sent identical feedback emails. At 6 months, participants had lost 6.6% of initial weight, compared to 0.4% in the wait-list group, and 43% of intervention participants had achieved a 5% or greater reduction in weight. This intervention was one of the first to show that delivering an intervention remotely through email, with semiautomated feedback from study staff, could be effective in producing clinically significant weight losses.

A study by Crane and colleagues used the semiautomated approach to deliver a 6-month weight loss program to 107 men (Crane, Lutes, Ward, Bowling, & Tate, 2015). Participants were randomized to the REFIT program (Rethinking Eating and FITness) or to a wait-list control group. REFIT was delivered via weekly contact during months 1–3, followed by monthly contact during months 4–6. The program started with two in-person groups followed by asynchronous online contacts for the remainder of the program. The study counselor emailed participants the link to an interactive survey module, which enabled weight loss and behavioral reporting, goal setting, and tailored feedback. Men in the intervention group lost 5.2% of their initial weight at 6 months, compared to 0.6% in the wait-list group. This study is notable in that the sample was entirely male, program utilization was very high (with participants completing 86% of the expected interactive survey modules), and utilization was associated with weight loss ($r = -.37$).

Mobile Phone

Interventions using text messages, mobile-based websites, and smartphone applications have the capability to reach many people, including those who have barriers to attending in-person programs. These interventions take advantage of the proliferation of mobile phones as part of everyday life, with 92% of Americans owning a cell phone and 68% owning a smartphone as of 2015 (Horrigan & Duggan, 2015; Rainie & Zickhur, 2015). The reliance on smartphones continues to rise, with the percentage of Americans who use smartphones exclusively to access the Internet increasing from 8% in 2013 to 13% in 2015. During that same time, broadband subscriptions declined from 70 to 67% (Horrigan & Duggan, 2015). Given that individuals generally take their cell phones wherever they go and rarely turn them off, using mobile methods to deliver intervention content, provide counseling, and collect self-monitoring data is a potentially cost-effective way to reach large populations of people.

The use of mobile phones in the delivery of weight loss interventions began with the use of text messaging, which had already been shown to be effective across a range of behaviors, including smoking cessation, physical activity, and diabetes self-management (Fjeldsoe, Marshall, & Miller, 2009; Head, Noar, Iannarino, & Grant Harrington, 2013). Efficacious components of these prior interventions included personal tailoring of messages and delivering messages in a random rather than fixed frequency (Head et al., 2013). Patrick et al. (2009) conducted one of the first studies to use a text-message-based intervention for weight loss, a 16-week study that randomized overweight adults to one of two groups: (1) an intervention that included text messages two to five times per day, printed materials, and monthly brief telephone calls from a health counselor; or (2) a comparison group that received monthly printed materials on weight control. Text messages were used for self-monitoring, prompts, and support for behavior change, and included topics such as goal setting for diet and physical activity and overcoming barriers. Tailoring of message frequency was integrated into the study by allowing users to specify the timing and number of text messages per day. At 16 weeks, the intervention group had lost 2.9 kg compared to 0.9 kg in the control group. Participants reported high satisfaction with the program and remained adherent to text messaging at the end of 16 weeks. This was the first evidence to suggest that an intervention delivered by text message could be feasible, acceptable to participants, and effective for weight loss.

Shapiro et al. (2012) tested a modified version of Patrick et al.'s (2009) program, in which adults who were overweight or obese were randomly assigned to an intervention group receiving daily text messages, but no monthly phone calls, or to a control group that received monthly e-newsletters. Participants received four text messages per day for the duration of the 12-month study, including prompts, tips, questions, and tailored graphical feedback. The study used behavioral strategies such as self-monitoring, goal setting, and problem solving. Text messages were tailored based on baseline eating behaviors. There were no differences in weight loss between the intervention and control groups at 6 or 12 months (–1.7 kg and –1.0 kg, respectively, at month 12). Text message adherence declined over time but was significantly associated with weight loss. Thus, the text message intervention was effective for those who continued to participate, but the program may have lacked components that kept participants engaged, such as some form of human counseling.

One additional randomized controlled trial (RCT) evaluated a 12-month program delivered entirely by text message, as compared to a control group (Haapala, Barengo, Biggs, Surakka, & Manninen, 2009). Intervention participants submitted their weight daily via text and, in response, were given a tailored caloric intake goal for the day based on their current weight, goal weight, and number of days left until the target goal weight date. Users were able to self-monitor their dietary intake and report their weight on a study website, but no counseling was provided outside of text message feedback. Weight loss in the intervention group was 4.5 kg at 12 months, which was significantly greater than the loss in the control group (–1.1 kg). Participant weight reporting and other contacts with the study declined over time, from 8.2 contacts per week in months 1–3 to 3.1 contacts per week in months 9–12. More frequent text messaging during the first 3 months of the program was associated with weight loss at 12 months.

Among the three text messaging studies just described, average weekly weight losses were highest in the 16-week study by Patrick et al. (2009). Research on behavioral interventions has demonstrated that human counseling is a key component for weight loss (Tate et al., 2006); thus the weight losses in the Patrick et al. (2009) study were likely aided by the addition of individual monthly telephone calls with study health counselors. Of note, participants in this study were able to change the frequency and timing of messages over the course of the study; participants in Haapala et al.'s (2009) study initiated text message contacts rather than receiving unprompted messages. In contrast, participants in the trial by Shapiro et al. (2012) received a fixed number of messages (four per day) for 1 year. It will be important to determine the frequency of text messages per day or week that is optimal and sufficient for weight loss, yet does not produce habituation, annoyance, or feelings of intrusion.

Smartphone-Delivered Interventions

With the increasing use of smartphones and the ability to easily disseminate smartphone programs, researchers have recently begun to study the feasibility and efficacy of using multiple features of smartphones to deliver weight loss interventions. An advantage to delivering intervention content and counseling exclusively using smartphones is the increased program flexibility for participants, who can access and participate in the intervention at any time. Smartphones can be used to deliver treatment through the use of mobile-based websites, native applications, text messaging, email, or telephone calls.

The first study to deliver a weight loss intervention entirely via smartphone, while also harnessing the advantages of modern wireless technology, was a 12-week RCT that compared a smartphone-based intervention, SmartLoss[SM], to a health education control group (Martin et al., 2015). At baseline, participants were given a calorie prescription and a graph displaying the weight loss that could be expected if they adhered to dietary and physical activity recommendations. Participants' weight and activity were remotely monitored using wirelessly transmitted accelerometers and scales, and graphical feedback was provided via email. Study counselors also provided feedback using email, text, or telephone, and implemented behavioral strategies (e.g., problem solving barriers to adherence) if participants were outside of their expected weight loss zone. At 12 weeks, participants in SmartLoss had lost 7.8 kg compared to 0.6 kg in the control group. This was the first study to demonstrate that an intervention delivered via smartphone with feedback from study counselors could result in significant weight loss.

An additional study randomized young adults who were overweight or obese to one of three groups for 24 months: a smartphone application group, a personal coaching plus smartphone group, or a control group (Svetkey et al., 2015). In the smartphone-only group, intervention content was delivered through a smartphone application that included goal setting; social support; prompts to self-monitor dietary intake, activity, and weight; and feedback on progress. The coaching plus smartphone group received intervention content in six weekly in-person group sessions and monthly telephone calls with a personal coach. The smartphone was used only for self-monitoring, and participants did not receive prompts to monitor. Both groups had digital scales that transmitted weights remotely to the study. At 6 months, the coaching plus smartphone group had lost significantly more weight than the control group (−3.1 kg vs. −1.1 kg), with no other significant differences between groups. At 12 months, however, no significant differences in weight loss were observed between any groups (−1.5 kg for smartphone only, −3.6 kg for coaching + smartphone, and −2.3 kg for control). The results of this study indicate that a smartphone-only treatment without personal or group counseling was not as effective at promoting initial weight loss (i.e., 6 months) as a hybrid treatment that combined in-person and telephone sessions with smartphone monitoring.

The small body of evidence on the use of smartphones and text messaging to deliver weight loss interventions demonstrates that these interventions were effective at producing weight loss, in comparison to control groups, when they included some form of interventionist feedback or brief counseling. To date, most smartphone-based programs appear to be less effective than in-person interventions. However, the modest weight losses can be clinically significant and remain impactful when considering the flexibility given to participants in accessing program content and the potential to increase treatment uptake by appealing to those who might not enroll in group treatment. Moreover, despite smaller weight losses, programs with greater automation and less human contact typically have a lower cost and staff burden, and have potential for dissemination and integration into programs that can reach large populations.

Social Media

Social media and social networking sites such as Twitter, Facebook, Instagram, and LinkedIn represent more recent technologies that have worldwide popularity, are commonly used in everyday life, and are continually being adopted by more users over time. Over the last decade, use of social networking sites by U.S. adults has increased nearly tenfold, from an estimated 7% in 2005 to 65% in 2015 (Perrin, 2015). Social media offer advantages similar to those of other remote delivery channels, such as minimizing time, costs, travel, and barriers to participation. Despite the increasing use of social media in the past decade, relatively little is known about the efficacy of social media as an independent method of delivery for weight loss interventions (Dahl, Hales, & Turner-McGrievy, 2016).

To date, two randomized trials with weight loss as the primary outcome have evaluated interventions that included general social networking sites as a main delivery channel or component of a larger intervention. In an 8-week pilot study, Napolitano and colleagues randomized 52 college students to a Facebook Plus, Facebook, or a wait-list control group (Napolitano, Hayes, Bennett, Ives, & Foster, 2013). Both intervention groups received access to a Facebook group (two separate groups for Facebook Plus and Facebook), through which intervention content was delivered, including polls and invitations to health-related events. Additionally, Facebook Plus participants received a digital scale, pedometer, weekly personalized feedback reports, and daily text messages regarding goal setting, self-monitoring, and social support. These participants also identified a "buddy" external to the study to provide support. The Facebook Plus group produced significantly more weight loss (−2.4 kg) than both the Facebook (−0.6 kg) and control groups (−0.2 kg). In the Facebook group, 24% of participants "liked" the study-related posts, and 41% commented or posted on the page at least once, compared to 22% in the Facebook Plus group who "liked" study-related posts and 78% who commented or posted on the page. This was the first pilot study to demonstrate the feasibility of delivering weight loss content to college students using Facebook. However, the results suggest that Facebook was effective only when supplemented with additional support and feedback from study staff.

In a 6-month randomized trial among 96 overweight adults, Turner-McGrievy and Tate (2011) used Twitter as a social support supplement to a podcast intervention that delivered content through a theory-based weight loss podcast. This podcast, which included nutrition and exercise information, instructions for setting goals, and a soap opera depicting weight loss experiences and expectations, had already been shown to be more effective at producing short-term weight loss than a publicly available weight loss podcast (Turner-McGrievy et al., 2009). Participants were randomized to a podcast-only group (Podcast) or to a group that received the podcast in addition to a mobile app for monitoring diet and activity, as well as Twitter interactions with a counselor and peers (Podcast + Mobile). Participants in both groups received two 15-minute podcasts per week in months 1–3, and two 5-minute mini-podcasts per week in months 4–6. Mean weight losses of 2.7% of initial weight were achieved in both groups at 6 months, suggesting no added effect of mobile self-monitoring and communication via Twitter in inducing weight loss. Despite encouragement to engage with Twitter daily, participants in the Podcast + Mobile group averaged two posts to Twitter per week, and posts declined over time. However, greater engagement with Twitter was associated with greater weight loss, such that every 10 posts was significantly associated with almost −0.5% weight loss (Turner-McGrievy & Tate, 2013). These studies suggest that maintaining user engagement and retention with social-media-based components in a weight loss intervention is a particular challenge. Leveraging the way that people currently use social media (e.g., enrolling groups of existing acquaintances) may facilitate better engagement with interventions over time (Maher et al., 2014). Thus, promoting user engagement with social media and online social networks within remotely delivered weight loss programs has the potential to improve outcomes and is worthy of future research efforts.

Summary and Future Directions

Advances in technology have enabled the evaluation of many alternative approaches to face-to-face weight management programs. Overall, interventions across a variety of remotely delivered approaches have demonstrated positive impact, with some achieving clinically significant weight loss outcomes. Those that included regular feedback from a trained interventionist, self-monitoring, and social support with other participants generally produced greater weight losses than programs that lacked these features. This finding is consistent with a prior review that found that counselor feedback, self-monitoring, social support, and use of a structured and individually tailored program were key components of technology-based intervention (Khaylis, Yiaslas, Bergstrom, & Gore-Felton, 2010). However, despite individual tailoring of some program components, there remains wide variability in treatment response between individuals. Efforts to identify why interventions are efficacious for some participants but not others, and to understand the characteristics of so-called responders and nonresponders to various obesity treatments, could facilitate the delivery of more personalized approaches that adapt to individual needs for support.

As technologies advance, opportunities will continuously emerge to utilize technology strategies for more efficient data capture, to identify nonresponders, and to adapt interventions so that they can be delivered more precisely and "just in time" when needed. Smartphones and wearable activity monitors now allow for the collection of large amounts of data that can be used to further specify and refine interventions. However, researchers must implement strategies that improve the efficiency and quality of interventions using these new technologies. Study designs used for building adaptive interventions include stepped care and sequential, multiple-assignment, randomized trials (SMART; Collins, Nahum-Shani, & Almirall, 2014). For more efficient development of remotely delivered interventions, a multiphase optimization strategy (MOST) that utilizes factorial designs can be applied to optimize multicomponent interventions for weight loss prior to evaluation (Collins,

Kugler, & Gwadz, 2015). Use of just-in-time adaptive interventions (JITAIs) is an emerging research method that capitalizes on the ability of mobile technology to continuously monitor an individual's status and context in real time, adapt moment to moment, and deliver the right type of intervention support for behavior change only when needed (e.g., prompt to weigh after 3 days without weighing; Nahum-Shani, Hekler, & Spruijt-Metz, 2015). To date, little research has used these newer approaches to evaluate remotely delivered weight loss treatments. As the health information and communication landscapes continue to rapidly evolve as a result of mobile technologies, novel interventions and rapid research approaches are needed to keep pace with these changes and to leverage them in implementing and disseminating weight loss treatments.

Acknowledgments

The authors gratefully acknowledge funding from the National Institute of Diabetes and Digestive and Kidney Diseases (Grant No. P30 DK056350) for the Nutrition and Obesity Research Center at the University of North Carolina, as well as the assistance provided by Lara Balian, Karen Hatley, and Sarah Mye.

References

Alamuddin, N., Bakizada, Z., & Wadden, T. A. (2016). Behavioral treatment of the patient with obesity. *Endocrinology and Metabolism Clinics of North America, 45*(3), 565–580.

Appel, L. J., Clark, J. M., Yeh, H. C., Wang, N. Y., Coughlin, J. W., Daumit, G., et al. (2011). Comparative effectiveness of weight-loss interventions in clinical practice. *New England Journal of Medicine, 365*(21), 1959–1968.

Bennett, G. G., Herring, S. J., Puleo, E., Stein, E. K., Emmons, K. M., & Gillman, M. W. (2010). Web-based weight loss in primary care: A randomized controlled trial. *Obesity, 18*(2), 308–313.

Collins, L. M., Kugler, K. C., & Gwadz, M. V. (2016). Optimization of multicomponent behavioral and biobehavioral interventions for the prevention and treatment of HIV/AIDS. *AIDS and Behavior, 20*(Suppl. 1), S197–S214.

Collins, L. M., Nahum-Shani, I., & Almirall, D. (2014). Optimization of behavioral dynamic treatment regimens based on the sequential, multiple assignment, randomized trial (SMART). *Clinical Trials, 11*(4), 426–434.

Crane, M. M., Lutes, L. D., Ward, D. S., Bowling, J. M., & Tate, D. F. (2015). A randomized trial testing the efficacy of a novel approach to weight loss among men with overweight and obesity. *Obesity, 23*(12), 2398–2405.

Dahl, A., Hales, S. B., & Turner-McGrievy, G. (2016). Integrating social media into weight loss interventions. *Current Opinion in Psychology, 9*, 11–15.

Digenio, A. G., Mancuso, J. P., Gerber, R. A., & Dvorak, R. V. (2009). Comparison of methods for delivering a lifestyle modification program for obese patients: A randomized trial. *Annals of Internal Medicine, 150*(4), 255–262.

Donnelly, J. E., Goetz, J. R., Gibson, C. A., Sullivan, D. K., Lee, R., Smith, B. K., et al. (2013). Equivalent weight loss for weight management programs delivered by phone and clinic. *Obesity, 21*(10), 1951–1959.

DPP Research Group. (2002). The Diabetes Prevention Program (DPP): Description of lifestyle intervention. *Diabetes Care, 25*(12), 2165–2171.

Fjeldsoe, B. S., Marshall, A. L., & Miller, Y. D. (2009). Behavior change interventions delivered by mobile telephone short-message service. *American Journal of Preventive Medicine, 36*(2), 165–173.

Flegal, K. M., Kruszon-Moran, D., Carroll, M. D., Fryar, C. D., & Ogden, C. L. (2016). Trends in obesity among adults in the United States, 2005 to 2014. *Journal of the American Medical Association, 315*(21), 2284–2291.

Gold, B. C., Burke, S., Pintauro, S., Buzzell, P., & Harvey-Berino, J. (2007). Weight loss on the web: A pilot study comparing a structured behavioral intervention to a commercial program. *Obesity (Silver Spring), 15*(1), 155–164.

Haapala, I., Barengo, N. C., Biggs, S., Surakka, L., & Manninen, P. (2009). Weight loss by mobile phone: A 1-year effectiveness study. *Public Health Nutrition, 12*(12), 2382–2391.

Harvey-Berino, J., West, D., Krukowski, R., Prewitt, E., VanBiervliet, A., Ashikaga, T., et al. (2010). Internet-delivered behavioral obesity treatment. *Preventive Medicine, 51*(2), 123–128.

Head, K. J., Noar, S. M., Iannarino, N. T., & Grant Harrington, N. (2013). Efficacy of text messaging-based interventions for health promotion: A meta-analysis. *Social Science and Medicine, 97*, 41–48.

Horrigan, J., & Duggan, M. (2015). Home broadband 2015. Retrieved from *www.pewinternet.org/2015/12/21/2015/Home-Broadband-2015*.

Jakicic, J. M., Marcus, B. H., Gallagher, K. I., Napolitano, M., & Lang, W. (2003). Effect of exercise duration and intensity on weight loss in overweight, sedentary women: A randomized trial. *Journal of the American Medical Association, 290*(10), 1323–1330.

Jeffery, R. W., Sherwood, N. E., Brelje, K., Pronk, N. P., Boyle, R., Boucher, J. L., et al. (2003). Mail and phone interventions for weight loss in a managed-care setting: Weigh-To-Be one-year outcomes. *International Journal of Obesity and Related Metabolic Disorders, 27*(12), 1584–1592.

Jensen, M. D., Ryan, D. H., Apovian, C. M., Ard, J. D., Comuzzie, A. G., Donato, K. A., et al. (2014). 2013 AHA/ACC/TOS guideline for the management of overweight and obesity in adults: A report of the American College of Cardiology/American Heart Association Task Force on Practice Guidelines and The Obesity Society. *Circulation, 129*(25, Suppl. 2), S102–S138.

Khaylis, A., Yiaslas, T., Bergstrom, J., & Gore-Felton, C. (2010). A review of efficacious technology-based weight-loss interventions: Five key components. *Telemedicine and e-Health, 16*(9), 931–938.

Knowler, W. C., Barrett-Connor, E., Fowler, S. E., Hamman, R. F., Lachin, J. M., Walker, E. A., et al. (2002). Reduction in the incidence of type 2 diabetes with lifestyle intervention or metformin. *New England Journal of Medicine, 346*(6), 393–403.

Look AHEAD Research Group. (2007). Reduction in weight and cardiovascular disease risk factors in individuals with type 2 diabetes: One-year results of the Look AHEAD Trial. *Diabetes Care, 30*(6), 1374–1383.

Maher, C. A., Lewis, L. K., Ferrar, K., Marshall, S., De Bourdeaudhuij, I., & Vandelanotte, C. (2014). Are health behavior change interventions that use online social networks effective?: A systematic review. *Journal of Medical Internet Research, 16*(2), e40.

Martin, C. K., Miller, A. C., Thomas, D. M., Champagne, C. M., Han, H., & Church, T. (2015). Efficacy of SmartLoss, a smartphone-based weight loss intervention: Results from a randomized controlled trial. *Obesity (Silver Spring), 23*(5), 935–942.

Micco, N., Gold, B., Buzzell, P., Leonard, H., Pintauro, S., & Harvey-Berino, J. (2007). Minimal in-person support as an adjunct to internet obesity treatment. *Annals of Behavioral Medicine, 33*(1), 49–56.

Nahum-Shani, I., Hekler, E. B., & Spruijt-Metz, D. (2015). Building health behavior models to guide the development of just-in-time adaptive interventions: A pragmatic framework. *Health Psychology, 34*(Suppl.), 1209–1219.

Napolitano, M. A., Hayes, S., Bennett, G. G., Ives, A. K., & Foster, G. D. (2013). Using Facebook and text messaging to deliver a weight loss program to college students. *Obesity (Silver Spring), 21*(1), 25–31.

National Institutes of Health. (1998). Clinical guidelines on the identification, evaluation, and treatment of overweight and obesity in adults—the evidence report. *Obesity Research, 6*(Suppl. 2), 51S–209S.

Patrick, K., Raab, F., Adams, M. A., Dillon, L., Zabinski, M., Rock, C. L., et al. (2009). A text message-based intervention for weight loss: Randomized controlled trial. *Journal of Medical Internet Research, 11*(1), e1.

Perrin, A. (2015). Social media usage: 2005–2015. Retrieved from *www.pewinternet.org/2015/10/08/social-networking-usage-2005-2015*.

Purcell, K. (2011). *Search and email still top the list of most popular online activities*. Retrieved from *www.pewinternet.org/2011/08/09/search-and-email-still-top-the-list-of-most-popular-online-activities*.

Rainie, L., & Zickhur, K. (2015). Americans' views on mobile etiquette. Retrieved from *www.pewinternet.org/2015/08/26/americans-views-on-mobile-etiquette*.

Rock, C. L., Flatt, S. W., Sherwood, N. E., Karanja, N., Pakiz, B., & Thomson, C. A. (2010). Effect of a free prepared meal and incentivized weight loss program on weight loss and weight loss maintenance in obese and overweight women: A randomized controlled trial. *Journal of the American Medical Association, 304*(16), 1803–1810.

Saperstein, S. L., Atkinson, N. L., & Gold, R. S. (2007). The impact of Internet use for weight loss. *Obesity Reviews, 8*(5), 459–465.

Shapiro, J. R., Koro, T., Doran, N., Thompson, S., Sallis, J. F., Calfas, K., et al. (2012). Text4Diet: A randomized controlled study using text messaging for weight loss behaviors. *Preventive Medicine, 55*(5), 412–417.

Sherwood, N. E., Jeffery, R. W., Welsh, E. M., VanWormer, J., & Hotop, A. M. (2010). The Drop It At Last (DIAL) Study: Six month results of a phone-based weight loss trial. *American Journal of Health Promotion, 24*(6), 378–383.

Steinberg, D. M., Tate, D. F., Bennett, G. G., Ennett, S., Samuel-Hodge, C., & Ward, D. S. (2013). The efficacy of a daily self-weighing weight loss intervention using smart scales and email. *Obesity (Silver Spring), 21*(9), 1789–1797.

Svetkey, L. P., Batch, B. C., Lin, P. H., Intille, S. S., Corsino, L., Tyson, C. C., et al. (2015). Cell phone intervention for you (CITY): A randomized, controlled trial of behavioral weight loss intervention for young adults using mobile technology. *Obesity (Silver Spring), 23*(11), 2133–2141.

Tate, D. F., Jackvony, E. H., & Wing, R. R. (2003). Effects of Internet behavioral counseling on weight loss in adults at risk for type 2 diabetes: A randomized trial. *Journal of the American Medical Association, 289*(14), 1833–1836.

Tate, D. F., Jackvony, E. H., & Wing, R. R. (2006). A randomized trial comparing human e-mail counseling, computer-automated tailored counseling, and no counseling in an Internet weight loss program. *Archives of Internal Medicine, 166*(15), 1620–1625.

Tate, D. F., Wing, R. R., & Winett, R. A. (2001). Using Internet technology to deliver a behavioral weight loss program. *Journal of the American Medical Association, 285*(9), 1172–1177.

Thomas, J. G., Leahey, T. M., & Wing, R. R. (2015). An automated internet behavioral weight-loss program by physician referral: A randomized controlled trial. *Diabetes Care, 38*(1), 9–15.

Turner-McGrievy, G. M., Campbell, M. K., Tate, D. F., Truesdale, K. P., Bowling, J. M., & Crosby, L. (2009). Pounds Off Digitally study: A randomized podcasting weight-loss intervention. *American Journal of Preventive Medicine, 37*(4), 263–269.

Turner-McGrievy, G. M., & Tate, D. F. (2011). Tweets, apps, and pods: Results of the 6-month Mobile

Pounds Off Digitally (Mobile POD) randomized weight-loss intervention among adults. *Journal of Medical Internet Research, 13*(4), e120.

Turner-McGrievy, G. M., & Tate, D. F. (2013). Weight loss social support in 140 characters or less: Use of an online social network in a remotely delivered weight loss intervention. *Translational Behavioral Medicine 3*(3), 287–294.

Wadden, T. A., Butryn, M. L., & Byrne, K. J. (2004). Efficacy of lifestyle modification for long-term weight control. *Obesity Resesarch, 12*(Suppl.), 151S–162S.

Wieland, L. S., Falzon, L., Sciamanna, C. N., Trudeau, K. J., Brodney, S., Schwartz, J., et al. (2012). Interactive computer-based interventions for weight loss or weight maintenance in overweight or obese people. *Cochrane Database of Systematic Reviews,* (8), Cd007675.

CHAPTER 29

Commercial Weight Loss Programs

Kimberly A. Gudzune
Jeanne M. Clark

Guidelines on weight management in adults from the American Heart Association/American College of Cardiology/The Obesity Society (AHA/ACC/TOS) recommend enrollment in a high-intensity, comprehensive lifestyle program for at least 6 months to achieve a 3–5% weight loss (Jensen et al., 2014). With this degree of weight loss, patients can lower blood glucose and triglycerides, and those at risk can prevent the development of type 2 diabetes mellitus. With additional weight loss, additional cardiovascular risk reduction benefits can occur, such as lowering blood pressure and low-density-lipoprotein (LDL) cholesterol, raising high-density-lipoprotein (HDL) cholesterol, and reducing the need for medications. The guidelines recommend that these programs include at least 14 in-person or group sessions led by a trained interventionist during the 6-month period and use behavioral strategies to encourage consumption of a lower-calorie diet and increased physical activity. The U.S. Preventive Services Task Force (USPSTF, 2012) recommends that similar elements be included in obesity counseling programs. Although a large body of evidence supports the recommendation of these programs, most practices do not offer such programs, and few weight loss programs in the community may meet these guidelines (Bloom, Mehta, Clark, & Gudzune, 2016). Therefore, clinicians may have difficulty finding an appropriate program to which they can refer their patients.

Commercial weight loss programs are available across the United States and provide nonmedical services, including individual or group counseling, menu and exercise planning, meal replacement products, and weight measurement monitoring to assist clients in losing weight. Over $2 billion is spent annually on such commercial weight loss services (IBISWorld, 2016). Therefore, commercial weight loss programs may be able to address this gap. The AHA/ACC/TOS guidelines suggest that some commercial-based programs may be recommended if there is peer-reviewed, published evidence of their efficacy and safety (Jensen et al., 2014). In this chapter, we review the evidence from randomized controlled trials (RCTs) of commercial weight loss programs (of 6 months or more) that provide high-intensity, comprehensive lifestyle interventions that include diet, physical activity, behavioral strategies, and support.

Weight Watchers

Weight Watchers is a high-intensity program in which individuals monitor their food intake by tracking "points"; track their physical activity; and participate in group, one-on-one, or online support sessions. Weight Watchers captures approximately 25% of the market share of the commercial weight loss services industry (IBISWorld, 2016). Relative to the other commercial programs reviewed in this chapter, Weight Watchers has the lowest costs (approximately $40 per month). However, clinicians should be aware that patients also need to factor in their costs for food in order to make a more appropriate price comparison with all other programs described in this chapter that use meal replacements (i.e., costs of these foods are included in the monthly estimates). A previous cost-effectiveness analysis, which did factor in food costs, found that Weight Watchers was the most cost-effective weight management strategy compared with other commercial programs (Finkelstein & Kruger, 2014).

RCTs showed that Weight Watchers participants achieved weight losses ranging from 3.6 to 7.3% of initial weight at 6 months and 3.1 to 5.5% at 12 months (Figure 29.1). These reductions were significantly greater than the control groups at both time points (between-group difference ≥ 3.6% loss at 6 months and ≥ 2.6% at 12 months; Gudzune et al., 2015). However, there was less difference between Weight Watchers and typical counseling interventions delivered in health care settings. When a trained psychologist delivered the counseling intervention, participants in this treatment arm had similar weight losses to those achieved by Weight Watchers participants (−5.4 kg compared to −6.0 kg at 48 weeks, respectively; Pinto, Fava, Hoffmann, & Wing, 2013). When compared to a counseling intervention delivered by a primary care physician, Weight Watchers participants lost more weight (Jolly et al., 2011). Participating in Weight Watchers clearly results in greater weight loss than doing nothing, and typically meets the AHA/ACC/TOS weight loss goal of a 3–5% sustained reduction or greater.

Several RCTs have reported cardiovascular disease (CVD) risk factor outcomes among Weight Watchers participants. In most trials, Weight Watchers participants achieved no significant between-group difference in systolic blood pressure and modest improvements in diastolic blood pressure (0.8–1.8 mmHg greater reduction) and lipids (3.5 mg/dL greater reduction in LDL cholesterol and 1.2 mg/dL greater increase in HDL cholesterol) outcomes relative to controls at 12 months (Mehta et al., 2016). Weight Watchers significantly lowered blood glucose more than the control group at 6 months; however, no significant between-group differences existed at 12 months (Chaudhry et al., 2016). Although these RCTs reported on CVD risk factors, it is important to note that they did not specifically recruit individuals with elevated CVD risk. As a result, the mean values for blood pressure, lipids, and blood glucose were all within the normal range at baseline, which may have diminished the magnitude of the program's effect on these outcomes. In addition, the degree of relative weight loss achieved with Weight Watchers may have been insufficient to result in substantial between-group differences in CVD risk factors. Recently, an RCT compared a modified version of Weight Watchers to a diabetes education program among individuals with pre-diabetes (Marrero et al., 2016). Weight Watchers participants had a significantly lower HbA1C than control participants at 6 months (−0.22% and −0.14%, respectively); however, this effect was attenuated and not statistically significant at 12 months, despite the Weight Watchers participants' achieving a significantly greater weight loss of approximately 5% of baseline body weight.

When reported, no serious adverse events occurred in trials of Weight Watchers' participants (Gudzune et al., 2015). No other harmful outcomes were reported in the trials.

In summary, Weight Watchers has clear evidence to support its efficacy in achieving sustained, modest weight losses; however, the program has only moderate benefits for CVD risk factor reduction within low-risk populations (Table 29.1). It is unclear whether greater CVD risk factor reduction might occur if this program were tested among populations with preexisting hypertension, dyslipidemia, or pre-diabetes.

Author, Year	Commercial Program	Mean % Weight Loss (95% CI)	Time Point (months)	Baseline N
Dansinger et al., 2005	Weight Watchers	3.6	6	40
Heshka et al., 2000	Weight Watchers	5.1	6	211
Johnston et al., 2013	Weight Watchers	5.0	6	147
Pinto et al., 2013	Weight Watchers	6.1	6	49
Truby et al., 2006	Weight Watchers	7.3 (5.7, 8.9)	6	58
Pinto et al., 2013	Weight Watchers	5.5	11	49
Dansinger et al., 2005	Weight Watchers	3.1	12	40
Heshka et al., 2003	Weight Watchers	4.6	12	211
Jebb et al., 2011	Weight Watchers	4.7	12	377
Jolly et al., 2011	Weight Watchers	3.7	12	100
Rock et al., 2007	Jenny Craig	7.8 (5.4, 10.2)	6	35
Rock et al., 2010	Jenny Craig	10.0	6	167
Rock et al., 2014	Jenny Craig	8.6 (7.3, 10.0)	6	74
Rock et al., 2007	Jenny Craig	7.1 (3.5, 10.7)	12	35
Rock et al., 2010	Jenny Craig	10.9 (9.7, 12.1)	12	167
Rock et al., 2014	Jenny Craig	7.4 (5.7, 9.1)	12	74
Foster et al., 2013	Nutrisystem	7.8	6	50
Anderson et al., 2011	HMR	13.9 (13.5, 14.4)	6	22
Wadden et al., 1998	OPTFAST	13.2 (11.0, 15.4)	5	25
Wadden et al., 2004	OPTFAST	12.0 (9.9, 14.1)	5	41
Wing et al., 1994	OPTFAST	16.1	6	45
Wadden et al., 2004	OPTFAST	8.6 (5.5, 11.7)	15	41
Davis et al., 2010	Medifast	7.8	9	

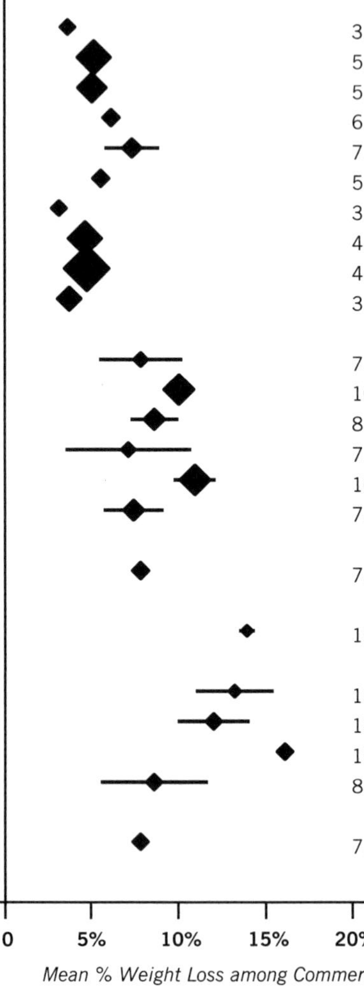

FIGURE 29.1. Mean percent reduction in initial weight achieved by commercial weight loss programs at 6 and 12 months. All data abstracted from results of RCTs of commercial weight loss programs with outcomes near the 6- and 12-month time points. Diamond size reflects the baseline sample size in the commercial weight loss program arm. Confidence intervals are presented when variance estimates were provided in the published study.

Jenny Craig

Jenny Craig encourages the use of prepackaged meal replacements as part of its programs, along with increased physical activity and counseling that may occur one-on-one, in groups, or online. The program's meal replacements have variable sodium and saturated fat levels (sodium range per item: 30–660 mg; saturated fat range per item: 0–4.0 g; Jenny Craig, 2016). In 2014, Jenny Craig had 13% of the market share of the commercial weight loss services industry (Gudzune et al., 2015); however, more recent market share data for this program are not available (IBISWorld, 2016). Including the cost of the Jenny Craig food, the program costs approximately $570 per month.

Jenny Craig participants achieved weight losses ranging from 7.8 to 10.0% of initial weight at 6 months and from 7.1 to 10.9% at 12 months (Figure 29.1). These reductions were significantly greater than control or counseling comparators at both time points (between-group difference ≥ 5.7% loss at 6 months and ≥ 4.9% at 12 months; Gudzune et al., 2015). Based on a meta-analysis of randomized trials, Jenny Craig participants typically lose 6.4 kg more than control participants at 12 months (Johnston et al., 2014).

Three RCTs have reported CVD risk factor outcomes among Jenny Craig participants. These individuals achieved modest improvements in blood pressure relative to a comparator group at 6 months (2.0–4.0 mmHg greater reduction in systolic blood pressure and 5.0–6.0 greater reduction in diastolic blood pressure); however, these benefits were not consistently sustained at 12 months (Mehta et al., 2016). This program did not result in greater reduction in LDL cholesterol relative to comparators, although program participants tended to have larger increases in HDL cholesterol relative to comparators (0.0–7.0 mg/dL greater increase in HDL cholesterol at 12 months; Mehta et al., 2016). No RCTs reported on the effect of Jenny Craig on blood glucose among individuals without diabetes mellitus. However, one RCT did test the effect of Jenny Craig among patients with type 2 diabetes. This intervention yielded significant reductions in HbA1C that were 0.4% greater than a comparator intervention (1-hour counseling session with dietitian followed by monthly calls or email) at 12 months and enabled a majority of individuals to reduce or stop their hypoglycemic medications (Chaudhry et al., 2016).

When reported, two deaths occurred among Jenny Craig participants (1% of participants), which were not attributed to participation in the program. One participant required cholecystectomy in one trial (3% of participants; Gudzune et al., 2015).

In summary, there is clear evidence to support Jenny Craig's efficacy in producing sustained, clinically significant weight loss. Additional evidence indicates that Jenny Craig may facilitate improvement in HbA1C and reduction in hypoglycemic medications among individuals with type 2 diabetes mellitus (Table 29.1). However, the program has few demonstrated benefits on other CVD risk factors. Given the potential weight loss and glycemic benefits, patients with type 2 diabetes mellitus may achieve substantial benefits from Jenny Craig.

TABLE 29.1. Summary of Outcomes for Selected Commercial Weight Loss Programs Relative to Comparator Conditions Included in Each Study

Program	Weight loss	Blood pressure	Lipids	Glucose
Weight Watchers (12-month outcomes)	≥ 3%	SBP ⊘ DBP ↓	LDL-c ↓ HDL-c ↑	⊘
Jenny Craig (12-month outcomes)	≥ 5%	⊘	LDL-c ⊘ HDL-c ↑	↓ A1C in DM
Nutrisystem (6-month outcomes)	6%	SBP ↓ DBP ⊘	⊘	↓ A1C in DM
HMR (6-month outcomes)	13%	Unknown	LDL-c ⊘ HDL-c unknown	↓ Glucose
OPTIFAST (6-month outcomes)	≥ 4%	SBP ↓ DBP ↓	⊘	↓ A1C in DM
Medifast (6-month outcomes)	2%	SBP ⊘ DBP ↓	⊘	Unknown

Note. A1C, hemoglobin A1C; DM, diabetes mellitus; HDL-c, high-density-lipoprotein cholesterol; LDL-c, low-density-lipoprotein cholesterol; ⊘, no difference; ↓, decrease; ↑, increase.

Nutrisystem

Similar to Jenny Craig, Nutrisystem encourages the partial use of prepackaged meal replacements along with exercise plans. Some versions may include access to advice from dietitians and counselors. Sodium and saturated fat levels in Nutrisystem's foods also vary (sodium range per item: 0–600 mg; saturated fat range per item: 0–7.0 g; Nutrisystem, 2016). Nutrisystem has approximately 21% of the market share (IBISWorld, 2016). Including the charges for the Nutrisystem food, the program costs approximately $280 per month.

Nutrisystem participants achieved an average weight loss of 7.8% of initial weight at 6 months in one trial among patients with type 2 diabetes (Figure 29.1), which was significantly greater than the comparator condition that participated in nine group counseling sessions over 6 months as part of a diabetes self-management education program (between-group difference of 5.7% loss at 6 months; Gudzune et al., 2015). Based on a meta-analysis of randomized trials, Nutrisystem participants typically lose 7.4 kg more than no-diet control groups at 6 months (Johnston et al., 2014). With respect to CVD outcomes, Nutrisystem reduced systolic blood pressure significantly more than counseling at 6 months (4.7 mmHg greater reduction), but showed no between-group differences in diastolic blood pressure, LDL cholesterol, or HDL cholesterol (Mehta et al., 2016). However, Nutrisystem did significantly reduce HbA1C by 0.3% more than counseling at 6 months in this trial of patients with type 2 diabetes (Chaudhry et al., 2016). Unfortunately, there have been no long-term (≥ 1 year) evaluations of Nutrisystem.

When reported, two serious adverse events (urinary retention with hematuria and myocardial infarction that occurred between screening and baseline visits) occurred among Nutrisystem participants in one trial (4% of participants; Gudzune et al., 2015). No other harmful outcomes were reported.

In summary, Nutrisystem has only preliminary evidence regarding its short-term weight loss efficacy and glycemic benefits (Table 29.1), given that only one trial has reported outcomes with this program at 6 months, and no trials have been conducted that follow participants to 12 months or beyond. Additional RCTs examining long-term outcomes with Nutrisystem are needed to consider routine referrals by clinicians.

Health Management Resources

Health Management Resources (HMR) promotes the use of meal replacement shakes and bars, along with increased physical activity and counseling that may occur in groups or via telephone coaching. HMR is frequently offered as part of a medically supervised weight loss program in which different calorie options are available; low-calorie (1,200–1,500 calories daily) and lower-calorie (fewer than 1,200 calories daily) may be offered. Including the cost of the HMR meal replacements, the program costs approximately $680 per month.

In one trial, participants prescribed a low-calorie version of HMR achieved an average loss of 13.9% of initial weight at 6 months (Figure 29.1), which was significantly greater than the counseling comparator that received three to four individual counseling sessions with a dietitian during the study period (between-group difference of 13.2% loss at 6 months; Gudzune et al., 2015). Another RCT found that a low-calorie version of HMR delivered with telephone group counseling was equivalent to the same program delivered with in-person group counseling (Donnelly et al., 2013). Weight losses at 6 months were 12.3% in the telephone group and 13.4% in the in-person group. HMR significantly lowered fasting blood glucose 10.4 mg/dL more than counseling at 6 months (Chaudhry et al., 2016), but no statistically significant between-group difference existed in LDL cholesterol (Mehta et al., 2016). No blood pressure or HDL cholesterol outcomes were reported. No long-term trials have evaluated HMR.

Among HMR participants, constipation occurred commonly (56% of participants; Gudzune et al., 2015). No trials reported on serious adverse events.

In summary, HMR has only preliminary evidence supporting its short-term weight loss efficacy and glycemic benefits (Table

29.1), given the single short-term trial. Clinicians should be aware that constipation occurs commonly among participants in this program. Additional RCTs of HMR that follow participants to 12 months or beyond are needed to consider routine referrals by clinicians.

OPTIFAST

OPTIFAST is used as part of medically supervised weight loss programs in which both low-calorie (1,000–1,500 calories daily) and very-low-calorie (≤ 800 calories daily) options may be offered. These programs use the OPTIFAST meal replacement shakes and bars along with increased physical activity and counseling that may occur in groups or one-on-one. Including the price of the OPTIFAST meal replacements, the program costs approximately $670 per month.

OPTIFAST participants achieved weight losses ranging from 12.0 to 16.1% of initial weight at 6 months and 8.6% at 15 months (Figure 29.1). Reductions were significantly greater than counseling and control conditions at 6 months (between-group difference ≥ 4% loss at 6 months), but not at 15 months in one trial (between-group difference = 2.3% at 12 months; Gudzune et al., 2015). With respect to CVD risk factors, only one RCT has reported these outcomes with a very-low-calorie version of OPTIFAST among patients with diabetes mellitus (Wing, Blair, Marcus, Epstein, & Harvey, 1994). OPTIFAST participants had lower blood pressure (3 mmHg for both systolic and diastolic blood pressure) and HbA1C (0.3%) than a counseling comparator at 6 months; however, LDL and HDL cholesterol were not improved (Chaudhry et al., 2016; Mehta et al., 2016).

When reported, four deaths had occurred among OPTIFAST participants in two trials (< 0.1% of participants; Gudzune et al., 2015). Biliary disorders, constipation, and hair loss occurred infrequently (0.1–0.2%, 0.3%, and 0.6–7.7%, respectively; Gudzune et al., 2015).

In summary, evidence from multiple RCTs supports OPTIFAST's short-term weight loss efficacy (Table 29.1). However, OPTIFAST has only preliminary evidence regarding its glycemic benefits among patients with type 2 diabetes, given that only a single trial has reported this outcome at 6 months. Furthermore, it is unclear whether participation in the OPTIFAST program improves other CVD risk factors. Additional RCTs of OPTIFAST that examine blood pressure, lipids, and glycemia at 12 months or beyond are needed to clarify the effect on these outcomes.

Medifast

Medifast also promotes the use of meal replacement products (shakes, bars, meals, and snacks) along with increased physical activity and counseling that may occur one-on-one or via online coaching. Medifast offers low-calorie (1,000–1,800 calories daily) options. Unlike HMR and OPTIFAST, Medifast is not typically provided as part of a medically supervised weight loss program; the product is sold direct to consumers. Medifast has approximately 12% of the market share (IBISWorld, 2016). Including the cost of the Medifast meal replacements, the program costs approximately $420 per month.

Medifast participants achieved an average weight loss of 7.8% of initial weight at 9 months in one trial (Figure 29.1), which was not significantly greater than a counseling control condition (between-group difference of 1.9% loss at 6 months; Gudzune et al., 2015). Medifast lowered diastolic blood pressure significantly more than counseling at 9 months (4.6 mmHg greater reduction), but did not significantly improve systolic blood pressure, LDL cholesterol, or HDL cholesterol (Mehta et al., 2016). This trial did not report any glycemic outcomes (Chaudhry et al., 2016). No long-term trials of Medifast have been published. When reported, no serious adverse events had occurred among Medifast participants (Gudzune et al., 2015). No other harms were reported.

In summary, Medifast has preliminary evidence regarding its short-term weight loss efficacy (Table 29.1); however, it is unclear whether the program has any benefits for CVD risk factors. Additional RCTs of Medifast that follow participants for 12 months or more and report effects on CVD risk factors are needed to consider routine referrals by clinicians.

Head-to-Head Comparisons of Commercial Weight Loss Programs

To date, most RCTs have compared commercial weight loss programs to control or counseling comparator groups. A head-to-head trial of different programs is the only methodology that is appropriate for directly comparing programs to determine whether one produces greater weight loss than another. Given that the studies with control or counseling comparators summarized above have differences in comparator groups and eligibility criteria, direct comparison of these programs is not appropriate using the current data. Few studies have directly compared commercial weight loss programs, and all trials to date have only reported outcomes at 3 months (Vakil et al., 2016). No long-term head-to-head trials comparing these programs exist, so it remains unclear whether or not the differences in weight loss achieved at 6 or 12 months, as reported above (e.g., 3% weight loss at 12 months for Weight Watchers vs. 7% weight loss at 12 months for Jenny Craig) are truly different.

Commercial Weight Loss Programs with Cancer Survivors

Given the association between obesity and increased risk of some types of cancer (Flegal, Graudbard, Williamson, & Gail, 2007), there is growing interest in weight loss among cancer survivors. In particular, breast cancer survivors with obesity have a 46% higher risk of cancer recurrence (Ewertz et al., 2011) and 40% greater odds of a second primary contralateral breast cancer as compared to normal-weight survivors (Li, Daling, Porter, Tang, & Malone, 2009). In the Nurses' Health Study, female breast cancer survivors who had body mass index (BMI) increases of ≥ 2 kg/m^2 had a 53% greater likelihood of recurrence compared with those whose BMI remained stable during a median follow-up of 9 years (Kroenke, Chen, Rosner, & Holmes, 2005). Given the popularity of commercial and proprietary weight loss programs among women (Cleland et al., 2001), many breast cancer survivors are likely to turn to these programs to lose weight.

To date, two RCTs have examined the weight loss efficacy of commercial programs among breast cancer survivors with overweight or obesity. One trial compared Weight Watchers to both control and counseling comparators; the control group only received printed materials on healthy nutrition, whereas the counseling group received intensive counseling by a dietitian (weekly sessions for the first 3 months, biweekly for the second 3 months, then monthly thereafter). As compared to control, women who participated in Weight Watchers lost more weight (between-group differences of –1.8% and –4.0% at 6 and 12 months, respectively; Djuric et al., 2002). However, women in the counseling group lost more weight than the Weight Watchers group at 6 and 12 months (between-group differences of 4.9% and 5.9%, respectively; Djuric et al., 2002). This trial did not report breast cancer recurrence outcomes. The other trial compared Curves to a control group. Curves encourages women to lose weight through physical activity at local centers, along with dietary change promoted during a 6-week nutrition course led by center staff. As compared to a control group, Curves participants lost significantly more weight at 6 months (between-group difference of –1.5%; Greenlee et al., 2013). No cases of breast cancer recurrence occurred in the Curves arm, and one recurrence occurred in the control. In summary, both Weight Watchers and Curves show preliminary success in achieving modest weight loss relative to control groups in female breast cancer survivors.

Other Commercial Programs

Many commercial weight loss programs include diet, physical activity, behavioral strategies, and support. However, they did not have any peer-reviewed, published, randomized controlled trials of their efficacy and safety that met the eligibility criteria for a recent systematic review (Gudzune et al., 2015). Table 29.2 lists these programs.

Alternatively, other commercial programs do have randomized controlled trials examining their efficacy (Table 29.2); however, they do not offer all elements of a comprehensive lifestyle intervention focused on weight loss (Jensen et al., 2014; U.S. Preventive Services Task Force, 2012). Despite this, evidence clearly supports the weight loss efficacy of the Atkins, Ornish, Volumetrics, and Zone diets. Atkins advises participants to eat a low-carbohydrate diet. Ornish is a CVD risk reduction program that emphasizes a low-fat vegetarian diet, exercise, stress management, and group support, which has been tested in patients with preexisting coronary heart disease. Volumetrics promotes eating less energy dense foods to lose weight. Zone encourages eating meals in which 40% of calories come from carbohydrates, 30% from protein, and 30% from fat. Relative to a no-diet comparator, at 12 months, Atkins resulted in a 6.4 kg greater weight loss, Ornish in a 6.6 kg greater loss, and Volumetrics and Zone both resulted in a 6.0 kg greater weight loss (Johnston et al., 2014). Although these programs have evidence to support their weight loss efficacy and therefore might be potentially considered as treatment options, clinicians should be aware that they do not have all of the components suggested in the USPSTF or AHA/ACC/TOS recommendations and are not all specifically designed to be weight loss programs.

Other Considerations Regarding Trials of Commercial Weight Loss Programs

The recent systematic reviews that synthesized the evidence regarding the effects of commercial weight loss programs on weight and CVD risk factors noted that the literature base has a high risk of bias (Chaudhry et al., 2016; Gudzune et al., 2015; Mehta et al., 2016; Vakil et al., 2016), particularly related to selection bias (based on inadequate generation of a randomized sequence), detection bias (based on lack of outcome assessor blinding), and attrition bias (due to high losses to follow-up and inadequate handling of missing data). To date, most trials that have been conducted were supported by the commercial programs that were evaluated, which could also alter interpretation or reporting of results. Clinicians should be aware that this body of literature has a high risk of bias and should take this factor into account, as appropriate, when interpreting the results and presenting this information to their patients.

TABLE 29.2. Index of Other Commercial Programs Not Discussed in This Chapter

Commercial weight loss programs that "meet guideline recommendations" but lack published RCTs	Commercial weight loss programs that "do not meet guideline recommendations" but have published RCTs
• Best Life • Body for Life • Dukan Diet • Flat Belly Diet • Ideal Protein • iDiet • Jillian Michaels • L.A. Weight Loss • Robard • South Beach Diet • Spark People • Taking Off Pounds Sensibly (TOPS)	• Atkins (self-directed with online support) • Biggest Loser Club (self-directed with online support) • eDiets (self-directed with online support) • Lose It! (self-directed with online support) • Ornish Spectrum (CVD risk reduction program) • SlimFast (self-directed with online support) • Volumetrics (self-directed without support) • The Zone (self-directed without support)

Note. For a program to meet guideline recommendations, the intervention must be an intensive and comprehensive lifestyle change program that focuses on weight loss. To be included in the recent systematic review (Gudzune et al., 2015), trials needed to be RCTs that lasted at least 3 months and compared a commercial program to control, counseling, or another commercial program. In addition, the trials needed to occur among overweight or obese adults, and the intervention needed to represent the program that would be available to the general public (e.g., programs tailored to a unique population such as the military or employer-based versions of the programs were excluded) and not focus on food addiction (e.g., Overeaters Anonymous).

The outcomes achieved in these RCTs also may overestimate the effect of the program, given that study participants typically represent the most motivated group, program fees are often waived with study participation, and study staff is often available to aid in retention. A study reporting retention of "real-world" participants in the Jenny Craig program reported that 22% of enrollees continued to participate in the program at 6 months and only 7% at 12 months (Finley et al., 2007). Finally, the benefits of modest weight loss on long-term CVD outcomes, such as myocardial infarction or stroke, remain unproven (Look AHEAD Research Group et al., 2013). Despite reduction in weight and CVD risk factors among individuals with type 2 diabetes at 1, 4, and 8 years in the Look AHEAD trial, no reduction in CVD events or mortality occurred in the weight loss intervention group.

Role of the Clinician with Commercial Weight Loss Programs

Clinicians commonly report barriers to providing weight loss counseling to their patients, including lack of training or experience (Bleich, Bennett, Gudzune, & Cooper, 2012; Kushner, 1995). Therefore, commercial weight loss programs that have evidence documenting their efficacy and safety may be a good referral option for clinicians to offer their patients with overweight and obesity. Not only can clinicians provide the referral, but the established relationship with the clinician, particularly in the primary care setting, provides opportunities for additional accountability for patients and support or "cheerleading" during follow-up visits (Bennett, Gudzune, Appel, & Clark, 2014). Patients lose significantly more weight when they have clinicians who take this supportive role and communicate the need to lose weight in a "judgment-free" way (Bennett et al., 2015; Gudzune, Bennett, Cooper, & Bleich, 2014). Clinicians can consider using the five A's behavior change strategy—assess, advise, agree, assist, arrange—to help guide assessment, counseling, referral, and follow-up. Using all five A's during a counseling session is important. Health care providers often fail to include assess, assist, or arrange (Alexander et al., 2011). Using the arrange step has been associated with greater patient weight loss than when the health care provider did not use this step (Alexander et al., 2011).

Insurance Coverage for Commercial Weight Loss Programs

The commercial weight loss services industry may experience increased referrals from clinicians, if the benefits coverage for obesity screening provided in the 2010 Patient Protection and Affordable Care Act continues (ACA; Congressional Budget Office, 2014). In January of 2018, Americans who obtain health insurance through the ACA federal exchanges receive coverage for all preventive services receiving grade A or B recommendations from the USPSTF, which include obesity screening and counseling. USPSTF-covered obesity counseling interventions are similar to those recommended by the AHA/ACC/TOS guidelines; thus, the commercial programs discussed in this chapter could potentially address this need. However, the future of the ACA and its benefits are unclear, and private insurance coverage for commercial weight loss services is not typical at this time. Clinicians should watch for changes in benefits coverage for these programs. In addition, clinicians can explore whether these programs may be offered as a benefit by patients' employers or suggest that patients consider putting funds aside in health savings accounts to help cover costs.

Conclusions

In conclusion, two commercial weight loss programs have demonstrated consistent weight loss efficacy at 12 months in multiple RCTs: Weight Watchers ($\geq 3\%$) and Jenny Craig ($\geq 7\%$). These weight loss programs also contain all elements of a comprehensive lifestyle intervention recommended by the AHA/ACC/TOS guidelines and USPSTF (Jensen et al., 2014; U.S. Preventive Services Task Force, 2012). Despite Weight Watchers' weight loss efficacy, limited improvement in CVD risk factors occurred, relative to control, with this program. This finding may be attributable to study populations having normal values of blood pressure and lipids at baseline, and/or the modest weight losses achieved may have been insufficient to result in substantial between-group differences in these outcomes. Jenny Craig showed significant reduction in HbA1C among patients with diabetes mellitus and improvement in HDL cholesterol, although the effects on blood pressure and LDL cholesterol showed little difference from the comparator. It should be noted that OPTIFAST demonstrated consistent weight loss efficacy at 6 months ($\geq 12\%$); however, only one trial examined outcomes beyond 12 months, at which time weight loss was no longer significantly different from the counseling control group. Nutrisystem, HMR, and Medifast each had only a single RCT that reported weight loss outcomes, and therefore we would consider their demonstrated weight loss efficacy to be preliminary at this time. Other commercial programs do not meet AHA/ACC/TOS and USPSTF recommendations, or have not demonstrated their efficacy and safety through published RCTs that test the program available to the general public. Clinicians might consider referring patients with CVD risk factors who wish to achieve a clinically significant weight loss of 5% or greater to Jenny Craig, whereas Weight Watchers may be an additional option for patients without comorbid conditions who have more modest weight loss goals (< 5% loss). Of course, patient preferences and finances should be taken into account during the discussion.

References

Alexander, S. C., Cox, M. E., Boling Turner, C. L., Lyna, P., Ostbye, T., Tulsky, J. A., et al. (2011). Do the five A's work when physicians counsel about weight loss? *Family Medicine, 43*(3), 179–184.

Anderson, J. W., Reynolds, L. R., Bush, H. M., Rinsky, J. L., & Washnock, C. (2011). Effect of a behavioral/nutritional intervention program on weight loss in obese adults: A randomized controlled trial. *Postgraduate Medicine, 123*(5), 205–213.

Bennett, W. L., Gudzune, K. A., Appel, L. J., & Clark, J. M. (2014). Insights from the POWER practice-based weight loss trial: A focus group study on the PCP's role in weight management. *Journal of General Internal Medicine, 29*(1), 50–58.

Bennett, W. L., Wang, N. Y., Gudzune, K. A., Dalcin, A. T., Bleich, S. N., Appel, L. J., et al. (2015). Satisfaction with primary care provider involvement is associated with greater weight loss: Results from the practice-based POWER trial. *Patient Education and Counseling, 98*(9), 1099–1105.

Bleich, S. N., Bennett, W. L., Gudzune, K. A., & Cooper, L. A. (2012). National survey of US primary care physicians' perspectives about causes of obesity and solutions to improve care. *BMJ Open, 2*(6), e001871.

Bloom, B., Mehta, A. K., Clark, J. M., & Gudzune, K. A. (2016). Guideline-concordant weight loss programs in an urban area are uncommon and difficult to identify through the Internet. *Obesity (Silver Spring), 24*(3), 583–588.

Chaudhry, Z. W., Doshi, R. S., Mehta, A. K., Jacobs, D. K., Vakil, R. M., Lee, C. J., et al. (2016). A systematic review of commercial weight loss programmes' effect on glycemic outcomes among overweight and obese adults with and without type 2 diabetes mellitus. *Obesity Reviews, 17*(8), 758–769.

Cleland, R., Graybill, D. C., Hubbard, V., Khan, L. K., Stern, J. S., Wadden, T. A., et al. (2001). Commercial weight loss products and programs: What consumers stand to gain and lose. *Critical Reviews in Food Science Nutrition, 41*(1), 45–70.

Congressional Budget Office. (2014). Updated estimates of the insurance coverage provisions of the Affordable Care Act. Retrieved June, 28, 2016, from www.cbo.gov/sites/default/files/cbofiles/attachments/45010-breakout-AppendixB.pdf.

Dansinger, M. L., Gleason, J. A., Griffith, J. L., Selker, H. P., & Schaefer, E. J. (2005). Comparison of the Atkins, Ornish, Weight Watchers, and Zone diets for weight loss and heart disease risk reduction: A randomized trial. *Journal of the American Medical Association, 293*(1), 43–53.

Davis, L. M., Coleman, C., Kiel, J., Rampolla, J., Hutchisen, T., Ford, L., et al. (2010). Efficacy of a meal replacement diet plan compared to a food-based diet plan after a period of weight loss and weight maintenance: A randomized controlled trial. *Nutrition Journal, 9*, 11.

Djuric, Z., DiLaura, N. M., Jenkins, I., Darga, L., Jen, C. K., Mood, D., et al. (2002). Combining weight loss counseling with the Weight Watchers plan for obese breast cancer survivors. *Obesity Research, 10*(7), 657–665.

Donnelly, J. E., Goetz, J., Gibson, C., Sullivan, D. K., Lee, R., Smith, B. K., et al. (2013). Equivalent weight loss for weight management programs delivered by phone and clinic. *Obesity (Silver Spring), 21*(10), 1951–1959.

Ewertz, M., Jensen, M. B., Gunnarsdottir, K. A., Hojris, I., Jakobsen, E. H., Nielsen, D., et al. (2011). Effect of obesity on prognosis after early-stage breast cancer. *Journal of Clinical Oncology, 29*(1), 25–31.

Finkelstein, E. A., & Kruger, E. (2014). Meta- and cost-effectiveness analysis of commercial weight loss strategies. *Obesity (Silver Spring), 22*(9), 1942–1951.

Finley, C. E., Barlow, C. E., Greenway, F. L., Rock,

C. L., Rolls, B. J., & Blair, S. N. (2007). Retention rates and weight loss in a commercial weight loss program. *International Journal of Obesity (London), 31*(2), 292–298.

Flegal, K. M., Graubard, B. I., Williamson, D. F., & Gail, M. H. (2007). Cause-specific excess deaths associated with underweight, overweight, and obesity. *Journal of the American Medical Association, 298*(17), 2028–2037.

Foster, G. D., Wadden, T. A., Lagrotte, C. A., Vander Veur, S. S., Hesson, L. A., Homko, C. J., et al. (2013). A randomized comparison of a commercially available portion-controlled weight loss intervention with a diabetes self-management education program. *Nutrition and Diabetes, 3,* e63.

Greenlee, H. A., Crew, K. D., Mata, J. M., McKinley, P. S., Rundle, A. G., Zhang, W., et al. (2013). A pilot randomized controlled trial of a commercial diet and exercise weight loss program in minority breast cancer survivors. *Obesity (Silver Spring), 21*(1), 65–76.

Gudzune, K. A., Bennett, W. L., Cooper, L. A., & Bleich, S. N. (2014). Perceived judgment about weight can negatively influence weight loss: A cross-sectional study of overweight and obese patients. *Preventive Medicine, 62,* 103–107.

Gudzune, K. A., Doshi, R. S., Mehta, A. K., Chaudhry, Z. W., Jacobs, D. K., Vakil, R. M., et al. (2015). Efficacy of commercial weight loss programs: An updated systematic review. *Annals of Internal Medicine, 162*(7), 501–512.

Heshka, S., Anderson, J. W., Atkinson, R. L., Greenway, F. L., Hill, J. O., Phinney, S. D., et al. (2003). Weight loss with self-help compared with a structured commercial program: A randomized trial. *Journal of the American Medical Association, 289*(14), 1792–1798.

Heshka, S., Greenway, F., Anderson, J. W., Atkinson, R. L., Hill, J. O., Phinney, S. D., et al. (2000). Self-help weight loss versus a structured commercial program after 26 weeks: A randomized controlled study. *American Journal of Medicine, 109*(4), 282–287.

IBISWorld. (2016). Weight loss services in the U.S. industry market research report. Retrieved June 28, 2016 from *www.ibisworld.com/industry/default.aspx?indid=1719.*

Jebb, S. A., Ahern, A. L., Olson, A. D., Aston, L. M., Holzapfel, C., Stoll, J., et al. (2011). Primary care referral to a commercial provider for weight loss treatment versus standard care: A randomised controlled trial. *Lancet, 378*(9801), 1485–1492.

Jenny Craig. (2016). Cuisine. Retrieved January 6, 2016 from *www.jennycraig.com/site/cuisine/cuisine.jsp.*

Jensen, M. D., Ryan, D. H., Apovian, C. M., Ard, J. D., Comuzzie, A. G., Donato, K. A., et al (2014). 2013 AHA/ACC/TOS guideline for the management of overweight and obesity in adults: A report of the American College of Cardiology/American Heart Association Task Force on Practice Guidelines and The Obesity Society. *Circulation, 129*(25, Suppl. 2), S102–S138.

Johnston, B. C., Kanters, S., Bandayrel, K., Wu, P., Naji, F., Siemieniuk, R. A., et al. (2014). Comparison of weight loss among named diet programs in overweight and obese adults: A meta-analysis. *Journal of the American Medical Association, 312*(9), 923–933.

Johnston, C. A., Rost, S., Miller-Kovach, K., Moreno, J. P., & Foreyt, J. P. (2013). A randomized controlled trial of a community-based behavioral counseling program. *American Journal of Medicine, 126*(12), e19–e24.

Jolly, K., Lewis, A., Beach, J., Denley, J., Adab, P., Deeks, J. J., et al. (2011). Comparison of range of commercial or primary care led weight reduction programmes with minimal intervention control for weight loss in obesity: Lighten Up randomised controlled trial. *BMJ, 343,* d6500.

Kroenke, C. H., Chen, W. Y., Rosner, B., & Holmes, M. D. (2005). Weight, weight gain, and survival after breast cancer diagnosis. *Journal of Clinical Oncology, 23*(7), 1370–1378.

Kushner, R. F. (1995). Barriers to providing nutrition counseling by physicians: A survey of primary care practitioners. *Preventive Medicine, 24*(6), 546–552.

Li, C. I., Daling, J. R., Porter, P. L., Tang, M. T., & Malone, K. E. (2009). Relationship between potentially modifiable lifestyle factors and risk of second primary contralateral breast cancer among women diagnosed with estrogen receptor-positive invasive breast cancer. *Journal of Clinical Oncology, 27*(32), 5312–5318.

Look AHEAD Research Group, Wing, R. R., Bolin, P., Brancati, F. L., Bray, G. A., Clark, J. M., et al. (2013). Cardiovascular effects of intensive lifestyle intervention in type 2 diabetes. *New England Journal of Medicine, 369*(24), 145–154.

Marrero, D. G., Palmer, K. N., Phillips, E. O., Miller-Kovach, K., Foster, G. D., & Saha, C. K. (2016). Comparison of commercial and self-initiated weight loss programs in people with prediabetes: A randomized control trial. *American Journal of Public Health, 106*(5), 949–956.

Mehta, A. K., Doshi, R. S., Chaudhry, Z. W., Jacobs, D. K., Vakil, R. M., Lee, C. J., et al. (2016). Benefits of commercial weight loss programs on blood pressure and lipids: A systematic review. *Preventive Medicine, 90,* 86–99.

Nutrisystem. (2016). Our food. Retrieved January 6, 2016, from *www.nutrisystem.com/jsps_hmr/catalog/menu/food.jsp.*

Pinto, A. M., Fava, J. L., Hoffmann, D. A., & Wing, R. R. (2013). Combining behavioral weight loss treatment and a commercial program: A randomized clinical trial. *Obesity (Silver Spring), 21*(4), 673–680.

Rock, C. L., Flatt, S. W., Pakiz, B., Taylor, K. S., Leone, A. F., Brelje, K., et al. (2014). Weight loss, glycemic control, and cardiovascular disease risk factors in response to differential diet composition in a weight loss program in type 2 diabetes: A randomized controlled trial. *Diabetes Care, 37*(6), 1573–1580.

Rock, C. L., Flatt, S. W., Sherwood, N. E., Karanja,

N., Pakiz, B., & Thomson, C. A. (2010). Effect of a free prepared meal and incentivized weight loss program on weight loss and weight loss maintenance in obese and overweight women: A randomized controlled trial. *Journal of the American Medical Association, 304*(16), 1803–1810.

Rock, C. L., Pakiz, B., Flatt, S. W., & Quintana, E. L. (2007). Randomized trial of a multifaceted commercial weight loss program. *Obesity (Silver Spring), 15*(4), 939–949.

Truby, H., Baic, S., deLooy, A., Fox, K. R., Livingstone, M. B., Logan, C. M., et al. (2006). Randomised controlled trial of four commercial weight loss programmes in the UK: Initial findings from the BBC "Diet Trials." *BMJ, 332*(7553), 1309–1314.

U.S. Preventive Services Task Force. (2012). Obesity in adults: Screening and management. Retrieved June 28, 2016, from *www.uspreventiveservicestaskforce.org/Page/Document/UpdateSummaryFinal/obesity-in-adults-screening-and-management*.

Vakil, R. M., Doshi, R. S., Mehta, A. K., Chaudhry, Z. W., Jacobs, D. K., Lee, C. J., et al. (2016). Direct comparisons of commercial weight loss programs on weight, waist circumference, and blood pressure: A systematic review. *BMC Public Health, 16*(1), 460.

Wadden, T. A., Considine, R. V., Foster, G. D., Anderson, D. A., Sarwer, D. B., & Caro, J. S. (1998). Short- and long-term changes in serum leptin dieting obese women: Effects of caloric restriction and weight loss. *Journal of Clinical Endocrinology and Metabolism, 83*(1), 214–218.

Wadden, T. A., Foster, G. D., Sarwer, D. B., Anderson, D. A., Gladis, M., Sanderson, R. S., et al. (2004). Dieting and the development of eating disorders in obese women: Results of a randomized controlled trial. *American Journal of Clinical Nutrition, 80*(3), 560–568.

Wing, R. R., Blair, E., Marcus, M., Epstein, L. H., & Harvey, J. (1994). Year-long weight loss treatment for obese patients with type II diabetes: Does including an intermittent very-low-calorie diet improve outcome? *American Journal of Medicine, 97*(4), 354–362.

CHAPTER 30

Treatment of Obesity in Community Settings

Delia S. West
Rebecca A. Krukowski
Chelsea A. Larsen

Obesity remains one of the most pressing public health problems facing the United States. If effective methods for achieving weight loss and reducing the health risks associated with obesity are to have a substantial impact on a population level, evidence-based treatment approaches will need to be transferred to community settings where they will be able to reach affected populations. The process of taking empirically validated interventions, developed for highly resourced and intensively monitored randomized controlled trials, and adapting them for implementation in real-world community settings (and testing the translated version to determine whether it retains potency in the community setting) is a critical step in disseminating obesity research (Mitchell, Prochazka, & Glasgow, 2016). This chapter reviews some of the important considerations in adapting evidence-based obesity interventions for community settings. We examine approaches that can serve as models for efforts to promote the diffusion of effective behavioral obesity interventions into community settings.

The Diabetes Prevention Program Lifestyle Balance Intervention

Many of the efforts to translate obesity research into community-based programs have focused on tailoring the Diabetes Prevention Program (DPP) Lifestyle Balance Program to the unique needs of community settings and/or target populations. The DPP was a multisite randomized clinical trial that examined whether a behavioral lifestyle intervention would prevent the development of type 2 diabetes among high-risk overweight and obese adults (Diabetes Prevention Program Research Group, 1999). The Lifestyle Balance intervention provided a "core" curriculum of 16 individual sessions followed by a maintenance intervention that combined individual and group contact, with periodic motivational campaigns to challenge participants to maintain weight loss and/or lose weight that might have been regained. The DPP lifestyle intervention produced an average weight loss of $6.9 \pm 4.5\%$ at the end of the core curriculum (Diabetes Prevention Program Research Group, 2004). The intervention group sustained greater weight losses and higher physical activity levels than the control group for 10 years (Knowler et al., 2009). Importantly, the intervention was effective across a wide range of ethnic minority groups and in both men and women (West, Prewitt, Bursac, & Felix, 2008). Further, the lifestyle intervention proved to be more effective than medication (i.e., metformin) in preventing diabetes (Diabetes Prevention Program Research Group, 2002a).

The strong success of the DPP Lifestyle Balance Program led to the Centers for Disease Prevention and Control (CDC) to adopt it as the cornerstone of their diabetes prevention efforts nationwide (Albright & Gregg, 2013). The DPP approach is now considered to be one of the gold-standard obesity treatment interventions. The availability of intervention materials to the research community and public health practitioners has encouraged the translation of the DPP lifestyle intervention into a range of community settings. Many of the community-based programs have evaluated the outcomes of these adapted versions. Although not all community-based behavioral obesity treatment programs are derivatives of the DPP Lifestyle program, most of those described in the scientific literature are based on social cognitive theory (Bandura, 1986), as is the DPP program, and share many of the same fundamental self-regulation strategies which are central to the DPP program (Diabetes Prevention Program Research Group, 2002a).

Critical Considerations in Adapting Lifestyle Interventions for Community Settings

Many of the adaptations of evidence-based weight loss programs for delivery in community settings are driven by cost considerations. Program-related costs for implementing the DPP Lifestyle Balance Program were estimated at $2,780 per individual over 3 years (Herman et al., 2003). Although the lifestyle intervention was demonstrated to be a cost-effective diabetes prevention approach relative to medication (Diabetes Prevention Program Research Group, 2002a), it is resource intensive. Not surprisingly, many of the adaptations made in community-based translations of the DPP lifestyle intervention are focused on reducing costs.

The most commonly reported adaptations made to the DPP lifestyle intervention for delivery in community settings pertain to the format of intervention sessions, the number of intervention sessions, and/or who delivers the intervention (Neamah, Sebert Kuhlmann, & Tabak, 2016). Although translations that have fewer substantive changes to the original DPP lifestyle protocol appear to produce greater weight losses, there do not seem to be particular modifications that, in and of themselves, markedly reduce the potency of DPP's Lifestyle Balance Program (Neamah et al., 2016).

Format of Treatment: Individual versus Group Delivery

Whether an intervention should be delivered in group or individual sessions is a key decision in the design of community-based obesity treatment. The DPP study implemented the lifestyle intervention in individual sessions, largely because it was difficult to identify large cohorts of individuals who satisfied the fairly extensive list of eligibility criteria for the clinical trial, and therefore it was not feasible to aggregate individuals into groups in a timely manner. Although practical limitations in the flow of participants precluded group administration in the original DPP Lifestyle Balance Program, community adaptations have not been similarly constrained. Group-based obesity treatment may actually be more effective for weight loss than individual delivery (Renjilian et al., 2001). Therefore, a common adaptation seen in community settings is administration of the program in group formats, with few communities electing to deliver the lifestyle program individually (see Table 30.1).

Intervention Duration and Contact Frequency

The optimal length and intensity of treatment for community-based treatment has not yet been established, although recent

TABLE 30.1. Community-Based Obesity Treatment Programs by Setting

Author (year)	N	Weight loss	Program format/length	Delivered by	Participants	Focus	Cost
Cooperative extension service offices							
Befort et al. (2010)	34	*At 6 months:* Group: −14.9 kg; individual: −9.5 kg; $p = .03$	In groups or individually by randomization; 16 weekly sessions + 4 biweekly sessions (6 months total)	Master's level dietitians and behaviorists	Overweight and obese rural women ages 22–65	Weight loss	Program costs: group: $203.73; individual: $382.26; Participant costs: group: $714.43; individual: $1,029.06
Perri et al. (2008)	298	*At 6 months:* −10 kg; *at 18 months (weight regain):* Face-to-face: +1.2 kg; phone-based: +1.2 kg; control: +3.7 kg	24 weekly group sessions + 26 biweekly individual contacts over 12 months (18 months total)	Family and consumer sciences agents or research staff	Overweight women ages 50–75 living in rural area	Weight loss	Total program + participant costs: face-to-face: $2,555; phone-based: $2,125; education control: $1,824
Perri et al. (2014)	612	*At 2 years:* control: −2.9%; low: −3.5%; moderate: −6.7%; high: −6.8%	*In groups:* Low: 8 weekly + 8 maintenance + 1 campaign; medium: 16 weekly + 16 maintenance + 2 campaigns; high: 24 weekly + 24 maintenance + 3 campaigns; control: 16 sessions of nutrition education (24 months total)	Cooperative extension services family and consumer science agents or research staff	Obese adults ages 21–75 living in rural area	Weight loss	Total cost: control: $13,233; low: $16,351; moderate: $19,426; high: $26,630 Cost per participant: control: $78; low: $111; moderate: $145; high: $165 Cost per kg lost: control: $28; low: $33; moderate: $22; high: $25
Church settings							
Krukowski et al. (2010)	34	*At 4 months:* Faith-tailored	16 weekly group sessions	Master's in public health	Overweight or obese church	Weight loss	Data not provided

Study	N	Results	Intervention	Interventionist	Population	Focus	
McNabb et al. (1997)	39	Int: −8.1 ± 4.1%; standard Int: −7.9 ± 4.2%; $p = .98$	14 weekly group sessions	student who was a member of the church	members ages 21 or older	Weight loss	Data not provided
Williams et al. (2013); Sattin et al. (2016)	604	*At 14 weeks*: Int: −4.5 kg; control: 0.9 kg; $p < .0001$		Lay health educators	Obese African American female church members	Weight loss	Data not provided
		At 12 weeks: Int: −2.62 kg; control: + 0.5 kg $p = .001$; *at 12 months*: Int: −2.39 kg; control: +0.47 kg; $p = .005$	12 weekly group sessions + 6 group booster sessions (12 months total)	Health professionals (72% were nurses) who were church members	Overweight or obese African Americans ages 20–64	Weight loss and diabetes prevention	Data not provided
Yanek et al. (2001)	529	*At 12 months*: Int: −0.49 kg; control: +0.38 kg; $p = .0008$	20 weekly group Int sessions + weekly support sessions for 7 months (12 months total)	Female African American health educators (study staff) and church lay leaders	African American women ages 40 and older	Cardiovascular health promotion for African American women	Data not provided
YMCAs							
Ackermann et al. (2008, 2011)	92	*At 12 months*: Int: −6%; control: −1.8%; $p = .008$; *at 28 months*: (72% of original DEPLOY sample continued in extended study): Int: −6% from baseline; control + Int: −3.6% from baseline	16 group sessions over 16 weeks + 12 group sessions over 8 months (12 months total); followed by both Int and control offered 5 weekly group sessions + 8 monthly group sessions	Trained YMCA staff	Overweight adults with elevated risk for Type 2 diabetes	Diabetes prevention through weight loss	Data not provided
Ackermann et al. (2014, 2015)	509	*At 12 months*: Proportion losing ≥ 5%: Int: 69 (32.4%); control: 29 (13.4%); $p < .001$	16 group sessions over 16–24 weeks + 6–7 monthly group sessions (12 months total)	Trained YMCA staff	Overweight low-income individuals (mostly minority) at elevated risk for Type 2 diabetes	Diabetes prevention through weight loss	Data not provided

(continued)

TABLE 30.1. (continued)

Author (year)	N	Weight loss	Program format/length	Delivered by	Participants	Focus	Cost
Fitzgibbon et al. (2005)	27 (cohort 1 in YMCA) 37 (cohort 2 in university)	At 20 weeks: Cohort 1 Int: +0.8%; control: +0.4% NS; cohort 2 Int: −4%; control: + 9%; $p < .01$	40 group sessions over 20 weeks	Research staff	Overweight African American women ages 35–65	Weight loss and breast health	Data not provided
Other community settings							
Barham et al. (2011) (worksite setting)	45	At 3 months: Int: −2.23 kg; control: +.73 kg; $p < .001$; at 12 months: 22.5% lost > 5%; 12.5% lost > 7%	12 weekly group sessions + 9 monthly group maintenance sessions (12 months total)	Nurses, dietician, physical therapist, psychologist	Overweight or obese employees at risk for diabetes or with diabetes	DPP-based weight loss	Data not provided
Katula et al. (2010); Blackwell et al. (2011); Katula et al. (2011); Lawlor et al. (2013) (diabetes education program sites)	301	At 12 months: Int: −7.1 kg; control: −1.4 kg; $p < .001$	24 weekly group sessions + 3 individual dietitian sessions + 18 monthly group sessions + 18 phone contacts (24 months total)	Community health workers with Type 2 diabetes	Overweight adults with pre-diabetes	Diabetes prevention through weight loss	Recruitment cost: $816 per participant randomized; lifestyle direct cost: $850 per participant
West et al. (2011); Krukowski et al. (2013) (senior centers)	228	At 4 months: Int: −3.8%; control: −2%; $p < .001$	12 weekly group sessions + 9 monthly group sessions	Lay health educators	Adults ≥ 60 years with BMI ≥ 30 and able to walk for exercise	Weight loss	Total per senior center: $2,731; per participant: $165; cost per kg lost: $45

Note. Int, intervention; NS, not significant.

data are beginning to inform these critical questions. The DPP lifestyle intervention was designed as 16 core sessions to be completed within 24 weeks, followed by a maintenance intervention over several years. Some community-based adaptations have kept the 16 core sessions, whereas others have reduced or expanded the program length (see Table 30.1). Increasing the number of weekly core sessions to 24 does not seem to produce significantly greater weight losses than are achieved with 16 sessions in a community-based program, but an 8-session core curriculum version produced significantly smaller weight losses than did either the 16- or 24-session versions (Perri et al., 2014). A 16-session "moderate-dose" intervention appears to be the preferred approach, given results that are comparable to those of the longer and more expensive 24-session version. There are no data yet to inform community planners and others whether the 12-session iteration used in many of the community adaptations achieves outcomes as robust as the 16-session version. Further, the available evidence supporting a 16-session program as preferred is from a program delivered by professionals within the cooperative extension services offices. Thus, it remains unclear whether this program duration "sweet spot" is similarly appropriate for other community settings or for programs delivered by individuals without the professional training of agents from cooperative extension.

The length of community-based obesity intervention programs varies considerably, largely based on whether a weight maintenance program is included. Many interventions do not include a weight loss maintenance element after the core "weight-loss induction" sessions, although some do (see Table 30.1). Maintenance programs lasting 6 months to 2 years have been described. One study directly examined the important question of whether there is value added by including a maintenance component and found that the addition of extended care effectively forestalled the weight regain that was observed without a maintenance component (Perri et al., 2008). Interestingly, this study also found that phone contacts were as beneficial as the more traditional face-to-face contact in sustaining weight losses. Furthermore, in a similar study that varied the intensity of the maintenance program, outcomes suggested that the high-intensity maintenance programs may not be necessary; a program that provided 16 phone-based maintenance sessions and two motivational campaigns promoted the same sustained weight losses as the more intensive program, which offered 24 maintenance sessions and three motivational campaigns (Perri et al., 2014). As might be expected, reducing the frequency of maintenance contact substantially reduces the costs (without sacrificing weight loss benefits) and will likely be welcome data to community-level program planners.

Intervention Delivery Personnel

Another key consideration in adapting the DPP Lifestyle Balance Program for community delivery is who will conduct the intervention. In the original DPP, each participant was assigned a "lifestyle coach" who was a health professional (i.e., registered dietitian, exercise physiologist, psychologist, or health educator). Similarly, many of the community-based interventions have used health professionals who bring particular expertise in skills related to weight management (see Table 30.1). However, translating efficacious lifestyle interventions to community settings can be challenging due to the high cost of health professionals and/or to the shortage of health professionals who can deliver the interventions, particularly in rural areas (Merwin, Hinton, Dembling, & Stern, 2003; Rosenblatt, Andrilla, Curtin, & Hart, 2006). Lay health educators (also known as community health workers, *promotoras*, etc.) provide one means of addressing these challenges in the community setting, and having these individuals deliver treatment may offer unique advantages (e.g., indigenous perspective on their community's culture, knowledge about community resources). Several studies successfully utilized lay health educators to deliver behavioral weight control programs in community settings and obtained clinically meaningful weight losses, although there are also examples of programs based on the DPP delivered by community members which did not achieve significant weight losses (Table 30.1).

Program Inclusion Criteria

Similar to the DPP, some community-based programs have recruited and enrolled overweight and obese participants at elevated risk of developing type 2 diabetes, based on impaired glucose tolerance, elevated blood glucose, and/or self-report risk assessment. Among these programs, the primary stated treatment goal is often diabetes prevention instead of (or in addition to) weight loss. However, other programs include individuals who are overweight or obese and do not require that participants also have prediabetes. These latter programs have a more specific focus on weight loss and may or may not examine changes in glucose or related outcomes. No data are available that suggest one treatment target or the other produces better weight loss outcomes in community settings.

Community-Based Obesity Treatment Program Elements

Treatment Goals

Goal setting is an important aspect of behavior change programs (Bandura & Simon, 1997). The DPP Lifestyle Balance Program established a weight loss goal of 7% of baseline weight, 150 minutes/week of physical activity, and fat intake goals, which were augmented with calorie goals if the fat goal alone was not sufficient to promote weight loss. Well-operationalized goals are a defining feature of evidence-based behavioral weight control programs and thus an important feature to be retained in community adaptations.

Weight Loss

Many community-based programs adopt the 7% weight loss goal that the DPP clinical trial demonstrated to be associated with prevention of type 2 diabetes (Diabetes Prevention Program Research Group, 2002b). However, some program adaptations provide a lower weight loss goal of 5%, a threshold that has been established as producing clinically meaningful health improvements (Williamson, Bray, & Ryan, 2015) (see Table 30.2).

Physical Activity

Many community-based weight loss programs also include an exercise goal, with most mirroring the DPP Lifestyle Balance Program and providing a target of 150 minutes/week. This exercise "dose" corresponds to general recommendations of physical activity levels that prevent weight gain but may not be sufficient to promote or sustain weight loss or weight maintenance (Donnelly et al., 2009). Although some community programs established slightly more ambitious exercise goals, they still fall short of the physical activity goals of 200–300 minutes/week that may be required to promote sustained weight loss (Donnelly et al., 2009). Perhaps of greatest concern, however, is the absence of exercise goals in a significant proportion of community adaptations of the DPP lifestyle intervention (Neamah et al., 2016), even though physical activity was a key target in the program and has health benefits independent of weight loss.

Dietary Intake

Most descriptions of community adaptations indicate that dietary goals were incorporated, with the majority providing both calorie and fat goals, although some provided only calorie goals; see Table 30.2). A few programs gave fat goals at the onset of treatment and added calorie goals only for individuals who failed to lose weight, as was done in the DPP Lifestyle Balance Program. Although it is unclear whether simultaneous goals for fat and calorie intake or progressive goals are more effective for promoting weight loss, clearly stated dietary goals are critical for changing eating habits. Specific and measurable goals, such as calorie and fat gram intake targets, can provide important self-regulation parameters against which to evaluate (and prompt modification of) eating behaviors. Dietary intake goals can be particularly effective when combined with self-monitoring to objectively track whether these goals are achieved.

TABLE 30.2. Treatment Elements of Community-Based Obesity Interventions

Author (year)	Goals					Additional components	Treatment fidelity
	Weight	Calorie	Fat	Exercise	Self-weighing		
Ackermann et al. (2008, 2011)	5–7%	Not noted	Not noted	15 MVPA	Not noted	Access to YMCA	Training, monthly telephone conferences, session logs, meetings
Ackermann et al. (2014, 2015)	5–7%	Yes	Yes	150 MVPA	Not noted	Access to YMCA, pedometer, measuring cups, food scales	Direct observation, training, tests
Barham et al. (2011)	5–7%	Not noted	Not noted	Not noted	Not noted	Pedometer, portion plate, measuring cups/spoons, library of exercise DVDs	Not noted
Befort et al. (2010)	10%	Yes	Not noted	Increase to 300 minutes/week of MVPA	Not noted	Prepackaged entrées and shakes for the first 16 weeks	Treatment manual, sessions audio-taped and 25% reviewed, checklist
Fitzgibbon et al. (2005)	Not noted	Cut 500 kcal/day	Not noted	Not noted	Not noted		Training
Katula et al. (2010); Blackwell et al. (2011); Katula et al. (2011); Lawlor et al. (2013)	5–7%	Yes	Not noted	≥ 180 minutes	Not noted	DVD series on nutrition and physical activity, goal setting, and problem solving	Meetings, direct observation
Krukowski et al. (2010)	7%	Yes	Yes	200 minutes	Not noted		Not noted
McNabb et al. (1997)	Not noted	Not noted	Yes	Not noted	Not noted		Training, direct observation
Perri et al. (2008)	Not noted	Yes	Not noted	30 minutes/day of walking	Not noted	Cooking demonstrations	Training
Perri et al. (2014)	Not noted	Yes	Not noted	30 minutes/day	Not noted	Campaigns, motivational incentives (e.g., water bottles, hats, T-shirts)	Training, weekly supervisory contacts by phone
West et al. (2011); Krukowski et al. (2013)	7%	Yes	Yes	150 MVPA	Not noted	Pedometers	Protocol, script, direct observation
Williams et al. (2013); Sattin et al. (2016)	7%	Yes	Yes	150 MET minutes/week	Not noted	Incentives (gift cards, pedometers, T-shirts)	Manual, scripts, direct observation
Yanek et al. (2001)	Not noted	Yes	Yes	30 minutes or more 5–7 days/week	Not noted		Training

Note. MVPA, moderate-to-vigorous physical activity; MET, metabolic equivalent.

Self-Monitoring and Interventionist Feedback

Self-monitoring, which is the systematic observation and recording of eating and exercise behaviors or body weight, is an important aspect of self-management. It contributed substantially to successful weight loss in the DPP (Diabetes Prevention Program Research Group, 2004), as well as in many other studies (see Burke, Wang, & Sevick, 2011). The DPP Lifestyle Balance Program used paper diaries for daily self-monitoring of fat, caloric intake, exercise, and weight. Many community-based programs have also provided paper diaries for dietary and exercise self-monitoring. Although no community-based studies have reported the use of electronic self-monitoring, it is expected that this medium will become increasingly common with the proliferation of technology-based tools and the ease of utilizing smartphones for real-time recording (as well as the ability to decrease printing costs if electronic tools are used instead of paper diaries). In addition, there are suggestions that technology-based approaches to self-monitoring may facilitate adherence and may even promote greater weight loss when coupled with feedback (Burke et al., 2012).

Although most community-based programs recommend self-monitoring of dietary intake and physical activity (if targeted), none report a goal of daily self-monitoring of weight. This behavior is emerging as an important component in effective weight management programs (Linde, Jeffery, French, Pronk, & Boyle, 2005; Shieh, Knisely, Clark, & Carpenter, 2016) and was included as an intervention recommendation in the original DPP Lifestyle Balance Program. It is unclear why community adaptations do not incorporate this potentially beneficial treatment component more routinely. Concerns about the potential for negative psychological impact with frequent self-weighing have been articulated, but data fail to substantiate these concerns (Steinberg et al., 2014).

Providing feedback on self-monitoring records is an effective, theory-derived behavioral technique that facilitates behavior change (Michie, Johnston, Francis, Hardeman, & Eccles, 2008); weekly feedback was a strong focus of the original DPP lifestyle program, as well as of community-level adaptations (Kramer et al., 2009). In their DPP-based program delivered in senior centers, West et al. (2011) offered a specific "recipe" in which reinforcement and affirmation of behaviors consistent with behavioral goals were sandwiched around the identification of potential areas for behavior change, providing feedback to shape new habits and to identify potential problems to be solved. Further, they identified an approach to training that entailed an experiential process in which interventionists in training completed the self-monitoring tasks themselves and then rehearsed providing constructive feedback (Krukowski et al., 2012). Despite the key role of feedback on self-monitoring to prompt behavior change, just a few community-based studies note that interventionists examined self-monitoring records or provided feedback on specific behaviors reported in the diaries. Thus, many community-based programs may have reduced the potential impact of self-monitoring for behavior change by not providing focused, behaviorally grounded performance feedback.

Other DPP Treatment Elements

The DPP lifestyle program used a "toolbox" approach that provided resources (e.g., additional sessions, running shoes, exercise videos, cooking classes, additional meal replacements) to address specific challenges encountered by a given individual, thereby facilitating diet or exercise behavior changes. Approximately $300 per participant was spent over 3 years for toolbox expenses in the lifestyle program (Diabetes Prevention Program Research Group, 2003), a cost that is likely beyond the available resources for most community-based programs. This cost may explain why none of the studies reviewed here included a formal toolbox.

Supervised physical activity sessions were another resource-intensive treatment component that was incorporated in the DPP lifestyle program; each clinical center offered sessions at least twice a week, with staffing costs estimated at approximately $100 per participant each year (Diabetes Prevention Program Research Group, 2003). It is not surprising that few of the community-based programs reviewed offered supervised exercise sessions. Programs delivered in settings such as the YMCA have the advantage of an existing infrastructure in which to provide exercise opportunities without necessarily paying for additional personnel, although it is unclear whether the adaptations in these settings offered supervised exercise group sessions to their participants or just gave them the opportunity to exercise at the facility. Furthermore, the importance of providing supervised exercise sessions is unclear, since there are some indications that it may be preferable to emphasize a home-based exercise program for weight management rather than a facility-based, supervised program (Perri, Martin, Leermakers, Sears, & Notelovitz, 1997).

A final element of the original DPP lifestyle intervention that may have contributed to the magnitude of weight loss achieved in that landmark study was the recommendation to use meal replacements (which were provided as part of the toolbox) or to use structured meal plans if individuals were experiencing difficulties with meeting weight loss goals. Meal replacements have been associated with increased weight losses of approximately 3 kg compared with interventions without meal replacements (Heymsfield, van Mierlo, van der Knaap, Heo, & Frier, 2003). Meal replacements are not commonly incorporated into community-based weight management programs despite the weight loss advantages they may provide, presumably because of the costs associated with providing them. A recent adaptation of a weight loss program translated from the Look AHEAD trial, which was based in part on the DPP lifestyle intervention, described a program in which meal replacements were prescribed rather than provided (Delahanty et al., 2015). In this clinic-based weight loss program for individuals with type 2 diabetes, meal replacements were not given to participants; rather, participants were advised to purchase and use them as part of a group-based intervention that produced an average 6.6% loss of initial weight at 6 months. This may well be a tenable approach for community settings that lack extensive resources, allowing programs to benefit from the weight loss advantages conferred by meal replacements without the costs associated with providing them. Structured meal plans also promote greater weight loss than is achieved using calorie targets only, without guidance on specific food selections; structured meal plans accompanied by grocery shopping lists produce comparable weight losses to those obtained when individuals are given the foods required for the specific menu suggestions (Wing et al., 1996).

Treatment Fidelity

Detailed descriptions of training protocols for implementing lifestyle interventions in community settings are relatively rare in the current literature, although some insights are available (Finch, Kelly, Marrero, & Ackermann, 2009; Krukowski et al., 2012). Most programs specify the length of the training (e.g., 2 hours, 2 days) but provide minimal detail about the content. Documented measures of treatment fidelity are even rarer. For programs that did report on treatment fidelity, the majority used a content checklist, *in vivo* observation, and/or audiotaped a random sample of sessions for supervision (see Table 30.2).

Community Settings

In general, only a limited number of evidence-based weight loss programs have been translated into community settings and described in the scientific literature with adequate outcome data to allow evaluation of their effect on weight change. Furthermore, no studies of which we are aware have directly compared the impact of equivalent lifestyle interventions deployed in different community settings to determine whether some settings are more effective than others for delivering behavioral weight control programs. Therefore, we consider different community settings in more detail below.

Faith-Based Settings

There is a rich tradition of weight management programs being translated into faith-based settings, particularly in African American churches, with some translations incorporating faith-related activities and others placing a standard weight control program in a church setting. Among these faith-based programs that provide objective measurement of weight outcomes and have a control group to permit comparisons, weight losses range from a minimal 0.5 kg (Yanek, Becker, Moy, Gittelsohn, & Koffman, 2001) to a modest 2.6 kg loss (Sattin et al., 2016), with little difference in outcomes between programs that lasted for a full year versus those that were shorter (Lancaster, Carter-Edwards, Grilo, Shen, & Schoenthaler, 2014). There are no descriptions of non-Christian faith-based weight loss programs in the literature, nor are there many descriptions of evidence-based weight loss programs delivered in Christian churches that are not predominantly African American. However, there are suggestions that translations of the DPP Lifestyle Balance Program into churches with largely white congregations appear promising (Krukowski, Lueders, Prewitt, Williams, & West, 2010).

Worksites

Worksite settings have also been considered as potentially viable venues for delivering obesity treatment within communities. However, there are few adaptations of programs like the DPP lifestyle intervention in workplace settings that provide data on objectively measured weight, and, among those that do, few have produced clinically meaningful weight loss (average weight losses of 1.3 kg; Anderson et al., 2009). Despite modest weight losses, some have argued that implementing obesity treatment within worksite settings may be advantageous, because it could possibly increase men's participation in weight loss interventions (Brace et al., 2015); men are often underrepresented in obesity treatment programs. Promising results were obtained in an initial translation of the DPP lifestyle program into a workplace, with average weight losses of 2.2 kg over 3 months and an intriguing suggestion that weight loss may improve job satisfaction (Barham et al., 2011).

YMCA

Several studies have examined a DPP-based intervention delivered by YMCA wellness instructors (Ackermann, Finch, Brizendine, Zhou, & Marrero, 2008; Ackermann et al., 2015). The YMCA was selected as a community partner because of the organization's broad reach within diverse communities across the country and its commitment to health promotion, as well as the potential for sustainability should the program prove effective. Instructors for these studies had an undergraduate degree in exercise science or equivalent training and had participated in a 16-hour structured training that incorporated readings, didactic presentations, and opportunities to demonstrate core competencies necessary for effective delivery of an interactive lifestyle program (Finch et al., 2009). Individuals who were both overweight and at elevated risk for type 2 diabetes were enrolled in the YMCA program, which focused on diabetes prevention (rather than weight loss alone). Those in the comparison group were offered health screenings, brief advice, and self-help materials to guide their weight loss efforts, whereas those in the DPP arm were provided with access to the group sessions, as well as these other resources. Importantly, participants in both sites had access to the YMCA and all of its health promotion activities to support their weight loss efforts (Ackermann et al., 2008).

In an initial pilot study, weight losses averaged 6% at 4–6 months and were significantly greater than the 2% average weight loss achieved by the individuals who were given screening and advice at the comparison site (Ackermann et al., 2008). Most (76%) of the participants who were offered the group lifestyle program attended at least one session, and those who came to at least one session attended an average of 75% of the 16 core sessions, suggesting that uptake in the program was strong if individuals were at all interested in attending. Among those in the pilot study who attended the subsequent maintenance program, weight losses were sustained for an additional 2 years (Ackermann et al., 2011).

A follow-up study replicated and extended the evaluation of this YMCA-based program into low-income, predominantly minority populations at elevated risk for type 2 diabetes (Ackermann et al., 2015). Individuals randomly assigned to the group-based program lost, on average. 2.3 kg more at 12 months than did those who were provided with standard advice for diabetes prevention and a single visit with a registered dietitian. Among those who actually completed at least 9 of the 16 group sessions, weight losses were markedly higher, with average reductions of 5.3 kg reported at 12 months (Ackermann et al., 2015).

Based on the positive outcomes in this series of studies, the YMCA organization has established a national initiative in collaboration with the CDC and now offers the DPP translation at over 200 YMCAs. However, the program is offered only to individuals at elevated risk for type 2 diabetes and not as a weight loss program for those who might be at elevated risk for other obesity-associated health complications. Thus, though an important resource for communities across the United States, the YMCA program does not fully address the need for evidence-based obesity treatment at a community level.

Partnering with the Cooperative Extension Service to Translate the DPP Lifestyle Balance Program

One of the more prominent community settings into which the DPP lifestyle program has been translated is the Cooperative Extension Service. This is a community-based agency with an explicit mission of promoting the health of families and communities and an infrastructure that extends throughout the country. Several studies have examined obesity treatment delivered in cooperative extension offices by family and consumer sciences agents (and other professionals with health-promotion-related degrees hired by research partners at the University of Florida). In one study, obese women were first enrolled in a 24-session weight loss program based on the DPP and were then randomized in a larger trial to an education-centered group or to 26-session biweekly weight loss maintenance programs, delivered either face-to-face or by phone (Perri et al., 2008). The 78% of women who completed the intervention achieved an average 6-month weight loss of 10 kg. These are among the largest weight losses achieved in community settings that have been reported in the literature. Further, the maintenance programs were successful in preventing regain, with 12-month mean weight regains of only 1.2 kg among participants receiving extended counseling either face-to-face or by phone, compared to a regain of 3.7 kg in the education control group. This finding underscores the importance of a maintenance program in community-based weight control and suggests that either delivery format can be beneficial. The investigators acknowledged that the degree of training and supervision provided to the cooperative extension service agents who delivered the intervention was intense and exceeded what might be available in most rural settings. Nonetheless, the strong outcomes over an extended period merit continued refinement to allow dissemination through the cooperative extension service in other states.

A Detailed Examination of a Lay-Led Community-Based Lifestyle Intervention

Senior centers represent another community venue that has the potential to broadly disseminate evidence-based obesity treatment because of their extensive infrastructure across the United States. Older adults have consistently been one of the subgroups who have responded well to weight control programs (Diabetes Prevention Program Research Group, 2004), and rates of obesity in this population group are high (Ogden, Carroll, Kit, & Flegal, 2014). One study implemented a group-based DPP adaptation in senior centers that had been randomized to receive a weight loss intervention and compared weight loss outcomes with centers randomized to a memory improvement intervention, which served as an attention control group (West et al., 2011). The Group Lifestyle Balance Program (Kramer et al., 2009) was modified to be delivered by trained lay health educators, who enrolled obese individuals ages 60 years or older in a 21-session weight management intervention (12 weekly sessions followed by 9 monthly sessions). Weight losses averaged 3.8% at 4 months among those in the weight loss intervention, using an intent-to-treat analysis, compared with only 0.2% in the comparison group (West et al., 2011). The 5% threshold of clinically significant weight loss was achieved by 38% of the participants in the lifestyle program and 24% of participants achieved the 7% DPP lifestyle weight loss goal. Attendance at intervention sessions averaged 76%. Importantly, weight losses increased to 4.2% at 1 year, with 37% of participants sustaining at least a 5% weight loss at 1 year. This lay health-educator-led adaptation compares favorably with the original DPP lifestyle program, in which approximately half the participants achieved the 7% weight loss goal after the core program and with other DPP adaptations delivered by community members, which reported average weight losses of 3.15% (Ali, Echouffo-Tcheugui, & Williamson, 2012).

This study trained 20 lay health educators to lead the intervention at eight senior centers. These individuals had no background in nutrition, exercise, or health care, but were invited by the senior center directors, who were guided with suggestions about characteristics of effective interventionists (i.e., an organized, responsible individual with experience speaking in front of a group). Predominantly well-educated overweight and obese women volunteered to serve as interventionists and lead the weight loss groups in their communities. Nonparticipating senior centers reported that the primary obstacles that precluded their participation in the study were concerns that they would be unable to identify an individual to deliver the weight loss program for the full year's duration and perceived barriers imposed by the time required for training lay leaders and program implementation (Felix et al., 2014). These obstacles reflect the tensions between community implementation and treatment outcomes; the longer the program, the more likely the participants are to achieve sustained weight control (Ali et al., 2012; Perri et al., 2008), but it may be more challenging to find community members available to commit to leading the intervention.

The training of lay health educators in the senior center program followed a structured protocol over 26 hours that covered the core elements of a goal-based behavioral weight control approach, including reviewing self-monitoring diaries and giving feedback (Krukowski et al., 2013). Experiential learning exercises and modeling and rehearsal of intervention delivery with corrective feedback were incorporated. Interestingly, the lay health educators lost 1.4% of initial weight at 4 months, even though weight loss was not an explicit goal for the group leaders (though it was for the participants). The group leaders' modeling of weight loss behaviors may have contributed to weight loss among the participants. However, the lay health educators had negligible weight loss at the 12-month assessment. In contrast, participants continued to lose weight from the 4-month to the 12-month assessment.

The program enrolled approximately a quarter of the eligible individuals already served by the senior centers (Felix et al., 2012), providing deep reach into the proportion of obese individuals who were eligible to participate at each community site, although approximately 23% of those who participated in the program were new senior center patrons (Felix et al., 2012). Community translations of evidence-based weight management programs seldom evaluate how successfully they engage their target population, despite calls to attend more closely to this important metric; greater emphasis on this element can inform whether interventions that are translated and delivered within communities are having a substantive impact on the obesity epidemic (Mitchell et al., 2016). The deep reach into the community achieved in this study may reflect the benefits of using community members to recruit for weight loss programs rather than having academic researchers enroll participants. Costs for the program compared favorably to the $1,399 per-person cost for the lifestyle intervention in the DPP trial (Diabetes Prevention Program Research Group, 2003), with total costs to implement the program at each senior center estimated at $2,731, or $165 per participant (Krukowski et al., 2013). The cost per kg lost in the study was $45. DPP trial data indicate that the risk of diabetes decreases 16% with each kg lost (Hamman et al., 2006).

In summary, this study provides evidence of the potential benefit of training lay health educators to effectively deliver a group-based weight control program to older adults to achieve meaningful weight loss outcomes in senior center settings. It suggests that extended reach can be obtained when using community members to engage eligible members of their own community. Some of the factors, however, which may promote greater weight loss efficacy (e.g., extended duration and a structured training) may present inherent challenges for the community to deliver, raising the question "What are the boundaries of effective evidence-based treatment that can be implemented by lay health educators?" However, in rural settings, such as those in which this program was embedded, lay health educators may be the most practical approach to dissemination into communities in need, given the scarcity of health care professionals and personnel with behavior change expertise in some rural regions. Further, in a review of DPP translations into real-world settings, Ali et al. (2012) concluded that there is no substantive difference in weight loss outcomes achieved by trained professionals and lay leaders. Therefore, lay educators from the community may represent an effective choice for other community settings as well.

Summary

There is a growing evidence base of empirically validated obesity treatment approaches delivered in community settings, with emerging data to guide important intervention design parameters. Community members, whether professionally educated or selected based on performance criteria, can be trained to deliver effective weight control programs. Modifications to interventions developed for highly resourced clinical trials can reduce the costs of administering obesity treatment programs within communities without sacrificing outcomes. Strong examples of effective community partners joining with academics in efforts to translate and disseminate obesity treatment exist, and more will surely follow as communities seek opportunities to confront the looming public health crisis that obesity presents.

References

Ackermann, R. T., Finch, E. A., Brizendine, E., Zhou, H., & Marrero, D. G. (2008). Translating the Diabetes Prevention Program into the community: The DEPLOY pilot study. *American Journal of Preventive Medicine, 35*(4), 357–363.

Ackermann, R. T., Finch, E. A., Caffrey, H. M., Lipscomb, E. R., Hays, L. M., & Saha, C. (2011). Long-term effects of a community-based lifestyle intervention to prevent type 2 diabetes: The DEPLOY extension pilot study. *Chronic Illness, 7*(4), 279–290.

Ackermann, R. T., Finch, E. A., Schmidt, K. K., Hoen, H. M., Hays, L. M., Marrero, D. G., et al. (2014). Rationale, design, and baseline characteristics of a community-based comparative effectiveness trial to prevent type 2 diabetes in economically disadvantaged adults: The RAPID study. *Contemporary Clinic Trials, 37*(1), 1–9.

Ackermann, R. T., Liss, D. T., Finch, E. A., Schmidt, K. K., Hays, L. M., Marrero, D. G., et al. (2015). A randomized comparative effectiveness trial for preventing type 2 diabetes. *American Journal of Public Health, 105*(11), 2328–2334.

Albright, A. L., & Gregg, E. W. (2013). Preventing type 2 diabetes in communities across the U.S.: The National Diabetes Prevention Program. *American Journal of Preventive Medicine, 44*(4, Suppl. 4), S346–S351.

Ali, M. K., Echouffo-Tcheugui, J., & Williamson, D. F. (2012). How effective were lifestyle interventions in real-world settings that were modeled on the Diabetes Prevention Program? *Health Affairs, 31*(1), 67–75.

Anderson, L. M., Quinn, T. A., Glanz, K., Ramirez, G., Kahwati, L. C., Johnson, D. B., et al. (2009). The effectiveness of worksite nutrition and physical activity interventions for controlling employee overweight and obesity: A systematic review. *American Journal of Preventive Medicine, 37*(4), 340–357.

Bandura, A. (1986). *Social foundations of thought and action: A social cognitive theory.* Englewood Cliffs, NJ: Prentice-Hall.

Bandura, A., & Simon, K. (1997). The role of proximal intentions in self-regulation of refractory behavior. *Cognitive Therapy and Research, 1*(3), 177–193.

Barham, K., West, S., Trief, P., Morrow, C., Wade, M., & Weinstock, R. S. (2011). Diabetes prevention and control in the workplace: A pilot project for county employees. *Journal of Public Health Management and Practice, 17*(3), 233–241.

Befort, C. A., Donnelly, J. E., Sullivan, D. K., Ellerbeck, E. F., & Perri, M. G. (2010). Group versus individual phone-based obesity treatment for rural women. *Eating Behaviors, 11*(1), 11–17.

Blackwell, C. S., Foster, K. A., Isom, S., Katula, J. A., Vitolins, M. Z., Rosenberger, E. L., et al. (2011). Healthy living partnerships to prevent diabetes: Recruitment and baseline characteristics. *Contemporary Clinical Trials, 32*(1), 40–49.

Brace, A. M., Padilla, H. M., DeJoy, D. M., Wilson, M. G., Vandenberg, R. J., & Davis, M. (2015). Applying RE-AIM to the evaluation of FUEL Your Life: A worksite translation of DPP. *Health Promotion Practice, 16*(1), 28–35.

Burke, L. E., Styn, M. A., Sereika, S. M., Conroy, M. B., Ye, L., Glanz, K., et al. (2012). Using mHealth technology to enhance self-monitoring for weight loss: A randomized trial. *American Journal of Preventive Medicine, 43*(1), 20–26.

Burke, L. E., Wang, J., & Sevick, M. A. (2011). Self-monitoring in weight loss: A systematic review of the literature. *Journal of the American Diet Association, 111*(1), 92–102.

Delahanty, L. M., Dalton, K. M., Porneala, B., Chang, Y., Goldman, V. M., Levy, D., et al. (2015). Improving diabetes outcomes through lifestyle change—A randomized controlled trial. *Obesity, 23*(9), 1792–1799.

Diabetes Prevention Program Research Group. (1999). The Diabetes Prevention Program: Design and methods for a clinical trial in the prevention of type 2 diabetes. *Diabetes Care, 22*(4), 623–634.

Diabetes Prevention Program Research Group. (2002a). The Diabetes Prevention Program (DPP): Description of lifestyle intervention. *Diabetes Care, 25*(12), 2165–2171.

Diabetes Prevention Program Research Group. (2002b). Reduction in the incidence of type 2 diabetes with lifestyle intervention or metformin. *New England Journal of Medicine, 346*(6), 393–403.

Diabetes Prevention Program Research Group. (2003). Costs associated with the primary prevention of type 2 diabetes mellitus in the Diabetes Prevention Program *Diabetes Care, 26*(1), 36–47.

Diabetes Prevention Program Research Group. (2004). Achieving weight and activity goals among Diabetes Prevention Program lifestyle participants. *Obesity Research and Clinical Practice, 12*(9), 1426–1434.

Donnelly, J. E., Blair, S. N., Jakicic, J. M., Manore, M. M., Rankin, J. W., & Smith, B. K. (2009). American College of Sports Medicine position stand: Appropriate physical activity intervention strategies for weight loss and prevention of weight regain for adults. *Medicine and Science in Sports and Exercise, 41*(2), 459–471.

Felix, H. C., Adams, B., Cornell, C. E., Fausett, J. K., Krukowski, R. A., Love, S. J., et al. (2014). Barriers and facilitators to senior centers participating in translational research. *Research on Aging, 36*(1), 22–39.

Felix, H. C., Adams, B., Fausett, J. K., Krukowski, R. A., Prewitt, T. E., & West, D. S. (2012). Calculating reach of evidence-based weight loss and memory improvement interventions among older adults attending Arkansas senior centers, 2008–2011. *Preventing Chronic Disease, 9*, E63.

Finch, E. A., Kelly, M. S., Marrero, D. G., & Ackermann, R. T. (2009). Training YMCA wellness instructors to deliver an adapted version of the Diabetes Prevention Program lifestyle intervention. *The Diabetes Educator, 35*(2), 224–228, 232.

Fitzgibbon, M. L., Stolley, M. R., Ganschow, P., Schiffer, L., Wells, A., Simon, N., et al. (2005). Results of a faith-based weight loss intervention for black women. *Journal of the National Medical Association, 97*(10), 1393–1402.

Hamman, R. F., Wing, R. R., Edelstein, S. L., Lachin, J. M., Bray, G. A., Delahanty, L., et al. (2006). Effect of weight loss with lifestyle intervention on risk of diabetes. *Diabetes Care, 29*(9), 2102–2107.

Herman, W. H., Brandle, M., Zhang, P., Williamson, D. F., Matulik, M. J., Ratner, R. E., et al. (2003). Costs associated with the primary prevention of type 2 diabetes mellitus in the Diabetes Prevention Program. *Diabetes Care, 26*(1), 36–47.

Heymsfield, S. B., van Mierlo, C. A., van der Knaap, H. C., Heo, M., & Frier, H. I. (2003). Weight management using a meal replacement strategy: Meta and pooling analysis from six studies. *International Journal of Obesity and Related Metabolic Disorders, 27*(5), 537–549.

Katula, J. A., Vitolins, M. Z., Rosenberger, E. L., Blackwell, C., Espeland, M. A., Lawlor, M. S., et al. (2010). Healthy living partnerships to prevent diabetes (HELP PD): Design and methods. *Contemporary Clinical Trials, 31*(1), 71–81.

Katula, J. A., Vitolins, M. Z., Rosenberger, E. L., Blackwell, C. S., Morgan, T. M., Lawlor, M. S., et al. (2011). One-year results of a community-based translation of the Diabetes Prevention Program: Healthy-living partnerships to prevent diabetes (HELP PD) project. *Diabetes Care, 34*(7), 1451–1457.

Knowler, W. C., Fowler, S. E., Hamman, R. F., Christophi, C. A., Hoffman, H. J., Brenneman, A. T., et al. (2009). 10-year follow-up of diabetes incidence and weight loss in the Diabetes Prevention Program outcomes study. *Lancet, 374*(9702), 1677–1686.

Kramer, M. K., Kriska, A. M., Venditti, E. M., Miller, R. G., Brooks, M. M., Burke, L. E., et al. (2009). Translating the Diabetes Prevention Program: A comprehensive model for prevention training and program delivery. *American Journal of Preventive Medicine, 37*(6), 505–511.

Krukowski, R. A., Lensing, S., Love, S., Prewitt, T. E., Adams, B., Cornell, C. E., et al. (2012). Training of lay health educators to implement an evidence-based behavioral weight loss intervention in rural senior centers. *The Gerontologist, 53*(1), 162–171.

Krukowski, R. A., Lueders, N. K., Prewitt, T. E., Williams, D. K., & West, D. S. (2010). Obesity treatment tailored for a Catholic faith community: A feasibility study. *Journal of Health Psychology, 15*(3), 382–390.

Krukowski, R. A., Pope, R. A., Love, S., Lensing, S., Felix, H. C., Prewitt, T. E., et al. (2013). Examination of costs for a lay health educator-delivered translation of the Diabetes Prevention Program in senior centers. *Preventive Medicine, 57*(4), 400–402.

Lancaster, K. J., Carter-Edwards, L., Grilo, S., Shen, C., & Schoenthaler, A. M. (2014). Obesity interventions in African American faith-based organizations: A systematic review. *Obesity Reviews, 15*(Suppl. 4), 159–176.

Lawlor, M. S., Blackwell, C. S., Isom, S. P., Katula, J. A., Vitolins, M. Z., Morgan, T. M., et al. (2013). Cost of a group translation of the Diabetes Prevention Program: Healthy living partnerships to prevent diabetes. *American Journal of Preventive Medicine, 44*(4, Suppl. 4), S381–S389.

Linde, J. A., Jeffery, R. W., French, S. A., Pronk, N. P., & Boyle, R. G. (2005). Self-weighing in weight gain prevention and weight loss trials. *Annals of Behavioral Medicine, 30*(3), 210–216.

McNabb, W., Quinn, M., Kerver, J., Cook, S., & Karrison, T. (1997). The PATHWAYS church-based weight loss program for urban African American women at risk for diabetes *Diabetes Care, 20*(10), 1518–1523.

Merwin, E., Hinton, I., Dembling, B., & Stern, S. (2003). Shortages of rural mental health professionals. *Archives of Psychiatric Nursing, 17*(1), 42–51.

Michie, S., Johnston, M., Francis, J., Hardeman, W., & Eccles, M. (2008). From theory to intervention: Mapping theoretically derived behavioural determinants to behaviour change techniques. *Journal of Applied Psychology, 57*(4), 660–680.

Mitchell, N. S., Prochazka, A. V., & Glasgow, R. E. (2016). Time to RE-AIM: Why community weight loss programs should be included in academic obesity research. *Preventing Chronic Disease, 13*, E37.

Neamah, H. H., Sebert Kuhlmann, A. K., & Tabak, R. G. (2016). Effectiveness of program modification strategies of the Diabetes Prevention Program: A systematic review. *The Diabetes Educator, 42*(2), 153–165.

Ogden, C. L., Carroll, M. D., Kit, B. K., & Flegal, K. M. (2014). Prevalence of childhood and adult obesity in the United States, 2011-2012. *Journal of the American Medical Association, 311*(8), 806–814.

Perri, M. G., Limacher, M. C., Durning, P. E., Janicke, D. M., Lutes, L. D., Bobroff, L. B., et al. (2008). Extended-care programs for weight management in rural communities: The treatment of obesity in underserved rural settings (TOURS) randomized trial. *Archives of Internal Medicine, 168*(21), 2347–2354.

Perri, M. G., Limacher, M. C., von Castel-Roberts, K., Daniels, M. J., Durning, P. E., Janicke, D. M., et al. (2014). Comparative effectiveness of three doses of weight-loss counseling: Two-year findings from the rural LITE trial. *Obesity, 22*(11), 2293–2300.

Perri, M. G., Martin, A. D., Leermakers, E. A., Sears, S. F., & Notelovitz, M. (1997). Effects of group- versus home-based exercise in the treatment of obesity. *Journal of Consulting and Clinical Psychology, 65*(2), 278–285.

Renjilian, D. A., Perri, M. G., Nezu, A. M., McKelvey, W. F., Shermer, R. L., & Anton, S. D. (2001). Individual versus group therapy for obesity: Effects of matching participants to their treatment preferences. *Journal of Consulting and Clinical Psychology, 69*(4), 717–721.

Rosenblatt, R. A., Andrilla, C. A., Curtin, T., & Hart, L. (2006). Shortages of medical personnel at community health centers: Implications for planned expansion. *Journal of the American Medical Association, 295*(9), 1042–1049.

Sattin, R. W., Williams, L. B., Dias, J., Garvin, J. T., Marion, L., Joshua, T. V., et al. (2016). Community trial of a faith-based lifestyle intervention to prevent diabetes among African-Americans. *Journal of Community Health, 41*(1), 87–96.

Shieh, C., Knisely, M. R., Clark, D., & Carpenter, J. S. (2016). Self-weighing in weight management interventions: A systematic review of literature. *Obesity Research and Clinical Practice, 10*(5), 493–519.

Steinberg, D. M., Tate, D. F., Bennett, G. G., Ennett, S., Samuel-Hodge, C., & Ward, D. S. (2014). Daily self-weighing and adverse psychological outcomes: A randomized controlled trial. *American Journal of Preventive Medicine, 46*(1), 24–29.

West, D. S., Bursac, Z., Cornell, C. E., Felix, H. C., Fausett, J. K., Krukowski, R. A., et al. (2011). Lay health educators translate a weight-loss intervention in senior centers: A randomized controlled trial. *American Journal of Preventive Medicine, 41*(4), 385–391.

West, D. S., Prewitt, T. E., Bursac, Z., & Felix, H. C. (2008). Weight loss of black, white, and Hispanic men and women in the Diabetes Prevention Program. *Obesity, 16*(6), 1413–1420.

Williams, L. B., Sattin, R. W., Dias, J., Garvin, J. T., Marion, L., Joshua, T., et al. (2013). Design of a cluster-randomized controlled trial of a Diabetes Prevention Program within African-American churches: The fit body and soul study. *Contemporary Clinical Trials, 34*(2), 336–347.

Williamson, D. A., Bray, G. A., & Ryan, D. H. (2015). Is 5% weight loss a satisfactory criterion to define clinically significant weight loss? *Obesity, 23*(12), 2319–2320.

Wing, R. R., Jeffery, R. W., Burton, L. R., Thorson, C., Nissinoff, K. S., & Baxter, J. E. (1996). Food provision vs structured meal plans in the behavioral treatment of obesity. *International Journal of Obesity and Related Metabolic Disorders, 20*(1), 56–62.

Yanek, L. R., Becker, D. M., Moy, T. F., Gittelsohn, J., & Koffman, D. M. (2001). Project Joy: Faith-based cardiovascular health promotion for African American women. *Public Health Reports, 116*(Suppl. 1), 68–81.

CHAPTER 31

Alternative Behavioral Weight Loss Approaches
Acceptance and Commitment Therapy and Motivational Interviewing

Meghan L. Butryn
Leah M. Schumacher
Evan M. Forman

Behavioral weight loss is the first line of treatment for obesity (Jensen et al., 2014). As described by Gomez-Rubalcava, Stabbert, and Phelan (Chapter 20, this volume), this approach produces clinically significant improvements in weight, health, and quality of life. However, there is marked variability among participants in short-term efficacy, and long-term maintenance of weight loss is suboptimal. Investigators are continuing to develop innovative forms of behavioral treatment in the hopes of improving short- and long-term outcomes. Increasingly, these innovations are rooted in the recognition that initiating and sustaining weight-related behavior change is quite difficult for most individuals, and that specialized intervention tools may be necessary to help them attain the level of motivation and commitment required for lifestyle modification. Two treatments that have emerged as especially strong fits for this need are motivational interviewing (MI) and acceptance and commitment therapy (ACT). Although MI and ACT can each be delivered as stand-alone interventions, the greatest promise of these approaches lies in their integration with a traditional behavioral treatment package. In this way, behavior modification skills may be viewed as necessary but not sufficient for many individuals attempting weight loss. MI and ACT have the potential to bridge the gaps that remain when individuals experience ambivalence, discomfort, or discouragement during the course of lifestyle modification. This chapter describes the theoretical underpinnings of MI and ACT and summarizes the evidence evaluating their efficacy.

Motivational Interviewing

Description of Theory

MI is a directive, client-centered counseling approach (Miller & Rollnick, 2002). The overarching goals of MI are to help individuals identify, articulate, and increase their intrinsic motivation for change, because it is believed that individuals will be most successful in initiating and sustaining changes to their behavior when change serves personally relevant goals and values and the individuals are the primary advocates for change (Miller & Rollnick, 2002). There are two active components of MI (Miller & Rose, 2009). First, as displayed in Figure 31.1, the interpersonal spirit of MI is characterized by collaboration, evocation, and autonomy. Expressing empathy for individuals by offering acceptance and accurate understanding is also critical to MI's approach (Miller & Rollnick, 2002). Second, MI involves the use of specific therapeutic strategies and techniques that aim to elicit and reinforce arguments for change (i.e., "change talk") from individuals (Miller & Rose, 2009). Drawing from Bem's (1967) self-perception theory and Festinger's (1957) theory of cognitive dissonance, MI posits that behavior change can be facilitated by increasing individuals' verbalizations for change and decreasing talk that focuses on sustaining current behavior (i.e., resistance or "sustain talk"; Miller & Rollnick, 2002; Miller & Rose, 2009). Once motivation for change has been articulated, MI seeks to strengthen individuals' commitment to change by helping them develop concrete plans for the future (Miller & Rollnick, 2002).

Description of Clinical Approach When Applied to Obesity

Many individuals find that the behaviors necessary for weight loss and weight loss maintenance (e.g., ongoing restriction of calorie intake, self-monitoring of food intake and weight, engagement in a high level of physical activity) require a tremendous amount of effort and often involve a sense of deprivation. Consequently, individuals may experience ambivalence about these behavioral changes. MI may be particularly well suited to address these challenges, in that it normalizes and explores ambivalence about change in a nonconfrontational manner and helps individuals to identify and set goals that are consistent with personal values and that enhance motivation for change.

MI has been used to treat obesity in individuals of all ages and in various stages of change, as well as in obesity treatment programs of differing intensities. For example, MI has been used in primary care settings to aid individuals in identifying obesity as a problem and to enhance initial motivation for change, as well as in high-intensity, formal weight loss and weight loss maintenance programs to enhance treatment engagement and success. Key principles that characterize an MI approach across these settings include expressing empathy, developing discrepancy (i.e., highlighting the gap between individuals' goals or values and their current behaviors), rolling with resistance (i.e., viewing resistance as a sign that the individual views the situation differently and adjusting one's approach accordingly, rather than directly confronting resistance), and supporting self-efficacy (Miller & Rollnick, 2002). Table 31.1 provides examples of specific ways in which these principles can be utilized to en-

MI Approach	MI-Inconsistent Approach
Collaboration. The client–counselor relationship is a partnership in which the individual's experiences and perspectives are respected.	*Confrontation.* The counselor seeks to override the individual's presumably flawed perspective and to convince him or her to see a certain perspective that the counselor believes is more accurate.
Evocation. Insights and motivation for change are elicited from the individual. The individual's own goals and values are explored.	*Education.* The individual is perceived to lack key knowledge, insight, or skills. The counselor thus tries to provide these to the individual.
Autonomy. The individual is free to choose whether or not to change and what changes to make. The individual's right to self-direction is respected.	*Authority.* The counselor tells the individual what to do or not do in a prescriptive or didactic manner.

FIGURE 31.1. Key components of the spirit of MI. Adapted with permission from Miller and Rollnick (2002).

TABLE 31.1. Motivational Interviewing (MI) Principles, Strategies, and Examples to Enhance Motivation for Lifestyle Modification

MI principle	Strategies	Examples
Express empathy	• Use reflective statements and summaries to validate the difficulty of changing eating behavior and increasing physical activity.	• "Reducing your sweet intake has been very difficult."
	• Communicate acceptance and understanding to the individual.	• "You're working incredibly hard to exercise 3 days per week."
Develop discrepancy	• Use open-ended questions to explore individuals' goals and values related to weight loss.	• "Why is it important to you to lose weight?" • "How would your life be better if your health improved?"
	• Use objective data and feedback to nonjudgmentally frame the discrepancy between current behavior and expressed goals.	• "Your initial goal was to lose 15 pounds, and you have lost 8 pounds so far."
Roll with resistance	• Explore the costs and benefits of both change and the status quo.	• "What would be the benefits of eating out less? What would be the not-so-good parts?"
	• Use strategic summaries of ambivalence to tip the decisional balance toward change.	• "While you don't like logging your eating, you know this helped you lose 20 pounds in the past."
Support self-efficacy	• Elicit and strengthen confidence talk and self-motivational statements.	• "What has allowed you to be successful with restaurant eating in the past?"
	• Leave the majority of planning for behavior change to the individual, with only subtle shaping by the counselor.	• "You want to exercise more. What would you like to do this week? What will help you meet that goal?"
	• Avoid direct persuasion when offering information or advice.	• "Is it okay if I share some information about how to calculate calories with you?"
	• Emphasize the individual's own resourcefulness.	• "You've been cooking for years and know that you can create some tasty, lower-calorie recipes."

hance lifestyle modification (DiLillo, Siegfried, & West, 2003; Miller & Rollnick, 2002). MI techniques can also promote effective goal setting, as plans for change are self-chosen based on personally held goals. As described below, MI strategies have been incorporated into many behavioral weight loss programs, and standard behavioral weight loss treatment and MI share several common features, such as a strong emphasis on goal setting. Key differences between standard behavioral treatment and MI include MI's unique approach to handling ambivalence about and resistance to change, as well as its strong emphasis on self-directed change.

Efficacy

Research on the use of MI in the treatment of obesity has increased substantially in recent years. A recent meta-analysis examined randomized controlled trials (RCTs) of behavior change interventions that utilized MI for adults with overweight or obesity (Armstrong et al., 2011). The intervention group from each study included in the meta-analysis differed from the comparison group only in the use of MI, allowing for examination of the unique benefit conferred by MI. Interventions ranged in duration from 3 to 18 months; comparison groups varied in format and included standard care, education, attention control, and no treatment. Results revealed a beneficial effect of MI on weight outcomes, with a greater reduction in body weight observed among individuals who received MI compared to controls (weighted mean difference = –1.47 kg; Armstrong et al., 2011). A systematic review also was conducted to examine RCTs that used MI for weight loss among adults in primary care settings (Barnes & Ivezaj, 2015). This review found limited benefit of MI, with more than half of the included studies finding no significant differences in weight loss among individuals who received MI relative to controls. As these and the findings below highlight, MI shows promise for use in obesity treatment, but the evidence regarding its efficacy is mixed.

Behavioral Weight Loss Programs for Adults

MI is a component of the larger treatment package used in many behavioral weight loss programs (e.g., Diabetes Prevention Program Research Group, 2002; Look AHEAD Research Group, 2006). Several studies have examined the unique effect of adding MI to moderate- to high-intensity behavioral weight loss treatment programs. These studies have yielded mixed but overall promising results. MI has produced greater weight loss or improved adherence to behavioral recommendations (e.g., self-monitoring) in a majority of studies (see Table 31.2). In the largest RCT to examine the additive effect of MI in behavioral weight loss, participants with type 2 diabetes who received the behavioral weight loss intervention with MI lost nearly twice as much weight at 18 months compared to those who received behavioral treatment alone (West, DiLillo, Bursac, Gore, & Greene, 2007). A motivation-focused weight loss maintenance program that used MI also appeared to be a viable alternative to a more traditional skills-based weight loss maintenance program, as similar weight losses were observed with the two interventions (West et al., 2011). Additionally, MI delivered prior to enrollment in behavioral treatment programs may enhance program retention (Goldberg & Kiernan, 2005).

Although there is some support for a beneficial effect of MI as an additive component of in-person behavioral treatment, MI appears to confer less benefit beyond the effects of behavioral treatment alone when treatment is delivered in nontraditional modalities. For example, greater improvements in eating-related outcomes were reported by individuals who received a six-session guided self-help behavioral weight loss treatment with two sessions of MI relative to those who received the same guided self-help program plus two traditional motivation-focused sessions. However, significant differences in weight loss were not observed (DiMarco, Klein, Clark, & Wilson, 2009). Similar weight losses were also observed among individuals who received an online behavioral weight loss program either with or without an MI-focused, facilitated chatroom (Webber, Tate, & Bowling, 2008).

In Primary Care Settings

As previously noted, research concerning the efficacy of MI among adults with obesity encountered in primary care settings has been mixed (Barnes & Ivezaj, 2015; Wadden, Butryn, Hong, & Tsai, 2014). Although a majority of RCTs of MI in primary care settings have not demonstrated improved weight loss outcomes relative to control conditions, approximately half of such studies have shown that a minority of participants achieved clinically meaningful (i.e., ≥ 5%) weight losses (Barnes & Ivezaj, 2015). Differential findings across primary care studies may be partially attributable to factors such as differences in treatment duration, provider type and training, and intervention fidelity (Barnes & Ivezaj, 2015). Notably, many studies of MI in primary care have used comparison conditions that did not control for treatment contact, limiting conclusions that can be drawn about the unique benefits conferred by MI. Indeed, the first RCT to employ an attention-control intervention when examining the efficacy of an MI intervention delivered in primary care observed superior outcomes for the attention-control intervention relative to both the web-based MI intervention and treatment as usual (Barnes, White, Martino, & Grilo, 2014). Additional research is needed to ascertain under what circumstances MI is an effective treatment for obesity in primary care settings.

TABLE 31.2. RCTs examining the independent effect of MI among Adults with Overweight or Obesity Enrolled in Group-Based Behavioral Weight Loss Treatment

Study (author and year)	Sample	Treatment length	MI condition	Comparison condition	Main findings
Befort et al. (2008)	44 African American women	16 weeks	Culturally tailored BWL program + four sessions of MI	Culturally tailored BWL program + four health education sessions	No significant differences in weight loss between MI ($M = -2.6$ kg) and control ($M = -3.2$ kg) condition.
Carels et al. (2007)	55 sedentary adults experiencing difficulties with weight loss during a BWL program	24 weeks	BWL program + MI sessions provided until participant was on track with weight loss target (stepped care model)	Participants who failed to meet weight loss targets and continued group treatment as usual, without MI	MI participants lost significantly more weight ($M = -4.8$ kg) than control participants ($M = -2.1$ kg). MI participants also engaged in greater weekly exercise (+68 minutes/week).
Smith, Heckmeyer, Kratt, & Mason (1997)	22 women ages 50 or older	16 weeks	BWL program + three MI sessions	BWL program only	No significant differences in weight loss between MI ($M = -5.5$ kg) and control ($M = -4.5$ kg) condition. However, MI group had significantly better attendance, food diary completion, and glucose control.
West et al. (2007)	217 women with Type 2 diabetes being treated with medication	18 months	BWL program + five MI sessions	BWL program + five health education sessions	MI group lost significantly more weight at 6 ($M = -4.7$ kg), 12 ($M = -4.8$ kg), and 18 months ($M = -3.5$ kg) compared to controls ($M = -3.1$ kg, -2.7 kg, and -1.7 kg, respectively).

Note. BWL, behavioral weight loss.

Treatment of Childhood and Adolescent Obesity

A small number of RCTs has examined MI as a stand-alone intervention or as an adjunct to treatment for childhood and adolescent obesity. Although one study demonstrated that the addition of MI sessions to a comprehensive adolescent obesity treatment program increased treatment attendance and adherence to behavioral recommendations (Bean et al., 2015), MI generally has not improved weight loss among children and adolescents (MacDonell, Brogan, Naar-King, Ellis, & Marshall, 2012; Resnicow, Taylor, Baskin, & McCarty, 2005; Walpole, Dettmer, Morrongiello, McCrindle, & Hamilton, 2013). Some research indicates that MI delivered in primary care settings, either alone or as part of a larger treatment package, may help prevent future weight gain among adolescents (Taveras et al., 2011). However, these benefits may not be well maintained over time (Broccoli et al., 2016).

Conclusions and Future Directions

MI is widely used in obesity treatment, and, although the research support for this approach is somewhat mixed, MI appears to have the potential to improve outcomes in some populations and settings. MI confers the greatest benefit for improving adherence to behavioral recommendations and increasing weight loss when used as an adjunct to comprehensive in-person behavioral weight loss programs for adults, with additional mean weight losses of 1–2 kg reported in multiple studies. However, the addition of MI to behavioral weight loss treatment programs delivered in nontraditional modalities (e.g., online, guided self-help) does not appear to meaningfully improve weight loss beyond that observed when treatment is delivered in these formats without MI. Although positive effects of MI have been observed in several studies among adults in primary care settings and among children and adolescents, a majority of studies have observed null effects of MI in these populations. Additional research is needed to determine why MI may be most effective when used with higher-intensity programs for adults. The variability in outcomes across these populations may reflect differences in factors such as treatment dose and treatment fidelity. For instance, greater treatment duration, use of treatment fidelity measures, having weight as a primary outcome, and inclusion of an attention control are all factors that have been associated with better outcomes (Armstrong et al., 2011; Barnes & Ivezaj, 2015). It is also possible that individuals who enroll in comprehensive, high-intensity lifestyle modification programs differ meaningfully from individuals who participate in less intensive programs (e.g., in initial motivation for change), and that differences in treatment outcomes are influenced by sample characteristics.

Key limitations of past research on the use of MI for obesity treatment include great heterogeneity in the amount and quality of MI training for treatment providers, limited examination of MI treatment fidelity and dose, failure to isolate the effects of MI from other treatment components, and limited use of active comparison groups. Given the need for scalable obesity interventions and the potential for MI to be delivered by a variety of providers (e.g., nurses), future research that addresses these limitations is warranted.

Acceptance and Commitment Therapy

Description of Theory

ACT is a form of behavioral treatment that, like MI, can be used to provide assistance with particular challenges of weight control. Behavioral treatments can be conceptualized as evolving from their most traditional form, focused on classical conditioning and operant learning, to those that have incorporated a strong emphasis on cognition, to the current generation of "third-wave" therapies (Hayes, 2004). Widely researched third-wave therapies include ACT, relational frame theory, dialectical behavior therapy, and mindfulness-based approaches. Third-wave approaches are unique in their focus on fostering acceptance of internal experiences while simultaneously encouraging adaptive behavior (Herbert & Forman, 2013). Typically, these approaches attend closely to the context in which behavior occurs. This section focuses on the theory and evidence for ACT and related acceptance-based treatments, because this third-wave approach offers the greatest amount of evidence supporting its use for weight loss. The primary goal of acceptance-based treatment is to enhance psychological flexibility, which allows individuals to persist in or change behavior in a manner consistent with their own values and goals (McCracken & Morley, 2014). When psychological flexibility is low, internal experiences such as thoughts, feelings, sensations, or urges may have an undue, maladaptive influence on behavior. ACT encourages individuals to experiment with new ways of relating and responding to internal experiences, and to adopt an agenda such that changing one's internal experience is not a precondition for changing behavior (Forman & Herbert, 2009; Hayes, Strosahl, & Wilson, 1999).

Description of Clinical Approach When Applied to Obesity

There are various ways in which the theory underlying ACT can be translated into treatment protocols for weight loss. The clinical approach described here is drawn from the protocol that has the strongest evidence for efficacy: acceptance-based behavioral treatment (Forman & Butryn, 2016; Forman et al., 2016). In this protocol, principles from ACT are integrated with traditional behavioral treatment goals within the traditional behavioral treatment structure. In this group-based program, each session begins with a private measurement of weight by the clinician. When the group convenes, each participant reports his or her average calorie intake, physical activity minutes, and days of self-monitoring since the previous session. The curriculum then uses structured activities and guided discussion to review and teach a particular weight control skill. Experiential exercises and metaphors are typically used to teach acceptance-based concepts. Deliberate practice via homework assignments is emphasized between sessions. Many components of behavioral treatment are retained in this protocol because they are viewed as necessary for efficacy (e.g., clinician and participant monitoring of weight loss, prescriptions for calorie intake and physical activity, and use of principles such as goal setting and stimulus control). Ultimately, the use of acceptance-based strategies in such a protocol is designed to facilitate adherence to diet and exercise prescriptions. In contrast, other clinicians may use an approach to treating obesity in which ACT principles are primary rather than teaching them through a traditional behavioral weight loss framework (Lillis, Hayes, Bunting, & Masuda, 2009; Lillis & Kendra, 2016). In that alternative approach, weight loss is not necessarily an explicit treatment goal, and thus evaluating the efficacy of such an application of ACT is more complicated.

Core Acceptance-Based Behavioral Skills

In acceptance-based behavioral weight loss treatment (Forman & Butryn, 2016; Forman et al., 2016), individuals are oriented to a unifying conceptual framework referred to as "Control what you can, accept what you can't." This framework encourages deliberate choices with regard to one's weight control behaviors, while accepting that there are limits to how much one can change the internal experiences that precede or follow from such behaviors. Individuals are taught to use strategies that can make healthy eating and physical activity easier and more automatic, such as stimulus control (e.g., keep tempting foods out of the house) and social support (e.g., plan to meet a partner for morning walks). At the same time, they are asked to embrace the reality that no "magic bullet" exists that will make weight control effortless or consistently comfortable. Rather, individuals are educated about the biological and environmental factors that create internal experiences that at times feel uncomfortable, such as a hedonic drive for palatable food or a desire to avoid physical activity. Many individuals enter weight loss treatment with the understandable wish that the program will make behavior change much more comfortable than it has been in the past. Individuals are prompted to feel a sense of "creative hopelessness" about this possibility. They are encouraged to abandon an agenda in which behavior change is dependent on ideal internal experiences and instead consider an agenda in which they move forward with behavior change regardless of internal experiences.

As evidenced by this overarching framework, a core component of treatment is fostering a stance of acceptance toward the uncomfortable internal experiences that are commonly encountered as part of long-term weight control efforts. Such experiences may include thoughts, feelings, urges, or physical sensations, and may be related to eating behavior, physical activity, or other weight control behaviors such as self-monitoring of weight or eating. For example, individuals may feel an urge to eat a donut that is sitting on a conference room table; experience fatigue or boredom during exercise or have the thought that another activity would be more enjoyable than exercise; or be tempted to avoid writing down the calories from an indulgent meal or feel anxious about stepping on the scale. The goal of treatment is not to resign oneself to the unhealthy behavior that such internal experiences may be prompting (e.g., eating the donut, skipping or ending a bout of exercise, or avoiding the food record or scale). Rather, individuals learn to tolerate—without judgment—uncomfortable thoughts, feelings, urges, and sensations, recognizing that they are a natural part of the human weight control experience. When ACT is used in other domains of behavior change, treatment may focus on internal experiences that are acutely distressing or aversive, such as feelings of panic. As applied to obesity, a broader framework is used that incorporates acceptance of less acute experiences, such as perceived deprivation, hedonic sacrifice, and the particular type of discomfort that can be experienced when forgoing a more pleasurable option for one that is perceived as less pleasurable. For example, when contemplating the choice of grilled chicken salad versus pizza for dinner, many individuals would not describe their internal experience at that moment as frank distress, but would agree that anticipation of forgoing the more palatable food can feel uncomfortable.

Individuals build on their attitude of acceptance by exhibiting willingness in their behaviors. Willingness is the core way of demonstrating psychological flexibility; a high level of willingness positions individuals to choose behaviors based on their values, rather than allowing internal experiences to dictate behavior. Many individuals entering treatment will find that in their previous attempts at weight loss, they had a low level of psychological flexibility, in that internal experiences such as hunger, cravings, or energy level powerfully dictated their eating and activity choices. ACT clinicians validate this "old" approach as a normative human response, while at the same time building self-efficacy for change. Willingness is framed as a "muscle" or "skill" that can be mastered through deliberate practice. Building willingness skills gives individuals the ability to choose behaviors that are consistent with their values and long-term goals, regardless of how pleasurable or uncomfortable they may feel in the short term. Ultimately, individuals strive to separate internal experiences from behavior.

Mindful decision making is framed as a tool that orients individuals toward flexible action. By having greater awareness of cues for behavior, individuals may in turn have less automatic reactions to such cues. Individuals learn to attend to, observe, and describe internal experiences without judgment, often recognizing that what is being "offered up" by the mind or body is a natural response to internal or external stimuli (e.g., a drive to consume palatable food). Such mindful awareness then allows individuals to deploy their willingness skills and make deliberate decisions based on long-term goals and values.

Mindful awareness of values is also a critical component of treatment. Individuals engage in activities, discussions, and exercises in order to develop greater clarity about what is most important to them. For example, they are asked to think deeply about what it means to them personally to be living a rich and full life. Individuals are also asked to consider the ways in which healthy eating, physical activity, and weight control will allow them to pursue fulfillment in the domains that are most important to them. Throughout treatment, individuals are encouraged to develop a heightened awareness of how their weight-related behaviors do or do not move them in the direction of living a valued life. Values awareness is critical for sustaining the effort required by willingness.

Efficacy

A number of studies have been conducted to evaluate the efficacy of acceptance-based interventions. These studies vary in format from analogue studies that are highly controlled but limited in focus and generalizability, to uncontrolled studies that have no active comparison intervention, to RCTs. In the following material, we discuss the body of evidence for interventions that meet our definition of "acceptance-based behavioral weight loss treatments," that is, those that at least loosely integrate ACT and behavioral weight loss concepts. Methods and results are summarized in Table 31.3. We note that we do not include traditional mindfulness (e.g., "mindful eating") interventions in this review, and that previous reviews have determined that such interventions do not produce weight loss (Katterman, Kleinman, Hood, Nackers, & Corsica, 2014).

Analogue Studies

Analogue studies use controlled laboratory conditions to test the initial efficacy and/or mechanisms of action for a focal intervention component. For example, two such studies investigated the efficacy of strategies for coping with food cravings (based on the premise that refraining from food cravings was an analogue for successful weight control). In the first study, regular chocolate eaters were asked to abstain from chocolate consumption for 48 hours. In addition, they were asked to keep a transparent box of Hershey's kisses with them at all times for 48 hours. Prior to the abstinence challenge, participants were randomized to receive one of two 75-minute interventions: a cognitive-behavioral intervention drawn from a standard behavioral weight loss protocol (Brownell, 2004) or an acceptance-based intervention adapted from ACT (Hayes et al., 1999). The acceptance training resulted in lower craving intensity and higher abstinence rates among those participants most susceptible to food stimuli (Forman et al., 2007). Equivalent results were obtained in a similar study with overweight participants who abstained from sweets for 72 hours (Forman, Hoffman, Juarascio, Butryn, & Herbert, 2013). Another study with similar methods randomized participants to thought suppression instruction, defusion instruction (an acceptance-based strategy to step back and see thoughts, feelings, and cravings as mental processes), or no instruction (Hooper, Sandoz, Ashton, Clarke, & McHugh, 2012). Participants who received either instruction showed improved chocolate abstinence across 6 days, and those who received the acceptance training showed the least consumption at a final lab taste test. Another study attempted to isolate the effect of an acceptance-based intervention for cravings by adding it to an existing weight loss treatment (Alberts, Mulkens, Smeets, & Thewissen, 2010). Participants in the weight loss treatment were randomized to receive the standard version of the treatment or a version with an additional acceptance-based cravings intervention. Those receiving the acceptance-based component reported reduced food cravings, but there was no difference in weight loss. Overall, results from analogue studies offer support for the efficacy of treatment components that teach psychological acceptance, both in terms of subjective experience and eating behavior.

Uncontrolled Trials

Trials conducted without a control group leave open the possibility that observed effects are not attributable to particular aspects of treatment. However, they do offer preliminary tests of effectiveness as well as opportunities to evaluate the acceptability and feasibility of a new treatment. As such, uncontrolled trials have established the potential promise of acceptance-based behavioral treatment. For example, participants who were enrolled in a 12-week, group-based, acceptance-based behavioral treatment (ABT) for weight loss achieved a mean weight loss of 8.1% (7.9 kg) at posttreatment and 10.1% (9.8 kg) at a 6-month follow-up (Forman, Butryn, Hoffman, & Herbert, 2009). A 24-session trial of ABT produced a 12.0 kg weight loss (and excellent weight loss maintenance at follow-up) among overweight individuals with disinhibited eating (who are known to exhibit reduced response to standard behavioral treatment; Niemeier, Leahey, Palm Reed, Brown, & Wing, 2012). In a small sample of cardiac patients, ABT

TABLE 31.3. Efficacy of Acceptance-Based Treatments (ABT) for Weight Loss

Study	Methods	Results
Analogue studies		
Forman et al. (2007)	Regular chocolate eaters (N = 98) were asked to carry a transparent box of chocolates for 48 hours, but not to eat any chocolate. Randomized to ABT or standard CBT training for coping with cravings.	ABT resulted in lower craving intensity and chocolate consumption among those most susceptible to food stimuli.
Alberts, Mulkens, Smeets, & Thewissen (2010)	Individuals in a weight loss group were randomized to an additional 7 weeks of acceptance-based intervention for managing cravings, or to a control.	Participants in the acceptance of cravings group reported significantly lower cravings for food, but weight loss was equivalent.
Forman, Hoffman, Juarascio, Butryn, & Herbert (2013)	Overweight participants (N = 48) who regularly ate sweets were asked to keep a transparent box of sweets for 72 hours, but not to eat any sweets. Randomized to ABT or standard CBT training for coping with cravings.	ABT coping strategies resulted in lower cravings and reduced consumption, particularly for those who demonstrated greater susceptibility to the presence of food and reported a tendency to engage in emotional eating.
Hooper, Sandoz, Ashton, Clarke, & McHugh (2012)	Participants (N = 54) were randomized to one of three conditions: thought suppression instruction, defusion instruction, or no instruction. Participants were then asked to refrain from eating chocolate for a 6-day period.	Both active interventions were equally effective during the 6-day abstinence period, but participants in the acceptance-based condition showed reduced rebound eating at a final, lab-based chocolate taste test.
Uncontrolled studies		
Forman, Butryn, Hoffman, & Herbert (2009)	Overweight participants (N = 19) were assigned to a 12-week ABT for weight control.	Participants exhibited a mean weight loss of 8.1% (7.9 kg) at posttreatment and 10.1% (9.8 kg) at 6-month follow-up.
Niemeier, Leahey, Palm Reed, Brown, & Wing (2012)	Overweight participants with disinhibited eating (N = 21) participated in a 24-week ABT weight loss intervention.	Weight loss at 3-month follow-up averaged 12.1 kg.
Goodwin, Forman, Herbert, Butryn, & Ledley (2012)	Patients just treated for cardiac events/conditions (N = 16) were entered into a four-session ABT intervention.	Patients experienced clinically significant decreases in weight (M = 0.9 kg/week) and calorie, saturated fat, and sodium intake, and increases in physical activity.
Bradley, Forman, Sarwer, Butryn, & Herbert (2013)	Patients 1.5 to 4 years postbariatric surgery who were regaining weight (N = 8) participated in a 10-week ABT group intervention.	Weight regain was stopped, with a mean total body weight *loss* of 3.6% at post treatment.
Bradley et al. (2015)	Patients ≥ 1.5 years postbariatric surgery who were regaining weight (N = 16) participated in a 10-week ABT web-based intervention.	Patients experienced a mean weight change of –5.1%.

(continued)

TABLE 31.3. *(continued)*

Study	Methods	Results
Randomized controlled trials		
Lillis, Hayes, Bunting, & Masuda (2009)	Individuals who had completed a weight loss program in the community (N = 84) were randomized to a 6-hour ACT-based workshop or to a wait-list control.	The workshop produced a 1.5% weight *loss* by the 3-month follow-up, whereas the wait list resulted in a 0.3% *gain*.
Tapper et al. (2009)	Overweight women (N = 62) were randomized to four 2-hour ACT workshops or to a control condition.	Those assigned to the ACT workshop exhibited greater reductions in BMI at 6 months (−0.54 vs. −0.04 kg/m^2) and greater increases in physical activity (+2.2 vs. −0.6 bouts/week) compared to controls.
Katterman, Goldstein, Butryn, Forman, & Lowe (2014)	University students (N = 58) were randomized to 8 hours of an ABT weight gain prevention intervention or an assessment-only control.	At the 1-year follow-up, ABT participants demonstrated a −0.47 kg/m^2 change in BMI, compared to +0.74 kg/m^2 for controls.
Forman, Butryn, et al. (2013)	Overweight participants (N = 128) were randomized to receive 30 sessions of group-based ABT or gold-standard CBT treatment over the course of 40 weeks.	At 15 months (6 months posttreatment), weight loss was somewhat greater for those receiving ABT, but the advantage of ABT was especially pronounced when delivered by weight control experts (11.0 vs. 4.8%), and for participants with particular vulnerabilities (e.g., 11.2% vs. 4.6% for those higher in depression).
Forman et al. (2016)	Overweight participants (N = 190) were randomized to 25 sessions of ABT or standard behavioral treatment over 1 year.	At 1 year, participants assigned to ABT lost more weight (13.3%) than did those assigned to standard treatment (9.8%).
Weineland, Hayes, & Dahl (2012)	Postbariatric surgery patients (N = 39) were randomized to either an ACT-based in-person plus Internet intervention or to treatment as usual.	Relative to the control condition, ACT participants demonstrated gains in quality of life and body satisfaction; disordered eating did not differ significantly at follow-up. Weight outcomes were not evaluated.

Note. ABT, acceptance-based behavioral treatment; CBT, cognitive-behavioral therapy; BMI, body mass index.

produced clinically significant decreases in weight (M = 0.9 kg/week) and intake of calories, saturated fat, and sodium (Goodwin, Forman, Herbert, Butryn, & Ledley, 2012). Two small open trials of ABT for individuals who had received bariatric surgery revealed that patients who were on a weight gain trajectory stopped and reversed this weight gain when ABT was delivered in person (Bradley et al., 2016) or online (Bradley et al., 2015). Collectively, these five studies strongly suggest that ABT is a feasible, acceptable, and effective method of achieving weight loss across a range of samples.

RCTs

A number of RCTs of ACT-related weight loss treatments have been conducted. These trials can be divided into those that used a gold-standard treatment in a comparison condition and those that did not. In the latter category, individuals who had already completed a community-based weight loss program (e.g., Weight Watchers) were randomized to a 6-hour ACT-based workshop or to a wait list. The workshop resulted in an additional 1.5% weight loss at 3 months, relative to a 0.3% weight gain among wait-list controls (Lillis et al., 2009). Another workshop study randomized women to four 2-hour ACT sessions or to a control condition. Compared to controls, those assigned to the ACT workshop exhibited greater reductions in body mass index (BMI) at 6 months (−0.54 vs. −0.04 kg/m^2) and greater increases in physical activity (+2.2 vs. −0.6 bouts/week; Tapper et al., 2009). A weight gain prevention study randomized university students to either 8 hours of ABT or an assessment-only control condition. ABT resulted in a 0.47 kg/m^2 decrease in BMI at 1-year follow-up versus a gain of 0.74 kg/m^2 for control participants (Katterman, Goldstein, Butryn, Forman, & Lowe, 2014). Bariatric surgery patients who were assigned to an ACT-based in-person plus Internet intervention demonstrated improved quality of life and decreased body dissatisfaction compared to those assigned to treatment as usual; body weight was not measured (Weineland, Hayes, & Dahl, 2012).

To our knowledge, only two trials have compared ABT to a gold-standard behavioral weight loss treatment. In one, overweight participants ($N = 128$) were randomized to either a 40-week, group-based ABT or to standard behavioral weight loss treatment (Forman, Butryn, et al., 2013). The core components of behavioral treatment were present and equivalent in the two conditions, and the treatments prescribed equivalent calorie intake, physical activity, and weight loss goals. At the final 15-month assessment (i.e., 6-month follow-up), participants assigned to ABT and standard behavioral treatment lost 9.2% and 7.4%, respectively ($p = .37$). However, an advantage of ABT was present under certain conditions. For example, weight losses were larger for those receiving ABT (11.0%) than for those who received standard treatment (4.8%) when the treatments were administered by weight control experts as opposed to graduate student trainees. Also, ABT resulted in considerably greater weight losses for those who showed elevated mood disturbance, responsivity to food cues, or disinhibited eating. In a follow-up study, participants with overweight and obesity ($N = 190$) were randomized to 25 sessions (delivered over 1 year) of ABT or standard behavioral treatment (Forman et al., 2016). Participants assigned to ABT achieved a significantly greater 12-month weight loss (13.3%) than did those assigned to standard treatment (9.8%). ABT participants were also more likely to maintain a ≥ 10% weight loss at 12 months (64.0 vs. 48.9% of participants). In contrast to several previous studies, no evidence of treatment moderators was found (i.e., the advantage of ABT appeared to be similar across subtypes of participants). Results also supported the mediating role of autonomous motivation and psychological acceptance of food-related urges (Forman et al., 2016).

Conclusions and Future Directions

Collectively, these results indicate that ABT is an effective weight loss treatment, and one RCT suggests that it may even be more effective than the current gold-standard behavioral treatment. However, several areas of future research are indicated. First, additional randomized trials comparing ABT to gold-standard treatment should be conducted, preferably by a variety of research labs. Second, studies that determine the extent to which treatment effects persist beyond in-person meetings should also be conducted. A related line of research could investigate methods that effectively extend the effects of ABT into the long term, such as booster sessions, online modules, phone contacts, text messages, and smartphone apps. In addition, it is important to identify whether there are certain individuals who are especially well suited (or especially nonresponsive) to ABT. The current findings are mixed in this regard. A relatively new and applicable approach to treatment-matching research involves comparing outcomes for participants who show a lack of response to a first-line treatment and then remain in the same treatment or are switched to a different treatment (e.g., ABT; Sherwood et al., 2016). Finally, it is critical that future studies investigate the mechanisms of action through which ABT exerts its effects. Doing so will enable modification of ABT in order to enhance its potency. This line of research may require the development of new methods of measurement, as much of the extant work relies on self-report measures, which are known to be unreliable.

References

Alberts, H. J., Mulkens, S., Smeets, M., & Thewissen, R. (2010). Coping with food cravings. Investigating the potential of a mindfulness-based intervention. *Appetite, 55*(1), 160–163.

Armstrong, M., Mottershead, T., Ronksley, P., Sigal, R., Campbell, T., & Hemmelgarn, B. (2011). Motivational interviewing to improve weight loss in overweight and/or obese patients: A systematic review and meta-analysis of randomized controlled trials. *Obesity Reviews, 12*(9), 709–723.

Barnes, R., & Ivezaj, V. (2015). A systematic review of motivational interviewing for weight loss among adults in primary care. *Obesity Reviews, 16*(4), 304–318.

Barnes, R., White, M. A., Martino, S., & Grilo, C. M. (2014). A randomized controlled trial comparing scalable weight loss treatments in primary care. *Obesity, 22*(12), 2508–2516.

Bean, M., Powell, P., Quinoy, A., Ingersoll, K., Wickham, E., & Mazzeo, S. (2015). Motivational interviewing targeting diet and physical activity improves adherence to paediatric obesity treatment: Results from the MI values randomized controlled trial. *Pediatric Obesity, 10*(2), 118–125.

Befort, C. A., Nollen, N., Ellerbeck, E. F., Sullivan, D. K., Thomas, J. L., & Ahluwalia, J. S. (2008). Motivational interviewing fails to improve outcomes of a behavioral weight loss program for obese African American women: A pilot randomized trial. *Journal of Behavioral Medicine, 31*(5), 367–377.

Bem, D. J. (1967). Self-perception: An alternative interpretation of cognitive dissonance phenomena. *Psychological Review, 74*(3), 183–200.

Bradley, L. E., Forman, E. M., Kerrigan, S., Butryn, M. L., Herbert, J. D., & Sarwer, D. B. (2016). A pilot study of an acceptance-based behavioral intervention for weight regain after bariatric surgery. *Obesity Surgery, 26*(10), 2433–2441.

Bradley, L. E., Forman, E. M., Kerrigan, S. G., Goldstein, S. P., Butryn, M. L., Thomas, J. G., et al. (2015). A pilot study to assess feasibility, acceptability, and effectiveness of a remotely-delivered intervention to address weight regain after bariatric surgery. *Surgery for Obesity and Related Diseases, 11*(6, Suppl.), S55.

Bradley, L. E., Forman, E. M., Sarwer, D. B., Butryn, M. L., & Herbert, J. D. (2013, November). *A role for acceptance-based interventions to stop weight regain in bariatric surgery patients.* Paper presented at the Obesity Society annual convention, Atlanta.

Broccoli, S., Davoli, A. M., Bonvicini, L., Fabbri, A., Ferrari, E., Montagna, G., et al. (2016). Motivational interviewing to treat overweight children: 24-month follow-up of a randomized controlled trial. *Pediatrics, 137*(1), 1–10.

Brownell, K. D. (2004). *The LEARN Program for weight management* (10th ed.). Dallas: American Health.

Carels, R. A., Darby, L., Cacciapaglia, H. M., Konrad, K., Coit, C., Harper, J., et al. (2007). Using motivational interviewing as a supplement to obesity treatment: A stepped-care approach. *Health Psychology, 26*(3), 369.

Diabetes Prevention Program Research Group. (2002). The Diabetes Prevention Program (DPP) description of lifestyle intervention. *Diabetes Care, 25*(12), 2165–2171.

DiLillo, V., Siegfried, N. J., & West, D. S. (2003). Incorporating motivational interviewing into behavioral obesity treatment. *Cognitive and Behavioral Practice, 10*(2), 120–130.

DiMarco, I. D., Klein, D. A., Clark, V. L., & Wilson, G. T. (2009). The use of motivational interviewing techniques to enhance the efficacy of guided self-help behavioral weight loss treatment. *Eating Behaviors, 10*(2), 134–136.

Festinger, L. (1957). *A theory of cognitive dissonance*. Evanston, IL: Row Petersen.

Forman, E. M., & Butryn, M. L. (2016). *Effective weight loss: An acceptance-based behavioral approach*. New York: Oxford University Press.

Forman, E. M., Butryn, M. L., Hoffman, K. L., & Herbert, J. D. (2009). An open trial of an acceptance-based behavioral intervention for weight loss. *Cognitive and Behavioral Practice, 16*(2), 223–235.

Forman, E. M., Butryn, M. L., Juarascio, A. S., Bradley, L. E., Lowe, M. R., Herbert, J. D., et al. (2013). The mind your health project: A randomized controlled trial of an innovative behavioral treatment for obesity. *Obesity, 21*(6), 1119–1126.

Forman, E. M., Butryn, M. L., Manasse, S. M., Crosby, R. D., Goldstein, S. P., Wyckoff, E. P., et al. (2016). Acceptance-based versus standard behavioral treatment for obesity: Results from the mind your health randomized controlled trial. *Obesity (Silver Spring), 24*(10), 2050–2056.

Forman, E. M., & Herbert, J. D. (2009). New directions in cognitive behavior therapy: Acceptance-based therapies. In W. O'Donohue & J. E. Fisher (Eds.), *General principles and empirically supported techniques of cognitive behavior therapy* (pp. 77–101). Hoboken, NJ: Wiley.

Forman, E. M., Hoffman, K. L., Juarascio, A. S., Butryn, M. L., & Herbert, J. D. (2013). Comparison of acceptance-based and standard cognitive-based coping strategies for craving sweets in overweight and obese women. *Eating Behaviors, 14*(1), 64–68.

Forman, E. M., Hoffman, K. L., McGrath, K. B., Herbert, J. D., Brandsma, L. L., & Lowe, M. R. (2007). A comparison of acceptance-and control-based strategies for coping with food cravings: An analog study. *Behaviour Research and Therapy, 45*(10), 2372–2386.

Goldberg, J. H., & Kiernan, M. (2005). Innovative techniques to address retention in a behavioral weight-loss trial. *Health Education Research, 20*(4), 439–447.

Goodwin, C. L., Forman, E. M., Herbert, J. D., Butryn, M. L., & Ledley, G. S. (2012). A pilot study examining the initial effectiveness of a brief acceptance-based behavior therapy for modifying diet and physical activity among cardiac patients. *Behavior Modification, 36*(2), 199–217.

Hayes, S. (2004). Acceptance and commitment therapy, relational frame theory, and the third wave of behavioral and cognitive therapies. *Behavior Therapy, 35*(4), 639–665.

Hayes, S., Strosahl, K. D., & Wilson, K. G. (1999). *Acceptance and commitment therapy*: New York: Guilford Press.

Herbert, J. D., & Forman, E. M. (2013). Caution: The differences between CT and ACT may be larger (and smaller) than they appear. *Behavior Therapy, 44*(2), 218–223.

Hooper, N., Sandoz, E. K., Ashton, J., Clarke, A., & McHugh, L. (2012). Comparing thought suppression and acceptance as coping techniques for food cravings. *Eating Behaviors, 13*(1), 62–64.

Jensen, M. D., Ryan, D. H., Hu, F. B., Stevens, F. J., Hubbard, V. S., Stevens, V. J., et al. (2014). 2013 AHA/ACC/TOS guideline for the management of overweight and obesity in adults: A report of the American College of Cardiology/American Heart Association Task Force on Practice Guidelines and The Obesity Society. *Journal of the American College of Cardiology, 63*(25, Pt. B), 2985–3023.

Katterman, S. N., Goldstein, S. P., Butryn, M. L., Forman, E. M., & Lowe, M. R. (2014). Efficacy of an acceptance-based behavioral intervention for weight gain prevention in young adult women. *Journal of Contextual Behavioral Science, 3*(1), 45–50.

Katterman, S. N., Kleinman, B. M., Hood, M. M., Nackers, L. M., & Corsica, J. A. (2014). Mindfulness meditation as an intervention for binge eating, emotional eating, and weight loss: A systematic review. *Eating Behaviors, 15*(2), 197–204.

Lillis, J., Hayes, S., Bunting, K., & Masuda, A. (2009). Teaching acceptance and mindfulness to improve the lives of the obese: A preliminary test of a theoretical model. *Annals of Behavioral Medicine, 37*(1), 58–69.

Lillis, J., & Kendra, K. E. (2016). Designing and implementing mindfulness- and acceptance-based interventions for weight control: Models and considerations. In A. Haynos, E. Forman, M. Butryn, & J. Lillis (Eds.), *Mindfulness and acceptance for treating eating disorders and weight concerns: Evidence based interventions* (pp. 169–183). Oakland, CA: Context Press.

Look AHEAD Research Group. (2006). The Look AHEAD study: A description of the lifestyle intervention and the evidence supporting it. *Obesity, 14*(5), 737.

MacDonell, K., Brogan, K., Naar-King, S., Ellis, D., & Marshall, S. (2012). A pilot study of motivational interviewing targeting weight-related behaviors in overweight or obese African American adolescents. *Journal of Adolescent Health, 50*(2), 201–203.

McCracken, L. M., & Morley, S. (2014). The psychological flexibility model: A basis for integration and progress in psychological approaches to chronic pain management. *Journal of Pain, 15*(3), 221–234.

Miller, W., & Rollnick, S. (2002). *Motivational interviewing: Preparing people for change*. New York: Guilford Press.

Miller, W., & Rose, G. S. (2009). Toward a theory of motivational interviewing. *American Psychologist, 64*(6), 527.

Niemeier, H. M., Leahey, T., Palm Reed, K., Brown, R. A., & Wing, R. R. (2012). An acceptance-based behavioral intervention for weight loss: A pilot study. *Behavior Therapy, 43*(2), 427–435.

Resnicow, K., Taylor, R., Baskin, M., & McCarty, F. (2005). Results of Go Girls: A weight control program for overweight African-American adolescent females. *Obesity Research, 13*(10), 1739–1748.

Sherwood, N. E., Butryn, M. L., Forman, E. M., Almirall, D., Seburg, E. M., Crain, A. L., et al. (2016). The BestFIT trial: A SMART approach to developing individualized weight loss treatments. *Contemporary Clinical Trials, 47*, 209–216.

Smith, D. E., Heckemeyer, C. M., Kratt, P. P., & Mason, D. A. (1997). Motivational interviewing to improve adherence to a behavioral weight-control program for older obese women with NIDDM: A pilot study. *Diabetes Care, 20*(1), 52–54.

Tapper, K., Shaw, C., Ilsley, J., Hill, A. J., Bond, F. W., & Moore, L. (2009). Exploratory randomised controlled trial of a mindfulness-based weight loss intervention for women. *Appetite, 52*(2), 396–404.

Taveras, E. M., Gortmaker, S. L., Hohman, K. H., Horan, C. M., Kleinman, K. P., Mitchell, K., et al. (2011). Randomized controlled trial to improve primary care to prevent and manage childhood obesity: The High Five for Kids study. *Archives of Pediatrics and Adolescent Medicine, 165*(8), 714–722.

Wadden, T. A., Butryn, M. L., Hong, P. S., & Tsai, A. G. (2014). Behavioral treatment of obesity in patients encountered in primary care settings: A systematic review. *Journal of the American Medical Association, 312*(17), 1779–1791.

Walpole, B., Dettmer, E., Morrongiello, B. A., McCrindle, B. W., & Hamilton, J. (2013). Motivational interviewing to enhance self-efficacy and promote weight loss in overweight and obese adolescents: A randomized controlled trial. *Journal of Pediatric Psychology, 38*(9), 944–953.

Webber, K. H., Tate, D. F., & Bowling, J. M. (2008). A randomized comparison of two motivationally enhanced internet behavioral weight loss programs. *Behaviour Research and Therapy, 46*(9), 1090–1095.

Weineland, S., Hayes, S., & Dahl, J. (2012). Psychological flexibility and the gains of acceptance-based treatment for post-bariatric surgery: Six-month follow-up and a test of the underlying model. *Clinical Obesity, 2*(1–2), 15–24.

West, D. S., DiLillo, V., Bursac, Z., Gore, S. A., & Greene, P. G. (2007). Motivational interviewing improves weight loss in women with type 2 diabetes. *Diabetes Care, 30*(5), 1081–1087.

West, D. S., Gorin, A. A., Subak, L. L., Foster, G., Bragg, C., Hecht, J., et al. (2011). A motivation-focused weight loss maintenance program is an effective alternative to a skill-based approach. *International Journal of Obesity, 35*(2), 259–269.

CHAPTER 32

Behavioral Economics and Weight Management

Mitesh S. Patel
Kevin G. M. Volpp

About 40% of premature mortality can be attributed to our health behaviors (McGinnis, Williams-Russo, & Knickman, 2002; Schroeder, 2007). For example, physical inactivity and poor diet are major contributing factors to obesity and other leading causes of morbidity and mortality (Lee et al., 2012). Even though most people know that these behaviors are bad for their health, they have difficulty changing their habits. Most of these behaviors are related to daily choices such as what to eat or whether to exercise and for how long.

Recognizing that there are many reasons people don't take action to improve their health, behavior change experts have focused efforts on changing both individual behaviors and environments in ways that will support health (Glanz & Bishop, 2010). Similarly, policymakers have instituted strategies targeted at individual behavior, such as incentives, and environmental strategies, such as mandated food labeling. For example, Section 2705 of the Affordable Care Act allows employers to provide incentives of up to 50% of total premiums based on outcomes such as reduced body mass index (BMI), lowered blood pressure or cholesterol, and smoking cessation, an approach that could put as much as $300 billion worth of employee health incentives in play annually (Volpp, Asch, Galvin, & Loewenstein, 2011; Madison, Schmidt, & Volpp, 2013).

Many of the approaches being used have built-in limitations, having been designed around the pervasive view that health care decisions are rationally based economic transactions and that rational people will dispassionately assess the net present value of the costs and benefits of alternative paths and pursue the best path forward. When incentives are used, there is often an assumption that all that matters is the magnitude of the incentives and that the design, feedback frequency, saliency, and framing do not matter. These approaches seem generally well suited to support the health of people who behave as economists assume they will behave but might be less effective in supporting the health of broader populations. Public health programs, including those involving financial incentives, would likely be more effective if designed based not on how perfectly rational people should make health decisions, but rather on how real people actually do make them (Loewenstein, Brennan, & Volpp, 2007).

Embracing a Behavioral Economic Framework

Behavioral economics is a field that differs in its approach from standard traditional economics (Table 32.1). Behavioral economics incorporates principles from psychology to help understand why individuals make decisions that are not in line with longer-term health goals. Instead, individuals often deviate from these goals in a predictable manner based on a common set of decision errors (Table 32.2). For example, individuals tend to be more motivated by immediate rather than delayed gratification (O'Donoghue & Rabin, 2000), and by losses rather than gains (Kahneman & Tversky, 1979). They also tend to avoid the feeling of regret (Zeelenberg & Pieters, 2004). These insights reveal that the design and delivery of an incentive have an important impact on its effectiveness. Behavioral economists have proposed an *asymmetric paternalism* approach to public policy (Loewenstein et al., 2007). This approach is paternalistic in attempting to help individuals achieve their own goals, in effect protecting them from themselves, in contrast with conventional forms of regulation designed to prevent individuals from harming others. Asymmetric paternalism differs from "heavy-handed" paternalism in attempting to protect people without limiting their freedom of choice. It is asymmetric in the sense of helping individuals who are prone to making irrational decisions, while not restricting the freedom of choice of those who make informed, deliberate decisions. For example, arranging the presentation of food in a cafeteria line so that the healthy foods appear first is likely to increase the amount of healthy foods chosen, without depriving those who want the unhealthy foods of the opportunity to purchase them (Thaler & Sunstein, 2003). People who believe that individuals behave optimally should not object to asymmetric paternalism because it does not limit freedom, whereas those who accept the limits of human rationality should actively endorse such measures.

Traditional economics justifies seemingly suboptimal decisions as reflections of some implied but hidden rational choices, whereas behavioral economics sees our seemingly suboptimal decisions as errors. Many people have trouble dieting, exercising, and saving money, and are prone to procrastination even when the cumulative consequences are severe (Loewenstein et al., 2007). Many commercial enterprises exploit these decision errors. Credit card companies and automobile manufacturers lure new customers with "$0 down" and fleeting but tempting teaser rates of "0% interest," playing on the common propensity to focus on the present rather than on the future. Banks earn revenue by

TABLE 32.1. Traditional versus Behavioral Economics

Traditional economics	Behavioral economics
Core theory: Expected utility maximization	Core theory: Prospect theory
Assumes perfect rationality	Recognizes that people make decision errors
Starting-point independent	Assessment depends on the starting point
Framing doesn't matter	Framing affects assessment even when utilities are the same
Stable preferences	Time-inconsistent preferences
People discount the future at constant rates	People discount the near future to a greater degree and have time-inconsistent discounting
Intervene only when my actions adversely affect others (negative externalities)	Consider interventions when people will harm their future selves (internalities)
Regulations and policies generally geared to protecting people from the actions of others	Regulations and policies often geared to protecting people from themselves

TABLE 32.2. Key Decision Errors and Suggestions for Addressing Them

Present-biased preferences	Feedback needs to be relatively immediate
Nonlinear probability weighting	Probabilistic rewards (lotteries) can be efficient ways to motivate.
Overoptimism and loss aversion	Getting people to precommit and put money at risk is an effective motivational tool.
Peanuts effect	Delivering rewards in bundles avoids dispensing many small rewards.
Narrow bracketing	Framing rewards in terms of effort per day is preferable to offering them per month or year.
Regret aversion	Utilizing anticipated regret can augment motivation.
Defaults/status quo bias	Setting defaults/using power of choice architect to create environments can shift the path of least resistance to favor healthy choices
Rational world bias	Recognize that simply providing information and assuming people will act rationally likely won't result in the desired behaviors.

charging high fees (generally not prominent in program descriptions) for minor mistakes such as account overdrafts or breaches of minimum balance rules. States market lottery tickets that return $0.45 on the dollar and promote these games in ways that ignore probabilities, with messages such as "You can't win if you don't play."

The promise of behavioral economics for population health is that many of the same messages, incentives, and choice structures that effectively lure people into situations where they may be exploited can be redirected to attract them to healthier choices that improve their long-term well-being. Decision errors affect policymakers as well, with broader ramifications for the types of policies that are developed and adopted.

Early Evidence on Using Behavioral Economics to Facilitate Weight Loss

Efforts using financial incentives to combat obesity began in the 1970s with seminal works by Bob Jeffery (Jeffery, Thompson, & Wing, 1978; Jeffrey, Gerber, Rosenthal, & Lundquist, 1983). Jeffery's early work was motivated by an observation from an earlier study in which participants deposited money and other valuables with a therapist and signed contracts stating that the return of valuables was contingent on progress toward prespecified goals. Even though participants received no training in weight loss or maintenance strategies, they lost an average of 14.5 kg (Mann, 1972). This small initial study lacked control groups and long-term follow-up but provided interesting proof of concept.

In the first study of deposit or precommitment contracts by Jeffery et al. (1978), participants who responded to an advertisement for a weight loss program were informed that study participation required a deposit of $200 (1974 dollars), which would be fully refunded contingent on satisfactory weight loss. After an 11-session, 10-week program, those who received incentives for losing weight or for limiting calories lost significantly more weight than those who received incentives for attending sessions. Of the participants in the former two groups, 70% lost more than 6.8 kg (15 pounds). The major limitation to this approach was that only 15% of the prospective participants who responded to the initial newspaper advertisement enrolled in the study, suggesting that deposit contracts that require participants to commit substantial funds up front are very effective for people who agree to participate, but that this requirement likely deters a substantial portion of high-risk participants from entering.

A subsequent study tested the effects on weight loss of deposit contracts of $30,

$150, or $300, with the deposits returned based on either individual or group weight loss over 15 weeks (Jeffrey et al., 1983). Participants in the intervention group could win $1, $5, or $10 per pound lost, up to a maximum cumulative weight loss of 2 pounds per week (either individual or group average). Mean weight loss was large in all three groups but did not differ significantly based on contract size. However, the proportion that reached the goal of 13.6 kg (30 pounds) weight loss was significantly higher in the larger incentive groups.

Because it is more difficult to lose larger amounts of weight, the investigators also tested whether a deposit contract with increasing payments ($5, $10, $20, $40, $75) for each 5-pound increment of weight loss would be more effective than offering $30 for each 5-pound increment of weight loss (Jeffrey, Bjornson-Benson, Rosenthal, Kurth, & Dunn, 1984). Participants in both conditions were also offered a maintenance program requiring $100 deposit, returned in $25 increments for attendance at follow-up visits every 3 months. The increasing contract resulted in qualitatively larger weight losses during the weight loss phase, but the maintenance program did not prevent weight gain, possibly because the magnitude of the deposit contract for maintenance was small, with feedback only every 3 months.

Jeffrey et al. (1993) found that paying participants for weight loss using direct payments was less effective than deposit contracts. In a randomized trial, the authors found that cash payments of up to $25 per week for making 100% of proportional progress toward the goal, $12.50 for 50% of goal, and $2.50 for not gaining weight did not result in greater weight loss in the payment group than among control subjects.

Studies that have shown no effects on either initial weight loss or maintenance typically used incentives of small magnitude or targeted behaviors, such as attendance at weight loss programs, that in and of themselves do not ensure weight loss (Jeffrey, Wing, Thorson, & Burton, 1998). In recent years, weight loss incentives have become a common feature in programs used by employers and health plans, and there have been a variety of start-ups focused on creating incentive-based programs online to potentially help people lose weight.

Recent and Emerging Evidence on Using Behavioral Economics to Facilitate Weight Loss

Over the past decade, our group has conducted a series of studies evaluating approaches that incorporate insights from behavioral economics into incentives designed to promote weight loss. Many of these studies were randomized controlled trials and were conducted in real-world settings, including wellness programs, and with diverse patient populations.

In a 16-week weight loss study, 57 participants with obesity in a Veterans Affairs medical center clinic were randomly assigned to a control group or to one of two financial incentive programs (Volpp et al., 2008). Participants in the incentive groups were asked to lose 7.3 kg (16 pounds) over the 16-week study and were given a daily weight target. In one incentive group, participants were offered a daily regret lottery, in which they were eligible for an approximately one in five chance of winning $10, or a one in 100 chance of winning $100, but only if they had met their weight loss target on the previous day. A regret lottery uses the concept of anticipated regret by informing participants whether they won and whether they would have won if they had met their goal. In the second incentive group, participants were offered a deposit contract in which they could contribute between $0.01 and $3.00 that would be returned and matched 1:1 with a $3.00 per day bonus for each day that they met their weight goal. After 16 weeks, participants in the control group had lost an average of 1.8 kg. Compared to the control group, the two incentive groups had lost significantly more weight, with a mean weight loss of 6.0 kg in the regret lottery group ($p = .02$) and 6.4 kg in the deposit contract group ($p < .01$) (Figure 32.1). About half of those in the incentive groups met their 7.3 kg (16 pounds) weight loss goal, compared to only about 10% of those in the control group. Participants were followed for an additional 3 months (framed

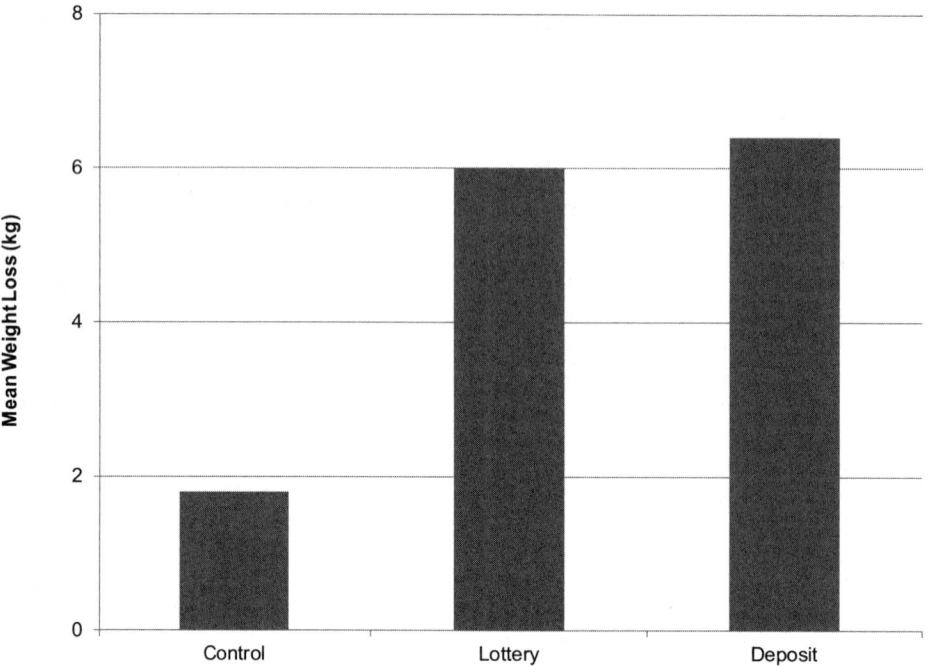

FIGURE 32.1. Weight loss in financial incentive groups compared to control after the 16-week intervention. Based on Volpp et al. (2008).

as a maintenance period), and while the incentive groups still lost more weight than the control group (i.e., the regret lottery group lost 4.2 kg, the deposit contract group lost 2.8 kg, and the control group lost 2.0 kg), differences were no longer statistically significant (Figure 32.2). This study demonstrated that financial incentives could be designed using insights from behavioral economics to promote weight loss in the short term and that evaluation of incentives over longer periods was needed.

In a follow-up study, 66 participants were randomly assigned to a control group or one of two deposit contract incentive groups in a 32-week weight loss program (John et al., 2011). Participants in both deposit contract groups could contribute between $0.01 and $3.00 per day and get their money back, plus a 1:1 match if they met their daily weight loss goal. The two groups differed only in that one group was told that weeks 25–32 were for "weight loss maintenance," whereas the other group was told it was a 32-week weight loss study. After 32 weeks, participants in the control group had lost a

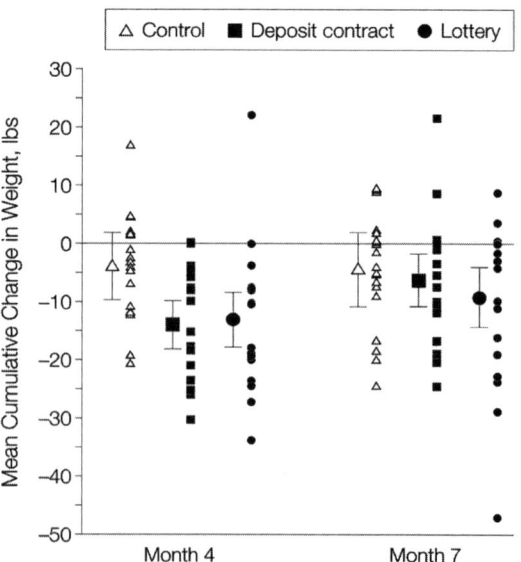

FIGURE 32.2. Weight loss by arm in control and incentive groups from enrollment to the end of 7 months. Data from Volpp et al. (2008).

mean of 0.5 kg, whereas participants in the incentive groups had lost significantly more, with a mean weight loss of 4.0 kg ($p = .04$) (no difference between intervention arms). Participants were followed for 9 additional months and differences were no longer significant, with the control group losing a mean of 0.1 kg, and the participants in the deposit contract groups losing a mean of 0.5 kg ($p = .76$) (Figure 32.3).

Although both of these studies suggest that financial incentives promote weight loss, many employers use premium adjustments (increases or decreases to health insurance payments) as their standard approach to using financial incentives for health promotion. There is little evidence evaluating the effectiveness of this practice. To examine this approach, we conducted one of the first prospective clinical trials of the effectiveness of premium-based financial incentives to promote weight loss (Patel, Asch, Troxel, et al., 2016). We enrolled 197 employees with a BMI of 30 kg/m^2 or greater in a workplace wellness program and gave them a goal of losing 5% of their initial weight over the next year. Weight scales were made available at several locations within the workplace, and participants were encouraged to use them as often as they wished. Participants were randomly assigned to a control group with no other intervention or to one of three financial incentive groups. Two intervention groups were offered a premium reduction of $550 if they achieved their weight loss goal by 1 year. The "delayed" group would receive the premium adjustment in the following year, spread across each pay period. The "immediate" group would have their premiums adjusted as soon as the weight loss goal was met. A third intervention group was offered a daily lottery with about a one in five chance of winning $10 and a one in 100 chance of winning $100. To be eligible

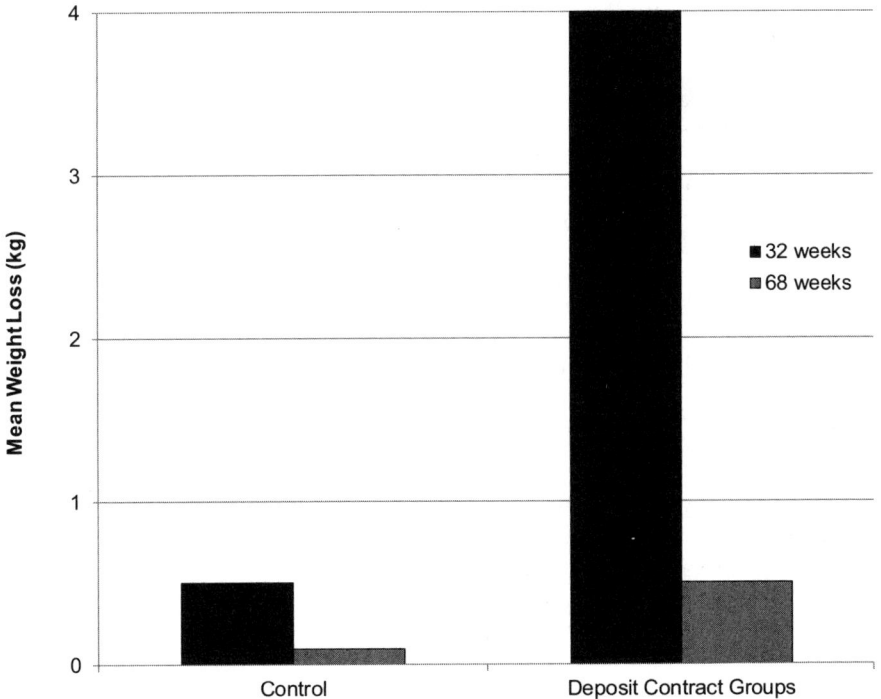

FIGURE 32.3. Mean weight losses at 32 and 68 weeks of participants randomly assigned to (1) control group; (2) deposit contract (DC) group that was informed that the 32-week intervention was divided into weight loss and weight loss maintenance; and (3) DC group that was only informed of one 32-week phase of treatment. Participants were followed up 36 weeks after treatment termination (i.e., week 68). From John et al. (2011).

to win each day, participants had to weigh in and be on track to lose 5% of their initial weight loss by 6 months, with maintenance for the subsequent 6 months. Unlike our prior studies, we were not able to provide regret feedback on occasions when participants won the lottery but did not weigh in, because we did not have employee schedules, and it was unclear if their not weighing in was due to nonadherence or to a day off. After 1 year in the program, on average, none of the intervention approaches showed a significant degree of weight loss. The control group gained < 0.1 kg, the delayed premium adjustment group lost 0.5 kg, the immediate premium adjustment group lost 0.6 kg, and the lottery incentive group lost 0.5 kg. On average, employees did not use the workplace weight scales often. The proportion of participants in the control group and both premium adjustment groups who weighed in at least once a week dropped from nearly 50% at the beginning of the study to 10% by week 6. The frequency of weekly weigh-ins in the daily lottery group began at near 90% and steadily declined to 25% by 6 months.

The relative ineffectiveness of premium-based financial incentives is not surprising, given their design (Patel, Asch, & Volpp, 2016). Such incentives are typically hidden in paychecks that are directly deposited in bank accounts and may go unnoticed by the individual. While a $550 incentive seems like a large amount, it is only $20 in each biweekly paycheck. Typically, these incentives are administered on an all-or-nothing basis, contingent on meeting a specific threshold, such as a BMI ≤ 25 kg/m^2, meaning that those who are close to the goal will try hard, but those who are further away have little chance of succeeding. Most employers use premium adjustments to deploy financial incentives because the infrastructure to do so is already in place, despite the fact that the evidence on their effectiveness in unknown. This study suggests that the standard approach of using premium-based incentives is not effective and that employers should consider alternatives.

Our group has demonstrated successful approaches for using financial incentives within the employer setting by using cash or check payments instead of premium adjustments. In one study, 105 employees were randomly assigned to a control arm, an individual incentive arm, or a group incentive arm for a 24-week weight loss program (Kullgren et al., 2013). All participants were given the goal of losing 0.4 kg each week and were asked to weigh in at work each month. Participants in the individual incentive arm could receive $100 at each weigh-in if they met their monthly weight goal. Participants in the group incentive arm were told that $500 would be split among five employees, but only those who met their monthly weight goal would receive a share of the money. After 24 weeks, the control arm had lost a mean of 0.5 kg. Participants in the individual incentive arm had lost a mean of 1.7 kg, but this loss was not significantly different from the control group ($p = .34$). However, the group incentive arm lost 4.8 kg, which was significantly more than the control group ($p = < .01$). After an additional 12 weeks of follow-up, the control group had a mean weight loss of 0.3 kg. The individual incentive arm had a mean weight loss of 0.8 kg, which was not different from control. However, the group incentive arm had a mean weight loss of 3.4 kg, which was still significantly different from the control condition ($p = .02$) (Kullgren et al., 2013).

In another study, we randomly assigned 281 overweight and obese adults to a control group or to one of three incentive groups for a 13-week physical activity program (Patel, Asch, Rosin, et al., 2016). All participants tracked their daily step counts using their smartphones and were given the goal of achieving 7,000 steps per day. Participants in each of the three incentive arms were offered the same magnitude incentive, $1.40 per day, and were told that accumulated earnings would be sent via a check at the end of each month. However, the incentive in each group was framed differently. In the standard gain incentive group, participants were told that they could earn $1.40 each day they achieved the goal. In the regret lottery incentive group, participants were in a daily regret lottery in which they had about a one in five chance of winning $5 and a one in 100 chance of winning $50, which averages to about $1.40 per day. In the loss-framing incentive group, participants were told at the beginning of each month that $42 had been placed in a virtual account and that they would lose $1.40 each day the goal was not achieved. During the 13-week intervention, participants in the control arm achieved their daily step goal about 30% of the time. Participants in the standard gain incentive and regret lottery incentive achieved the goal 35% and 36% of the time, respectively, but neither group was significantly different from the control group. However, in the loss-framing group, participants achieved the goal 45% of the time, a 50% relative increase, which was significantly greater than the control arm ($p = .001$). This study demonstrated how loss framing can be used to motivate behavior change. It is also one of the first studies to do so without requiring participants to put their own money at risk using a deposit contract. This aspect of the study is important because there is evidence that fewer people are willing to engage in deposit-contract-based incentives than in reward-based incentives (Halpern et al., 2015)

Our group has several other studies that are currently in the field or in press for publication. In one study, we are testing how differing degrees of employer-based matching of deposit contracts affects participation rates. Another study, in collaboration with Weight Watchers, is evaluating how differing degrees of employer subsidization of the cost of Weight Watchers membership (between 50% and 100%) affect enrollment, ongoing participation, and weight loss. In a second study with Weight Watchers, incentives are being evaluated for their role in facilitating the maintenance of weight loss. In addition, we are beginning to test how insights from behavioral economics could be incorporated into programs that focus more on social incentives, by asking participants to form teams with family members or friends and to participate in a gamification-based intervention that incorporates insights from behavioral economics.

Summary

Health behaviors play an important role in weight management and overall health. A growing body of evidence demonstrates that individuals typically do not make decisions using standard economic frameworks and instead have predictably irrational tendencies in regards to their decisions, behaviors, and habits. Public and private sector efforts to improve programs focused on weight management could benefit from incorporating insights from behavioral economics to design incentives that address predictable barriers to behavior change.

References

Glanz, K., & Bishop, D. B. (2010). The role of behavioral science theory in development and implementation of public health interventions [Review]. *Annual Review of Public Health, 31,* 399–418.

Halpern, S. D., French, B., Small, D. S., Saulsgiver, K., Harhay, M. O., Audrain-McGovern, J., et al. (2015). Randomized trial of four financial-incentive programs for smoking cessation. *New England Journal of Medicine, 372*(22), 2108–2117.

Jeffery, R. W., Bjornson-Benson, W. M., Rosenthal, B. S., Kurth, C. L., & Dunn, M. M. (1984). Effectiveness of monetary contracts with two repayment schedules of weight reduction in men and women from self-referred and population samples. *Behavior Therapy, 15,* 273–279.

Jeffery, R. W., Gerber, W. M., Rosenthal, B. S., & Lindquist, R. A. (1983). Monetary contracts in weight control: Effectiveness of group and individual contracts of varying size. *Journal of Consulting and Clinical Psychology, 51*(2), 242–248.

Jeffery, R. W., Thompson, P. D., & Wing, R. R. (1978). Effects on weight reduction of strong monetary contracts for calorie restriction or weight loss. *Behaviour Research and Therapy, 16*(5), 363–369.

Jeffery, R. W., Wing, R. R., Thorson, C., & Burton, L. R. (1998). Use of personal trainers and financial incentives to increase exercise in a behavioral weight-loss program. *Journal of Consulting and Clinical Psychology, 66*(5), 777–783.

Jeffery, R. W., Wing, R. R., Thorson, C., Burton, L. R., Raether, C., Harvey, J., et al. (1993). Strengthening behavioral interventions for weight loss: A randomized trial of food provision and monetary incentives. *Journal of Consulting and Clinical Psychology, 61*(6), 1038–1045.

John, L., Loewenstein, G., Troxel, A., Norton, L., Fassbender, J., & Volpp, K. G. (2011). Financial incentives for extended weight loss: A randomized, controlled trial. *Journal of General Internal Medicine, 26*(6), 621–626.

Kahneman, D., & Tversky, A. (1979). Prospect theory: An analysis of decision under risk. *Econometrica, 47*(2), 263–291.

Kullgren, J. T., Troxel, A. B., Loewenstein, G., Asch, D. A., Norton, L. A., Wesby, L., et al. (2013). Individual- versus group-based financial incentives for weight loss: A randomized, controlled trial. *Annals of Internal Medicine, 158*(7), 505–514.

Lee, I. M., Shiroma, E. J., Lobelo, F., Puska, P., Blair,

S. N., & Katzmarzyk, P. T. (2012). Impact of physical inactivity on the world's major non-communicable diseases. *Lancet, 380,* 219–229.

Loewenstein, G., Brennan, T., & Volpp, K. G. (2007). Asymmetric paternalism to improve health behaviors. *Journal of the American Medical Association, 298*(20), 2415–2417.

Madison, K., Schmidt, H., & Volpp, K. G. (2013). Smoking, obesity, health insurance, and health incentives in the Affordable Care Act. *Journal of the American Medical Association, 310*(2), 143–144.

Mann, R. A. (1972). The behavior-therapeutic use of contingency contracting to control an adult behavior problem: Weight control. *Journal of Applied Behavior Analysis, 5*(2), 99–109.

McGinnis, J. M., Williams-Russo, P., & Knickman, J. R. (2002). The case for more active policy attention to health promotion. *Health Affairs, 21*(2), 78–93.

O'Donoghue, T., & Rabin, M. (2000). The economics of immediate gratification. *Journal of Behavioral Decision Making, 13*(2), 233–250.

Patel, M. S., Asch, D. A., Rosin, R., Small, D. S., Bellamy, S. L., Heuer, J., et al. (2016). Framing financial incentives to increase physical activity among overweight and obese adults: A randomized, controlled trial. *Annals of Internal Medicine, 164*(6), 385–394.

Patel, M. S., Asch, D. A., Troxel, A. B., Fletcher, M. A., Osman-Koss, R., Brady, J. L., et al. (2016). Premium-based financial incentives did not promote workplace weight loss in a

Patel, M. S., Asch, D. A., & Volpp, K. G. (2016, March 6). Paying employees to lose weight. Retrieved from *www.nytimes.com/2016/03/06/opinion/sunday/paying-employees-to-lose-weight.html.*

Schroeder, S. A. (2007). We can do better: Improving the health of the American people. *New England Journal of Medicine, 357*(12), 1221–1228.

Thaler, R. H., & Sunstein, C. R. (2003). Libertarian paternalism. *American Economic Review, 93*(2), 175–179.

Volpp, K. G., Asch, D. A., Galvin, R., & Loewenstein, G. (2011). Redesigning employee health incentives: Lessons from behavioral economics. *New England Journal of Medicine, 365*(5), 388–390.

Volpp, K. G., John, L. K., Troxel, A. B., Norton, L., Fassbender, J., & Loewenstein, G. (2008). Financial incentive-based approaches for weight loss: A randomized trial. *Journal of the American Medical Association, 300*(22), 2631–2637.

Zeelenberg, M., & Pieters, R. (2004). Consequences of regret aversion in real life: The case of the Dutch postcode lottery. *Organizational Behavior and Human Decision Processes, 93,* 155–168.

CHAPTER 33

Nonsurgical Interventional Modalities for the Treatment of Obesity

Jacqueline M. Soegaard Ballester
Casey H. Halpern
Noel N. Williams
Kristoffel R. Dumon

Obesity remains a significant problem in the United States, as more than one-third of the American population is obese (Ogden, Carroll, Kit, & Flegal, 2014). Currently, bariatric surgery is the best-known treatment for morbid obesity (body mass index [BMI] > 40 or BMI > 35 with comorbidities). For patients with morbid obesity, multiple meta-analyses have shown bariatric surgery to be more effective than diet and exercise or pharmacological treatment (Gloy et al., 2013). However, the costs associated with bariatric surgery are prohibitive, which may be one reason why, worldwide, less than 1% of patients with morbid obesity who qualify for bariatric surgery actually receive it (Angrisani et al., 2015; Buchwald & Oien, 2013). Evidently, to increase access to treatment for the remainder of the morbidly obese and obese populations, as well as alleviate the financial burden of bariatric surgery, alternate modalities are needed. Nonsurgical interventional modalities present increasingly promising and exciting options for the treatment of obesity.

Recently, the U.S. Food and Drug Administration (FDA) approved the first nonsurgical interventional therapies for obesity. Three intragastric balloon systems were approved for use in patients with a BMI of 30–40 kg/m². Additionally, the AspireAssist system for gastric aspiration was approved on June 14, 2016 for use in patients with a BMI of 35–55 kg/m². Finally, several endoscopic gastric suturing techniques have been developed using both FDA-approved endoscopic devices and devices undergoing clinical trials for FDA approval.

The current nonsurgical interventional modalities for the treatment of obesity can be divided into six main categories: (1) space-occupying devices, (2) restrictive procedures, (3) bypass liners, (4) aspiration therapy, (5) electrical stimulation, and (6) other therapies. These categories are listed along with the associated devices in Table 33.1 and represented visually in Figure 33.1. Notable outcomes for selected devices, as reported in the pivotal clinical trial or largest study of each treatment, are shown in

Figure 33.2. At the end of the chapter, Appendix 33.1 lists detailed outcomes for the three FDA-approved balloons and the one FDA-approved aspiration therapy device. Appendix 33.2 provides links to webpages containing images of each type of treatment discussed in this chapter. In the following sections, selected examples of each treatment approach are described in turn.

These devices and approaches can be used as primary treatments for obesity, as bridge therapies to bariatric surgery, or as revisional treatments after bariatric surgery (Chiang & Ryou, 2016). This chapter provides gastrointestinal surgeons, endoscopists, and other readers with a comprehensive overview of nonsurgical interventional modalities for the primary treatment of obesity. Hopefully, these modalities will increase flexibility in tailoring multimodality treatment approaches to each individual patient and help address the current vastly unmet needs among patients with obesity and morbid obesity.

TABLE 33.1. Devices Associated with Nonsurgical Interventional Treatments for Obesity

Procedure	Device
	Space-occupying devices
Intragastric balloons	
FDA status: approved	ORBERA; ReShape Dual Balloon; Obalon
FDA status: not approved	Elipse; Heliosphere; Silimed Gastric Balloon; Endball; Adjustable Totally Implantable Intragastric Prosthesis (ATIIP)—Endogast; Ulllorex
Other space-occupying therapies	TransPyloric Shuttle; Full Sense Device; SatiSphere
	Restrictive procedures
Endoscopic sleeve gastroplasty	Apollo OverStitch
Primary obesity surgery endoluminal (POSE)	Incisionless Operating Platform (IOP); G-Cath EZ Suture Anchor Delivery Catheter
Endoscopic gastroplasty	EndoCinch; RESTORe Suturing System
Transoral gastroplasty	TOGA System
Articulating circular endoscopic stapling procedure	ACE stapler
	Bypass liners
Duodenal–jejunal bypass liner	EndoBarrier
Gastro–duodeno–jejunal bypass liner	ValenTx
Aspiration therapy	AspireAssist System
	Electrical stimulation
Gastric stimulation[a]	Enterra System; abiliti system; DIAMOND System
Vagal blockade[a]	Enteromedics Maestro Rechargeable System
	Other therapies
Magnet compression anastomoses	Incisionless Anastomotic System (IAS)
Duodenal mucosal resurfacing	Revita
Intragastric botulinum toxin-A	

[a]Currently requires open or laparoscopic placement.

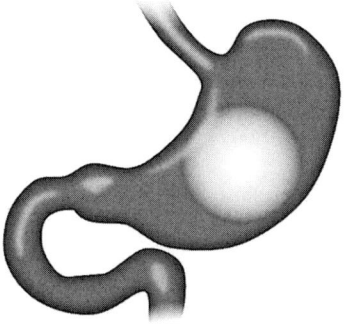

A. Space-Occupying Device
(Single Balloon System Depicted)

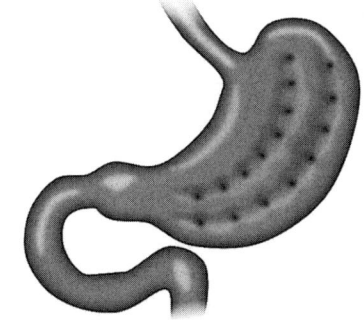

B. Restrictive Procedure
(Endoscopic Sleeve Gastroplasty Depicted)

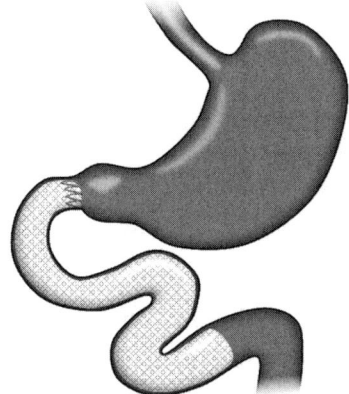

C. Bypass Liner
(Endobarrier System Depicted)

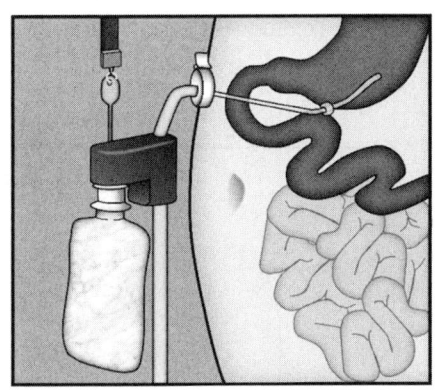

D. Aspiration Therapy

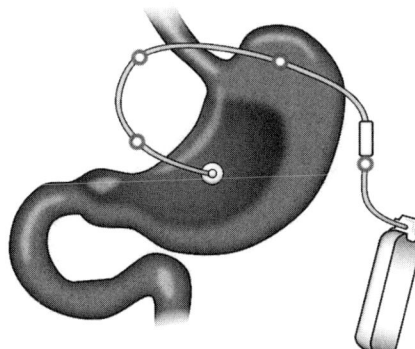

E. Gastric Stimulation

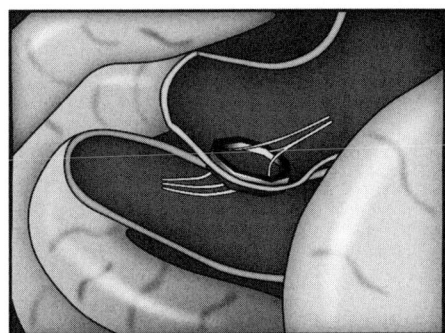

F. Magnetic Compression Bypass Anastomosis
(Incisionless Anastomotic System Depicted)

FIGURE 33.1. Visual representations of selected nonsurgical interventional treatments for obesity.

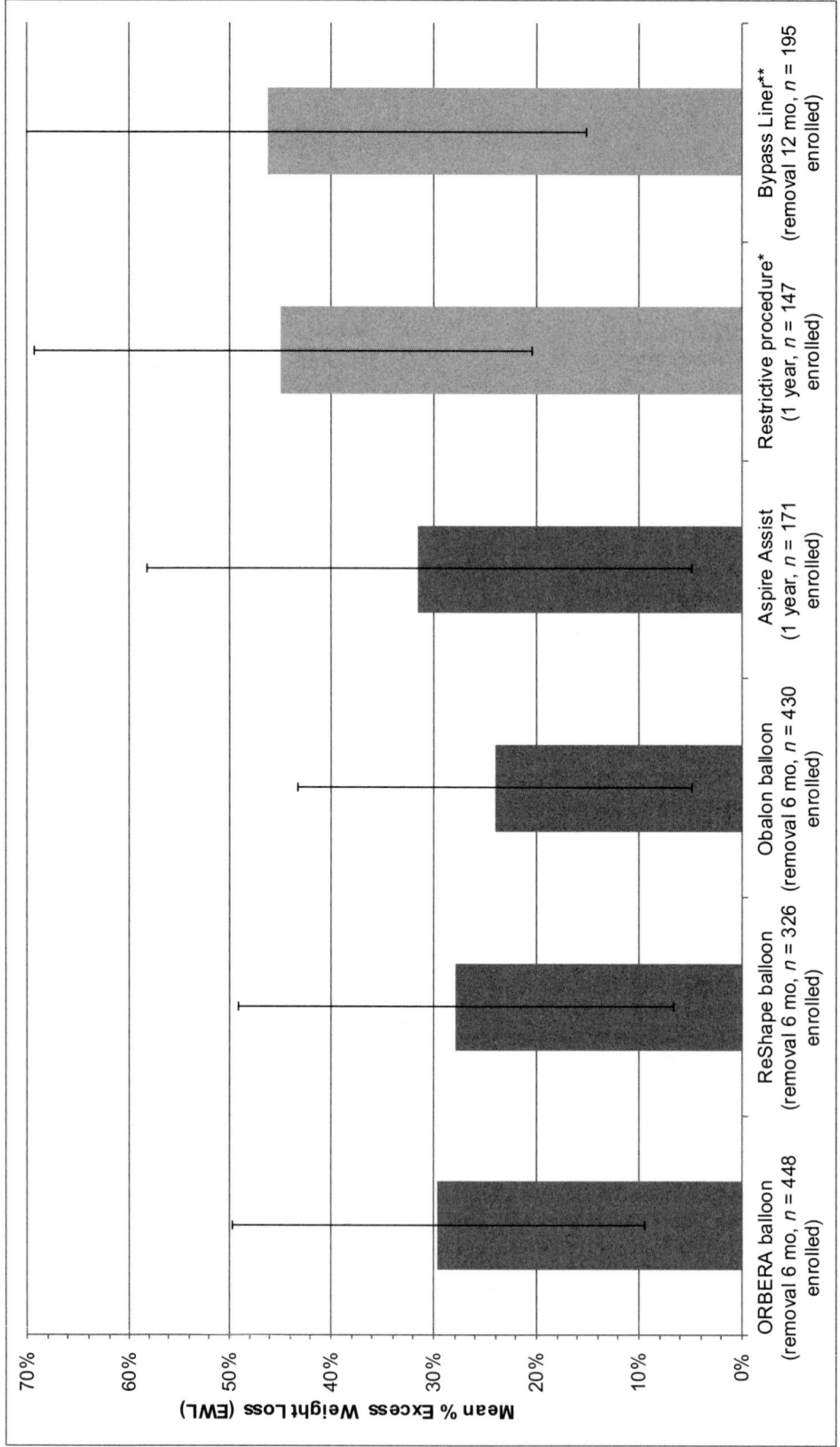

FIGURE 33.2a. Mean ± *SD* % EWL for select nonsurgical procedures as reported in the pivotal clinical trial that resulted in FDA approval (for FDA-approved devices, dark gray bars) or in the largest study of each (for non-FDA-approved devices, light gray bars). Data label refers to the time point of measurement of % EWL. Removal means upon removal of device. *% EWL 1 year after primary obesity surgery Endoluminal (POSE) procedure. **% EWL upon removal of the EndoBarrier duodenal–jejunal bypass liner.

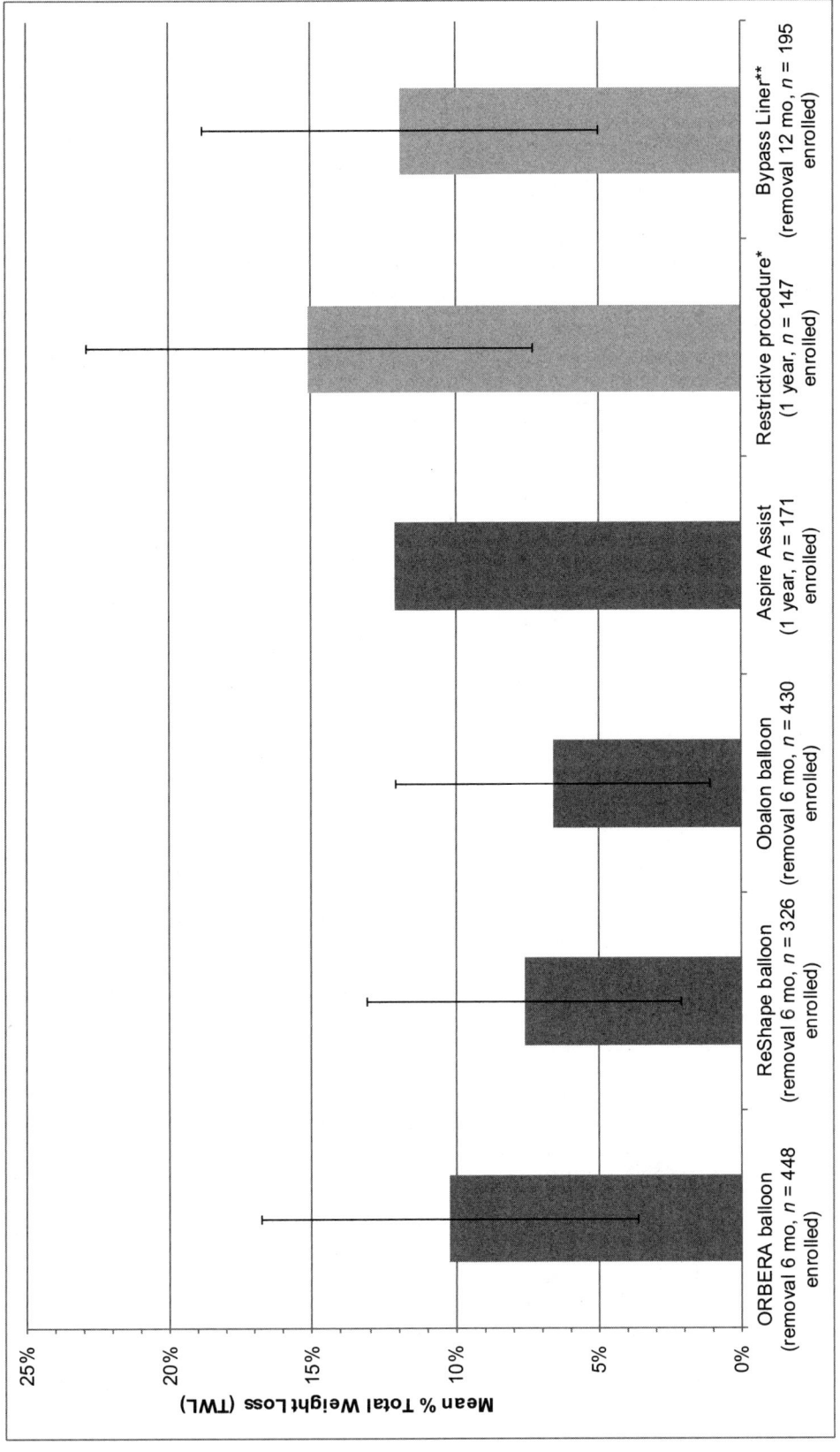

FIGURE 33.2b. Mean ± SD % TWL for select nonsurgical procedures, as reported in the pivotal clinical trial that resulted in FDA approval (for FDA-approved devices, dark gray bars) or in the largest study of each (for non-FDA-approved devices, light gray bars). Data label refers to the time point of measurement of % TWL. Removal means upon removal of device. *% TWL 1 year after primary obesity surgery Endoluminal (POSE) procedure. **% TWL upon removal of the EndoBarrier duodenal–jejunal bypass liner.

Space-Occupying Devices

Intragastric Balloons

Intragastric balloons are endoscopically placed air-, helium-, or fluid-filled silicone balloons that sit in the stomach and occupy space that could otherwise be filled by food. The FDA currently requires that these balloons be removed 6 months after implantation (U.S. FDA, 2015a). Failure to do so could potentially increase the chance of balloon deflation, which could lead to complications such as device migration and bowel obstruction (Öztürk, Akinci, & Kurt, 2010).

Some balloons consist of a single spherical or ovular shape (Figure 33.3a), whereas others consist of two connected spheres (Figure 33.3b). The single balloons are typically 500–750 ml (range: 250–950 ml) in size. The only dual balloon on the market (the ReShape Integrated Dual Balloon System) consists of two connected 450-ml balloons. Most balloons are placed endoscopically under light sedation, whereas others are swallowed (along with an attached inflation catheter) as a pill (e.g., Obalon, Elipse, Ullorex). Of these, the Obalon system is approved for placement of up to three balloons simultaneously. Another balloon system (Spatz3) includes a retractable inflation tube that allows for balloon volume adjustments after initial placement and is being investigated for removal 12 months after implantation. Whereas most balloons require endoscopic removal after completion of therapy, the Elipse balloon contains a self-releasing valve that can be set to open at a predetermined endpoint, thereby emptying the balloon and allowing it to be excreted from the body.

Studies have found intragastric balloons to be safe and effective in the short term. Typical complications include nausea, vomiting, and stomach pain that resolve within 72 hours. More serious adverse events include balloon migration and bowel perforation due to the break and distal passage of a balloon's safety ring, which can be life-threatening (Al-Zubaidi, Alghamdi, Alzobydi, Dhiloon, & Qureshi, 2015; Öztürk, Yavuz, & Atalay, 2015). In most studies, percent excess weight loss (% EWL) at the time of device removal ranges from 30 to 50% (Genco et al., 2015; Lopez-Nava, Bautista-Castaño, Jimenez-Baños, & Fernandez-Corbelle, 2015; Ponce, Quebbemann, & Patterson, 2013). However, few studies have performed long-term follow-up after balloon removal, and there are reports of weight regain following the removal (Kotzampassi, Grosomanidis, Papakostas, Penna, & Eleftheriadis, 2012).

The three intragastric balloons currently approved by the FDA for the treatment of obesity are the ORBERA balloon (P140008, approved August 5, 2015), the ReShape Dual Balloon system (P140012, approved July 28, 2015), and the Obalon balloon (P160001, approved September 8, 2016) (U.S. FDA, 2015a, 2016a).

ORBERA Intragastric Balloon System (FDA Status: Approved)

The ORBERA Intragastric Balloon System (Apollo EndoSurgery, Austin, Texas), formerly known as the BioEnterics Intragastric Balloon (BIB), is a spherical silicone balloon that is placed endoscopically in the gastric fundus and inflated using 500–750 ml of saline (Kumar, 2015). The ORBERA balloon was studied in a meta-analysis of 3,608 patients. The median % EWL upon removal of the device 6 months after implantation was 32.1 (95% confidence interval [CI] 26.9–37.4), and the median percent total body weight loss (% TWL) was 12.2 (95% CI 10–14.3). Four percent (4.2%) of the patients required early removal, 0.8% reported adverse events (nausea, vomiting, and bowel obstruction), and 0.1% reported gastric perforations (Imaz, Martínez-Cervell, García-Álvarez, Sendra-Gutiérrez, & González-Enríquez, 2008).

The FDA approved the ORBERA balloon in August 2015 after the pivotal multicenter randomized IB-005 trial, which compared treatment with the ORBERA balloon for 6 months against lifestyle intervention alone (A Study of BioEnterics® Intragastric Balloon [BIB®]) System to Assist in the Weight Management of Obese Subjects; ClinicalTrials.gov identifier: NCT00730327; $N = 448$ enrolled). Upon device removal at 6 months, patients in the balloon group achieved a significantly greater EWL than controls (29.6 ± 20.2% vs. 9.5 ± 14.4%) and a greater % TWL (10.2 ± 6.6% vs. 3.3 ± 5.0%). Six months after device removal, EWL and

TWL had decreased to 22.1 ± 22.5% and 7.6 ± 7.5%, respectively. Of the 125 patients in the balloon arm, 10% experienced serious adverse events, and 18.8% required early removal due to device intolerance or adverse events (U.S. FDA, 2015b).

One study evaluated the long-term effects of ORBERA. One hundred and twenty-two patients completed 5 years of follow-up. Among these patients, mean EWL was 58 ± 19% upon removal at 6 months, 39 ± 14% 1 year after removal, 25 ± 8% 2 years after removal, and 17 ± 8% at 5 years follow-up. Mean TWL was 30 ± 9 kg upon removal, 21 ± 8 kg 1 year after removal, 14 ± 7 kg 2 years after removal, and 9 ± 6 kg 5 years after removal (Kotzampassi et al., 2012; TWL was not given as a percent). To contex-

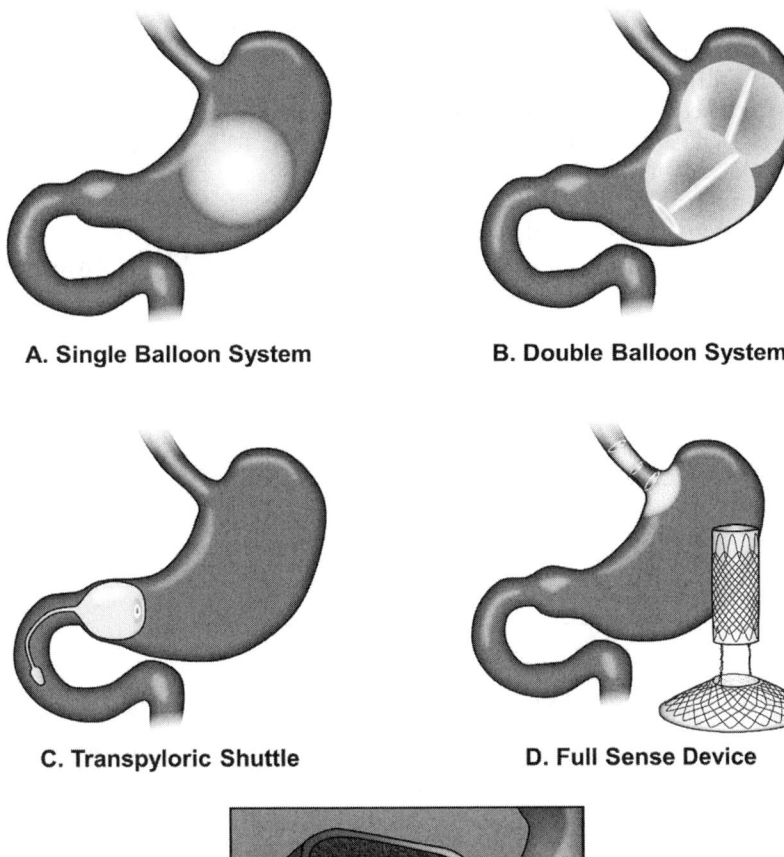

FIGURE 33.3. Visual representations of selected intragastric space-occupying devices for the treatment of obesity.

tualize the efficacy of this system, we compared the 5-year weight loss outcomes of the ORBERA balloon against outcome data for Roux-en-Y gastric bypass (RYGB), the current gold standard in weight loss surgery, as depicted in Figure 33.4 (Obeid et al., 2016).

Some investigators have tried treatment via successive or extended balloon placements. The initial study evaluating the use of successive balloons placed a second balloon in 19 patients (16% of participants in a prospective, nonrandomized multicenter study) at the patients' own requests. The results showed a significant reduction in the effectiveness of the second consecutive balloon and no weight loss effect from subsequent balloon placements (Dumonceau et al., 2010). After removal of the first balloon ($n = 19$), EWL (mean, interquartile range [IQR]) was 49 (27–61) % and TWL (mean, IQR in kg) was 15 (12–23) kg. After removal of the second balloon, EWL dropped to 30 (2.4–42) and TWL to 9.0 (1.0–13) kg. At final follow-up, there was no significant difference between the single and repeat treatment groups.

In contrast, a subsequent prospective randomized study ($N = 100$) revealed significantly greater weight loss among patients randomized to balloon removal at 6 months followed by a subsequent 6-month balloon placement 1 month thereafter (51.9 ± 24.6 % EWL), compared to patients randomized to balloon removal at 6 months followed by 7 months of diet therapy (25.1 ± 26.2 % EWL; Genco et al., 2010). Another study that followed patients with balloons left in place for longer than 6 months suggested a nonsignificant trend toward continued weight loss until the 14-month mark (Genco et al., 2015). Consistent with these findings, the FDA has not yet approved the

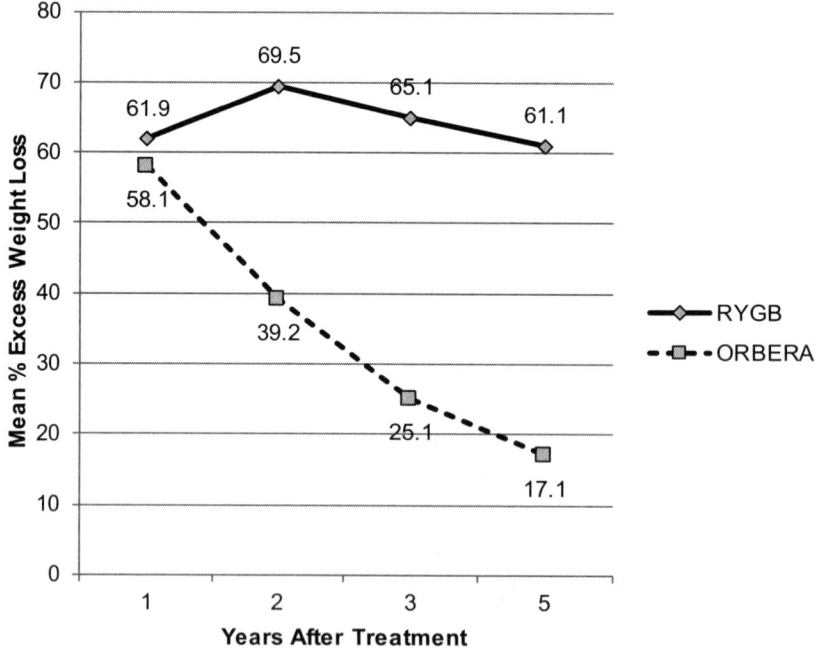

FIGURE 33.4. Five-year postinterventional weight loss comparison. ORBERA balloon: $n = 122$ (Kotzampassi, Grosomanidis, Papakostas, Penna, & Eleftheriadis, 2012); Roux-en-Y gastric bypass (RYGB): $n = 134$ (Obeid et al., 2016). For balloon patients, "treatment" refers to device implantation; for RYGB patients, "treatment" refers to surgery. From Neylan, Dempsey, Tewksbury, Williams, and Dumon (2016). Endoscopic treatments of obesity: A comprehensive review. *Surgery for Obesity and Related Diseases, 12*(5), 1108–1115. Copyright © 2016 Elsevier. Reprinted by permission.

ORBERA for use in successive implantations or for implantations lasting longer than 6 months.

The ORBERA is the best-studied intragastric balloon and has been evaluated in the context of super-super obesity (BMI ≥ 60 kg/m²; Zerrweck et al., 2012), metabolic effects (Forlano et al., 2010), dietary counseling (Tai et al., 2013), and mental health (Deliopoulou, Konsta, Penna, Papakostas, & Kotzampassi, 2013).

ReShape Dual Balloon System (FDA Status: Approved)

The ReShape Dual Balloon System (ReShape Medical, San Clemente, California) balloon consists of two closely attached, independently filled balloons that hold a combined 900 ml of saline (Figure 33.3b). The purpose of the dual design is to prevent migration if one balloon deflates. The ReShape Integrated Dual Balloon System was evaluated in the pivotal FDA REDUCE trial (A Prospective, Randomized Multicenter Study to Evaluate the Safety and Efficacy of the ReShape Duo Intragastric Balloon System in Obese Subjects; ClinicalTrials.gov identifier: NCT01673698; N = 326 enrolled). Upon balloon removal, 24 weeks after insertion, mean EWL was 27.9 ± 21.3 and TWL was 7.6 ± 5.5 (n = 167). Twenty-four weeks after removal (n = 136), the mean EWL dropped to 18.8% (Ponce et al., 2015; SD and TWL not given). Gastric ulceration was observed in approximately 35% of patients, which is higher than the approximately 0.1% rate of ulceration in ORBERA patients (Imaz et al., 2008). However, a modification was made to the ReShape Duo device during the trial, and the postmodification ulceration rate was 10% (Ponce et al., 2015).

A smaller controlled European study of 30 patients randomized 21 patients to ReShape Dual Balloon therapy for 24 weeks. The mean EWL and TWL (range, SD not given) upon balloon removal were 31.8% and 8.4%, respectively. At 48 weeks (24 weeks after device removal), the balloon group (n = 20) maintained 64% of their excess weight loss (Abu-Dayyeh, Sarmiento, Rajan, Vázquez-Sequeiros, & Gostout, 2014; Ponce et al., 2013).

Obalon Balloon System (FDA Status: Approved)

The Obalon Balloon System (Obalon Therapeutics, Carlsbad, California) consists of a swallowable capsule containing a collapsed, radio-opaque balloon attached to a thin inflation catheter. Using the catheter, the balloon is inflated with gas to its 250-ml capacity once the capsule has been swallowed and its position has been confirmed radiographically. This system is approved for placement of up to three balloons for up to 6 months, at which point the balloons must be deflated and removed endoscopically.

The Obalon System was evaluated in the pivotal SMART (Six Month Adjunctive Weight Reduction Therapy; ClinicalTrials.gov identifier: NCT02235870) prospective double-blinded randomized multicenter trial, which compared placement of up to three Obalon balloons with sham capsules (N = 430). At balloon removal (24 weeks after insertion), mean ± SD % EWL was 24.1 ± 19.2 and % TWL was 6.6 ± 5.1 for patients in the treatment arm (n = 198). However, 24 weeks after removal, patients who had lost weight at the 24-week endpoint had regained 3.2 ± 14.9 % EWL, or 0.9 ± 4.1 % TWL (n = 171). Eight percent of patients (n = 32/419) failed to swallow any capsules. Only one serious device- or procedure-related adverse event was reported (ulceration and gastrointestinal [GI] bleeding). One balloon (0.1% of 985) was found to be deflated during retrieval, but it had not migrated beyond the pylorus (U.S. FDA, 2016b).

Ellipse Intragastric Balloon System (FDA Status: Not Approved, Clinical Trial Underway)

The Elipse Intragastric Balloon System (Allurion Technologies, Wellesley, Massachusetts) is a collapsed balloon encased in a degradable capsule attached to a long, thin, removable delivery catheter. After the capsule has been swallowed and the balloon is located in the stomach, the catheter is used to fill the balloon with saline to its 550 ml capacity. The Elipse contains a self-releasing valve that opens at a preset time point, emptying the balloon and allowing it to be excreted from the body.

A recent abstract reported on a prospective multicenter study of 34 patients who had an Elipse balloon in place for 4 months. All patients were able to swallow the capsules, and all balloons were excreted at the 4-month mark, at which time patients were found to have achieved 37.2 % EWL and 9.5 % TWL (*SD* not reported). Ninety-three percent of the weight loss was maintained at 6-month follow-up (Chuttani et al., 2016). The Elipse balloon is now also undergoing a randomized, multicenter ENLIGHTEN clinical trial (a Randomized, Multi-Center, Phased, Pivotal Safety and Efficacy Study Comparing the Elipse™ Gastric Balloon System vs. Sham for the Treatment of Obese Adults; ClinicalTrials.gov identifier: NCT03261453).

Other Space-Occupying Devices

TransPyloric Shuttle (FDA Status: Not Approved)

The TransPyloric Shuttle (BAROnova, Goleta, California) is an endoluminally delivered, dumbbell-shaped device consisting of a large silicone sphere connected by a flexible catheter to a smaller cylindrical sphere (Figure 33.3c). The smaller sphere enters the duodenal bulb with peristalsis, which pulls the larger sphere to the pylorus and intermittently occludes the pylorus, delaying gastric emptying. One trial enrolled 20 patients and reported a 6-month (n = 10) mean % EWL of 41.0 ± 21.1 and % TWL of 14.5 ± 5.8, with two patients requiring early removal due to persistent gastric ulceration (Marinos, Eliades, Raman Muthusamy, & Greenway, 2014). The TransPyloric Shuttle is undergoing investigation in the ongoing randomized sham-controlled multicenter ENDObesity II trial (ENDObesity® II Study: TransPyloric Shuttle® System for Weight Loss; ClinicalTrials.gov identifier: NCT02518685).

Full Sense Device (FDA Status: Not Approved)

The Full Sense (Baker, Foote, Kemmeter, Walburn LLC, Grand Rapids, Michigan) device is a covered metal stent that is endoscopically placed across the gastroesophageal junction (Figure 33.3d). Theoretically, it induces satiety and fullness by placing pressure on the distal esophagus and gastric cardia. It has not been studied in a published clinical trial (Abu-Dayyeh et al., 2014; ASGE/ASMBS Task Force on Endoscopic Therapy, 2011).

SatiSphere (FDA Status: Not Approved, Trial Terminated Due to Safety Concerns)

The SatiSphere (EndoSphere, Columbus, Ohio) consists of a wire that runs through several mesh spheres that sit in the lumen of the distal stomach and duodenum in a "string-of-pearls" configuration (Figure 33.3e). It is designed to slow the transit of food. One study that evaluated 21 SatiSphere patients was prematurely terminated due to high migration rates; the device migrated in 10 patients, requiring two laparoscopic operations (Sauer et al., 2013).

Restrictive Procedures

Endoscopic Sleeve Gastroplasty

With this procedure, the Apollo OverStitch (Apollo EndoSurgery, Austin, Texas) is used to place full-thickness stitches in a manner designed to mimic sleeve gastrectomy. Closely spaced sutures are placed through the gastric wall from the prepyloric antrum to the gastroesophageal (GE) junction, effectively isolating a tubular lumen from the rest of the stomach volume (Abu Dayyeh, Rajan, & Gostout, 2013). The OverStitch is an FDA-approved endoscopic suturing device.

The largest published study (N = 20) reported a 6-month mean % EWL of 53.9 ± 26.3 and % TWL of 17.8 ± 7.5, with very few complications (Lopez-Nava, Galvão, da Bautista-Castaño, et al., 2015). A subsequent abstract from the same researchers reported on a multicenter study of 242 patients, in which the mean % TWL was 16.8 ± 6.4, 18.2 ± 10.1, and 19.8 ± 11.6 at 6, 12, and 18 months postprocedure, respectively (n = 137, 53, and 30, respectively). Five patients experienced serious complications, including two perigastric fluid collections requiring antibiotics and percutaneous drainage, a splenic laceration resulting in self-limited bleeding, a pulmonary embolism, and a pneumoperitoneum and pneumothorax requiring chest-tube placement (Lopez-Nava et al.,

2016). This procedure is being evaluated in the United States in the multicenter PROMISE trial (Primary Obesity Multicenter Incisionless Suturing Evaluation: The PROMISE Trial; ClinicalTrials.gov identifier: NCT01662024). Unpublished trial results reported on the trial website for the 15 subjects completing the study indicate that 12 months following the procedure, the mean % EWL was 70.8 (range 62.8–78.8) and the mean % TWL was 18.1 (range 15.8–20.4).

Primary Obesity Surgery Endoluminal

The Incisionless Operating Platform (USGI Medical, San Clemente, California) is used to create 8–10 full-thickness tissue plications in the gastric fundus, in two parallel ridges, until the fundic apex is brought down to the level of the GE junction (Kumar, 2015; Mathus-Vliegen, 2014). The largest study of this technique enrolled 147 patients and reported a 1 year (n = 116) mean % EWL of 44.9 ± 24.4 and % TWL of 15.1 ± 7.8, with very few complications (Lopez-Nava, Bautista-Castaño, Jimenez, de Grado, & Fernandez-Corbelle, 2015). This procedure was evaluated in the United States in the large (N = 377 enrolled) randomized sham-controlled multicenter ESSENTIAL trial (A Randomized, Subject and Evaluator-Blinded, Parallel-Group, Multicenter Clinical Trial Using an Endoscopic Suturing Device (G-Cath EZ™ Suture Anchor Delivery Catheter) For Primary Weight Loss; ClinicTrials.gov identifier: NCT01958385). Ultimately, 332 subjects were randomized to the active (n = 221) and sham (n = 111) groups, with the active group achieving a mean %TWL of 4.95 ± 7.04 at 12 months compared to 1.38 ± 5.58 in the sham group (p = 0.2256). While there was no significant difference between the two groups for this primary endpoint, the active group did have a significantly higher %EWL at 6 and 12 months of 22.3 and 16.0, respectively (SD not given), compared to 13.6 and 4.19 for the sham group. Moreover, a subgroup analysis revealed a not-significant higher rate of resolution or improvement in diabetes in 56.25% of diabetic patients in the active group (n = 9/15) compared to 10.00% of diabetic patients in the sham group (n = 1/10) (Sullivan et al., 2017)

Endoscopic Gastroplasty

This procedure uses the EndoCinch Suturing System (Davol/C.R.Bard, Warwick, Rhode Island), a vacuum-based, superficial thickness suturing system, to perform an endoluminal vertical gastroplasty. The largest study enrolled 64 patients and reported a 1-year (N = 59) mean % EWL of 58.1 ± 19.9, with no serious adverse events (TWL data not given; Fogel, De Fogel, Bonilla, & De La Fuente, 2008).

An updated version of the EndoCinch is capable of full-thickness tissue suturing and is called the RESTORe Suturing System (Davol/C.R.Bard, Warwick, Rhode Island). It was evaluated in one study that enrolled 18 patients and reported a 1-year (n = 14) mean % EWL of 27.7 ± 21.9 and TWL of 11 ± 10 kg. However, this study also identified lack of durability in the suture plications, with 83.3% of patients found to have partial or full plication release at 1 month postendoscopy (Brethauer, Chand, Schauer, & Thompson, 2012). It is currently unclear to what extent this technology is being further developed.

Transoral Gastroplasty

This procedure uses the transoral gastroplasy (TOGA) system (Satiety Inc., Palo Alto, California), a vacuum-based device that employs suction to gather and staple full-thickness bites of gastric tissue to create a sleeve along the lesser curvature of the stomach in a manner similar to surgical vertical banded gastroplasty (Abu-Dayyeh et al., 2014; Kumar, 2015). The largest published multicenter study enrolled 67 patients and reported a 1-year (n = 53) mean % EWL of 38.7 ± 17.1 and TWL of 19.5 ± 9.2 kg, with serious adverse events in two cases. Notably, 25 patients were found to have gaps in the staple line on endoscopy at 12 months follow-up (Familiari et al., 2011). This procedure is being evaluated in the United States in a randomized sham-controlled multicenter trial (Transoral Gastroplasty for the Treatment of Morbid Obesity [TOGA]; ClinicalTrials.gov identifier: NCT00661245). Currently, it is unclear whether this technology is being further developed.

Articulating Circular Endoscopic Stapling

The articulating circular endoscopic (ACE) stapler (Boston Scientific Corporation, Natick, Massachusetts) is an endoscopic stapler with a head capable of 360-degree rotation and complete retroflexion. It has been used to create eight plications in the fundus, which reduces gastric volume. Additionally, two plications are made in the antrum in order to delay gastric emptying. One study that evaluated use of the ACE stapler enrolled 17 patients and found a 1-year (N = 15) median (IQR) EWL of 34.9 (17.8–46.6) and a median TWL of 15.3% (IQR not given) with an acceptable safety profile (Verlaan et al., 2015). There were no issues of plication durability.

Bypass Sleeves

Duodenal–Jejunal Bypass Liner

The duodenal–jejunal bypass liner (DJBL) involves the implantation of the EndoBarrier (GI Dynamics, Lexington, Massachusetts), a 60-cm Teflon sleeve, for 6–12 months. The sleeve is implanted into the duodenal bulb and then extends 60 cm into the small bowel, allowing food to bypass the duodenum and proximal jejunum (Figure 33.5a). Pancreaticobiliary secretions move along the outside of the device to the jejunum (Abu-Dayyeh et al., 2014; Kumar, 2015).

The largest completed randomized controlled multicenter trial enrolled 77 patients and reported a mean (IQR) EWL of 32.0 (22.0–46.7) and TWL of 10.0 (6.8–12.3) upon removal of the device at 6 months (n = 33). The mean (IQR) EWL was 19.8 (10.6–45.0) and TWL was 5.8 (2.8–11.1) 6 months after device removal (n = 31; Koehestanie et al., 2014). More recently, a 195-patient cohort study in which 185 patients successfully underwent implantation reported a mean ± SD EWL of 46.3% (± 31.1) and TWL of 11.9% (± 6.9) at the time of device removal at 12 months. Notably, 17% of patients experienced significant adverse events, and 31% of patients required early explantation due to either adverse events or inability to tolerate the device (Betzel et al., 2017). Due to a high incidence of hepatic abscesses (four cases discovered among 325 subjects) observed in the EndoBarrier pivotal trial (Safety and Efficacy of EndoBarrier in Subjects with Type 2 Diabetes Who Are Obese (ENDO); ClinicalTrials.gov identifier: NCT01728116), the trial was prematurely terminated (GI Dynamics, n.d.-a). Nevertheless, after reviewing the safety and efficacy data and preparing a revised clinical

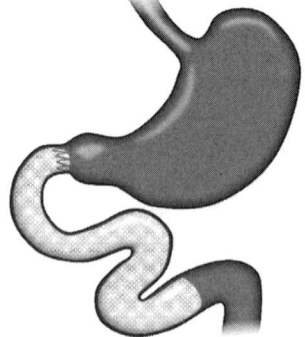

A. Duodenal–jejunal Bypass Liner

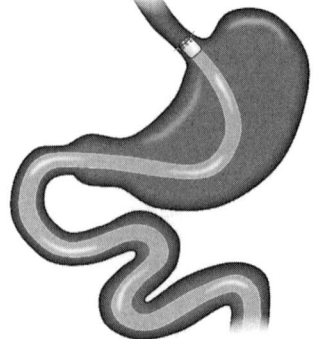

B. Gastro–duodenal–jejunal Bypass Liner

FIGURE 33.5. Visual representation of two bypass liner devices. Whereas the EndoBarrier (A) bypasses the duodenum and proximal jejunum, the ValenTx system (B) is anchored at the gastroesophageal junction and allows food to also bypass the stomach.

algorithm, GI Dynamics plans to continue pursuing FDA approval for the EndoBarrier device (GI Dynamics, n.d.-b).

Gastro–Duodeno–Jejunal Bypass Liner

The gastro–duodeno–jejunal bypass liner ValenTx (ValenTx, Maple Grove, Minnesota) is a 120-cm fluoropolymer sleeve that requires both endoscopic and laparoscopic implantation. It is laparoscopically anchored at the gastroesophageal junction, from which it extends 120 cm into the small intestine, allowing food to bypass the stomach, duodenum, and proximal jejunum (Abu-Dayyeh et al., 2014, Figure X.5b). It thus seeks to recreate the restrictive and malabsorptive aspects of post-RYGB physiology. The only study of this device to publish 1-year weight loss data (N = 10) reported 35.9% EWL (range, SD, and TWL not given; Sandler et al., 2015). At the time of this writing, the device was not FDA approved.

Aspiration Therapy

The distinctive feature of aspiration therapy is the insertion of a gastrostomy tube, known as the A-tube, into the patient's stomach. The patient then uses this tube to evacuate 30% of each meal that he or she consumes 20 minutes after consumption. Currently, the AspireAssist device (Aspire Bariatrics, King of Prussia, Pennsylvania) is the only FDA-approved device for this procedure.

An initial study (N = 22) reported a mean % EWL of 40.8 ± 19.8 (range 9.7–77.2%) and % TWL of 14.8 ± 6.3 (range 2.8–26.7%) after 6 months' use (Forssell & Norén, 2014). Following a pivotal 52-week randomized controlled multicenter PATHWAY trial (N = 171), this device was approved by the FDA (P150024) on June 14, 2016 for use in patients with a BMI of 35–55 kg/m^2 (Chiang & Ryou, 2016; Thompson et al., 2016; U.S. FDA, 2016a). Exclusion criteria for the trial included preexisting eating disorders such as bulimia nervosa, night eating disorder, and binge-eating disorder. Patients who underwent aspiration therapy and lifestyle counseling (n = 111) had a 31.5 ± 26.7% EWL and 12.1% TWL at 52 weeks, compared to 9.8 ± 15.5 % EWL in those receiving lifestyle counseling alone. Although there was a 3.6% (95% CI 0.1%–7.1%) rate of serious adverse events (including peritonitis and gastric ulceration), no patients were found to have developed an eating disorder at 52 weeks.

Electrical Stimulation

Gastric Stimulation

Acute retrograde gastric electrical stimulation (RGES) is a process in which electrodes are endoscopically placed in the stomach in order to simulate satiety (Zhang, Du, Fang, Yao, & Chen, 2014). One study (N = 16) found a significantly reduced caloric intake among patients who received this treatment, but did not examine weight loss as an outcome (Behary & Kumbhari, 2015).

The use of low-amplitude, high-frequency stimulation to induce vagal blockade has also been shown to promote satiety and support weight loss (Štimac, Klobučar Majanović, & Ličina, 2016). Both of these methods use devices (Enterra System, abiliti system; Enteromedics Maestro Rechargeable System, etc.) that require open or laparoscopic surgery for implantation. However, attempts to develop endoscopically implantable gastric electrodes or vagal pacing leads are currently underway (Abu-Dayyeh et al., 2014). At the time of this writing, no endoscopically implantable gastric stimulation devices were FDA approved for the treatment of obesity.

Deep Brain Stimulation

Beyond focusing on peripheral neuromuscular targets, other researchers are investigating the role of modulating central hunger and reward pathways using deep brain stimulation (DBS; Ho et al., 2015). Potential target areas identified via human neuroimaging and animal models include the lateral hypothalamus and ventromedial hypothalamus—known to regulate feeding and satiety, respectively—as well as the nucleus accumbens within the mesolimbic dopamine reward pathways. Weight loss and changes in feeding behavior and resting metabolism have been observed in early animal and human studies of DBS, yet much further research is needed to validate this approach

(Whiting et al., 2013). Nevertheless, DBS remains an exciting new avenue of inquiry into the mechanisms of and treatments for aberrant neurological activity that may underlie refractory obesity (Halpern et al., 2013). Initial human studies will likely involve patients who have been unable to lose weight using gold-standard definitive bariatric approaches.

Other Therapies

Magnetic Compression Anastomoses

The incisionless anastomotic system (IAS; GI Windows, West Bridgewater, Massachusetts) uses pairs of self-assembling, hexagonal magnets placed endoscopically that create magnetic compression anastomoses upon coupling (e.g., gastrojejunostomies, gastroileostomies, jejunoileostomies; Figure 33.6). This results in a dual-path enteral anatomy that can bypass absorptive capacity for bariatric purposes or circumvent gastrointestinal obstructions (Kumar, 2015; Ryou et al., 2011). Beyond bypass, another theory behind this technology's applicability to the treatment of obesity is that nutrient delivery to the distal small bowel will induce an ileal brake phenomenon, which will decrease food intake (ASGE Bariatric Endoscopy Task Force, et al., 2015a).

Porcine studies using endoscopy, simultaneous endoscopy/colonoscopy, and simultaneous endoscopy and open surgery to deploy the self-assembling magnets have demonstrated consistently successful creation of leak-free enteroenteric anastomoses (gastrojejunostomies, jejunocolostomies, and jejunoileostomies, respectively) within 10 days (Ryou et al., 2011; Ryou, Agoston, & Thompson, 2016; Ryou, Aihara, & Thompson, 2016). In two of these studies, magnets were spontaneously expulsed within 12 days, and a subsequent 3-month follow-up revealed widely patent anastomoses and no significant formation of intraabdominal adhesions (Ryou, Agoston, et al., 2016; Ryou, Aihara, et al., 2016). Most notably, in one study, the five pigs that underwent jejunocolonic bypass had experienced significant weight loss compared to controls (mean weight at 3 months = 45 kg vs. 78 kg, respectively; Ryou, Agoston, et al., 2016).

More recent human feasibility studies using IAS placed under simultaneous enteroscopy and colonoscopy (using endoscopic and fluoroscopic guidance with laparoscopic assistance as needed) to create jejunoilesostomies in 10 patients similarly found that leak-free anastomoses were formed within approximately 1 week. All magnets were painlessly excreted within 23 days of placement without obstruction. Anastomoses were found to be patent during 2- and 6-month follow-up endoscopies. At 6 months, patients had a mean EWL of 28.3% and a mean TWL of 10.6%, with a trend toward normalization of HbA1C and serum glucose in diabetic and pre-diabetic patients (Machytka, Buzga, Lautz, et al., 2016; Machytka, Buzga, Ryou, Lautz, & Thompson, 2016). At the time of this writing, neither this approach nor the two others discussed in this section were FDA approved.

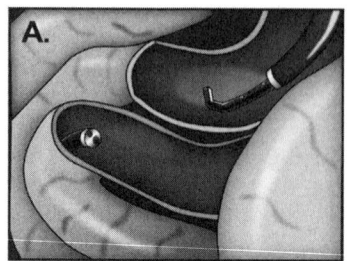 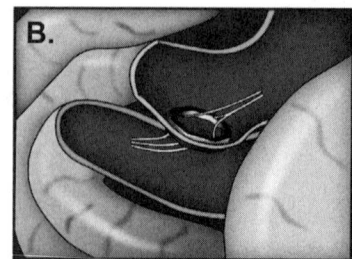 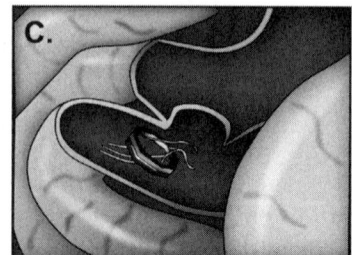

FIGURE 33.6. The GI Windows' incisionless anastomotic system (IAS) works via the coupling of pairs of endoscopically deployed, self-assembling magnets (A, B) to create a compression anastomosis that bypasses a portion of the GI tract (C).

Duodenal Mucosal Resurfacing

Revita duodenal mucosal resurfacing (DMR; Fractyl Laboratories, Lexington, Massachusetts) uses superficial mucosal thermal ablation to reset diseased duodenal enteroendocrine cells and restore crucial signaling pathways. It accomplishes thermal ablation either through the use of radiofrequency (ASGE Bariatric Endoscopy Task Force, ASGE Technology Committee, Abu Dayyeh, Edmundowicz, et al., 2015) or through the use of a recirculating hot-water-filled balloon (Kumbhari, Oberbach, & Nimgaonkar, 2015). A recently published trial reported on 39 diabetic patients (HbA1C > 7.5% on at least one antidiabetic medication) who underwent DMR (Rajagopalan et al., 2016). The patients, who had a mean baseline HbA1C of 9.6 ± 1.4% and a mean baseline BMI of 30.8 ± 3.5 kg/m^2, achieved as much as a 2.5% reduction in HbA1C at 3 months when undergoing long-segment treatment. Although the study focused primarily on glycemic metrics, the investigators noted a reported weight loss of 3.9 ± 0.5 kg at 3 months and 2.5 ± 0.1 kg at 6 months (% EWL and % TWL not reported; Chiang & Ryou, 2016b; Rajagopalan et al., 2016). Further targeted study is needed to understand the utility of this modality for primary weight loss outcomes.

Intragastric Botulinum Toxin Injections

This procedure involves the injection of botulinum toxin-A into the gastric antrum and/or fundus. By inhibiting the release of acetylcholine at the neuromuscular junction, the injection leads to local paralysis of the gastric muscle, which is thought to inhibit antral motility and delay gastric emptying (Štimac et al., 2016). Treatment effects typically last 3–6 months (Kumbhari et al., 2015). A meta-analysis including 115 patients performed pre- and postintervention comparisons that showed significant decrease in body weight after the injection of botulinum toxin A; moreover, patients treated with botulinum toxon-A had significantly greater decrease in body weight compared to patients injected with placebo. The meta-analysis did not report the percent of body weight lost (Bang et al., 2015).

Summary

Over the last few years, there has been a massive expansion in the number and variety of nonsurgical interventional modalities for the treatment of obesity. We described 17 devices in detail, four of which have been approved by the FDA for the treatment of obesity within the last 2 years (the ORBERA, Reshape, and Obalon intragastric balloons and the AspireAssist aspiration therapy system; U.S. FDA, 2015a, 2016) and at least three of which are currently undergoing active pivotal clinical trials. All three balloons present similar prospects for success, with relatively high safety profiles and, in the case of Obalon, with the benefit of not requiring procedural placement. However, it should be noted that the FDA released an alert in August 2017 when it began investigating five deaths occurring within one month of liquid-filled balloon placement (U.S. FDA, 2017). With encouraging initial data, postapproval studies for the newly approved AspireAssist will look particularly at long-term outcomes related to gastrostomy site complications and disordered eating behaviors (U.S. FDA, 2016).

The involvement of the American Society for Metabolic and Bariatric Surgery (ASMBS) and the American Society for Gastrointestinal Endoscopy (ASGE) will be critical in directing the clinical development of these new technologies and treatment approaches. The ASMBS and the ASGE have jointly defined minimum thresholds to be met for a new, primary endoscopic treatment of obesity to be considered appropriate for incorporation into clinical practice. These thresholds include a minimum of 25% EWL at the 12-month timemark in patients with a BMI ≥ 35 kg/m^2, as well as a maximum 5% risk of serious adverse events (ASGE/ASMBS Task Force on Endoscopic Therapy, 2011; ASGE Bariatric Endoscopy Task Force, ASGE Technology Committee, Abu Dayyeh, Kumar, et al., 2015). Our review has suggested promising early results for the ORBERA balloon: 30–50% EWL upon device removal, with nausea, vomiting, and stomach pain as the most common complications, and a serious adverse event rate of approximately 1%. This profile is in accordance with a recent meta-analysis, which found that the ORBERA balloon meets the ASMBS/ASGE minimum threshold requirements (ASGE Bariatric Endoscopy Task Force, ASGE Technology Committee, Abu Dayyeh, Kumar, et al., 2015). Further, the 12% TWL reported in the meta-analysis of the ORBERA balloon compares favorably to weight loss observed from pharmacological treatment (Yanovski & Yanovski, 2014) and meets the recommendations set forth for adoption of endoscopic bariatric therapies in the ASMBS/ASGE white paper (ASGE/ASMBS Task Force on Endoscopic Therapy, 2011). The other nonsurgical interventional treatments are not established enough to warrant comparison to the ASMBS/ASGE thresholds.

Although these position statements provide important standards for the field, as new interventional treatments enter the market, we must consider not only comparative safety and efficacy with respect to weight loss outcomes, but also the longitudinal cost-effectiveness of the course of treatment and the impact on weight-related medical comorbidities (Davis & Kroh, 2016). This consideration becomes even more important as less-invasive procedures and devices—used as primary, bridge, or revision therapies—play an increasing role in the chronic management of obesity across the spectrum of disease severity and along the course of patients' lifespans (Chiang & Ryou, 2016b). One concerning feature of the intragastric balloons and other reversible therapies is the evidence indicating that the weight loss effect of the balloon diminishes over time (Kotzampassi et al., 2012). Short-lived weight loss and/or need for repeated treatment detract from the appeal of nonsurgical interventional treatments as a cost-effective alternative to bariatric procedures.

These considerations highlight the need for each of the endoscopic treatments of obesity to be offered as part of an individualized, comprehensive, multidisciplinary weight management program (ASGE/ASMBS Task Force on Endoscopic Therapy, 2011). Patients must be counseled on the expected outcomes, possible risks, and economic burden of the different therapies, and they should have regular contact with their physician and nutritionist throughout the course of their treatment (Davis & Kroh, 2016). Behavior modification is an important part of nonsurgical interventional treatment and should be included as such.

Although nonsurgical interventions for obesity are still in the early stages of development, recent findings show promise and suggest that this field will continue to actively evolve in the immediate future. Further study is needed, focusing on long-term outcomes and cost-effectiveness. The next decade will challenge us to define the place that these approaches should occupy in the continuum of treatment as we aim to bridge gaps and increase access for patients with obesity. These novel approaches should not be viewed as a "quick fix" or a "magic bullet," but rather as part of an all-encompassing, multidisciplinary behavior modification program.

References

Abu Dayyeh, B. K., Rajan, E., & Gostout, C. J. (2013). Endoscopic sleeve gastroplasty: A potential endoscopic alternative to surgical sleeve gastrectomy for treatment of obesity. *Gastrointestinal Endoscopy, 78*(3), 530–535.

Abu-Dayyeh, B. K., Sarmiento, R., Rajan, E., Vázquez-Sequeiros, E., & Gostout, C. J. (2014). Endoscopic treatments of obesity and metabolic disease: Are we there yet? *Revista Espanola de Enfermedades Digestivas: Organo Oficial de La Sociedad Espanola de Patologia Digestiva, 106*(7), 467–476.

Al-Zubaidi, A. M., Alghamdi, H. U., Alzobydi, A. H., Dhiloon, I. A., & Qureshi, L. A. (2015). Bowel perforation due to break and distal passage of the safety ring of an adjustable intra-gastric balloon: A potentially life-threatening situation. *World Journal of Gastrointestinal Endoscopy, 7*(4), 429–432.

Angrisani, L., Santonicola, A., Iovino, P., Formisano, G., Buchwald, H., & Scopinaro, N. (2015). Bariatric surgery worldwide 2013. *Obesity Surgery, 25*(10), 1822–1832.

ASGE/ASMBS Task Force on Endoscopic Therapy. (2011). A pathway to endoscopic bariatric therapies. *Surgery for Obesity and Related Diseases, 7*(6), 672–682.

ASGE Bariatric Endoscopy Task Force, ASGE Technology Committee, Abu Dayyeh, B. K., Edmundowicz, S. A., Jonnalagadda, S., Kumar, N., et al. (2015a). Endoscopic bariatric therapies. *Gastrointestinal Endoscopy, 81*(5), 1073–1086.

ASGE Bariatric Endoscopy Task Force, ASGE Technology Committee, Abu Dayyeh, B. K., Kumar, N., Edmundowicz, S. A., Jonnalagadda, S., et al. (2015b). ASGE Bariatric Endoscopy Task Force systematic review and meta-analysis assessing the ASGE PIVI thresholds for adopting endoscopic bariatric therapies. *Gastrointestinal Endoscopy, 82*(3), 425–438.e5.

Bang, C. S., Baik, G. H., Shin, I. S., Kim, J. B., Suk, K. T., Yoon, J. H., et al. (2015). Effect of intragastric injection of botulinum toxin A for the treatment of obesity: A meta-analysis and meta-regression. *Gastrointestinal Endoscopy, 81*(5), 1141–1149.

Behary, J., & Kumbhari, V. (2015). Advances in the endoscopic management of obesity. *Gastroenterology Research and Practice, 2015*, 1–9.

Betzel, B., Homan, J., Aarts, E. O., Janssen, I. M. C., de Boer, H., Wahab, P. J., et al. (2017). Weight reduction and improvement in diabetes by the duodenal–jejunal bypass liner: A 198 patient cohort study. *Surgical Endoscopy, 31*(7), 2881–2891.

Brethauer, S. A., Chand, B., Schauer, P. R., & Thompson, C. C. (2012). Transoral gastric volume reduction as intervention for weight management: 12-month follow-up of TRIM trial. *Surgery for Obesity and Related Diseases, 8*(3), 296–303.

Buchwald, H., & Oien, D. M. (2013). Metabolic/bariatric surgery worldwide 2011. *Obesity Surgery, 23*(4), 427–436.

Chiang, A. L., & Ryou, M. (2016). Endoscopic treatment of obesity. *Current Opinion in Gastroenterology, 32*(6), 487–491.

Chuttani, R., Machytka, E., Raftopoulos, I., Bojkova, M., Kupka, T., Buzga, M., et al. (2016). The first procedureless gastric balloon for weight loss: Final results from a multi-center, prospective study evaluating safety, efficacy, metabolic parameters, quality of life, and 6-month follow-up. *Gastroenterology, 150*(4, Suppl. 1), S26.

Davis, M., & Kroh, M. (2016). Novel endoscopic and surgical techniques for treatment of morbid obesity: A glimpse into the future. *Surgical Clinics of North America, 96*(4), 857–873.

Deliopoulou, K., Konsta, A., Penna, S., Papakostas, P., & Kotzampassi, K. (2013). The impact of weight loss on depression status in obese individuals subjected to intragastric balloon treatment. *Obesity Surgery, 23*(5), 669–675.

Dumonceau, J. M., François, E., Hittelet, A., Mehdi, A. I., Barea, M., & Deviere, J. (2010). Single vs repeated treatment with the intragastric balloon: A 5-year weight loss study. *Obesity Surgery, 20*(6), 692–697.

Familiari, P., Costamagna, G., Bléro, D., Le Moine, O., Perri, V., Boskoski, I., et al. (2011). Transoral gastroplasty for morbid obesity: A multicenter trial with a 1-year outcome. *Gastrointestinal Endoscopy, 74*(6), 1248–1258.

Fogel, R., De Fogel, J., Bonilla, Y., & De La Fuente, R. (2008). Clinical experience of transoral suturing for an endoluminal vertical gastroplasty: 1-year follow-up in 64 patients. *Gastrointestinal Endoscopy, 68*(1), 51–58.

Forlano, R., Ippolito, A. M., Iacobellis, A., Merla, A., Valvano, M. R., Niro, G., et al. (2010). Effect of the BioEnterics intragastric balloon on weight, insulin resistance, and liver steatosis in obese patients. *Gastrointestinal Endoscopy, 71*(6), 927–933.

Forssell, H., & Norén, E. (2014). A novel endoscopic weight loss therapy using gastric aspiration: Results after 6 months. *Endoscopy, 47*(1), 68–71.

Genco, A., Cipriano, M., Bacci, V., Maselli, R., Paone, E., Lorenzo, M., et al. (2010). Intragastric balloon followed by diet vs intragastric balloon followed by another balloon: A prospective study on 100 patients. *Obesity Surgery, 20*(11), 1496–1500.

Genco, A., Maselli, R., Frangella, F., Cipriano, M., Forestieri, P., Delle Piane, D., et al. (2015). Intragastric balloon for obesity treatment: Results of a multicentric evaluation for balloons left in place for more than 6 months. *Surgical Endoscopy, 29*(8), 2339–2343.

GI Dynamics. (n.d.-a). ENDO trial placed on enrollment hold (updated March 5, 2015). Retrieved November 3, 2016, from *www.gidynamics.com/media-press-release.php?id=139*.

GI Dynamics. (n.d.-b). GI Dynamics announces topline results from U.S. pivotal clinical trial of EndoBarrier® therapy (the ENDO trial). Retrieved December 14, 2016, from *www.gidynamics.com/media-press-release.php?id=151*.

Gloy, V. L., Briel, M., Bhatt, D. L., Kashyap, S. R., Schauer, P. R., Mingrone, G., et al. (2013). Bariatric surgery versus non-surgical treatment for obesity: A systematic review and meta-analysis of randomised controlled trials. *BMJ (Clinical Research Ed.), 347*, f5934.

Halpern, C. H., Tekriwal, A., Santollo, J., Keating, J. G., Wolf, J. A., Daniels, D., et al. (2013). Amelioration of binge eating by nucleus accumbens shell deep brain stimulation in mice involves D2 receptor modulation. *Journal of Neuroscience, 33*(17), 7122–7129.

Ho, A. L., Sussman, E. S., Pendharkar, A. V., Azagury, D. E., Bohon, C., & Halpern, C. H. (2015). Deep brain stimulation for obesity: Rationale and approach to trial design. *Neurosurgical Focus, 38*(6), E8.

Imaz, I., Martínez-Cervell, C., García-Álvarez, E. E., Sendra-Gutiérrez, J. M., & González-Enríquez, J. (2008). Safety and effectiveness of the intragastric balloon for obesity: A meta-analysis. *Obesity Surgery, 18*(7), 841–846.

Koehestanie, P., de Jonge, C., Berends, F. J., Janssen, I. M., Bouvy, N. D., & Greve, J. W. M. (2014). The effect of the endoscopic duodenal–jejunal bypass liner on obesity and type 2 diabetes mellitus: A multicenter randomized controlled trial. *Annals of Surgery, 260*(6), 984–992.

Kotzampassi, K., Grosomanidis, V., Papakostas, P., Penna, S., & Eleftheriadis, E. (2012). 500 intragastric balloons: What happens 5 years thereafter? *Obesity Surgery, 22*(6), 896–903.

Kumar, N. (2015). Endoscopic therapy for weight loss: Gastroplasty, duodenal sleeves, intragastric balloons, and aspiration. *World Journal of Gastrointestinal Endoscopy, 7*(9), 847–859.

Kumar, N. (2016). Weight loss endoscopy: Development, applications, and current status. *World Journal of Gastroenterology, 22*(31), 7069–7079.

Kumbhari, V., Oberbach, A., & Nimgaonkar, A. (2015). Primary endoscopic therapies for obesity and metabolic diseases. *Current Opinion in Gastroenterology, 31*(5), 351–358.

Lopez-Nava, G., Bautista-Castaño, I., Jimenez, A., de Grado, T., & Fernandez-Corbelle, J. P. (2015). The Primary Obesity Surgery Endolumenal (POSE) procedure: One-year patient weight loss and safety outcomes. *Surgery for Obesity and Related Diseases, 11*(4), 861–865.

Lopez-Nava, G., Bautista-Castaño, I., Jimenez-Baños, A., & Fernandez-Corbelle, J. P. (2015). Dual intragastric balloon: Single ambulatory center Spanish experience with 60 patients in endoscopic weight loss management. *Obesity Surgery, 25*(12), 2263–2267.

Lopez-Nava, G., Galvão, M. P., da Bautista-Castaño, I., Jimenez, A., De Grado, T., & Fernandez-Corbelle, J. P. (2015). Endoscopic sleeve gastroplasty for the treatment of obesity. *Endoscopy, 47*(5), 449–452.

Lopez-Nava, G., Sharaiha, R. Z., Neto, M. G., Kumta, N. A., Topazian, M., Shukla, A., et al. (2016). Endoscopic sleeve gastroplasty for obesity: A multicenter study of 242 patients with 18 months follow-up. *Gastroenterology, 150*(4), S26.

Machytka, E., Buzga, M., Lautz, D. B., Ryou, M., Simonson, D., & Thompson, C. C. (2016). 103 a dual-path enteral bypass procedure created by a novel incisionless anastomosis system (IAS): 6-month clinical results. *Gastroenterology, 150*(4, Suppl.), S26.

Machytka, E., Buzga, M., Ryou, M., Lautz, D. B., & Thompson, C. C. (2016). 1139 endoscopic dual-path enteral anastomosis using self-assembling magnets: First-in-human clinical feasibility. *Gastroenterology, 150*(4, Suppl.), S232.

Marinos, G., Eliades, C., Raman Muthusamy, V., & Greenway, F. (2014). Weight loss and improved quality of life with a nonsurgical endoscopic treatment for obesity: Clinical results from a 3- and 6-month study. *Surgery for Obesity and Related Diseases, 10*(5), 929–934.

Mathus-Vliegen, E. M. H. (2014). Endoscopic treatment: The past, the present and the future. *Best Practice and Research Clinical Gastroenterology, 28*(4), 685–702.

Neylan, C. J., Dempsey, D. T., Tewksbury, C. M., Williams, N. N., & Dumon, K. R. (2016). Endoscopic treatments of obesity: A comprehensive review. *Surgery for Obesity and Related Diseases, 12*(5), 1108–1115.

Obeid, N. R., Malick, W., Concors, S. J., Fielding, G. A., Kurian, M. S., & Ren-Fielding, C. J. (2016). Long-term outcomes after Roux-en-Y gastric bypass: 10- to 13-year data. *Surgery for Obesity and Related Diseases, 12*(1), 11–20.

Ogden, C. L., Carroll, M. D., Kit, B. K., & Flegal, K. M. (2014). Prevalence of childhood and adult obesity in the United States, 2011–2012. *Journal of the American Medical Association, 311*(8), 806–814.

Öztürk, A., Akinci, Ö. F., & Kurt, M. (2010). Small intestinal obstruction due to self-deflated free intragastric balloon. *Surgery for Obesity and Related Diseases, 6*(5), 569–571.

Öztürk, A., Yavuz, Y., & Atalay, T. (2015). A case of duodenal obstruction and pancreatitis due to intragastric balloon. *Balkan Medical Journal, 32*(3), 323–326.

Ponce, J., Quebbemann, B. B., & Patterson, E. J. (2013). Prospective, randomized, multicenter study evaluating safety and efficacy of intragastric dual-balloon in obesity. *Surgery for Obesity and Related Diseases, 9*(2), 290–295.

Ponce, J., Woodman, G., Swain, J., Wilson, E., English, W., Ikramuddin, S., et al. (2015). The REDUCE pivotal trial: A prospective, randomized controlled pivotal trial of a dual intragastric balloon for the treatment of obesity. *Surgery for Obesity and Related Diseases, 11*(4), 874–881.

Rajagopalan, H., Cherrington, A. D., Thompson, C. C., Kaplan, L. M., Rubino, F., Mingrone, G., et al. (2016). Endoscopic duodenal mucosal resurfacing for the treatment of type 2 diabetes: 6-month interim analysis from the first-in-human proof-of-concept study. *Diabetes Care, 39*(12), 2254–2261.

Ryou, M., Agoston, A. T., & Thompson, C. C. (2016). Endoscopic intestinal bypass creation by using self-assembling magnets in a porcine model. *Gastrointestinal Endoscopy, 83*(4), 821–825.

Ryou, M., Aihara, H., & Thompson, C. C. (2016). Minimally invasive entero-enteral dual-path bypass using self-assembling magnets. *Surgical Endoscopy, 30*(1), 4533–4538.

Ryou, M., Cantillon-Murphy, P., Azagury, D., Shaikh, S. N., Ha, G., Greenwalt, I., et al. (2011). Smart Self-Assembling MagnetS for ENdoscopy (SAMSEN) for transoral endoscopic creation of immediate gastrojejunostomy (with video). *Gastrointestinal Endoscopy, 73*(2), 353–359.

Sandler, B. J., Rumbaut, R., Swain, C. P., Torres, G., Morales, L., Gonzales, L., et al. (2015). One-year human experience with a novel endoluminal, endoscopic gastric bypass sleeve for morbid obesity. *Surgical Endoscopy, 29*(11), 3298–3303.

Sauer, N., Rösch, T., Pezold, J., Reining, F., Anders, M., Groth, S., et al. (2013). A new endoscopically implantable device (SatiSphere) for treatment of obesity—efficacy, safety, and metabolic effects on glucose, insulin, and GLP-1 levels. *Obesity Surgery, 23*(11), 1727–1733.

Štimac, D., Klobučar Majanović, S., & Ličina, M. (2016). Recent trends in endoscopic management of obesity. *Surgical Innovation, 23*(5), 525–537.

Sullivan, S., Swain, J. M., Woodman, G., Antonetti, M., De La Cruz-Muñoz, N., Jonnalagadda, S. S., et al. (2017). Randomized sham-controlled trial evaluating efficacy and safety of endoscopic gastric plication for primary obesity: The ESSENTIAL trial. *Obesity, 25*(2), 294–301.

Tai, C. M., Lin, H. Y., Yen, Y. C., Huang, C. K., Hsu, W. L., Huang, Y. W., et al. (2013). Effectiveness of intragastric balloon treatment for obese patients: One-year follow-up after balloon removal. *Obesity Surgery, 23*(12), 2068–2074.

Thompson, C. C., Dayyeh, B. K. A., Kushner, R., Sullivan, S., Schorr, A. B., Amaro, A., et al. (2016). 381 the AspireAssist is an effective tool in the treatment of class II and class III obesity: Results of a one-year clinical trial. *Gastroenterology, 150*(4, Suppl.), S86.

U.S. FDA. (2015a). Medical devices cleared or approved by FDA in 2015. Retrieved November 3, 2016, from *www.fda.gov/MedicalDevices/ProductsandMedicalProcedures/DeviceApprovalsandClearances/Recently-ApprovedDevices/ucm430692.htm*.

U.S. FDA. (2015b). PMA P140008: FDA summary of safety and effectiveness data (SSED). Retrieved from *www.accessdata.fda.gov/cdrh_docs/pdf14/P140008B.pdf*.

U.S. FDA. (2016a). AspireAssist—PMA P150024: FDA summary of safety and effectiveness data (SSED). Retrieved from *www.accessdata.fda.gov/cdrh_docs/pdf15/p150024b.pdf*.

U.S. FDA. (2016b). Medical devices cleared or approved by FDA in 2016. Retrieved November 3, 2016, from *www.fda.gov/MedicalDevices/ProductsandMedicalProcedures/DeviceApprovalsandClearances/Recently-ApprovedDevices/ucm494389.htm*.

U.S. FDA. (2016c). Obalon Balloon System–PMA P160001: FDA summary of safety and effectiveness data (SSED). Retrieved from *www.accessdata.fda.gov/cdrh_docs/pdf16/P160001b.pdf*.

U.S. FDA. (2017). Liquid-filled Intragastric Balloon Systems: Letter to healthcare providers— Potential risks. Retrieved March 6, 2018, from *www.fda.gov/Safety/MedWatch/SafetyInformation/SafetyAlertsforHumanMedicalProducts/ucm570916.htm*.

Verlaan, T., Paulus, G. F., Mathus-Vliegen, E. M. H., Veldhuyzen, E. A. M. L., Conchillo, J. M., Bouvy, N. D., et al. (2015). Endoscopic gastric volume reduction with a novel articulating plication device is safe and effective in the treatment of obesity (with video). *Gastrointestinal Endoscopy, 81*(2), 312–320.

Whiting, D. M., Tomycz, N. D., Bailes, J., de Jonge, L., Lecoultre, V., Wilent, B., et al. (2013). Lateral hypothalamic area deep brain stimulation for refractory obesity: A pilot study with preliminary data on safety, body weight, and energy metabolism. *Journal of Neurosurgery, 119*(1), 56–63.

Yanovski, S. Z., & Yanovski, J. A. (2014). Long-term drug treatment for obesity: A systematic and clinical review. *Journal of the American Medical Association, 311*(1), 74–86.

Zerrweck, C., Maunoury, V., Caiazzo, R., Branche, J., Dezfoulian, G., Bulois, P., et al. (2012). Preoperative weight loss with intragastric balloon decreases the risk of significant adverse outcomes of laparoscopic gastric bypass in super-super obese patients. *Obesity Surgery, 22*(5), 777–782.

Zhang, Y., Du, S., Fang, L., Yao, S., & Chen, J. D. Z. (2014). Retrograde gastric electrical stimulation suppresses calorie intake in obese subjects. *Obesity, 22*(6), 1447–1451.

APPENDIX 33.1. Detailed Outcomes of FDA-Approved Nonsurgical Interventional Treatments Of Obesity

Study	Outcomes
	ORBERA Balloon
Imaz, Martínez-Cervell, García-Álvarez, Sendra-Gutiérrez, & González-Enríquez (2008)	$N = 3,608$ 32.1% EWL, 12.2% TWL at balloon removal at 6 months 4.2% early balloon removal 2 deaths
U.S. Food and Drug Administration (2015)	$N = 448$ 29.6% EWL, 10.2% TWL at ballon removal at 6 months 26.5% EWL, 9.1% TWL at 3 months postremoval 22.1% EWL, 7.6% TWL at 6 months postremoval 10% serious adverse effects 18.8% early balloon removal zero deflations/migrations, ulcerations, or deaths
Kotzampassi, Grosomanidis, Papakostas, Penna, & Eleftheriadis (2012)	$N = 122$ 58.1% EWL at removal at 6 months 57.9% EWL 6 months postremoval 39.2% EWL 12 months postremoval 25.1% EWL 24 months postremoval 17.1% EWL 60 months postremoval
Dumonceau et al. (2010)	$N = 19$ 49.3% EWL upon first balloon removal at 6 months 18.2% additional EWL upon second balloon removal
Zerrweck et al. (2012)	$N = 60$, BMI > 60kg/m^2 11.2% EWL at removal at 6 months
	ReShape Dual Balloon
Ponce et al. (2015)	$N = 326$ 27.9% EWL, 7.6% TBWL at removal ($n = 167$) 18.8% EWL 24 weeks after removal (TWL not given) ($n = 136$) 35% ulceration initially, 10% postmodification
Ponce, Quebbemann, & Patterson (2013)	$N = 21$ 31.8% EWL, 8.4% TBWL at removal at 24 weeks 64% of EWL maintained 24 weeks postremoval Zero deflations, migrations, or removals
	Obalon Balloon
U.S. Food and Drug Administration (2016b)	$N = 430$ 24.1% EWL, 6.6% TWL at balloon removal at 24 weeks 3.2% EWL, 0.9% TWL regained 24 weeks postremoval 8% failed to swallow capsuled ($n = 32$) One balloon (0.1% of 985) found to be deflated but not migrated at retrieval
	AspireAssist
Forssell & Norén (2014)	$N = 22$ 40.8% EWL, 14.8% EWL after 6 months of usage
Thompson et al. (2016); U.S. Food and Drug Administration (2016a)	$N = 171$ 31.5% EWL, 12.1% TWL at 52 weeks 3.6% serious adverse events (i.e., peritonitis, gastric ulceration) No subjects found to develop eating disorder

Note. EWL, excess weight loss; TWL, total weight loss; BMI, body mass index.

APPENDIX 33.2. Web Addresses for Images of and Information on Nonsurgical Interventional Treatments of Obesity

Device	Link
ORBERA	www.orbera.com
ReShape Dual Balloon	https://reshapeready.com
Obalon	www.obalon.com
Elipse	http://allurion.com/the-elipse-gastric-balloon
TransPyloric Shuttle	https://baronova.com/technology/baronova-products
Full Sense device	www.bfkw.org
SatiSphere	www.endosphereinc.com
Apollo OverStitch	http://apolloendo.com/overstitch
Incisionless Operating Platform (used in POSE procedure)	http://usgimedical.com/eos/index.htm
RESTORe Suturing System	Not available
TOGA system	Not available
ACE stapler	Not available
EndoBarrier	www.endobarrier.com/physician/how-it-works
ValenTx gastro–duodeno–jejunal bypass liner 3	www.valentx.com/technology.php
AspireAssist	www.aspirebariatrics.com/about-the-aspireassist
Incisionless Operating System (for magnetic compression anastomoses)	www.giwindows.com/main-pages/product
Revita	www.fractyl.com/our-focus/#revita-dmr

CHAPTER 34

Treatment of Eating Disorders in Persons with Obesity

Carlos M. Grilo

This chapter provides an overview of the current status of treatments for eating disorders in persons with obesity. The primary focus is the literature regarding the treatment of binge-eating disorder (BED), a formal eating disorder strongly associated with obesity in epidemiological and clinical samples. Controlled treatment research has produced strong empirical support for the acute effectiveness and long-term durability of two specialist psychological treatments: cognitive-behavioral therapy (CBT) and interpersonal psychotherapy (IPT). Treatment research has also produced empirical support for an additional specialist psychological treatment, dialectical behavior therapy (DBT), for guided-self-help versions of CBT, and for behavioral weight loss treatments for BED. Controlled treatment research has also produced empirical support for the short-term effectiveness of specific medications and for specific combinations of pharmacotherapy with either CBT or behavioral weight loss (BWL) approaches. This chapter addresses the implications of these findings about BED for informing clinical practice and future research, including emerging applications to patients who undergo bariatric surgery.

Eating Disorders and Obesity

Eating disorders and obesity represent two important public problems (i.e., psychiatric and medical diagnoses, respectively) associated with high rates of morbidity and mortality. Eating disorders have a low prevalence rate that is generally thought to be relatively stable (Zachrisson, Vedul-Kjelsas, Gotestam, & Mykletun, 2008; Mohler-Kuo, Schnyder, Dermota, Wei, & Milos, 2016), whereas obesity shows a high and increasing prevalence rate (Flegal, Carroll, Ogden, & Curtin, 2010). Certain forms of eating disorders and disordered eating show strong associations with obesity in epidemiological studies both nationally (Hudson, Hiripi, Pope, & Kessler, 2007) and internationally (Kessler et al., 2013). Interestingly, despite the associations between obesity and eating disorders, the rising prevalence of obesity is not accompanied by a rise in eating disorders (Zachrisson et al., 2008), although the comorbidity of eating disorders and obesity appears to be increasing (Darby, Hay, Mond, Quirk, Buttner, & Kennedy, 2009).

BED, a new formal diagnosis in the fifth edition of the *Diagnostic and Statistical Manual of Mental Disorders* (DSM-5;

American Psychiatric Association, 2013), is strongly associated with obesity and with elevated risk for psychiatric and medical comorbidities. BED is also associated with psychosocial problems, as determined in epidemiological studies (Hudson et al., 2007; Kessler et al., 2013). BED is defined by recurrent binge eating (i.e., loss of control while eating large quantities of food), marked distress about the binge eating, and the absence of inappropriate weight compensatory behaviors such as purging or laxative misuse. BED differs from other eating disorders and obesity (Allison, Grilo, Masheb, & Stunkard, 2006; Grilo, Crosby, et al., 2009). Research has consistently found that treatment-seeking persons with both BED and obesity differ from their peers with obesity who do not have BED (Grilo et al., 2008). Given the profile of BED in persons with obesity, effective interventions would ideally address the following clinical targets: binge eating, eating disorder psychopathology, associated psychological distress (e.g., elevated depression levels), and obesity or excess weight. The emerging treatment literature reviewed in this chapter evolved, in large part, based on adaptations of treatments for bulimia nervosa and obesity. The literature has varied considerably in how comprehensively it has considered the multidimensional needs of persons with both BED and obesity.

Psychological Treatments for BED

Two specific psychological "specialist" treatments—CBT and IPT—have received consistently strong empirical support. CBT, the most extensively studied approach, and IPT for BED are based on methods initially developed and empirically supported for the treatment of bulimia nervosa.

CBT

CBT for BED, based on cognitive-behavioral and restraint models of binge eating (Fairburn, Cooper, & Shafran, 2003; Fairburn, 2008), focuses initially on normalizing and structuring eating patterns (i.e., regular routine of meals and snacks to decrease unhealthy dietary restriction and chaotic eating). CBT employs self-monitoring techniques to identify external and internal triggers for binge eating and teaches specific goal-setting and problem-solving techniques to prevent binge eating, all the while reestablishing normalized eating. CBT then focuses on identifying and modifying maladaptive cognitions (i.e., to address the importance or "overvaluation" of shape/weight and other body image and psychological concerns) using cognitive restructuring and behavioral experiments.

CBT is a focused, short-term, manualized intervention that is delivered in 12–24 weeks, either individually or in small groups. It has consistently demonstrated effectiveness relative to a variety of control and comparison conditions. Research has found that CBT reliably produces binge-eating abstinence in roughly 50–60% of patients with BED. CBT produces robust improvements in eating disorder psychopathology and associated psychological functioning, including depression, but does not produce weight loss. CBT's effects on binge eating and eating disorder pathology are consistently superior to those for various controls, such as active treatment comparisons, including antidepressant medications (Grilo, Masheb, & Wilson, 2005) and BWL (Grilo, Masheb, Wilson, Gueorguieva, & White, 2011). However, CBT has not differed significantly from IPT (Wilfley et al., 2002). CBT outcomes are durable, with studies reporting good maintenance (roughly 50% binge-eating abstinence rates) through 12 months (Grilo et al., 2011; Grilo, Crosby, Wilson, & Masheb, 2012) and through 48 months (Hilbert et al., 2012) after finishing treatment. The longer-term outcomes for CBT are superior to those for pharmacotherapy with antidepressants (Grilo, Crosby, et al., 2012; Ricca et al., 2001) and BWL (Grilo et al., 2011) but not to IPT (Hilbert et al., 2012). Although on average CBT does not result in weight loss in patients with BED, binge abstinence is associated with weight loss (Grilo, Masheb, & Salant, 2005; Masheb, Dorflinger, Rolls, Mitchell, & Grilo, 2016). Long-term follow-up studies have reported stable weight (Hilbert et al., 2014), suggesting that CBT may interrupt weight gain trajectories and protect against future weight gain (Masheb, White, & Grilo, 2013).

A substantial body of research has found

that certain self-help formats of CBT for BED can be effective and scalable methods of treatment (Wilson & Zandberg, 2012). Unguided self-help (i.e., patient self-directed use of a self-care book containing the essentials of CBT) and guided-self-help (i.e., following a self-care CBT-based book supported and guided by a therapist in brief focused meetings) methods have received empirical support in a number of controlled trials (Peterson, Mitchell, Crow, Crosby, & Wonderlich, 2009; Striegel-Moore et al., 2010). Research has generally favored guided over pure self-help (Wilson & Zandberg, 2012). Guided self-help has demonstrated "treatment specificity" relative to active controls (Grilo & Masheb, 2005), and one study reported excellent durability of outcomes (roughly 60% abstinence from binge eating) through 24 months of follow-up (Wilson, Wilfley, Agras, & Bryson, 2010). These findings suggest that elements of CBT for BED can be effectively and broadly disseminated and may not be limited by the need for "specialist" CBT clinicians. This finding is important for a number of reasons: (1) The availability of "specialist" CBT clinicians is limited, (2) many patients with BED may not have the necessary financial resources to pay for specialized care, and (3) some persons with BED may prefer to work on the eating/weight problems themselves or be unwilling to seek professional help. Research has demonstrated that guided self-help CBT can be effectively delivered by generalist (i.e., nonspecialist) clinicians (Striegel-Moore et al., 2010; Wilson et al., 2010) and can be cost-effective in large health-care organizations (Lynch et al., 2010).

IPT

IPT for BED (Wilfley et al., 2002), based on interpersonal models of binge eating, evolved from IPT methods initially found to be effective for major depression and subsequently adapted for bulimia nervosa (BN). IPT focuses on helping patients in four primary domains: interpersonal deficits, role conflicts, role transitions, and loss/grief. IPT for BED focuses on helping patients to better tolerate and more effectively express feelings and to improve interpersonal relationships and psychosocial functioning. IPT generally does not target eating behaviors or pathology directly, nor does it utilize CBT techniques. It follows research findings that interpersonal stressors and perceived psychosocial ineffectiveness result in using binge eating as a (maladaptive) coping method to regulate or suppress negative emotions or manage stress. Over time, continued binge eating results in greater distress and shame, contributes to worsening interpersonal function and social isolation, and produces weight gain.

IPT is a focused, short-term, manualized intervention that is generally delivered in 16–24 weeks, either individually or in small groups. It has demonstrated short- and long-term outcomes that are generally comparable to CBT (Wilfley et al., 2002; Wilson et al., 2010). For example, IPT results in binge-eating abstinence rates of approximately 65%, along with robust improvements in both eating disorder pathology and psychological functioning. IPT for BED has demonstrated strong maintenance and excellent durability of outcomes following the short-term intervention. For example, Wilson et al. (2010) reported a 65% binge-eating abstinence rate at a 24-month follow-up. A second study reported 54% binge-eating abstinence at a 12-month follow-up (Wilfley et al., 2002) and 77% at a 48-month follow-up (Hilbert et al., 2012). The IPT longer-term binge-eating outcomes do not differ from those reported for CBT (Hilbert et al., 2012) but are superior to those reported for BWL (Wilson et al., 2010). Although IPT does not produce weight loss, follow-up studies suggest that both IPT and CBT may stabilize and prevent future weight gain in patients with BED.

DBT

Another psychological "specialist" treatment, DBT, has received promising initial empirical support for treating BED. DBT for BED is a focused, manualized therapy initially developed and empirically supported for treating emotional and behavioral dysregulation problems (i.e., borderline personality disorder, suicidality, substance abuse). It has produced promising outcomes in controlled trials. DBT conceptualizes binge-eating behaviors as attempts to cope with or to escape from distress. DBT focuses on teaching patients to help tolerate negative emotions and to learn more adaptive methods to regulate affect (e.g., mindfulness skills, distress tolerance, and emotional regulation). A recent randomized controlled trial (RCT; Safer, Robinson, & Jo, 2010) found that DBT, delivered in a group setting, was superior to an active group comparison therapy (ACGT) for reducing binge eating at posttreatment but not at the 12-month follow-up (although both interventions were associated with high rates of binge-eating abstinence: 64% in DBT and 56% in ACGT). Clinically, DBT appears to hold promise for complex patients with high impulsivity and difficulties with emotional dysregulation (Robinson & Safer, 2012).

BWL Treatment for BED

A variety of BWL approaches have also been evaluated for treating BED in persons with obesity. It is worth noting that the early research literature on BWL (and other "weight loss" methods) was quite mixed and led to debate regarding whether BWL was contraindicated, given concerns that dietary restriction might exacerbate binge eating (Wilson, Grilo, & Vitousek, 2007). However, not only has research demonstrated that structured BWL methods do not worsen binge eating, but RCTs have produced findings suggesting that BWL is an effective treatment for BED. RCTs have reported that BWL results in binge-eating abstinence rates (roughly 50%) that are comparable to those achieved by CBT methods at posttreatment and through 12 months of follow-up (Grilo et al., 2011; Wilson et al., 2010). BWL has the potential advantage over CBT and IPT of producing greater weight loss through 12 months of follow-up. Longer-term follow-ups, however, suggest that weight regain may occur over time. By 24 months, BWL is no longer associated with greater weight loss than either CBT or IPT treatments, which, in turn, show higher binge-eating abstinence rates. Grilo et al. (2011) found that a sequential approach, in which CBT (4 months) was delivered first, followed by BWL (6 months), was not superior to either CBT-only or BWL-only interventions through 12 months of follow-up.

Thus, manualized lifestyle BWL is a viable and effective treatment for BED (Grilo et al., 2011; Wilson et al., 2010). This finding is important because this "generalist" intervention is widely available. It can be delivered by a broader range of health care providers and is less costly than "specialist" treatments such as CBT and IPT. Indeed, a recent study (Grilo & White, 2013) reported that BWL for BED produced good outcomes (roughly 50% binge-eating abstinence rates through 6 months of follow-up) at a community mental health center serving socioeconomic status (SES)-disadvantaged, Spanish-speaking-only Latina/o patients with complex psychiatric problems.

Pharmacological Treatments for BED

Presently, there is only one FDA-approved medication for BED. In 2015, the FDA-approved lisdexamfetamine dimesylate (LDX) for the treatment of "moderate-to-severe BED" after an initial large Phase II RCT (McElroy, Hudson, et al., 2015) and two Phase III RCTs (McElroy, Hudson, et al., 2016). Researchers found that LDX (50–70 mg/day) was significantly superior to placebo in each of the three 11-week studies. McElroy, Hudson, et al. (2015) reported that binge-eating abstinence rates for LDX were superior to placebo (Study 1: 40 vs. 14%; Study 2: 36 vs. 13%). McElroy, Mitchell, et al. (2016) reported additional findings favoring LDX over placebo for several broader behavioral and psychological outcomes (e.g., reduced obsessive–compulsive symptoms). Presently, longer-term follow-up data are not available; thus, the longer-term durability of the effects remains unknown, as does the salient clinical question of whether or not to continue the medication. It is important to emphasize that the product labeling for LDX, which is classified as a DEA-controlled substance, includes a "Limitation of Use" (i.e., it is not indicated for weight loss, its effects on obesity are unknown, and similar classes of medication have been associated with cardiovascular adverse events) and a "Warning" (i.e., central nervous system [CNS] stimulants have a high potential for abuse/dependence).

Reas and Grilo (2014, 2015) recently reviewed 22 RCTs testing the effectiveness of a number of other medications for BED, either alone, relative to placebo, or in combination with psychological or behavioral interventions. Medications tested in randomized placebo-controlled trials included various antidepressants (Arnold, 2002; Grilo, Masheb, & Wilson, 2005; Leombruni et al., 2008; Hudson et al., 1998; Guerdjikova et al., 2008, 2012; White & Grilo, 2013); antiepileptic agents (McElroy et al., 2003; McElroy, Hudson, et al., 2007; Guerdjikova et al., 2009; McElroy et al., 2006); anti-obesity agents (Golay et al., 2005); and anticraving agents (McElroy et al., 2011, 2013).

The RCTs that tested medications varied considerably in methods. Most had limited sample sizes, all were of short duration (ranging from 8 to 24 weeks) and tested only acute treatment effects, and very few reported follow-up data. Thus, little is known regarding optimal length of treatment, maintenance or durability of the acute treatment outcomes, or the risk of relapse after medication discontinuation. The Reas and Grilo (2014, 2015) reviews, like other critical reviews and meta-analyses (Brownley, Peat, La Via, Bulik, 2015; Brownley et al., 2016; McElroy, Guerdjikova, Mori, & Keck, 2015; NICE, 2004), have converged in suggesting that certain medications have short-term efficacy relative to placebo for treating BED. Certain specific medications are superior to placebo for helping patients to reduce the frequency of or achieve abstinence from binge eating, and certain medications are superior to placebo for producing weight loss (albeit generally modest) over the short term. To date, except for LDX (which is *not* recommended for weight loss per the product labeling), only one medication—topiramate—has been shown to reliably produce substantial reductions in *both* binge eating and weight over the short term in patients with BED (McElroy et al., 2003, McElroy, Hudson, et al., 2007). Topiramate, however, is associated with a complex adverse event profile, and research has reported high rates of medication discontinuation attributed to side effects (McElroy et al., 2004).

There are almost no data on the longer-term effects of pharmacotherapy for BED. Unlike the research literature on pharmacotherapy for obesity, which tends to follow a clinical model of chronic management for energy regulation, the BED pharmacotherapy literature has generally followed a short-term acute intervention model. The few available data suggest that antidepressant medications are inferior to CBT in follow-up studies after treatment completion (Grilo, Crosby, et al., 2012; Ricca et al., 2001), and that topiramate (the only medication to date that reduces both binge eating and weight other than LDX) has extremely high dropout rates during longer-term maintenance therapy (McElroy et al., 2004). One study of an anti-obesity medication (sibutramine), which was subsequently withdrawn from the market, reported significant acute weight loss during treatment and weight regain once the medication was stopped (Grilo et al., 2014). Thus, important questions regarding effective pharmacotherapy for BED, such as optimal length of treatment, longer-term outcomes, whether to discontinue medication, and risk and timing of relapse await future empirical investigation.

Psychological and Behavioral Treatments Combined with Pharmacotherapy

Since many patients do not benefit sufficiently from the various medications tested to date or from the available psychological and behavioral treatments for BED, research has evaluated the potential utility of *combining* psychological and pharmacological treatment for BED. Grilo, Reas, and Mitchell (2016) reviewed all 11 RCTs published to date that have tested combination treatments for BED. The combination studies varied quite substantially in methods. Overall, the RCTs were relatively small (sample sizes ranged from 52 to 116), tested interventions ranging from 8 to 36 weeks, and all but two studies (Claudino et al., 2007; Golay et al., 2005) included follow-up evaluations (ranging from 3 to 24 months). The RCT designs and medications included *unblinded* tests of adding five medications: desipramine (Agras, Telch, & Arnow, 1994); imipramine (Laederach-Hofmann et al.,

1999); fluoxetine and fluvoxamine (Ricca et al., 2001); and zonisamide (Ricca et al., 2009). They also included *double-blinded* trials of four different medications added to either CBT or BWL treatments: fluoxetine in two trials (Devlin et al., 2005, Grilo, Masheb, & Wilson, 2005); orlistat in three trials (Grilo & White, 2013; Golay et al., 2005; Grilo, Masheb, & Salant, 2005); topiramate (Claudino et al., 2007); and sibutramine (Grilo, Masheb, White, et al., 2014).

Overall, based on the 11 relevant RCTs performed to date, the evidence suggests that the strategy of combining medications with either CBT or BWL treatments has generally not enhanced outcomes. Table 34.1 summarizes this literature. Combining medications with either CBT or BWL treatments results in superior binge-eating outcomes compared to pharmacotherapy alone but does *not* produce significantly improved outcomes compared to either CBT or BWL delivered alone. To date, one anti-obesity medication (orlistat) statistically improved weight losses (Grilo, Masheb, & Salant, 2005), albeit minimally, and only one medication (topiramate, an antiepileptic) significantly improved CBT outcomes for both binge eating and weight loss (Claudino et al., 2007).

Claudino et al. (2007) reported that the addition of topiramate to CBT resulted in significantly greater binge-eating abstinence rates than placebo (84 vs. 61%, respectively, based on 1-week endpoint analysis) and in significantly greater weight loss (−6.8 kg vs. −0.9 kg, respectively). The addition of topiramate to CBT, however, did not result in significantly greater reductions in binge-eating frequency, eating disorder pathology, or depression than placebo. Although Claudino et al. (2007) had only 19% attrition in their 21-week study, the only longer-term maintenance study of topiramate reported a 68% discontinuation rate associated with adverse events and difficulties tolerating the medication (McElroy et al., 2004).

Predictors, Moderators, and the Process of Change

Although a number of approaches have received empirical support for treating BED, as reviewed above, even the most effective treatments result in a substantial minority of patients continuing to have troublesome symptoms, and most patients achieve only minimal weight loss. Investigators have explored predictors and moderators of treatment outcomes, hoping to identify specific patient characteristics that could inform rationale prescription to specific treatments as a way to improve outcomes. However, reliable predictors and (especially) moderators of treatments for BED have been difficult to identify. Recent studies have suggested that patients with greater eating disorder psychopathology (Wilson et al., 2010), and specifically those with heightened overvaluation of shape/weight (Grilo, Masheb, & Crosby, 2012), may require or benefit more from specialized treatments such as CBT and IPT, rather than BWL or medication approaches.

Although research has yet to identify "mediators" of treatment outcomes—which would inform refinement of treatment methods (Wilson et al., 2007)—a series of studies have found that "rapid response" to treatment has specific reliable prognostic significance across different treatments. Overall, except for CBT—where rapid response does not predict different important long-term outcomes—studies have reported that patients who fail to show a rapid response to either BWL (Grilo, White, et al., 2012; Masheb & Grilo, 2007) or to medications (Grilo, Masheb, & Wilson, 2006; Grilo et al., 2015) are unlikely to start improving with continued treatment. Patients with BED who exhibit a rapid response to BWL are especially likely to achieve good outcomes in both binge eating and weight loss (Grilo, White, et al., 2012; Masheb & Grilo, 2007). Figure 34.1 shows the differential prognostic significance of early rapid response in patients treated with CBT versus BWL (Grilo, White, et al., 2012). These findings led Grilo and colleagues to suggest a possible "stepped-care" approach of starting with BWL (a widely available treatment) and switching those patients who do not evidence a rapid response after a month to a specialist treatment (CBT or IPT) and/or add pharmacotherapy. This strategy is the focus of a current National Institutes of Health (NIH)-funded RCT (clinical trial registry: NCT00516919).

TABLE 34.1. Randomized Controlled Trials Testing Combined Psychological and Pharmacological Treatments for BED

Study	Treatment	Sample size (total)	Treatment length (weeks)	Attrition (%)	Percent abstinent (at FUP)	Frequency of binge-eating	Weight loss
Agras et al. (1994)	a. BWL-only b. CBT/BWL c. CBT/BWL–desipramine	109	40	a. 27 b. 17 c. 23	a. 19, 14 b. 37, 28 c. 41, 32	*Binge days weekly* a. 4.5 to 1.5 to 2.0 b. 4.4 to 1.2 to 1.7 c. 5.1 to 0.9 to 1.5	*Weight loss (kg)* a. 3.7 to 4.2 b. 1.6 to 0[a] c. 6.0 to 4.8[b]
Laedrach-Hofmann et al. (1999)	a. Counseling b. Imipramine	31	6	a. 6 b. 7	NA	*Binge episodes weekly* a. 7.1 to 5.3 to 7.2 b. 7.1 to 2.5 to 4.1	*Weight loss (kg)* a. +0.2 to +2.2 b. 2.2 to 5.1[a]
Ricca et al. (2001)	a. CBT b. CBT + Fluoxetine c. CBT + Fluvoxamine d. Fluoxoetine e. Fluvoxamine	108	24	a. 15 b. 27 c. 22 d. 24 e. 27	NA	*Binge episodes monthly* a. 18 to 8.0 to 8.0[d,e] b. 17 to 6.0 to 7.0[d,e] c. 18.0 to 8.0 to 8.0[d,e] d. 20.0 to 19.0 to 21.0 e. 20.0 to 18.0 to 18.0	*BMI* NA Reported significantly reduced at post-tx and FUP for three CBT conditions but not for either Fluoxetine or Fluvoxamine.
Devlin et al. (2005); Devlin et al. (2007)	a. Fluoxetine b. Placebo c. CBT d. CBT + Fluoxetine All given concurrently with BWL	108	20	a. 31 b. 48 c. 40 d. 25	Main effect for CBT assignment: 62 vs. 33%[b] No main effect for Fluoxetine assignment: 52 vs. 41% No CBT by Fluoxetine interaction	*Binge episodes monthly* a. 16.4 to 4.9 b. 15.4 to 6.0 c. 17.1 to 3.7 d. 16.1 to 2.2 *Note:* At post-tx and 2-yr FUP, the addition of CBT to BWL significantly enhanced reduction in binge-eating frequency and binge remission versus BWL without CBT.	*Weight (kg) (baseline to post)* a. 113.8 to 111.9 b. 113.5 to 111.1 c. 116.5 to 114.6 d. 116.9 to 112.8 *Note:* At post-tx and FUP, no significant main effects for either CBT or medication.
Golay et al. (2005)	a. Orlistat + diet b. Placebo + diet	89	24	a. 11 b. 29	a. NA b. NA	*Binge episodes weekly* a. 5.4 to 1.0 b. 6.2 to 1.7	*Percent weight loss* a. 7.4% loss b. 2.3% loss[a]

Study	Treatment	N	Weeks	% Dropout	% Abstinent	Binge outcome	Weight/BMI outcome
Grilo, Masheb, & Salant (2005)	a. Orlistat + CBT guided-self-help b. Placebo + CBT guided-self-help	50	12	a. 24 b. 20	a. 64, 52 b. 36[a], 52	*Binge episodes monthly* a. 16.4 to 3.2 to 3.4 b. 13.5 to 3.6 to 2.8	*Percent achieving 5% loss* a. 36%, 32% b. 8%[a], 8%[a]
Grilo, Masheb, & Wilson (2005); Grilo, Crosby, Wilson, & Masheb (2012)	a. Fluoxetine b. Placebo c. CBT + placebo d. CBT + Fluoxetine	108	16	a. 22 b. 15 c. 21 d. 23	a. 22, 4 b. 26, NA c. 61[a,b], 36[a] d. 50[a,b], 27[a]	*Binge episodes monthly* a. 17.9 to 10.4 to 10.4 b. 13.2 to 7.2 to NA c. 16.6 to 2.3 to 4.6[a,b] d. 16.5 to 4.3 to 4.6[a,b]	*Weight loss (lbs.)* *(at post-tx and FUP)* a. 4.8 to 1.5 b. NA c. 5.0 to 9.8 d. 5.6 to 4.1
Claudino et al. (2007)	a. CBT + topiramate b. CBT + placebo	73	21	a. 19 b. 28	a. 84 b. 61[a]	*Binge episodes weekly* a. 4.2 to 0.0 b. 3.4 to 0.3	a. 6.8 kg b. 0.9 kg[a]
Ricca et al. (2009)	a. CBT b. CBT + zonisamide	52	24	a. 33 b. 50	NA	*Binge episodes monthly* a. 5.0 to 2.0 to 3.0 b. 5.0 to 2.0 to 2.0[a]	*BMI* a. 39.2 to 38.4 to 38.9 b. 38.4 to 36.7[a] to 36.5[a]
Grilo & White (2013)	a. BWL + orlistat b. BWL + placebo	40	16	a. 30 b. 25	a. 60, 50 b. 70, 50	a. NA b. NA	*BMI* a. 39.0 to 37.9 to 37.6 b. 37.2 to 36.0 to 36.7
Grilo et al. (2014)	a. Sibutramine b. Placebo c. CBT self-help + placebo d. CBT self-help + sibutramine	104	16	a. 27 b. 15 c. 12 d. 16	a. 39, 19, 19 b. 30, 41, 37 c. 24, 40, 40 d. 23, 50, 42	*Binge episodes monthly* a. 22.4 to 5.0 to 4.9 to 5.8 b. 21.1 to 5.3 to 5.7 to 6.7 c. 14.6 to 6.4 to 3.6[a,b] to 4.9 d. 16.9 to 3.6 to 3.9 to 3.0	*BMI* a. 39.4 to 38.4[c,d] to 38.7 to 39.3 b. 39.3 to 39.6[c,d] to 38.8 to 39.5 c. 36.5 to 35.9[a,b] to 35.3 to 35.4 d. 37.8 to 35.6[a,b] to 36.0 to 36.5

Note. BMI, body mass index; FUP, follow-up; BWL, behavioral weight loss; CBT, cognitive-behavioral therapy; NA, data not available; tx, treatment.
* $p < .05$; ** $p < .001$. Superscripts denote significant group differences between treatments.

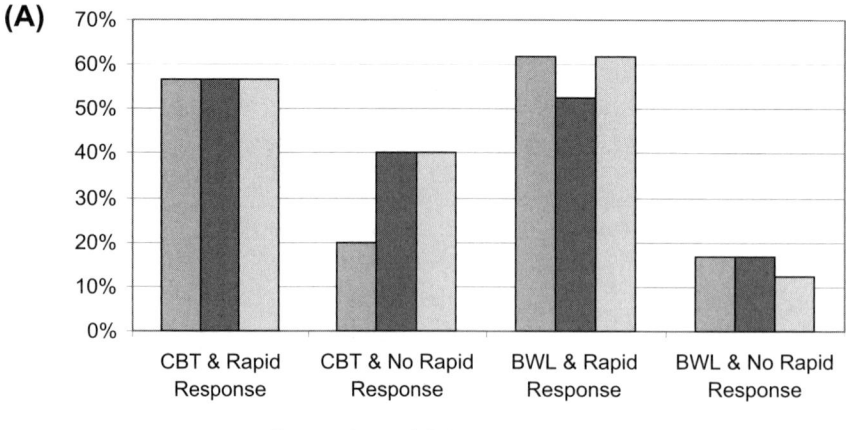
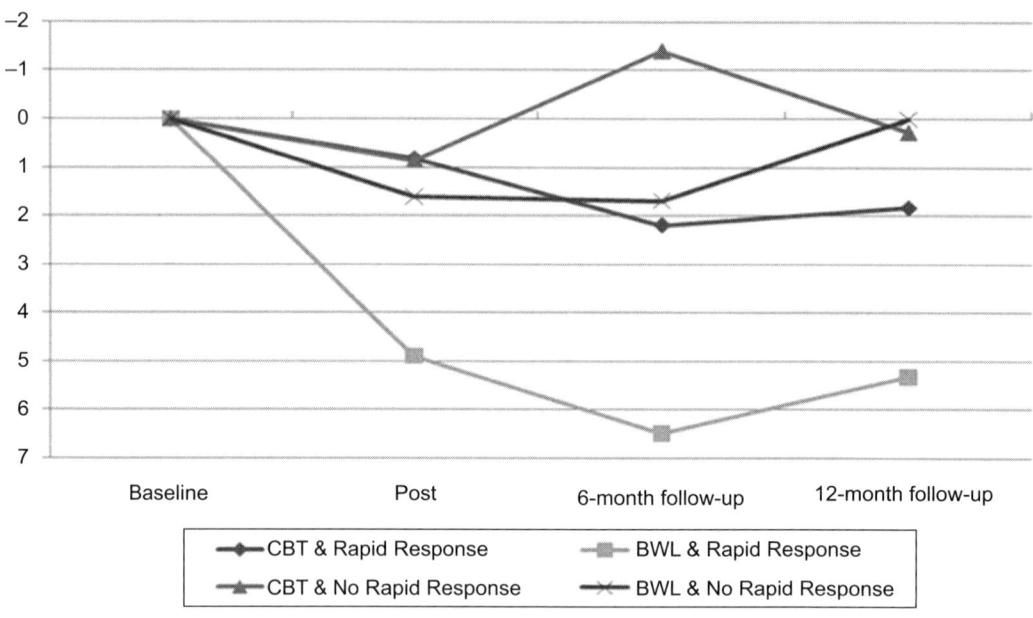

FIGURE 34.1. Prognostic significance of rapid response to BWL and CBT for BED. (A) The proportion (i.e., percentage) of participants with rapid response versus without rapid response that achieved abstinence from binge eating at posttreatment, 6-month, and 12-month follow-up assessments for BWL and CBT. (B) The percentage weight loss (y-axis shows estimated marginal means) by participants with rapid response versus without rapid response throughout the course of treatment and follow-ups (x-axis) for BWL and CBT. Adapted and based on data from Grilo, White, Wilson, Gueorguieva, and Masheb (2012). Rapid response predicts 12-month post-treatment outcomes in binge eating disorder: Theoretical and clinical implications. *Psychological Medicine, 42*(4), 807–817. Copyright © 2012 Elsevier. Adapted by permission.

Disordered Eating and Bariatric Surgery

A growing literature on identifying and treating disordered eating in patients with obesity is emerging from the study of severely obese persons who seek (and undergo) bariatric surgery. Many patients with severe obesity who seek bariatric surgery experience difficulties with binge eating preoperatively (Wadden et al., 2011; White, Kalarchian, Masheb, Marcus, & Grilo, 2010) and "loss of control" eating postoperatively (White al., 2010). Whereas binge eating prior to bariatric surgery has generally not predicted poorer weight loss outcomes (Wadden et al., 2011; White et al., 2010; Chao et al., 2016), disordered eating behaviors postoperatively appear to be a negative prognostic indicator (Devlin et al., 2016; Meany, Conceicao, & Mitchell, 2014; White et al., 2010). The emerging intervention literature consists of a few relatively small trials of brief behavioral, cognitive, and nutritional interventions adapted from the BWL and CBT literatures for obesity and BED. Critical reviews of the preliminary evidence have converged in suggesting the potential effectiveness of behavioral and cognitive interventions delivered after bariatric surgery (Beck, Johannsen, Stoving, Mehlsen, & Zachariae, 2012; Kalarchian & Marcus, 2015; Rudolph & Hilbert, 2013).

Future Research Directions

Longer-term and larger studies are needed to establish, more definitively, the role of pharmacotherapy for BED, including, most importantly, its durability and approaches to longer-term maintenance. Recently, four new anti-obesity medications or medication combinations (phentermine/topiramate, lorcaserin, naltrexone/bupropion, and liraglutide) have been approved by the FDA for treating obesity, but none has been evaluated for BED either as a monotherapy or in combination with CBT or BWL. Larger studies with greater diversity and generalizability (Thompson-Brenner et al., 2013) are needed to perform adequately powered analyses of mediators of outcomes. These data would inform how best to refine existing treatments, and analyses of moderators of outcomes would inform improved treatment prescription or "matching." Finding ways to effectively produce weight loss and longer-term weight control in patients with BED remains a major challenge. Methods for broader dissemination and training of clinicians in evidence-based methods represent additional challenges.

Acknowledgment

Preparation of this chapter was supported, in part, by National Institutes of Health Grant Nos. K24 DK070052, R01 DK49587, and R01 DK098492.

References

Agras, W. S., Telch, C. F., & Arnow, B. (1994). Weight loss, cognitive-behavioral, and desipramine treatments in binge eating disorder: An additive design. *Behavior Therapy, 25*(2), 225–238.

Allison, K. C., Grilo, C. M., Masheb, R. M., & Stunkard, A. J. (2006). Binge eating disorder and night eating syndrome: A comparative study of disordered eating. *Journal of Consulting and Clinical Psychology, 73*(6), 1107–1115.

American Psychiatric Association. (2013). *Diagnostic and statistical manual of mental disorders* (5th ed.). Arlington, VA: Author.

Arnold, L. M., McElroy, S. L., Hudson, J. I., Welge, J. A., Bennett, A. J., & Keck, P. E. (2002). A placebo-controlled, randomized trial of fluoxetine in the treatment of binge-eating disorder. *Journal of Clinical Psychiatry, 63*(11), 1028–1033.

Beck, N., Johannsen, M., Stoving, R., Mehlsen, M., & Zachariae, R. (2012). Do postoperative psychotherapeutic interventions and support groups influence weight loss following bariatric surgery?: A systematic review and meta-analysis of randomized and non-randomized trials. *Obesity Surgery, 22*(11), 1790–1797.

Brownley, K. A., Berkman, N. D., Peat, C. M., Lohr, K. N., Cullen, K. E., Bann, C. M., et al. (2016). Binge-eating disorder in adults: A systematic review and meta-analysis. *Annals of Internal Medicine, 165*(6), 409–420.

Brownley, K. A., Peat, C. M., La Via, M., & Bulik, C. M. (2015). Pharmacological approaches to the management of binge eating disorder. *Drugs, 75*(1), 9–32.

Chao, A. M., Wadden, T. A., Faulconbridge, L. F., Sarwer, D. B., Webb, V. L., Shaw, J. A., et al. (2016). Binge-eating and the outcome of bariatric surgery in a prospective observational study: Two-year results. *Obesity, 24*(11), 2327–2333.

Claudino, A. M., de Oliveira, I. R., Appolinario, J. C., Cordas, T. A., Duchesne, M., Sichieri, R., et al.

(2007). Double-blind, randomized, placebo-controlled trial of topiramate plus cognitive-behavior therapy in binge-eating disorder. *Journal of Clinical Psychiatry, 68*(9), 1324–1332.

Darby, A., Hay, P., Mond, J., Quirk, F., Buttner, P., & Kennedy, L. (2009). The rising prevalence of comorbid obesity and eating disorder behaviors from 1995 to 2005. *International Journal of Eating Disorders, 42*(2), 104–108.

Devlin, M. J., Goldfein, J. A., Petkova, E., Jiang, H., Raizman, P. S., Wolk, S., et al. (2005). Cognitive behavioral therapy and fluoxetine as adjuncts to group behavioral therapy for binge eating disorder. *Obesity Research, 13*(6), 1077–1088.

Devlin, M. J., Goldfein, J. A., Petkova, E., Liu, L., & Walsh, B. T. (2007). Cognitive behavioral therapy and fluoxetine for binge eating disorder: Two-year follow-up. *Obesity, 15*, 1702–1709.

Devlin, M. J., King, W. C., Kalarchian, M. A., White, G. E., Marcus, M. D., Garcia, L., et al. (2016). Eating pathology and experience and weight loss in a prospective study of bariatric surgery patients: 3-year follow-up. *International Journal of Eating Disorders, 49*(12), 1058–1067.

Fairburn, C. G. (2008). *Cognitive behavior therapy and eating disorders*. New York: Guilford Press.

Fairburn, C. G., Cooper, Z., & Shafran, R. (2003). Cognitive behavior therapy for eating disorders: A "transdiagnostic" theory and treatment. *Behaviour Research and Therapy, 41*(5), 509–528.

Flegal, K. M., Carroll, M. D., Ogden, C. L., & Curtin, L. R. (2010). Prevalence and trends in obesity among U.S. adults, 1999–2008. *Journal of the American Medical Association, 303*(3), 235–241.

Golay, A., Laurent-Jaccard, A., Habicht, F., Gachoud, J. P., Chabloz, M., Kammer, A., et al. (2005). Effect of orlistat in obese patients with binge eating disorder. *Obesity Research, 13*(10), 1701–1708.

Grilo, C. M., Crosby, R. D., Masheb, R. M., White, M. A., Peterson, C. B., Wonderlich, S. A., et al. (2009). Overvaluation of shape and weight in binge eating disorder, bulimia nervosa, and sub-threshold bulimia nervosa. *Behaviour Research and Therapy, 47*(8), 692–696.

Grilo, C. M., Crosby, R. D., Wilson, G. T., & Masheb, R. M. (2012). 12-month follow-up of fluoxetine and cognitive behavioral therapy for binge eating disorder. *Journal of Consulting and Clinical Psychology, 80*(6), 1108–1113.

Grilo, C. M., Hrabosky, J. I., White, M. A., Allison, K. C., Stunkard, A. J., & Masheb, R. M. (2008). Overvaluation of shape and weight in binge eating disorder and overweight controls: Refinement of a diagnostic construct. *Journal of Abnormal Psychology, 117*(2), 414–419.

Grilo, C. M., & Masheb, R. M. (2005). A randomized controlled comparison of guided self-help cognitive behavioral therapy and behavioral weight loss for binge eating disorder. *Behaviour Research and Therapy, 43*(11), 1509–1525.

Grilo, C. M., Masheb, R. M., & Crosby, R. D. (2012). Predictors and moderators of response to cognitive behavioral therapy and medication for the treatment of binge eating disorder. *Journal of Consulting and Clinical Psychology, 80*(5), 897–906.

Grilo, C. M., Masheb, R. M., & Salant, S. L. (2005). Cognitive behavioral therapy guided self-help and orlistat for the treatment of binge eating disorder: A randomized, double-blind, placebo-controlled trial. *Biological Psychiatry, 57*(3), 1193–1201.

Grilo, C. M., Masheb, R. M., White, M. A., Gueorguieva, R., Barnes, R. D., Walsh, B. T., et al. (2014). Treatment of binge eating disorder in racially and ethnically diverse obese patients in primary care: Randomized placebo-controlled clinical trial of self-help and medication. *Behaviour Research and Therapy, 58*, 1–9.

Grilo, C. M., Masheb, R. M., & Wilson, G. T. (2005). Efficacy of cognitive behavioral therapy and fluoxetine for the treatment of binge eating disorder: A randomized, double-blind, placebo-controlled trial. *Biological Psychiatry, 57*(3), 301–309.

Grilo, C. M., Masheb, R. M., Wilson, G. T., Gueorguieva, R., & White, M. A. (2011). Cognitive-behavioral therapy, behavioral weight loss, and sequential treatment for obese patients with binge-eating disorder: A randomized controlled trial. *Journal of Consulting and Clinical Psychology, 79*(5), 675–685.

Grilo, C. M., Reas, D. L., & Mitchell, J. E. (2016). Combining pharmacological and psychological treatments for binge eating disorder: Current status, limitations, and future directions. *Current Psychiatry Reports, 18*(6), 55.

Grilo, C. M., & White, M. A. (2013). Orlistat with behavioral weight loss for obesity with versus without binge eating disorder: Randomized placebo-controlled trial at a community mental health center serving educationally and economically disadvantaged Latino/as. *Behaviour Research and Therapy, 51*(3), 167–175.

Grilo, C. M., White, M. A., Masheb, R. M., & Gueorguieva, R. (2015). Predicting meaningful outcomes to medication and self-help treatments for binge eating disorder in primary care: The significance of rapid response. *Journal of Consulting and Clinical Psychology, 83*(2), 387–394.

Grilo, C. M., White, M. A., Wilson, G. T., Gueorguieva, R., & Masheb, R. M. (2012). Rapid response predicts 12-month post-treatment outcomes in binge eating disorder: Theoretical and clinical implications. *Psychological Medicine, 42*(4), 807–817.

Guerdjikova, A. I., McElroy, S. L., Kotwal, R., Welge, J. A., Nelson, E., Lake, K., et al. (2008). High-dose escitalopram in the treatment of binge-eating disorder with obesity: A placebo-controlled monotherapy trial. *Human Psychopharmacology, 23*(1), 1–11.

Guerdjikova, A. I., McElroy, S. L., Welge, J. A., Nelson, E., Keck, P. E., & Hudson, J. I. (2009). Lamotrigine in the treatment of binge-eating disorder with obesity: A randomized, placebo-controlled monotherapy trial. *International Clinical Psychopharmacology, 24*(3), 150–158.

Guerdjikova, A. I., McElroy, S. L., Winstanley, E. L., Nelson, E. B., Mori, N., McCoy, J., et al. (2012).

Duloxetine in the treatment of binge eating disorder with depressive disorders: A placebo-controlled trial. *International Journal of Eating Disorders, 45*(2), 281–289.

Hilbert, A., Bishop, M. E., Stein, R. I., Tanofsky-Kraff, M., Swenson, A. K., Welch, R. R., et al. (2012). Long-term efficacy of psychological treatments for binge eating disorder. *British Journal of Psychiatry, 200*(3), 232–237.

Hudson, J. I., Hiripi, E., Pope, H. G., & Kessler, R. C. (2007). The prevalence and correlates of eating disorders in the National Comorbidity Survey Replication. *Biological Psychiatry, 61*(3), 348–358.

Hudson, J. I., McElroy, S. L., Raymond, N. C., Crow, S., Keck, P. E., Jr., Carter, W. P., et al. (1998). Fluvoxamine in the treatment of binge-eating disorder: A multicenter placebo-controlled, double-blind trial. *American Journal of Psychiatry, 155*(12), 1756–1762.

Kalarchian, M. A., & Marcus, M. D. (2015). Psychosocial interventions pre and post bariatric surgery. *European Eating Disorders Review, 23*(6), 457–462.

Kessler, R. C., Berglund, P. A., Chiu, W. T., Deitz, A. C., Hudson, J. I., Shahly, V., et al. (2013). The prevalence and correlates of binge eating disorder in the World Health Organization World Mental Health Surveys. *Biological Psychiatry, 73*(9), 904–914.

Laederach-Hofmann, K., Graf, C., Horber, F., et al. (1999). Imipramine and diet counseling with psychological support in the treatment of obese binge eaters: A randomized, placebo-controlled double-blind study. *International Journal of Eating Disorders, 26*(3), 231–244.

Leombruni, P., Piero, A., Lavagnino, L., Brustolin, A., Campisi, S., & Fassino, S. (2008). A randomized, double-blind trial comparing sertraline and fluoxetine 6-month treatment in obese patients with binge eating disorder. *Progress in Neuropsychopharmacology and Biological Psychiatry, 32*(6), 1599–1605.

Lynch, F. L., Striegel-Moore, R. H., Dickerson, J. F., Perrin, N., Debar, L., Wilson, G. T., et al. (2010). Cost-effectiveness of guided self-help treatment for recurrent binge eating. *Journal of Consulting and Clinical Psychology, 78*(3), 322–333.

Masheb, R. M., Dorflinger, L. M., Rolls, B. J., Mitchell, J. E., & Grilo, C. M. (2016). Binge abstinence is associated with reduced energy intake after treatment in patients with binge disorder and obesity. *Obesity, 24*(12), 2491–2496.

Masheb, R. M., & Grilo, C. M. (2007). Rapid response treatment outcomes in binge eating disorder: Implications for stepped care. *Journal of Consulting and Clinical Psychology, 75*(4), 639–644.

Masheb, R. M., White, M. A., & Grilo, C. M. (2013). Substantial weight gains are common prior to treatment-seeking in obese patients with binge eating disorder. *Comprehensive Psychiatry, 54*(7), 880–884.

McElroy, S. L., Arnold, L. M., Shapira, N. A., Keck, P. E., Jr., Rosenthal, N. R., Karim, M. R., et al. (2003). Topiramate in the treatment of binge eating disorder associated with obesity: A randomized, placebo-controlled trial. *American Journal of Psychiatry, 160*(2), 255–261.

McElroy, S. L., Guerdjikova, A. I., Blom, T. J., Crow, S. J., Memisoglu, A., Silverman, B. L., et al. (2013). A placebo-controlled pilot study of the novel opioid receptor antagonist ALKS-33 in binge eating disorder. *International Journal of Eating Disorders, 46*(3), 239–245.

McElroy, S. L., Guerdjikova, A., Kotwal, R., Welge, J. A., Nelson, E. B., Lake, K. A., et al. (2007). Atomoxetine in the treatment of binge-eating disorder: A randomized placebo-controlled trial. *Journal of Clinical Psychiatry, 68*(3), 390–398.

McElroy, S. L., Guerdjikova, A. I., Mori, N., & Keck, P. E. (2015). Psychopharmacologic treatment of eating disorders: Emerging findings. *Current Psychiatry Reports, 17*(5), 35.

McElroy, S. L., Guerdjikova, A. I., Winstanley, E. L., O'Melia, A. M., Mori, N., McCoy, J., et al. (2011). Acamprosate in the treatment of binge eating disorder: A placebo-controlled trial. *International Journal of Eating Disorders, 44*(1), 81–90.

McElroy, S. L., Hudson, J. I., Capece, J. A., Beyers, K., Fisher, A. C., & Rosenthal, N. R. (2007). Topiramate for the treatment of binge eating disorder associated with obesity: A placebo-controlled study. *Biological Psychiatry, 61*(9), 1039–1048.

McElroy, S. L., Hudson, J., Ferreira-Cornwell, M. C., Radewonuk, J., Whitaker, T., & Gasior, M. (2016). Lisdexamfetamine dimesylate for adults with moderate to severe binge eating disorder: Results of two pivotal phase 3 randomized controlled trials. *Neuropsychopharmacology, 41*(5), 1251–1260.

McElroy, S. L., Hudson, J. I., Mitchell, J. E., Wilfley, D., Ferreira-Cornwell, M. C., Gao, J., et al. (2015). Efficacy and safety of lisdexamfetamine for treatment of adults with moderate to severe binge-eating disorder: A randomized clinical trial. *JAMA Psychiatry, 72*(3), 235–246.

McElroy, S. L., Kotwal, R., Guerdjikova, A. I., Welge, J. A., Nelson, E. B., Lake, K. A., et al. (2006). Zonisamide in the treatment of binge eating disorder with obesity: A randomized controlled trial. *Journal of Clinical Psychiatry, 67*(12), 1897–1906.

McElroy, S. L., Mitchell, J. E., Wilfley, D., Gasior, M., Ferreira-Cornwell, M. C., McKay, M., et al. (2016). Lisdexamfetamine dimesylate effects on binge eating behavior and obsessive–compulsive and impulsive features in adults with binge eating disorder. *European Eating Disorder Review, 24*(3), 223–231.

McElroy, S. L., Shapira, N. A., Arnold, L. M., Keck, P. E., Rosenthal, N. R., Wu, S. C., et al. (2004). Topiramate in the long-term treatment of binge-eating disorder associated with obesity. *Journal of Clinical Psychiatry, 65*(11), 1463–1469.

Meany, G., Conceicao, E., & Mitchell, J. E. (2014). Binge eating, binge eating disorder, and loss of control eating: Effects on weight outcomes after bariatric surgery. *European Eating Disorder Review, 22*(2), 87–91.

Mohler-Kuo, M., Schnyder, U., Dermota, P., Wei, W., & Milos, G. (2016). The prevalence, correlates, and help-seeking of eating disorders in Switzerland. *Psychological Medicine, 1*(13), 1–10.

NICE. (2004). Eating disorders: Core interventions in the treatment and management of anorexia nervosa, bulimia nervosa, and related eating disorders. *NICE Clinical Guideline No. 9*.

Peterson, C. B., Mitchell, J. E., Crow, S. J., Crosby, R. D., & Wonderlich, S. A. (2009). The efficacy of self-help group treatment and therapist-led group treatment for binge eating disorder. *American Journal of Psychiatry, 166*(12), 1347–1354.

Reas, D. L., & Grilo, C. M. (2014). Current and emerging drug treatments for binge eating disorder. *Expert Opinion in Emerging Drugs, 19*(1), 99–142.

Reas, D. L., & Grilo, C. M. (2015). Pharmacological treatment of binge eating disorder: Update review and synthesis. *Expert Opinion in Pharmacotherapy, 16*(10), 1463–1478.

Ricca, V., Castellini, G., Lo Sauro, C., Rotella, C. M., & Faravelli, C. (2009). Zonisamide combined with cognitive behavioral therapy in binge eating disorder: A one-year follow-up study. *Psychiatry, 6*(11), 23–28.

Ricca, V., Mannucci, E., Mezzani, B., Moretti, S., Di, B. M., Bertelli, M., et al. (2001). Fluoxetine and fluvoxamine combined with individual cognitive-behaviour therapy in binge eating disorder: A one-year follow-up study. *Psychotherapy and Psychosomatics, 70*(6), 298–306.

Robinson, A. H., & Safer, D. L. (2012). Moderators of dialectical behavior therapy for binge eating disorder: Results from a randomized controlled trial. *International Journal of Eating Disorders, 45*(4), 597–602.

Rudolph, A., & Hilbert, A. (2013). Post-operative behavioural management in bariatric surgery: A systematic review and meta-analysis of randomized controlled trials. *Obesity Reviews, 14*(4), 292–302.

Safer, D. L., Robinson, A. H., & Jo, B. (2010). Outcome from a randomized controlled trial of group therapy for binge eating disorder: Comparing dialectical behavior therapy adapted for binge eating to an active comparison group therapy. *Behavior Therapy, 41*(1), 106–120.

Striegel-Moore, R. H., Wilson, G. T., DeBar, L., Perrin, N., Lynch, F., Rosselli, F., et al. (2010). Cognitive behavioral guided self-help for the treatment of recurrent binge eating. *Journal of Consulting and Clinical Psychology, 78*(3), 312–321.

Thompson-Brenner, H., Franko, D. L., Thompson, D. R., Grilo, C. M., Boisseau, C. L., Roehrig, J. P., et al. (2013). Race/ethnicity, education, and treatment parameters as moderators and predictors of outcome in binge eating disorder. *Journal of Consulting and Clinical Psychology, 81*(4), 710–721.

Wadden, T. A., Faulconbridge, L. F., Jones-Corneille, L. R., Sarwer, D. B., Fabricatore, A. N., Thomas, J. G., et al. (2011). Binge eating disorder and the outcome of bariatric surgery at one-year: A prospective observational study. *Obesity, 19*(6), 1220–1228.

White, M. A., & Grilo, C. M. (2013). Buproprion for overweight women with binge eating disorder: A randomized, double-blind, placebo-controlled trial. *Journal of Clinical Psychiatry, 74*(4), 400–406.

White, M. A., Kalarchian, M. A., Masheb, R. M., Marcus, M. D., & Grilo, C. M. (2010). Loss of control over eating predicts outcomes in bariatric surgery patients: A prospective 24-month follow-up study. *Journal of Clinical Psychiatry, 71*(2), 175–184.

Wilfley, D. E., Welch, R. R., Stein, R. I., Spurrell, E. B., Cohen, L. R., Saelens, B. E., et al (2002). A randomized comparison of group cognitive-behavioral therapy and group interpersonal psychotherapy for the treatment of overweight individuals with binge-eating disorder. *Archives of General Psychiatry, 59*(8), 713–721.

Wilson, G. T., Grilo, C. M., & Vitousek, K. M. (2007). Psychological treatment of eating disorders. *American Psychologist, 62*(3), 199–216.

Wilson, G. T., Wilfley, D. E., Agras, W. S., & Bryson, S. W. (2010). Psychological treatments of binge eating disorder. *Archives of General Psychiatry, 67*(1), 94–101.

Wilson, G. T., & Zandberg, L. J. (2012). Cognitive-behavioral guided self-help for eating disorders: Effectiveness and scalability. *Clinical Psychology Review, 32*(4), 343–357.

Zachrisson, H. D., Vedul-Kjelsas, E., Gotostam, K. G., & Mykletun, A. (2008). Time trends in obesity and eating disorders. *International Journal of Eating Disorders, 41*(8), 673–680.

CHAPTER 35

Obesity and Body Image Dissatisfaction

David B. Sarwer
Colleen M. Tewksbury
Heather M. Polonsky

Dissatisfaction with physical appearance and body image is a common experience for individuals living in Westernized cultures. Body image dissatisfaction is frequently reported by those who have excess body weight. This dissatisfaction can affect both self-esteem and quality of life. Body image dissatisfaction is also believed to be the motivational catalyst for a range of appearance-enhancing behaviors, including weight loss efforts. This chapter provides an overview of the relationship between body image and obesity. The chapter begins with an overview of the development and refinement of the psychological construct of body image. This includes a discussion of definitions and theoretical models of the construct. Psychometric measures to assess body image are described. An overview of the etiology of body image, with a focus on severity and clinical significance, is detailed. The chapter concludes with a discussion of changes in body image with weight loss, as well as the role that psychotherapeutic interventions and cosmetic surgical procedures can play in addressing weight-related body image concerns.

The Psychological Construct of Body Image

Understanding of the psychological construct of body image begins with an awareness and appreciation of the role physical appearance plays in daily life. This issue has always been of great interest to philosophers and writers, business executives and marketing professionals, as well as anyone who has ever fallen in love. In the early 1970s, social psychologists began to formally study how an individual's physical appearance affects his or her social relationships. Early studies in this area focused on the role of physical attractiveness in romantic partner selection (Hatfield & Sprecher, 1986). Over time, researchers investigated the impact of physical appearance on a range of interpersonal interactions. This now substantial body of research has repeatedly demonstrated that individuals who are more physically attractive are judged or perceived in a more favorable light than less attractive individuals (Hatfield & Sprecher, 1986; Patzer, 2007). More attractive individuals are often believed to have more positive personality characteristics than their less attractive peers. For example, more attractive individuals are rated as being more intelligent, friendlier, and kinder than individuals who are less attractive. Studies also suggest that more attractive individuals receive preferential treatment in a variety of social situations across their lifespan (Aharon et al., 2001; Patzer, 2007). Whereas many of these studies focused specifically on facial appearance, others have focused on more global assessments of attractiveness or discrete issues such as height and weight. Not surprisingly, lean individuals are perceived to be more attractive than those who are overweight or obese (Etcoff, 2011).

As research on the role of physical appearance in interpersonal relationships evolved, other scholars focused on the "internal" view of physical appearance: body image (Cash & Smolak, 2011). The earliest work in this area was undertaken by neurologists trying to identify the basic elements of the mind–body relationship. Stunkard and Mendelson (1967) were the first to report that some individuals with obesity—particularly those with childhood onset of obesity and those who experienced unwanted comments about their weight—experienced body image dissatisfaction (Stunkard & Mendelson, 1967). It wasn't until the 1980s and 1990s that research on body image exploded. Using cognitive-behavioral theory as a foundation, investigators proposed new theoretical models of body image and conducted high-quality empirical research that rapidly advanced the field (Cash, 2012; Cash & Smolak, 2011). Much of the early work in the area of body image focused on the weight and shape concerns of individuals with anorexia nervosa and bulimia nervosa. However, as the global obesity problem grew in the 1990s, the body image concerns of individuals with excess body weight garnered more attention (Sarwer, Thompson, & Cash, 2005).

Definitions and Theoretical Models of Body Image

We all have a sense of our own body image—how we think, feel, and behave in response to our physical appearance. However, when the multidimensional nature of body image is considered, articulation of a concise definition of body image becomes challenging. Cash and Pruzinsky (1990) defined *body image* as the perceptions, thoughts, and feelings associated with the body and bodily experience. This definition captured the multidimensional nature of body image, including not only the manner in which an individual objectively appears to others (e.g., tall or short, large or small), but also the manner in which a body moves in time and space. These physical perceptions subsequently interact with thoughts and feelings about the features of one's appearance. Unfortunately, this definition does not specifically highlight body image behaviors, such as grooming habits and clothing selection, as well as more profound behaviors, such as physical changes from weight gain or loss.

Within a decade of Cash and Pruzinsky's definition, another text identified 13 different terms that were used interchangeably with *body image,* as experts in the field struggled to agree on a common definition of the construct (Thompson, Heinberg, Altabe, & Tantleff-Dunn, 1999). In an effort to return the field to a more straightforward definition, Cash and Smolak (2011) described body image as the "psychological experience of embodiment." This succinct description leaves the reader with a sense of the important role that body image plays in quality of life, self-esteem, and the overall human experience.

Much of our understanding of body image comes from a cognitive-behavioral theoretical model (Cash & Smolak, 2011). This model describes the perceptual, cognitive, affective, and behavioral aspects of body image; it also accounts for historical and proximal influences of the construct. In brief, historical influences include an individual's physical characteristics (and changes to them), personality traits (that may place an individual "at risk" to be overly concerned about his or her body image), interpersonal experiences (such as appearance-focused teasing), and cultural socialization. Proximal influences include cognitive processing of appearance-specific information from the environment that, along with more general cognitive processes, lends "meaning" to situations and events in daily life.

These historical and proximal variables influence two fundamental body image attitudes. The first is body image investment: the amount of time and energy—cognitive, emotional, and behavioral—an individual spends on his or her appearance. The second is body image evaluation: the degree to which an individual is satisfied or dissatisfied with his or her appearance. The interaction of the degree of investment in one's appearance and the degree of (dis)satisfaction influence subsequent body image behavior. Both attitudes are believed to fall along a continuum. Individuals who are both highly invested and highly dissatisfied with their appearance are most likely to engage in behaviors to change their appearance (Sarwer, Pertschuk, Wadden, & Whitaker, 1998). However, it is important to realize that there are contextual elements that can affect judgment of body image investment and satisfaction. Clothing is one such element. Many individuals will use oversized or loose-fitting clothing to camouflage their excess weight; others will avoid clothing options, such as shorts and bathing suits, which would display their excess weight or cellulite to others. Given the rapid growth of clothing options and accessories that can enhance body shape (e.g., Spanx) now available, it's quite likely that the degree of body image dissatisfaction varies when an individual is dressed or undressed (Sarwer & Polonsky, 2016).

Assessment of Body Image

A number of research methods can be used to assess body image (Cash, 2011). The earliest research in the area relied heavily on clinical interviews of patients' experiences with their bodies. The growth of body image scholarship over the past several decades was accompanied by the development of a large collection of psychometric measures to assess body image concerns (Thompson et al., 1999). These include measures of weight satisfaction, appearance satisfaction, and size perception (Thompson et al., 1999). The Body Shape Questionnaire has been widely used by researchers interested in assessing the body image concerns of individuals with eating disorders (Cooper, Taylor, Cooper, & Fairburn, 1987). The measure was subsequently used in several of the first studies of body image in persons with obesity. Other measures of disordered eating, such as the Eating Disorder Examination, also assess weight and shape concerns specifically related to eating behavior (Cooper & Fairburn, 1987). The Body Image Quality of Life Inventory assesses the positive and negative impact of body image on various aspects of life satisfaction (Cash & Fleming, 2002). The measure has been used in some studies of persons with obesity who have undergone weight loss.

Perhaps the most widely used body image assessment has been the Multidimensional Body–Self Relationship Questionnaire (MBSRQ; Cash, 2000). This 69-item self-report measure includes 10 subscales that assess individuals' attitudes and dispositions concerning their physical selves. In recent years, a shorter 34-item version of the measure, which includes the Appearance Subscales, has been developed and is often used in place of the larger measure. Unfortunately, the MBSRQ does not allow for an assessment of the body image concerns associated with discrete features of appearance. It also was not designed to specifically assess changes with weight loss.

Recently, a number of psychometric measures have been developed that are specifically designed to assess the body image and quality-of-life concerns in persons who experience a change in their physical appearance. The measure most relevant to the field of obesity is the BODY-Q. The BODY-Q measures three domains, including overall appearance, health-related quality of life, and experience of health care (Klassen et al., 2016). The measure has great potential to enhance understanding of changes in body image with weight loss.

The Etiology of Body Image Dissatisfaction

Prevalence of Body Image Dissatisfaction

Estimates of the prevalence of body image dissatisfaction have largely come from population surveys found in either magazines or, more recently, Internet-based surveys. Perhaps the most noteworthy of these is the 1996 Body Image Survey from *Psychology Today* magazine (Garner, 1997). The survey of magazine readers found that the majority of women (56%) and almost half (43%) of men were dissatisfied with their overall appearance. More recent population-based studies, as well as Internet-based surveys hosted on highly trafficked websites, have found similar results (Frederick, Jafary, Gruys, & Daniels, 2012).

Clearly, there are a number of problems with relying on magazine and Internet surveys for reliable prevalence data. Such surveys are frequently affected by sample biases that call into question the representativeness of the sample and, ultimately, the validity of the findings. Nevertheless, studies that used sampling strategies to ensure a more representative sample of the American population have found similar levels of body image dissatisfaction (Cash & Henry, 1995). Thus, most body image scholars agree that body image dissatisfaction is a ubiquitous problem among individuals living in Westernized cultures.

Although body image dissatisfaction is largely universal, it varies across different groups of individuals. Women are typically far more dissatisfied with their body image than are men (Schwartz & Brownell, 2004). Differences also exist across ethnic groups; African and Hispanic American women typically report less body image dissatisfaction than European American women (Franko & Roehrig, 2011). Body image dissatisfaction also appears to be related to degree of acculturation. Some evidence suggests that as Asian and Hispanic American individuals acculturate to American customs, body image dissatisfaction increases to mirror that of European Americans (Kawamura, 2011; Schooler & Lowry, 2011).

Specificity of Body Image Dissatisfaction

Body image dissatisfaction can be global or specific. As noted above, large percentages of individuals report dissatisfaction with their overall appearance. The greatest dissatisfaction with appearance is associated with excess body weight (Sarwer, Wadden, & Foster, 1998). Given the scope of the world's obesity problem, this observation is not particularly surprising. Among women with obesity, 47% reported that they were most dissatisfied with their waist and abdomen, whereas only 10% reported dissatisfaction with their overall body (Sarwer, Wadden, Pertschuk, & Whitaker, 1998). Additionally, 42% of women who were of average body weight indicated that they were most dissatisfied with their waist and abdomen, suggesting that dissatisfaction with the waistline may be independent of actual body weight.

Severity of Body Image Dissatisfaction

Body image dissatisfaction is believed to fall along a continuum. On one end of this continuum are individuals who are highly satisfied with their physical appearance. Results of the body image surveys would suggest that these individuals are a minority; there likely are very few individuals who evaluate their appearance regularly and, over time, do not experience at least some modest dissatisfaction with changes associated with aging or weight gain. Most individuals likely experience some degree of body image dissatisfaction, which is believed to be the motivational catalyst for appearance-enhancing behaviors, including weight loss (Sarwer, Lavery, & Spitzer, 2012).

Excess body weight is associated with greater body image dissatisfaction (Schwartz & Brownell, 2004; van den Berg, 2012). Across studies, there is a modest to strong correlation between body mass and body image dissatisfaction for children and adolescents, although the relationship is typically stronger for females than males. Among adults, the association between body mass index (BMI) and body image dissatisfaction exists for women and men who are overweight or who have class 1 obesity, as well as those with more extreme obesity (Sarwer, Dilks, & Spitzer, 2011). Greater body image dissatisfaction in persons with obesity has been associated with lower health- and weight-related quality of life, lower self-esteem, and greater depressive symptoms (Foster, Wadden, & Vogt, 1997; Grilo, Wilfley, Brownell, & Rodin, 1994; Sarwer, Wadden, & Foster, 1998).

Although body image dissatisfaction may be normative, some individuals report body image dissatisfaction that negatively affects their daily behavior. For example, a significantly greater percentage of women with obesity, compared to those without obesity, reported, on more than half of the days of the month, camouflaging their obesity with clothing, changing their posture or body movements, avoiding looking at their bodies, and becoming upset when thinking about their appearance (Sarwer, Wadden, & Foster, 1998). Others experience great shame related to their body size and weight, either because of their own self-consciousness or because of the experience of weight-related discrimination and bias (Sarwer, Fabricatore, Eisenberg, Sywulak, & Wadden, 2008). Severe body image dissatisfaction is a symptom of a number of formally recognized psychiatric disorders. These disorders include gender dysphoria and depression, as well as eating disorders and body dysmorphic disorder (American Psychiatric Association, 2013). Individuals with these conditions should likely be referred for assessment and treatment by a mental health professional prior to undertaking treatment for obesity (Sarwer, Allison, & Dilks, 2016).

Improvements in Body Image

Improvements in Body Image with Weight Loss

Individuals who lose weight typically experience improvements in several areas of psychosocial functioning (Allison & Sarwer, 2016; Sarwer et al., 2011; Still, Sarwer, & Blankenship, 2014). Body image is no exception. Individuals who lose modest amounts of weight with lifestyle modification or pharmacotherapy typically report improvements in body image (Sarwer, Dilks & Spitzer, 2011). In most cases, these improvements are independent of the magnitude of weight loss. Participation in regular exercise, independent of weight loss, has also been associated with improvements in body image (Campbell & Hausenblas, 2009)

Numerous studies have also found significant improvements in body image following bariatric surgery (Kolotkin, Crosby, Williams, Hartley, & Nicol, 2001; Sarwer, Bishop-Gilyard, & Carvajal, 2014; Sarwer, Spitzer, et al., 2014; Sarwer et al., 2013). For example, both men and women who underwent bariatric surgery as part of the Longitudinal Assessment of Bariatric Surgery (LABS) Consortium, reported significant improvements in body image at the end of the first postoperative year and after losing approximately 30% of their initial weight (Sarwer, Spitzer, et al., 2014; Sarwer et al., 2013). These individuals also reported significant improvements in quality of life and depressive symptoms; women reported statistically significant improvements in sexual functioning, whereas men did not. Improvements in body image were well maintained over the first 4 postoperative years, even as some individuals began to regain weight (Sarwer, Spitzer, et al., 2014; Sarwer et al., 2013).

Improvements in Body Image with Body-Contouring Surgery

Many individuals with excess body weight turn to cosmetic surgery to improve their body shape and body image. Abdominoplasty and liposuction (of the midsection) are among the most commonly performed body-contouring surgical procedures (American Society for Aesthetic Plastic Surgeons, 2015). Both are typically performed on patients who are either modestly overweight or of average body weight but are concerned about their body shape. They also are performed on patients who have lost massive amounts of weight (typically after bariatric surgery), sometimes in combination with arm lifts, thigh lifts, and lower body lifts.

According to the American Society for Aesthetic Plastic Surgeons, liposuction is the most popular cosmetic surgical procedure (American Society for Aesthetic Plastic Surgeons, 2015), with 414,335 patients undergoing the procedure in 2016. Although the specific area of the body treated via liposuction varies by patient, female patients most often seek lateral thigh and hip procedures, whereas men request abdominal—"love handle"—procedures. Abdominoplasty is also common, with 180,717 patients receiving this procedure in 2014 (American Society for Aesthetic Plastic Surgeons, 2015).

Patients often hold a number of misconceptions regarding the procedures' uses and outcomes. Liposuction patients often erroneously believe that the procedure will result in substantial weight loss, and that fat deposits will never return to the site of treatment (Sarwer, Didie, & Gibbons, 2006). In reality, patients experience modest weight losses, typically 1 or 2 kg, (Giese, Bulan, Commons, Spear, & Yanovski, 2001), and no changes in obesity-related metabolic outcomes (Hernandez et al., 2011; Klein et al., 2004). Many patients experience weight regain within a year of the procedure (Hernandez et al., 2011). Abdominoplasty patients, by contrast, experience larger initial weight losses (attributed to the removal of larger amounts of fat as well as some muscle and skin), and 70% experienced a 5% decrease in BMI 1 year after surgery (Fuller, Nguyen, & Moulton-Barrett, 2013).

Regardless of the magnitude of weight loss, most patients report high levels of satisfaction following these procedures (Saariniemi et al., 2014; Swanson, 2012). Many also report improvements in psychosocial functioning. In a study of 360 liposuction and abdominoplasty patients, 85.8% reported improved self-esteem, and 69.6% reported improved quality of life postoperatively (Swanson, 2012). Other studies have also demonstrated a reduction in body image dissatisfaction following both surgery types. One study found a reduced risk of eating disorders following liposuction, although methodological limitations of the study raise concerns about the validity of the results (Saariniemi, Salmi, Peltoniemi, Charpentier, & Kuokkanen, 2015).

Ellison and colleagues recently authored a detailed review of the literature on body contouring, specifically following the massive weight loss seen after bariatric surgery (Ellison, Steffen, & Sarwer, 2015). The vast majority of individuals who have undergone bariatric surgery report experiencing excess skin (Ellison et al., 2015; Kitzinger, Abayev, Pittermann, Karle, Bohdjalian, et al., 2012). The abdominal region is the area of greatest concern, followed by the breasts/chest, upper arms, thighs, and rear/buttocks (Kitzinger, Abayev, Pittermann, Karle, Kubiena, et al., 2012; Klopper, Kroese-Deutman, & Berends, 2014). The body areas that develop excess skin do not differ by surgery type, gender, age, time elapsed since surgery, pre-weight-loss surgery BMI, or postoperative weight loss (Giordano, Victorzon, Stormi, & Suominen, 2014). Higher levels of reported dissatisfaction with excess skin were found among women, adolescents, patients achieving a greater magnitude of BMI change, and patients with higher current BMI (Giordano et al., 2014; Staalesen, Fagevik Olsen, & Elander, 2013; Steffen et al., 2012).

This loose, hanging skin can affect physical functioning. Approximately 60% of patients report that excess hanging skin has resulted in problematic skin conditions (e.g., itching, rashes, chafing, ulcers, worsening of existing skin disease) (Kitzinger, Abayev, Pittermann, Karle, Bohdjalian, et al., 2012; Kitzinger, Abayev, Pittermann, Karle, Kubiena, et al., 2012; Mitchell et al., 2008). Up to 90% report that the hanging skin results in functional impairment. Specifically, patients reported pain and interference with their ability to find appropriate clothing, maintain personal hygiene, and engage in physical activity or sexual behavior (Klopper et al., 2014; Staalesen et al., 2013; van der Beek, Te Riele, Specken, Boerma, & van Ramshorst, 2010).

The vast majority of patients who undergo bariatric surgery desire body-contouring surgery (Staalesen et al., 2013; Steffen et al., 2012), with the abdomen being the most desired region for surgical treatment (Giordano et al., 2014). Several demographic and psychosocial factors have been found to predict requests for body-contouring surgery. Younger individuals and those who are divorced are more likely to undergo body contouring (Gusenoff, Messing, O'Malley, & Langstein, 2008; Singh et al., 2012). Individuals further removed from their weight loss are also more likely to undergo surgery (Gusenoff et al., 2008). Additionally, the degree of BMI change from pre- to postbariatric surgery was found to predict interest in surgery (de Zwaan et al., 2014; Gusenoff et al., 2008; Singh et al., 2012), with reported odds ratios being such that a 1 kg/m^2 decrease in BMI from presurgery to 1 year postsurgery translated into a 12% increase in likelihood of obtaining body-contouring surgery (Singh et al., 2012). A recent study found that individuals who underwent body-contouring surgery had lost a higher percentage of total weight and excess weight compared to those who did not undergo surgery (de Zwaan et al., 2014).

Patients who undergo body-contouring surgery are typically satisfied with the results (Song et al., 2006). Nearly all patients reported that they would undergo body-contouring surgery again (96%) and would recommend it to a friend or relative (92%) (Larsen et al., 2007). Patients often report improvements in several domains of quality of life, including pain, skin problems, and physical limitations that were caused by excess skin (Al-Hadithy, Welbourn, Aditya, Stewart, & Soldin, 2014). Significant improvements in the quality-of-life domains of work ability, physical activity, and sexual activity from postbariatric to post-body-contouring surgery time points have also been reported (Modarressi, Balague, Huber, Chilcott, & Pittet-Cuenod, 2013). Individuals undergoing body-contouring surgery were more likely to report being physically active and advancing in their careers (Al-Hadithy et al., 2014). One long-term follow-up study found that individuals who underwent body-contouring surgery experienced significant improvement in intimacy, mental well-being, physical appearance, and physical and social functioning (van der Beek, Geenen, de Heer, van der Molen, & van Ramshorst, 2012). Other studies have reported improvements in body image (Cintra et al., 2008; Lazar, Clerc, Deneuve, Auquit-Auckbur, & Milliez, 2009). The highest rates of satisfaction following body-contouring surgery were found in the breast, hip, and buttock regions, with lower rates of satisfaction with the thighs (Cintra et al., 2008; de Zwaan et al., 2014; Klopper et al., 2014; Song et al., 2006).

Improvements in Body Image without Weight Loss

Prior to the recognition of obesity as a significant public health issue, several groups of investigators studied the efficacy of improving body image in overweight and obese persons without weight loss. This work evolved from the belief that caloric restriction for weight loss could contribute to the development of disordered eating, and that greater body image acceptance could lead to healthier eating and weight loss. In one of the first such studies, Roughan and colleagues reported significant improvements in body image, as well as improvements in self-esteem and depression, following a program designed to promote weight acceptance and decrease overeating (Roughan, Seddon, & Vernonroberts, 1990). Polivy and Herman (1992) found that after a 10-week "undieting" program, women with obesity reported improvements in self-esteem and depression, but did not report improvements in body image.

Rosen and colleagues subsequently developed a cognitive-behavioral body image therapy program specifically tailored for women who were overweight or obese (Rosen, Orosan, & Reiter, 1995). The program was typically administered in a group format for 8 weeks. Participants were taught about the origins of body image development and shown how negative body image attitudes are learned and maintained through sociocultural influences and personal experiences. The intervention was combined with a standard lifestyle modification intervention and compared to the weight loss treatment alone. Throughout treatment, participants experienced modest changes in weight and reported improvements in body image and self-esteem. At the 3-month follow-up, the combined group experienced only a 0.4 kg weight regain compared to a 4 kg regain for the weight-control-alone condition. Furthermore, although the difference only approached statistical significance, the combined condition also reported lower body image dissatisfaction. At 1 year, the combined group experienced only a 2.2 kg weight regain compared to a 6.8 kg regain for the weight-control-alone group. Although this difference was not statistically significant, it suggests that the combination of behavioral weight control strategies and body image therapy may improve weight maintenance.

Cognitive-behavioral strategies to improve body image are now frequently included in lifestyle modification curricula, either during the active weight loss phase of treatment or as a behavioral lesson to help promote successful weight maintenance. Some individuals with obesity who have managed to lose and maintain their weight loss will also enter into individual psychotherapy with a mental health professional to address long-standing body image issues. This psychotherapeutic aspect can be an important element of addressing the psychosocial burden of obesity. However, in the presence of extreme obesity and/or significant weight-related comorbidities, it can be difficult to justify a cognitive-behavioral approach to improve body image without an accompanying approach to reduce weight and improve physical health.

Conclusions

Over the last several decades, there has been a greater understanding of the role of physical appearance and body image in daily life. A now large body of research has suggested that individuals who are more attractive are judged more favorably, and also receive preferential treatment in a variety of interpersonal interactions across the lifespan. Studies that have investigated body size and shape have reached similar conclusions—individuals of average body weight are seen and treated more positively than those who have excess body weight.

The psychological construct of body image is a useful foundation for understanding an individual's experience of his or her body in relation to the social world. Similar to research on the psychological aspects of physical appearance, scholarship on body image has grown rapidly in the last several decades. Much of this work originated from the body image concerns seen in persons with eating disorders. More recently, body image has become a routinely assessed construct in studies of a range of weight loss treatments.

Excess body weight is associated with body image dissatisfaction, and is believed to motivate both weight loss efforts—improvements in diet, increases in physical activity, pharmacotherapy, and bariatric surgery—as well as body-contouring procedures, such as liposuction and abdominoplasty. The limited amount of research conducted on the psychosocial characteristics and functioning of individuals who present for these procedures has suggested few differences from other aesthetic surgery patients. Postoperative studies have suggested that most patients are satisfied with their outcomes. These observations have also been seen in persons who seek body-contouring procedures after the massive weight loss that typically follows bariatric surgery.

At the same time, it is clear that even individuals of a normal body weight and those who are modestly overweight are dissatisfied with the impact of excess adiposity on their appearance. Whereas this dissatisfaction used to be attributed to "trivial vanity," we have come to learn that how we feel about our appearance plays an important role in our self-esteem and quality of life. Both are important, yet often overlooked, aspects of our functioning and well-being. In recent years, psychosocial functioning has come to play a more central role in patient-centered health care, with improvements in quality of life, self-esteem, body image, and other psychological constructs now seen as important criteria in evaluating the benefits of a medical treatment such as weight loss.

References

Aharon, I., Etcoff, N., Ariely, D., Chabris, C. F., O'Connor, E., & Breiter, H. C. (2001). Beautiful faces have variable reward value: fMRI and behavioral evidence. *Neuron, 32*(3), 537–551.

Al-Hadithy, N., Welbourn, R., Aditya, H., Stewart, K., & Soldin, M. (2014). A preliminary report on the development of a validated tool for measuring psychosocial outcomes for massive weight loss patients. *Journal of Plastic, Reconstructive, and Aesthetic Surgery, 67*(11), 1523–1531.

Allison, K. C., & Sarwer, D. B. (2016). Body image disturbance during pregnancy and the postpartum period. In A. Wenzel (Ed.), *The Oxford handbook of perinatal psychology* (pp. 231–251). New York: Oxford Library of Psychology.

American Psychiatric Association. (2013). *Diagnostic and statistical manual of mental disorders* (5th ed.). Arlington, VA: Author.

American Society for Aesthetic Plastic Surgeons. (2017). 2016 Cosmetic surgery national data bank statistics. Available at *www.surgery.org/sites/default/files/ASAPS-Stats2016.pdf*.

Campbell, A., & Hausenblas, H. A. (2009). Effects of exercise interventions on body image: A meta-analysis. *Journal of Health Psychology, 14*(6), 780–793.

Cash, T. F. (2000). *Multidimensional Body–Self Relations Questionnaire*. New York: Springer.

Cash, T. F. (2011). Crucial considerations in the assessment of body image. In T. F. Cash & L. Smolak (Eds.), *Body image: A handbook of science, practice, and prevention* (2nd ed., pp. 129–137). New York: Guilford Press.

Cash, T. F. (2012). *Encyclopedia of body image and human appearance* (Vol. 2). London: Academic Press.

Cash, T. F., & Fleming, E. C. (2002). The impact of body image experiences: Development of the Body

Image Quality of Life Inventory. *International Journal of Eating Disorders, 31*(4), 455–460.

Cash, T. F., & Henry, P. E. (1995). Women's body images: The results of a national survey in the USA. *Sex Roles, 33*(1–2), 19–28.

Cash, T. F., & Pruzinsky, T. (1990). *Body images: Development, deviance, and change.* New York: Guilford Press.

Cash, T. F., & Smolak, L. (2011). *Body image: A handbook of science, practice, and prevention* (2nd ed.). New York: Guilford Press.

Cintra, W., Jr., Modolin, M. L., Gemperli, R., Gobbi, C. I., Faintuch, J., & Ferreira, M. C. (2008). Quality of life after abdominoplasty in women after bariatric surgery. *Obesity Surgery, 18*(6), 728–732.

Cooper, P. J., Taylor, M. J., Cooper, Z., & Fairburn, C. G. (1987). The development and validation of the Body Shape Questionnaire. *International Journal of Eating Disorders, 6*(4), 485–494.

Cooper, Z., & Fairburn, C. (1987). The Eating Disorder Examination: A semi-structured interview for the assessment of the specific psychopathology of eating disorders. *International Journal of Eating Disorders, 6*(1), 1–8.

de Zwaan, M., Georgiadou, E., Stroh, C. E., Teufel, M., Kohler, H., Tengler, M., et al. (2014). Body image and quality of life in patients with and without body contouring surgery following bariatric surgery: A comparison of pre- and post-surgery groups. *Frontiers in Psychology, 18*(5), 1310.

Ellison, J. M., Steffen, K. J., & Sarwer, D. B. (2015). Body contouring after bariatric surgery [Review]. *Euopean Eating Disorders Review Journal, 23*(6), 479–487.

Etcoff, N. (2011). *Survival of the prettiest: The science of beauty.* New York: Anchor.

Foster, G. D., Wadden, T. A., & Vogt, R. A. (1997). Body image in obese women before, during, and after weight loss treatment. *Health Psychology, 16*(3), 226.

Franko, D. L., & Roehrig, J. P. (2011). African American body images. In T. F. Cash & L. Smolak (Eds.), *Body image: A handbook of science, practice, and prevention* (2nd ed., pp. 221–228). New York: Guilford Press.

Frederick, D. A., Jafary, A. M., Gruys, K., & Daniels, E. A. (2012). Surveys and the epidemiology of body image dissatisfaction. In T. F. Cash (Ed.), *Encyclopedia of body image and human appearance* (pp. 766–774). London: Elsevier.

Fuller, J. C., Nguyen, C. N., & Moulton-Barrett, R. E. (2013). Weight reduction following abdominoplasty: A retrospective case review pilot study. *Plastic and Reconstructive Surgery, 131*(2), 238e–244e.

Garner, D. M. (1997). The 1997 Body Image Survey results. *Psychology Today, 30*(1), 30–44.

Giese, S. Y., Bulan, E. J., Commons, G. W., Spear, S. L., & Yanovski, J. A. (2001). Improvements in cardiovascular risk profile with large-volume liposuction: A pilot study. *Plastic and Reconstructive Surgery, 108*(2), 510–519; discussion 520–521.

Giordano, S., Victorzon, M., Stormi, T., & Suominen, E. (2014). Desire for body contouring surgery after bariatric surgery: Do body mass index and weight loss matter? *Aesthetic Surgery Journal, 34*(1), 96–105.

Grilo, C. M., Wilfley, D. E., Brownell, K. D., & Rodin, J. (1994). Teasing, body image, and self-esteem in a clinical sample of obese women. *Addictive Behaviors, 19*(4), 443–450.

Gusenoff, J. A., Messing, S., O'Malley, W., & Langstein, H. N. (2008). Temporal and demographic factors influencing the desire for plastic surgery after gastric bypass surgery. *Plastic and Reconstructive Surgery, 121*(6), 2120–2126.

Hatfield, E., & Sprecher, S. (1986). *Mirror, mirror: The importance of looks in everyday life.* Albany: State University of New York Press.

Hernandez, T. L., Kittelson, J. M., Law, C. K., Ketch, L. L., Stob, N. R., Lindstrom, R. C., et al. (2011). Fat redistribution following suction lipectomy: Defense of body fat and patterns of restoration. *Obesity (Silver Spring), 19*(7), 1388–1395.

Kawamura, K.Y. (2011). Asian American body images. In T. F. Cash & L. Smolak (Eds.), *Body image: A handbook of science, practice, and prevention* (2nd ed., pp. 229–236). New York: Guilford Press.

Kitzinger, H. B., Abayev, S., Pittermann, A., Karle, B., Bohdjalian, A., Langer, F. B., et al. (2012). After massive weight loss: Patients' expectations of body contouring surgery. *Obesity Surgery, 22*(4), 544–548.

Kitzinger, H. B., Abayev, S., Pittermann, A., Karle, B., Kubiena, H., Bohdjalian, A., et al. (2012). The prevalence of body contouring surgery after gastric bypass surgery. *Obesity Surgery, 22*(1), 8–12.

Klassen, A. F., Cano, S. J., Alderman, A., Soldin, M., Thoma, A., Robson, S., et al. (2016). The BODY-Q: A patient-reported outcome instrument for weight loss and body contouring treatments. *Plastic and Reconstructive Surgery Global Open, 4*(4), 679–684.

Klein, S., Fontana, L., Young, V. L., Coggan, A. R., Kilo, C., Patterson, B. W., et al. (2004). Absence of an effect of liposuction on insulin action and risk factors for coronary heart disease. *New England Journal of Medicine, 350*(25), 2549–2557.

Klopper, E. M., Kroese-Deutman, H. C., & Berends, F. J. (2014). Massive weight loss after bariatric surgery and the demand (desire) for body contouring surgery. *European Journal of Plastic Surgery, 37*(2), 103–108.

Kolotkin, R. L., Crosby, R. D., Williams, G. R., Hartley, G. G., & Nicol, S. (2001). The relationship between health-related quality of life and weight loss. *Obesity Research, 9*(9), 564–571.

Larsen, M., Polat, F., Stook, F. P., Oostenbroek, R. J., Plaisier, P. W., & Hesp, W. L. (2007). Satisfaction and complications in post-bariatric surgery abdominoplasty patients. *Acta Chirurgiae Plasticae, 49*(4), 95–98.

Lazar, C. C., Clerc, I., Deneuve, S., Auquit-Auckbur, I., & Milliez, P. Y. (2009). Abdominoplasty after major weight loss: Improvement of quality of life and psychological status. *Obesity Surgery, 19*(8), 1170–1175.

Mitchell, J. E., Crosby, R. D., Ertelt, T. W., Marino, J. M., Sarwer, D. B., Thompson, J. K., et al. (2008). The desire for body contouring surgery after bariatric surgery. *Obesity Surgery, 18*(10), 1308–1312.

Modarressi, A., Balague, N., Huber, O., Chilcott, M., & Pittet-Cuenod, B. (2013). Plastic surgery after gastric bypass improves long-term quality of life. *Obesity Surgery, 23*(1), 24–30.

Patzer, G. L. (2007). *Why physically attractive people are more successful: The scientific explanation, social consequences, and ethical problems.* New York: Edwin Mellen Press.

Polivy, J., & Herman, C. P. (1992). Undieting: A program to help people stop dieting. *International Journal of Eating Disorders, 11*(3), 261–268.

Rosen, J. C., Orosan, P., & Reiter, J. (1995). Cognitive-behavior therapy for negative body-image in obese women. *Behavior Therapy, 26*(1), 25–42.

Roughan, P., Seddon, E., & Vernonroberts, J. (1990). Long-term effects of a psychologically based group program for women preoccupied with body-weight and eating behavior. *International Journal of Obesity, 14*(2), 135–147.

Saariniemi, K. M., Salmi, A. M., Peltoniemi, H. H., Charpentier, P., & Kuokkanen, H. O. (2015). Does liposuction improve body image and symptoms of eating disorders? *Plastic Reconstructive Surgery Global Open, 3*(7), e461.

Saariniemi, K. M., Salmi, A. M., Peltoniemi, H. H., Helle, M. H., Charpentier, P., & Kuokkanen, H. O. (2014). Abdominoplasty improves quality of life, psychological distress, and eating disorder symptoms: A prospective study. *Plastic Surgery International, 2014*, 1–4.

Sarwer, D. B., Allison, K. C., & Dilks, R. J. (2016). Clinical assessment of lifestyle behavioral factors during weight loss treatment. In J. I. Mechanick & R. F. Kushner (Eds.), *Lifestyle medicine* (pp. 55–64). New York: Springer.

Sarwer, D. B., Bishop-Gilyard, C. T., & Carvajal, R. (2014). Quality of Life. In C. D. Still, D. B. Sarwer, & J. Blankenship (Eds.), *The ASMBS textbook of bariatric surgery* (Vol. 2, pp. 19–24). New York: Springer.

Sarwer, D. B., Didie, E. R., & Gibbons, L. M. (2006). Cosmetic surgery of the body. In D. B. Sarwer et al. (Eds.), *Psychological aspects of reconstructive and cosmetic plastic surgery: Clinical, empirical, and ethical perspectives.* Philadelphia: Lippincott Williams & Wilkins.

Sarwer, D. B., Dilks, R. J., & Spitzer, J. C. (2011). Weight loss and changes in body image. In T. F. Cash & L. Smolak (Eds.), *Body image: A handbook of science, practice, and prevention* (2nd ed., pp. 369–377). New York: Guilford Press.

Sarwer, D. B., Fabricatore, A. N., Eisenberg, M. H., Sywulak, L. A., & Wadden, T. A. (2008). Self-reported stigmatization among candidates for bariatric surgery. *Obesity (Silver Spring), 16*(Suppl.), S75–S79.

Sarwer, D. B., Lavery, M., & Spitzer, J. C. (2012). A review of the relationships between extreme obesity, quality of life, and sexual function. *Obesity Surgery, 22*(4), 668–676.

Sarwer, D. B., Pertschuk, M. J., Wadden, T. A., & Whitaker, L. A. (1998). Psychological investigations in cosmetic surgery: A look back and a look ahead. *Plastic and Reconstructive Surgery, 101*(4), 1136–1142.

Sarwer, D. B., & Polonsky, H. M. (2016). Body image and body contouring procedures. *Aesthetic Surgery Journal, 36*, 1039–1047.

Sarwer, D. B., Spitzer, J. C., Wadden, T. A., Mitchell, J. E., Lancaster, K., Courcoulas, A., et al. (2014). Changes in sexual functioning and sex hormone levels in women following bariatric surgery. *JAMA Surgery, 149*(1), 26–33.

Sarwer, D. B., Spitzer, J. C., Wadden, T. A., Rosen, R. C., Mitchell, J. E., Lancaster, K., et al. (2013). Sexual functioning and sex hormones in persons with extreme obesity and seeking surgical and nonsurgical weight loss. *Surgery for Obesity and Related Diseases, 9*(6), 997–1007.

Sarwer, D. B., Thompson, J. K., & Cash, T. F. (2005). Body image and obesity in adulthood. *Psychiatry Clinics of North America, 28*(1), 69–87.

Sarwer, D. B., Wadden, T. A., & Foster, G. D. (1998). Assessment of body image dissatisfaction in obese women: Specificity, severity, and clinical significance. *Journal of Consulting and Clinical Psychology, 66*(4), 651–654.

Sarwer, D. B., Wadden, T. A., Pertschuk, M. J., & Whitaker, L. A. (1998). Body image dissatisfaction and body dysmorphic disorder in 100 cosmetic surgery patients. *Plastic and Reconstructive Surgery, 101*(6), 1644–1649.

Schooler, D., & Lowry, L. (2011). Hispanic/Latino body images. In T. F. Cash & L. Smolak (Eds.), *Body image: A handbook of science, practice, and prevention* (2nd ed., pp. 237–243). New York: Guilford Press.

Schwartz, M. B., & Brownell, K. D. (2004). Obesity and body image. *Body Image, 1*(1), 43–56.

Singh, D., Zahiri, H. R., Janes, L. E., Sabino, J., Matthews, J. A., Bell, R. L., et al. (2012). Mental and physical impact of body contouring procedures on post-bariatric surgery patients. *Eplasty, 2012*(12), e47.

Song, A. Y., Rubin, J. P., Thomas, V., Dudas, J. R., Marra, K. G., & Fernstrom, M. H. (2006). Body image and quality of life in post massive weight loss body contouring patients. *Obesity (Silver Spring), 14*(9), 1626–1636.

Staalesen, T., Fagevik Olsen, M., & Elander, A. (2013). Experience of excess skin and desire for body contouring surgery in post-bariatric patients. *Obesity Surgery, 23*(10), 1632–1644.

Steffen, K. J., Sarwer, D. B., Thompson, J. K., Mueller, A., Baker, A. W., & Mitchell, J. E. (2012). Predictors of satisfaction with excess skin and desire for body contouring after bariatric surgery. *Surgery for Obesity and Related Diseases, 8*(1), 92–97.

Still, C. D., Sarwer, D. B., & Blankenship, J. (2014).

The ASMBS textbook of bariatric surgery. New York: Springer.

Stunkard, A., & Mendelson, M. (1967). Obesity and the body image: 1. Characteristics of disturbances in the body image of some obese persons. *American Journal of Psychiatry, 123*(10), 1296–1300.

Swanson, E. (2012). Prospective outcome study of 360 patients treated with liposuction, lipoabdominoplasty, and abdominoplasty. *Plastic and Reconstructive Surgery, 129*(4), 965–978.

Thompson, K. J., Heinberg, L. J., Altabe, M. N., & Tantleff-Dunn, S. (1999). *Exacting beauty: Theory, assessment, and treatment of body image disturbance*. Washington, DC: American Psychological Association.

van den Berg, P. (2012). Body weight and body image in children and adolescents. In T. F. Cash (Ed.), *Encyclopedia of body image* (pp. 270–274). London: Elsevier.

van der Beek, E. S., Geenen, R., de Heer, F. A., van der Molen, A. B., & van Ramshorst, B. (2012). Quality of life long-term after body contouring surgery following bariatric surgery: Sustained improvement after 7 years. *Plastic and Reconstructive Surgery, 130*(5), 1133–1139.

van der Beek, E. S., Te Riele, W., Specken, T. F., Boerma, D., & van Ramshorst, B. (2010). The impact of reconstructive procedures following bariatric surgery on patient well-being and quality of life. *Obesity Surgery, 20*(1), 36–41.

CHAPTER 36

Obesity, Weight Management, and Self-Esteem

Carol A. Johnson

> To lose confidence in one's body
> is to lose confidence in one's self.
> —SIMONE DE BEAUVOIR

Webster's Dictionary defines self-esteem as confidence and satisfaction in oneself (Webster's Online Dictionary, 2015). The stigma associated with obesity often strips people defined as *obese* of both of these experiences. This is truly unfortunate, because stigmatization cripples the lives of these individuals in a variety of ways. Even more unfortunate is the fact that the negative assumptions made about overweight people stem from beliefs that are often inaccurate or incorrect. Not only are people with above-average weight regarded as physically unattractive, but they are also assumed to be lacking in character. They are bombarded daily with messages implying that they are unacceptable, undesirable, unmotivated, undisciplined—*un*-everything. Is it any wonder that many end up with severely wounded self-esteem?

The role of body size as an indicator of moral character stems from a variety of developments in the fields of medicine, psychology, culture, and fashion that converged in the 1940s and 1950s. Whereas amply fleshed people were formerly regarded as cheerful, well adjusted, productive, and prosperous, today they are viewed as individuals with no control over their voracious appetites. Women feel that unless they wear a single-digit dress size, they are fat.

The labels assigned to larger people go far beyond size. People looking at an overweight person make countless assumptions about that person, based solely on his or her size and weight. It is assumed that he or she is lazy, stupid, slothful, and unclean. It is somewhat amazing—and praiseworthy—that people viewed as overweight manage to function at all, given the barrage of negative messages and feedback that they encounter daily from society and the media. Pumping up the self-esteem of larger people is an especially difficult task. Those who have been heavy since childhood have been exposed to years of "fat bashing." Most have been led to believe that the only way they can repair their self-esteem is by losing weight—and not just by losing a modest amount of weight. Most admit they would not be satisfied with anything less than achieving their "ideal weight." The idea that they can maintain high self-esteem while still "amply proportioned" seems downright ludicrous to many larger people. They have been conditioned by our society to believe that they are not entitled to self-esteem unless they are thin. This is perhaps the most unfortunate consequence of stigmatization, because most larger people will never reach an "ideal weight," until science has a better understanding of obesity and more effective treatments have been developed. So what do they do until that time?

This chapter is devoted to a discussion of obesity and self-esteem and specifically to what health professionals can do to help their larger patients elevate their self-esteem without first having to lose weight.

Relationship between Obesity and Self-Esteem

It seems necessary to draw a distinction between self-esteem, body image satisfaction, and psychological health, because the research treats them as different concepts. In terms of self-esteem, Harter (1999) found that perceptions of appearance and self-worth are inextricably linked, such that perceived appearance consistently emerges as the strongest single predictor of self-esteem among both male and female adolescents. A meta-analysis by Miller and Downey (1999) demonstrated that being "heavy weight" is negatively correlated with self-esteem. However, effect sizes were much larger for studies based on self-perceived weight than those based on actual weight. Effect sizes were also larger for women than for men, and for samples of people in weight loss treatment programs than for samples of people who were recruited from general populations.

However, in at least one study of college students, no statistically significant relationship was found between body mass index (BMI) and self-esteem (Malkemus, Shipman, & Thomas, 2008). In a study of obese and nonobese women by Sarwer, Wadden, and Foster (1998), the two groups did not differ on self-reported symptoms of depression or self-esteem, although the vast majority of obese women demonstrated body image dissatisfaction related to their obesity. Hill (2010) concluded that the relationship between obesity and self-esteem is relatively modest. Most research demonstrates a relationship between body dissatisfaction and lower self-esteem. Lowery et al. (2005) found that self-esteem was consistently related to body image dissatisfaction, and findings from another study indicated that body dissatisfaction and self-esteem were strongly related among nearly all groups of adolescents (van den Berg, Mond, Eisenberg, Ackard, & Neumark-Sztainer, 2010).

Regarding psychological health, Carr, Friedman, and Jaffe (2007) found that whereas many studies revealed a negative relationship between body weight and psychological well-being, others showed either a positive or nonsignificant association (i.e., there was not a consistent, statistically significant relationship between obesity and psychological outcomes). They concluded that excessive body weight is not necessarily distressing—to the contrary, when a diverse range of obesity-related stressors were controlled, obese persons actually enjoyed better psychological health than their thinner peers. Friedman and Brownell (1995) reviewed the psychological correlates of obesity and found that studies comparing obese and non-obese persons have generally failed to find differences in global aspects of psychological functioning. McElroy, Kotwal, Malhotra, and Nemeroff (2004) found that most overweight and obese persons in the community did not have mood disorders. On the other hand, Simon et al. (2006) observed positive associations—albeit modest—between obesity and a range of mood and anxiety disorders in a nationally representative sample of the United States. Other investigators also found that women reported higher levels of depressive symptoms if they experienced loved ones being embarrassed by their weight, and men reported lower levels of self-esteem if they were disparaged by their sons (Puhl & Brownell, 2006).

What are the factors that at least put a "dent" in the self-esteem of above-average weight individuals?

- There is an expectation that larger people should have poor self-esteem and that only by losing weight can they gain self-esteem, self-confidence, and self-respect. This expectation acts as a self-fulfilling prophecy. Larger people are expected to have low self-esteem, which leads them to develop low self-esteem based on these expectations (Miller, 1998). Typically, advertisements for diet programs make use of "before" and "after" photos of their "successful" customers. These ads usually feature the now-thin customer lamenting that before the diet, she had little regard for herself; but now that she has lost weight, she is overflowing with self-esteem and self-confidence. The message to people who are still above average weight is that they could not possibly feel good about themselves until they too have shed their excess pounds (and if they do claim to feel good about themselves in their larger bodies, they are accused of self-deception).

• The popular assumption is that larger people lack self-discipline and don't care about themselves or their appearance. The person with above-average weight often hears questions such as "Don't you care about yourself?"; "Aren't you concerned about your health?"; "Don't you care what you look like?" Once again, the assumption that larger individuals don't care about themselves (or else they would lose weight) takes a toll on self-esteem.

• Diet failures are regarded as personal failures. When a person fails to lose weight or loses and regains weight, the "failure" is generally viewed as the fault of the dieter rather than the flawed process of dieting or the fact that science does not yet fully understand the condition of obesity. Dieters blame and chastise themselves for being weak and lacking "willpower." They view themselves as "failures." These feelings of failure go hand in hand with low self-esteem.

• Our Western culture generally considers fatness to be unattractive. Not only are larger people regarded as physically unappealing, they are also presumed to have other undesirable traits, based solely on their size. The word *fat* often gets strung together with other negative adjectives. When larger individuals are repeatedly exposed to these types of negative messages, their self-esteem suffers.

• Size discrimination abounds in our society. The constant barrage of antifat messages from the media, criticism and insults from others, social rejection, weight-related job discrimination, and comedians telling fat jokes all take a heavy toll on the self-esteem of larger people. One very powerful aspect of size discrimination is invisibility—that is, the fact that larger women are significantly underrepresented in popular women's magazines, in movies, or on TV. The message being transmitted to these women is that they are unacceptable for viewing. No one wants to see them. Researchers have found that more frequent stigmatization is correlated with lower self-esteem (Annis, Cash, & Hrabosky, 2004; Carr & Friedman, 2005; Friedman et al., 2005). Little by little, this seems to be changing, and we are seeing larger people represented more frequently in the entertainment industry.

• Perhaps the ultimate sadness for larger people is that they tend not to identify with other overweight people. Self-rejection becomes group rejection. This is borne out by the fact that children as young as 6 years of age have been found to label silhouettes of obese youngsters as lazy, stupid, cheats, lies, and ugly (Staffieri, 1967). But even more troublesome is that these judgments were made by obese youngsters themselves. One's self-esteem is deeply injured when a child regards others like him- or herself with disgust. Most overweight people do not feel that they will be lifelong members of the obese population. They think of themselves as "temporarily fat," a belief that discourages group solidarity and cohesion. One of the reasons that diverse racial/ethnic populations have been able to make major strides toward equality and acceptance is that they do not think of themselves as temporarily "black" or temporarily "brown." More importantly, they do not regard their race or ethnicity as an unacceptable characteristic.

• Wang, Brownell, and Wadden (2004) found that unlike other minority group members, overweight individuals do not appear to hold more favorable attitudes toward in-group members. The overweight individuals studied were found to hold strong, consistently negative implicit associations about being overweight, and they exhibited no preference for in-group members. Another study found a significant degree of antifat bias among all weight groups, including obese persons themselves (Schwartz, Vartanian, Nosek, & Brownell, 2006).

Variables That Affect Self-Esteem and Body Image

Gender

Studies have shown that males are much less likely than women to suffer from poor body image (Feingold & Mazzella, 1998). In one study, boys were as likely to want to be heavier as lighter, whereas very few girls desired to be heavier. Only girls associated body dissatisfaction with the concept of self-esteem. Male self-esteem was not affected by body dissatisfaction (Furnham, Badmin, & Sneade, 2002). Similar findings were reported by Pingitore, Spring, and Garfield (1997) in a study of college-age men and women. The men were much less likely to use weight as a determinant of self-esteem. In one study, obese men actually exhibited better mental health than normal-weight men, whereas obese women reported poorer mental health than normal-weight women (Magallares & Pais-Ribeiro, 2012).

Binge Eating

It is critical for physicians and other health professionals to differentiate between obese women with binge-eating disorder (BED) and obese women who do not typically binge. Research studies show that women who engage in binge-eating behavior have much lower self-esteem and will probably need much more support and guidance in working to improve their self-esteem. It has been found that:

- BED is a risk factor for depression, low self-worth (Steinbeck, 2009), self-discrimination (Rudolph & Hilbert, 2014), and affective disorders (Linde, Jeffrey, Levy, Pronk, & Boyle, 2004).
- Bingers, regardless of weight category, suffered higher levels of depression and anxiety and lower levels of self-esteem than non-bingers, regardless of weight category. In fact, obese nonbingers were indistinguishable on these variables from normal-weight nonbingers (Webber, 1994).
- Overweight girls who do not report eating-disordered attitudes and behaviors also do not report more depressive symptoms (Erickson, Robinson, Haydel, & Killen, 2000).
- Binge eating is associated with higher lifetime prevalence of major depression, panic disorder, phobias, and alcohol dependence. Obese women with BED scored higher on neuroticism and symptom scales measuring depression and anxiety/phobia (Bulik, Sullivan, & Kendler, 2002).
- College women with BED had significantly greater levels of eating, weight, and shape concerns, and lower levels of appearance satisfaction and self-esteem than the non-binge-eating group (Herbozo, Schaefer, & Thompson, 2015).

Once again, it is important in evaluating patients to determine whether there is a problem with binge eating. If there is, it may be advisable to refer the patient to a practitioner who specializes in treating BED.

Age of Onset

Studies have shown that a negative body image is more common in those with childhood or adolescent onset of obesity (Sarwer et al., 1998; Wardle, Waller, & Fox, 2002). Persons with early-onset obesity also report greater body dissatisfaction than those with adult-onset obesity (Grilo, Wilfley, Brownell, & Rodin, 1994). Furthermore, when those with adult-onset obesity reach a socially accepted weight, they tend to be satisfied with their appearance. This is not so with early-onset individuals, many of whom appear unsatisfied with their bodies, even if they succeed in maintaining a nearly normal body weight. This is most likely related to the fact that the body image construct develops at an early age and is fairly well entrenched by the time the child enters adolescence (Adami et al., 1998). Strauss (2000) found that obese 9- to 10-year-olds did not express differences in self-esteem from their nonoverweight counterparts. However, when examining 13- to 14-year-olds, there was a difference in self-esteem between overweight adolescents and their healthy-weight peers. Therefore, when evaluating obese patients, it may be important to inquire about their age of onset.

Ethnicity

Ethnicity also plays a role in shaping the self-esteem and body image of obese persons. Many studies have shown that excess weight does not significantly affect the self-esteem of African Americans. Chugh, Friedman, Clemow, and Ferrante (2013) found that African American women displayed greater self-confidence and a more positive body image than European American women, who often expressed low self-esteem and depression concerning their weight. African American participants mostly attributed their personal self-respect to their family values and identification with other female family members who were overweight or obese. In another study, self-esteem scores were similar among minority children regardless of their weight status (Wong, Mikhail, Ortiz, & Smith, 2014). Although the prevailing view in popular culture and the psychological literature is that European American women have greater body dissatisfaction than women of color, at least one study has challenged this belief. In a meta-analysis conducted by Grabe and Hyde (2006), the authors concluded that European American women and women of color differ only slightly in terms of body dissatisfaction.

Treatment Seekers

Results of a variety of studies indicated that overweight/obese treatment seekers were generally more impaired than overweight/obese nontreatment seekers on measures of psychological disturbance and quality of life (Kolotkin, Crosby, & Williams, 2002; Fitzgibbon, Stolley, & Kirschenbaum, 1993; Foster & Kendall, 1994; Fontaine, Bartlett, & Barofsky, 2000). Research in community samples suggests that despite moderate levels of body dissatisfaction, few obese children are depressed or have low self-esteem (Wardle, 2005). Taken together, these results remind us to avoid making generalizations about obese persons as a group, and to pay close attention to treatment-seeking status when drawing conclusions about obese individuals.

Criticism by Family Members

Parental and family criticism of weight is associated with decreased self-esteem (Unikel Santoncini et al., 2012; Taylor et al., 2006). In one study, overweight and obese women were surveyed regarding the most common interpersonal sources of weight stigma in their lives. Participants were provided with a list of 22 different individuals and asked how often each individual had stigmatized them because of their weight. Family members were the most frequent source of weight stigma, reported by 72% of participants (Puhl & Brownell, 2006). In another study, parental weight talk, particularly from mothers, was associated with a number of disordered-eating behaviors. Mothers' dieting was associated with girls' unhealthy and extreme weight control behaviors. In no instances were family weight talk and dieting variables associated with better outcomes for girls (Neumark-Sztainer et al., 2010).

Do Health Professionals Contribute to Their Patients' Poor Self-Esteem?

Although it may not be intentional, the attitudes and remarks of health professionals can injure the self-esteem of larger people. Implicit and explicit antifat bias appears to be as pervasive among physicians as it is among most people in society (Sabin, Marini, & Nosek, 2012). Physicians may become exasperated when patients are advised to lose weight and fail to do so. The experience is equally exasperating for above-average-weight patients who, fearful of being "scolded," may start avoiding doctor visits. This is definitely not a good outcome, as preventive care may be delayed until problems reach an acute stage. The larger patient may feel that "even my doctor doesn't like me," causing his or her self-esteem to plummet further.

Research shows that some physicians and other health professionals view patients with above-average weight with disdain, and may even make insulting remarks to them. As early as 1969, Maddox and Leiderman found that more than half of physicians described their obese patients as weak-willed (60%), ugly (54%), or awkward (55%). In a 2003 study, more than 50% of physicians who responded viewed obese patients as awkward, unattractive, ugly, and noncompliant. The authors concluded that "Primary care physicians view obesity as largely a behavioral problem and share our broader society's negative stereotypes about the personal attributes of obese persons" (p. 1168; Foster et al., 2003). Teachman and Brownell (2001) found that health professionals associated overweight people with negative attributes such as "bad" and "lazy," and thin people with positive attributes such as "good" and "motivated." Schwartz, Chambliss, Brownell, Blair, and Billington (2003) found that health professionals endorsed both the implicit and explicit stereotypes that fat people are lazy, stupid, and worthless.

Things do not seem to have improved significantly. More recently, researchers measured the antifat bias of almost 400,000 people, including more than 2,000 physicians. They found that physicians' implicit and explicit attitudes about weight followed the same antifat biases seen in large population samples. They concluded that *implicit and explicit antifat bias is as pervasive among physicians as it is among most people in society* (Sabin et al., 2012). Tomiyama et al. (2015) compared levels of bias in obesity specialists between 2001 and 2013. Although implicit antifat attitudes appeared to decrease from 2001 to 2013, explicit antifat attitudes increased. (Tomiyama et al. define explicit as "consciously accessible anti-fat attitudes," and implicit as "attitudes that are activated outside of conscious awareness" [p. 46].) Saguy (2013) has coined the term "size profiling" to refer to the assumption that a person has—or will develop—a particular ailment because he or she is heavy. Such profiling, Saguy claims, leads to false positives (i.e., people being either overtreated for conditions they may not have or undertreated for conditions that they do have).

Even more recently, Phelan et al. (2015) found that many health care providers still hold strong negative attitudes and stereotypes about people with obesity. Another study found that implicit and explicit weight bias is common among first-year medical students. Explicit attitudes were more negative toward obese people than toward racial minorities, gays, lesbians, and poor people (Phelan et al., 2014). How do larger people feel about the way they are treated in medical settings? In a study by Rand and MacGregor (1990), morbidly obese patients were asked a series of questions about how they had been treated by various members of society. One such item was, "I have been treated disrespectfully by the medical profession because of weight." Only 6% of patients responded "never," whereas 79% responded either "usually" or "always." In a later study by Wadden et al. (2000), the majority of obese women did not report being treated disrespectfully or insensitively by their physicians when weight management was discussed. Additional research has suggested that higher patient BMIs are associated with lower physician respect (Huizinga, Cooper, Bleich, Clark, & Beach, 2009). Gudzune, Huizinga, and Cooper (2011) found few differences in ratings of the patient–provider relationship for overweight and obese respondents when compared to respondents with a normal-range BMI. However, in an experiment using audiotapes of patient visits, these same researchers found that as BMI increased, patients were significantly more likely to overestimate physician respect (Gudzune, Huizinga, Beach, & Cooper, 2012). The tapes showed that although doctors provided the same basic information to all patients, including those who were overweight, they were far less empathic with the overweight group.

The mental health profession is not immune to this type of prejudice. The discipline of psychology commonly assumes that larger people are emotionally stunted and that they eat to compensate for a variety of problems. However, studies have failed to uncover greater degrees of psychopathology in obese women who are not suffering from BED. Psychologist Eleanor Webber (1994) cautions her colleagues to examine their own prejudices and to advocate for a reduction in the tendency to stereotype obese people in terms of presumed psychological characteristics. Disrespectful treatment can lead people with above-average weight to avoid going to the doctor. Drury and Louis (2002) found that an increase in BMI was associated with an increase in the delay/avoidance of health care. Weight-related reasons for delaying/avoiding health care included having gained weight since the last health care visit, not wanting to get weighed on the provider's scale, and knowing they would be told to lose weight.

In another study, obese women reported that they delayed cancer-screening tests.

Factors contributing to this avoidance included disrespectful treatment, embarrassment at being weighed, negative attitudes of providers, unsolicited advice to lose weight, and medical equipment that was too small to be functional. The percentage of women who reported these barriers increased as the women's BMIs increased (Amy, Aalborg, Lyons, & Keranen, 2006). In a review of English language journal articles published between 1990 and 2012 that addressed the question "Is being overweight or obese an unrecognized factor in healthcare avoidance?," a positive relationship was found between obesity and health care avoidance (McGuigan & Wilkinson, 2015).

Consequences of Poor Self-Esteem

Poor self-esteem can have significant and harmful consequences for the overweight person. Among these consequences are the following:

- *Postponement of life.* People who are waiting to be thin postpone all sorts of activities because they feel that they will be much better equipped to handle major life challenges in a slim body. They avoid social events, career opportunities, travel, relationships—even buying attractive clothes. They especially avoid activities such as going shopping or going to the beach, where they feel as if they are being observed (Hughes & Degher, 1993). These individuals literally put their lives "on hold." Researchers have found that many larger people use this type of avoidance behavior to disengage from negative feedback, which, over time, may result in chronic disengagement in multiple areas of living (Major & Schmader, 1998). The danger in this type of behavior is that the majority of overweight people are probably not going to achieve the weight they would consider "ideal" for moving ahead with their lives, given the present status of our knowledge about obesity and its treatment. This means that if they continue to put their lives on hold, there is a good chance they will never achieve many of their goals and aspirations.

- *Poor choices and decisions.* Larger people often feel inferior, which leads them to make poor choices and decisions in many areas of their lives, especially when it comes to romantic relationships. Larger women, in particular, may be so grateful for any attention paid to them by a potential romantic partner that they settle for relationships that are far from ideal. They may even come to feel that they are not deserving of a quality relationship. The same phenomenon can occur in other areas, such as employment, although job discrimination against the obese may have as much to do with this as personal feelings of inferiority. Nevertheless, lacking self-confidence, larger individuals may avoid life opportunities that involve any sort of challenge, risk, or chance for advancement. In young people, it has been found that obese adolescents with self-esteem difficulties are more likely to engage in risky behaviors such as smoking and drinking alcohol (Strauss, 2000).

- *Sabotage of good relationships.* Relationships can suffer even when one partner does not object to the other partner's ample weight. A larger woman may be heard to exclaim, "What could he possibly see in me? Why would he want someone like me?" The larger wife with shaky self-esteem may not want to accompany her husband to social gatherings. She may avoid going places with her children. Her family may become frustrated with her, not because of her weight, but because of her unhappiness with herself and how it affects them.

- *The "doormat" syndrome.* Many larger people become "people pleasers," wanting everyone to like them. They feel that they have to, in essence, pull extra duty to make up for their excess pounds. They may allow people to take advantage of them and find it difficult to be assertive in their responses.

The Importance of Self-Esteem to Effective Weight Management

Positive self-esteem and effective weight management should exist as a partnership. Common sense would seem to dictate that people with high self-regard have a vested interest in taking good physical care of themselves. Conversely, those with low self-esteem have little motivation to practice good self-care. Self-loathing constitutes a shaky foundation for the development of a healthy lifestyle.

Some experts believe it is a myth that weight loss is the only way you can come to accept your body. It has been suggested that people who need to lose weight in order to improve their health should separate the goals of weight loss and body acceptance. Body image expert Thomas Cash (1997) believes that the ability to lose weight may be strengthened by first learning to have a positive relationship with one's imperfect body. When University of Vermont researchers studied obese persons following a group body image therapy program, they found that participants showed great improvement in how they felt about their bodies—without reductions in their weight (Cash, 1997). Another 12-week group body image program produced the same type of positive results. The participants indicated that the exploration of related cultural issues and information about normal eating and set points had the greatest influence on changes in their attitudes and behaviors (Ciliska, 1998). More recently, an international team of researchers found that diet success can depend on how much you love your body—whatever shape it is—not how much you hate it. Their results showed a strong correlation between improvements in body image, especially in reducing anxiety about other peoples' opinions, and positive changes in eating behavior. The authors concluded, "Results suggest that improving body image, particularly by reducing its salience in one's personal life, might play a role in enhancing eating self-regulation during weight control. Accordingly, future weight loss interventions could benefit from proactively addressing body image-related issues as part of their protocols." (Carraça et al., 2011, p. 1).

Helping Individuals with Obesity Achieve Better Self-Esteem

Crocker, Cornwell, and Major (1993) concluded that individuals who attribute mistreatment to another person's anti-obese prejudice are less likely to experience negative psychological consequences than are persons with obesity who internalize negative stereotypes and attribute their negative experiences to an enduring personal trait. The latter individuals are far more likely to suffer psychological distress. However, there has not been much scientific research on how to improve the self-esteem of people with above-average weight. The popular prejudices cited earlier are probably contributing factors and beg the question, "Why bother?" Losing weight will improve their self-esteem, so why bother investing resources in research that will teach them how to feel better about themselves while they still occupy larger bodies? The ideal solution would be to eliminate size prejudice, but as Quinn and Crocker (1998) pointed out:

> Research on the stigmatized may be criticized for focusing too much on what to change about the stigmatized and not enough on how to change the culture. Although we would like to see the culture changed such that being overweight and feeling overweight is no longer stigmatizing, there is little evidence that our culture is moving in that direction. (p. 141)

For now, overweight individuals will probably have to take responsibility for cultivating their own self-esteem, but how do they do that? There is a small body of research directed at identifying which characteristics distinguish overweight people with good self-esteem from those with poor self-esteem. Some researchers have tried to identify and define what makes some larger people more *resilient* to the psychological distress caused by the stigma of being overweight. Some of the major findings that distinguish overweight individuals with good self-esteem from those with low self-esteem include the following:

- Those who are more resilient realize that not all outcomes are deserved and not all things (including weight) are under personal control. The idea that personal responsibility governs all aspects of our lives can be harmful when applied to weight, because it leads people to believe that diet failures are personal failures. This is not to suggest that personal responsibility should be abdicated. It simply means that there is a point when some people realize that, despite their very best efforts, the desired outcome may not be achievable and that this is not their "fault." Many diseases cannot be cured, not because the patient did anything wrong, but because medical science has not yet discovered how to effectively treat and cure them. Amato, Crocker, and Major (1995) found that overweight women who received information on uncontrollable aspects of obesity were better able to attribute rejection to weight prejudice, not their own failing. However, this knowledge did not necessarily improve their self-regard. The authors concluded:

> Believing that weight is controllable may be a double-edged sword. On one hand, it encourages overweight people to interpret rejection as revealing prejudice, instead of a personal failing, and this protects self-esteem. On the other hand, it may create a sense of powerlessness or hopelessness about the prospect of weight loss.

In one study, the most vulnerable children were those who believed that they were responsible for their above-average weight (an internal cause, i.e., overeating or not exercising enough). More positive self-esteem was seen in children with above-average weight who attributed their weight to an external cause (i.e., medical grounds or a familial predisposition), and those children who did not believe that their weight influenced the outcome of their social interactions (Pierce & Wardle, 1997).

- Does providing information on the uncontrollability of obesity reduce stigma and prejudice toward obese persons? One of the experiments in a study by Puhl, Schwartz, and Brownell (2005) found that reading about the uncontrollable causes of obesity did decrease beliefs that obesity is caused by personally controllable factors. But does this information reduce bias? Informing study participants that obesity is caused mainly by genetic factors did not result in lower bias (Teachman, Gapinski, Brownell, Rawlins, & Jeyaram, 2003). Anesbury and Tiggemann (2000) found that providing children with information on the uncontrollability of weight was successful in reducing the amount of controllability that children assigned to obesity, but it was not successful in reducing negative stereotyping of the obese. In a more recent study, information about weight controllability had no effect on levels of prejudice in either the controllable or uncontrollable conditions (Thorsteinsson, Loi, & Breadsell, 2016).

- Larger individuals show greater resilience to weight-based prejudice when they are able to blame the bias and prejudice of critics rather than themselves. Those who are able to avoid being stigmatized may protect their self-esteem by accusing their critics of being prejudiced rather than taking the blame for the negative attitudes directed against them. Thus, an overweight person who fails to get a job might conclude that the potential employer is prejudiced against fat people rather than concluding that he or she did not interview well.

- Resilience is greater among overweight individuals who are able to reject or ignore society's dictates about acceptable body weight. Some racial/ethnic groups have been successful at doing this. White women rated large women, especially large white women, lower on attractiveness, intelligence, job success, relationship success, happiness, and popularity than they did average or thin women. By contrast, black women did not show the same denigration of large women, and this was especially true when they were rating large black women (Hebl & Heatherton, 1998). In another study, Parker and colleagues observed that black girls focused on factors such as personal style and presentation in addition to body size/weight when evaluating their attractiveness (Parker et al., 1995). This multifaceted definition of beauty may promote both a greater investment in appearance and greater satisfaction with overall appearance regardless of body weight.

- Resilience intensifies in those who do not base their self-regard on others' approval. Individuals whose self-esteem is highly dependent on receiving praise and approval from others are vulnerable to low self-esteem when they fail to receive positive evaluations. Basing one's self-esteem on these reflected appraisals is especially risky and leads to self-esteem that is transient and fluctuates depending on what sort of feedback one is receiving from others (Quinn & Crocker, 1998). Those who can tune all this out and build their self-esteem from self-appraisal and self-knowledge will find that their self-esteem rests on solid ground. Finally, resilient overweight people do not view other overweight individuals with dislike or disgust. They have not internalized the negative stereotypes about overweight people. Research by Crandall (1994) on "anti-fat attitudes" showed that fat and lean people were equally likely to have antifat attitudes. Disliking overweight people when one is a member of the group seems risky for self-esteem, especially given the actual difficulty of ever leaving the group (Quinn & Crocker, 1998).

Advice to Health Professionals

What can health professionals do to make sure they are not contributing to poor self-esteem in persons of above-average weight (see Table 36.1)? What can be done in the context of the medical setting to assure that larger patients are treated with respect, compassion, and understanding? The National Task Force on the Prevention and Treatment of Obesity (2002) concluded:

> Physicians may be concerned that encouraging self-acceptance in obese patients will undermine efforts aimed at producing weight loss that can significantly improve health. Self-acceptance, however, need not imply complacency or the failure to heed well-founded advice about reducing health risks of obesity. A more constructive view is to focus on promoting self-acceptance and lifestyle changes aimed at improving health behaviors. Encouraging patients to lead as full and active a life as possible, regardless of their body weight or success at weight control, may help patients make positive changes such as increasing physical activity. (p. 87)

Additional suggestion for health professionals include the following:

- Consider that patients may have had negative experiences with other health professionals regarding their weight, and approach patients with sensitivity. Recognize that many patients have already tried to lose weight repeatedly.

- Recognize the complex etiology of obesity and communicate this to colleagues and patients. Avoid the stereotype that obesity is attributable to personal willpower. Make sure that you stay up-to-date on the contemporary obesity research. Providers who understand the complex web of causality have more positive attitudes about patients with obesity (O'Brien, Puhl, Latner, Mir, & Hunter, 2010). Be sure your entire staff is educated. Consider offering your staff members training in obesity sensitivity.

- Listen carefully to the patient's presenting problem(s) independent of weight, and don't attribute every health problem to excess weight. Consider this statement from an article in a VA newsletter: "You could walk in with an ax sticking out of your head and they [medical professionals] would tell you your head hurt because you're fat" (U.S. Department of Veterans Affairs, 2015). Explore all causes of presenting problems. Although obesity may be a contributing factor in conditions such as hypertension, diabetes, and joint problems, many thin people have high blood pressure, back problems, knee problems, and the like.

- Don't assume that the larger patient is simply eating too much. Some may be, but many are not. On the other hand, it is important to determine whether the patient is suffering from BED, in which case he or she may need to be referred to an eating disorder specialist.

- Give the same advice to obese patients as you would to nonobese patients presenting with the same types of problems. Don't just say, "Lose weight and come back in 6 months." If medication is warranted (and would be prescribed for a thin person with the same problem), write a prescription. Weight management can still be part of the overall treatment plan, but at least the benefits of medication can begin immediately.

- Don't blame the patient for a less than desired outcome. There is still a great deal to learn about obesity, and the patient can't be blamed for that.

- Focus on overall health and non-weight-related outcomes, such as improvement in blood pressure, glycemic control, or lipid values. Given the poor prognosis for the long-term management of obesity, clinicians and health care providers need to expand their foci to include strategies other than weight management alone (Jeffery et al., 2000).

TABLE 36.1. The Terminology of Weight

What terms are most commonly used?

1. *Obese, overweight:* The medical profession has traditionally preferred to use the terms *obese* and *overweight* probably because they can be quantified. The most common way to find out whether you're overweight or obese is to figure out your body mass index (BMI). BMI is an estimate of body fat. According to the CDC:
   - ☐ If your BMI is between 25 and < 30 kg/m², it falls within the overweight range.
   - ☐ If your BMI is ≥ 30 kg/m², it falls within the obese range.

   The problem is that the word *obese* has an unpleasant ring to it and has become offensive to many larger people. The label *morbidly obese* is even more odious. The term *overweight* causes some to ask, "Over *whose* weight?" What is *overweight* for one person may constitute a healthy weight for another person.

2. *Fat:* Some size-acceptance advocates prefer to be referred to as *fat*. They are determined to remove the stigma and negativity from this word, but despite their well-intended efforts, many larger people still do not want to be called *fat*. The history of negative connotations that often accompanies this word is too long and painful.

3. *Large, big, heavy:* These words are more neutral and acceptable in popular jargon, but may pose difficulties in the medical setting because they are not quantifiable.

What does the research say?

Volger et al. (2012) sought to identify terms that obese individuals who were treated in primary care would find the most and least acceptable for describing their excess weight. Ratings of 11 terms used to describe excess weight were transformed into a 5-point scale, ranging from "very desirable" to "very undesirable." The term *fatness* was rated as significantly more undesirable than all other descriptors. The terms *excess fat, large size, obesity,* and *heaviness* were rated as significantly more undesirable than the remaining terms, which included *weight problem, BMI,* and *excess weight*. In contrast, the term *weight* was viewed as the most desirable term for characterizing excess weight. In another study of public preferences and perceptions of weight-based terminology, the terms *morbidly obese, fat,* and *obese* were rated as the most undesirable, stigmatizing, and blaming (Puhl, Peterson, & Luedicke, 2013). Practitioners may want to consider broaching the topic using more patient-friendly terms such as *weight, BMI, weight problem,* or *excess weight*.

Some additional alternatives

1. *Above-average weight:* Physicians could consider saying, "Your weight is above average for your height and build." It is a nonjudgmental term and also has a mathematical basis.

2. *Healthy weight:* More and more, patients are being advised to strive for a "healthy weight" as opposed to an "ideal weight." Ideal weights have traditionally been based on height–weight charts and leave no room for individual differences based on genetics and physiology. For many larger people, these "ideal weights" are neither attainable nor maintainable. Research has shown that a "healthy weight" can often be achieved with a weight loss of 5–10%. Rather than setting arbitrary weight loss goals, the physician and his or her patient can act as partners in determining what would constitute a "healthy weight" for that individual patient.

Note. It is likely that personal preferences of patients will vary, so it can be helpful to ask them about preferred terms before discussing body weight issues. CDC, Centers for disease Control and Prevention.

- Congratulate and praise patients for making healthy changes no matter what the scale says. The patient who has not yet achieved a significant weight change, but is making incremental behavior changes, needs encouragement and recognition. For example, congratulate patients for lowering their HbA1C, even though they have not lost any significant amount of weight.

- Don't set a goal weight for the next visit. If the patient hasn't reached it, he or she may not return. Patients who are told to lose a specified amount of weight and aren't able to achieve it often are afraid to come back. Rather than focusing on "ideal" weights, talk to the patient about "healthy" weights, and the fact that even a 5–10% loss can confer significant health benefits. Avoidance of further weight gain can also be a goal.

- Create a supportive health care environment with large, armless chairs in waiting and exam rooms, and appropriately sized medical equipment and patient gowns. There is nothing more humiliating to larger patients than being given gowns that don't cover them. Use a large blood pressure cuff when appropriate. For more information on finding appropriately sized medical equipment, contact the Rudd Center for Food Policy & Obesity at rudd.center@uconn.edu or phone 860/380-1000.

- Do not insist on weighing larger patients. Some patients avoid medical care because they fear being weighed, and because of their concerns about negative comments that are sometimes made. If a larger patient comes in with a sore throat, there may be no need to obtain a weight. Of course, there are situations, such as preparation for anesthesia, that require weighing. Even then, the patient can always be given the option of "not looking."

- Fitness may ameliorate some of the health risks associated with obesity (Blair & Brodney, 1999; Lee, Blair, & Jackson, 1999). Although obese patients may be reluctant to engage in physical activity because of discomfort or embarrassment, physicians can encourage slow, gradual increases in physical activity. A brochure entitled "Active at Any Size," written for very large persons and containing tips for becoming more active, is available from the Weight-Control Information Network at 800/860-8747 or healthinfo@niddk.nih.gov.

- Because weight loss outcomes are often so poor, some physicians are reluctant to discuss weight or weight management at all. However, the concern is that most practitioners, according to their patients, offer little or no guidance for weight management (Wadden et al., 2000). Ask your overweight patients if they want to discuss their weight. This gives them a chance to tell you about their past efforts. You can tell them that the research on obesity is still progressing, that some factors are uncontrollable, but that there is still a lot they can do to improve their health. The National Task Force on the Prevention and Treatment of Obesity (2002) recommends soliciting permission to discuss weight issues; asking about the patient's weight history and how excess weight has affected his or her life; and being careful to communicate a nonjudgmental attitude that distinguishes between the weight problem and the patient with the problem (National Task Force on the Treatment and Prevention of Obesity, 2002).

- Consider posting a mission statement that includes "size acceptance" as one of your values.

- Tell your patients that they don't need to lose one pound to be worthwhile people, deserving of love, respect, and self-esteem.

Finally, an important resource for health care providers who would like to learn more about weight bias and stigma is the Rudd Center for Food Policy & Obesity at the University of Connecticut (*www.uconn-ruddcenter.org*). If you go to their website, click on "What We Do" and then on "Weight Bias and Stigma."

A Final Note to Health Professionals

Physicians and other health professionals are in a unique position to help overweight and obese people repair their self-esteem. You are the authority. You have credibility. You can give your patients accurate information about issues of size and weight. You can tell them that it's not their fault. You can explain to them that science is still searching for answers. You can help them to develop a healthy lifestyle, and let them know that effective weight management doesn't have to mean losing huge amounts of weight. You can teach them that their weight is not a measure of their self-worth. You, perhaps more than anyone, can help them restore their self-esteem to good health!

References

Adami, G. F., Gandolfo, P., Campostano, A., Meneghelli, A., Ravera, G., & Scopinaro, N. (1998). Body image and body weight in obese patients. *International Journal of Eating Disorders, 24*, 299–306.

Amato, M., Crocker, J., & Major, B. (1995, August). *The stigma of being overweight and self-esteem: The role of perceived control.* Paper presented at the annual meeting of the American Psychological Association, New York.

Amy, N. K., Aalborg, A., Lyons, P., & Keranen, L. (2006). Barriers to routine gynecological cancer screening for White and African-American obese women. *International Journal of Obesity, 30*(1), 147–155.

Anesbury, T., & Tiggemann, T. (2000). An attempt to reduce negative stereotyping of obesity in children by changing controllability beliefs. *Health Education Research, 15*, 145–152.

Annis, N. M., Cash, T. F., & Hrabosky J. I. (2004). Body image and psychosocial differences among stable average weight, currently overweight, and formerly overweight women: The role of stigmatizing experiences. *Body Image, 1*(2), 155–167.

Blair, S. N., & Brodney, S. (1999). Effects of physical inactivity and obesity on morbidity and mortality: Current evidence and research issues. *Medicine and Science in Sports and Exercise, 31*(11, Suppl.), 646–662.

Bulik, C., Sullivan, P., & Kendler, K. (2002). Medical and psychiatric morbidity in obese women with and without binge eating. *International Journal of Eating Disorders, 32*(1), 72–78.

Carr, D., & Friedman, M. A. (2005). Is obesity stigmatizing?: Body weight, perceived discrimination, and psychological well-being in the United States. *Journal of Health and Social Behavior, 46*(3), 244–259.

Carr, D., Friedman, M., & Jaffe, K. (2007). Understanding the relationship between obesity and positive and negative affect: The role of psychosocial mechanisms. *Body Image, 4*(2), 165–177.

Carraça, E. V., Silva, M. N., Markland, D., Vieira, P. N., Minderico, C. S., Sardinha, L. R., et al. (2011). Body image change and improved eating self-regulation in a weight management intervention in women. *International Journal of Behavioral Nutrition and Physical Activity, 8*, 75.

Cash, T. F. (1997). *The body image workbook*. Oakland, CA: New Harbinger.

Chugh, M., Friedman, A. M., Clemow, L. P., & Ferrante, J. M. (2013). Women weigh in: Obese African American and White women's perspectives on physicians' roles in weight management. *Journal of the American Board of Family Medicine, 26*(4), 421–428.

Ciliska, D. (1998). Evaluation of two nondieting interventions for obese women. *Western Journal of Nursing Research, 20*, 119–135.

Crandall, C. S. (1994). Prejudice against fat people: Ideology and self-interest. Journal of *Personality and Social Psychology, 66*, 882–894.

Crocker, J., Cornwell, B., & Major, B. (1993). The stigma of overweight: Affective consequences of attributional ambiguity. *Journal of Personality and Social Psychology, 64*, 60–70.

Drury, C. A., & Louis, M. (2002). Exploring the association between body weight, stigma of obesity, and health care avoidance. *Journal of the American Academy of Nurse Practitioners, 14*(12), 554–561.

Erickson, S. J., Robinson, T. N., Haydel, K. F., & Killen, J. D. (2000). Are overweight children unhappy?: Body mass index, depressive symptoms, and overweight concerns in elementary school children. *Archives of Pediatrics and Adolescent Medicine, 154*(9), 931–935.

Feingold, A., & Mazzella, R. (1998). Gender differences in body image are increasing. *Psychological Science, 9*(3), 190–195.

Fitzgibbon, M. L., Stolley, M. R., & Kirschenbaum, D. S. (1993). Obese people who seek treatment have different characteristics than those who do not seek treatment. *Health Psychology, 12*, 342–345.

Fontaine, K. R., Bartlett, S. J., & Barofsky, I. (2000). Health-related quality of life among obese persons seeking and not currently seeking treatment. *International Journal of Eating Disorders, 27*, 101–105.

Foster, G. D., & Kendall, P. C. (1994). The realistic treatment of obesity. *Clinical Psychology Review, 14*, 701–736.

Foster, G. D., Wadden, T. A., Makris, A. P., Davidson, D., Sanderson, R. S., Allison, D. B., et al. (2003). Primary care physicians' attitudes about obesity and its treatment. *Obesity Research, 11*(10), 1168–1177.

Friedman, K. E., Reichmann, S. K., Costanzo, P. R., Zelli, A., Ashmore, J. A., & Musante, G. J. (2005). Weight stigmatization and ideological beliefs: Relation to psychological functioning in obese adults. *Obesity Research, 13*(5), 907–916.

Friedman, M. A., & Brownell, K. D. (1995). Psychological correlates of obesity: Moving to the next research generation. *Psychological Bulletin, 117*, 3–20.

Furnham, A., Badmin, N., & Sneade, I. (2002). Body image dissatisfaction: Gender differences in eating attitudes, self-esteem, and reasons for exercise. *Journal of Psychology: Interdisciplinary and Applied, 136*(5), 581–596.

Grabe, S., & Hyde, J. S. (2006). Ethnicity and body dissatisfaction among women in the United States: A meta-analysis. *Psychological Bulletin, 132*(4), 622–640.

Grilo, C. M., Wilfley, D. E., Brownell, K. D., & Rodin, J. (1994). Teasing, body image, and self-esteem in a clinical sample of obese women. *Addictive Behaviors, 19*(4), 443–450.

Gudzune, K. A., Huizinga, M. M., Beach, M. C., & Cooper, L. A. (2012). Obese patients overestimate physicians' attitudes of respect. *Patient Education and Counseling, 88*(1), 23–28.

Gudzune, K. A., Huizinga, M. M., & Cooper, L. A. (2011). Impact of patient obesity on the patient–provider relationship. *Patient Education and Counseling, 85*(3), e322–e325.

Harter, S. (1999). *The construction of the self: A developmental perspective*. New York: Guilford Press.

Hebl, M. R., & Heatherton, T. F. (1998). The stigma of obesity in women: The difference is black and white. *Personality and Social Psychology Bulletin, 24*, 417–426.

Herbozo, S., Schaefer, L., & Thompson, J. K. (2015). A comparison of eating disorder psychopathology, appearance satisfaction, and self-esteem in overweight and obese women with and without binge eating. *Eating Behaviors, 17*, 86–89.

Hill, A. (2010). Psychosocial issues in obese children and adults. In D. Crawford, R. W. Jeffery, K. Ball, & J. Brug (Eds.), *Obesity epidemoiology: From aetiology to public health* (pp. 59–73). Oxford, UK: Oxford University Press.

Hughes, G., & Degher, D. (1993). Coping with a deviant identity. *Deviant Behavior, 14,* 297–315.

Huizinga, M. M., Cooper, L. A., Bleich, S. N., Clark, J. M., & Beach, M. C. (2009). Physician respect for patients with obesity: Brief report. *Journal of General Internal Medicine, 24,* 1236.

Jeffery, R. W., Epstein, L. H., Wilson, G. T., Drewnowski, A., Stunkard, A. J., & Wing, R. R. (2000). Long-term maintenance of weight loss: Current status. *Health Psychology, 19,* 5–16.

Kolotkin, R. L., Crosby, R. D., & Williams, R. G. (2002). Health-related quality of life varies among obese subgroups. *Obesity Research, 10*(8), 748–756.

Lee, C. D., Blair, S. N., & Jackson, A. S. (1999). Cardiorespiratory fitness, body composition, and all-cause and cardiovascular disease mortality in men. *American Journal of Clinical Nutrition, 69,* 373–380.

Linde, J. A., Jeffery, R. W., Levy, R. L., Pronk, N. P., & Boyle, R. G. (2004). Binge eating disorder, weight control self-efficacy, and depression in overweight men and women. *International Journal of Obesity and Related Metabolic Disorders, 28,* 418–425.

Lowery, S. E., Robinson Kurpius, S. E., Befort, C., Blanks, E. H., Sollenberger, M. S., Foley Nicpon, M., et al. (2005). Body image, self-esteem, and health-related behaviors among male and female first-year college students. *Journal of College Student Development, 46,* 612–623.

Maddox, G. L., & Leiderman, V. R. (1969). Overweight as a social disability with medical implications. *Journal of Medical Education, 44,* 215–220.

Magallares, A., & Pais-Ribeiro, J. L. (2014). Mental health and obesity: A meta-analysis. *Applied Research in Quality of Life, 9*(2), 295–308.

Major, B., & Schmader, T. (1998). Coping with stigma through psychological disengagement. In J. K. Swim & C. Stangor (Eds.), *Prejudice: The target's perspective* (pp. 219–241). San Diego, CA: Academic Press.

Malkemus, L. A., Shipman, L. M., & Thomas, C. J. (2008). The relationship between body mass index and self-esteem in female college students. *Undergraduate Research Journal for the Human Sciences, 7.* Retrieved from *www.kon.org/urc/v7/malkemus.html.*

McElroy, S. L., Kotwal, R., Malhotra, S., & Nemeroff, C. B. (2004). Are mood disorders and obesity related?: A review for the mental health professional. *Journal of Clinical Psychiatry, 65,* 634–651.

McGuigan, R. D., & Wilkinson, J. M. (2015). Obesity and healthcare avoidance: A systematic review. *AIMS Public Health, 2*(1), 56–63.

Miller, C. T. (1998). What is lost by not losing?: Losses related to body weight. In J. H. Harvey (Ed.), *Perspectives on loss: A sourcebook* (pp. 253–264). Philadelphia: Brunner/Mazel.

Miller, C. T., & Downey, K. T. (1999). A meta-analysis of heavyweight and self-esteem. *Personality and Social Psychology Review, 3,* 68–84.

National Task Force on the Prevention and Treatment of Obesity. (2002). Medical care for obese patients: Advice for health care professionals. *American Family Physician, 65*(1), 81–88.

Neumark-Sztainer, D., Bauer, K. W., Friend, S., Hannan, P. J., Story, M., & Berge, J. (2010). Family weight talk and dieting: How much do they matter for body dissatisfaction and disordered eating behaviors in adolescent girls? *Journal of Adolescent Health, 47*(3), 270–276.

O'Brien, K. S., Puhl, R. M., Latner, J. D., Mir, A. S., & Hunter, J. A. (2010). Reducing anti-fat prejudice in preservice health students: A randomized trial. *Obesity, 18,* 2138–2144.

Parker, S., Nichter, M., Nichter, M., Vuckovic, N., Sims, C., & Ritenbaugh, C. (1995). Body image and weight concerns among African-American and white adolescent females: Differences that make a difference. *Human Organization, 54,* 103–114.

Phelan, S. M., Burgess, D. J., Yeazel, M. W., Hellerstedt, W. L., Griffin, J. M., & van Ryn, M. (2015). Impact of weight bias and stigma on quality of care and outcomes for patients with obesity. *Obesity Reviews, 16,* 319–326.

Phelan, S. M., Dovidio, J. F., Puhl, R. M., Burgess, D. J., Nelson, D. B., Yeazel, M. W., et al. (2014). Implicit and explicit weight bias in a national sample of 4,732 medical students: The medical student CHANGES study. *Obesity, 4,* 1201–1208.

Pierce, J. W., & Wardle, J. (1997). Cause and effect beliefs and self-esteem of overweight children. *Journal of Child Psychology and Psychiatry and Allied Disciplines, 38,* 645–650.

Pingitore, R., Spring, B., & Garfield, D. (1997). Gender differences in body satisfaction. *Obesity Research, 5*(5), 402–409.

Puhl, R. M., & Brownell, K. D. (2006). Confronting and coping with weight stigma: An investigation of overweight and obese adults. *Obesity, 14,* 1802–1815.

Puhl, R. M., Peterson, J. L., & Luedicke, J. (2013). Motivating or stigmatizing?: Public perceptions of weight-related language used by health providers. *International Journal of Obesity, 37*(4), 612–619.

Puhl, R. M., Schwartz, M. B., & Brownell, K. D. (2005). Impact of perceived consensus on stereotypes about obese people: A new approach for reducing bias. *Health Psychology, 24,* 517–525.

Quinn, D., & Crocker, J. (1998). Vulnerability to the affective consequences of the stigma of overweight. In J. K. Swim & C. Stangor (Eds.), *Prejudice: The target's perspective* (pp. 125–143). San Diego, CA: Academic Press.

Rand, C. S., & MacGregor, A. M. (1990). Morbidly obese patients' perceptions of social discrimination before and after surgery for obesity. *Southern Medical Journal, 83,* 1390–1395.

Rudolph, A., & Hilbert, A. (2015). A novel measure to assess self-discrimination in binge-eating disorder and obesity. *International Journal of Obesity, 39*(2), 368–370.

Sabin, J., Marini, M., & Nosek, B. (2012). Implicit and explicit anti-fat bias among a large sample of medical doctors by BMI, race/ethnicity and gender. *PLOS ONE, 7*(11), e48448.

Saguy, A. (2013, January 25). How "size profiling" harms overweight patients [OpEd]. The Washington Post. Retrieved from *www.washingtonpost.com/opinions/how-size-profiling-harms-overweight-patients/2013/01/25/7dc9ed3a-602e-11e2-b05a-605528f6b712_story.html?utm_term=.826a39329645*.

Sarwer, D. B., Wadden, T. A., & Foster, G. D. (1998). Assessment of body image dissatisfaction in obese women: Specificity, severity and clinical significance. *Journal of Consulting and Clinical Psychology, 66*, 651–654.

Schwartz, M. B., Chambliss, H. O., Brownell, K. D., Blair, S. N., & Billington, C. (2003). Weight bias among health professionals specializing in obesity. *Obesity Research, 11*(9), 1033–1039.

Schwartz, M. B., Vartanian, L. R., Nosek, B. A., & Brownell, K. D. (2006). The influence of one's own body weight on implicit and explicit anti-fat bias. *Obesity, 14*(3), 440–447.

Simon, G. E., Von Korff, M., Saunders, K., Miglioretti, D. L., Crane, P. K., van Belle, G., et al. (2006). Association between obesity and psychiatric disorders in the U.S. adult population. *Archives of General Psychiatry, 63*, 824–830.

Staffieri, J. R. (1967). A study of social stereotypes of body image in children. *Journal of Personality and Social Psychology, 7*, 101–104.

Steinbeck, K. (2009). Childhood obesity: Consequences and complications. In P. G. Kopelman, I. D. Caterson, & W. H. Dietz (Eds.), *Clinical obesity in adults and children* (pp. 392–407). Hoboken, NJ: Wiley-Blackwell.

Strauss, R. S. (2000). Childhood obesity and self-esteem. *Pediatrics, 105*(1), e15.

Taylor, C. B., Bryson, S., Celio Doyle, A. A., Luce, K. H., Cunning, D., Abascal, L. B., et al. (2006). The adverse effect of negative comments about weight and shape from family and siblings on women at high risk for eating disorders. *Pediatrics, 118*(2), 731–738.

Teachman, B. A., & Brownell K. D. (2001). Implicit anti-fat bias among health professionals: Is anyone immune? *International Journal of Obesity and Related Metabolic Disorders, 25*(10), 1525–1531.

Teachman, B. A., Gapinski, K. D., Brownell, K. D., Rawlins, M., & Jeyaram, S. (2003). Demonstrations of implicit anti-fat bias: The impact of providing causal information and evoking empathy. *Health Psychology, 22*, 68–78.

Thorsteinsson, E. B., Loi, N. M., & Breadsell, D. (2016). The effect of weight controllability beliefs on prejudice and self-efficacy. *PeerJ, 4*, e1764.

Tomiyama, A. J., Finch, L. E., Belsky, A. C., Buss, J., Finley, C., Schwartz, M. B., et al. (2015). Weight bias in 2001 versus 2013: Contradictory attitudes among obesity researchers and health professionals. *Obesity, 23*(1), 46–53.

Unikel Santoncini, C., Martín Martín, V., Juárez García, F., González-Forteza, C., Nuño Gutiérrez, B. (2012). Disordered eating behaviors and body weight and shape: Relatives' criticism in overweight and obese 15- to 19-year-old females. *Journal of Health Psychology, 18*(1), 75–85.

U.S. Department of Veterans Affairs. (2015). Do doctors dislike overweight patients?: Probing the roots and results of obesity bias in health care. Research News from the U.S. Department of Veterans Affairs. *VA Research Currents*. Available at *www.research.va.gov/currents/0815-2.cfm*.

van den Berg, P. A., Mond, J., Eisenberg, M., Ackard, D., & Neumark-Sztainer, D. (2010). The link between body dissatisfaction and self-esteem in adolescents: Similarities across gender, age, weight status, race/ethnicity, and socioeconomic status. *Journal of Adolescent Health, 47*, 290–296.

Volger, S., Vetter, M. L., Dougherty, M., Panigrahi, E., Egner, R., Webb, V., et al. (2012). Patients' preferred terms for describing their excess weight: Discussing obesity in clinical practice. *Obesity, 20*(1), 147–150.

Wadden, T. A., Anderson, D. A., Foster, G. D., Bennett, A., Steinberg, C., & Sarwer, D. B. (2000). Obese women's perceptions of their physicians' weight management attitudes and practices. *Archives of Family Medicine, 9*, 854–860.

Wang, S. S., Brownell, K. D., & Wadden, T. A. (2004). The influence of the stigma of obesity on overweight individuals. *International Journal of Obesity, 28*, 1333–1337.

Wardle, J. (2005). The impact of obesity on psychological well-being. *Best Practice and Research in Clinical Endocrinology and Metabolism, 19*(3), 421–440.

Wardle, J., Waller, J., & Fox, E. (2002). Age of onset and body dissatisfaction in obesity. *Addictive Behaviors, 27*(4), 561–573.

Webber, E. M. (1994). Psychological characteristics of binging and nonbinging obese women. *Journal of Psychology, 128*, 339–351.

Webster's Online Dictionary. (2015). Retrieved from *www.merriam-webster.com*.

Wong, W. W., Mikhail, C., Ortiz, C. L., & Smith, E. O. (2014). Body weight has no impact on self-esteem of minority children living in inner city, low-income neighborhoods: A crosssectional study. *BMC Pediatrics, 14*(1), 14–19.

PART VII
Childhood Obesity and Obesity Prevention

CHAPTER 37

The Development of Childhood Obesity

Tanja V. E. Kral
Robert I. Berkowitz

Today, 42 million infants and young children worldwide are affected by overweight and obesity (World Health Organization, 2016). Obesity at a young age puts children at increased risk of premature onset of serious chronic diseases such as type 2 diabetes, cardiovascular disease, certain cancers, osteoarthritis, and sleep apnea (Office of the Surgeon General, 2010). Data from the Bogalusa Heart Study showed that 61% of overweight 5- to 10-year-olds already carried at least one risk factor for heart disease, and 26% of them had two or more risk factors (Freedman, Dietz, Srinivasan, & Berenson, 1999). For the first time, the current generation of children in the United States may not live as long as their parents due to the negative effects of obesity on health and longevity (Olshansky et al., 2005). Obesity not only leads to a decreased lifespan, but has also been shown to be associated with a decreased quality of life (Buttitta, Iliescu, Rousseau, & Guerrien, 2014; Griffiths, Parsons, & Hill, 2010). Children with obesity are at risk of being teased and bullied by their peers, which can adversely affect their psychological, social, and academic development and lead to decreased self-esteem, negative body image, and depression. This chapter provides an overview of current prevalence rates of obesity among U.S. children and discusses select early-life risk factors, genetic and environmental influences, and behavioral phenotypes that have been implicated in the development of the disease.

Prevalence of Childhood Obesity and Tracking into Adulthood

Childhood obesity rates have tripled in the last 30 years and have reached an all-time high, with 17.4% of U.S. children and adolescents between the ages of 2 and 19 years being considered obese (body mass index [BMI] for age ≥ 95th percentile; Ogden & Carroll, 2010; Skinner, Perrin, & Skelton, 2016). Recent data also confirm that there has been a statistically significant increase in all classes of obesity, including severe obesity, despite continued clinical and policy efforts to prevent childhood obesity. In 2013–2014, nearly 10% of adolescents met criteria for class 2 obesity (≥ 120% of the 95th percentile or BMI ≥ 35 kg/m^2), and nearly 5%

also met criteria for class 3 obesity (≥ 140% of the 95th percentile or BMI ≥ 40 kg/m²). Youth with severe obesity are of particular concern, as they are at increased risk of developing cardiometabolic comorbidities (Skinner, Perrin, Moss, & Skelton, 2015).

There are significant racial and socioeconomic disparities in obesity rates, with minority children and youth from low-income households being disproportionately affected by the disease. Based on data from the 2011–2012 National Health and Nutrition Examination Survey (NHANES), 20.2% non-Hispanic black and 22.4% Hispanic youth, ages 2–19 years, were considered obese, compared with 14.1% of non-Hispanic white youth (Ogden, Carroll, Kit, & Flegal, 2014). Further, rates of severe obesity (BMI for age ≥ 99th percentile) were approximately 1.7 times higher among youth from families with greater poverty, compared with youth from families of higher socioeconomic status (Skelton, Cook, Auinger, Klein, & Barlow, 2009).

Development of obesity during early childhood is a public health concern not only because it puts children at increased risk for adverse health outcomes, but also because obesity during childhood has been shown to track into adulthood. Data from a retrospective cohort study showed that the probability of being obese as a young adult (i.e., ages 21–29) increased with the age of the obese child and was higher at all child ages, ranging from 1 to 17 years, for children who exceeded the 95th percentile for BMI for age (Whitaker, Wright, Pepe, Seidel, & Dietz, 1997). More specifically, after 6 years of age, the probability of being obese as a young adult exceeded 50% for obese children as compared with 10% for nonobese children. For older youth, there is a 70% chance that an overweight adolescent will be overweight or obese as an adult.

The tracking of childhood obesity into adulthood is a severe public health concern that calls for early prevention efforts. Over the past few decades, great progress has been made in the identification of early-life risk factors that are associated with childhood obesity. Some of these risk factors come into play during early childhood or even earlier, before the baby is born.

Early-Life Risk Factors

Maternal Prepregnancy BMI, Gestational Weight Gain, and Parental Weight Status

Parental weight status and maternal weight status, in particular, have been identified as important predictors of offspring weight status during early childhood. One of these risk factors concerns the weight status at which expecting mothers enter pregnancy. A landmark longitudinal study of growth and development followed infants who were born at high or low risk of obesity on the basis of maternal prepregnancy body weight (Berkowitz, Stallings, Maislin, & Stunkard, 2005). Infants who were born to mothers who, before pregnancy, were overweight or obese were classified as "high risk"; infants who were born to mothers who were normal weight prepregnancy were classified as "low risk." As early as age 4 years old, high-risk children, when compared to low-risk children, showed a significantly greater body weight, BMI, waist circumference, and lean body mass. By age 6, high-risk children differed significantly in all weight- and adiposity-related outcomes from low-risk children, including differences in fat mass, percent body fat, and the sum of four skinfold thicknesses. At the age of 6, 10 of the 33 (30.3%) high-risk children were considered overweight or obese compared with 1 of 37 (2.7%) low-risk children (odds ratio [OR]: 15.7). These between-group differences in weight and adiposity outcomes persisted over time and point to important metabolic, genetic, and environmental influences affecting child growth patterns.

Maternal weight status at the outset of pregnancy is not the only factor that can influence child weight outcomes. Data are also emerging that identify gestational weight gain over the course of the pregnancy as an important determinant of infants' birth weight and subsequent weight development (Lau, Liu, Archer, & McDonald, 2014; Woo Baidal et al., 2016). A woman's prepregnancy weight status determines how much weight she should gain during pregnancy. The higher a woman's weight is entering pregnancy, the less weight she needs to gain over the course of the pregnancy (Institute of Medicine, 2009). An analysis based on cross-sectional, population-based data from the 2010/2011 Pregnancy Risk Assessment Monitoring System showed that maternal prepregnancy BMI was strongly associated with weight gain that exceeded the Institute of Medicine's (IOM) recommendations (Deputy, Sharma, Kim, & Hinkle, 2015). Overweight women and those with class 1 obesity (BMI 30.0–34.9 kg/m^2) showed the highest prevalence (~64%) of excessive gestational weight gain and were nearly three times as likely to exceed the weight gain recommendations compared with normal-weight women. Excess gestational weight gain during pregnancy, in turn, has been identified as an early risk factor for obesity in the offspring during early childhood. Based on data from a prospective cohort study, exceeding the IOM gestational weight gain recommendations was associated with a 46% increase in odds of having an overweight or obese child at ages 2–5 years (Sridhar et al., 2014).

One potential mechanism underlying the association between maternal weight status (before and during pregnancy) and childhood obesity involves in utero fetal programming by nutritional stimuli (Taylor & Poston, 2007). Fetal programming *in utero* postulates that fetuses may adapt to the supply (deficit or abundance) of nutrients crossing the placenta, and these adaptations may permanently change fetuses' physiology and metabolism, which in turn may represent the origins of later life diseases and morbidity.

Parental weight status continues to exert a pronounced effect on offspring weight outcomes once the child is born. Data from a prospective cohort study showed that children of mothers with obesity were at a threefold increased risk of developing obesity during childhood (Strauss & Knight, 1999). Evidence is also emerging that suggests that parental obesity continues to exert its effect on offspring weight outcomes beyond childhood into adulthood. In a landmark study, Whitaker et al. (1997) showed that both obese and nonobese children, ages 1–17, were at greater risk for obesity as adults if at least one parent was obese. Their data further indicated that parental obesity more than doubled the risk of adult obesity among both obese and nonobese children under 10 years of age.

Weight- and Nutrition-Related Risk Factors during Early Infancy

The first months of life have been identified as a critical period in infancy for the development of obesity. Both the rate at which infants gain weight during the first year and early feeding practices can have important implications for their weight development during childhood and later adulthood.

Rapid weight gain during the first 6–12 months of an infant's life has been shown to confer an increased risk of obesity. Specifically, a meta-analysis by Druet et al. (2012) showed that each +1 unit increase in weight standard deviation scores between 0 and 1 year of age conferred a twofold higher risk of childhood obesity and a 23% higher risk of adult obesity. Proposed mechanisms that may underlie the association between rapid weight gain and an increased obesity risk involve early feeding practices (e.g., breastfeeding vs. formula feeding), early expression of a genetic predisposition to excess weight gain (Stettler, Kumanyika, Katz, Zemel, & Stallings, 2003), hyperphagic eating traits (e.g., vigorous sucking behavior; Stunkard, Berkowitz, Stallings, & Schoeller, 1999), and long-term changes in hypothalamic appetite regulating centers and insulin secretion (Plagemann et al., 1999; Waterland & Garza, 2002).

The American Academy of Pediatrics (2012) recommends exclusive breastfeeding during an infant's first 6 months of life. Data from the Centers for Disease Control and Prevention (CDC) National Immunization Survey indicated that 43.3% of infants born in 2012 were breastfed exclusively for 3 months and only 21.9% were breastfed exclusively for 6 months (Centers for Disease Control and Prevention, 2016). Some, but not all studies, have pointed to a potentially protective effect of breastfeeding on the development of overweight and obesity during childhood (Marseglia et al., 2015). A meta-analysis by Arenz and colleagues showed that initiation of breastfeeding resulted in a modest but significant overall reduced risk of childhood obesity (OR: 0.78) (Arenz,

Ruckerl, Koletzko, & von Kries, 2004). The data further showed that for each month of breastfeeding (up to 9 months), the odds of child overweight decreased by 4%. Several mechanisms have been proposed that may be implicated in the association between breastfeeding and a modest reduction in risk of later overweight and obesity. Breastfeeding, when compared with formula feeding, may confer a protective effect on excess weight gain by promoting infants' self-regulation of energy intake and/or by promoting more favorable metabolic outcomes (Bartok & Ventura, 2009). Formula-fed infants have been shown to have higher protein and total energy intakes and differences in the release of pancreatic and gut hormones, including higher plasma levels of insulin, which can stimulate fat deposition (Heinig, Nommsen, Peerson, Lonnerdal, & Dewey, 1993; Lucas et al., 1980; Whitehead, 1995).

The timing in which solid foods are introduced has also been identified as a potential risk factor for overweight and obesity during childhood, particularly among formula-fed infants (Huh, Rifas-Shiman, Taveras, Oken, & Gillman, 2011). However, a recent longitudinal analysis of 1,181 youths who participated in the Infant Feeding Practices Study II refuted this association (Barrera, Perrine, Li, & Scanlon, 2016). Results of this study showed that the odds of obesity among infants introduced to solids at < 4 months of age, compared to those introduced between 4 and 6 months of age, was not significantly associated with subsequent obesity when controlling for maternal and child characteristics.

In summary, several early-life risk factors have been identified that pose an increased risk for later obesity in the offspring. Some of these risk factors are conferred by parents and include their own weight status and early feeding practices, whereas others pertain to characteristics of the child and include early growth patterns and behavioral traits. Children's body weight and eating behaviors are tightly regulated by a complex interplay of both genetic and environmental factors. There is growing evidence that suggests that a genetic susceptibility interacts with factors in children's early environment to predispose some children to overeating and excess weight gain.

Heredity

Human body weight and body composition are highly heritable. Genetic factors are estimated to explain between 70 and 80% of the variance in child and adolescent BMI (Maes, Neale, & Eaves, 1997). Single gene mutations associated with extreme obesity are rare, affecting less than 5% of individuals with severe obesity (Ranadive & Vaisse, 2008). A recent genomewide association meta-analysis of 14 studies identified two novel loci (i.e., *OLFM4* at 13q14 and *HOXB5* at 17q21) that were associated with common early-onset childhood obesity (Bradfield et al., 2012) (Figure 37.1). More common than single gene mutations are gene variants (polymorphisms) in candidate genes that have a functional role in regulating central and peripheral pathways controlling energy balance. Many of these candidate genes encode hormones, peptides, and neurons that are implicated in the regulation of hunger, fullness, and food intake. Examples of such a gene polymorphism are the variants of the fat mass and obesity-associated gene (*FTO*), which has been shown to play an important role in the regulation of food intake, satiety, body weight, and fat mass in children and adolescents (Bradfield et al., 2012; Cecil, Tavendale, Watt, Hetherington, & Palmer, 2008; Wardle et al., 2008). For example, a study by Wardle and colleagues with preschool children from the Twin Early Development Study (TEDS) showed that children with higher-risk (AA) *FTO* alleles consumed significantly more snacks in the absence of hunger when compared to children with a more protective (TT) genotype, an effect that was independent of children's weight status (Wardle, Llewellyn, Sanderson, & Plomin, 2009).

Evidence is also emerging that suggests that several behavioral traits, including hyperphagic eating traits that may lead to excess weight gain in children, are shared among nuclear family members and are heritable. For example, heritability has been established in children for the rate of eating (heritability estimate $[h^2]$ = 62%; Llewellyn, van Jaarsveld, Boniface, Carnell, & Wardle, 2008), food cue (h^2 = 75%), satiety (h^2 = 63%) responsiveness (Carnell, Haworth, Plomin, & Wardle, 2008), and eating in the

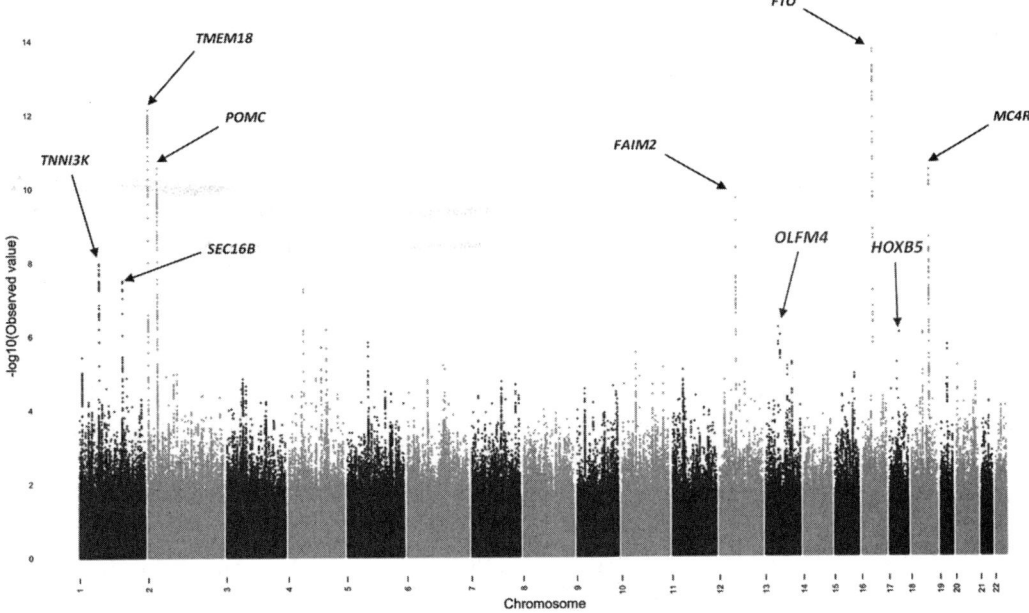

FIGURE 37.1. Manhattan plot of the results from a meta-analysis of genomewide association studies (GWAS) for childhood obesity for loci that achieved genomewide significance ($p < 5 \times 10-8$). From Bradfield, Taal, Timpson, Scherag, Lecoeur, Warrington, et al. (2012). A genome-wide association meta-analysis identifies new childhood obesity loci. *Nature Genetics, 44*(5), 526–531. Reprinted by permission from Macmillan Publishers Ltd. Copyright © 2012 Macmillan Publishers Ltd.

absence of hunger (EAH; $h^2 = 51\%$; Fisher et al., 2007). In a seminal study by Faith and colleagues, 36 monozygotic (MZ) and 18 dizygotic (DZ) twins consumed an *ad libitum* lunch in the laboratory, during which they could freely select from a variety of foods and beverages at a multi-item buffet (Faith, Rha, Neale, & Allison, 1999). The results of this study showed that MZ twins were more similar in caloric intake than DZ twins, with genetic variations accounting for 24–33% of variance in age- and sex-adjusted total caloric intake at the meal. Similarly, in a study conducted in weight-discordant siblings, overweight and obese siblings showed poorer caloric compensation (i.e., inaccurate adjustments in intake at a test meal in response to changes in the energy density [ED; kcal/g] of a compulsory preload) and significantly more eating EAH when compared to their normal-weight siblings (Kral et al., 2012). Data from this study also showed familial associations for both eating traits that were significant for full siblings but not for half-siblings, which suggests that genetic influences may underlie both of these eating traits.

Together, these examples illustrate that the regulation of body weight and energy intake in children is partly under genetic control. Although genetic predispositions may increase some children's susceptibility to overeating and excess weight gain, evidence also suggests that aspects of the obesogenic food environment can greatly affect children's food choices and consumption behaviors.

Obesogenic Food Environment

The current food environment offers easy access to large portions of inexpensive, energy-dense foods and beverages. Based on data from the NHANES, food purchases at stores and full- and quick-service restaurants accounted for approximately 85% of daily calories consumed among youth between 6 and 19 years of age (Drewnowski & Rehm, 2013). A recent analysis based on intercept surveys of children's purchases outside urban corner stores further showed that youth in grades 4–6 shop at corner stores frequently and purchase energy-dense snacks and sugar-sweetened beverages that average 357 calories for a total cost of just $1.07 (Borradaile et al., 2009) (Figure 37.2). The relatively inexpensive cost of energy-dense foods and sugar-sweetened beverages often results from pricing strategies that promote the sale of large food portions. Food retailers commonly structure meal prices in such a way that the per unit cost of foods and beverages is lowest for larger portion sizes—a strategy known as value size pricing (Vermeer, Alting, Steenhuis, & Seidell, 2010).

The portion size of foods and beverages has been identified as a risk factor for increased energy intake in both children and adults (Rolls, 2010). Laboratory-based experimental studies have shown that children as young as 2 years of age significantly increased their energy intake when larger portions of a main entrée were served (Birch, Savage, & Fisher, 2015; Fisher, 2007). Data from a study by Kral and colleagues with 8- to 10-year old children further showed that when the portion size of a sugar-sweetened beverage that was served at a meal was doubled from 10 fluid ounces to 20 fluid ounces, calories consumed from that beverage increased by 33% (Kral, Remiker, Strutz, & Moore, 2014). Current estimates suggest that children ages 2–12 years consume as many as 30% of their daily calories from salty and sugary snacks, and up to 40% when sugar-sweetened beverages are added in (Bleich & Wolfson, 2015; Piernas & Popkin, 2010). There is strong epidemiological and experimental evidence for the independent roles of sugar-sweetened beverage intake (DeBoer, Scharf, & Demmer, 2013; Malik, Pan, Willett, & Hu, 2013; Malik, Schulze, & Hu, 2006) and increased snacking frequency (Barlow, 2007; Davis et al., 2007; Kuhl, Clifford, & Stark, 2012; Larson & Story, 2013) in the promotion of excess weight gain and obesity in children and adolescents. Therefore, a sustained exposure to large portions of these types of energy-dense foods and beverages can lead to excess weight gain in children.

Children who reside in lower-income neighborhoods may be especially affected by the obesogenic environment, in part because impoverished neighborhoods are often characterized by an overabundance of high-en-

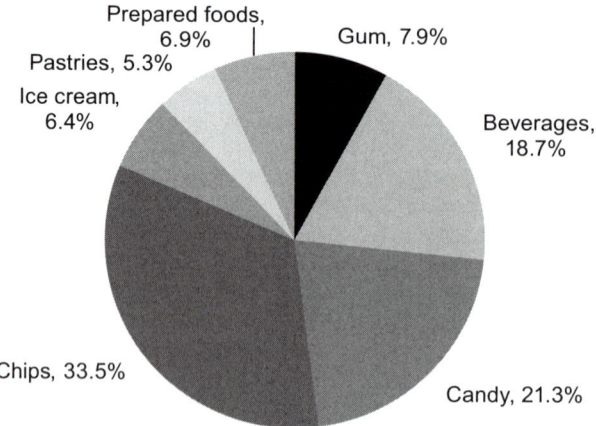

FIGURE 37.2. Total items (by type of item) purchased in urban corner stores by children in grades 4–6. Data based on 833 intercept surveys conducted before and after school. Reproduced with permission from Borradaile, Sherman, Vander Veur, McCoy, Sandoval, Nachmani, et al. (2009). Snacking in children: The role of urban corner stores. *Pediatrics, 124*(5), 1293–1298. Copyright © 2009 the American Academy of Pediatrics.

ergy, nutrient-poor foods (i.e., food swamp), while providing less access to a full-service supermarket or large grocery store (i.e., food desert). Additionally, high rates of poverty have been shown to adversely affect children's weight outcomes. Based on nationally representative data from NHANES, rates of severe obesity (BMI for age ≥ 99th percentile) were 1.7 times higher among youth from families with greater poverty, compared with youth from families of higher socioeconomic status (Skelton et al., 2009). One of the factors that has been implicated in the relationship between poverty and obesity is food insecurity. *Food insecurity* refers to the "limited or uncertain availability of nutritionally adequate and safe foods or limited or uncertain ability to acquire acceptable foods in socially acceptable ways" (Expert Panel, 1990, p. 1,598). Food insecurity may increase the odds of obesity due to a variety of factors, including limited resources; limited access to healthy, affordable foods; cycles of food deprivation and overeating; fewer opportunities for physical activity; greater exposure to marketing of energy-dense food products; and higher levels of stress, anxiety, and deprivation (Hartline-Grafton, 2015).

In summary, a sustained exposure to obesogenic food environments in which large portions of foods and beverages are readily available and easily accessible can shape children's food choices and consumption patterns in profound ways. Children not only learn about consumption and (oversized) portion size norms, but they may adopt eating behaviors that disrupt their energy intake regulation. Energy-dense, nutrient-poor foods and snacks, as well as sugar-sweetened drinks, are often heavily marketed to children and their families. Brownell and Battle Horgen (2004) provide a thorough review of the influence of the food industry, as well as food marketing and advertising campaigns, on shaping unhealthy food and beverage consumption behaviors in children.

Eating Phenotypes

Experimental research has identified several behavioral traits in children that are linked to overeating and excess weight gain (Fisher & Kral, 2008; French, Epstein, Jeffery, Blundell, & Wardle, 2012; Kral & Faith, 2009). These behavioral traits are believed to be shaped by an interaction between biology (genetics) and factors in children's early environment (nurture). One characteristic that many of these behavioral traits have in common is that they are believed to disrupt children's internal regulation of hunger and fullness. Early ingestive behavior research suggested that humans are born with an innate ability to regulate energy intake. In a classic experiment by Fomon and colleagues, two groups of male infants, ages 6 and 16 weeks, were fed infant formulas that differed in ED (67 kcal/dl vs. 133 kcal/dl) (Fomon, Filer, Thomas, Rogers, & Proksch, 1969). The study showed that the quantity consumed by infants fed the high-ED formula was substantially less compared to the quantity consumed by infants fed the low-ED formula. Energy intakes (expressed as kcal/kg) did not differ significantly between the two feeding groups, which suggests that infants were able to compensate for the greater or lesser ED by adjusting the amounts of formula consumed.

Young children's ability to regulate energy intake appears to deteriorate with age, as they become more exposed to and influenced by food and social cues in the environment. The use of certain caregiver feeding practices has also been shown to have the potential to impair children's self-regulation of energy intake. For example, studies that investigated individual differences in children's ability to regulate energy intake showed that poorer caloric compensation ability was associated with increased child weight status (Johnson & Birch, 1994; Kral et al., 2012), increased child age (Cecil et al., 2005), and overly controlling parental feeding practices (e.g., food restriction; Tripicchio et al., 2014).

Another eating phenotype that has been associated with overeating and excess weight gain in children is EAH, which refers to children's susceptibility to eating when satiated in response to the presence of palatable, energy-dense snack foods (Cutting, Fisher, Grimm-Thomas, & Birch, 1999). EAH is a behavioral eating trait that increases short-term energy intake (Fisher & Birch, 1999b, 2000) and is associated with an increased risk of overweight in children (Fisher & Birch, 2002; Fisher et al., 2007; Kral et al., 2012). The trait appears to be stable during childhood (Birch, Fisher, & Davison, 2003; Fisher & Birch, 2002), heritable (Fisher et al., 2007), and is increased in children whose caregivers use restrictive feeding practices and increased monitoring (Birch et al., 2003; Fisher & Birch, 1999a).

Besides behavioral traits that reflect low avoidance tendencies such as impaired satiety, additional traits reflect high approach tendencies toward food, which can emerge early in life. For example, the vigor of infant sucking behavior has been identified as an early predictor of increased weight status and adiposity during early childhood. In a longitudinal study for growth and development, infants born at high risk for obesity on the basis of maternal prepregnancy BMI showed significant differences in nutritive sucking behavior when compared to infants born at low risk for obesity (Stunkard et al., 1999). When feeding infants either received breast milk or their customary formula from a nutritive sucking apparatus, high-risk infants showed significantly greater total intakes (150g ± 57 vs. 123g ± 48), total number of sucks (920 ± 559 sucks vs. 620 ± 293 sucks), and higher sucking rates (0.75 sucks/sec ± 0.25 vs. 0.59 sucks/sec ± 0.26) than low-risk infants. Nutrient sucking behavior and daily energy intake at 3 months of age explained ~17% of the variability in infants' weight, weight for length, body fat, fat-free mass, and skinfold thickness at 12 months of age. When the same cohort of children was studied several years later, investigators assessed the association between children's rate of eating during a test meal in the laboratory and their weight status. The results indicated that a higher rate of eating at 4 years of age, expressed as mouthfuls of food per minute, predicted child overweight status at 6 years of age, as well as excess weight gain from ages 4 to 6 years (Berkowitz et al., 2010).

In sum, several behavioral traits have been identified that are believed to be shaped both by genes and the environment, and can lead to excess calorie intake and weight gain during early childhood. We note, however, that the relationship between behavioral eating traits and children's early upbringing and environment is believed to be bidirectional. That is, caregivers and the greater environment may help shape child eating traits, but caregivers may also be responding to children's individual traits, and/or children themselves may be seeking out food environments that meet their individual appetitive predispositions (Carnell & Wardle, 2008).

Energy Expenditure

Physical Activity and Sedentary Behavior

The association between physical activity, sedentary behaviors, and adiposity in youth has been studied extensively. Common assumptions postulate that overweight/obese children and adolescents spend less time in moderate-to-vigorous physical activity (MVPA) and more time in sedentary activities compared to their normal-weight peers, but data supporting these differences are mixed. Several studies, especially those examining child behaviors in the free-living environment, showed lower levels of physical activity and MVPA in overweight and obese children (Colley et al., 2011; Lazzer et al., 2003). Other studies, however, failed to find a negative association between body fat and physical activity (Wilks, Besson, Lindroos, & Ekelund, 2011) or found that overweight and obese youth were expending as much, if not more, energy than lean youth due to the higher metabolic cost of movement (Maffeis, Zaffanello, Pinelli, & Schutz, 1996). Evidence also points to potential sex and age differences in physical activity behaviors among youth of different weight statuses (Belcher et al., 2010; Colley et al., 2011). For example, data from the Canadian Health Measures Survey (CHMS) indicated that overweight and obese youth did not differ significantly in amounts of time spent in sedentary behavior, but overweight and obese boys, but not girls, engaged in significantly less MVPA per day than normal-weight children (Colley et al., 2011).

Metabolic Rate

There has also been considerable interest in whether low metabolic rate, perhaps because of more efficient energy utilization, may be a risk factor for the development of obesity in infancy and early childhood. Early data by Roberts and colleagues showed that infants who were born to mothers with obesity, and who had a low total energy expenditure (TEE) at 3 months of age, became overweight at age 1 year, whereas infants who were born to mothers with or without obesity and who had a higher TEE did not (Roberts, Savage, Coward, Chew, & Lucas, 1988). No significant associations between children's resting energy expenditure (REE) and obesity were reported in this study.

However, other studies failed to show a relationship between low TEE and the development of obesity. For example, a longitudinal study of 38 infants who were born to normal-weight mothers and 40 infants who were born to mothers with obesity found no relationship between TEE and REE and infant body weight and weight gain at 1 year of age (Stunkard et al., 1999). Data from the same cohort of children also failed to show a significant association between TEE during the first 6 years of life and child BMI for age percentile, BMI z-score, and percent body fat at age 8 (Zinkel et al., 2016). Data from other studies showed that TEE and postprandial REE were not related to fat mass in preschool children (Goran et al., 1995) and preadolescents (Goran et al., 1998), providing further evidence that a low TEE may play a limited role in the development of obesity during infancy and childhood.

Summary

In summary, there are multiple, complex routes to the development of overweight and obesity in children. For many of these routes, genetic predispositions interact with factors in the environment to affect children's eating and physical activity behaviors and weight development. New evidence suggests that risk factors for childhood obesity emerge even before a child is born, which calls for early prevention efforts. Given the severe physical and mental health risks associated with childhood obesity, concerted efforts are needed by many partners, including government and industry, to address this complex public health problem.

References

American Academy of Pediatrics. (2012). Breastfeeding and the use of human milk. *Pediatrics, 129*, e827–e841.

Arenz, S., Ruckerl, R., Koletzko, B., & von Kries, R. (2004). Breast-feeding and childhood obesity: A systematic review. *International Journal of Obesity and Related Metabolic Disorders, 28*(10), 1247–1256.

Barlow, S. E. (2007). Expert committee recommendations regarding the prevention, assessment, and treatment of child and adolescent overweight and obesity: Summary report. *Pediatrics, 120*(Suppl. 4), S164–S192.

Barrera, C. M., Perrine, C. G., Li, R., & Scanlon, K. S. (2016). Age at introduction to solid foods and child obesity at 6 years. *Childhood Obesity, 12*(3), 188–192.

Bartok, C. J., & Ventura, A. K. (2009). Mechanisms underlying the association between breastfeeding and obesity. *International Journal of Pediatric Obesity, 4*(4), 196–204.

Belcher, B. R., Berrigan, D., Dodd, K. W., Emken, B. A., Chou, C. P., & Spruijt-Metz, D. (2010). Physical activity in U.S. youth: Effect of race/ethnicity, age, gender, and weight status. *Medicine and Science in Sports and Exercise, 42*(12), 2211–2221.

Berkowitz, R. I., Moore, R. H., Faith, M. S., Stallings, V. A., Kral, T. V., & Stunkard, A. J. (2010). Identification of an obese eating style in 4-year-old children born at high and low risk for obesity. *Obesity (Silver Spring), 18*(3), 505–512.

Berkowitz, R. I., Stallings, V. A., Maislin, G., & Stunkard, A. J. (2005). Growth of children at high risk of obesity during the first 6 y of life: Implications for prevention. *American Journal of Clinical Nutrition, 81*(1), 140–146.

Birch, L. L., Fisher, J. O., & Davison, K. K. (2003). Learning to overeat: Maternal use of restrictive feeding practices promotes girls' eating in the absence of hunger. *American Journal of Clinical Nutrition, 78*(2), 215–220.

Birch, L. L., Savage, J. S., & Fisher, J. O. (2015). Right sizing prevention: Food portion size effects on children's eating and weight. *Appetite, 88*, 11–16.

Bleich, S. N., & Wolfson, J. A. (2015). U.S. adult and child snacking patterns among sugar-sweetened beverage drinkers and non-drinkers. *Preventive Medicine, 72*, 8–14.

Borradaile, K. E., Sherman, S., Vander Veur, S. S., McCoy, T., Sandoval, B., Nachmani, J., et al. (2009). Snacking in children: The role of urban corner stores. *Pediatrics, 124*(5), 1293–1298.

Bradfield, J. P., Taal, H. R., Timpson, N. J., Scherag, A., Lecoeur, C., Warrington, N. M., et al. (2012). A genome-wide association meta-analysis identifies new childhood obesity loci. *Nature Genetics, 44*(5), 526–531.

Brownell, K., & Battle Horgen, K. (2004). *Food fight: The inside story of the food industry, America's* obesity crisis, and what we can do about it. New York: McGraw-Hill.

Buttitta, M., Iliescu, C., Rousseau, A., & Guerrien, A. (2014). Quality of life in overweight and obese children and adolescents: A literature review. *Quality of Life Research, 23*(4), 1117–1139.

Carnell, S., Haworth, C. M., Plomin, R., & Wardle, J. (2008). Genetic influence on appetite in children. *International Journal of Obesity (London), 32*(10), 1468–1473.

Carnell, S., & Wardle, J. (2008). Appetitive traits and child obesity: Measurement, origins and implications for intervention. *Proceedings of the Nutrition Society, 67*(4), 343–355.

Cecil, J. E., Palmer, C. N., Wrieden, W., Murrie, I., Bolton-Smith, C., Watt, P., et al. (2005). Energy intakes of children after preloads: Adjustment, not compensation. *American Journal of Clinical Nutrition, 82*(2), 302–308.

Cecil, J. E., Tavendale, R., Watt, P., Hetherington, M. M., & Palmer, C. N. (2008). An obesity-associated *FTO* gene variant and increased energy intake in children. *New England Journal of Medicine, 359*(24), 2558–2566.

Centers for Disease Control and Prevention. (2016). Breastfeeding among U.S. children born 2002–2012. Retrieved July 29, 2016, from *www.cdc.gov/breastfeeding/data/nis_data/index.htm*.

Colley, R. C., Garriguet, D., Janssen, I., Craig, C. L., Clarke, J., & Tremblay, M. S. (2011). Physical activity of Canadian children and youth: Accelerometer results from the 2007 to 2009 Canadian Health Measures Survey. *Public Health Reports, 22*(1), 15–23.

Cutting, T. M., Fisher, J. O., Grimm-Thomas, K., & Birch, L. L. (1999). Like mother, like daughter: Familial patterns of overweight are mediated by mothers' dietary disinhibition. *American Journal of Clinical Nutrition, 69*(4), 608–613.

Davis, M. M., Gance-Cleveland, B., Hassink, S., Johnson, R., Paradis, G., & Resnicow, K. (2007). Recommendations for prevention of childhood obesity. *Pediatrics, 120*(Suppl. 4), S229–S253.

DeBoer, M. D., Scharf, R. J., & Demmer, R. T. (2013). Sugar-sweetened beverages and weight gain in 2- to 5-year-old children. *Pediatrics, 132*(3), 413–420.

Deputy, N. P., Sharma, A. J., Kim, S. Y., & Hinkle, S. N. (2015). Prevalence and characteristics associated with gestational weight gain adequacy. *Obstetrics and Gynecology, 125*(4), 773–781.

Drewnowski, A., & Rehm, C. D. (2013). Energy intakes of U.S. children and adults by food purchase location and by specific food source. *Nutrition Journal, 12,* 59.

Druet, C., Stettler, N., Sharp, S., Simmons, R. K., Cooper, C., Smith, G. D., et al. (2012). Prediction of childhood obesity by infancy weight gain: An individual-level meta-analysis. *Paediatric and Perinatal Epidemiology, 26*(1), 19–26.

Expert Panel. (1990). Core indicators of nutritional state for difficult-to-sample populations. *Journal of Nutrition, 120*(11, Suppl.), 1559–1600.

Faith, M. S., Rha, S. S., Neale, M. C., & Allison, D. B. (1999). Evidence for genetic influences on human energy intake: Results from a twin study using measured observations. *Behavior Genetics, 29*(3), 145–154.

Fisher, J. O. (2007). Effects of age on children's intake of large and self-selected food portions. *Obesity (Silver Spring), 15*(2), 403–412.

Fisher, J. O., & Birch, L. L. (1999a). Restricting access to foods and children's eating. *Appetite, 32*(3), 405–419.

Fisher, J. O., & Birch, L. L. (1999b). Restricting access to palatable foods affects children's behavioral response, food selection, and intake. *American Journal of Clinical Nutrition, 69*(6), 1264–1272.

Fisher, J. O., & Birch, L. L. (2000). Parents' restrictive feeding practices are associated with young girls' negative self-evaluation of eating. *Journal of the American Dietetic Association, 100*(11), 1341–1346.

Fisher, J. O., & Birch, L. L. (2002). Eating in the absence of hunger and overweight in girls from 5 to 7 y of age. *American Journal of Clinical Nutrition, 76*(1), 226–231.

Fisher, J. O., Cai, G., Jaramillo, S. J., Cole, S. A., Comuzzie, A. G., & Butte, N. F. (2007). Heritability of hyperphagic eating behavior and appetite-related hormones among Hispanic children. *Obesity (Silver Spring), 15*(6), 1484–1495.

Fisher, J. O., & Kral, T. V. (2008). Super-size me: Portion size effects on young children's eating. *Physiology and Behavior, 94*(1), 39–47.

Fomon, S. J., Filer, L. J., Jr., Thomas, L. N., Rogers, R. R., & Proksch, A. M. (1969). Relationship between formula concentration and rate of growth of normal infants. *Journal of Nutrition, 98*(2), 241–254.

Freedman, D. S., Dietz, W. H., Srinivasan, S. R., & Berenson, G. S. (1999). The relation of overweight to cardiovascular risk factors among children and adolescents: The Bogalusa Heart Study. *Pediatrics, 103*(6, Pt. 1), 1175–1182.

French, S. A., Epstein, L. H., Jeffery, R. W., Blundell, J. E., & Wardle, J. (2012). Eating behavior dimensions: Associations with energy intake and body weight—a review. *Appetite, 59*(2), 541–549.

Goran, M. I., Carpenter, W. H., McGloin, A., Johnson, R., Hardin, J. M., & Weinsier, R. L. (1995). Energy expenditure in children of lean and obese parents. *American Journal of Physiology, 268*(5, Pt. 1), E917–E924.

Goran, M. I., Shewchuk, R., Gower, B. A., Nagy, T. R., Carpenter, W. H., & Johnson, R. K. (1998). Longitudinal changes in fatness in white children: No effect of childhood energy expenditure. *American Journal of Clinical Nutrition, 67*(2), 309–316.

Griffiths, L. J., Parsons, T. J., & Hill, A. J. (2010). Self-esteem and quality of life in obese children and adolescents: A systematic review. *International Journal of Pediatric Obesity, 5*(4), 282–304.

Hartline-Grafton, H. (2015). Understanding the connections: Food insecurity and obesity. Retrieved from *http://frac.org/pdf/frac_brief_understanding_the_connections.pdf*.

Heinig, M. J., Nommsen, L. A., Peerson, J. M., Lonnerdal, B., & Dewey, K. G. (1993). Energy and protein intakes of breast-fed and formula-fed infants during the first year of life and their association with growth velocity: The DARLING Study. *American Journal of Clinical Nutrition, 58*(2), 152–161.

Huh, S. Y., Rifas-Shiman, S. L., Taveras, E. M., Oken, E., & Gillman, M. W. (2011). Timing of solid food introduction and risk of obesity in preschool-aged children. *Pediatrics, 127*(3), e544–e551.

Institute of Medicine. (2009). *Weight gain during pregnancy: Reexamining the guidelines.* Washington, DC: National Academies Press.

Johnson, S. L., & Birch, L. L. (1994). Parents' and children's adiposity and eating style. *Pediatrics, 94*(5), 653–661.

Kral, T. V., Allison, D. B., Birch, L. L., Stallings, V. A., Moore, R. H., & Faith, M. S. (2012). Caloric compensation and eating in the absence of hunger in 5- to 12-y-old weight-discordant siblings. *American Journal of Clinical Nutrition, 96*(3), 574–583.

Kral, T. V., & Faith, M. S. (2009). Influences on child eating and weight development from a behavioral genetics perspective. *Journal of Pediatric Psychology, 34*(6), 596–605.

Kral, T. V., Remiker, A. M., Strutz, E. M., & Moore, R. H. (2014). Role of child weight status and the relative reinforcing value of food in children's response to portion size increases. *Obesity (Silver Spring), 22*(7), 1716–1722.

Kuhl, E. S., Clifford, L. M., & Stark, L. J. (2012). Obesity in preschoolers: Behavioral correlates and directions for treatment. *Obesity (Silver Spring), 20*(1), 3–29.

Larson, N., & Story, M. (2013). A review of snacking patterns among children and adolescents: What are the implications of snacking for weight status? *Childhood Obesity, 9*(2), 104–115.

Lau, E. Y., Liu, J., Archer, E., & McDonald, S. M. (2014). Maternal weight gain in pregnancy and risk of obesity among offspring: A systematic review. *Journal of Obesity, 2014*, 524939.

Lazzer, S., Boirie, Y., Bitar, A., Montaurier, C., Vernet, J., Meyer, M., et al. (2003). Assessment of energy expenditure associated with physical activities in free-living obese and nonobese adolescents. *American Journal of Clinical Nutrition, 78*(3), 471–479.

Llewellyn, C. H., van Jaarsveld, C. H., Boniface, D., Carnell, S., & Wardle, J. (2008). Eating rate is a heritable phenotype related to weight in children. *American Journal of Clinical Nutrition, 88*(6), 1560–1566.

Lucas, A., Sarson, D. L., Blackburn, A. M., Adrian, T. E., Aynsley-Green, A., & Bloom, S. R. (1980). Breast vs bottle: Endocrine responses are different with formula feeding. *Lancet, 1*(8181), 1267–1269.

Maes, H. H., Neale, M. C., & Eaves, L. J. (1997). Genetic and environmental factors in relative body weight and human adiposity. *Behavior Genetics, 27*(4), 325–351.

Maffeis, C., Zaffanello, M., Pinelli, L., & Schutz, Y. (1996). Total energy expenditure and patterns of activity in 8–10-year-old obese and nonobese children. *Journal of Pediatric Gastroenterology and Nutrition, 23*, 256–261.

Malik, V. S., Pan, A., Willett, W. C., & Hu, F. B. (2013). Sugar-sweetened beverages and weight gain in children and adults: A systematic review and meta-analysis. *American Journal of Clinical Nutrition, 98*(4), 1084–1102.

Malik, V. S., Schulze, M. B., & Hu, F. B. (2006). Intake of sugar-sweetened beverages and weight gain: A systematic review. *American Journal of Clinical Nutrition, 84*(2), 274–288.

Marseglia, L., Manti, S., D'Angelo, G., Cuppari, C., Salpietro, V., Filippelli, M., et al. (2015). Obesity and breastfeeding: The strength of association. *Women Birth, 28*(2), 81–86.

Office of the Surgeon General. (2010). *The Surgeon General's vision for a healthy and fit nation.* Retrieved from *www.ncbi.nlm.nih.gov/books/NBK44660/pdf/Bookshelf_NBK44660.pdf.*

Ogden, C. L., & Carroll, M. D. (2010). *Prevalence of obesity among children and adolescents: United States, trends 1963–1965 through 20007–2008.* Retrieved from *www.cdc.gov/nchs/data/hestat/obesity_child_07_08/obesity_child_07_08.htm.*

Ogden, C. L., Carroll, M. D., Kit, B. K., & Flegal, K. M. (2014). Prevalence of childhood and adult obesity in the United States, 2011–2012. *Journal of the American Medical Association, 311*(8), 806–814.

Olshansky, S. J., Passaro, D. J., Hershow, R. C., Layden, J., Carnes, B. A., Brody, J., et al. (2005). A potential decline in life expectancy in the United States in the 21st century. *New England Journal of Medicine, 352*(11), 1138–1145.

Piernas, C., & Popkin, B. M. (2010). Trends in snacking among U.S. children. *Health Affairs (Millwood), 29*(3), 398–404.

Plagemann, A., Harder, T., Rake, A., Voits, M., Fink, H., Rohde, W., et al. (1999). Perinatal elevation of hypothalamic insulin, acquired malformation of hypothalamic galaninergic neurons, and syndrome x-like alterations in adulthood of neonatally overfed rats. *Brain Research, 836*(1–2), 146–155.

Ranadive, S. A., & Vaisse, C. (2008). Lessons from extreme human obesity: Monogenic disorders. *Endocrinology and Metabolism Clinics of North America, 37*(3), 733–751.

Roberts, S. B., Savage, J., Coward, W. A., Chew, B., & Lucas, A. (1988). Energy expenditure and intake in infants born to lean and overweight mothers. *New England Journal of Medicine, 318*(8), 461–466.

Rolls, B. J. (2010). Plenary Lecture 1: Dietary strategies for the prevention and treatment of obesity. *Proceedings of the Nutrition Society, 69*(1), 70–79.

Skelton, J. A., Cook, S. R., Auinger, P., Klein, J. D., & Barlow, S. E. (2009). Prevalence and trends of severe obesity among U.S. children and adolescents. *Academic Pediatrics, 9*(5), 322–329.

Skinner, A. C., Perrin, E. M., Moss, L. A., & Skelton, J. A. (2015). Cardiometabolic risks and severity of obesity in children and young adults. *New England Journal of Medicine, 373*(14), 1307–1317.

Skinner, A. C., Perrin, E. M., & Skelton, J. A. (2016). Prevalence of obesity and severe obesity in U.S. children, 1999–2014. *Obesity (Silver Spring), 24*(5), 1116–1123.

Sridhar, S. B., Darbinian, J., Ehrlich, S. F., Markman,

M. A., Gunderson, E. P., Ferrara, A., et al. (2014). Maternal gestational weight gain and offspring risk for childhood overweight or obesity. *American Journal of Obstetrics and Gynecology, 211*(3), 259, e1–e8.

Stettler, N., Kumanyika, S. K., Katz, S. H., Zemel, B. S., & Stallings, V. A. (2003). Rapid weight gain during infancy and obesity in young adulthood in a cohort of African Americans. *American Journal of Clinical Nutrition, 77*(6), 1374–1378.

Strauss, R. S., & Knight, J. (1999). Influence of the home environment on the development of obesity in children. *Pediatrics, 103*(6), e85.

Stunkard, A. J., Berkowitz, R. I., Stallings, V. A., & Schoeller, D. A. (1999). Energy intake, not energy output, is a determinant of body size in infants. *American Journal of Clinical Nutrition, 69*(3), 524–530.

Taylor, P. D., & Poston, L. (2007). Developmental programming of obesity in mammals. *Experimental Physiology, 92*(2), 287–298.

Tripicchio, G. L., Keller, K. L., Johnson, C., Pietrobelli, A., Heo, M., & Faith, M. S. (2014). Differential maternal feeding practices, eating self-regulation, and adiposity in young twins. *Pediatrics, 134*(5), e1399–e1404.

Vermeer, W. M., Alting, E., Steenhuis, I. H., & Seidell, J. C. (2010). Value for money or making the healthy choice: The impact of proportional pricing on consumers' portion size choices. *European Journal of Public Health, 20*(1), 65–69.

Wardle, J., Carnell, S., Haworth, C. M., Farooqi, I. S., O'Rahilly, S., & Plomin, R. (2008). Obesity associated genetic variation in *FTO* is associated with diminished satiety. *Journal of Clinical Endocrinology and Metabolism, 93*(9), 3640–3643.

Wardle, J., Llewellyn, C., Sanderson, S., & Plomin, R. (2009). The *FTO* gene and measured food intake in children. *International Journal of Obesity (London), 33*(1), 42–45.

Waterland, R. A., & Garza, C. (2002). Early postnatal nutrition determines adult pancreatic glucose-responsive insulin secretion and islet gene expression in rats. *Journal of Nutrition, 132*(3), 357–364.

Whitaker, R. C., Wright, J. A., Pepe, M. S., Seidel, K. D., & Dietz, W. H. (1997). Predicting obesity in young adulthood from childhood and parental obesity. *New England Journal of Medicine, 337*(13), 869–873.

Whitehead, R. G. (1995). For how long is exclusive breast-feeding adequate to satisfy the dietary energy needs of the average young baby? *Pediatric Research, 37*(2), 239–243.

Wilks, D. C., Besson, H., Lindroos, A. K., & Ekelund, U. (2011). Objectively measured physical activity and obesity prevention in children, adolescents and adults: A systematic review of prospective studies. *Obesity Reviews, 12*(5), e119–e129.

Woo Baidal, J. A., Locks, L. M., Cheng, E. R., Blake-Lamb, T. L., Perkins, M. E., & Taveras, E. M. (2016). Risk factors for childhood obesity in the first 1,000 days: A systematic review. *American Journal of Preventative Medicine, 50*(6), 761–779.

World Health Organization. (2016). Childhood overweight and obesity. Retrieved from *www.who.int/end-childhood-obesity/facts/en*.

Zinkel, S. R., Berkowitz, R. I., Stunkard, A. J., Stallings, V. A., Faith, M., Thomas, D., et al. (2016). High energy expenditure is not protective against increased adiposity in children. *Pediatric Obesity, 11*(6), 528–534.

CHAPTER 38

Prevention of Obesity in Youth

Findings from Controlled Trials

Hannah G. Lawman
Alexis C. Wojtanowski
Gary D. Foster

The upward trend in obesity prevalence in U.S. youth (ages 2–19 years) has plateaued during the last decade. However, the prevalence remains high at 17.0% as of 2011–2014, and trends vary by age group (Ogden et al., 2016). As seen in Figure 38.1, from 1988–1994 to 2011–2014 the prevalence of obesity increased and then declined in early childhood (ages 2–5 years) to 9.4%, increased then remained stable in ages 6–11 years at 17.4%, and increased in 12- to 19-year-olds to 20.6% (Ogden et al., 2016). Globally, childhood obesity rates are rising, particularly in developing countries (Malik, Willett, & Hu, 2013). Childhood obesity has significant negative impacts on physical and psychological health (Pulgarón, 2013).

Given the tracking of childhood obesity to adult obesity (Singh, Mulder, Twisk, Van Mechelen, & Chinapaw, 2008) and the modest long-term success of behavioral treatments for obesity (Wadden, Webb, Moran, & Bailer, 2012), significant attention has been directed toward the prevention of obesity in youth. The treatment of childhood obesity has largely been addressed in clinical settings, whether through behavioral (Balantekin, Wilfley, & Epstein, Chapter 39, this volume), pharmacological (Berkowitz & Chao, Chapter 40, this volume), or surgical approaches (Beamish & Inge, Chapter 41, this volume). This chapter focuses on studies that targeted the prevention of childhood obesity in community settings (e.g., child care, schools, and community centers) with a focus on randomized controlled trials (RCTs). This is a narrative review, since comprehensive or systematic reviews of the literature on the prevention of childhood obesity already exist (Wang et al., 2013). All studies reviewed in the current chapter reported at least one relative-weight measure such as obesity prevalence, remission or incidence of obesity, body mass index (BMI), waist circumference, percent body fat, or BMI z-score. Studies that included only health behavior outcomes (e.g., dietary intake, physical activity) or obesity-related clinical outcomes (e.g., blood pressure) but not weight outcomes were not reviewed, in order to narrow the focus to interventions that directly affect obesity. In some cases, novel trials that were quasi-controlled are included. The chapter is organized around three age groups: early childhood (birth–5 years), childhood (ages 6–12 years), and adolescence (ages 13–17 years).

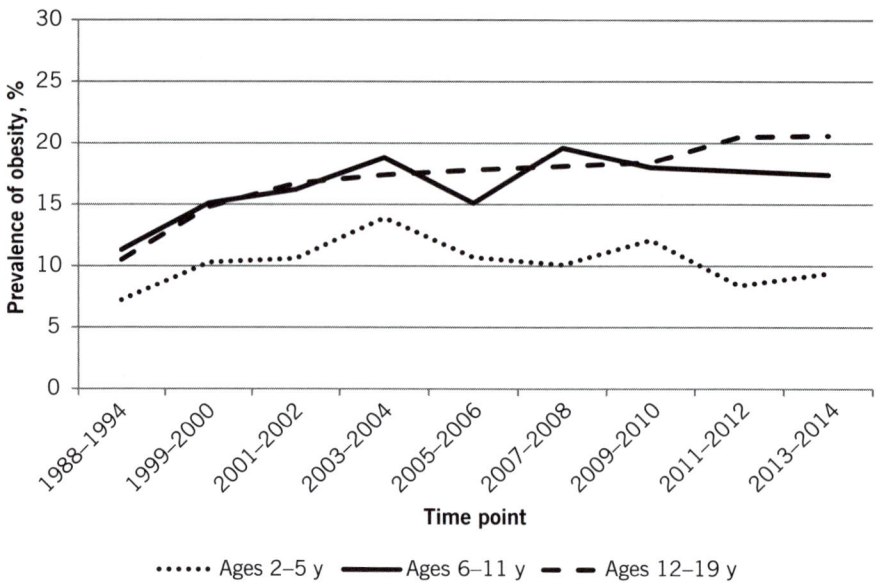

FIGURE 38.1. Trends in obesity prevalence among children and adolescents in the United States, 1988–1994 through 2013–2014. Based on data from Ogden et al. (2016).

Obesity Prevention Trials in Preschool-Age Children (Birth–5 Years)

Community-based obesity prevention programs in preschool-age children have predominantly focused on the early childhood education and child care settings. These interventions can be grouped into two main types: interventions that specifically target weight-related behaviors (e.g., a focused nutrition and physical activity intervention at child care centers) and interventions that promote early childhood education in general, without a specialized emphasis on eating and activity (e.g., Head Start).

Targeted Interventions

Studies that have focused specifically on obesity-related behaviors have used a variety of techniques to improve nutrition and physical activity within child care settings. The Hip-Hop to Health Jr. efficacy trial used teacher training with weekly supervision meetings, nutrition education puppet shows, and songs with exercise routines. The study also included culturally relevant foods, music, and recipes (Fitzgibbon et al., 2005). Approximately 400 predominantly black preschoolers (ages 3–5 years) from 12 Head Start programs in Chicago participated in the RCT. Six of the preschools were randomized to the weight control intervention and six to a general health education control group. The preschoolers in the weight control group received Hip-Hop to Health Jr., a 14-week intervention, and engaged in 40-minute lessons three times per week that consisted of 20 minutes focused on healthy eating and 20 minutes of physical activity. The lessons were delivered by highly trained visiting educators. Parents in those schools were sent weekly newsletters with content that mirrored that week's classroom lessons and a homework assignment that helped parents with behavioral methods (e.g., self-monitoring, problem solving).

Those in the general health education control group also had 14 weeks of programming, but there was only one 20-minute lesson per week, and the topics were focused on a variety of health concepts (e.g., dental health, seat belt safety, how 911 works). Two-year follow-up results of this efficacy trial showed significantly smaller increases in BMI and BMI z-score in the intervention group compared to the control group (0.54 vs. 1.08 kg/m², respectively; Fitzgibbon et al., 2005). When this successful trial was adapted to an effectiveness RCT and implemented with school teachers in 18 Chicago Head Start preschools (N = 618 children, 94% black), there was no difference between intervention and control groups in BMI and BMI z-score at 14 weeks (Fitzgibbon et al., 2011). Another translation of Hip-Hop to Health Jr. with 331 Latino children in 12 preschools, also in Chicago, similarly showed no changes in BMI or BMI z-score at 2-year follow-up (Fitzgibbon et al., 2006).

The TigerKids RCT enrolled over 2,000 5- to 6-year-old children from 64 kindergarten classes in four regions of Germany (Bayer et al., 2009). The kindergartens were randomized in a 2:1 ratio to intervention or assessment-only control. The children in 42 kindergartens (2,089 children) received TigerKids. The 1-year intervention included informational modules with songs, increased fruits and vegetables throughout the day, encouragement to drink water instead of sugar-sweetened beverages (SSBs), and newsletters and a website to provide teachers and families with additional information. Twenty-two kindergartens (1,125 children) were assessment-only controls. One cluster of 1,318 children was assessed after approximately 6 months, and a second cluster of 1,340 students was assessed after approximately 18 months. Neither cluster showed significant differences in the prevalence of overweight and obesity between the intervention and control groups.

More recent trials have also not found effects on BMI. The CHILE (Child Health Initiative for Lifelong Eating and Exercise) RCT in New Mexico enrolled 1,898 children in 16 Head Start programs. Eight Head Start programs received a 2-year multifaceted lifestyle intervention that included individual, social, community, and policy targets (Davis et al., 2016). Components included curriculum for kids; quarterly professional development training with teachers and food service staff; policy changes to food preparation techniques; family engagement; and partnerships with local health care providers and a local grocery store to emphasize healthy eating and physical activity, while also increasing access to healthy foods and recipes while shopping. The other eight Head Start programs were assessment-only controls. After 2 years, there were no significant differences in BMI z-score between the intervention and control group. One RCT in Switzerland randomized 40 preschool classes in 30 schools (N = 652 children) in a one-to-one ratio to a multidimensional intervention or assessment-only control. The culturally tailored intervention included a physical activity classroom program; a curriculum on nutrition, screen time, and sleep; and class environment changes that promoted physical activity, such as equipment and games (e.g., climbing walls, hammocks, balls, stilts, a "movement corner"). There was no difference between intervention and control groups on BMI, but there were small differences between groups in percentage body fat (−1.1%) and waist circumference (−1.0 cm) (Puder et al., 2011).

In summary, RCTs that have evaluated specifically targeted physical activity and healthy eating changes in child care centers have shown very little effect on weight-based outcomes. Systematic reviews of traditional obesity prevention RCTs in child care settings (Wang et al., 2013) and RCTs with preschool-age children across settings (Ling, Robbins, & Wen, 2016; Monasta et al., 2011) reveal a similar lack of effects.

General Early-Childhood Education

In addition to targeted interventions that occur in child care settings, there has been a parallel focus on how general early-childhood education itself could impact obesity without any supplemental or specific nutrition and physical activity programming. Such an approach is appealing because of its easier scalability (no special training, use of existing staff and curriculum, etc.). Head Start participation is a popular example, but there are no RCTs that examine the effect of Head Start on weight (U.S. Department of Health and Human Services, Administration for Children and Families, 2010). There are two small-scale RCTs that investigated the effect of high-intensity (e.g., 2 years with daily interactive education, weekly 90-minute home visits, teachers with master's degrees) early-childhood education programs: the Perry Preschool Program (Muennig, Schweinhart, Montie, & Neidell, 2009) and the Carolina Abecedarian Project (Campbell et al., 2014). Although these trials provided long-term follow-ups (37 years and ~30 years, respectively), their small sample sizes ($N = 66–103$), multiple hypothesis testing, and differential attrition greatly limit their utility in determining effectiveness. Neither program showed a benefit of general early-childhood education on obesity prevalence or BMI, despite intensive intervention. This limited literature suggests that early childhood education programs do not impact childhood obesity.

Taken together, these studies suggest that community-based obesity prevention programs in early childhood do not affect weight outcomes. Where effects have been found in efficacy trials (Fitzgibbon et al., 2005), they have not translated to effectiveness trials (Fitzgibbon et al., 2011), or effects were so small that their clinical impact is questionable (Puder et al., 2011). Early childhood programs may have benefits on outcomes that are not weight-based (e.g., health behaviors, academic outcomes), but any claims about obesity prevention are without empirical support.

Obesity Prevention Trials in Childhood (6–12 Years)

As the social–ecological model in Figure 38.2 depicts, food and activity decisions are influenced by many multilevel factors. Once children reach school age, their environments broaden. They are learning, eating, and playing in many more places, including schools, summer camps, community centers, local businesses, and in the family home (U.S. Department of Health and Human Services & U.S. Department of Agriculture, 2015).

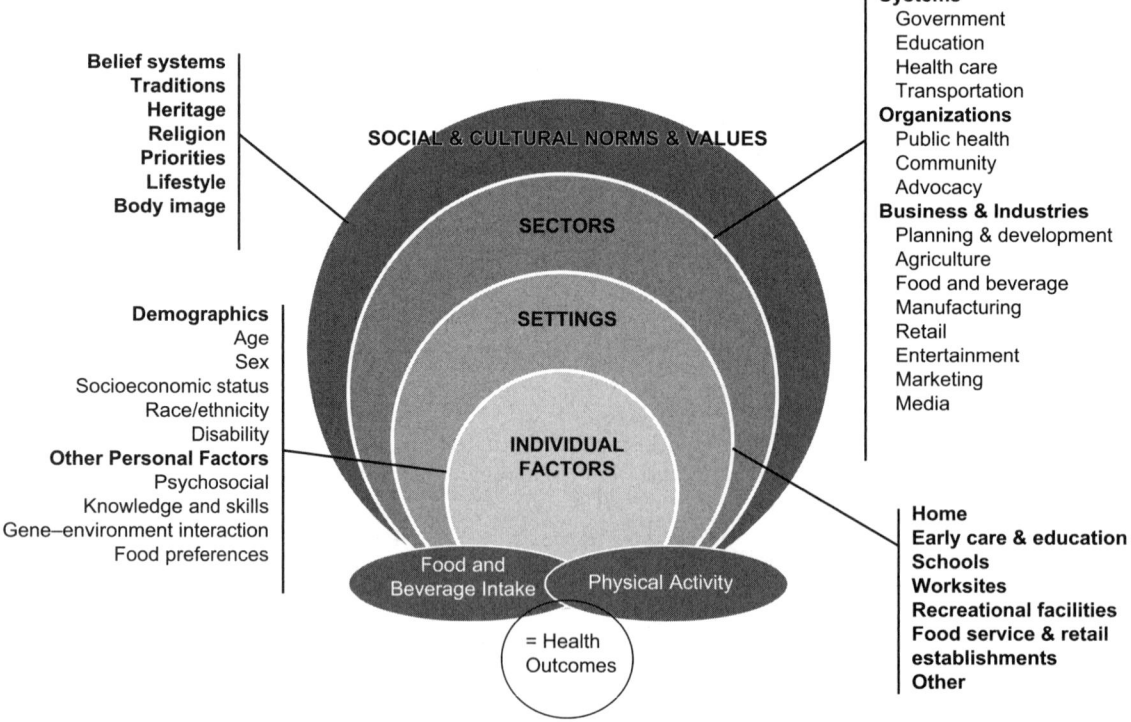

FIGURE 38.2. A social–ecological model for food and physical activity decisions. Based on Figure 3-1 from the U.S. Department of Health and Human Services and U.S. Department of Agriculture (2015).

School-Based Obesity Prevention Interventions

As Table 38.1 demonstrates, the majority of research to date has focused on schools, although obesity prevention interventions have been evaluated across many settings. Given the amount of time that children spend in schools, it seems intuitive that childhood obesity prevention programs would focus on the school environment as an important lever in altering eating and activity habits. Meta-analytic studies of school-based RCTs have shown inconsistent effects on weight (Brown & Summerbell, 2009; Cook-Cottone,

TABLE 38.1. Comparative Effectiveness of Childhood Obesity Prevention Interventions across Settings

Setting	Intervention	Conclusion	SOE
School	Diet	Benefit	Moderate
	Physical activity	Benefit	Moderate
	Combination	No conclusion, inconsistent results	Insufficient
School–home	Diet	Not enough evidence to reach conclusion	Insufficient
	Physical activity	Benefit	High
	Combination	Benefit	Moderate
School–home–community	Physical activity	Not enough evidence to reach conclusion	Insufficient
	Combination	Benefit	High
School–community	Diet	Not enough evidence to reach conclusion	Insufficient
	Physical activity	Not enough evidence to reach conclusion	Insufficient
	Combination	Benefit	Moderate
School–CHI	Physical activity	No conclusion, inconsistent results	Insufficient
	Combination	No conclusion, inconsistent results	Insufficient
School–home–CHI	Combination	Not enough evidence to reach conclusion	Insufficient
Home	Diet	Not enough evidence to reach conclusion	Insufficient
	Combination	No benefit	Low
Home–school–community	Combination	Not enough evidence to reach conclusion	Insufficient
Home–PC–CHI	Combination	Not enough evidence to reach conclusion	Insufficient
PC	Combination	Not enough evidence to reach conclusion	Insufficient
CC	Combination	No benefit	Low
	Physical activity	Not enough evidence to reach conclusion	Insufficient
Community	Physical activity	Not enough evidence to reach conclusion	Insufficient
Community–school	Combination	Benefit	Moderate
Community–school–home	Combination	Not enough evidence to reach conclusion	Insufficient
Community–home	Combination	No conclusion, high risk of bias studies	Insufficient
Community–home–PC–CC	Combination	Not enough evidence to reach conclusion	Insufficient

Note. Combination, combination of diet and physical activity intervention; CHI, consumer health information; CC, child care; PC, primary care; SOE, strength of evidence. Reprinted from Wang et al. (2013). Reprinted by permission.

Feeley, & Baran, 2009; Gonzalez-Suarez, Worley, Grimmer-Somers, & Dones, 2009; Katz, O'Connell, Njike, Yeh, & Nawaz, 2008; Sobol-Goldberg, Rabinowitz, & Gross, 2013; Wang et al., 2013). To illustrate the range of school-based studies, three traditional, comprehensive, large-scale school-based RCTs that were not found effective are described (Bright Start, CATCH, and HEALTHY), as well as two that did show positive effects (MATCH; Lazorick, Fang, & Crawford, 2016; Cao, Wang, & Chen, 2015).

The Bright Start study was an RCT that enrolled more than 400 American Indian kindergarten children from 14 schools on the Pine Ridge Reservation in South Dakota (Story et al., 2012). The schools were randomized to the Bright Start intervention or assessment-only controls. The intervention started in kindergarten and lasted through the end of first grade. Bright Start included activities focused on physical activity, healthy eating, and family engagement. The physical activity component aimed to increase physical activity to at least 60 minutes of moderate-to-vigorous physical activity (MVPA) per day, and consisted of nature walks, in-class "action breaks," and active recess, incorporating American Indian music and Lakota words throughout. The healthy eating component focused on increasing fruits and vegetables and decreasing SSBs and high-fat foods. This component was implemented primarily through the school cafeteria offerings and serving style (e.g., offer 1% milk before 2% milk) and the replacement of classroom snack rewards with nonfood rewards. Families were engaged through three family nights that provided behavioral messages regarding physical activity, healthy eating, and limiting screen time. The primary outcomes were BMI, percentage of body fat, and prevalence of overweight and obesity. At the end of first grade, there were no significant differences between the intervention and control students in BMI or percentage body fat. However, Bright Start did significantly decrease the incidence of overweight in the intervention group compared to the control group (13.4 vs. 24.8%), though there was not a significant change in the corresponding prevalence of obesity.

In the early 1990s, the CATCH (Child and Adolescent Trial for Cardiovascular Health) RCT enrolled 5,106 third through fifth graders (69.0% white) in 96 schools across the United Schools (Luepker et al., 1996). The 56 schools randomized to the intervention group received CATCH, a comprehensive 3-year program focused on both the school and family environments. The school-based components focused on all parts of the day. For food service, the total fat content of meals was lowered to 30%, saturated fat content to 10%, and sodium to 600–1,000 mg, while maintaining participation in school meal programs and retaining taste. For physical education (PE) classes, PE specialists were trained in ways to increase the amount of enjoyable MVPA to 40% of the class. For classroom curricula, over 50 lessons were dedicated to skill development around eating behaviors and physical activity habits. The family-based component consisted of 19 activity packets (that could not be completed without adult participation) sent home to complement the classroom lessons and "family fun nights" at the school to highlight healthy snacks, healthy recipes, and fun games. The 40 control schools were assessment-only and received the usual health lessons, PE classes, and food service. Despite the successful implementation of CATCH (intervention schools increased the MVPA in PE classes and decreased the energy intake from fat in school lunches compared to control schools), the changes in food intake and physical activity were modest, and there were no significant differences in weight, BMI, or skinfolds between the intervention and control students.

From 2006 to 2009, the HEALTHY study enrolled more than 4,600 sixth graders (54.2% Hispanic, 18.0% black) from 42 schools across the United States (HEALTHY Study Group, 2010). The 21 intervention schools received a 3-year multicomponent intervention, HEALTHY (*www.healthystudy.org*), which focused on nutrition, physical activity, behavioral knowledge and skills, and communications and social marketing. The nutrition component focused on the quantity and quality of the food served throughout the school, including in the cafeteria, vending machines, classroom celebrations, and school stores. This component also promoted single-serving-size packages; water instead of SSBs; and increased servings of fruits, vegetables, and legumes. The physical activity intervention focused on increasing the amount of MVPA time in PE classes by training the teachers in class management and motivation techniques and outlining sports-based units. The behavior intervention used brief classroom activities (FLASH: fun learning activities for student health) and family outreach to increase self-awareness, knowledge, and behavioral skills such as goal-setting and self-monitoring. Lastly, the communication strategy consisted of schoolwide campaigns featuring student-generated media that reflected the themes of choice, strength, and balance. These media prominently featured students from the participating schools. The other 21 schools served as assessment-only controls.

At the end of the 3 years, there was a decrease in the primary outcome, the combined prevalence of overweight and obesity, in both the intervention and control groups. However, there was no difference between groups. There were significantly greater reductions in the weight-related secondary outcomes of BMI z-score and percentage of students with waist circumference in the 90th percentile or higher, and a nearly significant greater reduction in prevalence of obesity ($p = .05$) in intervention students when compared to controls. In a preplanned subgroup analysis of students who started out the study as overweight/obese (49.5% of total sample), those in intervention schools had significantly greater decreases in the prevalence of overweight and obesity compared to the control schools (16.5 vs. 15.9%).

More consistently positive results come from a smaller and quasi-experimental study of the MATCH (Motivating Adolescents with Technology to Choose Health) intervention from 2009 (Lazorick, Fang, & Crawford, 2016). The study showed significant differences in the weight trajectories of intervention and control students 4 years after the short-term intervention. The 14-week MATCH intervention was provided to a convenience sample of 189 seventh-grade students (63% black) in two schools. The intervention consisted of 26 teacher-delivered lessons focused on making healthy eating and physical activity choices, supplemented by the use of technology (e.g., web-based tools to plot BMI and dietary intake) and small, nonfood incentives (e.g., water bottles, pens, pedometers). As seen in Figure 38.3, compared to 173 students in one assessment-only control school, the intervention group had significantly smaller increases in BMI (2.66 vs. 4.03 kg/m^2), greater decreases in BMI z-score (–0.15 vs. 0.04 kg/m^2), lower incidence of obesity (13 vs. 39%), and greater remission of overweight to healthy weight (40 vs. 26%) 4 years postintervention.

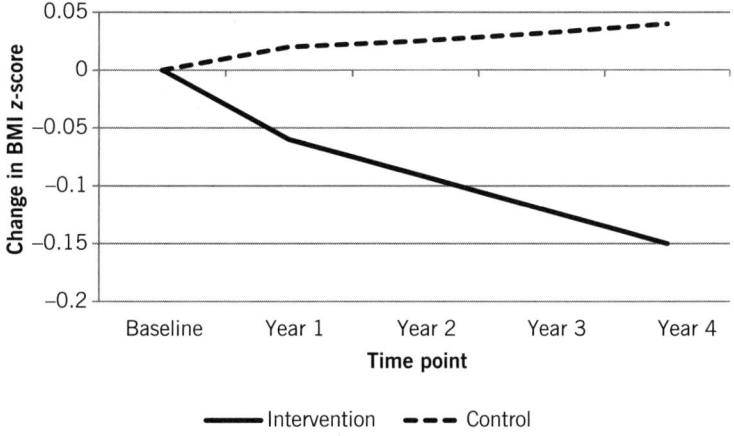

FIGURE 38.3. Change at 4-year follow-up in BMI z-score, MATCH intervention and control groups. Based on data from Lazorick, Fang, and Crawford (2016) and Lazorick, Fang, Hardison, and Crawford (2015).

In 2015, Cao, Wang, and Chen published the results of an RCT that evaluated a family–individual–school-based (FIS) intervention that focused on connecting the family and school environments. The study enrolled 2,446 first-grade students from 14 primary schools in Shanghai, China. Seven schools were randomized to receive a 3-year intervention that encouraged health education, dietary intervention, and exercise intervention in both the school and family environments. The health education component relied on obesity-related health information delivered through the school newspaper, class meetings, brochures, and teacher-led seminars attended by the parents and students. The school reduced the fat content of their food and increased the availability of fruits and vegetables as part of the dietary intervention. Additionally, the teachers advised students on eating rates and snacking, and parents were sent materials on healthy eating habits for children. The exercise component focused on opportunities for activity at school (e.g., 20-meter music shuttle runs two to three times per week and at least 1 hour of physical activity time each school day) and at home (e.g., sent a jump rope home with each child). The other seven schools were assessment-only controls. After 3 years, the students in the intervention schools had significantly greater reductions in the prevalence of overweight and obesity, lower odds of developing overweight or obesity, and greater decreases in BMI z-score compared to the control group.

Multiple review articles (Sobol-Goldberg et al., 2013; Wang et al., 2013; Katz et al., 2008) have attempted to look across studies to determine which characteristics make some large school-based interventions successful whereas others have no effect. However, the conclusions offered by these reviews are mixed. Some reviewers (Sobol-Goldberg et al., 2013; Wang et al., 2013) have suggested that greater efficacy was associated with interventions that focused on both nutrition and physical activity and lasted at least 1 year. In addition, interventions that incorporated hands-on activities and printed materials throughout the school day—including in classroom lessons, the school cafeteria, and PE classes—appear to be more successful (Katz et al., 2008; Wang et al., 2013). Others have suggested the importance of parental support (Sobol-Goldberg et al., 2013; Katz et al., 2008). There are, however, significant exceptions to these generalizations, as the large, well-controlled studies described above demonstrate. Thus, it remains unclear why some complex, schoolwide, long-term interventions fail and simpler, shorter-term interventions succeed (Brown & Summerbell, 2009). It is important to note that even in studies with effects, the effect size is modest (effect size = 0.076; Sobol-Goldberg et al., 2013; Wang et al., 2013).

Although it is not clear how to move forward with comprehensive school-based interventions focused on nutrition and physical activity, some smaller school-based studies have shown promising results by focusing on simple interventions. For example, an RCT by Robinson (1999) enrolled 192 third and fourth graders from two San Jose, California elementary schools and found that an 18 lesson, 6-month sedentary behavior intervention did affect obesity. The one school randomized to the intervention implemented a program specifically targeting reducing television viewing, video game use, and videotape use, without promoting active behaviors as replacements. The regular classroom teachers incorporated the 30- to 50-minute lessons into the standard curriculum and taught the children to self-monitor their screen time, challenged them to a "television turnoff," and had them set weekly screen time goals. Additionally, the parents were provided with an electronic television time manager and newsletters that suggested strategies for limiting television, videotape, and video game use for the entire family. There were no intervention components focused on changing eating or physical activity. The other school was an assessment-only control.

Postintervention, intervention students experienced significantly greater reductions in BMI, skinfold thickness, waist circumference, and waist-to-hip ratio compared to controls. Although this approach has increasing relevance due to the high levels of screen time youth access (Henry J. Kaiser Family Foundation, 2010), it also has more challenges given the greater use of energy-saving devices among children since 1999. Despite this challenge, creatively addressing screen time may be an effective approach to obesity prevention in youth (Liao, Liao, Durand, & Dunton, 2014). This approach has the potential to influence both sides of the energy balance equation through increased energy expenditure and decreased energy intake from reduced exposure to food advertising and eating in front of the television, via stimulus control principles.

In another "simple" intervention, James, Thomas, Cavan, and Keer (2004) focused on reducing the consumption of carbonated ("fizzy") drinks. Six hundred sixty-four middle high school students (ages 7 to 11 years) from six primary schools in southwest England formed 29 clusters that were randomized to intervention or control. Randomization was clustered at the class level and blinded to school or grade. Fifteen clusters received four 60-minute sessions over 1 school year focused on the association between sugar consumption and health (overall and dental), including a music challenge to create a song or rap with a healthy message. Fourteen clusters were assessment-only control. At 12 months, there were no significant differences between groups in BMI or BMI z-score. However, there was a reduction in the number of students with overweight and obesity in the intervention schools compared to an increase in the control schools.

Similarly, in a quasi-experimental study, Schwartz, Leardo, Aneja, and Elbel (2016) focused on the impact of installing water jets (large clear water jugs with chilled water and a push lever for quick dispensing) in 1,227 New York public elementary and middle schools serving 1,065,562 students. From 2008–2009 to 2012–2013, ~40% of the schools received a water jet whereas 60% of schools did not. The water jugs were significantly associated with a reduction in BMI and a reduced likelihood of being overweight. These simple approaches are in contrast to the traditional comprehensive diet and physical activity interventions, but may produce modest improvements in weight.

Other Community-Based Obesity Prevention Interventions

Researchers are beginning to examine other community-based settings that children frequent, outside of schools, as venues for obesity prevention and treatment interventions. Some representative studies from other possible settings, including corner stores, summer day camps, YMCAs, and neighborhoodwide initiatives, are reviewed.

In urban areas, many schools are located in the middle of the neighborhoods. Many students walk to school, providing them with multiple opportunities to purchase snacks and beverages from corner stores on their way. Corner stores are generally defined as stores with less than 10 employees and less than 1,000 feet of floor space. They primarily sell cigarettes, prepackaged foods, and SSBs that are high in energy and low in nutritive value. A 2012 systematic review (Gittelsohn, Rowan, & Gadhoke, 2012) identified 16 trials of small-store interventions located primarily in minority and low-income neighborhoods. The interventions most often focused on increasing the availability of healthier food (e.g., fruits and vegetables), increasing point-of-purchase promotions (e.g., shelf labels and posters), and community engagement. However, most of these studies (15 out of 16) only sampled adults and all (16 out of 16) used self-report surveys instead of direct observations.

The Snackin' Fresh study was the first and, to date, only RCT of a corner store intervention that used direct observation of purchases and focused on purchases by children (Lent et al., 2014). From 2008 to 2010, 10 schools and their nearby corner stores (N = 24) were randomly assigned to the Snackin' Fresh intervention or an assessment-only control. Nearly 800 fourth, fifth, and sixth graders (54% black, 22.9% Hispanic) were followed for 2 years. Snackin' Fresh was implemented in both schools and corner stores. The school-based intervention consisted of seven 45-minute classroom-based education lessons delivered by a Snackin' Fresh teacher. The lessons focused on various skills, including identifying healthier choices in the corner store, self-monitoring consumption, goal setting, and label reading. The corner store intervention asked owners to increase the availability and promotion of healthier items (e.g., grouping single-serving-size packages together with increased signage), while also providing fruit salads in refrigerated barrels as well as bottled water, all of which were Snackin' Fresh branded. The intervention also included a branded social marketing campaign that included banners, small giveaways, a website, comic book, and video.

Throughout the 2 years, research staff approached students outside of the 24 corner stores and collected 2,215 anonymous "intercepts," or short interviews, in which they asked the student to show them what they had purchased that day. The staff recorded each item's name, size, and the total amount of money spent, which were later connected to a nutrition database to calculate the nutritional content per intercept. Each intercept was equal to one corner store visit by one student, who may have had more than one item. At baseline, students spent an average of $1.07 for two items, most often chips, candy, and SSBs, that added up to ~350 calories per purchase (Borradaile et al., 2009). As Figure 38.4 illustrates, Snackin' Fresh did not result in significant changes in weight (BMI, BMI percentile, or BMI z-score) or energy content per corner store purchase, and there were no differences between control and intervention students at year 1 or year 2 (Lent et al., 2014).

Although not an RCT, Ontario, Canada's single-center, single-cohort (36 families) feasibility trial of the Children's Health and Activity Modification Program (CHAMP) highlights the potential of summer day camp as a place for intervention (Burke et al., 2015). CHAMP was a multicomponent, 4-week, family-based intervention for children with obesity delivered by trained counselors at community facilities (e.g., YMCA, Western University's Canadian Centre for Activity and Aging). Children attended a summer day camp on weekdays and had daily group-based physical activity, behavioral modification counseling, and dietary counseling. The family members (parents and/or guardians only) attended weekly group-based educational sessions on Saturdays. After the 1-month intervention, 2-hour booster sessions were offered every other month for 1 year. The children's BMI z-score decreased significantly postintervention, and the changes were sustained at the 6-month follow-up. This trial highlights that summer camps, with the benefits of full-day attendance, group interaction and support, and leadership opportunities, are a potentially effective setting for childhood obesity interventions. However, the lack of a control group limits interpretation.

Another approach, more based on treatment than prevention, is to move traditional clinic-based obesity treatment to community centers. The 16-week JOIN for ME intervention, developed and evaluated in a single-arm 18-month study (Foster et al., 2012), was delivered to the parents and children together through weekly group-based sessions at YMCAs. The intervention focused on be-

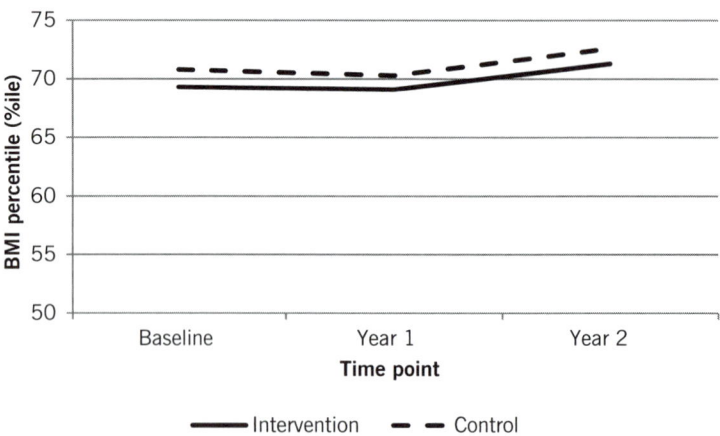

FIGURE 38.4. Change in BMI percentile, Snackin' Fresh intervention and control group. Based on data from Lent et al. (2014).

havioral strategies for weight management that included goal setting, self-monitoring, calorie targets, reducing screen time, and increasing physical activity. In a small RCT (Trost, Sundal Foster, Lent, & Vojta, 2014), 41 child–parent dyads in the control group received the JOIN for ME program alone, whereas 34 child–parent dyads in the intervention group attended the JOIN for ME program and also received an active gaming (e.g., Xbox Kinect) device with games. Control participants received the Kinect device after the intervention period. As illustrated by Figure 38.5, after 4 months, both the intervention and control groups had significant reductions in relative weight. However, the intervention group achieved twice the reduction in percentage overweight and BMI z-score as the control group. The intervention group also had significantly greater increases in MVPA than did controls.

Some of the most ambitious interventions have chosen to focus on multiple settings within the community, enacting changes in policies, systems, the built environment, and institutions. There have not been any RCTs in this area, but a few natural experiments raise interesting possibilities. One of the first natural experiments to be evaluated was in Somerville, Massachusetts. Shape Up Somerville was a 2-year, nonrandomized, controlled trial in 2003–2005 that aimed to improve energy balance by increasing physical activity and the availability of healthy foods (Economos et al., 2013). For the purpose of evaluation, Somerville (the intervention community) was paired with two sociodemographically matched control communities. In all, 30 public schools (10 intervention, 20 control) and 1,721 first-, second-, and third-grade children participated.

Shape Up Somerville engaged many community groups (e.g., parents, teachers, city departments, restaurants, and the media) and was designed to influence every part of an early elementary school student's day, from the school cafeteria to classroom lessons and after-school clubs. Changes in food service included highlighting a different fruit or vegetable each month, reducing the availability of ice cream, displaying nutrition information, and developing vegetarian recipes. In the classroom, teachers (including art and PE teachers) delivered health curriculum through the HEAT (Healthy Eating and Active Time) Club with lessons on healthy snacking, increasing activity, decreasing screen time, and increasing the consumption of healthy foods. Students could continue the HEAT Club activities through a 26-lesson after-school program that incorporated cooking, varied sports (from yoga to soccer), and field trips to local farms. Outside of the school environment, restaurants could earn "Shape Up Approved" status

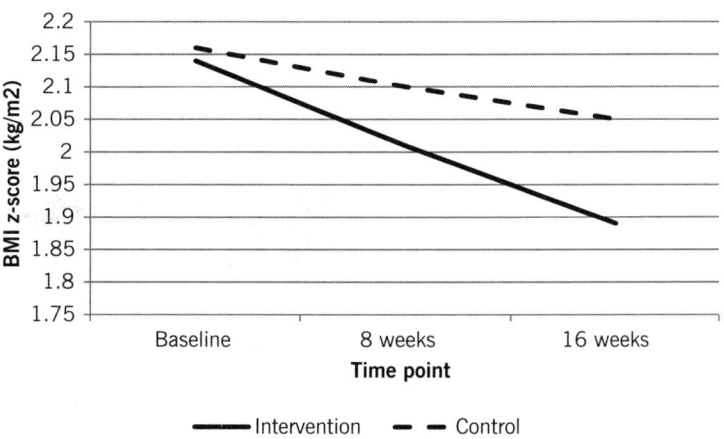

FIGURE 38.5. Change in BMI z-score, JOIN for ME intervention and control group. Based on data from Trost, Sundal, Foster, Lent, and Vojta (2014).

if they offered healthier items in portion-controlled sizes, and a community walking committee worked on creating "Safe Routes to School" maps, fixed up bike racks, and repainted crosswalks.

After 2 years, Somerville children had significantly greater decreases in BMI z-score (0.06 kg/m^2), reductions in the prevalence of overweight/obesity, and increases in the remission of obesity compared to controls. In 2011, without external funding or design help from researchers, community leaders (business leaders, faith communities, schools, government officials, and local health professionals) from Mebane, North Carolina started the Mebane on the Move intervention. Modeled after Shape Up Somerville, Mebane on the Move aimed to increase physical activity and decrease obesity in the resident children (Benjamin Neelon et al., 2015). The intervention focused exclusively on physical activity and promoted increased movement through multiple channels, including walking and running clubs at the elementary schools and in the community; free community exercise programs at the recreation center; portable play equipment sent to low-income families through home-delivery food-assistance programs; and walking paths (sidewalks, crosswalks, and walking trails with motivational signage) installed throughout town. A similar community 96 miles from Mebane was recruited to serve as a comparison. Although the intervention was provided to all residents, physical activity and weight data were collected from 64 Mebane children (ages 5–11 years, 76.6% white) and 40 children (ages 5 to 11 years, 85.0% white) from the comparison town. At the 1-year follow-up, Mebane children had greater increase in MVPA (1.3 minutes/hour) and had significantly decreased their BMI z-score (0.5 kg/m^2) compared to control children.

Although more recent research on school-based obesity prevention programs have sometimes shown small positive effects on obesity (Lazorick et al., 2016; James et al., 2004; Scwhartz et al., 2016), traditional, school-based, randomized-controlled obesity prevention trials have generally not shown effects on weight-based outcomes. Communitywide interventions may hold promise, but there is no evidence for many broadly promoted programs with the goal of obesity prevention. Studies like JOIN for ME (Trost et al., 2014), CHAMP (Burke et al., 2015), and Shape Up Somerville (Economos et al., 2013) show potential for scalability due to their community-based settings, reliance on trained community staff, and promising benefits on weight-related outcomes. However, there is insufficient evidence to draw conclusions on community-based programs outside of schools (Bleich, Segal, Wu, Wilson, & Wang, 2013). It is likely that in community-based settings, few would object to efforts to improve the adoption of healthy behaviors such as increased physical activity, increased water consumption, and increased consumption of fruits and vegetables, even in the known absence of benefits to obesity prevention. However, this would require a shift in commonly used language and rationale, and it should be noted that effect sizes for health behavior interventions are also small (Cushing, Brannon, Suorsa, & Wilson, 2014).

Obesity Prevention Trials in Adolescence (13–17 Years)

Few community-based studies have been conducted with adolescents, and almost all have been conducted in school settings. One noteworthy RCT is the COPE Healthy Lifestyle TEENS Program (COPE: Creating Opportunities for Personal Empowerment; TEEN: Thinking, Emotions, Exercise, Nutrition; Melnyk et al., 2013). This intervention (N = 11 high schools, N = 779 students, ages 14–16 years) consisted of a 15-week, 15-session health education curriculum that emphasized cognitive-behavioral skill building and nutrition and physical activity information, taught by school staff. The control group received an attention control Healthy Teens program that focused on safety and common health topics such as road safety, dental care, skin care, and immunizations. At postintervention, small but significantly greater improvements were seen in BMI (COPE Healthy Lifestyles TEENS = 24.57 kg/m^2, Healthy Teens = 24.77 kg/m^2) as well as other outcomes (i.e., physical activity, social skills, academic performance in the health course, and alcohol use) in the intervention compared to control group. As seen in Figure 38.6, at 6 months postintervention, significant between-group improvements were sustained in BMI (COPE Healthy Lifestyles TEENS = 24.72 kg/m², Healthy Teens = 25.05 kg/m²) and overweight prevalence in intervention (44% at baseline; 41% at 6-month follow-up) compared to control group participants (41% at baseline; 43% at follow-up). These findings are in contrast to other traditional, large-scale obesity prevention trials in adolescents. Other school-based RCTs, including the New Moves trial (N = 12 schools), the Trial of Activity in Adolescent Girls (TAAG; N = 36 schools), and the Nutrition and Enjoyable Activity for Teen Girls trial (NEAT; N = 12 schools) have not found significant improvements in BMI or percent body fat compared to assessment-only controls (Lubans et al., 2012; Neumark-Sztainer et al., 2010; Webber et al., 2008). The main difference between COPE Healthy Lifestyles TEENS and these trials is that COPE included a novel, broader focus that incorporated social skills and mental health, whereas the other large trials were focused only on obesity prevention.

Another novel, school-based RCT was conducted in France. This trial compared a traditional school-based environmental intervention (i.e., increasing the availability and promotion of healthy foods and physical activity) to reduce overweight and obesity with a different approach that consisted of screening and facilitating access to health care services (PRALIMAP intervention; Bonsergent et al., 2013). The screening and care strategy included school nurses referring students who were overweight/obese to local community-based networks of overweight and obesity management specialists (physicians, dietitians, psychologists, and sports educators). A third education approach emphasized nutrition and physical activity education curriculum. Each of the 24 schools was randomized to receive or not receive each of the three strategies (i.e., a 2 × 2 × 2 factorial design), and over 3,500 students (grades 10 and 11) were followed for 2 years.

Although the effect sizes were very small (0.11 lower increase in BMI; 0.04 greater decrease in BMI z-score, 1.7% greater decrease in overweight/obesity prevalence than controls), the 12 schools that received the screening and care approach showed a sig-

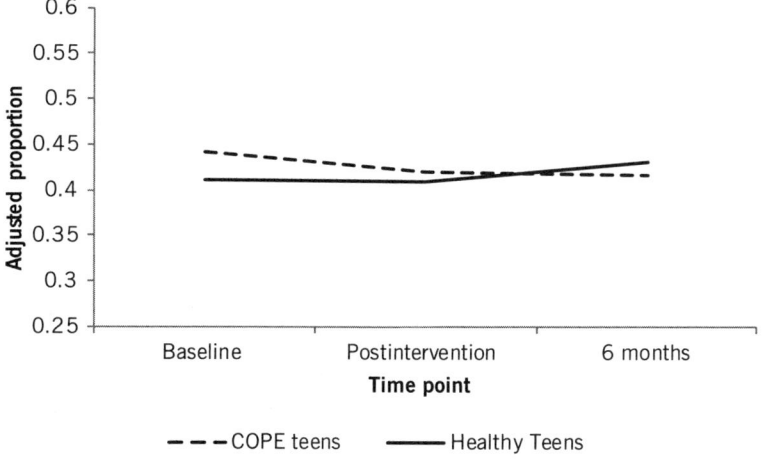

FIGURE 38.6. Percentage of overweight for the COPE and Healthy Teens groups across time. Reprinted from Melnyk, Jacobson, Kelly, Belyea, Shaibi, Small, et al. (2013). Promoting healthy lifestyles in high school adolescents: A randomized controlled trial. *American Journal of Preventive Medicine, 45*(4), 407–415. Copyright © 2013, with permission from Elsevier. Melnyk et al. (2013). Reprinted by permission.

nificantly greater decrease in the prevalence of overweight/obesity (–2.27%) after 2 years compared to those that did not (–0.56%). In this study, and consistent with other traditional school-based obesity prevention programs, the schools that utilized education and environmental approaches were no more effective than schools that received no intervention. This screening and care approach is novel and promising compared to traditional school-based obesity prevention programs aiming to educate students and improve the school environment. However, the integration with health care services may present additional challenges in the United States.

There are few community-based interventions in adolescents outside of school settings. The island of Tonga, with an exceptionally high obesity prevalence, was the setting for a 3-year quasi-experimental study of a community-based health promotion intervention among adolescents (Fotu et al., 2011). The intervention strategies included social marketing campaigns, community capacity building, and grassroots activities to promote healthy eating and physical activity. However, both intervention and control groups had an increased prevalence of adolescent obesity after 3 years, and there were no differences in weight between groups.

National surveillance data on trends in adolescent obesity show a very small but continued increase over the last 20 years (Ogden et al., 2016). School-based obesity prevention programs for adolescents are less common than programs for children ages 6–12 years, but generally show similar null or modest effects. These findings emphasize the need for creative strategies for adolescents. Reviews of studies with adolescents have also concluded that the evidence for school-based obesity prevention programs is weaker for adolescents than for 6- to 12-year-old children, and that they generally have not shown improvements in BMI (Sobol-Goldberg et al., 2013). One review suggests that effectiveness may increase with older adolescents and young adults (i.e., up to 24 years of age; Stice, Shaw, & Marti, 2006); however, not enough community-based trials in younger versus older adolescents have been conducted to assess this possibility.

Summary of the Evidence and Conclusions

Obesity prevention in youth has been targeted to all ages, ranging from before birth (Vinter, Jensen, Ovesen, Beck-Nielsen, & Jørgensen, 2011) to adolescence (Melnyk et al., 2013) across many settings, including primary care, child care, home- and school-based, and community or environmental approaches (Wang et al., 2013). The studies reviewed in this chapter reveal little evidence that childcare-, school-, and community-based obesity prevention programs are effective at changing weight-related outcomes in youth. This conclusion is consistent with several reviews (Bleich et al., 2013; Kropski, Keckley, & Jensen, 2008; Wang et al., 2013), including one that estimated that only 21% of obesity prevention programs resulted in significant positive effects (Stice et al., 2006). The empirical evidence from traditional interventions targeting diet and physical activity for the goal of obesity prevention is scant. It is possible that these strategies are necessary but not sufficient. Promising approaches may include targeting sedentary behavior, water and carbonated beverage consumption, and integrating mental health and specialized health care into interventions, although these approaches require much more extensive empirical validation. While some newer and/or one-component trials suggest improvements to weight using these strategies (e.g., James et al., 2004; Schwartz et al., 2016; Bonsergent et al., 2013; Melnyk et al., 2013), the effect sizes are modest, and additional evidence is needed.

Stice et al. (2006) point out that although modest effects demonstrate the difficulty of changing health behaviors related to obesity, modest effects are also observed with many other public health problems that relate to behavior change. Effect sizes for prevention programs for HIV, eating disorders, substance abuse, and smoking are all similar and modest (r's range from .05 to .12) in comparison to obesity prevention ($r = .04$; Stice et al., 2006). Despite null or inconsistent effects on weight, youth obesity prevention programs may have benefits to health behaviors. Many trials reviewed in this chapter had some positive impact on secondary outcomes (e.g., fruit and vegetable intake, physical activity). However, in the absence of changes to weight, which are relatively easy to measure objectively, health behavior changes are difficult to interpret given their frequently self-reported nature and the fact that they are typically tested in the context of multiple comparisons. It is important to emphasize that, to date, scientific evidence from controlled trials of the effectiveness of school- and community-based programs in youth largely lacks any demonstration of impact on weight outcomes.

References

Bayer, O., von Kries, R., Strauss, A., Mitschek, C., Toschke, A. M., Hose, A., et al. (2009). Short- and mid-term effects of a setting based prevention program to reduce obesity risk factors in children: A cluster-randomized trial. *Clinical Nutrition (Edinburgh, Scotland), 28*(2), 122–128.

Benjamin Neelon, S. E., Namenek Brouwer, R. J., Ostbye, T., Evenson, K. R., Neelon, B., Martinie, A., et al. (2015). A community-based intervention increases physical activity and reduces obesity in school-age children in North Carolina. *Childhood Obesity, 11*(3), 297–303.

Bleich, S. N., Segal, J., Wu, Y., Wilson, R., & Wang, Y. (2013). Systematic review of community-based childhood obesity prevention studies. *Pediatrics, 132*(1), 201.

Bonsergent, E., Agrinier, N., Thilly, N., Tessier, S., Legrand, K., Lecomte, E., et al. (2013). Overweight and obesity prevention for adolescents: A cluster randomized controlled trial in a school setting. *American Journal of Preventive Medicine, 44*(1), 30–39.

Borradaile, K. E., Sherman, S., Vander Veur, S. S., McCoy, T., Sandoval, B., Nachmani, J., et al. (2009). Snacking in children: The role of urban corner stores. *Pediatrics, 124*(5), 1293–1298.

Brown, T., & Summerbell, C. (2009). Systematic review of school-based interventions that focus on changing dietary intake and physical activity levels to prevent childhood obesity: An update to the obesity guidance produced by the National Institute for Health and Clinical Excellence. *Obesity Reviews, 10*(1), 110–141.

Burke, S. M., Shapiro, S., Petrella, R. J., Irwin, J. D., Jackman, M., Pearson, E. S., et al. (2015). Using the RE-AIM framework to evaluate a community-based summer camp for children with obesity: A prospective feasibility study. *BioMed Central Obesity, 2*(21), 1–10.

Campbell, F., Conti, G., Heckman, J. J., Moon, S. H., Pinto, R., Pungello, E., et al. (2014). Early childhood investments substantially boost adult health. *Science, 343*(6178), 1478–1485.

Cao, Z. J., Wang, S. M., & Chen, Y. A. (2015). Randomized trial of multiple interventions for childhood obesity in China. *American Journal of Preventive Medicine, 48*(5), 552–560.

Cook-Cottone, C., Casey, C. M., Feeley, T. H., & Baran, J. (2009). A meta-analytic review of obesity prevention in the schools: 1997–2008. *Psychology in the Schools, 46*(8), 695–719.

Cushing, C. C., Brannon, E. E., Suorsa, K. I., & Wilson, D. K. (2014). Systematic review and meta-analysis of health promotion interventions for children and adolescents using an ecological framework. *Journal of Pediatric Psychology, 39*(8), 949–962.

Davis, S. M., Myers, O. B., Cruz, T. H., Morshed, A. B., Canaca, G. F., Keane, P. C., et al. (2016). CHILE: Outcomes of a group randomized controlled trial of an intervention to prevent obesity in preschool Hispanic and American Indian children. *Preventive Medicine, 89*, 162–168.

Economos, C. D., Hyatt, R. R., Must, A., Goldberg, J. P., Kuder, J., Naumova, E. N., et al. (2013). Shape Up Somerville two-year results: A community-based environment change intervention sustains weight reduction in children. *Preventive Medicine, 57*(4), 322–327.

Fitzgibbon, M. L., Stolley, M. R., Schiffer, L., Braunschweig, C. L., Gomez, S. L., Van Horn, L., et al. (2011). Hip-Hop to Health Jr. obesity prevention effectiveness trial: Post-intervention results. *Obesity (Silver Spring), 19*(5), 994–1003.

Fitzgibbon, M. L., Stolley, M. R., Schiffer, L., Van Horn, L., KauferChristoffel, K., & Dyer, A. (2005). Two-year follow-up results for Hip-Hop to Health Jr.: A randomized controlled trial for overweight prevention in preschool minority children. *Journal of Pediatrics, 146*(5), 618–625.

Fitzgibbon, M. L., Stolley, M. R., Schiffer, L., Van Horn, L., KauferChristoffel, K., & Dyer, A. (2006). Hip-Hop to Health Jr. for Latino preschool children. *Obesity, 14*(9), 1616–1625.

Foster, G. D., Sundal, D., McDermott, C., Jelalian, E., Lent, M. R., & Vojta, D. (2012). Feasibility and preliminary outcomes of a scalable, community-based treatment of childhood obesity. *Pediatrics, 130*(4), 652–659.

Fotu, K. F., Millar, L., Mavoa, H., Kremer, P., Moodie, M., Snowdon, W., et al. (2011). Outcome results for the Ma'alahi Youth Project, a Tongan community-based obesity prevention programme for adolescents. *Obesity Reviews, 12*(Suppl. 2), 41–50.

Gittelsohn, J., Rowan, M., & Gadhoke, P. (2012). Interventions in small food stores to change the food environment, improve diet, and reduce risk of chronic disease. *Preventing Chronic Disease, 9*, E59.

Gonzalez-Suarez, C., Worley, A., Grimmer-Somers, K., & Dones, V. (2009). School-based interventions on childhood obesity: A meta-analysis. *American Journal of Preventive Medicine, 37*(5), 418–427.

HEALTHY Study Group. (2010). A school-based intervention for diabetes risk reduction. *New England Journal of Medicine, 363*(5), 443–453.

Henry J. Kaiser Family Foundation. (2010, January 20). Generation M2: Media in the lives of 8- to

18-year-olds. Retrieved October 13, 2016, from http://kff.org/other/event/generation-m2-media-in-the-lives-of.

James, J., Thomas, P., Cavan, D., & Keer, D. (2004). Preventing childhood obesity by reducing consumption of carbonated drinks: Cluster randomized controlled trial. *British Medical Journal (Clinical Research Edition), 328*(7450), 1237.

Katz, D. L., O'Connell, M., Njike, V. Y., Yeh, M. C., & Nawaz, H. (2008). Strategies for the prevention and control of obesity in the school setting: Systematic review and meta-analysis. *International Journal of Obesity (London), 32*(12), 1780–1789.

Kropski, J. A., Keckley, P. H., & Jensen, G. L. (2008). School-based obesity prevention programs: An evidence-based review. *Obesity, 16*(5), 1009–1018.

Lazorick, S., Fang, X., & Crawford, Y. (2016) The MATCH Program: Long-term obesity prevention through a middle school based intervention. *Childhood Obesity, 12*(2), 103–112.

Lazorick, S., Fang, X., Hardison, G. T., & Crawford, Y. (2015) Improved body mass index measures following a middle school-based obesity intervention: The MATCH Program. *Journal of School Health, 85*(10), 680–687.

Lent, M. R., Vander Veur, S. S., McCoy, T. A., Wojtanowski, A. C., Sandoval, B., Sherman, S., et al. (2014). A randomized controlled study of a healthy corner store initiative on the purchases of urban, low-income youth. *Obesity (Silver Spring), 22*(12), 2494–2500.

Liao, Y., Liao, J., Durand, C. P., & Dunton, G. F. (2014). Which type of sedentary behavior intervention is more effective at reducing body mass index in children?: A meta-analytic review. *Obesity Reviews, 15*(3), 159–168.

Ling, J., Robbins, L. B., & Wen, F. (2016). Interventions to prevent and manage overweight or obesity in preschool children: A systematic review. *International Journal of Nursing Studies, 53*, 270–289.

Lubans, D. R., Morgan, P. J., Okely, A. D., Dewar, D., Collins, C. E., Batterham, M., et al. (2012). Preventing obesity among adolescent girls: One-year outcomes of the nutrition and enjoyable activity for teen girls (NEAT girls) cluster randomized controlled trial. *Archives of Pediatrics and Adolescent Medicine, 166*(9), 821–827.

Luepker, R. V., Perry, C. L., McKinlay, S. M., Nader, P. R., Parcel, G. S., Stone, E. J., et al. (1996). Outcomes of a field trial to improve children's dietary patterns and physical activity: The Child and Adolescent Trial for Cardiovascular Health—CATCH collaborative group. *Journal of the American Medical Association, 275*(10), 768–776.

Malik, V. S., Willett, W. C., & Hu, F. B. (2013). Global obesity: Trends, risk factors and policy implications. *Nature Reviews Endocrinology, 9*(1), 13–27.

Melnyk, B. M., Jacobson, D., Kelly, S., Belyea, M., Shaibi, G., Small, L., et al. (2013). Promoting healthy lifestyles in high school adolescents: A randomized controlled trial. *American Journal of Preventive Medicine, 45*(4), 407–415.

Monasta, L., Batty, G. D., Macaluso, A., Ronfani, L., Lutje, V., Bavcar, A., et al. (2011). Interventions for the prevention of overweight and obesity in preschool children: A systematic review of randomized controlled trials. *Obesity Reviews, 12*(5), e107–e118.

Muennig, P., Schweinhart, L., Montie, J., & Neidell, M. (2009). Effects of a prekindergarten educational intervention on adult health: 37-year follow-up results of a randomized controlled trial. *American Journal of Public Health, 99*(8), 1431–1437.

Neumark-Sztainer, D. R., Friend, S. E., Flattum, C. F., Hannan, P. J., Story, M. T., Bauer, K. W., et al. (2010). New Moves: Preventing weight-related problems in adolescent girls. *American Journal of Preventive Medicine, 39*(5), 421–432.

Ogden, C. L., Carroll, M. D., Lawman, H. G., Fryar, C. D., Kruszon-Moran, D., Kit, B. K., et al. (2016). Trends in obesity prevalence among children and adolescents in the United States, 1988–1994 through 2013–2014. *Journal of the American Medical Association, 315*(21), 2292–2299.

Puder, J. J., Marques-Vidal, P., Schindler, C., Zahner, L., Niederer, I., Bürgi, F., et al. (2011). Effect of multidimensional lifestyle intervention on fitness and adiposity in predominantly migrant preschool children (Ballabeina): Cluster randomised controlled trial. *British Medical Journal, 343*, d6195.

Pulgarón, E. R. (2013). Childhood obesity: A review of increased risk for physical and psychological co-morbidities. *Clinical Therapeutics, 35*(1), A18–A32.

Robinson, T. N. (1999). Reducing children's television viewing to prevent obesity: A randomized controlled trial. *Journal of the American Medical Association, 282*(16), 1561–1567.

Schwartz, A. E., Leardo, M., Aneja, S., & Elbel, B. (2016). Effect of a school-based water intervention on child body mass index and obesity. *JAMA Pediatrics, 170*(3), 220–226.

Singh, A. S., Mulder, C., Twisk, J. W., Van Mechelen, W., & Chinapaw, M. J. (2008). Tracking of childhood overweight into adulthood: A systematic review of the literature. *Obesity Reviews, 9*(5), 474–488.

Sobol-Golberg, S., Rabinowitz, J., & Gross, R. (2013). School-based obesity prevention programs: A meta-analysis of randomized controlled trials. *Obesity, 21*(12), 2422–2428.

Stice, E., Shaw, H., & Marti, C. N. (2006). A meta-analytic review of obesity prevention programs for children and adolescents: The skinny on interventions that work. *Psychological Bulletin, 132*(5), 667–691.

Story, M., Hannan, P. J., Fulkerson, J. A., Rock, B. H., Smyth, M., Arcan, C., et al. (2012). Bright Start: Description and main outcomes from a group-randomized obesity prevention trial in American Indian children. *Obesity (Silver Spring), 20*(11), 2241–2249.

Trost, S. G., Sundal, D., Foster, G. D., Lent, M. R., & Vojta, D. (2014). Effects of a pediatric weight management program with and without active video games: A randomized trial. *JAMA Pediatrics, 168*(5), 407–413.

U.S. Department of Health and Human Services, Administration for Children and Families. (2010). Head Start impact study: Final report. Retrieved October 13, 2016, from *http://eric.ed.gov/?id=ED507845*.

U.S. Department of Health and Human Services & U.S. Department of Agriculture. (2015). 2015–2020 Dietary guidelines for Americans (8th ed.). Retrieved October 13, 2016, from *http://health.gov/dietaryguidelines/2015/guidelines*.

Vinter, C. A., Jensen, D. M., Ovesen, P., Beck-Nielsen, H., & Jørgensen, J. S. (2011). The LiP (Lifestyle in Pregnancy) study. *Diabetes Care, 34*(12), 2502–2507.

Wadden, T. A., Webb, V. L., Moran, C. H., & Bailer, B. A. (2012). Lifestyle modification for obesity: New developments in diet, physical activity, and behavior therapy. *Circulation, 125*(9), 1157–1170.

Wang, Y., Wu, Y., Wilson, R. F., Bleich, S., Cheskin, L., Weston, C., et al. (2013). Childhood obesity prevention program: Comparative effectiveness review and meta-analysis. *Comparative Effectiveness Review No. 115*. Retrieved October 13, 2016, from *www.effectivehealthcare.ahrq.gov/reports/final.cfm*.

Webber, L. S., Catellier, D. J., Lytle, L. A., Murray, D. M., Pratt, C. A., Young, D. R., et al. (2008). Promoting physical activity in middle school girls: Trial of activity for adolescent girls. *American Journal of Preventive Medicine, 34*(3), 173–184.

CHAPTER 39

Behavioral Treatment of Obesity in Youth

Katherine N. Balantekin
Denise E. Wilfley
Leonard H. Epstein

The childhood obesity epidemic is a pressing public health concern; approximately 31.8% of U.S. children have either overweight or obesity (Ogden, Carroll, Kit, & Flegal, 2014). Childhood obesity represents a considerable cost to society through increased health care burden and associated spending (Finkelstein, Trogdon, Cohen, & Dietz, 2009). It has many negative health consequences, including both medical (e.g., increased risk of cardiovascular disease and type 2 diabetes) and psychosocial (e.g., bullying, weight-based teasing, and stigmatization) comorbidities that lead to a reduced quality of life (Dietz, 1998). Given that 82% of children with obesity become adults with obesity (Juonala et al., 2011), these health care costs and physical and psychological comorbidities are likely to persist into adulthood if the obesity is not treated.

Fortunately, when obesity is treated at an early age, due to the potential for height growth, relatively small weight losses can have a significant impact on weight status (Goldschmidt, Wilfley, Paluch, Roemmich, & Epstein, 2013). Children ages 8–9 years with a body mass index (BMI) above the 97th percentile for age and sex need to lose only 1.8 (girls) to 2.1 (boys) kg over 1 year to achieve a healthy weight, which is in contrast to the 5.5 (boys) to 7.6 (girls) kg weight loss necessary for a 12- to 13-year-old to reach a healthy weight. Furthermore, maintaining weight and preventing weight gain improve cardiovascular risk factors in children but not in adolescents (Reinehr, 2013). Early childhood intervention also allows healthy eating and physical activity habits to be established before children become entrenched in obesogenic patterns. Thus, early intervention is critical to promote a healthy weight and cardiovascular health in adulthood. In this chapter we (1) present current treatment recommendations for childhood obesity and provide a brief review of the literature in support of childhood obesity treatment; (2) describe the components of family-based behavioral treatments for childhood obesity; (3) discuss possible adjuncts to family-based behavioral treatments for childhood obesity; (4) summarize factors found to affect or predict the effectiveness of these treatments; and (5) explore future directions in the management of childhood obesity.

Current Treatment Recommendations

In 2010, the United States Preventive Services Task Force (USPSTF) issued recommendations that clinicians screen children ages 6 years and older for obesity and offer or refer them to intensive counseling and behavioral interventions to promote improvements in weight status (Barton, 2010). These recommendations were based upon the results of a rigorous scientific review that demonstrated the efficacy of comprehensive interventions of moderate (26–75 contact hours) to high (> 75 contact hours) intensity (Whitlock, O'Connor, Williams, Beil, & Lutz, 2010). The USPSTF defined treatments as comprehensive if they included dietary, physical activity, and behavioral counseling components (Barton, 2010). The USPSTF systematic review was updated in 2017, with recommendations staying consistent (O'Connor, Evans, Burda, Walsh, Eder, et al., 2017). Unfortunately, treatment for older children and adolescents with severe obesity and severe medical comorbidities is somewhat more complicated. For this population, the use of pharmacotherapy and/or surgery in combination with evidence-based behavioral weight loss treatment may be considered (Barlow & Committee, 2007; Kelly et al., 2013), though few studies have evaluated the long-term outcomes and safety of pharmacological and surgical treatments for obesity in youth. Adherence to lifestyle behavior changes is still necessary following weight loss surgery and to potentiate the success of pharmacotherapy (Berkowitz, Wadden, Tershakovec, & Cronquist, 2003), and thus children who meet the criteria for these more invasive interventions should still participate in intensive, multicomponent interventions.

Review of the Literature

These recommendations and guidelines are supported by a significant body of research demonstrating the potency of intensive, multicomponent lifestyle interventions in inducing weight loss in children and in reducing medical and psychological comorbidities associated with obesity, as compared to no-treatment, education-only, or single-component conditions. Amount (or duration) of treatment contact has also been found to be a consistent predictor of long-term weight outcomes in children (Janicke et al., 2014). Furthermore, the inclusion of parents or caregivers in the treatment of childhood obesity improves weight loss outcomes in comparison to interventions that target only the child. In fact, interventions with a family-based component result in a 6% greater mean reduction in percent overweight compared to those without this component (Young, Northern, Lister, Drummond, & O'Brien, 2007). Moreover, a systematic review that examined the impact of session format found that interventions that included individual family sessions achieved a greater magnitude of weight loss than those with only group sessions (Hayes, Altman, Coppock, Wilfley, & Goldschmidt, 2015). A representative sample of these reviews and meta-analyses and their main findings are summarized in Table 39.1.

Family-Based Behavioral Interventions in Obesity Treatment

Family-based behavioral weight loss treatment (FBT) is a multicomponent behavioral weight control intervention developed and refined by Leonard Epstein, Denise Wilfley, and colleagues (Epstein, Paluch, Roemmich, & Beecher, 2007; Wilfley, Stein, et al., 2007). FBT targets both children and parents and is considered a first-line treatment for this population (Wilfley, Kass, & Kolko, 2011). FBT is effective at improving weight status in both the short and long term (Epstein, Valoski, Wing, & McCurley, 1994; Wilfley, Stein, et al., 2007), and has been shown to ameliorate other obesity-related comorbidities, such as improving cardiometabolic risk factors and psychological well-being (Gunnarsdottir et al., 2014; Ho et al., 2012).

Given the large age range of children affected by the USPSTF recommendation, it is important to acknowledge that FBT will need to be adapted to be developmentally appropriate for the targeted child. For example, children of different ages will differ in their cognitive abilities; capacities for

TABLE 39.1. Relevant Reviews and Meta-Analyses of Childhood Obesity Treatment Studies

Author	Type of review and number of studies	Target population	Conclusions
Altman & Wilfley (2015)	Systematic review of 53 studies	Children and adolescents (2–18 years) with overweight or obesity	This review found that multicomponent treatments that include a parent component are the most efficacious.
Epstein, Paluch, et al. (2007)	Targeted systematic review of eight studies	Children (5–12 years) with overweight or obesity	This review demonstrates a consistent pattern of weight loss results across efficacy studies across time—an important step in preparing interventions for translation to wider-spread clinical care.
Hayes et al. (2015)	Systematic review of 22 studies	Children and adolescents (2–18 years) with overweight or obesity	This review found that behavioral interventions that include individual family sessions achieve a greater magnitude of weight loss than those with only group sessions.
Ho et al. (2012)	Systematic review of 38 RCTs	Children and adolescents ($\leq$ 18 years) with overweight or obesity	This review concluded that weight loss was greater when the duration of treatment was longer than 6 months.
Janicke et al. (2014)	Meta-analysis of 20 RCTs	Children and adolescents ($\leq$ 19 years) with overweight or obesity	This meta-analysis found that dose (duration, number of sessions, time in treatment) was positively related to effect size, and that individual and in-person comprehensive family interventions were associated with larger effect sizes.
Whitlock et al. (2010)	Targeted systematic review of 16 studies	Children and adolescents (5–18 years) with overweight or obesity	This review confirmed that comprehensive moderate- to high-intensity behavioral interventions can be effective at producing significant weight loss in children.
Wilfley, Tibbs, et al. (2007)	Meta-analysis of 14 RCTs	Children ($\leq$ 19 years) with overweight	This meta-analysis concluded that lifestyle interventions produce significant changes in weight status in the short term, with evidence suggesting that results persist in the long term.
Young et al. (2007)	Meta-analysis of 16 studies	Children (5–12 years) with overweight or obesity	This meta-analysis found that interventions with a family-component achieve a greater magnitude of weight loss than those using an alternative treatment approach.

self-regulation; social networks; and how they respond to parents, teachers, and peers. Although the majority of studies have been conducted with children in middle childhood (Epstein, Paluch, et al., 2007), FBT has also been successfully adapted for use with both preschoolers (Quattrin et al., 2012) and adolescents (Jelalian et al., 2010).

To improve a child's weight status, FBT targets modification of energy balance behaviors (i.e., decreasing energy intake and increasing energy expenditure) through the use of behavioral treatment techniques and the active involvement of a parent or caregiver. In FBT, the parent or caregiver, who often also has overweight or obesity, is charged with both changing his or her own energy balance behaviors, as well as supporting the child in these endeavors. Furthermore, the parent or caregiver is encouraged to engineer the home environment so that it promotes these behaviors for the entire family. To facilitate long-term weight loss maintenance, treatment contact is extended to allow for the continued practice of behavioral change skills and the development of family and social networks in support of weight loss maintenance behaviors (Wilfley, Stein, et al., 2007). The components of FBT are described below and summarized in Table 39.2.

Key Components of FBT

Dietary Modification

There are three primary dietary modification goals in FBT: (1) decrease energy intake, (2) improve nutritional quality, and (3) shift food preferences toward healthier choices. To facilitate a decrease in energy intake while improving nutritional quality, FBT uses a family-friendly method of categorizing foods according to traffic light colors (Epstein & Squires, 1988). In addition, families learn to gradually adopt healthier eating habits through decreasing portion sizes; reducing intake of energy dense, low-nutrient-dense foods (red foods); increasing intake of lower-calorie, more nutritious foods (green foods); and regularly consuming three meals a day. To shift taste preferences from less nutritious to more nutritious food options, families are discouraged from swapping energy-dense foods with non- or low-calorie or fat substitutes (e.g., having frozen yogurt instead of ice cream) because these latter foods are typically processed to taste the same as their high-calorie alternative.

Appetitive traits, such as poor satiety responsiveness (Carnell & Wardle, 2008), high food reinforcement (Temple, Legierski, Giacomelli, Salvy, & Epstein, 2008), binge or loss-of-control eating (Tanofsky-Kraff et al., 2004), and impulsivity (Nederkoorn, Braet, Van Eijs, Tanghe, & Jansen, 2006) are heritable traits that may hinder treatment response. As a result, addressing these appetitive traits through early detection and targeted intervention is critical. Treatment helps address these traits by encouraging parents to help their children (1) regulate their portion sizes, (2) limit access to unhealthy foods to decrease temptation, (3) differentiate between hunger and emotional states, and (4) seek alternate activities other than eating if they are not hungry.

Energy Expenditure Modification

The primary energy expenditure goals in FBT are to increase moderate-to-vigorous physical activity and to decrease sedentary behaviors (e.g., nonschool or work-related screen time). The colors of the traffic light are also used to help families identify which activities to increase (*green*: moderate-to-vigorous physical activity) and to decrease (*red*: sedentary behaviors). Families are also encouraged to increase lifestyle activities such as using stairs instead of elevators, or walking or riding a bike to school rather than taking a car. Eating is a complementary behavior to sedentary behavior for many people (i.e., they both increase or decrease in the same direction); thus, decreasing time spent engaging in sedentary behaviors not only creates opportunities for greater time spent being physically active, but also decreases opportunities for eating (Epstein, Paluch, Gordy, & Dorn, 2000). Increasing physical activity not only facilitates weight change in the short term, it is also predictive of sustained weight change 10 years after participation in FBT (Epstein, Valoski, et al., 1994).

TABLE 39.2. Family-Based Behavioral Treatment Components

Goal	Strategies
Dietary modification	
Decrease energy intake	• Define appropriate calorie range. • Increase intake of green foods (i.e., highly nutritious, low-calorie dense foods). • Decrease intake of red foods (i.e., high-fat, high-sugar foods).
Energy expenditure modification	
Increase energy expenditure	• Increase physical activity (goal: 60 minutes/day, 5 days/week). • Decrease sedentary activity (goal: < 2 hours/day outside of school time).
Behavior modification	
Goal setting	• Dietary goals (e.g., < 15 red foods/week, calorie range 1,200–1,500). • Physical activity goals (e.g., > 60 minutes/day, reduce sedentary activity by 50%). • Weight goals (e.g., weight loss of 0.5 pounds/week).
Self-monitoring	• Record daily food intake (e.g., calorie intake, number of red foods, fruit and vegetable intake). • Record activity (e.g., time spent in moderate-to-vigorous activity and sedentary activity).
Reward systems	• Record weight (e.g., weekly weighing). • Rewards based on dietary and physical activity goal achievement. • Rewards based on weight achievement.
Stimulus control	• Engineer the home environment (i.e., increase availability of green foods and decrease availability of red foods) to increase weight loss success.
Parental involvement	
Shape home environment	• Make the healthy choice the easy choice in home through stimulus control.
Model healthy eating and activity	• Model healthy eating and physical activity behaviors.
Parenting skills	• Develop skills to support healthy lifestyle choices for family (e.g., problem-solve solutions).
Limit setting	• Parents set limits to help create structure around eating, activity, and sleep behaviors.
Goals	• Diet, physical activity, and weight goals are also set for parents.
Socioenvironmental contexts	
Peer level	• Parents help children establish healthy peer networks. • Teach techniques to help deal with weight-based teasing and improve body image and self-esteem.
Community level	• Families are encouraged to become advocates for increased access to healthy foods in their schools and communities. • Problem-solve ways to work with the built environment.

Behavior Change Strategies

Goal Setting

Goal setting is the process of creating specific, measurable, and realistic targets (i.e., goals) for behavior change. The frequency of goal setting is associated with sustained behavior change, and continued, frequent goal setting is an important component of weight maintenance (Nothwehr & Yang, 2007). All children and parents are given weight loss goals, but other goals are individualized to focus on specific behaviors most needing improvement. As the intervention progresses, goals change to accommodate participant progress.

Self-Monitoring

Goals are accompanied by self-monitoring, which allows one to observe and note progress in a methodical way. Those who participate in frequent self-monitoring are more aware of their energy balance behaviors and have more successful weight outcomes (Saelens et al., 2002). In FBT, both the parent and child are encouraged to participate in regular self-monitoring of weight-related behaviors, and parents are encouraged to help their child master this skill.

Reward Systems

The rationale behind the use of reward systems in behavior change comes from operant learning theory, which states that behavior that produces rewards will be continued and thus reinforced (Skinner, 1938). As such, using rewards is a powerful way to reinforce target behaviors. Although there are many rewards intrinsic to weight loss that can reinforce behavior change (e.g., the feeling of success that comes with weight loss, reduced teasing), these changes are often slow to manifest, and thus more immediate material rewards may be more effective at reinforcing new behaviors (Levy, Finch, Crowell, Talley, & Jeffery, 2007). For example, financial incentives have been effectively used in obesity treatment with adults (Jeffery, 2012); however, more research is needed in children. FBT often involves the use of incentive systems to help reinforce the targeted behaviors. To develop an incentive system, parents and children work together to determine appropriate and appealing rewards. Children earn points for achieving their goals and can exchange their points for rewards. Ideal rewards are those that increase social support and reinforce the targeted behaviors (e.g., park visit with friends).

Stimulus Control

Stimulus control is defined as using environmental enrichment to restructure the environment to increase the likelihood of engaging in desired behaviors (Terrace, 1966), and is a critical component of behavior change interventions for obesity (Young et al., 2007). Within a behavioral economics framework, people's choices to obtain commodities are influenced by the constraints placed on those commodities. As the constraints on the commodities change, so do choices. As such, stimulus control works by placing constraints on undesirable choices (i.e., red foods and activities) to help someone make the best choice by making the healthy choice (i.e., green food and activities) the easy choice. In FBT, it is necessary for parents to remove prompts for unhealthy foods and sedentary behaviors (e.g., removing chips and cookies from the home or from within easy reach for children, keeping videogame equipment on a high shelf in the closet) and to increase the prompts for healthy foods and physical activity (e.g., placing fruits in a basket on the kitchen counter, keeping sneakers by the door) in the home.

Family Involvement and Support

Family involvement is a critical component of FBT. Participating parents and caregivers are taught to systematically use behavioral principles and positive parenting approaches to help shape and support their child's weight change efforts. Children's weight-related behaviors exist in the context of their home and family environment. By including parents in their child's treatment, the goal is to capitalize on this parental influence to promote healthier behavior choices and maximize health outcomes for both parent and child. Parents are encouraged to create a healthy home environment and model healthy behaviors by purchasing healthier foods, planning healthier meals, developing a family-based reward system to reinforce healthy choices, participating in and encouraging increased physical activity, and using praise to reinforce healthy behaviors (Epstein, Paluch, Kilanowski, & Raynor, 2004). Parents are also taught how to use effective limit setting to help create structure and routines around eating, activity, and sleep behaviors.

Parents participating in FBT are encouraged to actively work toward changing their own weight status in addition to supporting their child's efforts. By including parents as active treatment targets, they can model the healthier eating and physical activity behaviors that are critical for weight loss success. According to social learning theory, modeling is a critical way for parents to socialize their children's behavior (Bandura, 1977). When children are learning new behavior, observing a key socialization agent (i.e., a parent) engage in this behavior reinforces it. In fact, children with overweight or obesity may be particularly sensitive to adult influence in the transmission of health behaviors (Frerichs, Araz, & Huang, 2013), underscoring the importance of active parental involvement in FBT. As such, parent weight loss is a positive predictor of child weight loss in FBT (Wrotniak, Epstein, Paluch, & Roemmich, 2004).

The Importance of Intervening across Time and Contexts

A child's weight-related dietary and physical activity behaviors are developed and maintained in the context of the family home as well as the broader community within which children and their families live, work, and play. Interventions that utilize a socioenvironmental approach are efficacious for weight loss because they extend the focus of behavior change beyond the individual to encompass the home, peer, and community contexts (Huang, Drewnowski, Kumanyika, & Glass, 2009). Bouton's work on context-specific extinction shows that when new weight control behaviors are acquired during the course of FBT, these new behaviors do not replace the old behaviors associated with weight gain but rather coexist with them (Bouton, 2002). Unfortunately, new behaviors are not very generalizable outside of the setting in which they were learned, and old behaviors are easily activated across the different contexts of our obesogenic world. As a result of this contextual influence on the acquisition and practice of energy balance behaviors, FBT takes a socioenvironmental or multilevel approach to behavior change to improve maintenance of weight losses over time (Wilfley et al., 2010). To address challenges to the maintenance of these new behaviors, FBT teaches families to plan for the different constraints or barriers to maintaining a healthy energy balance across these different levels of influence (e.g., learn how to identify and capitalize on facilitators for healthy living within peer networks and the community).

Peer Level

Peer interactions are naturally reinforcing to children, and good peer relationships have a positive influence on overall quality of life. When peers are supportive of healthy energy balance behaviors, weight loss maintenance efforts are enhanced (Salvy et al., 2007). Conversely, a lack of peer support for physical activity and healthy eating contributes to weight gain (Wilfley, Stein, et al., 2007). In FBT, heightened social problems (e.g., loneliness, jealousy, susceptibility to teasing) predict greater weight regain after FBT (Epstein, Klein, & Wisniewski, 1994), and children with higher levels of social problems have poorer weight loss maintenance (Wilfley, Stein, et al., 2007). These findings may be partially explained by the fact that youth who experience social problems or rejection may be more likely to use food as a coping mechanism (DeWall & Bushman, 2011) and less likely to engage in physical activity (Jefferson, 2006). These findings highlight the need to include training in prosocial techniques as part of treatment. Therefore, in FBT, families are encouraged to establish healthy peer networks and to disentangle socializing from unhealthy activities. In an effort to improve children's confidence in their ability to relate positively to peers, FBT also includes training in prosocial techniques for dealing with teasing and cognitive-behavioral techniques to improve body image and self-esteem.

Community Level

The community or built environment offers many opportunities as well as challenges to families participating in FBT. However, families are often unaware of the ways in which their communities affect their behavioral choices. The built environment influences children's weight loss success in FBT. Access to parks and open spaces predicted greater weight loss success at a 2-year follow-up, whereas reduced access to parks and greater access to supermarkets and convenience stores predicted poorer outcome (Epstein et al., 2012). In FBT, families engage in a number of activities to help increase their familiarity with how their built environment can both help and interfere with the establishment of healthy habits over the long term. Problem solving, goal setting, and stimulus control are techniques that families can use in FBT to better work around or with their built environments. In addition, families are encouraged to become advocates for increased access to healthy foods and activity choices in their schools, their work places, and other community settings. Families are encouraged to build a culture of health in their homes, in their relationships, and in their communities to provide support for the difficult challenge of healthy weight maintenance in our obesogenic world.

Adjuncts to Traditional Behavioral Interventions

Improving Executive Function

Executive function refers to a set of cognitive processes that help manage behavior, emotion, and thought with a consideration to future goals and outcomes (Bickel, Jarmolowicz, Mueller, Gatchalian, & McClure, 2012). Executive functioning, specifically the self-control aspect of it, has been identified as an individual difference that predicts long-term outcomes in personal finances, criminal behavior, and physical and psychological health (Moffitt et al., 2011). Skill deficits in executive functions have been documented in adolescents with obesity (Maayan, Hoogendoorn, Sweat, & Convit, 2011). The goal of executive functioning training is to improve impulse control and self-regulation skills in children, which may lead to decreases in impulsive eating behavior. In a recent trial, children with obesity in inpatient treatment were randomly assigned to receive executive function training or to a control group (Verbeken, Braet, Goossens, & Van der Oord, 2013). Children who received 25 40-minute executive functioning training sessions (working memory and inhibition training tasks delivered through a virtual reality game) showed improved weight loss maintenance compared to the control group. However, this difference was no longer significant at a 12-week follow-up assessment. This finding suggests that although executive functioning training may be a valuable adjunctive approach, additional research is needed to determine how to bolster and maintain these effects.

Improving Reinforcement Pathology

People allocate their limited resources to gain access to commodities within a system of variable constraint. Individual differences in factors such as food reinforcement (i.e., the motivation to eat) and impulsivity (i.e., decision making, the ability to inhibit responding) influence how individuals make these decisions.

Food Reinforcement

The reinforcing value of an item is defined as the motivation to obtain that item, and the relative reinforcing value of an item is defined as the motivation to obtain that item relative to another item. Reinforcement plays a fundamental role in choice; in a system with equal constraints, people often choose to engage in activities and behaviors that they find more reinforcing. Food is considered a primary reinforcer (i.e., does not need to be learned and is intrinsically motivating). Children with obesity find food more reinforcing than their peers without obesity (Temple, Legierski, Giacomelli, Salvy, & Epstein, 2008).

There are two ways to change the relative reinforcing value of something to shift choices away from the more reinforcing to the less reinforcing choice. The first way is to increase the reinforcing value of the alternative choice (e.g., by substituting a more reinforcing choice for the original alternative or by increasing the reinforcing value of the current alternative). It has been suggested that children with overweight/obesity consume more food not only because they find it more reinforcing but also because they do not have many alternatives to eating (Jacobs & Wagner, 1984). Time spent with peers may be a valuable alternative to eating, and therefore increasing a child's social network may increase the reinforcing value of peer relationships and thus help decrease eating (Epstein, Leddy, Temple, & Faith, 2007; Epstein, Salvy, Carr, Dearing, & Bickel, 2010). Given that there are many problems (e.g., bullying, ostracism) surrounding social situations for children with obesity, social skills training as part of FBT may help improve the reinforcing value of peer relationships, thus making it a more competitive alternative to high-energy-dense food.

The second way to decrease the reinforcing value of food is to increase the amount of work necessary to obtain the food—for example, in FBT, by engineering the environment so that one has to leave the house to obtain ice cream. Laboratory studies have shown that increasing the amount of work necessary to obtain the more reinforcing food caused the choice to shift to the alternative (Goldfield & Epstein, 2002), and that increasing the behavioral cost of gaining access to sedentary activities led to decreased time spent being sedentary and increased time spent being physically active (Epstein, Saelens, Myers, & Vito, 1997).

Compliance with dietary targets set in FBT may also reduce the reinforcing value of food. For example, both variety and fat content have been shown to influence the reinforcing value of food (Epstein, Leddy, et al., 2007). Thus, reducing both the variety of high-energy-dense foods consumed and the overall fat content of the diet may reduce the overall reinforcing value of food. In one treatment program, those who consumed the greatest variety of vegetables and the least variety of high-energy-dense foods lost the most weight (Raynor, Jeffery, Tate, & Wing, 2004). However, the reinforcing value of food was not specifically tested in that trial, and thus it is unclear whether changes in the reinforcing value of food contributed to treatment success.

Improving Impulsivity

The inability to delay gratification (i.e., high impulsivity) has been explored for its relation to obesity development and maintenance. The ability to delay gratification can be quantified by delay discounting (DD), or the tendency to discount large future rewards for smaller, immediate rewards (Bickel & Marsch, 2001). Research suggests that children with obesity are more likely to choose a small immediate food reward over a larger delayed food reward. In children the inability to delay gratification predicts greater subsequent weight gain (Francis & Susman, 2009) and poorer response to FBT (Best et al., 2012).

Improving DD is critical to ensuring successful behavior change necessary for weight loss, as many of the health benefits associated with weight loss treatment are not immediate. There are a number of interventions that have been shown to reduce DD, and many of these treatment methods and intervention targets are part of contemporary FBT (Best et al., 2012; Daniel, Stanton, & Epstein, 2013). For example, parental inconsistency in the use of short- and longer-term rewards can increase children's impulsive decisions (Schneider, Peters, Peth, & Büchel, 2014), but parents who are taught the proper use of contingency management to encourage working for future FBT goals may be able to reduce impulsive choices. Planning, which is a central skill taught to families in FBT, can reduce future discounting (Baird, Smallwood, & Schooler, 2011). FBT can teach families to provide alternatives to food, which improves treatment outcome (Best et al., 2012). Additionally, framing decisions in terms of future consequences, rather than immediate rewards—referred to as "pre-experiencing the future"—can be taught. This is called *episodic future thinking* (EFT), and is an adaptive cognitive process that allows humans to plan and make decisions about how to allocate time and effort to achieve future outcomes (Gilbert & Wilson, 2007). Failing to think about the future (prospection) when making decisions about the consequences of small immediate rewards versus larger delayed rewards may put one at the mercy of the immediate option. In FBT, we have adapted the use of EFT by teaching parents and children to simulate future events as they make decisions about small immediate rewards versus larger delayed rewards (Peters & Büchel, 2010). Research has shown a reduction in DD and in energy intake in children after training in EFT (Daniel, Said, Stanton, & Epstein, 2015).

Reinforcement Pathology

An imbalance in the interaction between these two systems (i.e., food reinforcement and impulsivity) may lead to eating behaviors that result in weight gain over time (Carr, Daniel, Lin, & Epstein, 2011). The combination of increased food reinforcement and increased impulsivity is called *reinforcement pathology*. Individuals with this combination of traits find food highly rewarding and are unable to inhibit their desire to consume food. In adults, the combination of high impulsivity and increased food reinforcement predicts increased intake (Appelhans et al., 2011). In FBT, children who show signs of reinforcement pathology have a blunted response to treatment (Best et al., 2012); thus, children with this combination of traits would benefit from the aforementioned adjuctive treatments in combination with FBT.

Treatment Modality and Setting

The majority of successful treatment studies for childhood obesity have been conducted in an individual or individual family format within a clinical research setting; however, additional delivery settings and formats are being explored. One way to increase availability of effective childhood obesity treatment would be to deliver treatment in a group format. However, a recent review of group-based childhood weight loss programs found that group-only treatment formats may not achieve clinically significant weight changes. Outcomes improved when treatment format was mixed (i.e., both individual and group sessions) (Hayes et al., 2015).

Another way to improve availability of FBT while preserving its potency would be to conduct FBT with individual families within primary care settings. Co-location is a model of coordinated health care that places a behavioral health care provider within the same location as the primary care physician. Preliminary research suggests that FBT interventionists can be successfully co-located within pediatric primary care practices and produce both child and parent weight losses (Quattrin et al., 2014). However, this study used an abbreviated form of FBT in terms of both treatment content and intensity. Although further research is needed to test the efficacy of full-dose FBT in primary care, the co-location of a behavioral health interventionist within primary care would allow pediatricians to more easily refer appropriate families to comprehensive behavioral treatment for weight loss within the familiar practice setting. Furthermore, co-location also would allow for easier coordination of care, which is important given the comorbidities associated with obesity.

Evaluating Treatment Success

Cutoffs for clinically meaningful weight loss have been suggested in the literature, with BMI z-score changes ≥ 0.25 defined as clinically significant (Ford, Hunt, Cooper, & Shield, 2010; Kalavainen, Utriainen, Vanninen, Korppi, & Nuutinen, 2012). Weight changes of this magnitude have been shown to improve cardiovascular risk factors (e.g., insulin sensitivity, total cholesterol, blood pressure) in children and adolescents (Ford et al., 2010; Kalavainen et al., 2012; Kolsgaard et al., 2011; Reinehr et al., 2016). FBT results in clinically meaningful weight losses. An examination of twenty-five years of FBT studies revealed that at 6 months after starting treatment, 80–85% of children had BMI z-score changes ≥ 0.5, with 67% of children maintaining BMI z-score changes ≥ 0.5 at 10 years (Epstein, Paluch, et al., 2007).

Percent overweight (i.e., percentage the child's BMI is above median for age and sex) is another metric used to measure changes in weight status in children; decreases ≥ 9 units in percent overweight are considered clinically significant. In one seminal study comparing FBT to a child-only treatment and a wait-list control group, participants in the FBT condition showed decreases in percent overweight (11.2 and 7.5 at 5 and 10 years, respectively), whereas participants in the child-only (+2.7 and +4.5), and control (+7.9 and +14.3) groups showed increases in percent overweight (Epstein, Valoski, Wing, & McCurley, 1990). In another study, 82% of children who received FBT achieved percent overweight reductions of ≥ 9 units, with an average reduction of 17.4 percentage points over 12 months (Wilfley, 2013).

Treatment success may also be defined as the percentage of children transitioning to a lower weight status (i.e., going from obesity to overweight, or from obesity to normal weight). In contemporary FBT studies, 6 months after starting FBT, an average of 33.2% of children no longer had obesity, with 8.8% of children transitioning to a normal-weight status (Epstein, Paluch, et al., 2007).

Conclusions and Future Directions

Evidence supports providing early intervention for obesity during childhood, as robust and sustainable changes can be made at this time. FBT for childhood obesity, a multicomponent treatment that intervenes across several socioenvironmental contexts, has demonstrated effectiveness in reducing weight and improving physiological and psychosocial outcomes in children and their parents. Given its reach beyond the target child, FBT may be a very cost-effective way to treat obesity across multiple generations. The potential for FBT's impact to generalize to other family members' health is an important area for future research. In addition, sustainable behavior change is associated with early treatment response; children who lost weight by Week 8 had the greatest likelihood of both short-term and sustained success (Goldschmidt et al., 2011). Future work should examine whether an adaptive treatment approach (i.e., increasing intensity, adding adjunctive treatment components) improves treatment success in early nonresponders.

Although FBT has proven to be effective for the treatment of childhood obesity, access to care remains a challenge. Barriers include time and cost of training providers in FBT delivery, lack of reimbursement for treatment, and limited specialty clinics to which providers can refer their patients (Simpson & Cooper, 2009). As insurers and medical service delivery systems shift toward a health care market that incentivizes prevention and the effective management of complex, multilevel diseases such as obesity, interventions such as FBT will be in demand to meet this need. In anticipation of this shift in the health care system, it will be necessary to determine how best to scale-up FBT for broader implementation without losing its potency. To achieve the broadest reach, professionals must be equipped to deliver FBT across multiple settings. One proposed approach to address this gap is creating regional centers of excellence in which FBT experts train center leaders to deliver FBT and supervise delivery (McHugh & Barlow, 2010). Such centers would have the potential to bridge the gap between treatment experts and interventionists to ensure proper delivery of FBT on a large scale.

References

Altman, M., & Wilfley, D. E. (2015). Evidence update on the treatment of overweight and obesity in children and adolescents. *Journal of Clinical Child and Adolescent Psychology, 44*(4), 521–537.

Appelhans, B. M., Woolf, K., Pagoto, S. L., Schneider, K. L., Whited, M. C., & Liebman, R. (2011). Inhibiting food reward: Delay discounting, food reward sensitivity, and palatable food intake in overweight and obese women. *Obesity, 19*(11), 2175–2182.

Baird, B., Smallwood, J., & Schooler, J. W. (2011). Back to the future: Autobiographical planning and the functionality of mind-wandering. *Consciousness and Cognition, 20*(4), 1604–1611.

Bandura, A. (1977). *Social learning theory*. New York: General Learning Press.

Barlow, S. E., & Expert Committee. (2007). Expert committee recommendations regarding the prevention, assessment, and treatment of child and adolescent overweight and obesity: Summary report. *Pediatrics, 120*(Suppl. 4), S164–S192.

Barton, M. (2010). Screening for obesity in children and adolescents: U.S. Preventive Services Task Force recommendation statement. *Pediatrics, 125*(2), 361–367.

Berkowitz, R. I., Wadden, T. A., Tershakovec, A. M., & Cronquist, J. L. (2003). Behavior therapy and sibutramine for the treatment of adolescent obesity: A randomized controlled trial. *Journal of the American Medical Association, 289*(14), 1805–1812.

Best, J. R., Theim, K. R., Gredysa, D. M., Stein, R. I., Welch, R. R., Saelens, B. E., et al. (2012). Behavioral economic predictors of overweight children's weight loss. *Journal of Consulting and Clinical Psychology, 80*(6), 1086–1096.

Bickel, W. K., Jarmolowicz, D. P., Mueller, E. T., Gatchalian, K. M., & McClure, S. M. (2012). Are executive function and impulsivity antipodes?: A conceptual reconstruction with special reference to addiction. *Psychopharmacology, 221*(3), 361–387.

Bickel, W. K., & Marsch, L. A. (2001). Toward a behavioral economic understanding of drug dependence: Delay discounting processes. *Addiction, 96*(1), 73–86.

Bouton, M. E. (2002). Context, ambiguity, and unlearning: Sources of relapse after behavioral extinction. *Biological Psychiatry, 52*(10), 976–986.

Carnell, S., & Wardle, J. (2008). Appetitive traits and child obesity: Measurement, origins and implications for intervention. *Proceedings of the Nutrition Society, 67*(4), 343–355.

Carr, K. A., Daniel, T. O., Lin, H., & Epstein L. H. (2011). Reinforcement pathology and nutrition. *Current Drug Abuse Reviews, 4*(3), 190–196.

Daniel, T. O., Said, M., Stanton, C. M., & Epstein, L. H. (2015). Episodic future thinking reduces delay discounting and energy intake in children. *Eating Behaviors, 18*, 20–24.

Daniel, T. O., Stanton, C. M., & Epstein, L. H. (2013). The future is now: Comparing the effect of episodic future thinking on impulsivity in lean and obese individuals. *Appetite, 71*, 120–125.

DeWall, C. N., & Bushman, B. J. (2011). Social acceptance and rejection: The sweet and the bitter. *Current Directions in Psychological Science, 20*(4), 256–260.

Dietz, W. H. (1998). Health consequences of obesity in youth: Childhood predictors of adult disease. *Pediatrics, 101*(Suppl. 2), 518–525.

Epstein, L. H., Klein, K. R., & Wisniewski, L. (1994). Child and parent factors that influence psychological problems in obese children. *International Journal of Eating Disorders, 15*(2), 151–158.

Epstein, L. H., Leddy, J. J., Temple, J. L., & Faith, M. S. (2007). Food reinforcement and eating: A multilevel analysis. *Psychological Bulletin, 133*(5), 884.

Epstein, L. H., Paluch, R. A., Gordy, C. C., & Dorn, J. (2000). Decreasing sedentary behaviors in treating pediatric obesity. *Archives of Pediatrics and Adolescent Medicine, 154*(3), 220–226.

Epstein, L. H., Paluch, R. A., Kilanowski, C. K., & Raynor, H. A. (2004). The effect of reinforcement or stimulus control to reduce sedentary behavior in the treatment of pediatric obesity. *Health Psychology, 23*(4), 371.

Epstein, L. H., Paluch, R. A., Roemmich, J. N., & Beecher, M. D. (2007). Family-based obesity treatment, then and now: Twenty-five years of pediatric obesity treatment. *Health Psychology, 26*(4), 381.

Epstein, L. H., Raja, S., Daniel, T. O., Paluch, R. A., Wilfley, D. E., Saelens, B. E., et al. (2012). The built environment moderates effects of family-based childhood obesity treatment over 2 years. *Annals of Behavioral Medicine, 44*(2), 248–258.

Epstein, L. H., Saelens, B. E., Myers, M. D., & Vito, D. (1997). Effects of decreasing sedentary behaviors on activity choice in obese children. *Health Psychology, 16*(2), 107.

Epstein, L. H., Salvy, S. J., Carr, K. A., Dearing, K. K., & Bickel, W. K. (2010). Food reinforcement, delay discounting and obesity. *Physiology and Behavior, 100*(5), 438–445.

Epstein, L. H., & Squires, S. (1988). *The stoplight diet for children: An eight-week program for parents and children.* New York: Little, Brown.

Epstein, L. H., Valoski, A., Wing, R. R., & McCurley, J. (1990). Ten-year follow-up of behavioral, family-based treatment for obese children. *Journal of the American Medical Association, 264,* 2519–2523.

Epstein, L. H., Valoski, A., Wing, R. R., & McCurley, J. (1994). Ten-year outcomes of behavioral family-based treatment for childhood obesity. *Health Psychology, 13*(5), 373.

Finkelstein, E. A., Trogdon, J. G., Cohen, J. W., & Dietz, W. (2009). Annual medical spending attributable to obesity: Payer- and service-specific estimates. *Health Affairs, 28*(5), w822–w831.

Ford, A. L., Hunt, L. P., Cooper, A., & Shield, J. P. (2010). What reduction in BMI SDS is required in obese adolescents to improve body composition and cardiometabolic health? *Archives of Disease in Childhood, 95*(4), 256–261.

Francis, L. A., & Susman, E. J. (2009). Self-regulation and rapid weight gain in children from age 3 to 12 years. *Archives of Pediatrics and Adolescent Medicine, 163*(4), 297–302.

Frerichs, L. M., Araz, O. M., & Huang, T. T. K. (2013). Modeling social transmission dynamics of unhealthy behaviors for evaluating prevention and treatment interventions on childhood obesity. *PL7OS ONE, 8*(12), e82887.

Gilbert, D. T., & Wilson, T. D. (2007). Prospection: Experiencing the future. *Science, 317*(5843), 1351–1354.

Goldfield, G. S., & Epstein, L. H. (2002). Can fruits and vegetables and activities substitute for snack foods? *Health Psychology, 21*(3), 299.

Goldschmidt, A. B., Stein, R. I., Saelens, B. E., Theim, K. R., Epstein, L. H., & Wilfley, D. E. (2011). Importance of early weight change in a pediatric weight management trial. *Pediatrics, 128*(1), e33–e39.

Goldschmidt, A. B., Wilfley, D. E., Paluch, R. A., Roemmich, J. N., & Epstein, L. H. (2013). Indicated prevention of adult obesity: How much weight change is necessary for normalization of weight status in children? *JAMA Pediatrics, 167*(1), 21–26.

Gunnarsdottir, T., Einarsson, S. M., Njardvik, U., Olafsdottir, A. S., Gunnarsdottir, A. B., Helgason, T., et al. (2014). Family-based behavioral treatment for obese children: Results and two year follow up. *Laeknabladid, 100*(3), 139–145.

Hayes, J. F., Altman, M., Coppock, J. H., Wilfley, D. E., & Goldschmidt, A. B. (2015). Recent updates on the efficacy of group-based treatments for pediatric obesity. *Current Cardiovascular Risk Reports, 9*(4), 1–10.

Ho, M., Garnett, S. P., Baur, L. A., Burrows, T., Stewart, L., Neve, M., et al. (2012). Effectiveness of lifestyle interventions in child obesity: Systematic review with meta-analysis. *Pediatrics, 130,* e1647–e1671.

Huang, T. T., Drewnowski, A., Kumanyika, S. K., & Glass, T. A. (2009). A systems-oriented multilevel framework for addressing obesity in the 21st century. *Preventing Chronic Disease, 6*(3), A82.

Jacobs, S. B., & Wagner, M. K. (1984). Obese and nonobese individuals: Behavioral and personality characteristics. *Addictive Behaviors, 9*(2), 223–226.

Janicke, D. M., Steele, R. G., Gayes, L. A., Lim, C. S., Clifford, L. M., Schneider, E. M., et al. (2014). Systematic review and meta-analysis of comprehensive behavioral family lifestyle interventions addressing pediatric obesity. *Journal of Pediatric Psychology, 39*(8), 809–825.

Jefferson, A. (2006). Breaking down barriers: Examining health promoting behaviour in the family. *Nutrition Bulletin, 31*(1), 60–64.

Jeffery, R. W. (2012). Financial incentives and weight control. *Preventive Medicine, 55,* S61–S67.

Jelalian, E., Lloyd-Richardson, E. E., Mehlenbeck, R. S., Hart, C. N., Flynn-O'Brien, K., Kaplan, J., et al. (2010). Behavioral weight control treatment with supervised exercise or peer-enhanced adventure for overweight adolescents. *Journal of Pediatrics, 157*(6), 923–928.

Juonala, M., Magnussen, C. G., Berenson, G. S., Venn, A., Burns, T. L., Sabin, M. A., et al. (2011). Childhood adiposity, adult adiposity, and cardiovascular risk factors. *New England Journal of Medicine, 365*(20), 1876–1885.

Kalavainen, M., Utriainen, P., Vanninen, E., Korppi, M., & Nuutinen, O. (2012). Impact of childhood obesity treatment on body composition and metabolic profile. *World Journal of Pediatrics, 8*(1), 31–37.

Kelly, A. S., Barlow, S. E., Rao, G., Inge, T. H., Hayman, L. L., Steinberger, J., et al. (2013). Severe obesity in children and adolescents: Identification, associated health risks, and treatment approaches—a scientific statement from the American Heart Association. *Circulation, 128,* 1689–1712.

Kolsgaard, M. L. P., Joner, G., Brunborg, C., Anderssen, S. A., Tonstad, S., & Andersen, L. F. (2011). Reduction in BMI z-score and improvement in cardiometabolic risk factors in obese children and adolescents: The Oslo Adiposity Intervention Study—a hospital/public health nurse combined treatment. *BMC Pediatrics, 11*(1), 1.

Levy, R. L., Finch, E. A., Crowell, M. D., Talley, N. J., & Jeffery, R. W. (2007). Behavioral intervention for the treatment of obesity: Strategies and effectiveness data. *American Journal of Gastroenterology, 102*(10), 2314–2321.

Maayan, L., Hoogendoorn, C., Sweat, V., & Convit, A. (2011). Disinhibited eating in obese adolescents is associated with orbitofrontal volume reductions and executive dysfunction. *Obesity, 19*(7), 1382–1387.

McHugh, R. K., & Barlow, D. H. (2010). The dissemination and implementation of evidence-based psychological treatments: A review of current efforts. *American Psychologist, 65*(2), 73.

Moffitt, T. E., Arseneault, L., Belsky, D., Dickson, N., Hancox, R. J., Harrington, H., et al. (2011). A gradient of childhood self-control predicts health, wealth, and public safety. *Proceedings of the National Academy of Sciences of the USA, 108*(7), 2693–2698.

Nederkoorn, C., Braet, C., Van Eijs, Y., Tanghe, A., & Jansen, A. (2006). Why obese children cannot resist food: The role of impulsivity. *Eating Behaviors, 7*(4), 315–322.

Nothwehr, F., & Yang, J. (2007). Goal setting frequency and the use of behavioral strategies related to diet and physical activity. *Health Education Research, 22*(4), 532–538.

O'Connor, E. A. (2016, November). *Systematic review of interventions to reduce excess weight in children and adolescents.* Paper presented at the annual meeting of The Obesity Society, New Orleans, LA.

Ogden, C. L., Carroll, M. D., Kit, B. K., & Flegal, K. M. (2014). Prevalence of childhood and adult obesity in the United States, 2011–2012. *Journal of the American Medical Association, 311*(8), 806–814.

Peters, J., & Büchel, C. (2010). Episodic future thinking reduces reward delay discounting through an enhancement of prefrontal–mediotemporal interactions. *Neuron, 66*(1), 138–148.

Quattrin, T., Roemmich, J. N., Paluch, R., Yu, J., Epstein, L. H., & Ecker, M. A. (2012). Efficacy of family-based weight control program for preschool children in primary care. *Pediatrics, 130*(4), 660–666.

Quattrin, T., Roemmich, J. N., Paluch, R., Yu, J., Epstein, L. H., & Ecker, M. A. (2014). Treatment outcomes of overweight children and parents in the medical home. *Pediatrics, 134*(2), 290–297.

Raynor, H., Jeffery, R., Tate, D. F., & Wing, R. (2004). Relationship between changes in food group variety, dietary intake, and weight during obesity treatment. *International Journal of Obesity, 28*(6), 813–820.

Reinehr, T. (2013). Lifestyle intervention in childhood obesity: Changes and challenges. *Nature Reviews. Endocrinology, 9*(10), 607–614.

Reinehr, T., Lass, N., Toschke, C., Rothermel, J., Lanzinger, S., & Holl, R. W. (2016). Which amount of BMI-SDS reduction is necessary to improve cardiovascular risk factors in overweight children? *Journal of Clinical Endocrinology and Metabolism, 101*(8), 3171–3179.

Saelens, B. E., Sallis, J. F., Wilfley, D. E., Patrick, K., Cella, J. A., & Buchta, R. (2002). Behavioral weight control for overweight adolescents initiated in primary care. *Obesity Research, 10*(1), 22–32.

Salvy, S.-J., Bowker, J. W., Roemmich, J. N., Romero, N., Kieffer, E., Paluch, R., et al. (2007). Peer influence on children's physical activity: An experience sampling study. *Journal of Pediatric Psychology, 33*(1), 39–49.

Schneider, S., Peters, J., Peth, J., & Büchel, C. (2014). Parental inconsistency, impulsive choice and neural value representations in healthy adolescents. *Translational Psychiatry, 4*(4), e382.

Simpson, L. A., & Cooper, J. (2009). Paying for obesity: A changing landscape. *Pediatrics, 123*(Suppl. 5), S301–S307.

Skinner, B. F. (1938). *The behavior of organisms: An experimental analysis.* New York: Appleton-Century-Crofts.

Tanofsky-Kraff, M., Yanovski, S. Z., Wilfley, D. E., Marmarosh, C., Morgan, C. M., & Yanovski, J. A. (2004). Eating-disordered behaviors, body fat, and psychopathology in overweight and normal-weight children. *Journal of Consulting and Clinical Psychology, 72*(1), 53.

Temple, J. L., Legierski, C. M., Giacomelli, A. M., Salvy, S.-J., & Epstein, L. H. (2008). Overweight children find food more reinforcing and consume more energy than do nonoverweight children. *American Journal of Clinical Nutrition, 87*(5), 1121–1127.

Terrace, H. S. (1966). Stimulus control. In W. K. Honig (Ed.), *Operant behavior: Areas of research and application* (pp. 271–344). New York: Appleton-Century-Crofts.

Verbeken, S., Braet, C., Goossens, L., & Van der Oord, S. (2013). Executive function training with game elements for obese children: A novel treatment to enhance self-regulatory abilities for weight-control. *Behaviour Research and Therapy, 51*(6), 290–299.

Whitlock, E. P., O'Connor, E. A., Williams, S. B., Beil, T. L., & Lutz, K. W. (2010). Effectiveness of weight management interventions in children: A targeted systematic review for the USPSTF. *Pediatrics, 125*(2), e396–e418.

Wilfley, D. E. (2013, November). *Lifestyle and family-based interventions in obesity.* Paper presented at the annual meeting of The Obesity Society, Atlanta, GA.

Wilfley, D. E., Buren, D. J., Theim, K. R., Stein, R. I., Saelens, B. E., Ezzet, F., et al. (2010). The use of biosimulation in the design of a novel multilevel weight loss maintenance program for overweight children. *Obesity, 18*(Suppl. 1), S91–S98.

Wilfley, D. E., Kass, A. E., & Kolko, R. P. (2011). Counseling and behavior change in pediatric obesity. *Pediatric Clinics of North America, 58*(6), 1403–1424.

Wilfley, D. E., Stein, R. I., Saelens, B. E., Mockus, D. S., Matt, G. E., Hayden-Wade, H. A., et al. (2007). Efficacy of maintenance treatment approaches for childhood overweight: A randomized controlled trial. *Journal of the American Medical Association, 298*(14), 1661–1673.

Wilfley, D. E., Tibbs, T. L., Van Buren, D., Reach, K. P., Walker, M. S., & Epstein, L. H. (2007). Lifestyle interventions in the treatment of childhood overweight: A meta-analytic review of randomized controlled trials. *Health Psychology, 26*(5), 521–532.

Wrotniak, B. H., Epstein, L. H., Paluch, R. A., & Roemmich, J. N. (2004). Parent weight change as a predictor of child weight change in family-based behavioral obesity treatment. *Archives of Pediatrics and Adolescent Medicine, 158*(4), 342–347.

Young, K. M., Northern, J. J., Lister, K. M., Drummond, J. A., & O'Brien, W. H. (2007). A meta-analysis of family-behavioral weight-loss treatments for children. *Clinical Psychology Review, 27*(2), 240–249.

CHAPTER 40

Pharmacological Treatment of Pediatric Obesity

Robert I. Berkowitz
Ariana M. Chao

Obesity in children and adolescents is a major public health problem in the United States. This condition is associated with medical and psychosocial problems, including lipid disorders, type 2 diabetes mellitus, hypertension, obstructive sleep apnea, and psychosocial distress, as discussed by Kral and Berkowitz (Chapter 37, this volume). There is a critical need for strategies and policies to prevent the development of childhood obesity.

Effective weight reduction therapies also are needed for children and adolescents who already are overweight or obese. Lifestyle modification generally results in modest reductions in measures of body mass index (BMI), and there is a clear tendency for relapse over time (Butryn et al., 2011). The addition of weight loss medication to lifestyle modification may significantly improve both the induction and maintenance of weight loss in adolescents, as discussed in a later section of this chapter (Berkowitz, Wadden, Tershakovec, & Cronquist, 2003; Berkowitz et al., 2006). Identifying the potential efficacy and safety of drug treatment for pediatric obesity is an important area of research.

This chapter provides an overview of medications approved by the U.S. Food and Drug Administration (FDA) for the management of obesity in youth. The chapter is necessarily brief because, at the time of this writing, only one medication (orlistat) is approved for use with adolescents. There have been no published reports of the results of pediatric trials of the four new weight loss medications that the FDA recently approved for use with adults.

The present chapter is not intended to provide medical advice regarding whether or not a specific pediatric patient should take medications. Patients are referred to their health care professionals for individual medical assessment and management. In addition, the treatment of pediatric obesity should utilize a staged and individualized approach (Barlow & Dietz, 2002). Weight loss medications may be useful as an adjunct to lifestyle modification programs in pediatric patients who have not made satisfactory progress with behavioral treatment alone or potentially to facilitate long-term maintenance of weight loss (Butryn et al., 2011). However, obesity medications have side effects and, as discussed later, long-term outcome data in pediatric populations are not available. Pharmacotherapy should be considered only for those most likely to benefit, with due consideration of the side effects and risks of the medications, as well as the severity of the patient's obesity, previous weight loss attempts, age, pubertal maturation, and comorbidities (Kelly, Fox, Rudser, Gross, & Ryder, 2016).

Orlistat: The Only FDA-Approved Medication for Pediatric Obesity

Currently, orlistat is the only FDA-approved weight loss medication that may be prescribed as an adjunct to lifestyle modification for youth ages 12 years and older who are obese (BMI ≥ 30 kg/m^2) or who are overweight (BMI ≥ 27 kg/m^2) and have one or more risk factors such as hypertension, type 2 diabetes mellitus, and/or lipid disorders (Genentech USA, Inc., South San Francisco, California; Genentech, 2016). Orlistat is prescribed at 120 mg three times daily, prior to consuming meals containing approximately 30% of calories from fat. The medication also is available over the counter as 60 mg, to be taken three times daily with meals. A daily multivitamin is recommended to provide vitamins A, D, E, and K because these fat-soluble vitamins may not be absorbed as well from the diet while taking orlistat. Vitamins should be taken 2 hours before or after a dose of orlistat.

Mechanisms

Orlistat is a reversible inhibitor of gastrointestinal lipases, which are involved in the breakdown of dietary fat (triglycerides). The medication blocks the absorption of approximately 30% of the fat contained in a meal. The excess fat is not digested or absorbed, but is instead excreted in stool, resulting in a reduction in overall absorption of ingested calories (Chanoine, Hampl, Jensen, Boldrin, & Hauptman, 2005; Genentech, 2016).

Safety and Side Effects

As described in the current drug labeling, the use of orlistat during pregnancy is contraindicated because of possible risks to the fetus. The primary side effects of the drug include excess oil in stool, resulting in fecal urgency with fatty/oily stool, oily evacuation, and fecal incontinence. In addition, the revised labeling of the drug reported that there are potential renal effects. There have been rare cases of oxalate nephrolithiasis and acute oxalate nephropathy with renal failure reported in orlistat-treated patients who were at risk for or had renal disease (Genentech, 2016). There also have been rare cases of hepatotoxicity, including liver injury with hepatocellular necrosis or acute hepatic failure, with some cases resulting in liver transplantation or death (Genentech, 2016). It is not clear whether orlistat was the cause of these adverse hepatic or renal events; however, these potential risks must be considered prior to prescribing orlistat to youth.

Pediatric Use

Orlistat produces modest weight loss in youth when added to a program of lifestyle modification. In the largest study to date (N = 539), youth ages 12–16 years were randomly assigned to orlistat (120 mg three times daily) or to placebo and instructed to consume a hypocaloric diet of conventional foods (with 30% of calories from fat) (Chanoine et al., 2005). At the end of 1 year, youth who received orlistat had a reduction in BMI of 0.55 kg/m^2, compared to an increase of 0.31 kg/m^2 for those on placebo (p = .001). In a responder analysis, 26.5% of youth who took orlistat attained a 5% reduction in BMI compared with 15.6% of those on placebo (p = .005). However, in this study, treatment with orlistat was not associated with significantly greater improvements in lipids, blood pressure, or glucose compared with placebo. Gastrointestinal side effects were significantly more common in the orlistat than in the placebo group.

A secondary analysis of this study examined the relationship between early response to treatment at week 12 and weight change at year 1 in adolescents treated with orlistat or placebo (Chanoine & Richard, 2011). The percentage change in weight at week 12 correlated with the 1-year reduction in weight (r^2 = .41) (p < .001) for all adolescents, regardless of treatment condition. For those who achieved a 5% weight loss at week 12, the amount of weight loss at the end of the study was similar in both the orlistat and placebo conditions. Those taking orlistat, however, were more than twice as likely to lose ≥ 5% of their weight by week 12, as were those on placebo. Orlistat helped more adolescents obtain a larger weight loss at week 12 and, thus, a larger weight loss at year 1. Based on this report, it is advised that use of orlistat should be continued after 12 weeks only in youth who have an early favorable response.

Discussion

Orlistat may facilitate clinically meaningful weight loss in adolescents who respond with at least a 5% or greater weight loss by week 12 of treatment. However, there are rare but serious adverse events associated with the use of orlistat, including liver and kidney problems. Thus, orlistat must be used with caution in adolescents with obesity. The medication should not be used beyond 12 weeks in nonresponders.

Medications Not Currently Approved for Pediatric Obesity but Approved for Adults with Obesity

In addition to orlistat, four medications—lorcaserin, liraglutide, phentermine/topiramate, and naltrexone/bupropion—are approved by the FDA for chronic weight management in adults. These medications are possible candidates for pediatric obesity if efficacy and safety data become available. Bray and Ryan (Chapter 21, this volume) have provided a thorough description of the mechanisms, safety, and efficacy of these four newly approved medications. The next sections of this chapter provide an update on the status of research on these medications in children and adolescents. Until these medications are approved for these populations, their use with youth (i.e., < 18 years of age) must be considered "off label."

Lorcaserin

Lorcaserin is a selective agonist of the serotonin 2C (5-HT_{2C}) receptor, developed for weight management in adults with obesity (Smith et al., 2010). It has a low level of activity at the 5-HT_{2B} receptors; increased activity at these receptors is thought to increase the risk of serotonin-related valvulopathy (Rothman et al., 2000). Stimulation of the 5-HT_{2C} receptors decreases eating through the neural proopiomelancortin (POMC) system (Lam et al., 2008).

Safety

Headache, dizziness, and nausea were more likely to be reported by adults on lorcaserin than by those in the placebo group; both conditions reported similar rates of serious adverse events (Smith et al., 2010). A multisite cardiovascular safety adult trial is ongoing and will provide further data regarding cardiac endpoints.

Pediatric Use

Pharmacokinetic studies of lorcaserin in children and adolescents are being conducted at the time of this writing, and a Phase III trial is being planned (ClinicalTrials.gov, 2014, 2015). However, there currently are no published trials of lorcaserin in children or adolescents, and, thus, use of this medication in youth is considered experimental.

Liraglutide

Liraglutide is a long-acting glucagon-like peptide-1 (GLP-1) agonist. It is an injectable, once-daily, self-administered medication (Blonde & Russell-Jones, 2009). In 2010, liraglutide 1.8 mg/day was approved by the FDA for adults with type 2 diabetes. In 2014, the medication was approved at 3.0 mg/day, combined with a reduced-calorie diet and increased physical activity, for chronic weight management in adults.

Safety

Nausea has been the most frequently reported adverse event with liraglutide 3.0 mg in adults, as well as diarrhea, constipation, vomiting, dyspepsia, abdominal pain, decreased appetite, headache, dizziness, and fatigue (Astrup et al., 2012). Increased lipase has also been seen among patients. The medication has a black-box warning pertaining to the risk of thyroid C-cell tumors, which have been seen in rats and mice. However, the risk of thyroid C-cell tumors in humans is unknown. Liraglutide is contraindicated in adults with a personal or family history of medullary thyroid carcinoma or in patients with multiple endocrine neoplasia syndrome type 2.

Pediatric Use

No randomized controlled trials of the use of liraglutide 3.0 mg for pediatric weight management have been published. Small, short-term studies of liraglutide 1.8 mg have been conducted in youth ages 10–17 years with type 2 diabetes (Klein et al., 2014; Petri, Jacobsen, & Klein, 2015). These trials demonstrated that the medication was well tolerated, with safety and pharmacokinetic profiles similar to those of adults. After 5 weeks, HbA1C was significantly lower in the liraglutide group than in placebo (–0.86 vs. 0.04%). However, groups did not differ in mean body weight change.

Phentermine Extended Release/Topiramate Extended Release

Phentermine extended release (ER) is a sympathomimetic, anorexigenic medication that is FDA-approved for the short-term (≤12 weeks) management of obesity in adults with a BMI ≥ 30 kg/m^2 or BMI ≥ 27 kg/m^2 with obesity-related comorbidities. This medication may reduce appetite by stimulating the release of norepinephrine or inhibiting adrenaline reuptake into the nerve terminals to cause early satiety (Bray & Greenway, 1999). Phentermine is pharmacologically related to amphetamine and has been designated a Schedule IV controlled substance to indicate a relatively low potential for abuse (Heal et al., 1998). Topiramate ER is FDA-approved for use as an antiepileptic (in persons ≥ 2 years of age) and for treatment of migraine headache (in persons ≥ 12 years of age). It is not approved as monotherapy for obesity in adults or children. The exact weight loss mechanisms of topiramate are unknown but are hypothesized to suppress appetite and improve satiety through enhancement of the inhibitory activity of gamma-aminobutyric acid (GABA), modulation of voltage-gated ion channels, inhibition of carbonic anhydrase, and/or inhibition of AMPA/kainite excitatory glutamate receptors (Allison et al., 2012).

In 2012, the FDA approved the combination of phentermine and topiramate ER (7.5 mg/46 mg or 15 mg/92 mg) for the treatment of adult obesity. Approval was based on findings that the combination of the two medications, used at low doses, produced equal or greater weight loss, and with a more favorable side-effect profile, than either drug used alone as a monotherapy (at the same dose) (Aronne et al., 2013). The combination is believed to better address the complex neural regulation of body weight than can a single medication.

Safety

In adult trials, the most common side effects of phentermine ER/topiramate ER are paresthesia, dizziness, dysgeusia, insomnia, constipation, and dry mouth. The treatment combination has also been associated with metabolic acidosis, depression, anxiety, cognitive effects (e.g., disturbed attention), increased heart rate, and kidney stones (Gadde et al., 2011). The medication has a warning of potential increased risk for orofacial clefts in neonates exposed to topiramate and requires effective contraception and monthly pregnancy tests for females of reproductive age. The medication is not recommended for patients with cardiovascular disease and is contraindicated in patients with glaucoma, hyperthyroidism, and within 14 days of treatment with monoamine oxidase inhibitors.

Pediatric Use

Results from randomized pediatric studies of phentermine ER/topirimate ER have not been reported. However, pharmacokinetic studies for adolescent obesity are currently ongoing (ClinicalTrials.gov, 2016). The combination of phentermine ER/topiramate ER is not recommended at this time. Similarly, the long-term safety and effectiveness of phentermine, as used alone in pediatric (or adult) patients, has not been established, although there have been some small short-term trials in youth (Lorber, 1966). Childhood obesity is a chronic condition and requires long-term treatment. Thus, the short-term use of phentermine as monotherapy in pediatric patients is not recommended.

Naltrexone Sustained Release/Bupropion Sustained Release

Naltrexone sustained release (SR) is an opioid antagonist and has minimum effect on weight loss on its own. Bupropion (SR) is an aminoketone approved for the treatment of depression and for smoking cessation in adults. It is a mild reuptake inhibitor of dopamine and norepinephrine. The combination of naltrexone and bupropion is based on the premise that naltrexone can block POMC neuron autoinhibition by endogenous opioids, whereas bupropion augments the anorexic alpha-melanocyte-stimulating hormone release (Greenway et al., 2010; Plodkowski et al., 2009). The combination of naltrexone SR/bupropion SR (32 mg/360 mg) was approved for use in adults by the FDA in 2012.

Safety

Nausea has been the most frequent adverse event with naltrexone SR/bupropion SR, along with constipation, headache, vomiting, dizziness, and insomnia. There is also concern about an increased risk of seizures with the use of bupropion (Greenway et al., 2010; Wadden et al., 2011). Naltrexone SR/bupropion SR also may increase blood pressure and pulse, or attenuate improvements in these, which are outcomes expected with weight loss. Thus, the combination should be prescribed only to patients with controlled hypertension, and blood pressure should be monitored in the early weeks of therapy. All antidepressants in the United States are required to carry a black-box warning of suicidality, and the combination's label includes this label. However, there was no signal of suicidality in Phase III studies.

Pediatric Use

No randomized controlled trials of naltrexone SR/bupropion SR conducted with pediatric patients have been published. Thus, this medication is not recommended for pediatric use until there are sufficient data on its long-term safety and efficacy in youth.

Use of Metformin in Youth with Obesity

Metformin is a biguanide antihyperglycemic agent that is FDA-approved for the treatment of diabetes mellitus in children older than 10 years. The ER formulations are approved for individuals older than 18 years. Metformin improves glucose tolerance in patients with type 2 diabetes and lowers both basal and postprandial plasma glucose by decreasing intestinal absorption of glucose, reducing hepatic glucose production, and increasing peripheral glucose uptake and utilization (Bailey & Turner, 1996; Brufani et al., 2011). Common side effects of metformin include diarrhea, nausea/vomiting, flatulence, asthenia, indigestion, abdominal discomfort, and headache (Park, Kinra, Ward, White, & Viner, 2009).

A number of randomized clinical trials have tested the efficacy of metformin in youth, although the majority of trials have been conducted with small samples, adolescents ages 12–19 years, and with a treatment duration of 6 months or less (Brufani et al., 2013). Among youth with obesity and without diabetes, after 6–12 months of treatment, metformin (1,000–2,000 mg/day) produced modest but significantly greater mean reductions in BMI than placebo or lifestyle intervention alone. Results from systematic reviews and meta-analyses revealed an overall placebo-subtracted reduction of 1.1–2.7 kg/m^2 for participants treated with metformin (Bouza, Lopez-Cuadrado, Gutierrez-Torres, & Amate, 2012; Brufani et al., 2013; Park et al., 2009). Metformin also has favorable effects on some metabolic parameters, although these results have been inconsistent in youth without diabetes. In a systematic review of metformin trials among youth without comorbidities (e.g., diabetes, metabolic syndrome, polycystic ovary syndrome), after treatment, fasting insulin decreased 9.94 μU/ml, and the mean homeostatic model assessment of insulin resistance score declined by 1.78. However, metformin yielded no improvements in lipid values (Bouza et al., 2012). Further research is needed regarding metformin's longer-term safety and efficacy in order to consider this medication for the treatment of pediatric obesity.

A Model for Combining Weight Loss Medication with Lifestyle Modification

We anticipate that some of the medications approved by the FDA (since 2012) for the chronic management of obesity in adults will eventually be approved for pediatric populations. In the event that they are, we strongly recommend that weight loss medications prescribed for youth be used as an adjunct to a high-intensity lifestyle modification program, which has been described by Balantekin, Wilfley, and Epstein (Chapter 39, this volume). Our recommendation is based on findings from two studies of sibutramine that combined this medication with an intensive family-based program of lifestyle modification. Sibutramine was removed from the marked in 2010 because of findings that it increased the risk of cardiovascular disease (CVD) morbidity and mortality in adults with a prior history of CVD (James et al., 2010). Nonetheless, the two studies provide a model of how future FDA-approved medications for youth can be used most effectively.

A total of 82 adolescents, ages 13–17 years with a BMI of 32–44 kg/m^2, participated in an initial, single-site randomized controlled trial (Berkowitz et al., 2003). All teens received a comprehensive family-based behavioral weight loss program delivered through detailed treatment manuals. In the first 6 months, participants attended 13 weekly group sessions, followed by six every-other-week group sessions. For the second 6 months, group sessions were held every other week from months 7–9 and monthly from months 10–12. Parents met separately in group sessions held on the same schedule as the adolescents' meetings. Adolescents were instructed to consume a 1,200–1,500 kcal/day diet of conventional foods, with approximately 30% from fat, 15% from protein, and the remainder from carbohydrate. They were prescribed an eventual goal of walking or engaging in similar aerobic activity for 120 minutes per week or more. Participants kept daily eating and activity logs that they submitted at each session. The content of the parents' sessions paralleled that of their children's sessions.

In this double-blind trial, half of the participants were randomly assigned to receive up to 15 mg/day of sibutramine and the other half to receive placebo. To facilitate participant retention, the study was converted to an open-label trial at month 7, and placebo-treated participants were given sibutramine. Those originally assigned to sibutramine continued to receive it for the full year.

At month 6, participants treated with behavior therapy plus sibutramine had achieved a mean reduction in initial BMI of 8.5%, compared to a significantly smaller 4.0% in participants who received behavior therapy plus placebo ($p = .002$). In the following 6-month open-label phase, adolescents who remained on sibutramine maintained their reduction in BMI of 8.6%, and those switched from placebo to sibutramine had a further reduction to 6.4% at month 12 (with no significant differences between groups at this time). Thus, adolescents initially treated with sibutramine reached their maximal weight loss by month 6 and maintained their weight loss at month 12, whereas those first treated with behavior therapy and placebo—with sibutramine added in the second phase—achieved additional weight loss at month 12.

Findings from our single-site study of behavior therapy and sibutramine were replicated in a multisite trial of 498 adolescents, confirming the effectiveness of this combined approach (Berkowitz et al., 2006). These collective findings lead us to believe that a lifestyle intervention typically should be used to induce weight loss with adolescents. Medication may be introduced later in treatment, both to induce further weight loss and/or to facilitate weight loss maintenance. Further studies in adolescents, using new medications, are needed to address the efficacy, timing, and maintenance of weight loss with pharmacological treatment.

Conclusion

There have been relatively few randomized controlled trials of weight loss medications in adolescents and fewer still in children. Orlistat is the only FDA-approved weight loss medication available for adolescents ages 12 years and older, but it is associated with only modest weight loss, gastrointestinal side effects, rare but potentially serious liver and renal disorders, and no improvement in cardiometabolic risk factors. Given these concerns, the use of orlistat is recommended with caution for the treatment of obesity in adolescents and only for long-term use in those who lose ≥ 5% of weight in the first 12 weeks. New medications have been approved for use in adults, including loracersin, liraglutide 3.0 mg, phentermine ER/topirimate ER, and bupropion SR/naltrexone SR. Long-term safety and efficacy trials of these medications clearly are needed as prescribed for children and adolescents. There is a pressing need for more treatment options for these age groups.

References

Allison, D. B., Gadde, K. M., Garvey, W. T., Peterson, C. A., Schwiers, M. L., Najarian, T., et al. (2012). Controlled-release phentermine/topiramate in severely obese adults: A randomized controlled trial (EQUIP). *Obesity, 20*(2), 330–342.

Aronne, L. J., Wadden, T. A., Peterson, C., Winslow, D., Odeh, S., & Gadde, K. M. (2013). Evaluation of phentermine and topirimate versus phentermine/topirimate extended-release in obese adults. *Obesity (Silver Spring), 21*, 2163–2171.

Astrup, A., Carraro, R., Finer, N., Harper, A., Kunesova, M., Lean, M., et al. (2012). Safety, tolerability, and sustained weight loss over 2 years with the once-daily human GLP-1 analog, liraglutide. *International Journal of Obesity, 36*(6), 843–854.

Bailey, C. J., & Turner, R. C. (1996). Metformin. *New England Journal of Medicine, 334*(9), 574–579.

Barlow, S. E., & Dietz, W. H. (2002). Management of child and adolescent obesity: Summary and recommendations based on reports from pediatricians, pediatric nurse practitioners, and registered dietitians. *Pediatrics, 110*(Suppl. 1), 236–238.

Berkowitz, R. I., Fujioka, K., Daniels, S. R., Hoppin, A. G., Owen, S., Perry, A. C., et al. (2006). Effects of sibutramine treatment in obese adolescents: A randomized trial. *Annals of Internal Medicine, 145*(2), 81–90.

Berkowitz, R. I., Wadden, T. A., Tershakovec, A. M., & Cronquist, J. L. (2003). Behavior therapy and sibutramine for the treatment of adolescent obesity: A randomized controlled trial. *Journal of the American Medical Association, 289*(14), 1805–1812.

Blonde, L., & Russell-Jones, D. (2009). The safety and efficacy of liraglutide with or without oral antidiabetic drug therapy in type 2 diabetes: An overview of the LEAD 1–5 studies. *Diabetes, Obesity and Metabolism, 11*(Suppl. 3), 26–34.

Bouza, C., Lopez-Cuadrado, T., Gutierrez-Torres, L., & Amate, J. (2012). Efficacy and safety of metformin for treatment of overweight and obesity in adolescents: An updated systematic review and meta-analysis. *Obesity Facts, 5*(5), 753–765.

Bray, G. A., & Greenway, F. L. (1999). Current and potential drugs for treatment of obesity. *Endocrine Reviews, 20*(6), 805–875.

Brufani, C., Crinò, A., Fintini, D., Patera, P. I., Cappa, M., & Manco, M. (2013). Systematic review of metformin use in obese nondiabetic children and adolescents. *Hormone Research in Paediatrics, 80*(2), 78–85.

Brufani, C., Fintini, D., Nobili, V., Patera, P. I., Cappa, M., & Brufani, M. (2011). Use of metformin in pediatric age. *Pediatric Diabetes, 12*(6), 580–588.

Butryn, M. L., Wadden, T. A., Rukstalis, M. R., Bishop-Gilyard, C., Xanthopoulos, M. S., Louden, D., et al. (2011). Maintenance of weight loss in adolescents: Current status and future directions. *Journal of Obesity, 2010*(2), 1–12.

Chanoine, J. P., Hampl, S., Jensen, C., Boldrin, M., & Hauptman, J. (2005). Effect of orlistat on weight and body composition in obese adolescents: A randomized controlled trial. *Journal of the American Medical Association, 293*(23), 2873–2883.

Chanoine, J. P., & Richard, M. (2011). Early weight loss and outcome at one year in obese adolescents treated with orlistat or placebo. *International Journal of Pediatric Obesity, 6*(2), 95–101.

ClinicalTrials.gov. (2014). Single dose study to determine the safety, tolerability, and pharmacokinetic properties of lorcaserin hydrochloride (BELVIQ) in obese adolescents from 12 to 17 years of age. Retrieved from *https://clinicaltrials.gov/ct2/show/NCT02022956*.

ClinicalTrials.gov. (2015). A single dose pharmacokinetic study of lorcaserin hydrochloride in obese pediatric subjects 6 to 11 years of age. Retrieved from *https://clinicaltrials.gov/ct2/show/NCT02398669*.

ClinicalTrials.gov. (2016). A pharmacokinetic study comparing VI-0521 with placebo in obese adolescents. Retrieved from *https://clinicaltrials.gov/ct2/show/NCT02714062?term=phentermine+topiramate&rank=8*.

Gadde, K. M., Allison, D. B., Ryan, D. H., Peterson, C. A., Troupin, B., Schwiers, M. L., et al. (2011). Effects of low-dose, controlled-release, phentermine plus topiramate combination on weight and associated comorbidities in overweight and obese adults (CONQUER): A randomised, placebo-controlled, phase 3 trial. *Lancet, 377*(9774), 1341–1352.

Genentech, I. (2016). Xenical (orlistat) prescribing information. Retrieved from *www.gene.com/download/pdf/xenical_prescribing.pdf*.

Greenway, F. L., Fujioka, K., Plodkowski, R. A., Mudaliar, S., Guttadauria, M., Erickson, J., et al. (2010). Effect of naltrexone plus bupropion on weight loss in overweight and obese adults (COR-I): A multicentre, randomised, double-blind, placebo-controlled, phase 3 trial. *Lancet, 376*(9741), 595–605.

Heal, D., Aspley, S., Prow, M., Jackson, H., Martin, K., & Cheetham, S. (1998). Sibutramine: A novel anti-obesity drug: A review of the pharmacological evidence to differentiate it from d-amphetamine and d-fenfluramine. *International Journal of Obesity and Related Metabolic Disorders, 22*(Suppl.), S18–S28; discussion S29.

James, W. P. T., Caterson, I. D., Coutinho, W., Finer, N., Van Gaal, L. F., Maggioni, A. P., et al. (2010). Effect of sibutramine on cardiovascular outcomes in overweight and obese subjects. *New England Journal of Medicine, 363*(10), 905–917.

Kelly, A., Fox, C., Rudser, K., Gross, A., & Ryder, J. (2016). Pediatric obesity pharmacotherapy: Current state of the field, review of the literature and clinical trial considerations. *International Journal of Obesity, 40*(7), 1043–1050.

Klein, D. J., Battelino, T., Chatterjee, D., Jacobsen, L. V., Hale, P. M., & Arslanian, S. (2014). Liraglutide's safety, tolerability, pharmacokinetics, and pharmacodynamics in pediatric type 2 diabetes: A randomized, double-blind, placebo-controlled trial. *Diabetes Technology and Therapeutics, 16*(10), 679–687.

Lam, D. D., Przydzial, M. J., Ridley, S. H., Yeo, G. S., Rochford, J. J., O'Rahilly, S., & Heisler, L. K. (2008). Serotonin 5-HT2C receptor agonist promotes hypophagia via downstream activation of melanocortin 4 receptors. *Endocrinology, 149*(3), 1323–1328.

Lorber, J. (1966). Obesity in childhood: A controlled trial of anorectic drugs. *Archives of Disease in Childhood, 41*(217), 309–312.

Park, M. H., Kinra, S., Ward, K. J., White, B., & Viner, R. M. (2009). Metformin for obesity in children and adolescents: A systematic review. *Diabetes Care, 32*(9), 1743–1745.

Petri, K. C. C., Jacobsen, L. V., & Klein, D. J. (2015). Comparable liraglutide pharmacokinetics in pediatric and adult populations with type 2 diabetes: A population pharmacokinetic analysis. *Clinical Pharmacokinetics, 54*(6), 663–670.

Plodkowski, R. A., Nguyen, Q., Sundaram, U., Nguyen, L., Chau, D. L., & St. Jeor, S. (2009). Bupropion and naltrexone: A review of their use individually and in combination for the treatment of obesity. *Expert Opinion on Pharmacotherapy, 10*(6), 1069–1081.

Rothman, R. B., Baumann, M. H., Savage, J. E., Rauser, L., McBride, A., Hufeisen, S. J., et al. (2000). Evidence for possible involvement of 5-HT2B receptors in the cardiac valvulopathy associated with fenfluramine and other serotonergic medications. *Circulation, 102*(23), 2836–2841.

Smith, S. R., Weissman, N. J., Anderson, C. M., Sanchez, M., Chuang, E., Stubbe, S., et al. (2010). Multicenter, placebo-controlled trial of lorcaserin for weight management. *New England Journal of Medicine, 363*(3), 245–256.

Wadden, T. A., Foreyt, J. P., Foster, G. D., Hill, J. O., Klein, S., O'Neil, P. M., et al. (2011). Weight loss with naltrexone SR/bupropion SR combination therapy as an adjunct to behavior modification: The COR-BMOD trial. *Obesity, 19*(1), 110–120.

CHAPTER 41

Bariatric Surgery in Adolescents with Severe Obesity

Andrew J. Beamish
Thomas H. Inge

The development of obesity has increasingly shifted toward childhood (Shah, D'Alessio, Ford-Adams, Desai, & Inge, 2016). Over one in five children globally is classified as overweight (Ng et al., 2014), and one in six children in the United States has obesity (Ogden, Carroll, Kit, & Flegal, 2014). Despite significant investment of effort and resources, effective strategies to address obesity—including its prevention and treatment—are lacking around the globe (NCD Risk Factor Collaboration, 2016; Kelly, Barlow, Rao, Inge, Hayman, Steinberger, et al., 2013). With this paucity of therapeutic options, the child with obesity is highly unlikely to become a normal-weight adult (Freedman et al., 2005) and likely faces a lifelong battle with excess weight and the myriad life-changing (Ebbeling, Pawlak, & Ludwig, 2002; Juonala et al., 2011), life-threatening (Pinhas-Hamiel & Zeitler, 2007), and life-shortening (Olshansky et al., 2005) comorbidities that can be expected to follow. Given the successful development of surgical programs in the adult population, with excellent outcomes across several decades (Sjöström, 2013), the introduction of surgery in adolescent obesity programs is increasingly offering hope of significant and apparently lasting improvement for adolescents with severe obesity. This chapter describes the emergence of adult bariatric surgical practice and explores its application to adolescents with severe obesity. We examine appropriate patient selection, the multidisciplinary team (MDT), surgical considerations, and patient outcomes, both favorable and detrimental.

History of Bariatric Surgery

The roots of bariatric surgery can be traced to the middle of the 20th century, when J. Howard Payne described the jejunocolic shunt (Payne, Dewind, & Commons, 1963). Involving the bypass of most of the small intestine, this radical procedure was extremely effective in achieving significant weight loss, but at the expense of markedly negative side effects. More than half of patients required reoperation to reestablish normal gastrointestinal anatomy, following the development of dehydrating diarrhea, profound nutritional deficiencies, and numerous other adverse outcomes (Payne et al., 1963).

Meanwhile, surgeons observed that weight loss and failure to regain weight were frequent consequences of existing gastrointestinal procedures that were performed to treat conditions unrelated to obesity, such as peptic ulceration (Warren & Meadows, 1949) and carcinoma of the stomach (Harnett, 1947). These undesirable weight loss effects were reappropriated to the expanding field of severe obesity, as Edward E. Mason reported in 1967. The new gastric bypass procedure involved bypassing most of the stomach in order to induce weight loss (Mason & Ito, 1967). This proved to be extremely effective, with the average weight loss at 12 months reported to be 44 kg (Mason & Ito, 1969). However, in these early days, an associated mortality above 8% made this a high-risk procedure by modern standards (Royal College of Surgeons of England/Department of Health, 2011).

Roux-en-Y gastric bypass (RYGB) is now the world's most commonly performed bariatric procedure, both in adolescents (Beamish, Johansson, et al., 2015) and adults (Angrisani et al., 2015). However, sleeve gastrectomy (SG) is rapidly gaining acceptance (Esteban Varela & Nguyen, 2015).

The first reports of RYGB performed on children and adolescents followed less than a decade after Mason's initial reports in adults (Randolph, Weintraub, & Rigg, 1974; Soper, Mason, Printen, & Zellweger, 1975). Interest in the potential benefits and risks of adolescent bariatric surgery reemerged in the early part of this century, yielding increasingly more data evaluating outcomes of more modern operations.

Much of the emerging literature highlights considerations that are specific to adolescents, whose growth and development may be incomplete. The potential for detrimental nutritional effects, coupled with the intended lifelong duration of action, raises concern regarding adequate bioavailability of key micronutrients. Long-term outcomes related to nutritional status after bariatric surgery and the potential effect upon micronutrient-dependent systems, such as blood and the skeleton, have not yet been adequately documented in this population. However, the adolescent already suffering from severe obesity is afforded limited options to improve his or her personal future health prospects, both near and distant. In these individuals, surgery can offer a uniquely effective therapeutic option to improve weight and cardiometabolic health and to decrease risk factors (Beamish, Johansson, & Olbers, 2015).

Patient Selection in Adolescents with Severe Obesity

Patient selection is crucially important in order to maximize the potential for benefit and minimize the risk of suboptimal or adverse outcomes. Selection criteria for adult bariatric surgery were developed at the 1991 NIH Consensus Development Program (National Institutes of Health, 1991), and have not received a major revision since. Consensus guidelines for adolescent bariatric surgery have been based upon the guidelines for adults (Pratt et al., 2009). Adolescent criteria also take account of the ongoing growth of adolescents, and investigators have demonstrated epidemiologically that the adult body mass index (BMI) definitions of 25 kg/m^2 for overweight and 30 kg/m^2 for obesity equate to values of 22 kg/m^2 and 27 kg/m^2 at age 13 years (Cole, Bellizzi, Flegal, & Dietz, 2000). Across adolescence, these values rise to meet adult definitions at 18 years (Cole et al., 2000). While evidence shows that both cardiovascular and metabolic risks rise when BMI for age is greater than the 99th percentile in adolescents (Freedman, Mei, Srinivasan, Berenson, & Dietz, 2007), this group includes all boys and most girls with a BMI exceeding 35 kg/m^2 (Freedman et al., 2007). For this reason, current guidelines follow criteria similar to the original NIH standards, recommending that adolescents should qualify for bariatric surgery if they have a BMI of 35 kg/m^2, accompanied by "serious" (major) comorbidity, or a BMI of 40 kg/m^2, accompanied by "other" (minor) comorbidity (Table 41.1). This guideline allows for a relatively more conservative selection with decreasing patient age. This guidance (Pratt et al., 2009) defines serious comorbidity as including type 2 diabetes mellitus (T2DM), pseudotumor cerebri, moderate or severe obstructive sleep apnea (OSA), or severe steatohepatitis. "Other" comorbidity includes dyslipidemia, hypertension, glucose intolerance, insulin resistance, mild OSA, impaired quality of life, and a number of other conditions (see Figure 41.1 and Table 41.1).

A number of additional prerequisites are generally followed. Individuals should be sufficiently well-developed physically, defined as having reached at least Tanner Stage IV, along with 95% growth attainment (Michalsky et al., 2012). Perhaps of greatest importance, the patient's family members or caregivers should demonstrate committed social support and a genuine understanding of the procedure and its risks and benefits, as should the patient. They should be able to fully comprehend the necessary short- and long-term lifestyle requirements in diet and meal intake (including nutritional supplementation) required by the adolescent, with realistic expectations for change (Table 41.2).

Psychosocial comorbidities are particularly common among adolescents with severe obesity (Herget, Rudolph, Hilbert, & Bluher, 2014). A history of such conditions is not an absolute contraindication, but psychosocial conditions must be under control and monitored by mental health profes-

TABLE 41.1. Comorbidity Examples for Patient Selection

Exceptional circumstances
- Life-threatening obesity-related comorbidities

Major comorbidity
- Type 2 diabetes mellitus
- Heart failure due to obesity
- Moderate–severe obstructive sleep apnea
- Benign intracranial hypertension

Minor comorbidity
- Impaired fasting glucose
- Impaired glucose tolerance
- Dyslipidemia
- Hypertension
- Steatohepatitis
- Mild obstructive sleep apnea
- Panniculitis
- Venous stasis
- Gastroesophageal reflux disease
- Urinary incontinence
- Weight-related joint disease
- Body size precluding ambulation
- Impaired activities of daily living
- Severe psychosocial morbidity

Note. See Figure 41.1 for the patient selection pathway.

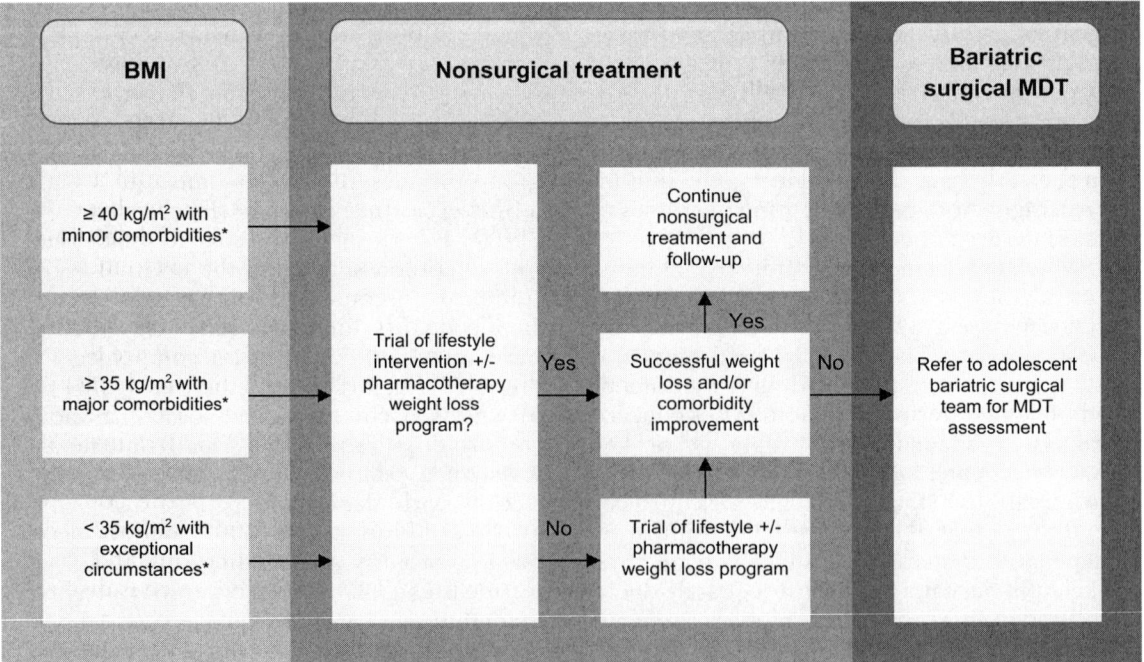

FIGURE 41.1. Inclusion pathway for adolescent bariatric surgery. *See Table 41.1 for clarification of minor or major comorbidity status and exceptional circumstances.

TABLE 41.2. Exclusion Criteria

Patient and family understanding
- Not fully committed to follow-up
- Unable to understand risks and benefits
- Unable to assent/consent as appropriate

Patient factors
- Treatable medical cause of obesity
- Skeletal immaturity (Tanner Stage ≤ III)
- Unstable psychiatric condition
- Ongoing addiction (alcohol, drugs, medication)

Note. See Figure 41.1 for the patient selection pathway.

sionals prior to and after surgery. Severe or unstable psychosis, major depression, or borderline personality disorder should be considered contraindications (Table 41.2), although formal discussion of individual circumstances should be undertaken by the MDT for these patients.

The MDT

All aspects of bariatric surgery for adolescents should be provided by an experienced MDT. This is consistent with existing guidance (Pratt et al., 2009) and is essential to enable effective evaluation, according to the above selection criteria, as well as optimization for surgery and preparation for its lifelong success. The inclusion of several central members of the MDT is recommended, consistent with guidance from the American Society for Metabolic and Bariatric Surgery (ASMBS; Michalsky et al., 2012), including either a pediatric surgeon with bariatric experience or a bariatric surgeon with pediatric experience, a pediatrician, dietitian, mental health specialist, physical therapist or exercise physiologist, and a dedicated clinical coordinator. A positive experience has been reported by employing a team of surgeons, incorporating the skills of both a bariatric surgeon and a pediatric surgeon simultaneously (Olbers et al., 2012).

The pediatrician should have specialist expertise in obesity medicine, endocrinology, gastroenterology, nutrition, or adolescent medicine. A family practitioner with experience in adolescent medicine is also appropriate. The dietitian should have experience in working with adolescents and the family unit. The mental health specialist could be a psychologist or psychiatrist with experience both in obesity and in the assessment of children or adolescents. The physical therapist or exercise physiologist should have specific experience in the provision of safe activity programs for youth with severe obesity. A coordinator is essential to the effective function of the team and to a positive outcome for the patient. This individual coordinates the overall care pathway of each patient within the service, acting as a trusted and accessible regular point of contact for the adolescent and their family. The coordinator, often an advanced practice nurse or social worker, may be key to ensuring that follow-up appointments are kept and that the patient adheres to treatment recommendations. Beyond the core MDT members, further expertise is often necessary across a wide breadth of specialties, including but not limited to endocrinology, cardiology, pulmonology, gynecology, gastroenterology, sleep disorders, and radiology.

Bariatric Surgical Procedures

The evolution of bariatric surgery across more than half a century has resulted in a range of available procedures, three of which dominate in adults and have been used in most reports of adolescent bariatric surgery. These are the RYGB, SG, and adjustable gastric band (AGB). RYGB has been the most commonly used thus far in adolescents, although the use of SG continues to increase and may outpace RYGB in the near future (Michalsky et al., 2012). Having emerged much more recently, SG and AGB are understandably supported by a thinner literature base than RYGB (Soper et al., 1975).

The earliest bariatric procedures involved bypassing portions of the gastrointestinal tract, and RYGB capitalizes on this concept, rearranging the gut to bypass almost all of the stomach, the entire duodenum, and up to 3 feet of the jejunum. The stomach is disconnected, but not excised, leaving only a small gastric pouch, measuring approximately 25 ml. The jejunum is anastomosed onto this pouch, approximately 50–100 cm distal to the ligament of Trietz, becoming the Roux limb beyond this gastrojejunal anastomosis. Proximal to the anastomosis, the jejunum is transected before being anastomosed a further 80–150 cm along the new Roux limb. Digestive juices pass through this biliary limb and jejuno–jejunal anastomosis to meet ingested food, as the Roux and biliary limbs converge to become a common channel.

Unlike RYGB, SG involves excision of a large part of the stomach. On the distal greater curvature, beginning approximately 5 cm proximal to the pylorus, multiple firings of a linear cutting stapler are deployed around a calibration bougie, progressing proximally until reaching the angle of His. Once complete, the remnant stomach is tubular in shape, resembling a sleeve and measuring approximately one-quarter of its original volume.

The AGB is the only procedure of the three that is considered reversible. It is less invasive than RYGB or SG, and involves the insertion of a synthetic device around the proximal stomach, permitting adjustable restriction of the passage of food and, as a result, limiting the volume of food that the individual can ingest. Adjustment of restriction is achieved by injection and withdrawal of saline into a balloon within the band, via a port situated within the anterior abdominal wall.

There is currently debate regarding which procedure should be used with adolescents, and decisions are based on the MDT's interpretation of an individual patient's circumstances, drawing on experience and evidence from surgery with adults. Adequately designed and powered prospective controlled trials are needed to compare the outcomes of existing procedures in adolescents (Beamish, 2016). A number of trials are ongoing in adults, including the BEST trial (Olbers, 2015) in Sweden (ClinicalTrials.gov: NCT02767505) and the By-Band-Sleeve trial (Rogers et al., 2014) in the United Kingdom (*isrctn.com*: ISRCTN00786323), both comparing long-term outcomes of RYGB and SG. The latter trial also includes AGB.

A 2013 meta-analysis of five small trials that compared outcomes after RYGB and SG in 396 adults reported that RYGB resulted in a greater percentage of excess weight loss and superior metabolic outcomes, including remission of T2DM and normalization of insulin levels, LDL and triglycerides levels, and insulin resistance (Li, Lai, Ni, & Sun, 2013). However, these favorable outcomes came at the expense of slightly greater risk of complications in RYGB.

Advocates of AGB often cite its reversibility and limited invasiveness as a main benefit (O'Brien et al., 2010). However, its mechanism of action is predominantly restrictive/obstructive, physically limiting the volume that individuals can consume. This is in contrast to RYGB, which primarily affects multiple axes of gut–brain signaling, thereby altering patterns of hunger and satiety. RYGB's proven effectiveness in reversing comorbidities and reducing weight in the long term in adults, coupled with a long record of safety, provide a strong argument for its proponents. However, as SG use increases (Inge et al., 2014; Michalsky et al., 2012), an increasing body of evidence suggests that its benefits in adolescents appear similar, at least in the short term, to those of RYGB (Beamish, Johansson, et al., 2015; Inge et al., 2015). There is evidence that nutritional deficiency occurs after bariatric surgery, although the extent appears to be similar following RYGB and SG (Moize et al., 2013).

Preoperative Workup

Potential surgical candidates must be formally assessed for their eligibility. This should incorporate not only an assessment of the individual's general physical health, comorbid diseases, and nutritional status, but also psychosocial elements such as motivation of both patient and family. These individuals must understand that major dietary changes and long-term follow-up care are required following surgery (Fried et al., 2007). Any identified comorbidities should be optimally managed with referral to allied specialists. Arrangements should be in place to allow assessment, when necessary, of metabolic and endocrine function, pulmonary function and sleep apnea, helicobacter pylori testing, body composition and bone density assessments, and indirect calorimetry.

Psychological evaluation is extremely important in this group because adolescent obesity is associated with a particularly high prevalence of anxiety, depressive symptoms, low quality of life, and low self-esteem (Jarvholm et al., 2015). Although many patients experience improvements in psychosocial health, as many as 19% of adolescents experience ongoing symptoms 2 years after RYGB (Jarvholm et al., 2015). Thorough discussion of these and other benefits and risks of surgery is essential in advance of any decision to operate. In addition, unreported psychosocial symptoms (e.g., depression, anxiety) should be screened for within the preoperative workup and treated as needed. Surgery should be deferred when necessary, and enhanced psychological follow-up and support should be provided to the most vulnerable individuals.

Adherence to a balanced very-low-calorie diet (e.g., 800 kcal/day) is advisable during the 2 weeks prior to surgery. The adult RYGB literature has shown this presurgical diet component to be associated with reduced postoperative complications and reduced perceived surgical technical difficulty (Van Nieuwenhove et al., 2011).

Perioperative Care

Surgery should be performed in a specialist unit, where the staff has adequate expertise and experience with bariatric surgery and perioperative care. Admission to the hospital on the day of surgery is usually appropriate, and preferably to an environment designed to suit adolescents, rather than younger pediatric age groups. There should be a standardized clinical pathway for these patients, which should follow that established for adults undergoing the same procedures (e.g., informal consent, thromboprophylaxis, preoperative checks).

After surgery, patients should be managed by personnel experienced in adolescent bariatric surgical care. Whereas AGB is often performed as an ambulatory procedure in adults, in this age group it is advisable to observe patients overnight in the hospital. Following the more invasive SG and RYGB procedures, routine analgesia and intravenous maintenance fluids are necessary during the first postoperative 24 hours, and regular small amounts (< 25 ml) of clear fluids are also encouraged, as tolerated. Beyond 24 hours, in the absence of any signs of a postoperative complication, a soft diet may be introduced in small amounts. If soft food is tolerated, discharge with reiteration of postoperative dietary advice is appropriate on post-operative day 2.

Radiological contrast studies are required only if there is clinical evidence of obstruction or significant impediment, such as regurgitation of saliva or disproportionate pain upon swallowing. Routine confirmation of adequate gastrointestinal throughput should rely upon clinical acumen in response to patient symptoms and signs.

Some abdominal discomfort in the first 24–36 hours is common and readily treated with analgesics. Patients and their families should be made aware of this prior to surgery so as to minimize the anxiety it may cause. Discomfort should diminish markedly within the first 2 days. Signs and symptoms of early complications include tachypnea, tachycardia, increased oxygen requirement, fever, regurgitation, excessive pain, decreased conscious level, and anxiety. Such symptoms should arouse suspicion of bleeding, gastric or intestinal obstruction, gastrointestinal leakage, or pulmonary embolus, and should warrant expeditious medical assessment by a senior member of the surgical team.

Dietary difficulties are common after discharge, and arrangements should be made for patients to contact a team member for advice and in case of medical problems. If emergent medical assessment is required in the first 48 hours, an experienced member of the bariatric team should be available to ensure that appropriate assessment and investigations are performed (and that unnecessary investigations are avoided). A routine telephone follow-up call from a member of the bariatric MDT within 48 hours of discharge is advised to ascertain whether recovery is proceeding as planned. Patients should have clear, easy-to-understand, written guidance explaining whom to contact (and under what circumstances) in the early postoperative period.

Postoperative Follow-Up

We advocate frequent follow-up in the early postoperative period, as often as weekly or every 2 weeks for 4–6 weeks. After this, follow up every 4–8 weeks is appropriate to 6 months, then every 3 months until completion of 2 postoperative years. With high rates of successful weight loss and comorbidity resolution, maintaining contact with patients is not always easy. Achieving the U.S. standard of follow-up of three-quarters of patients to a minimum of 5 years can prove difficult (Michalsky et al., 2011). This is potentially made more difficult in the adolescent population by the transfer of care to adult services as patients mature. Specific transitional arrangements should be made in advance (Michalsky et al., 2011), and preparation of the provider in a patient's medical home is important.

Outcomes

A large volume of data has reported weight loss and comorbidity resolution resulting from bariatric surgery in adults, as reviewed by Nor Hanipah, Aminian, and Schauer (Chapter 22, this volume). A recent meta-analysis by Chang et al. (2014) analyzed over 160,000 patients across 164 studies, 37 of which were randomized trials. At 1 year postsurgery, BMI had decreased between 11.8 and 13.5 kg/m^2, which was maintained at 5 years after surgery, when the reduction was between 11.4 and 14.3 kg/m^2. The increasing body of evidence from adolescents shows similar BMI reductions beyond 6 months of 11.6 kg/m^2 after AGB, 14.1 kg/m^2 after SG, and 16.6 kg/m^2 after RYGB. Recent long-term adolescent data suggest that the reduction in BMI can be maintained at 5 years (13.1 kg/m^2; Olbers et al., 2017) and even at 8 years (17.0 kg/m^2; Inge et al., 2017) after RYGB. An overview of improvements in BMI and comorbidity conditions following adolescent bariatric surgery is provided in Table 41.3 (Beamish, Johansson, et al., 2015). Figure 41.2 demonstrates change in BMI in the medium to long term from two robust studies, the Teen Longitudinal Assessment of Bariatric Surgery (Teen-LABS) study in the United States (Inge et al., 2015) and the Adolescent Morbid Obesity Surgery (AMOS) study in Europe (Olbers et al., 2017), which are discussed in more detail later in this chapter.

T2DM

The prevalence of T2DM increases in parallel with increasing BMI (Mokdad et al., 2003), and extensive evidence from 11 randomized trials in adults now documents the powerful effect of bariatric surgery in improving glucose homeostasis and in reversing T2DM (Schauer, Mingrone, Ikramuddin, & Wolfe, 2016). For many patients, bariatric surgery appears superior to all other therapeutic options. Remission has been reported in 33–90% of those with T2DM (Schauer et al., 2016), including some study participants with relatively low BMIs (< 35 kg/m^2

TABLE 41.3. Outcomes of Adolescent Bariatric Surgery by Procedure

Outcome	AGB	RYGB	SG	All procedures (95% CI)
BMI reduction (kg/m^2)	8.5–11.7	13.3–22.5	13.0–17.2	13.5 (11.9–15.1)
T2DM resolution (%)	80–100	67–100	0–68	0–100
Insulin resistance resolution (%)	44–77	100	50–96	44–100
Dyslipidemia resolution (%)	35–100	87–100	0–58	0–100
Hypertension resolution (%)	50–100	82–100	69–100	50–100
Obstructive sleep apnea resolution (%)	20–100	100	56–80	20–100
Polycystic ovarian syndrome resolution (%)	—	100	0	0–100

Note. CI, confidence interval.

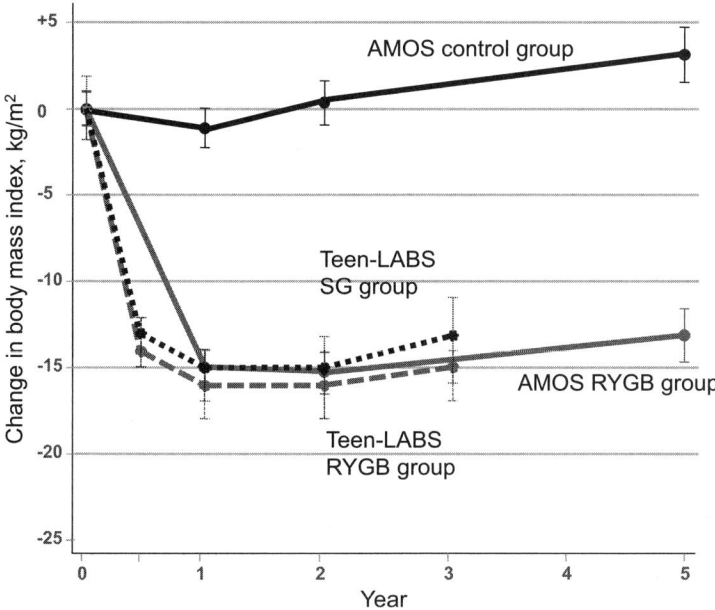

FIGURE 41.2. Change in BMI in the Teen Longitudinal Assessment of Bariatric Surgery (Teen-LABS) study (Inge et al., 2015) and the Adolescent Morbid Obesity Surgery (AMOS) study (Olbers et al., 2017).

and even < 30 kg/m²). Odds of remission appear higher when the diagnosis of T2DM is recent (Sjöstrom et al., 2014). In addition, bariatric surgery offers patients without diabetes protection from developing T2DM (Carlsson et al., 2012).

There is mounting evidence that T2DM behaves far more aggressively when its onset occurs during childhood than adult-onset T2DM. First-line therapies fail earlier in adolescents, and progression to the need for insulin occurs more rapidly (Beamish, D'Alessio, et al., 2015; Shah et al., 2016). With this in mind, it is perhaps even more noteworthy that studies of adolescents, although very limited to date, show T2DM resolution in 79–100% of cases following RYGB (Inge et al., 2015, 2017; Olbers et al., 2017; Paulus et al., 2015), 50–94% following SG (Inge et al., 2015; Paulus et al., 2015), and 100% following AGB (Paulus et al., 2015). These actual figures should be interpreted cautiously, as insufficient data exist to verify the true remission rates, and adult trials thus far suggest RYGB to be superior to SG for T2DM resolution, which in turn appears superior to AGB (Schauer et al., 2016).

Cardiovascular Disease

In addition to ameliorating BMI and T2DM, adolescent bariatric surgery improves a number of other cardiovascular risk factors, resolving hypertension in 50–100% of patients, dyslipidemia in 35–100%, and inflammation in 74% (Beamish & Olbers, 2015; Inge et al., 2017; Olbers et al., 2017; Paulus et al., 2015). Although data are not yet available for adolescents, cardiovascular events are significantly reduced in adults after bariatric surgery. These include a reduction, by around 50%, of the risk of stroke (odds ratio [OR] 0.46, 95% confidence interval [CI] 0.30–0.69), myocardial infarction (OR 0.54, 95% CI 0.41–0.70), and the composite endpoint of "all cardiovascular events" (OR 0.49, 95% CI 0.32–0.75) (Kwok et al., 2014). These benefits are likely to be replicated in adolescents, as cardiovascular risk factors identified in childhood have been shown to track into adulthood and translate into end-organ injury, an example being childhood dyslipidemia, which is predictive of greater adult carotid artery intima media thickness (Li et al., 2003; Raitakari et al., 2003).

There is also mounting evidence in the adult literature of an association between BMI and risk of a broad range of cancers. Overweight and obesity are associated with cancer of the breast, cervix, colon and rectum, endometrium, esophagus, gallbladder, kidney, liver, ovary, pancreas, stomach, and thyroid (Bhaskaran et al., 2014; Calle & Kaaks, 2004).

Following bariatric surgery, women who wish to become pregnant may benefit from increased fertility and reduced likelihood of gestational diabetes and eclampsia, alongside potentially reduced risk for adverse neonatal outcomes (Maggard et al., 2008). However, patients should be warned of these potential effects and advised that pregnancy in the first 2 years after surgery may carry additional risks. Patients should be offered contraception (Michalsky et al., 2012).

Risks and Concerns

Bariatric surgery is always accompanied by risk, but thanks to modern-day laparoscopic surgical techniques and perioperative practice, including early recovery pathways (Lemanu et al., 2013), its safety is well established in adults. Thirty-day mortality is now below 0.1%, a figure lower even than that of laparoscopic cholecystectomy (Sandblom, Videhult, Crona Guterstam, Svenner, & Sadr-Azodi, 2015; Sinha et al., 2013), despite the multiple comorbidities associated with obesity (Chang et al., 2014). Death within 30 days of adolescent bariatric surgery has been exceptionally rare thus far (Michalsky et al., 2013).

Bariatric surgery involves a specific risk of postoperative complications that require emergent reoperation, such as bleeding, gastrointestinal obstruction, and gastrointestinal leakage, the latter of which occurs where staple lines or anastomoses are created.

After RYGB, food passes directly from the small gastric pouch into the jejunum. The gastrojejunal anastomosis does not replicate the regulation of gastric outflow normally afforded by the pylorus, instead delivering digestive contents to the jejunum more rapidly. The early delivery of hyperosmolar nutrients into the jejunum can potentially lead to gastrointestinal symptoms such as abdominal pain, diarrhea, nausea, bloating, and vasomotor symptoms such as fatigue, palpitations, and hypotension, often described as the *dumping syndrome* (Banerjee, Ding, Mikami, & Needleman, 2013). Although these symptoms are unpleasant, this side effect provides a feedback mechanism, which most patients consider to be positive. It is generally controlled by simple dietary modification and helps patients to avoid eating particularly calorie-rich foods (Laurenius & Engstrom, 2016).

In the longer term, nutritional deficiency can present particular challenges. Obesity is associated with numerous vitamin and mineral deficiencies, which should be corrected in advance of surgery, but often persist or worsen postoperatively (Bal, Finelli, Shope, & Koch, 2012). A number of factors promote such deficiencies, including exclusion of relevant anatomical structures from digestion and the overgrowth of small intestinal bacteria (Bal et al., 2012). Nutritional deficiencies have caused concern regarding pregnancy and the preconception period, yet little is actually known about the prevalence of deficiencies during these times (Gadgil et al., 2014). It is particularly important to ensure that these topics are included in preoperative and follow-up discussions with female patients, who are also at significant risk of iron deficiency anemia following surgery (Alvarez-Leite, 2004), making compliance with supplementation important.

The skeleton of individuals with obesity generally has a greater bone mineral content and bone mineral density than that of normal-weight persons. Both of these measures decrease after bariatric surgery (Coates, Fernstrom, Fernstrom, Schauer, & Greenspan, 2004), although some reassurance is provided by reports on adolescents (Beamish, Gronowitz, et al., 2016; Kaulfers, Bean, Inge, Dolan, & Kalkwarf, 2011), which show that the abnormally dense bones generally reduce to normal levels over 2 years. Very few patients demonstrated abnormally low bone density or mineral content within this time. However, long-term data are crucial to determine the true implications for skeletal mass following bariatric surgery, particularly because adolescents will be exposed to the effects of surgery for longer than their adult counterparts. This is an important area for preoperative counseling, including the need for compliance with lifelong nutritional supplementation (Malinowski, 2006).

Finally, several anatomical consequences of bariatric procedures are relevant to future health and investigations. The RYGB has been shown to be technically feasible to reverse, without significant complication in the short term (Himpens, Dapri, & Cadiere, 2006), whereas the SG involves excision of a large portion of stomach, which is irreversible.

The use of gastroscopy (Braley, Nguyen, & Wolfe, 2002) and endoscopic cholangiography as diagnostic and therapeutic procedures can be rendered either more difficult, or even impossible, following bariatric surgery. As a result, novel techniques have been developed, such as double-balloon techniques, allowing enteroscopy after RYGB (Koornstra, 2008), and CT virtual gastroscopy (Brethauer et al., 2014) for use where gastroscopy is not possible. Prophylactic cholecystectomy was formerly undertaken to avoid gallstone disease (Guadalajara et al., 2006), although this is no longer recommended (Warschkow et al., 2013).

Our Experience with Adolescent Bariatric Surgery

Adolescent bariatric surgery has been investigated within the formal research projects of the Teen-LABS group in the United States and the AMOS group in Europe. The Teen-LABS study (Inge et al., 2007) is a prospective multicenter longitudinal study examining the outcomes of 242 adolescents undergoing RYGB or SG for obesity across five U.S. centers (*www.Teen-LABS.org*). The AMOS study (Olbers et al., 2012) is a national prospective multicenter nonrandomized controlled study comparing outcomes of 81 adolescents undergoing RYGB with 80 matched adolescents undergoing conservative treatment for obesity in Sweden. The longitudinal results of these two studies concur across most outcomes in their respective 3- and 5-year outcome reports (Inge et al., 2015; Olbers et al.,2017), and largely replicate those illustrated within the adult literature. Across almost a decade since their inception, these studies have offered valuable lessons for the management of adolescent obesity in surgical programs.

Both groups have experienced a high prevalence of mood-related psychosocial problems. In the Teen-LABS study almost 40% of subjects reported depressive symptoms in the clinically significant range at baseline, three to four times higher than national base rates (Zeller, Modi, Noll, Long, & Inge, 2009). In the AMOS study this figure was 27% (Jarvholm et al., 2012), although more than two-thirds (68%) had some degree of psychosocial impairment (Olbers et al., 2012), most commonly anxiety and mood disorders (Jarvholm et al., 2012). Both studies reported positive psychological outcomes following bariatric surgery, while emphasizing the psychosocial vulnerability of this population and the importance of careful monitoring and support.

Accurate measurement of adherence to routine nutritional supplementation is inherently difficult to achieve, making the literature in this area understandably thin. Adherence may be even more difficult to achieve in an adolescent population (Ziegler, Sirveaux, Brunaud, Reibel, & Quilliot, 2009) and was reported to be poor in two-thirds of patients in the AMOS study (Olbers et al., 2012), owing at least partly to apathy and/or acting out. Severe, potentially life-threatening nutritional deficiencies can arise, albeit rarely, after bariatric surgery. We have previously reported several cases of beriberi as a result of severe thiamine deficiency, necessitating prompt recognition and treatment (Towbin et al., 2004). Other nutritional deficiencies may have more insidious consequences. As noted, bone health remains an important area of unquantified risk in the long term after bariatric surgery. Although both the Teen-LABS and AMOS studies showed normalization of bone mineral content and density (Beamish et al., 2016; Kaulfers et al., 2011), a small proportion (< 5%) of patients had bone mineral density below the normal range (Beamish, Gronowitz, et al., 2016) at 2 years. Adherence to supplementation is likely more important in this subgroup, and bone health is an area of active, ongoing evaluation in both study cohorts. It remains to be seen whether the downward trajectory in bone density will continue or plateau at or near the expected range for weight and age in adolescents. Limited data from adults have emerged, showing a continued reduction in BMD between 2 and 5 years after RYGB, although the mean did not reach abnormally low levels (Raoof, Näslund, Rask, & Szabo, 2016). The emergence of specific complete supplements, combining all of the vitamins and minerals recommended after bariatric surgery (O'Kane et al., 2014), may help to improve adherence.

A majority (84%) of adults undergoing RYGB experience problems with excess skin as a result of major weight loss (Biorserud, Olbers, & Fagevik Olsen, 2011). Although practitioners had hoped that the younger skin of adolescents would be more likely to retain the body's contour, adolescents appear to be troubled by excess skin in similar numbers as adults, leading to similar proportions seeking body-contouring surgery (Staalesen et al., 2014). However, whereas there is a good correlation between the amount of excess skin and the severity of related symptoms, there is a very weak relationship between change in BMI and symptoms, making prediction of such problems difficult (Staalesen et al., 2014). This important and common consequence of major weight loss should be discussed with patients in advance of surgery.

A number of adolescents do not achieve significant weight loss; more than 1 in 10 lost < 10% of their BMI in both the Teen-LABS (Inge et al., 2015) and AMOS (Olbers et al., 2017) studies. This presents an important area for future work, since investigators do not yet understand why suboptimal weight loss occurs or how to improve the effects of surgery in this subgroup. The number of patients who did not reach a BMI < 35 kg/m^2 differed between the two studies (Teen-LABS, 45% vs. AMOS, 28%), most likely because of a marked difference in the baseline weight of the participants. Although all participants in both studies had severe obesity (BMI ≥ 35 kg/m^2) at baseline the mean BMI in the Teen-LABS cohort was 58.5 kg/m^2, whereas in the AMOS surgical patients it was only 45.5 kg/m^2. The existence of a strong dose-related increase in the prevalence of several obesity-related comorbid diseases, such as T2DM and hypertension (Beamish, Olbers, et al., 2016), coupled with a similar absolute BMI reduction between the two studies (Teen-LABS, −15 kg/m^2 vs. AMOS, −13 kg/m^2; see Figure 41.2), suggests that offering surgery in advance of adolescents reaching such an extreme BMI may be advantageous.

Summary and Conclusions

The rapidly growing literature on adolescent bariatric surgery demonstrates unparalleled weight loss and marked improvements in cardiometabolic health and quality of life, comparable with those reported in adults who have had surgery. However, surgical management is not without risk, and long-term studies are needed to further understand the effects of this surgery, both positive and negative, while actively seeking to optimize outcomes. It is essential that health care providers, patients, and their families consider the significant potential negative effects of surgery in the decision-making process.

Embedded in a comprehensive obesity program, led by a multidisciplinary specialist team, bariatric surgery represents an important and highly effective therapeutic option for the treatment of severe adolescent obesity. It is indicated in cases where obesity and its health consequences are severe, and nonsurgical options have been exhausted. As a result of the failure of existing prevention strategies, many adolescents are already suffering from severe obesity and its wide-ranging consequences. For these young people, surgery offers the potential of significant and sustainable health improvements in the absence of any other reliably effective treatment, and it may replace desperation with hope.

References

Alvarez-Leite, J. I. (2004). Nutrient deficiencies secondary to bariatric surgery. *Current Opinion in Clinical Nutrition and Metabolic Care, 7*(5), 569–575.

Angrisani, L., Santonicola, A., Iovino, P., Formisano, G., Buchwald, H., & Scopinaro, N. (2015). Bariatric surgery worldwide 2013. *Obesity Surgery, 25*(10), 1822–1832.

Bal, B. S., Finelli, F. C., Shope, T. R., & Koch, T. R. (2012). Nutritional deficiencies after bariatric surgery. *Nature Reviews Endocrinology, 8*(9), 544–556.

Banerjee, A., Ding, Y., Mikami, D. J., & Needleman, B. J. (2013). The role of dumping syndrome in weight loss after gastric bypass surgery. *Surgical Endoscopy, 27*(5), 1573–1578.

Beamish, A. J. (2016). Bariatric surgery for obese adolescents to prevent type 2 diabetes. *British Medical Journal, 353*, i2977.

Beamish, A. J., D'Alessio, D. A., & Inge, T. H. (2015). Controversial issues: When the drugs don't work, can surgery provide a different outcome for diabetic adolescents? *Surgery for Obesity and Related Diseases, 11*(4), 946–948.

Beamish, A. J., Gronowitz, E., Olbers, T., Flodmark, C. E., Marcus, C., & Dahlgren, J. (2017). Body composition and bone health in adolescents after Roux-en-Y gastric bypass for severe obesity. *Pediatric Obesity, 12*(3), 239–246.

Beamish, A. J., Johansson, S. E., & Olbers, T. (2015). Bariatric surgery in adolescents: What do we know so far? *Scandinavian Journal of Surgery, 104*(1), 24–32.

Beamish, A. J., & Olbers, T. (2015). Bariatric and metabolic surgery in adolescents: A path to decrease adult cardiovascular mortality. *Current Atherosclerosis Reports, 17*(9), 53.

Beamish, A. J., Olbers, T., Kelly, A. S., & Inge, T. H. (2016). Cardiovascular effects of bariatric surgery. *Nature Reviews Cardiology, 13*(12), 730–743.

Bhaskaran, K., Douglas, I., Forbes, H., dos-Santos-Silva, I., Leon, D. A., & Smeeth, L. (2014). Body-mass index and risk of 22 specific cancers: A population-based cohort study of 5.24 million UK adults. *Lancet, 384*(9945), 755–765.

Biorserud, C., Olbers, T., & Fagevik Olsen, M. (2011). Patients' experience of surplus skin after laparoscopic gastric bypass. *Obesity Surgery, 21*(3), 273–277.

Braley, S. C., Nguyen, N. T., & Wolfe, B. M. (2002). Late gastrointestinal hemorrhage after gastric bypass. *Obesity Surgery, 12*(3), 404–407.

Brethauer, S. A., Kothari, S., Sudan, R., Williams, B., English, W. J., Brengman, M., et al. (2014). Systematic review on reoperative bariatric surgery: American Society for Metabolic and Bariatric Surgery Revision Task Force. *Surgery for Obesity and Related Diseases, 10*(5), 952–972.

Calle, E. E., & Kaaks, R. (2004). Overweight, obesity and cancer: Epidemiological evidence and proposed mechanisms. *Nature Reviews Cancer, 4*(8), 579–591.

Carlsson, L. M., Peltonen, M., Ahlin, S., Anveden, A., Bouchard, C., Carlsson, B., et al. (2012). Bariatric surgery and prevention of type 2 diabetes in Swedish obese subjects. *New England Journal of Medicine, 367*(8), 695–704.

Chang, S. H., Stoll, C. R., Song, J., Varela, J. E., Eagon, C. J., & Colditz, G. A. (2014). The effectiveness and risks of bariatric surgery: An updated systematic review and meta-analysis, 2003–2012. *JAMA Surgery, 149*(3), 275–287.

Coates, P. S., Fernstrom, J. D., Fernstrom, M. H., Schauer, P. R., & Greenspan, S. L. (2004). Gastric bypass surgery for morbid obesity leads to an increase in bone turnover and a decrease in bone mass. *Journal of Clinical Endocrinology and Metabolism, 89*(3), 1061–1065.

Cole, T. J., Bellizzi, M. C., Flegal, K. M., & Dietz, W. H. (2000). Establishing a standard definition for child overweight and obesity worldwide: International survey. *British Medical Journal, 320*(7244), 1240–1243.

Ebbeling, C. B., Pawlak, D. B., & Ludwig, D. S. (2002). Childhood obesity: Public-health crisis, common sense cure. *Lancet, 360*(9331), 473–482.

Esteban Varela, J., & Nguyen, N. T. (2015). Laparoscopic sleeve gastrectomy leads the U.S. utilization of bariatric surgery at academic medical centers. *Surgery for Obesity and Related Diseases, 11*(5), 987–990.

Freedman, D. S., Khan, L. K., Serdula, M. K., Dietz, W. H., Srinivasan, S. R., & Berenson, G. S. (2005). The relation of childhood BMI to adult adiposity: The Bogalusa Heart Study. *Pediatrics, 115*(1), 22–27.

Freedman, D. S., Mei, Z., Srinivasan, S. R., Berenson, G. S., & Dietz, W. H. (2007). Cardiovascular risk factors and excess adiposity among overweight children and adolescents: The Bogalusa Heart Study. *Journal of Pediatrics, 150*(1), 12–17.e2.

Fried, M., Hainer, V., Basdevant, A., Buchwald, H., Deitel, M., Finer, N., et al. (2007). Inter-disciplinary European guidelines on surgery for severe obesity. *International Journal of Obesity, 31*(4), 569–577.

Gadgil, M. D., Chang, H. Y., Richards, T. M., Gudzune, K. A., Huizinga, M. M., Clark, J. M., et al. (2014). Laboratory testing for and diagnosis of nutritional deficiencies in pregnancy before and after bariatric surgery. *Journal of Womens Health, 23*(2), 129–137.

Guadalajara, H., Sanz Baro, R., Pascual, I., Blesa, I., Rotundo, G. S., Lopez, J. M., et al. (2006). Is prophylactic cholecystectomy useful in obese patients undergoing gastric bypass? *Obesity Surgery, 16*(7), 883–885.

Harnett, W. (1947). A statistical study of 1405 cases of cancer of the stomach. *British Journal of Surgery, 34*(136), 379–385.

Herget, S., Rudolph, A., Hilbert, A., & Bluher, S. (2014). Psychosocial status and mental health in adolescents before and after bariatric surgery: A systematic literature review. *Obesity Facts, 7*(4), 233–245.

Himpens, J., Dapri, G., & Cadiere, G. B. (2006). Laparoscopic conversion of the gastric bypass into a normal anatomy. *Obesity Surgery, 16*(7), 908–912.

Inge, T. H., Courcoulas, A. P., Jenkins, T. M., Michalsky, M. P., Helmrath, M. A., Brandt, M. L., et al. (2015). Weight loss and health status 3 years after bariatric surgery in adolescents. *New England Journal of Medicine, 374*(2), 113–123.

Inge, T. H., Jenkins, T. M., Xanthakos, S. A., Dixon, J. B., Daniels, S. R., Zeller, M. H., et al. (2017). Long-term outcomes of bariatric surgery in adolescents with severe obesity (FABS-5+): A prospective follow-up analysis. *Lancet Diabetes and Endocrinology, 5*(3), 165–173.

Inge, T. H., Zeller, M., Harmon, C., Helmrath, M., Bean, J., Modi, A., et al. (2007). Teen-Longitudinal Assessment of Bariatric Surgery: Methodological features of the first prospective multicenter study of adolescent bariatric surgery. *Journal of Pediatric Surgery, 42*(11), 1969–1971.

Inge, T. H., Zeller, M. H., Jenkins, T. M., Helmrath, M., Brandt, M. L., Michalsky, M. P., et al. (2014). Perioperative outcomes of adolescents undergoing bariatric surgery: The Teen-Longitudinal Assessment of Bariatric Surgery (Teen-LABS) study. *JAMA Pediatrics, 168*(1), 47–53.

Jarvholm, K., Karlsson, J., Olbers, T., Peltonen, M., Marcus, C., Dahlgren, J., et al. (2015). Two-year trends in psychological outcomes after gastric bypass in adolescents with severe obesity. *Obesity, 23*(10), 1966–1972.

Jarvholm, K., Olbers, T., Marcus, C., Marild, S., Gronowitz, E., Friberg, P., et al. (2012). Short-term psychological outcomes in severely obese adolescents after bariatric surgery. *Obesity, 20*(2), 318–323.

Juonala, M., Magnussen, C. G., Berenson, G. S., Venn, A., Burns, T. L., Sabin, M. A., et al. (2011). Childhood adiposity, adult adiposity, and cardiovascular risk factors. *New England Journal of Medicine, 365*(20), 1876–1885.

Kaulfers, A. M., Bean, J. A., Inge, T. H., Dolan, L. M., & Kalkwarf, H. J. (2011). Bone loss in adolescents after bariatric surgery. *Pediatrics, 127*(4), e956–e961.

Kelly, A. S., Barlow, S. E., Rao, G., Inge, T. H., Hayman, L. L., Steinberger, J., et al. (2013). Severe obesity in children and adolescents: Identification, associated health risks, and treatment approaches: A scientific statement from the American Heart Association. *Circulation, 128*(15), 1689–1712.

Koornstra, J. J. (2008). Double balloon enteroscopy for endoscopic retrograde cholangiopancreaticography after Roux-en-Y reconstruction: Case series and review of the literature. *Netherlands Journal of Medicine, 66*(7), 275–279.

Kwok, C. S., Pradhan, A., Khan, M. A., Anderson, S. G., Keavney, B. D., Myint, P. K., et al. (2014). Bariatric surgery and its impact on cardiovascular disease and mortality: A systematic review and meta-analysis. *International Journal of Cardiology, 173*(1), 20–28.

Laurenius, A., & Engstrom, M. (2016). Early dumping syndrome is not a complication but a desirable feature of Roux-en-Y gastric bypass surgery. *Clinical Obesity, 6*(5), 332–340.

Lemanu, D. P., Singh, P. P., Berridge, K., Burr, M., Birch, C., Babor, R., et al. (2013). Randomized clinical trial of enhanced recovery versus standard care after laparoscopic sleeve gastrectomy. *British Journal of Surgery, 100*(4), 482–489.

Li, J. F., Lai, D. D., Ni, B., & Sun, K. X. (2013). Comparison of laparoscopic Roux-en-Y gastric bypass with laparoscopic sleeve gastrectomy for morbid obesity or type 2 diabetes mellitus: A meta-analysis of randomized controlled trials. *Canadian Journal of Surgery, 56*(6), E158–E164.

Li, S., Chen, W., Srinivasan, S. R., Bond, M. G., Tang, R., Urbina, E. M., et al. (2003). Childhood cardiovascular risk factors and carotid vascular changes in adulthood: The Bogalusa Heart Study. *Journal of the American Medical Association, 290*(17), 2271–2276.

Maggard, M. A., Yermilov, I., Li, Z., Maglione, M., Newberry, S., Suttorp, M., et al. (2008). Pregnancy and fertility following bariatric surgery: A systematic review. *Journal of the American Medical Association, 300*(19), 2286–2296.

Malinowski, S. S. (2006). Nutritional and metabolic complications of bariatric surgery. *American Journal of Medical Science, 331*(4), 219–225.

Mason, E. E., & Ito, C. (1967). Gastric bypass in obesity. *Surgical Clinics of North America, 47*(6), 1345–1351.

Mason, E. E., & Ito, C. (1969). Gastric bypass. *Annals of Surgery, 170*(3), 329–339.

Michalsky, M., Kramer, R. E., Fullmer, M. A., Polfuss, M., Porter, R., Ward-Begnoche, W., et al. (2011). Developing criteria for pediatric/adolescent bariatric surgery programs. *Pediatrics, 128*(Suppl. 2), S65–S70.

Michalsky, M., Reichard, K., Inge, T., Pratt, J., Lenders, C., & American Society for Metabolic & Bariatric Surgery. (2012). ASMBS pediatric committee best practice guidelines. *Surgery for Obesity and Related Diseases, 8*(1), 1–7.

Michalsky, M., Teich, S., Rana, A., Teeple, E., Cook, S., & Schuster, D. (2013). Surgical risks and lessons learned: Mortality following gastric bypass in a severely obese adolescent. *Journal of Pediatric Surgery Case Reports, 1*(9), 321–324.

Moize, V., Andreu, A., Flores, L., Torres, F., Ibarzabal, A., Delgado, S., et al. (2013). Long-term dietary intake and nutritional deficiencies following sleeve gastrectomy or Roux-En-Y gastric bypass in a mediterranean population. *Journal of the Academy of Nutrition and Dietetics, 113*(3), 400–410.

Mokdad, A. H., Ford, E. S., Bowman, B. A., Dietz, W. H., Vinicor, F., Bales, V. S., et al. (2003). Prevalence of obesity, diabetes, and obesity-related health risk factors, 2001. *Journal of the American Medical Association, 289*(1), 76–79.

National Institutes for Health. (1991). NIH conference: Gastrointestinal surgery for severe obesity. *Annals of Internal Medicine, 115*(12), 956–961.

NCD Risk Factor Collaboration. (2016). Trends in adult body-mass index in 200 countries from 1975 to 2014: A pooled analysis of 1698 population-based measurement studies with 19.2 million participants. *Lancet, 387*(10026), 1377–1396.

Ng, M., Fleming, T., Robinson, M., Thomson, B., Graetz, N., Margono, C., et al. (2014). Global, regional, and national prevalence of overweight and obesity in children and adults during 1980–2013: A systematic analysis for the Global Burden of Disease Study 2013. *Lancet, 384*(9945), 766–781.

O'Brien, P. E., Sawyer, S. M., Laurie, C., Brown, W. A., Skinner, S., Veit, F., et al. (2010). Laparoscopic adjustable gastric banding in severely obese adolescents: A randomized trial. *Journal of the American Medical Association, 303*(6), 519–526.

Ogden, C. L., Carroll, M. D., Kit, B. K., & Flegal, K. M. (2014). Prevalence of childhood and adult obesity in the United States, 2011–2012. *Journal of the American Medical Assocation, 311*(8), 806–814.

O'Kane, M., Pinkney, J., Aasheim, E., Barth, J., Batterham, R., & Welbourn, R. (2014). *BOMSS guidelines on perioperative and postoperative biochemical monitoring and micronutrient replacement for patients undergoing bariatric surgery.* London: BOMSS.

Olbers, T. (2015). Bypass equipoise sleeve trial (BEST). Retrieved from *https://clinicaltrials.gov/ct2/show/NCT02767505*.

Olbers, T., Beamish, A. J., Gronowitz, E., Flodmark, C. E., Dahlgren, J., Bruze, G., et al. (2017). Laparoscopic Roux-en-Y gastric bypass in adolescents with severe obesity (AMOS): A prospective five-year Swedish nationwide study. *Lancet Diabetes and Endocrinology, 5*(3), 174–183.

Olbers, T., Gronowitz, E., Werling, M., Marlid, S., Flodmark, C. E., Peltonen, M., et al. (2012). Two-year outcome of laparoscopic Roux-en-Y gastric bypass in adolescents with severe obesity: Results from a Swedish Nationwide Study (AMOS). *International Journal of Obesity, 36*(11), 1388–1395.

Olshansky, S. J., Passaro, D. J., Hershow, R. C., Layden, J., Carnes, B. A., Brody, J., et al. (2005). A potential decline in life expectancy in the United States in the 21st century. *New England Journal of Medicine, 352*(11), 1138–1145.

Paulus, G. F., de Vaan, L. E., Verdam, F. J., Bouvy, N. D., Ambergen, T. A., & van Heurn, L. W. (2015). Bariatric surgery in morbidly obese adolescents: A systematic review and meta-analysis. *Obesity Surgery, 25*(5), 860–878.

Payne, J. H., Dewind, L. T., & Commons, R. R. (1963). Metabolic observations in patients with jejunocolic shunts. *American Journal of Surgery, 106*, 273–289.

Pinhas-Hamiel, O., & Zeitler, P. (2007). Acute and chronic complications of type 2 diabetes mellitus in children and adolescents. *Lancet, 369*(9575), 1823–1831.

Pratt, J. S., Lenders, C. M., Dionne, E. A., Hoppin, A. G., Hsu, G. L., Inge, T. H., et al. (2009). Best practice updates for pediatric/adolescent weight loss surgery. *Obesity, 17*(5), 901–910.

Raitakari, O. T., Juonala, M., Kahonen, M., Taittonen, L., Laitinen, T., Maki-Torkko, N., et al. (2003). Cardiovascular risk factors in childhood and carotid artery intima-media thickness in adulthood: The Cardiovascular Risk in Young Finns Study. *Journal of the American Medical Association, 290*(17), 2277–2283.

Randolph, J. G., Weintraub, W. H., & Rigg, A. (1974). Jejunoileal bypass for morbid obesity in adolescents. *Journal of Pediatric Surgery, 9*(3), 341–345.

Raoof, M., Näslund, I., Rask, E., & Szabo, E. (2016). Effect of gastric bypass on bone mineral density, parathyroid hormone and vitamin D: 5 years follow-up. *Obesity Surgery, 26*(5), 1141–1145.

Rogers, C. A., Welbourn, R., Byrne, J., Donovan, J. L., Reeves, B. C., Wordsworth, S., et al. (2014). The by-band study: Gastric bypass or adjustable gastric band surgery to treat morbid obesity: Study protocol for a multi-centre randomised controlled trial with an internal pilot phase. *Trials, 15*(1), 1–14.

Royal College of Surgeons of England/Department of Health. (2011). The higher risk general surgical patient: Towards improved care for a forgotten group. Retrieved from *www.rcseng.ac.uk/publications/docs/higher-risk-surgical-patient*.

Sandblom, G., Videhult, P., Crona Guterstam, Y., Svenner, A., & Sadr-Azodi, O. (2015). Mortality after a cholecystectomy: A population-based study. *HPB, 17*(3), 239–243.

Schauer, P. R., Mingrone, G., Ikramuddin, S., & Wolfe, B. (2016). Clinical outcomes of metabolic surgery: Efficacy of glycemic control, weight loss, and remission of diabetes. *Diabetes Care, 39*(6), 902–911.

Shah, A. S., D'Alessio, D., Ford-Adams, M. E., Desai, A. P., & Inge, T. H. (2016). Bariatric surgery: A potential treatment for type 2 diabetes in youth. *Diabetes Care, 39*(6), 934–940.

Sinha, S., Hofman, D., Stoker, D. L., Friend, P. J., Poloniecki, J. D., Thompson, M. M., et al. (2013). Epidemiological study of provision of cholecystectomy in England from 2000 to 2009: Retrospective analysis of hospital episode statistics. *Surgical Endoscopy, 27*(1), 162–175.

Sjostrom, L. (2013). Review of the key results from the Swedish Obese Subjects (SOS) trial: A prospective controlled intervention study of bariatric surgery. *Journal of Internal Medicine, 273*(3), 219–234.

Sjostrom, L., Peltonen, M., Jacobson, P., Ahlin, S., Andersson-Assarsson, J., Anveden, A., et al. (2014). Association of bariatric surgery with long-term remission of type 2 diabetes and with microvascular and macrovascular complications. *Journal of the American Medical Association, 311*(22), 2297–2304.

Soper, R. T., Mason, E. E., Printen, K. J., & Zellweger, H. (1975). Gastric bypass for morbid obesity in children and adolescents. *Journal of Pediatric Surgery, 10*(1), 51–58.

Staalesen, T., Olbers, T., Dahlgren, J., Fagevik Olsen, M., Flodmark, C. E., Marcus, C., et al. (2014). Development of excess skin and request for body-contouring surgery in postbariatric adolescents. *Plastic and Reconstructive Surgery, 134*(4), 627–636.

Towbin, A., Inge, T. H., Garcia, V. F., Roehrig, H. R., Clements, R. H., Harmon, C. M., et al. (2004). Beriberi after gastric bypass surgery in adolescence. *Journal of Pediatrics, 145*(2), 263–267.

Van Nieuwenhove, Y., Dambrauskas, Z., Campillo-Soto, A., van Dielen, F., Wiezer, R., Janssen, I., et al. (2011). Preoperative very low-calorie diet and operative outcome after laparoscopic gastric bypass: A randomized multicenter study. *Archives of Surgery, 146*(11), 1300–1305.

Warren, R., & Meadows, E. C. (1949). Subtotal gastrectomy or vagotomy for peptic ulcerations: Early results and postoperative symptoms. *New England Journal of Medicine, 240*(10), 367–372.

Warschkow, R., Tarantino, I., Ukegjini, K., Beutner, U., Guller, U., Schmied, B. M., et al. (2013). Concomitant cholecystectomy during laparoscopic Roux-en-Y gastric bypass in obese patients is not justified: A meta-analysis. *Obesity Surgery, 23*(3), 397–407.

Zeller, M. H., Modi, A. C., Noll, J. G., Long, J. D., & Inge, T. H. (2009). Psychosocial functioning improves following adolescent bariatric surgery. *Obesity, 17*(5), 985–990.

Ziegler, O., Sirveaux, M. A., Brunaud, L., Reibel, N., & Quilliot, D. (2009). Medical follow up after bariatric surgery: Nutritional and drug issues. General recommendations for the prevention and treatment of nutritional deficiencies. *Diabetes and Metabolism, 35*(6, Pt 2), 544–557.

CHAPTER 42

Using Public Policy to Address Obesity

Past, Present, and Future

Marlene B. Schwartz
Kelly D. Brownell

The rapid increase in the prevalence of obesity at the end of the 20th century led the World Health Organization (WHO) to declare a global obesity epidemic (World Health Organization, 1998). In the United States, the country that leads the world with the highest obesity rates, the epidemic "came quickly, with little fanfare, and was out of control before the nation noticed" (p. 3; Brownell & Horgen, 2004). When the first edition of this book was published, alarm about the rising rate of obesity in the United States was in the news. Researchers estimated approximately 325,000 annual deaths attributable to obesity (Allison, Fontaine, Manson, Stevens, & VanItallie, 1999), which was approaching the 400,000 annual deaths attributable to tobacco-related deaths at that time. The health care costs were estimated at $99.2 billion in 1995 (Wolf & Colditz, 1998). It was clear that the status quo was not going to turn the epidemic around, and a new approach was needed.

Although the majority of chapters in this volume are focused on obesity treatment, Horgen and Brownell's 2002 chapter made the case that treatment efficacy in studies was low, and treatment effectiveness for the general population was very low, because treatment is costly and available to a select few. Therefore, it was time to consider alternative responses to the obesity epidemic. They presented the argument that obesity rates were rising due to the pervasiveness of a toxic environment, and that a promising response would be to focus on prevention and public policy.

This revised chapter does not need to continue to make the case for confronting the toxic environment. Over the past 15 years there has been tremendous acceptance of the idea that we need to address obesity through public health approaches to improve the environment and influence the health of a population. Many changes have been made and there have been reports containing a glimmer of hope: slight decreases in the prevalence of obesity among young children and a plateau of obesity rates in older children (Ogden et al., 2016). Although it is not yet time to celebrate and declare victory, it is worth taking a moment to appreciate how far we have come and identify where public health efforts should be focused going forward.

The aim of this chapter is to review how the idea of confronting the toxic environment has evolved, the actions that have occurred, and opportunities to build momentum and promote future work. We address several of the recommendations that were made in the previous chapter: Increase awareness of the obesity epidemic, regulate food advertising to youth, improve the school nutrition environment, and tax unhealthy foods. Although not an exhaustive list of policy recommendations, the objective is to provide an overview of how much has been done to engage public policy in the effort to prevent obesity in the United States. We then review opportunities where obesity policies can be connected to other major social movements and conclude with recommendations for future research and advocacy.

Confronting the Toxic Environment

Increase Awareness of the Obesity Epidemic

An important goal in the early phases of policy development was to increase the public's awareness of the obesity epidemic. This goal was distinct from the goal of increasing awareness of the importance of maintaining a healthy weight—that was already understood. Obesity rates rose in the 1980s and 1990s in the face of tremendous pressure to be thin, and multiple industries focused on dieting and weight control. In the United States, health clubs, diet centers, and low-fat snacks fueled a $33-billion-a-year industry in the 1990s (Institute of Medicine, 1995). The common belief was that individuals were responsible for solving their own weight problems. This view needed to change in order to garner support for public policy changes.

In 2001, the Surgeon General reflected this view of collective responsibility when he called for a shift away from a simple focus on "personal responsibility" and toward a more comprehensive view of the role of the community in helping people maintain health:

> Many people believe that dealing with overweight and obesity is a personal responsibility. To some degree they are right, but it is also a community responsibility. When there are no safe accessible places for children to play or adults to walk, jog, or ride a bike, that is a community responsibility. When school lunchrooms or office cafeterias do not provide healthy and appealing food choices, that is a community responsibility. When new or expectant mothers are not educated about the benefits of breastfeeding, that is a community responsibility. When we do not require daily physical education in our schools, that is also a community responsibility. There is much we can and should do together. (U.S. Department of Health and Human Services, 2001).

The Surgeon General's comments were reinforced and repeated by many researchers and advocates in subsequent years. In public health circles, a set of maps created by the Centers for Disease Control and Prevention (CDC), which illustrated the rapid rise in obesity across the states starting in 1985, were shared at meetings and presentations. The graphic representation of the rapid rise in obesity rates from one year to the next was convincing evidence that something other than individual choices had to be at play, as there was no other indication that the American population had suddenly become irresponsible in other ways (Brownell et al., 2010).

The seriousness of the epidemic was reinforced by research documenting the range of health and psychological consequences of obesity, especially for children. More studies were conducted on the expected health care costs attributable to the epidemic to make a business case for addressing this problem. Then, a 2005 paper estimating changes in life expectancy due to the rise in obesity led to the often-cited statement that this generation of children is expected to live shorter lives than their parents (Olshansky et al., 2005). The idea that children would not live as long as their parents had lived hit a societal nerve. It became easier to make the case that as a nation, we needed to change the environment in order to protect our children.

Several signs have emerged to suggest that the population has changed its attitudes about the best way to approach the obesity epidemic in the United States. One indication of public attitudes is how the topic of obesity is framed in the media. In a study that compared television network news coverage of obesity in two 5-year time periods (1995–

1999 and 2005–2009), researchers found that overall coverage increased significantly, and there were changes in the types of stories (Gearhart, Craig, & Steed, 2012). Specifically, there was a significant decrease in stories that focused on individuals and specific events, an increase in stories that presented the issue of obesity in a broader social context, and an increase in featuring politicians in the news coverage. This finding is consistent with an increase in public awareness of public policy approaches to reducing obesity.

Another example of the change in thinking is the adoption of the social–ecological model as a standard tool in explaining the complex influences that contribute to the risk of obesity. See Figure 42.1 for an example from the CDC.

The different versions of the summary pages of the Dietary Guidelines for Americans provide another metric of how attitudes have changed. The 2005 guidelines highlighted the importance of physical activity as a way to maintain body weight, recommending that people "balance calories from foods and beverages with calories expended." In addition, the guidelines recommended that "to prevent gradual weight gain over time, make small decreases in food and beverage calories and increase physical activity" (USDA, 2005). By 2010 (USDA, 2005), the message for people who were overweight or obese directly acknowledged that less should be eaten: "Control total calorie intake to manage body weight. For people who are overweight or obese, this will mean consuming fewer calories from foods and beverages." In 2015 (USDA, 2015), the message about eating less of specific foods was spelled out: "Limit calories from added sugars and saturated fats and reduce sodium intake. Consume an eating pattern low in added sugars, saturated fats, and sodium. Cut back on foods and beverages higher in these components to amounts that fit within healthy eating patterns" (p. xii). Further, for the first time, one of the key messages was a public health message: "Support healthy eating patterns for all. Everyone has a role in helping to create and support healthy eating patterns in multiple settings nationwide, from home to school to work to communities" (p. xii).

A final piece of evidence that attitudes about obesity have changed is the increase in support for public policies to protect indi-

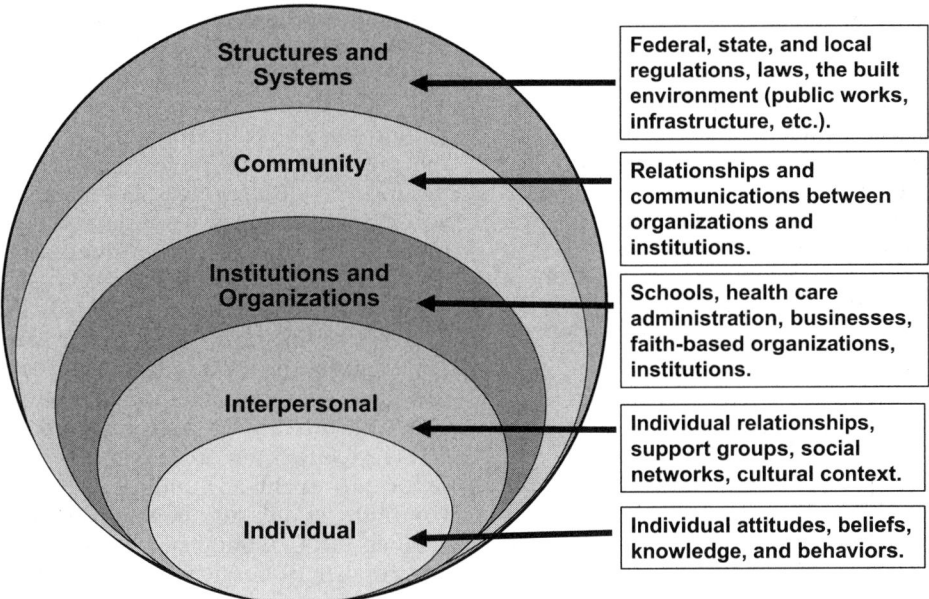

FIGURE 42.1. The social–ecological model. From *www.cdc.gov/nccdphp/dnpao/state-local-programs/health-equity/framing-the-issue.html*.

viduals with obesity from discrimination. As discussed by Puhl and Pearl (Chapter 10, this volume), the stigma associated with obesity is well documented, and there is strong evidence linking stigma experiences with stress and negative emotional and physical health consequences. Recent research suggests that there is growing public support for policies to protect people with obesity. Requiring policies that address weight-based bullying was supported by 90% of educators and 88% of parents (Puhl, Neumark-Sztainer, Bryn Austin, Suh, & Wakefield, 2016). Suh and colleagues also found that over 80% of parents supported strengthening policies to reduce weight stigma and discrimination, and there have been significant increases between 2011 and 2013 in parental support (over 82% agreement) to require television shows to positively portray children of diverse body sizes and show them eating healthy food and being physically active (Suh, Puhl, Liu, & Fleming Milici, 2014). During the same 2011–2013 time frame, another study documented that at least 75% of participants supported laws prohibiting weight discrimination in the workplace (Suh, Puhl, Liu, & Milici, 2014).

In sum, there is evidence that federal government agencies have accepted a public health view of obesity, and societal attitudes have shifted accordingly. It is possible that there is a connection between the acceptance of the view of obesity as a societal problem, the belief in the role of the toxic environment on poor diet, and the increased support for policies that protect obese children from bullying and obese adults from discrimination at work. When the responsibility for preventing obesity is shared by a community, the community also shares the responsibility for caring for those individuals who are affected by obesity.

Regulate Food Advertising Targeting Youth

Substantial progress has been made over the past 10 years in bringing attention to the problem of food marketing directed at children and teens. The Institute of Medicine's (2006) report, *Food Marketing to Children: Threat or Opportunity?*, addressed the nature, extent, and influence of food and beverage marketing on children and adolescents in the United States and concluded that there was strong evidence that exposure to marketing influenced food preferences, purchase requests, and short-term consumption for children ages 2–11 years. In 2009, the WHO commissioned a systematic review of the research on food marketing to children, which was then updated in 2013 (Cairns, Angus, Hastings, & Caraher, 2013). The authors concluded that predominantly low-nutrition foods were being marketed to children, and exposure to food marketing was influencing children's food preferences, purchases, consumption, and diet-related health. Experimental studies have found a significant relationship between exposure to television ads and increased food intake among children (Boyland et al., 2016; Harris, Bargh, & Brownell, 2009) and exposure to advergames (i.e., online games that feature branded characters and graphics) and increased consumption of unhealthy foods (Harris, Speers, Schwartz, & Brownell, 2012).

In response to the evidence that food marketing was contributing to the problem of poor diet among American children, Congress directed the federal government to create the Interagency Working Group (IWG) in 2009 with representatives from the CDC, the U.S. Federal Drug Administration (FDA), the Federal Trade Commission, and the U.S. Department of Agriculture (USDA). The IWG was tasked to review the evidence and propose a set of voluntary principles for the industry to use as a guide for marketing food to children ages 2–17 years. These voluntary principles were designed to promote stronger industry self-regulation, not government regulation. The IWG released a draft of strong nutrition standards (Federal Trade Commission, 2011). Organizations representing the food industry characterized the IWG recommendations as unreasonable and unrealistic (Hernandez & Kolish, 2011; McGlockton, 2011), and the industry reportedly spent $37 million to oppose the voluntary standards (Nestle, 2011). In December 2011, Congress effectively stopped any further discussion of the recommendations by specifically stating that no further work could be done by the IWG before a cost–benefit analysis was completed.

One key component of the industry defense against the IWG recommendations was that they had already created a self-regulation body. In 2009, the Better Business Bureau organized the Child Food and Beverage Advertising Initiative (CFBAI) (Council of Better Business Bureaus, 2016). The purpose of this organization is to "shift the mix of foods advertised to children under 12 to encourage healthier dietary choices and healthy lifestyles" (p. 1; Council of Better Business Bureaus, 2016). The group has made progressive changes over the years it has been in existence. In the beginning, any advertisement that included a message about physical activity was considered appropriate to marketing to children, and each participating company created its own nutrition standards. Some experts questioned the value of this, as companies tended to emphasize limiting nutrients that were not typically a problem in their product category (e.g., cereal companies set strict fat limits but more lenient sugar limits; a soup company set strong sugar limits but more lenient sodium limits). In 2011, a set of unified nutrition standards were adopted by all participating companies, and the same definition of "children's marketing" was adopted. Although advocates and marketing researchers have pushed for even stronger nutrition standards and less lenient definitions of child-directed marketing (Harris, Sarda, Schwartz, & Brownell, 2013), progress has been made from the food industry's perspective.

Research has evaluated the impact of CFBAI on marketing to children. Kunkel, Castonguay, and Filer (2015) compared ads in 2013 to ads from 2007 and evaluated the nutrition quality of the foods, using the U.S. Department of Health and Human Services "Go, Slow, Whoa" system. They found that although there were fewer food ads per hour in 2013 (6.4 vs. 8.5 ads/hour), there was no significant improvement in the nutritional quality; 80% of the ads were for foods in the poorest nutritional category. The authors attribute the lack of progress to weak nutrition standards and to the fact that not all companies participate in CFBAI.

A recent report using Nielsen data to examine food advertising on television between 2002 and 2015 showed that for children ages 2–11 years, exposure to food marketing on television has finally dropped below 2007 levels (Frazier & Harris, 2016) (see Figure 42.2). However, viewed in context of other age groups, it is evident that food ads on TV have recently dropped for all groups—including adults.

Although the decrease in marketing to children on TV may be a sign of progress, it may also be the consequence of companies reaching children and adolescents through digital media in addition to TV (Kelly, Vandevijvere, Freeman, & Jenkin, 2015). In many ways digital media is a greater threat to children and adolescents because parents cannot feasibly monitor or control their children's access. Traditional television commercials are understood by youth as marketing; other strategies that place the product in front of the child as part of the general environment are more subtle. A recent report found that half of the 2009 spending targeting children ages 2–11 years was spent on cross-promotions, which included media-character merchandising and tie-ins with TV programs, movies, videogames, and social media (Kraak & Story, 2016). For example, the character "Shrek" was originally introduced in a movie; however, he has also been represented in dozens of toys, featured in promotions for McDonald's Happy Meals, and eventually was featured in a special variety, "Ogre O's" of Kellogg's cereal.

Improve the School Environment

The school setting is arguably the greatest example of success in improving the nutrition environment. The nutrition standards for the National School Lunch Program, National School Breakfast Program, and competitive foods sold in schools have all been dramatically improved in the past 5 years as a result of the Healthy, Hunger-Free Kids Act 2010 (U.S. Department of Agriculture, 2012). For the first time in decades, this legislation required the USDA to bring the school meal programs into alignment with the United States dietary guidelines and returned the power to the USDA to regulate all foods sold during the school day on school grounds.

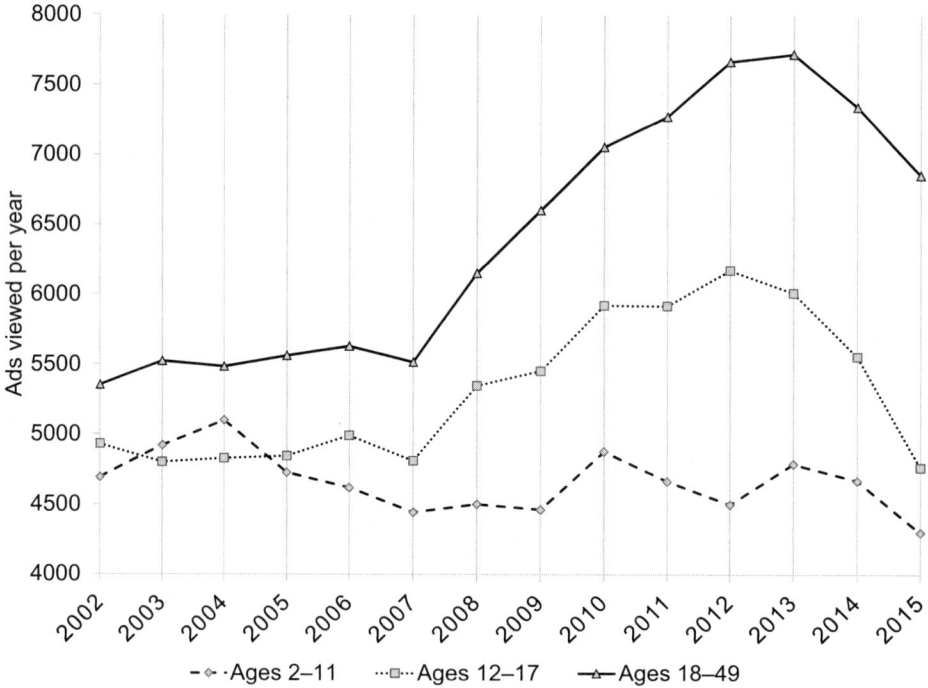

FIGURE 42.2. Changes in total TV food, beverage, and restaurant advertising viewed by children (ages 2–11), adolescents (ages 12–17), and adults (ages 18–49) from 2002 to 2015. From Frazier and Harris (2016). Reprinted by permission.

Beverages

The changes in the beverages sold in schools have been dramatic. In the late 1990s, the majority of high schools in the country had a vending machine that sold sugared soft drinks, and most districts had "pouring rights" contracts with one of the major soft drink companies (Brownell & Horgen, 2004). In 2003, California was the first state to pass legislation to limit the beverages and snacks that could be sold in schools. In 2006, Connecticut passed the first state law that prohibited the sale of any beverage other than water, 100% juice, and milk in all K–12 schools.

In 2006 the American Beverage Association (ABA) entered into a voluntary agreement with the Clinton Foundation and the American Heart Association to "change the mix" of beverages in schools by removing full-calorie sodas and increasing lower-calorie options. The ABA enlisted a researcher to evaluate its efforts and declared victory, saying that shipments of full-calorie soft drinks had declined by 97%, and that 90% fewer beverage calories were being delivered to schools than prior to their commitment (Wescott, Fitzpatrick, & Phillips, 2012). Although the fact that full-sugar soda had been banned from schools in several states during that same time frame may also have contributed to this success story, the important outcome was that students were significantly less likely to encounter soda at school. Finally, in 2014, all soda was officially restricted from schools nationwide when the USDA's Smart Snacks regulations were implemented (U.S. Department of Agriculture—Food and Nutrition Service, 2016).

Competitive Foods

The USDA's Smart Snacks regulations apply to food items, in addition to beverages, sold outside the school meals. All of these are called "competitive foods" because they essentially compete with the school lunch.

Most states that took on changing beverages in schools addressed snacks as well. By 2010, 27 states had some level of regulation for competitive foods that were permitted for sale in schools (Centers for Disease Control and Prevention, 2012). Notably, the nutrition regulations were not the same across states, which created a challenge for companies designing snacks to be sold in schools.

There is evidence that changing competitive food standards can have a positive influence on the nutrition environment in schools and metrics of student health. One national study documented that both state and district policies influence the availability of snacks and beverages in elementary schools (Chriqui, Turner, Taber, & Chaloupka, 2013). Another study compared students' dietary intake in a state with strong competitive food standards (California) to students in 14 states without any standards governing the sale of such foods and found that California high school students consumed on average 157 fewer calories in school per day than students in the comparison states (Taber, Chriqui, & Chaloupka, 2012). To assess the impact of state laws regulating competitive foods on student weight change, another analysis examined changes in body weight between fifth grade and eighth grade in a national dataset. It found that students in states with strong and comprehensive competitive food laws gained, on average, 0.25 fewer BMI units and were less likely to remain overweight or obese over time than students in states with no laws (Taber, Chriqui, Perna, Powell, & Chaloupka, 2012).

School Meals

The school meal standards for both breakfast and lunch have been updated progressively over the past few years. Although schools were given time to source new products and create new recipes, the changes were significant and posed a challenge to some school districts. The popular media coverage of the changes to the school meal program has been mixed (Confessore, 2014). The School Nutrition Association had a divided response to the changes, with some members in vocal support of the changes and others advocating to roll back the standards. Because First Lady Michelle Obama was a visible champion for school meal reform, many of the attacks became political. Further, there were specific segments of the food industry that were concerned about being able to sell their products in schools. The two groups that appeared to lobby Congress successfully were those that sought to protect potatoes and pizza sauce in the school meal program.

Despite the rocky start of implementing the new standards, nearly all districts in the nation now appear to be compliant with the new regulations. Further, recent evidence shows that the nutritional value of school lunches has improved substantially (Johnson, Podrabsky, Rocha, & Otten, 2016), students are eating more fruit, and plate waste has not increased (Cohen, Richardson, Parker, Catalano, & Rimm, 2014). There is reason to be optimistic that progress improving student nutrition will continue as the overall school food system becomes accustomed to the new regulations and students become more familiar with the healthier recipes.

Tax Unhealthy Foods

Taxation can encourage healthy eating by making it more expensive to eat unhealthy foods and, if the funds are used as subsidies, making it less expensive to eat healthy foods (Andreyeva, Chaloupka, & Brownell, 2011; Brownell et al., 2009). Jacobson and Brownell (2000) proposed the idea of using the funds raised by a tax to subsidize healthy food purchases—an idea that had not been implemented previously when cities or states had imposed small taxes on snack foods or soda (Jacobson & Brownell, 2000). Over the past 15 years, the idea of taxing foods at a rate large enough to make a difference in consumption has transitioned from a radical idea that no one thought was feasible to a mainstream concept that has now been considered seriously in many states and cities around the country. This transition is due to a combination of scientific evidence, advocacy, and lobbying.

In retrospect, there were a few key points that seemed to push the field forward. One was drawing an analogy between taxing tobacco and taxing food in order to give people a frame of reference for the idea that taxes could be used for public health purposes (Brownell & Warner, 2009). Another was testing the price elasticity of foods to determine whether increasing sugary drink prices, for example, would reliably decrease consumption. Economists have used both actual and simulated impact of prices on consumption and demand to do this work and have found that consumption and demand for sugary drinks is generally price-elastic (Andreyeva, Long, & Brownell, 2010; Colchero, Popkin, Rivera, & Ng, 2016; Powell, Chriqui, Khan, Wada, & Chaloupka, 2013). Next, the field narrowed the target to a tax on sugary drinks, as opposed to a tax on unhealthy foods in general. This decision was justified by the strength of the science concerning the harm associated with sugary drinks; it also made the entire endeavor feasible to implement in the retail system.

Once the target was clear, the battle to get a tax policy passed began. It became clear that the beverage companies were using the tobacco industry playbook (Brownell & Warner, 2009), which included the following:

- Focusing on personal responsibility as the cause of the nation's unhealthy diet.
- Raising fears that government action usurps personal freedom.
- Vilifying critics with totalitarian language, characterizing them as the food police, leaders of a nanny state, and even "food fascists," and accusing them of desiring to strip people of their civil liberties.
- Criticizing studies that hurt industry as "junk science."
- Emphasizing physical activity over diet.
- Stating that there are no good or bad foods; hence no food or food type (soft drinks, fast foods, etc.) should be targeted for change.
- Planting doubt when concerns are raised about the industry.

There have been campaigns to pass sugary drink taxes in several states and cities, and for several years, all of these efforts were defeated. However, in 2015, a ballot initiative in Berkeley, California passed, which was an important step. Although the beverage industry tried to paint it as an extreme policy is an atypical place in the country, a year later in 2016, another tax passed in Philadelphia, Pennsylvania (Nadolny, 2016). In November 2016, taxes passed in three cities in California; Boulder, Colorado; and Cook County, Illinois (Dardick, 2016; Jansen, 2016).

The research on the impact of taxes is being conducted now. So far, we know that the tax in Berkeley was passed on to the consumer, which alleviates the concern that the beverage industry or retailers would undermine the effect of the tax by absorbing it and keeping the sugary drinks at the same price as they were before (Falbe, Rojas, Grummon, & Madsen, 2015). Another recent study suggests that low-income individuals in Berkeley have decreased their consumption of the taxed products by 21%, whereas consumption increased by 4% in comparison cities (Falbe et al., 2016).

Time will tell the long-term impact of this policy change, but evidence to date is encouraging. It is also possible that the earned media exposure associated with the tax campaigns is its own public health initiative because it is educating the public about the harm associated with sugary drinks.

The Future Policy Landscape

Balancing the Tension between Personal and Social Responsibility

The tension between personal and social responsibility has been central to public policy discussions. Opponents of policy approaches such as taxes, restrictions on marketing or sales practices of food companies, and even informational efforts such as menu labeling, raise cries of a nanny state, big brother, and intrusive government, as mentioned previously. The implicit and often explicit assumption tied to these concerns is that personal responsibility is ignored.

It is possible to reconcile this tension (Brownell et al., 2010), and in fact this tension has been reconciled. Government has a long history of taking action to protect the health and well-being of its citizens in ways that support personally responsible behavior. Food safety standards help create a safer food supply, but consumers must play their role by handling and preparing foods in proper ways. Labels on clothing help inform consumers, who then make choices about what to purchase. Automobiles have seat belts, but drivers must assume responsibility for their use.

Because healthier default conditions support rather than undermine personal responsibility, this concept was clearly been embraced as policy once policy was passed to create better defaults (Brownell et al., 2010; Johnson & Goldstein, 2003; Thaler & Sunstein, 2008). There has been widespread change, showing that the United States and many other countries have addressed the question about whether government has a legitimate role in encouraging healthier diets and in preventing obesity. School nutrition standards, menu-labeling requirements, limiting trans fats in the food supply, pressure on food companies to reduce the marketing of unhealthy foods to children, and soda taxes are but a few of the initiatives that exemplify this conceptual view.

Thinking Ahead

Even taking into account the vagaries of which political party is in power at the local, state, and national levels, there is a clear trend toward harnessing public policy to address obesity prevention in particular and dietary change in general. We expect this trend to continue, and for initiatives now underway to expand. Tough nutrition standards for schools are now being considered for preschool and child care settings. A critical mass of soda taxes seems to have been reached to embolden new jurisdictions to take action. Work on the nation's dietary guidelines has led to reformulation of the food label and the impending addition of "added sugars" to the label.

It is difficult to predict trends in legislative and regulatory actions, as the composition of local, state, and federal legislatures and agencies change, but judging from precedents such as tobacco policy (Brandt, 2007; Warner, 2014), we would expect continued progress on such policy fronts. Soda taxes may be increased in places that have passed them already, and a broader range of food could be taxed in some locations. Food package labeling would improve by highlighting added sugars, and we hope a tested front-of-package system for this key information would be considered by legislators.

There also appears to be momentum for health-related institutions such as hospitals to set nutrition standards for what can be sold and served on their premises, and government facilities to do the same to protect the health of employees (Centers for Disease Control and Prevention, 2016).

We also expect progress on food marketing, particularly that directed at children. There are legal barriers to efforts to require such change because of the protection of commercial speech afforded businesses by the courts from the interpretation of the First Amendment of the U.S. Constitution. There is some relevant legal authority vested in state and local authorities, particularly in state attorneys general, to address marketing and matters such as portion-size regulations (Pomeranz & Brownell, 2011, 2012, 2014).

Finally, we believe that the future will bring tighter connection between parties working on obesity and nutrition policies with those working on other areas of food policy. For example, the cost, availability, and manufacturing of certain foods are heavily influenced by trade and agriculture policies, yet little connection occurs to link this information to work on obesity. Groups working to address hunger and food insecurity worldwide have, for the most part, not been connected to obesity policy. There are obvious places where linkage would be helpful. Nutrition standards for food banks and food pantries would ideally help address food insecurity and obesity simultaneously (Handforth, Hennink, & Schwartz, 2013). The link between early childhood malnutrition/stunting and later risk for obesity and diabetes is another connection (Prentice, 2006).

The lack of connection between individuals and organizations working on different areas of food policy exposes several key weaknesses in the current picture. One is that people working in the different areas do not learn from each other, and another is that the opportunity is missed to build much larger and stronger coalitions than now exist to argue for a common set of policies. As an example, there is great concern about increasing meat production and consumption around the world (Herrero et al., 2013). Those interested in public health nutrition are concerned about the associated calorie and saturated-fat consumption, but alone are not a strong enough voice to reverse these trends. Groups such as the National Resources Defense Council, Sierra Club, and sustainable agriculture groups underscore the impact of meat production on climate change. Other groups focus on how meat production is so water intensive. Were the nutrition, environmental, and agriculture groups to come together into a coalition to argue for policies that would curb meat consumption, the political might would far exceed what currently exists.

In sum, public policy offers the potential to reach the entire population of a city, state, or nation in ways that might help reduce the rates, progression, and economic and health impacts of obesity. Given that it is only in recent years that policies have entered the picture in legislative and regulatory circles, and in the past several years when most such policies have been enacted, data to know what work best and at what cost are just beginning to accumulate. Research to carefully evaluate the impact of policies and the processes by which they succeed or fail when proposed is an important need in the field. Our hope is that evidence-based approaches to policymaking will be the norm, and that as the evidence grows, a policy agenda for the nation will follow.

References

Allison, D. B., Fontaine, K. R., Manson, J. E., Stevens, J., & VanItallie, T. B. (1999). Annual deaths attributable to obesity in the United States. *Journal of the American Medical Association, 282*(16), 1530–1538.

Andreyeva, T., Chaloupka, F. J., & Brownell, K. D. (2011). Estimating the potential of taxes on sugar-sweetened beverages to reduce consumption and generate revenue. *Preventive Medicine, 52*(6), 413–416.

Andreyeva, T., Long, M. W., & Brownell, K. D. (2010). The impact of food prices on consumption: A systematic review of research on the price elasticity of demand for food. *American Journal of Public Health, 100*(2), 216–222.

Boyland, E. J., Nolan, S., Kelly, B., Tudur-Smith, C., Jones, A., Halford, J. C., et al. (2016). Advertising as a cue to consume: A systematic review and meta-analysis of the effects of acute exposure to unhealthy food and nonalcoholic beverage advertising on intake in children and adults. *American Journal of Clinical Nutrition, 103*(2), 519–533.

Brandt, A. M. (2007). *The cigarette century: The rise, fall, and deadly persistence of the product that defined America.* New York: Basic Books.

Brownell, K. D., Farley, T., Willett, W. C., Popkin, B. M., Chaloupka, F. J., Thompson, J. W., et al. (2009). The public health and economic benefits of taxing sugar-sweetened beverages. *New England Journal of Medicine, 361*(16), 1599–1605.

Brownell, K. D., & Horgen, K. B. (2004). *Food fight: The inside story of the food industry, America's obesity crisis, and what we can do about it.* New York: McGraw-Hill Education.

Brownell, K. D., Kersh, R., Ludwig, D. S., Post, R. C., Puhl, R. M., Schwartz, M. B., et al. (2010). Personal responsibility and obesity: A constructive approach to a controversial issue. *Health Affairs, 29*(3), 379–387.

Brownell, K. D., & Warner, K. E. (2009). The perils of ignoring history: Big Tobacco played dirty and millions died: How similar is Big Food? *Milbank Quarterly, 87*(1), 259–294.

Cairns, G., Angus, K., Hastings, G., & Caraher, M. (2013). Systematic reviews of the evidence on the nature, extent and effects of food marketing to children: A retrospective summary. *Appetite, 62,* 209–215.

Centers for Disease Control and Prevention. (2012). *Competitive foods and beverages in U.S. schools: A state policy analysis.* Atlanta, GA: U.S. Department of Health and Human Services.

Centers for Disease Control and Prevention. (2016). Healthy food service guidelines. Retrieved from *www.cdc.gov/obesity/strategies/food-serv-guide.html.*

Chriqui, J. F., Turner, L., Taber, D. R., & Chaloupka, F. J. (2013). Association between district and state policies and U.S. public elementary school competitive food and beverage environments. *JAMA Pediatrics, 167*(8), 714–722.

Cohen, J. F., Richardson, S., Parker, E., Catalano, P. J., & Rimm, E. B. (2014). Impact of the new U.S. Department of Agriculture school meal standards on food selection, consumption, and waste. *American Journal of Preventive Medicine, 46*(4), 388–394.

Colchero, M. A., Popkin, B. M., Rivera, J. A., & Ng, S. W. (2016). Beverage purchases from stores in Mexico under the excise tax on sugar sweetened beverages: Observational study. *British Medical Journal, 352,* h6704.

Confessore, N. (2014, October 7). How school lunch became the latest political battleground. *New York Times Magazine.*

Council of Better Business Bureaus. (2016). Children's food and beverage advertising initiative. Retrieved from *www.bbb.org/council/the-national-partner-program/national-advertising-review-services/childrens-food-and-beverage-advertising-initiative.*

Dardick, H. (2016, November 11). Cook County soda pop tax approved with Preckwinkle breaking tie vote. *Chicago Tribune.*

Falbe, J., Rojas, N., Grummon, A. H., & Madsen, K. A. (2015). Higher retail prices of sugar-sweetened beverages 3 months after implementation of an excise tax in Berkeley, California. *American Journal of Public Health, 105*(11), 2194–2201.

Falbe, J., Thompson, H. R., Becker, C. M., Rojas, N., McCulloch, C. E., & Madsen, K. A. (2016). Impact of the Berkeley excise tax on sugar-sweetened beverage consumption. *American Journal of Public Health, 106*(10), 1865–1871.

Federal Trade Commission. (2011). Interagency working group seeks input on proposed voluntary principles for marketing food to children. Retrieved from *www.ftc.gov/news-events/press-releases/2011/04/interagency-working-group-seeks-input-proposed-voluntary*.

Frazier, W. C., & Harris, J. L. (2016). *Trends in television food advertising to young people: 2015 update*. Hartford, CT: Rudd Center for Food Policy and Obesity.

Gearhart, S., Craig, C., & Steed, C. (2012). Network news coverage of obesity in two time periods: An analysis of issues, sources, and frames. *Health Communication, 27*(7), 653–662.

Handforth, B., Hennink, M., & Schwartz, M. B. (2013). A qualitative study of nutrition-based initiatives at selected food banks in the Feeding America network. *Journal of the Academy of Nutrition and Dietetics, 113*(3), 411–415.

Harris, J. L., Bargh, J. A., & Brownell, K. D. (2009). Priming effects of television food advertising on eating behavior. *Health Psychology, 28*(4), 404–413.

Harris, J. L., Sarda, V., Schwartz, M. B., & Brownell, K. D. (2013). Redefining "child-directed advertising" to reduce unhealthy television food advertising. *American Journal of Preventive Medicine, 44*(4), 358–364.

Harris, J. L., Speers, S. E., Schwartz, M. B., & Brownell, K. D. (2012). U.S. food company branded advergames on the internet: Children's exposure and effects on snack consumption. *Journal of Children and Media, 6*(1), 51–68.

Hernandez, M., & Kolish, E. (2011). Better Business Bureau child food and beverage advertising initiative general comments and comments on the proposed nutrition principles and marketing definitions for Interagency working group on food marketed to children: FTC Project No. P094513. Retrieved from *www.ftc.gov/sites/default/files/documents/public_comments/preliminary-proposed-nutrition-principles-guide-industry-self-regulatory-efforts-project-no.p094513-07845/07845-80012.pdf*.

Herrero, M., Havlik, P., Valin, H., Notenbaert, A., Rufino, M. C., Thornton, P. K., et al. (2013). Biomass use, production, feed efficiencies, and greenhouse gas emissions from global livestock systems. *Proceedings of the National Academy of Sciences of the USA, 110*(52), 20888–20893.

Institute of Medicine. (1995). *Weighing the options: Criteria for evaluating weight-management programs*. Washington, DC: National Academies Press.

Institute of Medicine. (2006). *Food marketing to children and youth: Threat or opportunity?* Washington, DC: National Academies Press.

Jacobson, M. F., & Brownell, K. D. (2000). Small taxes on soft drinks and snack foods to promote health. *American Journal of Public Health, 90*(6), 854–857.

Jansen, B. (2016, November 10). 4 cities vote to tax sugary drinks, soda. *USA Today*.

Johnson, D. B., Podrabsky, M., Rocha, A., & Otten, J. J. (2016). Effect of the Healthy Hunger-Free Kids Act on the nutritional quality of meals selected by students and school lunch participation rates. *JAMA Pediatrics, 170*(1), e153918.

Johnson, E. J., & Goldstein, D. (2003). Medicine: Do defaults save lives? *Science, 302*(5649), 1338–1339.

Kelly, B., Vandevijvere, S., Freeman, B., & Jenkin, G. (2015). New media but same old tricks: Food marketing to children in the digital age. *Current Obesity Reports, 4*(1), 37–45.

Kraak, V. I., & Story, M. (2016). The use of brand mascots and media characters: Opportunities for responsible food marketing to children. Retrieved from *http://healthyeatingresearch.org/wp-content/uploads/2016/03/her_mascot_3-22_FINAL-1.pdf*.

Kunkel, D. L., Castonguay, J. S., & Filer, C. R. (2015). Evaluating industry self-regulation of food marketing to children. *American Journal of Preventive Medicine, 49*(2), 181–187.

McGlockton, J. (2011). Comments of the National Restaurant Association on the Interagency Working Group on food marketed to children: General comments and proposed marketing definitions: FTC Project No. P094513. Retrieved from *www.ftc.gov/sites/default/files/documents/public_comments/preliminary-proposed-nutrition-principles-guide-industry-self-regulatory-efforts-project-no.p094513-07857/07857-80022.pdf*.

Nadolny, T. L. (2016, June 16). Soda tax passes; Philadelphia is first big city in nation to enact one. *Philadelphia Inquirer*.

Nestle, M. (2011). Congress caves in again: Delays IWG recommendations. Retrieved from *www.foodpolitics.com/2011/12/congress-caves-in-again-delays-iwg-recommendations*.

Ogden, C. L., Carroll, M. D., Lawman, H. G., Fryar, C. D., Kruszon-Moran, D., Kit, B. K., et al. (2016). Trends in obesity prevalence among children and adolescents in the United States, 1988–1994 through 2013–2014. *Journal of the American Medical Association, 315*(21), 2292–2299.

Olshansky, S. J., Passaro, D. J., Hershow, R. C., Layden, J., Carnes, B. A., Brody, J., et al. (2005). A potential decline in life expectancy in the United States in the 21st century. *New England Journal of Medicine, 352*(11), 1138–1145.

Pomeranz, J. L., & Brownell, K. D. (2011). Advancing public health obesity policy through state attorneys general. *American Journal of Public Health, 101*(3), 425–431.

Pomeranz, J. L., & Brownell, K. D. (2012). Portion sizes and beyond: Government's legal authority to regulate food-industry practices. *New England Journal of Medicine, 367*(15), 1383–1385.

Pomeranz, J. L., & Brownell, K. D. (2014). Can government regulate portion sizes? *New England Journal of Medicine, 371*(21), 1956–1958.

Powell, L. M., Chriqui, J. F., Khan, T., Wada, R., & Chaloupka, F. J. (2013). Assessing the potential effectiveness of food and beverage taxes and subsidies for improving public health: A systematic review of prices, demand, and body weight outcomes. *Obesity Reviews, 14*(2), 110–128.

Prentice, A. M. (2006). The emerging epidemic of obesity in developing countries. *International Journal of Epidemiology, 35*(1), 93–99.

Puhl, R. M., Neumark-Sztainer, D., Bryn Austin, S., Suh, Y., & Wakefield, D. B. (2016). Policy actions to address weight-based bullying and eating disorders in schools: Views of teachers and school administrators. *Journal of School Health, 86*(7), 507–515.

Suh, Y., Puhl, R., Liu, S., & Fleming Milici, F. F. (2014). Parental support for policy actions to reduce weight stigma toward youth in schools and children's television programs: Trends from 2011 to 2013. *Childhood Obesity, 10*(6), 533–541.

Suh, Y., Puhl, R., Liu, S., & Milici, F. F. (2014). Support for laws to prohibit weight discrimination in the United States: Public attitudes from 2011 to 2013. *Obesity (Silver Spring), 22*(8), 1872–1879.

Taber, D. R., Chriqui, J. F., & Chaloupka, F. J. (2012). Differences in nutrient intake associated with state laws regarding fat, sugar, and caloric content of competitive foods. *Archives of Pediatrics and Adolescent Medicine, 166*(5), 452–458.

Taber, D. R., Chriqui, J. F., Perna, F. M., Powell, L. M., & Chaloupka, F. J. (2012). Weight status among adolescents in states that govern competitive food nutrition content. *Pediatrics, 130*(3), 437–444.

Thaler, R. H., & Sunstein, C. R. (2008). *Nudge: Improving decisions about health, wealth, and happiness*. New Haven, CT: Yale University Press.

U.S. Department of Agriculture. (2005). Dietary Guidelines for Americans, 2005. Available at *https://health.gov/dietaryguidelines/dga2005/recommendations.htm*. Washington, DC: Author.

U.S. Department of Agriculture. (2010). Dietary Guidelines for Americans, 2010. Available at *www.cnpp.usda.gov/sites/default/files/dietaryguidelinesforamericans/PolicyDoc.pdf*.

U.S. Department of Agriculture. (2012). Nutrition standards in the national school lunch and school breakfast programs. *Federal Register, 77*(17), 4088–4167.

U.S. Department of Agriculture. (2015). Dietary Guidelines for Americans, 2015–2020. Available at *https://health.gov/dietaryguidelines/2015/resources/2015-2020_Dietary_Guidelines.pdf*. Washington, DC: Author.

U.S. Department of Agriculture Food and Nutrition Service. (2016, April 14). Healthier school day: Tools for schools—focusing on smart snacks. Retrieved from *www.fns.usda.gov/healthierschoolday/tools-schools-focusing-smart-snacks*.

U.S. Department of Health and Human Services. (2001). *The Surgeon General's call to action to prevent and decrease overweight and obesity*. Rockville, MD: Public Health Service, Office of the Surgeon General.

Warner, K. E. (2014). Tobacco control policies and their impacts: Past, present, and future. *Annals of the American Thoracic Society, 11*(2), 227–230.

Wescott, R. F., Fitzpatrick, B. M., & Phillips, E. (2012). Industry self-regulation to improve student health: Quantifying changes in beverage shipments to schools. *American Journal of Public Health, 102*(10), 1928–1935.

Wolf, A. M., & Colditz, G. A. (1998). Current estimates of the economic cost of obesity in the United States. *Obesity Research, 6*(2), 97–106.

World Health Organization. (1998). *Obesity: Preventing and managing the global epidemic*. Report of a WHO consultation on obesity, Geneva, June 3–5, 1997.

Author Index

Aalborg, A., 582
Abar, L., 14
Abayev, S., 570
Abbott, G. R., 151
Abbott, W. G. H., 42, 43
Abdelbaki, T. N., 387
Abrams, B., 139
Abrams, C., 101
Abu-Dayyeh, B. K., 539, 540–542, 545, 546
Abu-Elheiga, L., 56
Acevedo-Garcia, D., 140
Acheson, K. J., 42
Ackard, D., 577
Ackermann, R. T., 210, 293, 495, 499, 501, 502, 503
Adair, L. S., 255
Adami, G. F., 175, 579
Adams, K. M., 418
Adams, M. A., 144
Adams, T. D., 197, 198, 199, 201, 382, 385
Adan, R. A., 84, 85
Addy, C., 359
Adeyemo, A. A., 440
Aditya, H., 571
Adler, G., 298, 340
Adler, M. L., 9
Adler, N. E., 155
Admiraal, W. M., 448
Affenito, S., 175
Afshin, A., 141
Agarwal, S., 382

Agoston, A. T., 544
Agras, W. S., 172, 178, 236, 554, 556, 558
Aguiar, I. C., 383
Agus, M. S., 316
Aharon, I., 566
Ahima, R. S., 66
Ahmad, S., 65
Ahren, B., 30
Aihara, H., 544
Ainsworth, B., 261
Ainsworth, B. E., 107, 108
Ajslev, T. A., 80
Akabas, S. R., 247
Akinci, Ö. F., 536
Al, E., 140
Al Harakeh, A. B., 375, 378, 379
Al Snih, S., 232, 233, 234
Alamuddin, N., 259, 283, 337, 338, 340, 466
Alberga, A. S., 152
Albert, S. M., 123
Alberts, H. J., 516, 517
Albrecht, S. S., 140
Albright, A. L., 493
Albu, J. B., 125
Alegria, M., 155
Alessi, C., 123
Alexander, S. C., 488
Alfaris, N., 131
Algahim, M. F., 382
Alger, S., 43
Alghamdi, H. U., 536

Alhadeff, A. L., 27
Al-Hadithy, N., 571
Ali, M. K., 293, 504, 505
Ali, S., 158
Allan, J. D., 442
Allebrandt, K. V., 129
Allen, D. B., 69
Allen-Vercoe, E., 79
Alley, D. E., 159, 193
Allison, D. B., 65, 129, 158, 317, 355, 356, 427, 441, 442, 597, 639, 659
Allison, K. C., 153, 169, 171, 174, 175, 176, 177, 260, 261, 553, 569
Allshouse, J. E., 142
Almeida, L., 160
Almirall, D., 476
Alosco, M. L., 211
Alpert, M. A., 9
Alpert, S., 41
Altabe, M. N., 566
Alter, D. A., 3
Alting, E., 598
Altman, M., 139, 172, 623, 624
Alvarez-Crespo, M., 29
Alvarez-Leite, J. I., 652
Alverdy, J. C., 383
Alzobydi, A. H., 536
Al-Zubaidi, A. M., 536, 543
Amate, J., 640
Amato, M., 584
Ambrose, C., 79

Ambrosius, W. T., 236
Amianto, F., 171
Aminian, A., 284, 367, 369, 375, 379, 459, 650
Amonkar, M. M., 158
Amori, R. E., 360
Amy, N. K., 582
Andeersen, C. S., 80
Andersen, G. S., 175
Andersen, R. E., 261, 326
Andersen, T., 318
Anderson, D., 156
Anderson, D. A., 209, 441
Anderson, J. J., 236
Anderson, J. W., 318, 362, 482
Anderson, L. A., 155
Anderson, L. M., 502
Anderson, S. E., 156
Anderson, T. E., 41
Andersson, I., 175, 394
Andresen, M. A., 141
Andrews, S., 328
Andreyeva, T., 143, 159, 160, 665, 666
Andriacchi, T. P., 236
Andrilla, C. A., 497
Aneja, S., 613
Anesbury, T., 584
Anglin, K., 443
Angrisani, L., 370, 531, 645
Angus, K., 662
Annesi, J. J., 214
Annis, N. M., 578
Ansley, S. J., 69
Antognoli, E. L., 417
Anton, S. D., 215
Apovian, C. M., 247, 283, 299, 301, 349, 350, 357, 360, 362, 415, 454
Appel, L. J., 291, 294, 395, 398, 407, 456, 461, 468, 470, 488
Appelhans, B. M., 130, 631
Arab, L., 448
Araujo, J., 125
Aravani, A., 197
Araz, O. M., 628
Archer, E., 594
Ard, J., 444
Ard, J. D., 426
Arem, H., 124, 261
Arena, R., 246
Arenz, S., 595
Ariel-Donges, A. H., 294, 393
Armstrong, M., 268, 510, 513
Arnold, L. M., 556
Arnow, B., 556
Aronne, L., 349, 350
Aronne, L. J., 81, 243, 247, 253, 255, 257, 284, 358, 362, 639

Aronson, W., 15
Arora, T., 129, 131
Arsenijevic, D., 54
Arterburn, D. E., 201, 382, 386
Asakawa, A., 29
Asarnow, L. D., 130
Asch, D. A., 522, 527, 528
Ascherio, A., 9
Ashley, J. M., 457
Ashrafian, H., 385
Ashton, J., 516, 517
Astrup, A., 28, 54, 288, 309, 312, 313, 314, 315, 318, 354, 360, 638
Atalay, T., 536
Atkinson, N. L., 467
Atkinson, R. L., 158
Atlantis, E., 154
Aubin, H. J., 245
Audrain-McGovern, J., 124
August, M. A., 151
Augustin, L. S., 316
Auinger, P., 594
Aune, D., 6, 13, 14
Auquit-Auckbur, I., 571
Avenell, A., 289
Aversa, A., 212
Aveyard, P., 245, 401
Ayres, C. G., 418
Ayyad, C., 318
Azadbakht, L., 97

B

Baan, C. A., 140
Babu, A. R., 361
Babyak, M. A., 175
Bacak, S. J., 143
Backhed, F., 75, 76, 77, 78, 83
Bader, M. D., 143
Badmin, N., 579
Badylak, S. F., 233
Baer, H. J., 417
Baer, R. A., 330
Bahnson, J. L., 230
Bahr, R., 115, 116
Bailer, B. A., 605
Bailey, B. W., 131
Bailey, C. J., 640
Bain, S. C., 286
Baird, B., 630
Bajema, C. J., 8
Bakacs, E., 80
Baker, E. A., 143
Baker, M., 154
Baker, R., 418
Baker, R. C., 340
Bakizada, Z., 466

Bakizada, Z. M., 259, 283
Bal, B., 376, 378
Bal, B. S., 652
Balague, N., 571
Balantekin, K. N., 437, 605, 622, 641
Balasubramaniam, A., 28
Baldwin, K. M., 81
Balen, A. H., 15
Baler, R. D., 177
Bales, C. W., 233, 236
Baliunas, A. J., 236
Ball, K., 151, 330
Ballantyne, G. H., 28
Bandini, L. G., 298
Bandura, A., 337, 393, 493, 498, 628
Banerjee, A., 652
Bang, C. S., 545
Banks, M., 231
Banks, S., 129
Banks, W. A., 28, 29, 31
Baran, J., 610
Barbin, J. M., 209
Bardia, A., 417
Barendregt, J. J., 159
Barengo, N. C., 474
Bargh, J. A., 662
Barham, K., 496, 499, 502
Barlow, D. H., 632
Barlow, S. E., 594, 598, 623, 636, 644
Barnea, M., 126
Barnes, L. L., 232
Barnes, R., 511, 513
Barnes, R. D., 153
Barofsky, I., 158, 580
Baron, K. G., 127, 129, 130
Barone, M., 53
Barrachina, M. D., 26
Barreira, T. V., 111
Barrera, C. M., 596
Barrett, E., 80
Barrett-Connor, E., 229
Barrios, D. M., 432
Barrios, L., 430
Barry, D., 155
Bartels, L. K., 16
Bartelt, A., 56
Bartlett, S. J., 298, 580
Bartness, T. J., 28, 30
Bartok, C. J., 596
Barton, M., 623
Baskin, D. G., 30, 67
Baskin, M., 513
Bassett, D. R., 141, 327
Bassett, D. R., Jr., 107, 114
Bastian, B. A., 7
Bates, D. W., 417

Batterham, R. L., 28, 368
Battle Horgen, K., 599
Bauer, U. E., 186
Baum, C., 428
Baum, C. L., 159
Bauman, A., 114
Bauman, K., 438, 439
Baumann, M. H., 353
Baumeister, R. F., 171
Baumgartner, R. N., 236
Baur, L. A., 64
Baura, G. D., 30
Bautista-Castaño, I., 536, 541
Bayer, O., 607
Beach, A. M., 96, 98
Beach, M. C., 581
Beamish, A. J., 605, 644, 645, 648, 650, 651, 652, 653, 654
Bean, J. A., 652
Bean, M., 513
Bearon, L. B., 231
Beaulieu, K., 119
Beaumont, K., 31
Beck, A. T., 157, 209, 223, 253, 263, 341
Beck, N., 561
Becker, C., 152
Becker, D. M., 502
Beck-Nielsen, H., 618
Beebe, D. W., 126
Beecher, M. D., 623
Beeken, R. J., 161
Beers, E. A., 330
Befort, C. A., 494, 499, 512
Begg, D. P., 26, 30, 31
Beglin, S., 260
Behary, J., 543
Beil, T. L., 623
Beinfeld, M. C., 26
Bel, S., 124
Belcher, B. R., 600
Belkaid, Y., 84
Bell, E. A., 98
Bellizzi, M. C., 645
Bellocchio, L., 81
Belsky, D. W., 65
Belyea, M., 617
Belza, A., 315
Bem, D. J., 509
Bender, M. S., 448
Benedict, F. G., 46
Benjamin Neelon, S. E., 616
Bennett, C., 186
Bennett, G. G., 428, 447, 448, 468, 470, 475
Bennett, P. H., 440
Bennett, W. L., 413, 488
Benoit, S. C., 30
Bentley, T., 265

Berends, F. J., 570
Berenson, G. S., 593, 645
Berg, C., 259
Berger, K., 131
Berghuis, K. A., 224
Bergouignan, A., 256
Bergstrom, J., 476
Berkman, N. D., 172, 173
Berkowitz, R. I., 154, 161, 286, 299, 593, 594, 595, 600, 605, 623, 636, 641
Berman, S. R., 216
Bernstein, D. P., 266
Berrington de Gonzalez, A., 6, 7
Berry, E. M., 343
Berset, M., 151
Bes-Rastrollo, M., 43, 97
Bessard, T., 42
Bessesen, D. H., 362
Besson, H., 600
Best, J. R., 630, 631
Betzel, B., 542
Beydoun, M. A., 185
Beyer, R. E., 115
Bhaskaran, K., 652
Bhatti, J. A., 271
Bian, B., 417
Bianchini, F., 12
Bickel, W. K., 629, 630
Biedert, E., 214
Biener, A., 432
Bienias, J. L., 232, 232–233
Biggs, S., 474
Bigus, E., 157
Billington, C., 581
Billington, C. J., 30
Bindels, L. B., 77, 83
Biorserud, C., 654
Birch, D. W., 383
Birch, L. L., 96, 598, 599, 600
Birketvedt, G., 175
Bishaw, A., 438
Bishop, D. B., 522
Bishop-Gilyard, C. T., 569
Bixler, E. O., 130, 131
Bjorbaek, C., 31
Bjorge, T., 6, 8
Bjornson-Benson, W. M., 525
Björntorp, P., 150
Black, A. E., 46
Black, C., 143
Black, D. R., 233
Black, S., 153
Blackburn, G. L., 230
Blackman, A., 247
Blackwell, C. S., 496, 499
Blackwell, D. L., 438
Blaine, B. E., 268
Blair, E., 485

Blair, S. N., 112, 225, 228, 326, 581, 587
Blake, M., 171
Blakemore, A. I. F., 255
Blandford, A., 393
Blankenship, J., 569
Blansit, A., 330
Blatt, A. D., 98
Blaum, C. S., 232
Bleich, S. N., 100, 413, 418, 488, 581, 598, 616, 618
Blissmer, B., 152, 224, 225
Block, G., 258
Block, J. P., 100, 417, 418
Blomquist, K. K., 153
Blomqvist, A. G., 28
Blonde, L., 638
Bloom, B., 480
Bloom, S. R., 28
Bluher, S., 646
Blumenthal, D. M., 143
Blumenthal, J. A., 175
Blundell, J., 119
Blundell, J. E., 113, 118, 119, 353, 599
Blustein, J., 80
Bochukova, E. G., 66, 68
Bodenlos, J. S., 151
Boerma, D., 570
Bogardus, C., 41, 42, 44, 46, 48, 50, 54, 441
Boggiano, M. M., 28
Bohannan, B. J., 80
Bohdjalian, A., 570
Boldrin, M., 350, 637
Boldrin, M. N., 195, 301, 350, 459
Bolinder, J., 361
Bolognesi, A., 151, 153
Bond, D. S., 269, 326
Bond, K., 131
Boniface, D., 596
Bonilla, Y., 541
Bonnefond, A., 70
Bonnet, F., 158
Bonneux, L., 159
Bonomi, A. G., 45
Bonsergent, E., 618
Booth, T. L., 233
Borah, R., 129
Borders-Hemphill, V., 431
Bordi, P., 94
Börnhorst, C., 124
Borradaile, K. E., 598, 614
Borrel, G., 79
Borsheim, E., 115, 116, 118
Bos, G., 140
Boston, R. C., 174
Bosy-Westphal, A., 46, 54, 131

Bouchard, C., 39, 49, 52, 65, 70, 105, 106, 111, 216, 255, 258, 316, 349, 369, 376, 377, 380
Bouter, K. E., 83
Bouton, M. E., 628
Bouza, C., 640
Bowers, C. W., 28
Bowles, H. R., 108
Bowling, J. M., 344, 473, 511
Bowman, B. A., 186
Boxer, P., 160
Boyer, J. G., 212
Boyland, E. J., 353, 662
Boyle, C. N., 31
Boyle, R. G., 339, 500, 579
Brace, A. M., 502
Brach, J. S., 233, 235
Bracken, M. B., 15
Bradfield, J. P., 596, 597
Bradley, A. J., 360
Bradley, L. E., 517, 518
Braet, C., 625, 629
Brahler, E., 174
Braley, S. C., 653
Brancati, F. L., 230
Branch, L. G., 233
Brand, M. D., 54
Brandon, L. J., 47
Brandt, A. M., 667
Brannon, E. E., 616
Branscombe, N. R., 160
Brauer, P., 454
Brawley, L., 236
Braxton, D. F., 445, 446
Bray, G. A., 32, 42, 43, 47, 50, 52, 64, 97, 99, 227, 230, 247, 284, 299, 312, 313, 317, 349, 350, 352, 353, 359, 362, 369, 376, 377, 380, 458, 498, 638, 639
Breadsell, D., 584
Brennan, L., 156, 160
Brennan, L. K., 143
Brennan, T., 522
Brethauer, S., 369
Brethauer, S. A., 368, 370, 371, 375, 378, 379, 382, 383, 386, 387, 541, 653
Breusing, N., 131
Brewer, C. J., 15
Brewer, G., 269, 460
Breyer, B., 144
Briend, A., 141
Brindle, K. M., 54
Brinkworth, G. D., 210, 211, 212
Briss, P. A., 186
Brizendine, E., 502
Broccoli, S., 513
Brochu, P. M., 160
Brock, B., 31

Brock, J., 337
Brodie, D., 152
Brodney, S., 587
Brogan, K., 513
Brolin, R. E., 380
Brooks, G. A., 111, 115
Brooks, L., 85
Brouns, F., 114
Brouwer, E. M., 54
Brown, A., 236
Brown, D. R., 155
Brown, G. K., 209, 253
Brown, K. W., 330
Brown, L. M., 30
Brown, M., 18, 138
Brown, M. S., 28
Brown, P. J., 441
Brown, R. A., 516, 517
Brown, T., 609, 612
Brown, T. T., 140
Brown, W., 330
Brownell, K., 160, 599
Brownell, K. D., 143, 154, 155, 156, 157, 160, 161, 178, 286, 304, 337, 356, 516, 568, 577, 578, 579, 580, 581, 584, 659, 660, 662, 663, 664, 665, 666, 667
Brownley, K. A., 157, 556
Brownson, R. C., 143, 144, 155
Brozek, J., 52, 208
Brubaker, P. H., 231
Bruce, B., 235
Brufani, C., 640
Brug, J., 137
Brugere, J. F., 79
Brugger, U., 137
Brumpton, B., 150
Brunaud, L., 653
Bruni, O., 123
Brunstrom, J. M., 100
Bruusgaard, D., 342, 343
Bryan, J., 211
Bryn Austin, S., 662
Bryson, S. W., 172, 178, 554
Büchel, C., 630
Bucher, T., 98
Bucholtz, D. C., 447
Buchwald, H., 359, 371, 380, 382, 383, 531
Buckley, J. D., 210
Buckley, J. P., 330
Buckley, M. C., 387
Buehler, R., 141
Buescher, J. L., 28
Buffington, C. K., 131
Bulan, E. J., 570
Bulik, C., 579
Bulik, C. M., 157, 170, 171, 556

Bulow, J., 54
Buman, M., 108, 261
Bunker, C., 9
Bunting, K., 162, 330, 514, 518
Bunyan, D. P., 160
Burgess, S. M., 18
Burgoine, T., 143, 144
Buring, J., 261
Buring, J. E., 9, 112, 322
Burke, A., 99
Burke, L. E., 270, 338, 339, 340, 344, 500
Burke, S., 471
Burke, S. M., 614, 616
Burks, D. J., 30
Burnand, B., 81
Burney, B. O., 29
Burr, H., 114
Bursac, Z., 444, 493, 511
Burt, V., 8
Burton, J. H., 47
Burton, L. R., 525
Busch, C., 85
Busch, V., 130
Busetto, L., 200
Bushe, C. J., 360
Bushman, B. J., 628
Butler, B. A., 326, 340
Butryn, M., 265, 337, 339, 340
Butryn, M. L., 96, 249, 287, 330, 336, 338, 339, 340, 341, 393, 454, 466, 508, 511, 514, 516, 517, 518, 519, 636
Butte, N. F., 70
Buttitta, M., 593
Buttner, P., 552
Buysse, D. J., 216
Buzga, M., 544
Buzzell, P., 406, 471
Byard, T. D., 326
Byrne, K. J., 466
Byrne, N. M., 115
Byrne, S. M., 178
Byrnes, W. C., 116

C

Cacciapaglia, H. M., 403
Cachelin, F. M., 140
Cadiere, G. B., 653
Cahalin, L., 108, 261
Cai, J., 233
Cairns, G., 662
Calle, E. E., 652
Callister, R., 259
Calugi, S., 210
Calzo, J. P., 152
Camhi, S. M., 441

Author Index

Campbell, A., 569
Campbell, F., 608
Campostano, A., 175
Camps, S., 217
Cani, P. D., 77, 83, 84
Cannon, B., 82
Canoy, D., 8
Cao, J., 56
Cao, Z. J., 610, 612
Capers, P. L., 129
Caraher, M., 662
Cardinal, T. M., 256
Carels, R. A., 162, 395, 402, 403, 512
Carey, M., 263
Carey, M. P., 212
Carey, V. J., 9, 10
Carlsson, L. M., 385, 651
Carmelli, D., 65
Carnell, S., 65, 596, 600, 625
Carnethon, M. R., 140
Carnicelli, A., 380
Caro, J. F., 51
Carpenter, J. S., 500
Carpiniello, B., 157
Carr, D., 161, 577, 578
Carr, K. A., 630, 631
Carraça, E. V., 583
Carraway, M., 131
Carrel, A. L., 69
Carroll, J., 256, 330
Carroll, M. D., 3, 140, 185, 243, 349, 419, 453, 466, 503, 531, 552, 593, 594, 622, 644
Carson, T., 444
Carter, J. C., 178
Carter-Edwards, L., 446, 502
Carvajal, F., 177
Carvajal, R., 569
Casazza, K., 98, 267, 309, 310, 311
Cases, S., 56
Casey, C. M., 610
Cash, T. F., 214, 566, 567, 568, 578, 583
Caspersen, C. J., 261
Cassin, S. E., 178
Castellanos, V. H., 98
Castellarin, M., 79
Castellini, G., 170
Castro, G. C., 30
Catalano, P. J., 665
Catenacci, V. A., 324
Caudwell, P., 119
Cavadas, C., 28
Cavan, D., 613
Cawley, J., 18, 141, 432
Cecil, J. E., 65, 596, 599
Cedernaes, J., 126
Cefalu, W. T., 361

Cerhan, J. R., 7
Cerú-Björk, C., 175
Chabas, D., 131
Chai, S. Y., 31
Chaix, B., 144
Chakravorty, S., 125
Chalasani, N., 382, 383
Chaloupka, F. J., 665, 666
Chambliss, H. O., 581
Chamorro, R., 131
Champagne, C. M., 94, 99
Chan, C. B., 327
Chan, D. S., 14
Chan, J. M., 9, 10
Chand, B., 371, 541
Chang, S. H., 650, 652
Chang, V. W., 159, 193
Chanoine, J. P., 350, 353, 637
Chao, A. M., 561, 605, 636
Chao, H. L., 214
Chao, Y. H., 160
Chapman, C. D., 125
Chapman, I., 31
Chapman, S. L., 337, 340
Chapotot, F., 132
Chaput, J., 255, 265
Chaput, J. P., 131, 216, 316, 317
Charpentier, P., 570
Chaudhry, Z. W., 481, 483, 484, 485, 487
Cheatham, R. A., 210, 211
Chelikani, P. K., 28
Chen, C., 155
Chen, H. C., 56
Chen, J. D. Z., 543
Chen, M., 69
Chen, N., 56
Chen, S. H., 227
Chen, W. Y., 486
Chen, Y., 150
Chen, Y. A., 610, 612
Cheng, Y. J., 185
Chennareddygari, S., 382
Cherkin, D. C., 330
Chernikova, D. A., 80
Chew, B., 601
Chia, C. W., 27
Chia, S. C., 4
Chiang, A. L., 532, 543, 545, 546
Chida, Y., 151
Chikunguwo, S., 379
Chilcott, M., 571
Chinapaw, M. J., 4, 111, 605
Chiou, W. B., 160
Chiriboga, D. E., 151
Chirinos, J. A., 130
Cho, H. J., 358
Choi, J., 448
Chomontowska, H., 81

Chomsky, D. B., 81
Chow, S. C., 402
Chriqui, J. F., 665, 666
Christakis, N. A., 139, 262
Christensen, N. J., 54
Christian, J. G., 454, 455
Christin, L., 41, 50, 51
Christopoulos, A., 31
Christopoulos, G., 31
Christou, N., 197
Christou, N. V., 197, 200, 382, 385
Chrousos, G. P., 131
Chugh, M., 580
Church, T. S., 111, 114, 225, 228, 261, 323, 326, 330
Chuttani, R., 540
Cibula, D., 263, 457
Ciechomska, I., 81
Ciliska, D., 583
Cintra, W., Jr., 571
Cirona-Singh, A. A., 169, 177
Cizza, G., 132
Clapham, J. C., 54
Clar, C., 361
Clark, D., 500
Clark, D. O., 232
Clark, E. M., 447
Clark, J. E., 400
Clark, J. M., 15, 227, 291, 293, 298, 458, 480, 488, 581
Clark, J. T., 28
Clark, M. M., 265
Clark, V. L., 337, 511
Clarke, A., 516, 517
Clarke, D., 156
Clarke, S. F., 76
Clarke, T. C., 438
Claudino, A. M., 556, 557, 558
Clay-Williams, G., 441
Clegg, D. J., 30
Cleland, R., 486
Clement, K., 67
Clementi, G., 31
Clemow, L. P., 580
Clerc, I., 571
Clifford, C., 258
Clifford, L. M., 131, 598
Clifton, P. M., 210, 319
Clifton, R. G., 344
ClinicalTrials.gov, 638, 639
Close, K. L., 381
Coates, A., 129
Coates, P. S., 652
Cocores, J. A., 177
Cody, R. P., 380
Coen, P. M., 326
Coffeng, J., 114
Coffey, J. T., 159

Cohen, A. K., 139
Cohen, D. A., 336
Cohen, J. F., 665
Cohen, J. W., 18, 186, 622
Cohen, P., 156
Cohen, S., 267
Colbert, J. A., 419
Colby, S. L., 438, 439
Colchero, M. A., 666
Colditz, G. A., 3, 9, 10, 111, 330, 659
Cole, T. J., 46, 645
Coleman, K. J., 197, 198
Coletta, M., 96
Coletta, M. C., 337
Colles, S. L., 174
Colley, R. C., 600
Collier, D. N., 131
Collins, C. E., 259
Collins, H., 459
Collins, L. M., 476
Collins, R., 286
Combellick, J., 80
Commons, G. W., 570
Commons, R. R., 644
Conceicao, E., 561
Conceição, E., 153, 213
Conceição, E. M., 213
Condo, D., 319
Confessore, N., 665
Conklin, M. T., 94
Conroy, M. B., 340
Considine, R. V., 51
Convit, A., 629
Cook, D., 429
Cook, S. R., 594
Cook-Cottone, C., 609
Cooper, A., 631
Cooper, J., 632
Cooper, L. A., 413, 488, 581
Cooper, P. J., 213, 567
Cooper, R. S., 440
Cooper, Z., 213, 341, 393, 395, 400, 407, 553, 567
Coppock, J. H., 623
Corbin, W. R., 178
Cornelisse-Vermaat, J. R., 140
Cornier, M., 256
Cornoni-Huntley, J. C., 233
Cornwell, B., 583
Corona, E., 448
Corsica, J. A., 404, 516
Costa, P. T., Jr., 433, 434
Costello, E. K., 80
Costill, D. L., 111
Cotillard, A., 82
Cottrell, R. C., 186
Coughlin, J. W., 291
Coughlin, S. S., 340
Courcoulas, A. P., 302, 303, 381

Court, R., 361
Covasa, M., 25
Coward, W. A., 46, 601
Cowley, M. A., 28, 29
Cox, B. J., 155
Cox, L. M., 80
Cox, T., 267
Coyle, E. F., 111
Cozier, Y. C., 140
Cragg, S. E., 144
Craig, C., 661
Craig, C. L., 111, 144
Craig, P., 441, 442
Craighead, L. W., 459
Crandall, C. S., 585
Crane, M. M., 344, 469, 473
Crawford, A. G., 417
Crawford, D., 330
Crawford, Y., 610, 611
Crawley, J. N., 26
Creasy, S. A., 326, 327, 330
Crerand, C. E., 215, 253, 256, 257, 270, 337
Crimmins, E. M., 232
Crocker, J., 583, 584, 585
Crona Guterstam, Y., 652
Crönlein, T., 130
Cronquist, J. L., 623, 636
Crosby, R. D., 158, 159, 217, 262, 553, 554, 556, 557, 558, 569, 580
Crouter, S. E., 141
Crow, S. J., 554
Crum, R. M., 156
Cummings, D. E., 29, 368, 381
Cummings, J. H., 83
Cummins, S., 115, 144
Cunningham, J. J., 46
Curac, N., 114
Currie, P. J., 29
Curtin, L., 442
Curtin, L. R., 140, 552
Curtin, T., 497
Cushing, C. C., 616
Cussler, E. C., 405, 406
Cutler, D. M., 142
Cutting, T. M., 599
Cuzzolaro, M., 151, 153
Cypess, A. M., 54, 55
Cyr, H. N., 298
Cyrus, K., 157
Czira, M. E., 131

D

da Bautista-Castaño, I., 540
Daga, G. A., 171
Dahl, A., 475
Dahl, J., 518, 519

Dahlgren, G., 137
Dahmen, N., 131
Dailey, M. J., 83
D'Alessio, D., 644
D'Alessio, D. A., 651
Daling, J. R., 486
Dallal, G. E., 8
Dalle Grave, R., 210
Dalrymple, K. L., 156
Danforth, E., Jr., 50, 54
Daniel, T. O., 630, 631
Daniels, E. A., 568
Daniels, G. H., 286
Dansinger, M. L., 482
Dapri, G., 653
Darby, A., 552
Darby, L. A., 403
Dardennes, R., 177
Dardick, H., 666
Darling, H., 143
Darmon, N., 141
Dart, H., 3
Das, D., 208
Das, S. K., 211
Daston, S., 153
Date, Y., 28
Daughters, R. S., 26
Daumann, H., 85
Daumit, G., 291
Davey Smith, G., 139
Davidsen, L., 28
Davies, M. J., 159
Davis, C., 178, 236
Davis, K., 213
Davis, L. M., 482
Davis, M., 546
Davis, M. M., 598
Davis, N. J., 212
Davis, P., 454, 455
Davis, R. B., 186
Davis, S. M., 442, 607
Davis-Martin, P. D., 454, 455
Davison, K. K., 598, 600
Dawes, A. J., 157, 263, 271
Day, S. C., 215
de Beauvoir, S., 576
de Boer, M. R., 141
De Bourdeaudhuij, I., 140
De Fogel, J., 541
De Gaetano, A., 380
de Git, K. C., 84, 85
de Groot, M., 229
de Heer, F. A., 571
de Jong, F. H., 236
de Jonge, L., 47, 51
De Jonghe, B. C., 26
De La Fuente, R., 541
De Nunzio, C., 15
de Smith, A. J., 69
de Wit, L., 154

Author Index

de Zwaan, M., 170, 174, 176, 263, 570, 571
Dearing, K. K., 630
DeBoer, M. D., 130, 598
Decker, S. L., 428
DeFronzo, R. A., 9
Degher, D., 582
Deitel, M., 379
Del Mar, C., 341
Del Prete, E., 31
DeLaet, C., 159
Delahanty, L. M., 263, 457, 501
Delhanty, P. J., 29
Deliens, G., 132
Deliopoulou, K., 539
DelParigi, A., 81
Delzenne, N. M., 77
Dembling, B., 497
Demmer, R. T., 598
Dempsey, D. T., 302, 538
Deneuve, S., 571
Dengel, D. R., 330
Depner, C. M., 129, 130, 131
Deputy, N. P., 595
Dermota, P., 552
Derogar, M., 197, 199
Derogatis, L., 157
Derogatis, L. R., 212
Desai, A. P., 644
DeSalvo, K. B., 417
Després, J., 255
Despres, J. P., 52, 216
Dethlefsen, L., 80
Dettmer, E., 513
DeVita, P., 236
Devlin, M. J., 557, 558, 561
Devonport, T. J., 171
Dewey, K. G., 596
Dewey, M. E., 152
Dewind, L. T., 644
Dhiloon, I. A., 536
Di Chiara, G., 177
Di Pietro, L., 112
DiBonaventura, M., 18
Dickinson, L. M., 458
Dickson, S. L., 27
Didie, E., 286, 287
Didie, E. R., 569
Dietz, W., 18, 186, 622
Dietz, W. H., 8, 16, 163, 255, 298, 417, 593, 594, 636, 645
Diez-Roux, A. V., 143, 144, 216
Digenio, A. G., 459, 468, 470
Diggens, J., 171
Diliberti, N., 94
DiLillo, V., 510, 511
Dilks, R. J., 568, 569
DiMarco, I. D., 511
Dimitrova, A., 131
Dina, C., 65

Ding, S. A., 381
Ding, Y., 652
Dinges, D. F., 123, 125, 126, 127, 128, 129, 131, 216
Dinsa, G. D., 139
Dishman, R. K., 118
Ditschuneit, H. H., 298, 340
Dixon, J., 142
Dixon, J. B., 174, 302, 303, 379, 381, 383
Djousse, L., 112
Djousse, M. L., 322
Djuric, Z., 486
Do, D. P., 125
Dobal, M. T., 175
Dobbs, R., 93, 426
Doche, M. E., 69
Doi, S. A., 124, 131
Dolan, L. M., 652
Dölemeyer, R., 265
Dominguez-Bello, M. G., 80
Donahoo, W. T., 44, 47
Donat, M., 125
DonCarlos, L., 123
Dones, V., 610
Dong, C., 156
Donnelly, J. E., 113, 291, 323, 324, 326, 327, 329, 395, 398, 399, 407, 468, 471, 472, 484, 498
Dor, A., 16, 431
Dorflinger, L. M., 553
Dorn, J., 625
Dorner, T. E., 140
Dorrian, J., 129
Doshi, S., 360
Dossat, A. M., 27
Douglass, O. M., 403
Dovidio, J. F., 160, 161
Downey, K. T., 577
Downey, M., 304, 336, 425, 426, 430, 431
Drake, C. L., 125
Drapeau, V., 131, 175, 261
Drenowatz, C., 113
Drewnowski, A., 141, 142, 393, 598, 628
Dropleman, L. F., 209
Drucker, D. J., 27
Druet, C., 595
Drummond, J. A., 623
Drury, C. A., 581
Du, H., 81
Du, S., 543
Dubé, L., 140
Duca, F. A., 77
Duchmann, E. G., 209
Due, A., 312
Duerson, M. C., 367
Duggan, M., 473
Dulloo, A. G., 217

Dumon, K. R., 284, 302, 531, 538
Dumonceau, J. M., 538
Dunn, A. L., 144
Dunn, M. M., 525
Dunstan, D., 111
Dunstan, D. W., 111, 231, 232
Dunton, G. F., 613
Durand, C. P., 613
Durso, L. E., 160, 161, 262
Dushay, J., 360
Dutton, G. R., 16, 161, 394, 395, 407
Dvorak, R. V., 459, 470
Dyrby, C. O., 236
Dyrbye, L. N., 454
Dziura, J., 112

E

Earls, F., 139
Earnest, C. P., 225, 228, 261, 323, 326
Earp, J. A., 212
Eaton, W. W., 156
Eaves, L. J., 64, 596
Ebbeling, C. B., 52, 316, 317, 644
Ebbert, J. O., 94
Eberhardt, N. L., 47
Eccles, M., 500
Echouffo-Tcheugui, J., 293, 504
Eckburg, P. B., 78
Eckert, E. A., 316
Economos, C. D., 615, 616
Edmundowicz, S. A., 545
Edwards, C. A., 84
Edwards, P., 141
Edwards-Hampton, S. A., 426
Egan, K. B., 15
Egecioglu, E., 29
Egger, G., 137, 142
Egger, M., 11
Eichinger, M., 140
Eichler, K., 137
Eisenberg, M., 577
Eisenberg, M. H., 569
Ekelund, U., 50, 600
El Ghoch, M., 210
Elander, A., 570
Elangbam, C. S., 26
Elasy, T., 232
Elbel, B., 101, 613
Eldar, S., 369, 372, 379, 386
Elder, C. R., 131, 161, 263, 267
Elder, S. J., 65
Eleftheriadis, E., 536, 538
Elfering, A., 151
El-Hadi, M., 383
Elia, M., 46
Eliades, C., 540

Eliasson, A. H., 383
Elli, M., 75
Ellis, D., 513
Ellis, D. A., 328
Ellison, J. M., 215, 570
Ellison, M. C., 432
Ellison, N., 394
Ello Martin, J. A., 96
Ely, E. K., 202
Emery, C. F., 143
Emond, M., 26
Enerbäck, S., 55
Engel, A., 131
Engel, S., 271
Engel, S. G., 217
Engeland, A., 6
Engels, R. C., 150
Engstrom, M., 652
Enns, M. W., 155
Ensrud, K. E., 188
Epel, E. S., 155
Epstein, L., 107
Epstein, L. H., 330, 437, 485, 599, 605, 622, 623, 624, 625, 628, 629, 630, 631, 632, 641
Erbaugh, J., 157, 223
Erickson, S. J., 579
Ericsson, A. C., 77
Eriksen, D., 114
Eriksson, K. F., 188, 189, 191, 192
Erlichman, J., 112
Eschbach, K., 234
Esmaillzadeh, A., 97
Esparza, J., 440
Esposito, K., 188
Estaki, M., 82
Esteban Varela, J., 645
Etcoff, N., 566
Etherton, T., 314
Ettinger, A. S., 15
Evans, D. A., 232, 233
Evans, M., 227
Evans, R. K., 326
Even, C., 177
Everard, A., 79, 84
Evers, K. E., 458
Ewertz, M., 486
Expert Committee, 623
Eyler, A. A., 155

F

Fabricatore, A. N., 154, 209, 227, 257, 263, 269, 270, 286, 340, 569
Fabsitz, R. R., 65
Fagevik Olsen, M., 570, 654
Fahrenberg, J., 45

Fairburn, C., 567
Fairburn, C. G., 213, 236, 260, 341, 400, 553, 567
Faith, J. J., 82
Faith, M. S., 149, 150, 154, 156, 158, 160, 442, 597, 599, 630
Faivre, L., 70
Falbe, J., 666
Fallon, E. A., 152
Familiari, P., 541
Fan, J. X., 322
Fang, L., 543
Fang, X., 610, 611
Fang, Z., 126
Farese, R. V., Jr., 56
Farley, A., 245
Farooqi, I. S., 53, 64, 65, 66, 67, 68, 118, 255, 286
Farrell, T. M., 426
Fassino, S., 171
Fatima, Y., 124, 131
Faulconbridge, L. F., 29, 32, 161, 209, 299, 461
Faulkner, G. E. J., 142
Faulkner, G. P., 94
Faulkner, J. A., 115
Fava, J. L., 262, 481
Feeley, T. H., 610
Feeney, B. P., 141
Fehmann, H. C., 31
Feingold, A., 579
Feinle-Bisset, C., 83
Feldman, H. A., 316
Felitti, V. J., 265
Felix, E. L., 379
Felix, H. C., 444, 493, 504
Felson, D. T., 236
Felton, S., 457
Fenwick, E., 16
Ferguson, C., 16, 431
Ferguson, E. L., 141
Fernandez-Corbelle, J. P., 536, 541
Fernandez-Mendoza, J., 130, **131**
Fernstrom, J. D., 652
Fernstrom, M. H., 652
Ferrante, J. M., 580
Ferraro, K. F., 232, 233
Ferraro, R. T., 51
Ferris, S., 99
Ferrucci, L., 433
Ferry, R. J., 246
Ferster, C. B., 393
Festinger, L., 509
Fidler, M. C., 353
Field, A. E., 9, 153, 344
Fiery, M. F., 442
Filer, L. J., Jr., 599
Filiatrault, M. L., 131
Fillenbaum, G. G., 233

Finch, E. A., 501, 502, 627
Fine, J. T., 233
Finelli, F. C., 376, 652
Fink, L., 266
Finkelstein, E. A., 18, 142, 143, 186, 328, 481, 622
Finlayson, G., 119
Finley, C. E., 488
Finucane, M. M., 3
Fisher, A., 124
Fisher, J. O., 100, 597, 598, 599, 600
Fisher, W. P., 417
Fiske, L., 152
Fisler, J. S., 50
Fissinger, J. A., 116
Fitzgibbon, M., 442
Fitzgibbon, M. L., 157, 447, 496, 499, 580, 606, 607, 608
Fitzhugh, E. C., 114
Fitzpatrick, B. M., 664
Fjeldsoe, B. S., 473
Flak, J. N., 26
Flanagan, E., 426
Flanders, D., 194
Flap, H., 140
Flatt, J. P., 42, 43, 49, 51
Flechtner-Mors, M., 298, 340
Flegal, K. M., 3, 4, 6, 140, 185, 243, 349, 419, 453, 466, 486, 503, 531, 552, 594, 622, 644, 645
Fleming, E. C., 567
Fleming Milici, F. F., 662
Fletcher, P. C., 178
Flier, J. S., 31
Flint, A., 28
Flint, A. J., 7, 8
Flint, E., 115
Flint, S. W., 16
Flood, J. E., 97, 98
Flood-Obbagy, J. E., 97
Flores, M. R., 185, 294
Flores, Y. N., 448
Florez, H., 210
Florez, J. C., 342
Flum, D. R., 200, 379
Flynn, K. J., 442
Fobian, A. D., 129
Foerster, F., 45
Fogel, R., 541
Folsom, A. R., 9, 195, 261
Fomon, S. J., 599
Fontaine, K. R., 156, 158, 580, 659
Fontenot, K., 438
Ford, A. L., 631
Ford, E. S., 124
Ford, W. F., 159

Ford-Adams, M. E., 644
Foreyt, J. P., 299, 300, 458
Forlano, R., 539
Forman, E., 265
Forman, E. M., 287, 330, 508, 513, 514, 516, 517, 518, 519
Forouhi, N. G., 81, 143
Forrester, T. E., 440
Forssell, H., 302
Fortin, S. M., 29
Fortuyn, H. A., 131
Foster, D. O., 54
Foster, G. D., 94, 130, 155, 157, 253, 269, 286, 294, 298, 336, 343, 395, 403, 407, 441, 460, 461, 475, 482, 568, 569, 577, 580, 581, 605, 614, 615
Foster, J. A., 330
Foster-Schubert, K. E., 395, 401
Fothergill, E., 54, 461
Fotu, K. F., 618
Fournier, G., 52
Fowler, J. H., 139, 262
Fowler, J. S., 177
Fox, C., 637
Fox, E., 579
Francis, J., 500
Francis, L. A., 630
Franckle, R. L., 124
Franco, M., 195
Frank, L. D., 141
Franklin, B. A., 8
Franko, D. L., 175, 568
Frayling, T. M., 65
Frayn, K. N., 43
Frayo, R. S., 29
Frazier, A. L., 344
Frazier, W. C., 663, 664
Frederich, R. C., 318
Frederick, D. A., 568
Freedland, S. J., 15
Freedman, D. S., 593, 644, 645
Freedson, P., 108
Freeman, B., 663
French, S., 342
French, S. A., 94, 143, 195, 211, 339, 394, 500, 599
Frerichs, L. M., 628
Frey, G. C., 116
Fried, M., 648
Friedman, A. M., 580
Friedman, J. M., 64
Friedman, K. E., 578
Friedman, M., 577
Friedman, M. A., 154, 155, 157, 577, 578
Friedman, M. I., 51
Friedman, S., 177
Friedmann, J. M., 232, 233

Frier, H. I., 298, 501
Fries, J. F., 235
Frimel, T. N., 231, 232
Froguel, P., 255
Froidevaux, F., 51
Frost, G., 83
Froy, O., 126
Frühbeck, G., 349
Fryar, C. D., 3, 185, 243, 419, 453, 466
Frydman, M. L., 54
Fuerst, T., 236
Fuglestad, P. T., 258, 393
Fujimiya, M., 25
Fukuoka, Y., 448
Fuld, R., 29
Fuller, J. C., 570
Fulton, L., 76
Fumagalli, E., 139
Funk, K. L., 444
Furnham, A., 579
Fursland, A., 178

G

Gaci, N., 79
Gadde, K. M., 32, 176, 355, 356, 639
Gadgil, M. D., 652
Gadhoke, P., 613
Gaesser, G. A., 115
Gaffney, S., 157
Gagne, D. A., 177
Gail, M. H., 486
Galanos, A. N., 233
Galgani, J. E., 53
Galioto, R., 211
Gall, S., 257
Gallagher, C., 417, 429
Gallagher, D. A., 81, 393
Gallagher, K. I., 324, 325, 467
Gallant, A. R., 175, 261
Galobardes, B., 139, 141
Galuska, D. A., 155, 186
Galvão, M. P., 540
Galvin, R., 522
Gamborg, M., 80
Gandek, B., 217
Gang, C. H., 176
Gao, H. X., 381
Gapinski, K. D., 584
Garaulet, M., 126
Garcia, A., 160
García-Álvarez, E. E., 536
Garfield, D., 579
Gariepy, G., 155
Garner, D. M., 567
Garnett, S. P., 64

Garvey, W. T., 195, 196, 283, 287, 299, 301, 352, 356, 415, 416, 454
Garza, C., 595
Garza, C. A., 382
Gatchalian, K. M., 629
Gaudreau, P., 152
Gaukstern, J. E., 236
Gavin, A. R., 155
Gaziano, J. M., 9
Gazze, D., 31
Gearhardt, A. N., 178
Gearhart, S., 661
Geenen, R., 571
Geiss L. S., 185
Gelber, R. P., 9
Geliebter, A., 175, 213
Geller, F., 130
Gemelli, T., 70
Genco, A., 538
Genentech, I., 637
Genkinger, J. M., 11
Geoffroy, M. C., 156
Gerasimidis, K., 84
Gerber, R. A., 459, 470
Gerber, W. M., 524
Gerzoff, R. B., 194
Gewirtz, A., 75
Ghaderi, I., 426
Ghezel-Ahmadi, D., 131
Giacomelli, A. M., 625, 629
Gibbons, C., 119
Gibbons, L. M., 257, 569
Gibbs, J., 25
Gibson, E. L., 139, 151
Gibson, S., 186
Gibson-Smith, D., 155
Giese, S. Y., 570
Gigante, D. P., 152
Gilbert, D. T., 630
Gilhooly, C. H., 215
Gill, R. S., 371, 383
Gill J. A., 361
Gillman, M. W., 344, 596
Gilson, M., 132
Giltay E. J., 151
Ginsberg, H. N., 56
Giordano, S., 570
Giovannucci, E., 15
Gittelsohn, J., 502, 613
Giuliani, C., 233
Glaeser, E. L., 142
Glanz, K., 143, 522
Glasgow, R. E., 445, 449, 492
Glass, T. A., 628
Glassman, M., 427
Glatzle, J., 25
Gleaves, D. H., 209
Glik, D., 442

Glonti, K., 139
Gloy, V. L., 268, 531
Glozier, N., 217
Gluck, M. E., 151, 175, 176
Godin, G., 256
Goel, N., 125, 126, 127, 128, 129, 131
Goff, D. C., Jr., 231
Golay, A., 556, 557, 558
Gold, B. C., 468, 471
Gold, E. C., 406
Gold, M. S., 177
Gold, R. S., 467
Goldberg, J. H., 511
Goldfield, G., 152
Goldfield, G. S., 630
Goldman, N., 139
Goldschmidt, A. B., 152, 622, 623, 632
Goldsmith, C. A., 330
Goldstein, A. B., 141
Goldstein, D., 667
Goldstein, D. J., 461
Goldstein, J. L., 28
Goldstein, S. P., 518, 519
Goldstone, A. P., 69
Golley, R. K., 130
Golub, M. S., 9
Gomez-Marin, O., 261
Gomez-Rubalcava, S., 172, 288, 290, 299, 336, 508
Gong, Q., 124, 191
Gonissen, H., 217
González-Enríquez, J., 536
Gonzalez-Suarez, C., 610
Goodman, A. L., 75
Goodman, R. A., 186
Goodman, R. J., 330
Goodpaster, B. H., 324, 396, 401
Goodrich, J. K., 80, 81
Goodwin, C. L., 517, 518
Goodwin, J. S., 232, 234
Goossens, L., 629
Goran, M. I., 48, 441, 601
Gordon, J. I., 76, 78, 82
Gordon, J. R., 341
Gordon-Larsen, P., 144, 255
Gordy, C. C., 625
Gore, C. J., 115
Gore, S. A., 330, 511
Gore-Felton, C., 476
Gorin, A. A., 261, 340, 344, 396, 399, 402, 407
Goris, A. H., 45
Gormally, J., 153
Gortmaker, S. L., 16, 18
Goryakin, Y., 139
Gostout, C. J., 539, 540
Gotostam, K. G., 552

Gotschi, T., 115
Gould, R. A., 215
Gower, B. A., 115
Goyal, M., 330
Grabe, S., 580
Grace, M. K., 30
Graham, R., 415
Gramzow, R. H., 124
Granata, G. P., 47
Grandner, M., 216
Grandner, M. A., 124, 125
Grant, C., 129
Grant Harrington, N., 473
Graubard, B. I., 6, 486
Gray, J., 70
Gredysa, D. M., 172
Greenaway, M., 114
Greenburg, D. L., 383
Greene, L. F., 96
Greene, P. G., 511
Greenfield, J. R., 68
Greenfield, S., 415
Greenlee, H. A., 486
Greenspan, S. L., 652
Greenstein, R. J., 379
Greenway, F., 540
Greenway, F. L., 260, 352, 357, 359, 639, 640
Gregg, E. W., 185, 187, 194, 294, 359, 493
Gretebeck, R. J., 233
Grier, S. A., 442
Griffin, S., 144
Griffin, S. J., 143
Griffing, G. T., 176
Griffith, D. M., 447
Griffith, H. M., 418
Griffith, J., 442
Griffiths, L. J., 593
Grigoryan, Z., 80
Grill, H. J., 24, 25, 26, 29
Grilo, C. M., 153, 157, 171, 172, 261, 511, 552, 553, 554, 555, 556, 557, 558, 560, 561, 568, 579
Grilo, S., 446, 502
Grimmer-Somers, K., 610
Grimm-Thomas, K., 599
Grishin, N. V., 28
Grobbee, D. E., 236
Groesz, L. M., 461
Gronowitz, E., 652, 653
Grontved, A., 111
Grosomanidis, V., 536, 538
Gross, A., 637
Gross, R., 610
Grosse, Y., 12
Grouzmann, E., 28
Grummon, A. H., 666

Grunstein, R. R., 217
Grunwald, G. K., 313
Gruys, K., 568
Gu, Q., 8
Guadalajara, H., 653
Guaraldi, F., 80
Guccione, A. A., 236
Gudzune, K., 114
Gudzune, K. A., 292, 293, 298, 413, 458, 480, 481, 482, 483, 484, 485, 486, 487, 488, 581
Guelfi, J. D., 177
Gueorguieva, R., 171, 553, 560
Guerdjikova, A. I., 556
Guerra, M., 442
Guerrien, A., 593
Guh, D. P., 8, 9, 14, 15
Gunnarsdottir, T., 623
Gunstad, J., 211
Gunther, S., 418
Guo, F., 418
Guo, J. J., 417
Guralnik, J. M., 235
Gurubhagavatula, I., 125
Gusenoff, J. A., 570
Gutekunst, D. J., 236
Gutierrez-Torres, L., 640
Guyenet, S. J., 286
Gwadz, M. V., 477

H

Haack, M., 132
Haapala, I., 469, 474
Haditsch, B., 140
Haedt-Matt, A. A., 171
Haeusslein, E., 382
Haghighatdoost, F., 97
Hagins, M., 329, 330
Hagobian, T. A., 344
Haines, J., 131, 152
Haines, P. S., 233
Haire-Joshu, D., 344, 442, 443
Hajduk, C. L., 99
Halal, C. S., 124
Haldar, S., 4
Hale, B. C., 18
Hale, L., 125
Hales, C. M., 185
Hales, S. B., 475
Halford, J. C., 353
Hall, K. D., 41, 42, 43, 52, 310, 314
Hallersund, P., 382
Halperin, F., 381
Halpern, C. H., 284, 531, 544
Halpern, S. D., 529
Halverson, K. H., 98

Halyburton, A. K., 210, 211
Hamad, G., 383
Hamady, M., 75
Hamilton, J., 513
Hamilton, M., 262, 263
Hamman, R. F., 190, 504
Hammel, J. P., 386
Hammer, M., 432
Hammond, R. A., 3, 18, 139, 186
Hampl, S., 350, 637
Hampp, C., 431
Han, E., 431
Han, J. C., 70
Hand, G. A., 113
Hand, T. W., 84
Handforth, B., 667
Handjieva-Darlenska, T., 319
Hanipah, Z. N., 284, 302, 303, 367, 374, 459, 650
Hankey, C. R., 188, 359
Hankinson, A. L., 112
Hannan, L., 7
Hansberry, M. R., 232
Hansen, G. L., 101
Hardeman, W., 500
Harding, J. L., 151
Harding, M., 255
Hardt, S., 51
Hardy, L. L., 64
Harnett, W., 645
Harper, I. T., 44
Harper, J. A., 54
Harrington, C., 360
Harrington, D. M., 111
Harrington, M., 186, 195
Harris, J. A., 46
Harris, J. L., 368, 370, 387, 662, 663, 664
Harris, K. I., 94
Harris, M. A., 116
Harris, T., 188, 233
Harris, T. B., 236
Harris, V., 31
Harrold, J. A., 353
Harstra, A. V., 83
Hart, C. N., 125
Hart, L., 497
Harter, S., 577
Hartge, P., 7
Hartley, G. G., 569
Hartline-Grafton, H., 599
Hartmann-Boyce, J., 401
Hartz, A. J., 10, 236
Harvey, A. G., 130
Harvey, J., 485
Harvey-Berino, J., 292, 405, 406, 468, 471
Harvie, M., 311
Hashimi, M. W., 9

Hasin, D. S., 160
Haskell, W., 108
Haskell, W. L., 191
Hassan, M. K., 158
Hastings, G., 662
Hatfield, E., 565
Hatoum, I. J., 64, 68, 417
Hatzenbuehler, M. L., 160
Hauptman, J., 195, 301, 350, 459, 637
Hausenblas, H. A., 569
Haver, A. C., 28
Hawker, D. M., 341
Hawkes, C., 144
Haworth, C. M., 65, 596
Hay, D. L., 31
Hay, P., 552
Hayashi, K., 160
Haydel, K. F., 579
Hayes, J. F., 623, 624, 631
Hayes, M. R., 24, 25, 26, 27, 31
Hayes, S., 475, 513, 514, 516, 518, 519
Hayes, S. C., 162, 330
Hayes, T. M., 27
Hayman, L. L., 644
Haynes, S. N., 337
He, L., 360
Head, K. J., 473
Head, S., 175, 262
Heal, D., 639
Healy, G. N., 111
Heatherton, T. F., 171, 584
Heaton, P. C., 417
Hebebrand. J., 130
Hebert, J. R., 113
Hebert, P. R., 343, 443, 444
Hebl, M. R., 584
Heckemeyer, C. M., 512
Heeren, J., 56
Heianza, Y., 312
Heilbronn, L. K., 209
Heiman, M. L., 28
Heinberg, L. J., 566
Heinen, L., 143
Heinig, M. J., 596
Heiskanen, T. H., 158
Heitmann, B. L., 175
Hekler, E. B., 477
Heller, R. F., 11
Henandez, A. L., 212
Henderson, K. E., 157
Hendricks, E. J., 359
Heneghan, H. M., 369, 378, 382
Henry, C. J., 4
Henry, P. E., 568
Henschel, A., 52, 208
Hensrud, D., 330
Heo, M., 156, 158, 298, 501

Heppner, K. M., 29
Herbert, J. D., 513, 514, 516, 517, 518
Herbozo, S., 160, 579
Herbst, K. L., 461
Herget, S., 646
Herman, C. P., 94, 171, 571
Herman, W. H., 493
Hernandez, M., 662
Hernandez, T. L., 570
Herrero, M., 667
Herring, L., 268
Herzog, H., 28
Heshka, S., 293, 482
Hesselink, M. K., 55
Hester, C. M., 85
Hetherington, M. M., 65, 596
Heuchert, J. W. P., 209
Heuer, C., 262
Heuer, C. A., 16, 17, 160
Heymsfield, S. B., 6, 41, 53, 94, 288, 289, 293, 298, 299, 300, 304, 340, 367, 501
Hgah, W. Z. W., 211
Hicken, M. T., 156
Hiddinka, G. J., 417
Hilbert, A., 174, 553, 554, 561, 579, 646
Hildebrandt, M. A., 76
Hill, A., 577
Hill, A. J., 593
Hill, J. O., 81, 142, 227, 258, 268, 269, 313, 324, 330, 432, 457
Hills, A. P., 115
Hilton, J. M., 31
Himpens, J., 653
Hinkle, S. N., 595
Hinton, I., 497
Hirano, K., 85
Hiripi, E., 170, 552
Hirsch, J., 25, 41, 81, 393, 461
Hirschkowitz, M., 123
Hittelman, K. J., 115
Hjorth, M. F., 124, 312
Ho, A. L., 543
Ho, M., 623, 624
Hocking, M. P., 367
Hoffman, K. L., 516, 517
Hoffmann, D. A., 481
Hofker, M. H., 118
Hogenkamp, P. S., 125
Hoie, L. H., 342, 343
Holder, J. L., Jr., 70
Hollander, P., 357
Hollands, G. J., 98, 100
Hollenbeck, A. R., 124
Hollis, J. F., 343
Holmboe-Ottesen, G., 143
Holmes, M. D., 486

Holst, J. J., 26, 27, 28, 118
Holtan, S. G., 417
Holtermann, A., 114
Homberg, J. R., 150
Hong, P. S., 250, 454, 511
Hood, M. M., 516
Hoogendoorn, C., 629
Hooper, N., 516, 517
Hopkins, M., 119
Horgen, K. B., 659, 664
Horn, L. V., 127
Horowitz, M., 83
Horrigan, J., 473
Horta, B. L., 152
Horvath, P. J., 330
Hosoda, H., 28, 29
Hosokawa, P. W., 457
Hotop, A. M., 470
Houmard, J. A., 236
Housemann, R. A., 143
Houston, D. K., 233
Howarth, N. C., 99
Howden-Chapman, P., 144
Howell, A., 311
Howley, E. T., 106, 111
Hoyland, A., 218, 224
Hoyo, C., 13
Hrabosky J. I., 578
Hron, B. M., 316
Hsu, A., 393
Hu, F. B., 3, 4, 11, 111, 112, 259, 312, 317, 330, 598, 605
Huang, A. J., 212
Huang, T. T., 628
Huang, T. T. K., 628
Huang, W., 31
Huang, Z., 9
Huber, J. M., 94, 98
Huber, O., 571
Hubert, H., 235
Hudgel, D. W., 125
Hudson, J. I., 170, 552, 553, 555, 556
Huffman, K. M., 236
Hughes, G., 582
Huguet, N., 236
Huh, S. Y., 596
Huizinga, M. M., 581
Humes, K. R. J., 438, 439
Hunger, J. M., 160
Hunt, L. P., 631
Hunt, S. C., 385
Hunter, G. R., 115
Hunter, J. A., 585
Hurvitz, P. M., 141
Huskey, K. W., 186
Hussin, N. M., 211
Hutchesson, M. J., 259
Hutfless, S., 114

Hutson, M. A., 442
Huurre, A., 80
Hwang, R. F., 379
Hyde, J. S., 580
Hyde, R. T., 261

I

Iacovino, J. M., 172
Iannarino, N. T., 473
Ibrahim, M., 151
Ikramuddin, S., 302, 303, 381, 383, 650
Iliescu, C., 593
Imaz, I., 536, 539
Imperial, J., 132, 462
Inge, T. H., 605, 644, 648, 651, 652, 653, 654
Inoue, D., 85
Inzlicht, M., 330
Ip, E. H., 233
Ip, K., 268
Isasi, C. R., 212
Isidori, A. M., 212
Islam, N., 101
Israel, S., 65
Ito, C., 645
Iversen, C. L., 101
Ives, A. K., 475
Ivezaj, V., 153, 511, 513
Iyer, S., 143

J

Jackman, M. R., 256
Jackson, A. S., 587
Jackson, N., 124
Jackson, R. S., 66, 68
Jackson, S. E., 161
Jackvony, E. H., 472
Jacobs, D. R., 261
Jacobs, D. R., Jr., 107
Jacobs, S. B., 630
Jacobsen, L. V., 639
Jacobshagen, N., 151
Jacobson, M. F., 665
Jacques, P. F., 8, 156
Jaeger, L. F., 50
Jafary, A. M., 568
Jaffe, K., 577
Jakicic, J. M., 261, 288, 297, 322, 323, 324, 325, 326, 327, 328, 331, 339, 340, 343, 396, 401, 407, 467
Jakubiec-Puka, A., 81
Jakubowicz, D., 126
James, B. L., 95

James, J., 613, 616, 618
James, W. P., 32, 112, 299
James, W. P. T., 459, 641
Jangi, S., 419
Janicke, D. M., 623, 624
Janney, C., 324, 401
Jansen, A., 625
Jansen, B., 666
Janssen, I., 236
Jarlenski, M. P., 100
Jarmolowicz, D. P., 629
Jarosz, P. A., 175
Jarry, J. L., 268
Jarvholm, K., 649, 653
Jarvis, M. J., 159
Jaspan, J. B., 31
Jay, M., 418
Jean-Louis, G., 216
Jebb, S. A., 100, 293, 401, 482
Jefferson, A., 628
Jeffery, R., 261, 630
Jeffery, R. W., 99, 195, 211, 258, 324, 326, 339, 340, 341, 342, 343, 393, 394, 396, 399, 401, 404, 405, 468, 470, 500, 524, 525, 579, 585, 599, 627
Jeffrey, D. B., 337, 340
Jekabsons, M. B., 54
Jelalian, E., 625
Jenkin, G., 663
Jenkins, C. H., 343
Jenkins, K. R., 232
Jensen, C., 350, 637
Jensen, D. M., 618
Jensen, D. R., 56
Jensen, G. L., 232, 233, 618
Jensen, M. D., 47, 188, 208, 243, 253, 259, 268, 269, 283, 284, 286, 287, 288, 289, 290, 291, 292, 294, 298, 324, 330, 339, 341, 349, 350, 362, 371, 393, 400, 415, 437, 453, 461, 467, 480, 487, 488
Jéquier, E., 41, 42, 51, 81, 313
Jerome, C., 25
Jess, T., 80
Jeyaram, S., 584
Jia, H., 158
Jiang, F., 124
Jiang, L., 461
Jih, J., 140
Jimenez-Baños, A., 536, 541
Jo, B., 555
Johannsen, M., 561
Johannsen, N. M., 261, 323
Johanssen, D. L., 49, 52, 53
Johansson, S. E., 645, 648, 650
John, L., 526, 527
Johns, D. J., 401

Johnson, B. L., 197, 198
Johnson, C. A., 576
Johnson, C. M., 445, 446
Johnson, D. B., 665
Johnson, E. J., 667
Johnson, F., 99, 100
Johnson, J. A., 208
Johnson, S. L., 599
Johnson, S. P., 430
Johnson, T. D., 298, 340
Johnston, B. C., 403, 483, 484, 487
Johnston, C. A., 482
Johnston, M., 500
Johnstone, A. M., 99
Joinson, A., 328
Jolly, K., 481, 482
Jones, A. M., 64
Jones, D. A., 186
Jones, D. B., 430
Jones, I. R., 27
Jonnalagadda, S., 314
Jordan, J., 26
Jordan, R. C., 403
Jørgensen, J. S., 618
Jorgensen, R. S., 124
Josbeno, D. A., 326
Joseph, F., 330
Joshi, A. V., 158
Juarascio, A. S., 516, 517
Jumpertz, R., 82, 83, 84
Juonala, M., 11, 622, 644

K

Kaaks, R., 652
Kabat-Zinn, J., 330
Kaciroti, N., 256
Kaestner, R., 140
Kahan, S., 254, 372, 413, 417, 418
Kahl, K. G., 158
Kahlhöfer, J., 131
Kahlmeier, S., 115
Kahn, S. E., 31
Kahneman, D., 523
Kaholokula, J. K., 448
Kaiser, K. A., 129, 317
Kaiyala, K. J., 31
Kalarchian, M., 326
Kalarchian, M. A., 396, 399, 561
Kalavainen, M., 631
Kalebjian, R., 153
Kalfarentzos, F., 380
Kalkhoff, R. D., 10
Kalkwarf, H. J., 652
Kalra, P. S., 28
Kalra, S. P., 28
Kamarck, T., 267

Kamegai, J., 29
Kanfer, F. H., 393
Kang, E. M., 431
Kang, J., 94
Kang, J. C., 358
Kang, J. G., 358
Kang, J. H., 358
Kangawa, K., 28
Kanoski, S. E., 26, 29
Kanter, D., 314
Kantor, L. S., 142
Kapka, T., 289, 350, 454
Kaplan, J. M., 29
Kaplan, M. S., 236
Kaprio, J., 64, 195
Kara, S., 125
Karagianis, J., 360
Karimi, G., 97
Karle, B., 570
Karlsson, J., 343
Karmali, S., 371, 383
Karpiel, A. B., 26
Karschin, J., 131
Karson, A. S., 417
Kase, C., 265
Kashyap, P. C., 84
Kass, A. E., 623
Kastin, A. J., 31
Kasturi, K. S., 382
Katch, F. I., 111
Katch, V. L., 111
Katterman, S. N., 516, 518, 519
Katula, J. A., 496, 499
Katz, D. A., 158
Katz, D. L., 610, 612
Katz, S. H., 595
Katzmarzyk, P. T., 49, 105, 111, 124
Kaufmann, N. A., 343
Kaukua, J., 212, 224, 225, 235
Kaul, S., 314
Kaulfers, A. M., 652, 653
Kaushal, N., 137
Kautenburger, T., 85
Kawamura, K.Y., 568
Kay, K., 27
Kaye, S. A., 9
Kearney, W. B., 447
Keating, K. D., 317
Keck, P. E., 556
Keckley, P. H., 618
Keel, P. K., 171
Keer, D., 613
Kehagias, I., 380
Keire, D. A., 28
Keller, S. K., 223
Keller, U., 214
Kelley-Moore, J. A., 232
Kellogg, T. A., 380

Kelly, A., 637
Kelly, A. S., 360, 623, 644
Kelly, B., 663
Kelly, M. S., 501
Kelly, S., 617
Kelton, C. M., 417
Kempe, A., 458
Kemps, E., 211
Kenardy, J., 341
Kendall, P. C., 580
Kendler, K., 579
Kendler, K. S., 157, 170
Kendra, K. E., 514
Kennedy, L., 552
Kenney, G. M., 428
Kenney, M. A., 31
Kenney, W. L., 111
Kenny, G. P., 152
Keogh, J. B., 319
Keranen, L., 582
Kerbey, A. L., 112
Kern, A. S., 130
Kern, H. F., 26
Kerr, M. A., 101
Kershaw, K. N., 140
Kersting, A., 265
Kesman, R. L., 94, 98
Kessler, R. C., 170, 171, 552, 553
Keum, N., 158
Keyes, K. M., 160
Keys, A., 46, 52, 208
Khalsa, S. B. S., 330
Khan, M. J., 84
Khan, T., 666
Khaylis, A., 476
Khoo, J., 212
Khunti, K., 159
Kiefe, C., 155
Kiemle, G., 152
Kiernan, M., 396, 400, 401, 407, 511
Kikuchi, H., 125
Kilanowski, C. K., 628
Kilkus, J. M., 132, 462
Killen, J. D., 579
Kim, E. M., 30
Kim, J. S., 80
Kim, K., 131
Kim, K. K., 358
Kim, S. Y., 595
Kim, Y., 361
Kimura, I., 85
King, N. A., 64, 118
King, T. K., 265
King, W. C., 264, 271, 326, 331
Kinra, S., 640
Kirschenbaum, D. S., 157, 340, 580
Kissileff, H. R., 25

Kiszko, K., 101
Kit, B. K., 6, 349, 503, 531, 594, 622, 644
Kitzinger, H. B., 570
Kjøllesdal, M. R., 143
Klassen, A. F., 567
Klatzkin, R. R., 157
Klein, D. A., 511
Klein, D. J., 639
Klein, K. R., 628
Klein, S., 82, 231, 570
Kleinman, B. M., 516
Klem, M. L., 81, 324
Kline, G. A., 94
Kling, S. M., 94
Klobučar Majanović, S., 543
Klopper, E. M., 570, 571
Kneeland, E. T., 156
Knickman, J. R., 522
Knight, J., 595
Knight, R., 75, 76, 78
Knisely, M. R., 500
Knowler, W. C., 49, 188, 189, 341, 342, 385, 444, 466, 493
Knudsen, J., 261
Knuth, N. D., 51, 53, 309
Kocelak, P., 82
Koch, T. R., 376, 652
Kochanek, K. D., 7
Koelenc, M. A., 417
Koffman, D. M., 502
Kofman, M. D., 213
Kohlmeier, M., 418
Kojima, M., 28
Kolaczynski, J. W., 51
Koletzko, B., 596
Koleva, P. T., 80
Kolish, E., 662
Kolko, R. P., 623
Kolodinsky, J. M., 141
Kolotkin, R. L., 158, 159, 170, 212, 217, 262, 569, 580
Kolsgaard, M. L. P., 631
Kong, A., 447
König, H. H., 18, 140
Konner, M., 441
Konnopka, A., 18, 140
Konsta, A., 539
Konttinen, H., 150, 156
Konz, E. C., 318
Koornstra, J. J., 653
Kordari, P., 56
Korkeila, M., 195
Korppi, M., 631
Kosaka, K., 189, 190
Kosinski, M., 217, 223
Kosloski, K. D., 158
Kosloski, T., 217
Koster, A., 233, 235

Kostova, D., 428
Kotagal, S., 130
Kothari, S. N., 430
Kotwal, R., 577
Kotzampassi, K., 536, 537, 538, 539, 546
Kovacs, A., 77
Kovacs, P., 47
Kovacs, S. J., 261, 322
Kowalsky, R. J., 326
Kozak, L. P., 55
Kozyrskyi, A. L., 80
Kraak, V. I., 663
Kraemer, H. C., 175, 236
Krahn, L. E., 130
Krakoff, J., 151, 175
Kral, T. V., 93, 597, 598, 599, 600
Kral, T. V. E., 93, 100, 593, 636
Kramer, C. K., 284
Kramer, M. K., 500, 503
Kraschnewski, J. L., 417
Kratt, P. P., 512
Kraus, S., 330
Kraus, W. E., 236
Krause, K. M., 418
Kravitz, M., 442
Kremers, S. P. J., 138
Kreuter, M. W., 139, 447
Kris-Etherton, P. M., 98, 314
Kristeller, J. L., 330
Kristensen, P., 29
Kritchevsky, S., 233
Kroenke, C. H., 486
Kroenke, K., 263
Kroese-Deutman, H. C., 570
Kroh, M., 368, 379, 546
Kronenberg, H. M., 246
Kropski, J. A., 618
Krude, H., 66, 67
Kruger, E., 481
Kruger, J., 186
Krukowski, R. A., 290, 293, 336, 343, 492, 494, 496, 499, 500, 501, 502, 504
Kruszon-Moran, D., 3, 185, 243, 419, 453, 466
Kubiena, H., 570
Kublaoui, B. M., 70
Kubota, N., 30
Kuehnel, R. H., 257
Kugler, K. C., 477
Kuhl, E. S., 598
Kuhnen, P., 68
Kuller, L. H., 9
Kullgren, J. T., 528
Kulseng, B., 118
Kumanyika, S. K., 343, 437, 442, 443, 444, 455, 456, 595, 628

Kumar, N., 536, 541, 542, 544, 546
Kumar, R. B., 243, 253, 255, 257, 284
Kumbhari, V., 543, 545
Kuna, S. T., 188
Kunz, I., 51
Kuo, Y. F., 234
Kuokkanen, H. O., 570
Kupfer, D. J., 216
Kurt, M., 536
Kurth, C. L., 525
Kushner, R. F., 245, 254, 284, 299, 371, 372, 413, 418, 488
Kuzuya, T., 190
Kwok, C. S., 651
Kyle, T., 162
Kyle, T. K., 304, 336, 425

L

La Via, M., 556
Labad, J., 157
Lackey, M., 445, 446
Ladenheim, E. E., 26
Laderman, M., 155
Laederach-Hofmann, K., 556, 558
LaForgia, J., 115
Lahlou, N., 67
Lahmek, P., 245
Lai, D. D., 648
Laing, B. Y., 292
Lakerveld, J., 137, 139, 143
Lam, D. D., 638
Lamb, K. M., 159
Lambert, P. J., 430
Lamberts, S. W., 236
Lamerz, A., 174
Lampel, M., 26
Lancaster, K. J., 446, 502
Lang, C. C., 81
Lang, I. A., 235
Lang, T., 236
Lang, W., 227, 324, 325, 326, 327, 340, 343, 401, 467
Langellier, B. A., 442
Langford, J., 81
Langguth, B., 130
Langhammer, A., 150
Langhans, W., 30
Langstein, H. N., 570
Langwith, C., 16, 431
Laposky, A. D., 216
LaRose, J. G., 262, 268
Larsen, C. A., 290, 293, 336, 343, 492
Larsen, M., 571
Larsen, P. R., 246

Author Index

Larsen, T. M., 311, 312, 319
Larson, C. J., 430
Larson, C. L., 316
Larson, D. E., 47, 51
Larson, K., 46
Larson, N., 152, 598
Larson, N. I., 80, 124
Larsson, S. C., 13
Lasikiewicz, N., 218, 224
Laska, M. N., 124
Lasserre, A. M., 150
Latner, J., 155
Latner, J. D., 160, 161, 262, 585
Lau, D. C. W., 283, 285, 286
Lau, E. Y., 594
Lau, J., 360
Lauby-Secretan, B., 11, 12, 13
Lauer, J. B., 403
Launer, L. J., 188, 194, 233
Laurenius, A., 270, 652
Lauretti, J., 270
Lautz, D. B., 544
Lavery, M., 158, 568
Lavie, C. J., 261, 323
Lavori, P. W., 457
Lawlor, D. A., 139
Lawlor, M. S., 496, 499
Lawman, H. G., 336, 605
Lawton, C. L., 218, 224, 353
Lazar, C. C., 571
Lazorick, S., 610, 611, 616
Lazzer, S., 600
Le Chatelier, E., 86
Le Foll, C., 31
Le Roux, C., 260
le Roux, C. W., 196, 379
Leahey, T., 516, 517
Leahey, T. M., 262, 268, 294, 338, 397, 399, 407, 472
Lean, M. E., 188, 359
Lear, S. A., 114
Leardo, M., 613
Leblanc, C., 65
LeBlanc, E., 289
LeBlanc, E. S., 350, 454
Lebrun, C. E., 236
Lecoeur, C., 597
Lecoultre, V., 55
Leddy, J. J., 630
Lederman, S. A., 247
Ledikwe, J. H., 96, 97
Ledley, G. S., 517, 518
Lee, C. D., 432, 587
Lee, H. B., 156
Lee, H. Y., 77
Lee, I., 261, 322
Lee, I. M., 10, 112, 323, 522
Lee, J. S., 194, 428
Lee, K. R., 358

Leermakers, E. A., 326, 501
Legierski, C. M., 625, 629
Lehnert, T., 18, 140
Lei, H., 343
Leibel, R. L., 25, 41, 50, 53, 75, 81, 294, 393, 461
Leiderman, V. R., 580
Leidig, M. M., 316
Lemon, S. C., 151
Lennon, L., 195
Lent, M. R., 269, 287, 613, 614, 615
Leombruni, P., 556
Leon, A. S., 107
Leopold, L., 53
Leproult, R., 132
Lerma-Cabrera, J. M., 177
Leroux, J. S., 140
Lesage, A. D., 155
Leslie, W. S., 359, 361
Letizia, K. A., 256, 267, 294, 298, 343
Lettieri, C. J., 383
Leung, V., 212
Levine, A. S., 30
Levine, J. A., 44, 45, 47, 48, 50, 52, 111, 330
Levine, R., 3, 18, 186
Levitsky, D. A., 258
Levitt, E. B., 393
Levy, R. L., 404, 405, 579, 627
Lewis, K. H., 426
Ley, R. E., 78, 82, 83
Li, A. W., 330
Li, C. I., 486
Li, G., 190, 191
Li, H., 124
Li, J. F., 648
Li, K., 159
Li, L., 15, 156
Li, R., 596
Li, S., 651
Li, T. Y., 111, 330
Liakos, A., 361
Liang, G., 28
Liang, Z., 381
Liao, D., 130
Liao, J., 613
Liao, Y., 613
Libman, G., 178
Libotte, E., 98
Lichtman, S. W., 259, 298, 340
Ličina, M., 543
Lieberman, M., 197, 385
Lifson, N., 44
Lillioja, S., 41, 43, 51
Lillis, J., 162, 330, 514, 518, 519
Lilly, N., 27
Lin, H., 631

Lin, H. V., 85
Lin, J., 417, 431
Lin, J. S., 188
Lindberg, N. M., 448
Linde, J. A., 339, 500, 579
Lindgarde, F., 188, 189, 191, 192
Lindquist, R. A., 524
Lindroos, A. K., 600
Lindsay, J., 236
Lindström, J., 189, 342
Ling, J., 607
Linke, S. E., 461
Lipschutz, P. E., 257
Lissner, L., 286
Lister, K. M., 623
Little, B. B., 106
Little, T. J., 83
Littlewood, J. A., 100
Litvak, K., 351
Liu, C., 27, 260
Liu, F., 141
Liu, J., 69, 594
Liu, L., 56
Liu, S., 662
Liu, Y., 462
Livhits, M., 271
Livingstone, M. B., 101
Llewellyn, C., 596
Llewellyn, C. H., 596
Lochner, K. A., 140
Locke, A. E., 56, 65
Loewenstein, G., 522, 523
Loi, N. M., 584
Long, J. D., 653
Long, M. W., 143, 666
Long, S. K., 428
Lonnerdal, B., 596
Loomis, D., 12
Looney, S. M., 402
Loos, R. J., 65
Lopez, N., 428
Lopez-Cuadrado, T., 640
López-García, E., 258
Lopez-Legarrea, P., 177
Lopez-Nava, G., 536, 540, 541
Lorber, J., 639
Lorr, J., 209
Loth, K. A., 152
Louis, M., 581
Lourenco, S., 100
Lovasi, G. S., 442
Lovenheim, M. F., 255
Lovesky, M. M., 316
Loviselli, A., 157
Löwe, B., 263
Lowe, G. D., 188
Lowe, M. R., 96, 260, 518, 519
Lowery, S. E., 577
Lowry, L., 568

Lu, J. F., 158
Lu, L., 236
Lubans, D. R., 617
Lubetkin, E. I., 158
Lucas, A., 596, 601
Lucas, C., 459
Lucas, J. W., 438
Lucassen, E. A., 129
Ludman, E. J., 155
Ludwig, D. S., 51, 313, 316, 317, 644
Ludwig, W. W., 403
Lueders, N. K., 502
Luedicke, J., 163, 586
Luepker, R. V., 610
Luft, F. C., 51
Luke, A., 440
Lukwago, S. N., 447
Lumeng, J. C., 256
Lundberg, J. M., 28
Lundgren, J., 175, 261
Lundgren, J. D., 174, 175, 176, 177
Lupattelli, G., 55
Luppino, F. S., 150, 154
Lurie-Beck, J., 156
Luskey, K. L., 31
Lutes, L. D., 131, 344, 402, 473
Lutz, K. W., 623
Lutz, T. A., 31
Luzio, S. D., 27
Lycett, D., 245
Lyketsos, C. G., 156
Lynch, F. L., 554
Lynch, J. W., 139
Lynch, K., 343
Lyons, P., 582

M

Ma, J., 156, 157, 456, 457
Maas, I., 140
Maassen van den Brink, H., 140
Maayan, L., 629
Macartney, S., 438, 439
MacDonald, K. G., 200, 382
MacDonell, K., 513
Macfarlane, G. T., 83
Macfarlane, S., 83
MacGregor, A. M., 581
Macgregor, A. M., 174
Machado, V. H., 382
Machytka, E., 544
Maciejewski, M. L., 197, 209, 224
MacInnis, R. J., 7
Macintyre, S., 144
Mackay, D. F., 16
Mackenbach, J. D., 137, 139, 143, 144

Mackiewicz, U., 81
Mackintosh, R., 81
MacLean, P. S., 100, 256, 393
Madalosso, C. A., 383
Madans, J., 188, 233
Madhavan, S. S., 158
Madison, K., 522
Madsen, J., 54
Madsen, K. A., 666
Maersk, M., 317
Maes, H. H., 64, 596
Maffei, M., 53, 66
Maffeis, C., 600
Magal, M., 331
Magallares, A., 579
Maggard, M. A., 652
Magnusson, P. K., 64
Magwood, G. S., 343
Maher, C. A., 130, 476
Mahler, R. J., 9
Mai, X. M., 150
Maia, M., 379
Mainous, A. G., 430
Maislin, G., 594
Major, B., 160, 582, 583, 584
Majumdar, S. R., 208
Makovec, F., 26
Malcolm, R. J., 177
Malhotra, A., 106, 124
Malhotra, S., 577
Malik, V. S., 3, 259, 317, 598, 605
Malina, R. M., 106
Malinowski, S. S., 653
Malkemus, L. A., 577
Malone, K. E., 486
Mamun, A. A., 124, 131
Mancher, M., 415
Mancuso, J. P., 459, 470
Maness, L. M., 31
Manibay, E., 442
Mann, R. A., 524
Mannarino, E., 55
Manne, S., 417, 431
Manninen, P., 474
Manohar, C. U., 330
Manson, J. E., 6, 9, 10, 111, 330, 659
Mansoor, N., 314
Manuel, D. G., 186
Manzato, E., 151, 153
Maraldo, T. M., 177
Marathe, P. H., 381
Marcus, B. H., 324, 325, 401, 467
Marcus, M., 485
Marcus, M. D., 260, 561
Marinari, G. M., 175
Marini, M., 96, 580
Marinos, G., 540
Markides, K. S., 232, 234

Markwald, R. R., 125
Marlatt, G. A., 341
Marlatt, K., 330
Marlatt, K. L., 38, 259
Marrero, D., 224, 225, 229
Marrero, D. G., 293, 481, 501, 502
Marsch, L. A., 630
Marseglia, L., 595
Marsh, A. P., 233
Marsh, T., 18, 138
Marshall, A. L., 473
Marshall, H. M., 175
Marshall, K., 211
Marshall, N. S., 217
Marshall, S., 513
Marso, S. P., 196, 197, 286
Marteau, T. M., 100
Marti, C. N., 213, 618
Martin, A. D., 326, 501
Martin, B. W., 115
Martin, C. K., 171, 208, 209, 211, 212, 215, 216, 217, 225, 228, 310, 354, 469, 474
Martin-Diener, E., 115
Martinelli, C. E., 68
Martinez, I., 81
Martinez, J., 156
Martinez, V., 26
Martínez-Cervell, C., 536
Martinez-Gonzalez, M. A., 43
Martino, S., 511
Martins, C., 118, 119
Martos, R., 53
Martz, D. M., 442
Maruthur, N., 114
Masheb, R. M., 171, 553, 554, 556, 557, 558, 560, 561
Maslowski, K. M., 85
Mason, D. A., 512
Mason, E. E., 645
Mason, S., 265
Masuda, A., 162, 330, 514, 518
Mather, A. A., 155, 156
Mathew, J. L., 130
Mathiason, M. A., 255, 430
Mathis, C., 25
Mathurin, P., 383
Mathus-Vliegen, E. M. H., 541
Matricciani, L., 130
Matsuki, T., 85
Matsuo, H., 28
Matsuo, K., 13
Mattei, J., 99, 312
Matthews, C. E., 111, 124
Matthews, D. E., 53
Matthews, D. R., 249
Mattson, M. P., 106, 118
Maukonen, M., 129
Mayer, J., 113, 114

Mayer, L. E., 25
Mayer, R. R., 339
Mayo, K., 442
Mazda, T., 25, 26
Mazlan, N., 99
Mazzella, R., 579
Mazzeo, R. S., 116
Mbaiwa, S. E., 99
McAdoo, W. G., 403
McAllister, D. A., 403
McAllister, E. J., 25
McAlpine, D. A., 330
McArdle, W. D., 111
McCann, K. L., 398
McCann, M. T., 101
McCarty, F., 417, 513
McClelland, J. W., 231
McCloskey, C. A., 382
McClure, S. M., 629
McCorkle, S. K., 31
McCoy, T., 598
McCracken, L. M., 514
McCrady, S. K., 330
Mc-Crindle, B. W., 513
McCrory, M. A., 99
McCuen-Wurst, C., 153, 169, 260, 261
McCullough, P. A., 8
McCurley, J., 623, 632
McDermott, M. M., 235, 236
McDermott, T. M., 99
McDonald, J., 79
McDonald, S. M., 594
McElroy, S. L., 173, 555, 556, 557, 577
McEvoy, G. K., 351
McFarland, B. H., 236
McGinnis, J. M., 522
McGlinchey, E., 130
McGlockton, J., 662
McGuigan, R. D., 582
McGuire, M. T., 81, 324
McHorney, C. A., 158
McHugh, L., 516, 517
McHugh, P. R., 26
McHugh, R. K., 632
McKay, H. G., 445
McKay, L. D., 30
Mclain, J., 142
McNabb, W., 495, 499
McNair, D. M., 209
McNay, D. E. G., 84, 85
McNeil, J., 131
McNeill, L. H., 139
McPherson, K., 18, 138
McTiernan, A., 323
Mead, N., 380
Meadows, E. C., 645
Meany, G., 153, 213, 561

Mechanick, J. I., 270, 284, 372
Medeiros, M. D., 28
Meengs, J. S., 93, 94, 95, 97, 98, 100
Mehlsen, M., 561
Mehta, A. K., 480, 481, 483, 484, 485, 487
Mei, Z., 645
Meier, L. L., 151
Melanson, E. L., 44, 313
Melby, C. L., 116
Melhorn, S. J., 118
Mellor, D. D., 330
Melmed, S., 246
Melnyk, B. M., 616, 617, 618
Melzer, D., 235
Mendelson, M., 157, 223, 566
Mendes de Leon, C. F., 232, 233
Mermelstein, R., 267
Merriam, P. A., 448
Merrow, M., 129
Mertens, L., 143
Mertz, W., 41
Merwin, E., 497
Mesas, A. E., 258
Mesquita, D. N., 80
Messick, S., 215, 260
Messier, S. P., 188, 194, 230, 236
Messing, S., 570
Messroghli, L., 131
Mestdagh, R., 82
Metchnikoff, E., 75
Meter, K., 158
Meyer, K. A., 124
Meyerhoefer, C., 18, 432
Mhurchu, C. N., 142
Micco, N., 395, 399, 468, 471
Michalsen, A., 330
Michalsky, M., 646, 647, 648, 650, 652
Michel, Y., 442
Michener, J. L., 418
Michie, S., 500
Mickelsen, O., 52, 208
Mietlicki-Baase, E. G., 26, 27, 31
Mifflin, M. D., 46
Mikami, D. J., 652
Mikhail, C., 580
Mikhail, N., 9
Mikkelsen, P. B., 315
Miller, A. L., 130
Miller, C. T., 160, 577
Miller, G. D., 231, 232
Miller, G. J., 107
Miller, J., 351
Miller, J. M., 330
Miller, M. E., 233
Miller, N. P., 213
Miller, W., 508, 509, 510

Miller, W. M., 8
Miller, W. R., 458
Miller, Y. D., 473
Miller Wolman, D., 415
Milliez, P. Y., 571
Millman, J., 429
Milos, G., 552
Mingrone, G., 380, 381, 382, 650
Mintem, G. C., 152
Mir, A. S., 585
Miranda, W. R., 201
Mirza, A., 29
Mitchell, J. A., 124
Mitchell, J. E., 153, 213, 553, 554, 555, 556, 561, 570
Mitchell, N. S., 432, 449, 458, 492, 504
Mitchell, P. C., 75
Mitra, K. P., 113
Moate, P. J., 174
Mock, J., 157, 223
Modarressi, A., 571
Modi, A. C., 653
Moffitt, T. E., 629
Mohler-Kuo, M., 552
Moize, V., 648
Mokdad, A. H., 650
Mollet, A., 31
Monasta, L., 607
Mond, J., 155, 552, 577
Monda, K. L., 144
Monk, T. H., 216
Monsivais, P., 141, 142, 143, 144
Montague, C. T., 66
Montani, J. P., 217
Montie, J., 608
Moore, B. J., 247
Moore, R. H., 177, 598
Moore, R. L., 25
Moore, S., 140
Moore, S. C., 124
Moore, W., 329
Moorthy, M., 261
Mora, M., 212
Morabito, A., 386
Morais, J., 152
Moran, C. H., 605
Moran, T. H., 24, 25, 26, 83
Mordes, J., 260
Mordes, J. P., 27
Moreno, C., 177, 178
Morgan, L., 118
Mori, N., 556
Morin, P. C., 457
Morino, M., 379
Morland, K., 144
Morley, S., 514
Morrell, H. E. R., 160
Morris, E. L., 93

Morris, J. N., 107
Morris, M., 330
Morris, M. C., 232
Morris, S., 159
Morrongiello, B. A., 513
Moss, L. A., 594
Motamedi, S. M. K., 368
Mouchacca, J., 151
Moudon, A. V., 141
Moulin, P., 158
Moulton-Barrett, R. E., 570
Mourtakos, S. P., 344
Moustarah, F., 375, 378, 379
Moy, T. F., 502
Moyer, V. A., 288, 416, 453, 458
Mozaffarian, D., 141, 190
Mueller, E. T., 629
Mueller, N. T., 80
Muennig, P., 608
Mujahid, M. S., 143
Mulder, C., 4, 605
Mulkens, S., 516, 517
Muller, A., 174
Muller, M. J., 46, 54
Mummadi, R. R., 382, 383
Mundermann, A., 236
Muñoz-Pareja, M., 258
Munsch, S., 214
Munzberg, H., 31
Murawski, M. E., 341
Murphy, E. M., 53
Murphy, R., 80
Murphy, S. A., 343
Murphy, S. L., 7
Must, A., 8, 16, 156
Mustajoki, P., 212, 224, 225, 343
Mustian, M., 330
Myer, J. R., 26
Myers, C. A., 208
Myers, H., 330
Myers, M. D., 630
Myers, M. G., Jr., 81
Mykletun, A., 552
Myrissa, K., 218, 224

N

Naar-King, S., 513
Nachmani, J., 598
Nackers, L. M., 397, 402, 407, 516
Nadglowski, J., 162
Nadolny, T. L., 666
Naglak, M., 314
Nahum-Shani, I., 343, 476, 477
Napolitano, M., 324, 325, 467
Napolitano, M. A., 175, 469, 475
Narang, I., 130

Narayan, K. M., 185
Näslund, I., 654
Nassel, A. F., 449
Naumova, E. N., 156
Navarro Rosenblatt, D. A., 13, 14
Nawaz, H., 610
Neale, M. C., 64, 596, 597
Neamah, H. H., 493, 498
Neckerman, K. M., 442
Nedeltcheva, A. V., 125, 126, 132, 462
Nedergaard, J., 82
Nederkoorn, C., 625
Needham, B. L., 155
Needleman, B. J., 652
Neel, J. V., 38, 440
Neggers, S. J., 29
Neidell, M., 608
Nelson, M. R., 71
Nemeroff, C. B., 577
Nemeth, L. S., 343
Nestle, M., 93, 662
Netemeyer, R. G., 260
Neuhaus, M., 111, 143
Neumark-Sztainer, D., 124–125, 152, 343, 577, 580, 662
Neumark-Sztainer, D. R., 80, 617
Newlin, D. B., 403
Newman, A. B., 233
Newman, J. M., 268
Newsom, J. T., 236
Newsome, P. N., 15
Newton, R. L., Jr., 447
Newton, T., 152
Neylan, C. J., 302, 538
Nezami, B. G., 75
Nezami, B. T., 291, 344, 466
Nezin, L. E., 441
Nezu, A. M., 398, 404
Ng, M., 644
Ng, S. W., 114, 141, 666
Nguyen, C. N., 570
Nguyen, N. T., 379, 645, 653
Nguyen, T., 51
Ni, B., 648
NICE., 556
Nicholas A., 438
Nicholls, W., 171
Nicklas, B. J., 188
Nicklas, J. M., 186
Nicol, S., 569
Niego, S. H., 213
Niehoff, M. L., 28
Niemeier, H. M., 516, 517
Nienhuijs, S. W., 224
Nieuwdorp, M., 83
Nimgaonkar, A., 545
Niswender, K. D., 30

Nitka, D., 155
Njike, V. Y., 610
Noakes, M., 210
Noakes, T., 106
Noar, S. M., 473
Noda, M., 190
Noll, J. G., 653
Nommsen, L. A., 596
Nonaka, N., 28
Norat, T., 13, 14
Nordstrom, C. R., 16
Norén, E., 302
Norgren, R., 24, 25
Norris, S. L., 188
Northern, J. J., 623
Norton, E. C., 431
Nosek, B., 580
Nosek, B. A., 578
Notelovitz, M., 326, 501
Nothwehr, F., 627
Novak, S. A., 161
Nurnberger, J. I., 393
Nusselder, W. J., 159
Nuutinen, O., 631
Nwankwo, T., 8

O

Obarzanek, E., 343, 443
Obeid, N. R., 538
Oberbach, A., 545
O'Brien, J., 427
O'Brien, K. S., 585
O'Brien, P. E., 174, 648
O'Brien, R., 459
O'Brien, W. H., 337, 623
Ochner, C. N., 299, 432
Ockene, I. S., 448
O'Connell, M., 50, 610
O'Connor, E., 289, 350, 454
O'Connor, E. A., 623
Odoms-Young, A., 447
Odoms-Young, A. M., 447
O'Donoghue, T., 523
O'Donovan, D., 83
Ogawa, A., 31
Ogden, C. L., 3, 4, 140, 185, 243, 349, 419, 453, 466, 503, 531, 552, 593, 594, 605, 606, 618, 622, 644, 659
Ogilvie, D., 144
Ogilvie, R. P., 462
Oguma, Y., 10
Ogunleye, A. A., 19
Oh, W., 56
Ohmori, K., 233
Oien, D. M., 531

O'Kane, M., 654
Oken, E., 344, 596
Okubo, T., 82
Olbers, T., 645, 647, 648, 650, 651, 653, 654
Olds, T. S., 130
O'Leary, J. P., 367
Oliver, G., 139, 143
Oliver, L., 125
Olshansky, S. J., 593, 644, 660
Olszewski, P. K., 29
O'Malley, W., 570
Onat, A., 247
O'Neil, P. M., 177, 215, 353, 354
Onland-Moret, N. C., 118
Onyike, C. U., 156
O'Rahilly, S., 53, 255
Orchard, T. J., 286
O'Reardon, J. P., 175, 176, 177
Ornish, D., 191, 192
Orosan, P., 571
O'Rourke, P., 341
Orpana, H., 6
Ortega, A. N., 442
Ortinski, P. I., 27
Ortiz, C. L., 580
Ortman, J. M., 438, 439
Ory, M. G., 442
Oslin, D., 343
Ostbye, T., 212, 418
Osterholt, K. M., 99, 100
Ostir, G. V., 232
Osypuk, T. L., 140
Otahal, P., 257
O'Toole, P. W., 79
Otten, J. J., 665
Ottenbacher, K. J., 234
Otto, A. D., 326, 328
Otto, R. M., 330
Ottone, L., 171
Overby, D. W., 426
Overduin, J., 29
Ovesen, P., 618
Owen, N., 111
Owens, D. R., 27
Öztürk, A., 536

P

Pacanowski, C. R., 258
Pachucki, M. C., 255, 256
Padwal, R. S., 208
Paffenbarger, R. S., 261
Paffenbarger, R. S., Jr., 10
Pagoto, S., 263
Pagoto, S. L., 151, 447
Pais-Ribeiro, J. L., 579

Palm Reed, K., 516, 517
Palmer, C. N., 65, 596
Paluch, A. E., 113
Paluch, R. A., 622, 623, 624, 625, 628, 631, 632
Pamuk, E. R., 186, 194
Pan, A., 16, 150, 156, 158, 317, 598
Pan, Q., 229
Pan, X. R., 188, 189, 190
Panagiotopoulos, S., 380
Pang, Q., 15
Panter, J., 144
Panunzi, S., 380, 381
Papadaki, A., 319
Papadopoulos, S., 160
Papakostas, P., 536, 538, 539
Paradis, A., 256
Paraponaris, A., 159
Parikh, M., 381
Park, C. Y., 358
Park, D., 29
Park, M. H., 640
Park, S. W., 358
Park, Y. W., 358
Parker, E., 665
Parker, S., 584
Parks, B. W., 77
Parrino, C., 246
Parsons, J. K., 15
Parsons, M. J., 129
Parsons, T. J., 593
Patel, M. S., 246, 292, 522, 527, 528
Patel, S. R., 216
Patnode, C., 289
Patnode, C. D., 350, 454
Patrick, D. L., 209, 224
Patrick, K., 469, 473, 474
Patterson, E. J., 536
Patti, E. T., 398
Patzer, G. L., 565, 566
Paul-Ebhohimhen, V., 289
Paulus, G. F., 651
Pawlak, D. B., 644
Pawlow, L., 215
Pawlow, L. A., 177
Paxinos, G., 31
Paxton, S. J., 171
Payette, H., 152
Payne, J. H., 644
Pearce, L. R., 70
Pearl, R. L., 149, 161, 262, 263, 264, 266, 662
Pearson, E. S., 339
Peat, C. M., 556
Pedersen, S. D., 94, 98
Peerson, J. M., 596

Peeters, A., 159, 200
Peigneux, P., 132
Pejovic, S., 131
Pekkarinen, T., 212, 224, 225, 229, 343
Pelchat, M. L., 178
Pelkman, C. L., 98
Pell, J. P., 16
Pellegrini, C. A., 328
Pelleymounter, M. A., 53
Peltoniemi, H. H., 570
Penev, P., 125
Penev, P. D., 132, 462
Penna, S., 536, 538, 539
Penninx, B., 151
Pepe, M. S., 255, 594
Pera, V., 265
Percy, C., 229
Pereira, M. A., 339
Perez, A., 360
Perez, M., 157
Perez-Escamilla, R., 95, 96, 97
Perlis, M. L., 125
Perna, F. M., 665
Perreault, L., 190
Perri, M. G., 231, 289, 294, 326, 338, 341, 393, 397, 398, 400, 403, 404, 405, 406, 407, 494, 497, 499, 501, 503, 504
Perrin, A., 475
Perrin, E. M., 593, 594
Perrin, J. M., 16
Perrine, C. G., 596
Perry, C. D., 201
Pertschuk, M. J., 567, 568
Pérusse, L., 49, 64, 65, 70, 255, 256
Pescatello, L. S., 246
Peters, A. L., 461
Peters, J., 630
Peters, J. C., 258, 330
Peters, J. H., 26
Peters, J. L., 159
Petersen, L., 175
Peterson, C. B., 170, 554
Peterson, C. M., 47
Peterson, D. A., 78
Peterson, E. D., 8
Peterson, J. L., 163, 586
Peth, J., 630
Petri, K. C. C., 639
Petrin, C., 417, 428
Petry, N. M., 155
Phelain, J. F., 116
Phelan, S., 32, 81, 162, 172, 269, 288, 294, 336, 344, 508
Phelan, S. M., 163, 581
Phillips, E., 664

Phillips, R. J., 25
Phinney, S., 106
Piantadosi, C., 212
Pickering, R. P., 155, 156
Pieper, C. F., 233
Pierce, J. W., 584
Piernas, C., 598
Piers, A., 265
Pieters, R., 523
Pietrobelli, A., 156
Pietrzak, R. H., 155
Piette, J. D., 445
Pinelli, L., 600
Pingitore, R., 579
Pinhas-Hamiel, O., 644
Pinna, F., 157
Pintauro, S., 406, 471
Pinto, A. M., 481, 482
Pischon, T., 51
Pisetsky, E. M., 213
Pi-Sunyer, F. X., 352, 354, 415, 432
Pi-Sunyer, X., 196, 197, 210, 342, 444
Pittas, A. G., 360
Pittermann, A., 570
Pittet-Cuenod, B., 571
Piwek, L., 328
Plagemann, A., 595
Plasqui, G., 45
Pliner, P., 94
Plodkowski, R. A., 640
Plomin, R., 65, 596
Podrabsky, M., 665
Poehlman, E. T., 65
Poelman, M. P., 95
Pogoto, S. L., 428
Poirier, P., 188, 382
Pol, K., 318
Polivy, J., 94, 171, 571
Pollak, K. I., 417, 418
Pollert, G., 271
Polley, B. A., 326
Pollmächer, T., 131
Polonsky, H. M., 214, 565, 567
Polonsky, K., 246
Polonsky, W. H., 210
Polzien, K. M., 328
Pomeranz, J. L., 286, 429, 667
Ponce, J., 369, 536, 539
Pontiroli, A. E., 386
Pope, G., Jr., 170
Pope, H. G., 552
Popkin, B. M., 114, 141, 144, 598, 666
Porte, D., Jr., 30, 67
Porter, A. M., 161
Porter, P. L, 486

Post, R. E., 254, 417
Postmes, T., 160
Poston, L., 595
Poston, W. S., 459
Poston, W. S., II, 343
Potosky, A., 258
Potts, J. E., 360
Poulsen, S. K., 316
Pournaras, D., 260
Pouwels, S., 224
Powell, A. G., 247, 349, 350
Powell, K., 139
Powell, L. M., 665, 666
Power, C., 156
Powers, S. K., 111
Powley, T. L., 25
Prachand, V. N., 383
Pratley, R. E., 46
Pratt, J. S., 645, 647
Preiss, K., 156
Prelip, M. L., 442
Prentice, A. M., 46, 667
Prewitt, T. E., 440, 444, 493, 502
Price, R. A., 65, 156
Prigeon, R. L., 31
Prineas, R. J., 9
Printen, K. J., 645
Printz, C., 247
Prochaska, J. O., 458
Prochazka, A. V., 449, 492
Proenca, R., 53
Proksch, A. M., 599
Pronk, N. P., 339, 500, 579
Proper, K. I., 111, 114
Prud'homme, D., 152
Prus-Wisniewski, R., 299
Pruzinsky, T., 566
Pucher, J., 141
Puder, J. J., 607, 608
Puhl, R., 160
Puhl, R. M., 16, 17, 149, 160, 161, 162, 163, 262, 263, 264, 266, 577, 580, 584, 585, 586, 662
Pulcini, M. E., 161
Pulgarón, E. R., 605
Purcell, K., 472
Putnam, J. J., 142

Q

Qi, L., 312
Qi, Q., 65, 312
Quan, Y., 368
Quattrin, T., 625, 631
Quebbemann, B. B., 536
Quick, V., 152, 153
Quilliot, D., 653

Quinn, D., 583, 584, 585
Quirk, F., 552
Qureshi, L. A., 536

R

Raaijmakers, L. C., 224
Rabin, M., 523
Rabinowitz, J., 610
Rabkin, J., 382
Rahe, C., 131
Rai, M., 139
Rainie, L., 473
Raitakari, O. T., 651
Rajagopalan, H., 545
Rajan, E., 539, 540
Ramachandran, A., 189
Ramachandrappa, S., 66, 70
Raman Muthusamy, V., 540
Ramirez, R. R., 438
Ramos, E., 125
Ranadive, S. A., 596
Rand, C. S., 174, 581
Randal, E., 144
Randolph, J. G., 645
Rao, G., 644
Rao, M., 141, 142
Raoof, M., 654
Rardin, D., 153
Rask, E., 654
Rasmussen, F., 64
Ratcliffe, D., 394
Raudenbush, S. W., 139
Ravera, G., 175
Ravussin, E., 31, 38, 41, 42, 44, 45, 46, 47, 48, 49, 50, 51, 54, 55, 81, 209, 228, 259, 310, 440, 441
Ravussin, Y., 76, 80
Rawlins, M., 584
Ray, L., 232
Raynor, H., 630
Raynor, H. A., 94, 99, 100, 397, 402, 407, 628
Rayos, G. H., 81
Raza, F., 137
Reas, D. L., 556
Redding, C. A., 152, 458
Redekop, W. K., 159
Redman, L. M., 47, 209, 211, 215, 310
Reed, G. W., 258, 330
Reeve, J. R., Jr., 28
Rehkopf, D. H., 139
Rehm, C. D., 141, 598
Reibel, N., 653
Reid, K. J., 127, 130

Author Index

Reidelberger, R. D., 28
Reiff, C., 330
Reiman, D., 80
Reinehr, T., 622, 631
Reinhardt, M., 50, 53
Reinke, E., 116
Reis, L. O., 212
Reiter, J., 571
Rejeski, W. J., 188, 192, 194, 208, 223, 224, 225, 227, 228, 230, 231, 233, 236, 397, 401
Remely, M., 79
Remiker, A. M., 598
Renehan, A. G., 11
Renjilian, D. A., 289, 493
Reoch, J., 368
Resnicow, K., 513
Resta, O., 131
Retnakaran, R., 284
Retterstøl, K., 314
Reynolds, C. F., III, 216
Reynolds, K. D., 445
Reynolds, S. L., 232
Rha, S. S., 597
Rhoden, E. L., 212
Rhodes, R. E., 137
Ricca, V., 553, 556, 557, 558
Richard, M., 637
Richardson, M. T., 107
Richardson, S., 665
Rich-Edwards, J. W., 15
Rickman, A. D., 326
Ricks, K. M., 29
Ridaura, V. K., 77
Riebe, D., 246, 331
Riedel-Heller, S., 18, 140
Riediger, T., 31
Rifas-Shiman, S. L., 344, 596
Rigg, A., 645
Riis, J., 100
Rimm, A. A., 10
Rimm, E. B., 9, 11, 316
Ringel, J. S., 159
Rising, R., 42, 43, 44, 46, 125
Rissanen, A., 195
Rissel, C., 114, 115
Ristow, B., 382
Ritenbaugh, C., 441
Ritter, R. C., 24, 25, 26
Rivera, J. A., 666
Ritz, C., 312
Robbins, L. B., 607
Roberts, D. L., 454
Roberts, R., 155
Roberts, S. B., 99, 601
Robertson, D. S., 51
Robertson, R. J., 326
Robinson, A. H., 555

Robinson, E., 98
Robinson, S. M., 29
Robinson, T. N., 579, 612
Robinson, W. R., 125
Robles, G., 31
Rocha, A., 665
Rock, C. L., 95, 291, 293, 468, 471, 482
Rodgers, B., 155
Rodgers, R. J., 32
Rodin, J., 568, 579
Rodman, J., 268
Rodriguez, D., 124
Rodríguez-Artalejo, F., 258
Roe, L. S., 93, 94, 95, 96, 97, 98, 100
Roehrborn, C. G., 14
Roehrig, J. P., 568
Roehrs, T., 125
Roemmich, J. N., 330, 622, 623, 628
Roenneberg, T., 129
Rogers, C. A., 648
Rogers, P. J., 258
Rogers, R. J., 261, 322, 326, 328
Rogers, R. R., 599
Rogers, S., 418
Rogula, T., 379
Rojas, N., 666
Rollnick, S., 458, 508, 509, 510
Rollo, M. E., 259
Rolls, B. J., 93, 94, 95, 96, 97, 98, 99, 100, 393, 553, 598
Romach, E. H., 26
Romeo, S., 197, 199
Romer, J., 29
Romundstad, P., 150
Ronel, N., 178
Ronti, T., 55
Rooney, B. L., 255
Root, T. L., 176
Rose, G., 186
Rose, G. S., 509
Rosella, L. C., 186
Rosen, E. D., 55
Rosen, J. C., 571
Rosenbaum, M., 25, 41, 50, 53, 54, 75, 81, 294, 393, 461
Rosenbaum, S., 428
Rosenberg, I. H., 236
Rosenberg, M., 157
Rosenberger, P. H., 157
Rosenblatt, R. A., 497
Rosenheck, R., 259
Rosenkilde, M., 113, 117, 119
Rosen-Reynosos, M., 155, 156
Rosenstein, L., 156
Rosenstock, J., 360

Rosenthal, B. S., 524, 525
Rosenthal, R. J., 386
Rosin, R., 528
Rosner, B., 11, 486
Ross, R., 105, 108, 236, 261, 326
Rossier, M. M., 31
Rössner, S., 175, 394
Rosthoj, S., 114
Roth, J. D., 31
Roth, T., 125
Rothman, A. J., 393
Rothman, R. B., 353, 359, 638
Rothwell, N. J., 47
Rotnitzky, A., 10
Roubenoff, R., 236
Roughan, P., 571
Rouhani, M. H., 97
Rousseau, A., 593
Rowan, M., 613
Rowe, S., 100
Roy, H., 51
Roy, M., 152
Roy, P., 113
Rubin, C. J., 215
Rubin, R. R., 188, 210, 224, 226, 229, 230
Rubino, F., 284, 303, 369, 371, 379, 380, 381
Ruckerl, R., 596
Rudolph, A., 561, 579, 646
Rudser, K., 637
Rueda-Clausen, C. F., 19
Ruiz-Lozano, T., 130
Rumley, A., 188
Rumpel, C., 188, 233
Rundle, A., 329
Rungby, J., 31
Rupley, D. C., Jr., 10
Rupp, K., 342
Rupprecht, L. E., 27, 31
Rupprecht, R., 130
Rushing, P. A., 31
Russell, R., 99
Russell-Jones, D., 638
Rutan, G., 9
Rutledge, T., 461, 462
Rutters, F., 129
Ruttimann, J., 105
Ryan, A. S., 188
Ryan, C. L., 438, 439
Ryan, D., 187, 358
Ryan, D. A., 327
Ryan, D. H., 209, 284, 299, 349, 359, 457, 458, 498
Ryan, L., 313
Ryan D. H., 638
Ryder, J., 637
Rydin, S., 403

Ryff, C. D., 161
Ryou, M., 532, 543, 544, 545, 546

S

Saariniemi, K. M., 570
Sabin, J., 580, 581
Sackner-Bernstein, J., 314
Sacks, F. M., 99, 312, 315, 339, 397, 403, 407
Sadhasivam, S., 430
Sadr-Azodi, O., 652
Sadry, S. A., 27
Saelens, B. E., 627, 630
Safer, D. L., 555
Saguy, A., 581
Sahoo, T., 69
Sahu, A., 28
Said, M., 631
Saito, M., 55
Saito, T., 189, 190
Saito, Y., 232
Salamone, L., 236
Salant, S. L., 553, 557, 558
Salbe, A. D., 175
Saliba, B., 159
Sallinen, B. J., 131
Sallis, J. F., 144
Salmi, A. M., 570
Salvatori, G., 80
Salvy, S. J., 625, 628, 629, 630
Sampalis, F., 197, 385
Sampalis, J. S., 197, 199, 385
Sampson, R. J., 139
Samuel-Hodge, C. D., 445, 446
Sanchez, C. E., 95
Sanchez, L. E., 156
Sánchez-Pernaute, A., 368
Sandblom, G., 652
Sande, E., 56
Sanderson, S., 596
Sanders-Thompson, V., 447
Sandoval, B., 598
Sandoz, E. K., 516, 517
Sands-Lincoln, M., 124
Sane, T., 212, 224, 225
Sanghvi, A., 310
Saperstein, S. L., 467
Sarda, V., 262, 663
Sareen, J., 155
Sarink, D., 101
Saris, W. H., 54, 112, 114, 313
Sarmiento, R., 539
Sarr, M. G., 376
Sarwer, D. B., 155, 158, 213, 214, 257, 270, 271, 299, 517, 565, 566, 567, 568, 569, 577, 579

Satov, T., 175
Sattin, R. W., 495, 499, 502
Sauer, N., 540
Savage, J., 601
Savage, J. S., 96
Savoy, S., 160
Saxena, S. K., 430
Sayon-Orea, C., 43
Scanlon, K. S., 596
Schachter, L. M., 383
Schaefer, L., 579
Schaefer, L. M., 160
Scharf, R. J., 130, 598
Scharrer, E., 31
Schauberger, C. W., 255
Schauer, P., 379
Schauer, P. R., 284, 286, 302, 303, 367, 368, 369, 371, 372, 374, 375, 378, 379, 380, 381, 382, 383, 386, 387, 459, 541, 650, 651, 652
Schaumberg, K., 265
Schele, E., 84
Scherag, A., 597
Schiffelers, S. L., 54
Schindler, J., 101
Schirmer, B., 368, 372, 378, 383, 387
Schleusner, S. J., 330
Schlögl, M., 50
Schmader, T., 582
Schmalz, D. L., 161
Schmid, T. L., 141, 394
Schmidhauser, S., 137
Schmidt, H., 522
Schmitt, M. T., 160
Schmitz, K. H., 124
Schmitz, N., 155
Schmitz, O., 31
Schneider, B., 430
Schneider, K. L., 151
Schneider, S., 630
Schnorr, S. L., 79, 81
Schnyder, U., 552
Schoeller, D., 132
Schoeller, D. A., 45, 132, 161, 298, 462, 595
Schoenthaler, A. M., 446, 502
Schofield, W. N., 46
Schooler, D., 568
Schooler, J. W., 630
Schopfer, E. A., 124
Schram, C. A., 175
Schrauwen, P., 46, 54, 82
Schrenk, D., 85
Schroeder, D. R., 94
Schroeder, S. A., 522
Schuit, A. J., 141

Schuld, A., 130
Schulsinger, F., 65
Schulz, L. O., 440
Schulze, M. B., 259, 598
Schumacher, L. M., 287, 508
Schutz, Y., 41, 42, 43, 51, 81, 217, 600
Schvey, N. A., 160, 161
Schwartz, A. E., 613, 616, 618
Schwartz, G. J., 25, 26
Schwartz, M. B., 143, 155, 156, 304, 568, 578, 581, 584, 659, 662, 663, 667
Schwartz, M. W., 30, 31, 66, 67, 81, 286
Schwartz, R. S., 50
Schweinhart, L., 608
Sciamanna, C. N., 417
Scoccianti, C., 12
Scopinaro, N., 175, 369
Scott, J. A., 80
Scott, K. M., 155
Scully, I. D., 124
Seagle, H. M., 324
Sears, S., 330
Sears, S. F., 326, 400, 501
Sebert Kuhlmann, A. K., 493
Seddon, E., 571
Sedlock, D. A., 116
Seeley, R. J., 30, 81
Segal, J., 114, 616
Segal, K. R., 459
Seger, J. C., 416
Seidah, N. G., 68
Seidel, K. D., 255, 594
Seidell, J. C., 140, 141, 598
Seimon, R. V., 312
Selman, C., 115
Semmer, N. K., 151
Sen, S., 382
Sendra-Gutiérrez, J. M., 536
Seo, S., 70
Sepah, S. C., 461
Serdula, M. K., 186
Sesso, H., 261
Sesso, H. D., 9, 10, 112, 322, 323
Sethi, M., 369
Setiawan, V. W., 13
Severo, M., 125
Sevick, M. A., 340, 500
Sexton, P. M., 31
Shafran, R., 553
Shah, A. S., 644, 651
Shah, S. M., 25
Shahar, S., 211
Shai, I., 315, 316
Shaibi, G., 617
Shaikh, M. G., 84

Shanafelt, T. D., 454
Shang, E., 265
Shaper, A. G., 195
Shapiro, J. M., 142
Shapiro, J. R., 469, 473, 474
Shapiro, R. M., 403
Sharkey, J. R., 233
Sharma, A. J., 595
Sharma, A. M., 19, 51, 245, 284, 371
Shatenstein, B., 152
Shaw, H., 618
Shaw, K., 341
Shaw, M., 139
Shaw Tronieri, J. A., 253, 284, 287, 301
Shechter, A., 125
Sheer, J. L., 428
Shelmet, J. J., 43
Shemilt, I., 100
Shen, C., 446, 502
Shen, H. C., 212
Shephard, R. J., 106, 261
Sherbourne, C. D., 158, 262
Shermak, M. A., 387
Sherman, K. J., 330
Sherman, S., 598
Sherman, S. A., 261, 322, 329, 330
Sherwood, N., 261
Sherwood, N. E., 258, 324, 326, 343, 401, 417, 468, 470, 519
Shieh, C., 500
Shield, J. P., 631
Shihab, H. M., 9
Shikany, J. M., 317
Shimizu, H., 379
Shioda, S., 28
Shipman, L. M., 577
Shiroma, E., 261
Shiroma, E. J., 323
Sholinsky, P., 65
Shook, R. P., 112, 113, 117
Shope, T. R., 652
Shugar, S. L., 328
Shungin, D., 65
Shuto, Y., 29
Siahpush, M., 236
Siegfried, N. J., 510
Siegrist, M., 98
Siener, C., 231
Siervo, M., 211
Sigal, R. J., 152
Silva, A. P., 28
Silventoinen, K., 64
Simasko, S. M., 26
Simon, G. E., 155, 577
Simon, K., 498

Simonds, S. E., 68
Simoni, M., 151, 153
Simonsick, E. M., 233
Simonson, D., 544
Simpson, L. A., 632
Sinacore, D. R., 231
Sinfield, P., 418
Singh, A. S., 4, 111, 605
Singh, D., 570
Singh, G., 141
Singh, M., 125
Singh-Franco, D., 31, 360
Sinha, M. K., 51
Sinha, S., 652
Sirey, J. A., 156
Sirikul, B., 115
Siri-Tarino, P. W., 312
Sirveaux, M. A., 653
Sjoholm, K., 197, 198
Sjöström, C. D., 286
Sjöström, L., 195, 197, 198, 199, 200, 286, 301, 350, 359, 380, 381, 382, 385, 386, 644, 651
Skarupski, K. A., 233
Skelton, J. A., 64, 593, 594, 599
Skilton, M. R., 158
Skinner, A. C., 64, 593, 594
Skinner, B. F., 337, 627
Skinner, J. S., 326
Slade, P. D., 152
Slentz, C. A., 236, 326
Slezak, J. M., 417
Slocumb, N., 130
Sloth, B., 28
Small, L., 617
Smallwood, J., 630
Smeets, M., 516, 517
Smiley, D. L., 28
Smith, A., 448
Smith, B. R., 379, 387
Smith, C., 141
Smith, C. F., 339
Smith, D. E., 512
Smith, E. O., 580
Smith, G. D., 6
Smith, G. P., 25
Smith, L. P., 141
Smith, S. J., 56
Smith, S. R., 47, 51, 301, 352, 353, 359, 638
Smith, U., 55
Smolak, L., 566
Sneade, I., 579
Snih, S. A., 159
Snitker, S., 47, 50, 54, 441
Snyder, W. S., 42
Sobal, J., 139, 140
Sobol, A. M., 16

Sobol-Golberg, S., 610, 612, 618
Soegaard Ballester, J. M., 284, 302, 531
Sogari, P. R., 212
Sogg, S., 270
Soldin, M., 571
Soler, J. T., 9
Soler, R. E., 143
Solomon, T. E., 28
Sondag, C., 271
Sone, H., 192
Song, A. Y., 570, 571
Sonne-Holm, S., 16
Sonneville, J. R., 153
Sonntag, D., 18, 140
Sonoyama, K., 82
Soo, R. M., 79
Sood, G. K., 382
Soper, R. T., 645, 647
Sorensen, T. I., 16, 65, 80, 195
Sorensen, T. I. A., 175
Soukup, J. R., 417
Sowemimo, O. A., 200
Spaeth, A. M., 123, 125, 126, 127, 128, 129, 130, 131, 216
Spalding, K. L., 255
Sparto, P. J., 326
Speakman, J. R., 38, 48, 50, 84, 85, 115, 117
Spear, S. L., 570
Specken, T. F., 570
Specter, S. E., 142
Spector, I. P., 212
Speers, S. E., 662
Spence, M., 94, 402
Sperry, S. D., 124
Spevak, P. A., 403
Spiegel, K., 125, 126
Spiegelman, B. M., 55
Spitzer, J. C., 158, 568, 569
Spitzer, R. L., 171, 263
Spitznagel, M. B., 211
Spraul, M., 46, 50, 51
Sprecher, S., 565
Spring, B., 579
Spruijt-Metz, D., 477
Spyropoulos, C., 380
Squires, S., 625
Sridhar, S. B., 595
Srinivasan, S., 75
Srinivasan, S. R., 593, 645
Staalesen, T., 570, 654
Stabbert, K., 172, 288, 336, 508
Staffieri, J. R., 578
Stagaman, K., 80
Staiano, A. E., 111
Stallings, V. A., 594, 595
Stampfer, M. J., 9, 11

Stanton, C. M., 630, 631
Stark, L. J., 598
Stearns, S. C., 431
Steed, C., 661
Steenhuis, I. H., 100, 598
Steer, R. A., 209, 253, 263
Steeves, E. A., 402
Steeves, J. A., 114
Steffen, K., 271
Steffen, K. J., 215, 570
Stein, L. J., 30
Stein, R. I., 623, 625, 628
Steinbeck, K., 579
Steinberg, C., 299
Steinberg, D. M., 292, 428, 469, 472, 500
Steinberg, E., 415
Steinberg, L., 212
Steinberg, M. B., 246
Steinberger, J., 644
Steinig, J., 265
Stelmach-Mardas, M., 97
Stenholm, S., 233
Steptoe, A., 151
Stern, S., 497
Sternberg, J. A., 294
Sternfeld, B., 107
Sternlieb, B., 330
Stettler, N., 595
Stevens, J., 144, 233, 659
Stevens, S. D., 160
Stevens, V. J., 188, 343, 443, 444, 448
Stewart, A. L., 212
Stewart, K., 571
Stewart, T. M., 213, 214
Stice, E., 213, 618
Still, C. D., 569
Štimac, D., 543, 545
Stitt, F. W., 107
Stock, M. J., 47
Stocks, T., 312
Stolley, M. R., 157, 447, 580
Stone, M. A., 159
St-Onge, M. P., 125, 126
Stormi, T., 570
Story, M., 598, 610, 663
Story, M. T., 80
Stothard, E. R., 129
Stoving, R., 561
Straif, K., 12
Strath, S. J., 107
Strauss, J., 79
Strauss, R. S., 579, 582, 595
Strazzullo, P., 8
Striegel-Moore, R. H., 174, 175, 178, 442, 554
Stronegger, W. J., 140
Strosahl, K. D., 514

Strutz, E. M., 598
Stuart, J. A., 54
Stuart, R. B., 336
Stubbs, R. J., 99
Stuckey, H. L., 417
Stukel, T. A., 186
Stumbo, P. J., 259
Stunkard, A., 566
Stunkard, A. J., 16, 65, 139, 140, 144, 154, 157, 171, 174, 175, 176, 177, 215, 253, 260, 294, 459, 553, 594, 595, 600, 601
Sturm, R., 159
Sturmey, P., 337
Stutzmann, F., 68
Su, Y. P., 233
Subak, L. L., 212
Subramanian, S., 139
Suchard, M. A., 340
Suchindran, C. M., 255
Suglia, S. F., 125
Suh, Y., 160, 662
Suhrcke, M., 139
Sullivan, P., 579
Sullivan, P. F., 157, 170
Sullivan, S., 541
Sumithran, P., 81, 243, 294, 303, 432
Summerbell, C., 609, 612
Sun, K. X., 648
Sun, Q., 150, 156
Sundal, D., 615
Sundborn, G., 140
Sunstein, C. R., 523, 667
Suominen, E., 570
Suorsa, K. I., 616
Surakka, L., 474
Surkan, P. J., 97
Susman, E. J., 630
Susulic, V. S., 54
Sutin, A. R., 161, 433, 434
Sutton, E. F., 47
Sutton, S. M., 343
Svenner, A., 652
Svensson, P., 264, 271
Svetkey, L. P., 338, 342, 405, 406, 407, 444, 445, 469, 475
Swain, R. M., 441
Swain J. F., 316
Swanson, E., 570
Swartz, A. M., 107
Swartz, D. E., 379
Sweat, V., 629
Swift, D. L., 261, 323, 329
Swinburn, B., 137, 141, 142
Swinburn, B. A., 48, 258
Syngal, S., 188
Sywulak, L. A., 569
Szabo, E., 654

T

Taal, H. R., 597
Tabak, R., 344
Tabak, R. G., 493
Taber, D. R., 665
Tache, Y., 26
Taegtmeyer, H., 382
Tagliabue, A., 75
Taheri, S., 129, 131
Tai, C. M., 539
Takahashi, M., 125
Takala, I., 343
Takemura, N., 82
Talebpour, A., 368
Talebpour, M., 368, 387
Talley, N. J., 627
Talwalkar, A., 417
Tam, C. S., 55
Tamayo, A., 140
Tan, E., 16, 431
Tanaka, K., 125
Tandon, R., 177, 178
Tang, M. T., 486
Tanghe, A., 625
Tanofsky-Kraff, M., 172, 625
Tantleff-Dunn, S., 566
Tapia Granados, J. A., 141, 142
Tapper, K., 518, 519
Tasali, E., 125, 132
Tataranni, P. A., 46, 47, 50, 54
Tate, D. F., 99, 291, 292, 324, 326, 328, 344, 396, 399, 401, 407, 466, 468, 469, 472, 473, 476, 511, 630
Tatemoto, K., 28
Tatone-Tokuda, F., 125
Tavendale, R., 65, 596
Taveras, E. M., 513, 596
Taverno Ross, S. E., 342–343
Taylor, C. B., 580
Taylor, H. L., 52, 208
Taylor, M. J., 213, 567
Taylor, P. D., 595
Taylor, R., 513
Te Riele, W., 570
Teachman, B. A., 584
Tehrani, A. B., 75, 84
Teismann, H., 131
Teixeira, P. J., 214, 344
Telch, C. F., 556
Telöken, C., 212
Temple, J. L., 625, 629, 630
ten Hoor, F., 114
Teng, N. I. M. F., 211, 216
ter Bogt, N. C., 455, 456
Teras, L. R., 11
Terra, J., 158
Terracciano, A., 161, 433

Terrace, H. S., 627
Tershakovec, A. M., 623, 636
Teubner, B. J., 28, 30
Teufel-Shone, N. I., 448
Tewksbury, C. M., 214, 302, 538, 565
Thaler, J. P., 243
Thaler, R. H., 523, 667
Than, N. N., 15
Thangaratinam, S., 251
Thanos, P. K., 177
Thearle, M. S., 151
Theriault, G., 52
Thewissen, R., 516, 517
Thier, S. L., 260
Thivel, D., 130
Thodiyil, P. A., 378
Tholin, S., 174, 175, 176
Thomas, C. J., 577
Thomas, D., 449
Thomas, D. M., 25, 41
Thomas, J. G., 96, 269, 294, 469, 472
Thomas, L. N., 599
Thomas, P., 613
Thompson, A. M., 225, 228
Thompson, C. C., 541, 543, 544
Thompson, D., 175
Thompson, D. L., 114, 141
Thompson, J. K., 160, 566, 579
Thompson, K. J., 566, 567
Thompson, P. D., 246, 524
Thompson, T. J., 185, 194
Thompson, W. G., 417
Thompson-Brenner, H., 531
Thomson, C. A., 131
Thorndike, A. N., 143
Thorp, A. A., 111, 143, 261
Thorson, C., 525
Thorsteinsson, E. B., 584
Thorwart, M. L., 98
Thun, M., 194
Tian, J., 257
Tibbs, T. L., 624
Tiggemann, M., 211
Tiggemann, T., 584
Timpson, N. J., 65, 597
Titze, S., 140
Tobias, D. K., 314
Toledo, K., 227
Tolson, K. P., 70
Tomasi, D., 177
Tomiyama, A. J., 159, 161, 210, 581
Tomuta, N., 212
Tong, L., 56
Tonn, P., 131
Toor, P., 131
Torgerson, J. S., 195, 196, 301, 350, 353

Toshinai, K., 29
Tottey, W., 79
Toubro, S., 315
Traversy, G., 265
Treadwill, T., 161
Tremblay, A., 49, 52, 65, 70, 131, 216, 255, 316
Trief, P. M., 263, 267, 457
Tripicchio, G. L., 599
Trogdon, J. G., 18, 186, 622
Troiano, R., 108
Trost, S. G., 615, 616
Troxel, A. B., 527
Truby, H., 118, 482
Tsai, A. G., 159, 250, 267, 293, 298, 299, 311, 336, 343, 432, 453, 454, 455, 456, 457, 458, 511
Tschop, M., 28, 29
Tschop, M. H., 32
Tse, C. K., 262
Tse-Hwei, J. C., 152
Tsenkova, V. K., 161
Tsourosm, A. D., 141
Tsuda, S., 430
Tsujimoto, G., 85
Tuck, M. L., 9
Tudor-Locke, C., 108, 327
Tuna, M., 186
Tunceli, K., 159
Tuomilehto, J., 188, 189, 359
Turek, V. F., 31
Turk, M. W., 340
Turnbaugh, P. J., 76, 78, 80, 82, 83
Turner, A. J., 28
Turner, L., 665
Turner, M., 417
Turner, R. C., 640
Turner-McGrievy, G., 475
Turner-McGrievy, G. M., 340, 469, 476
Tussing-Humphreys, L. M., 447
Tverdal, A., 6
Tversky, A., 523
Twentyman, C. T., 403
Twisk, J. W., 4, 605
Tynelius, P., 64
Tyson, M., 11

U

Uebelacker, L. A., 330
Ujcic-Voortman, J. K., 140
Ul-Haq, Z., 16
Unger, R. H., 31
Unick, J. L., 267, 324, 343, 448
Unikel Santoncini, C., 580
Ursell, L. K., 75

Utriainen, P., 631
Utzinger, L. M., 213
Uusitupa, M., 190, 191, 192

V

Vadiveloo, M., 99
Vahidi, H., 368
Vaisse, C., 596
Vakil, R. M., 486, 487
Valencia, M. E., 440
Valezi, A. C., 382
Valle, C. G., 291, 466
Valoski, A., 623, 625, 632
Valrie, C. R., 131
van Baak, M. A., 54
van Binsbergen, J. J., 417
Van Cauter, E., 125, 216
van den Berg, P., 152, 568
van den Berg, P. A., 577
van der Beek, E. S., 570, 571
van der Klaauw, A. A., 66, 286
van der Knaap, H. C., 298, 501
van der Lely, A. J., 29
van der Molen, A. B., 571
Van der Oord, S., 629
van der Schouw, Y. T., 118, 236
van Dillen, S. M. E., 417
van Doorslaer, E., 139
Van Dorsten, B., 227
Van Eijs, Y., 625
van Erp-Baart, M. A., 114
van Gemert, W., 224, 226, 229
van Jaarsveld, C. H., 596
van Lenthe, F., 143
van Marken Lichtenbelt, W. D., 54, 55, 82
Van Mechelen, W., 605
van Mechelen, W., 4, 111, 114
van Mierlo, C. A., 298, 501
Van Nieuwenhove, Y., 649
van Oostveen, Y., 139
van Ramshorst, B., 570, 571
van Reedt Dortland, A., 151
van Sluijs, E. M., 50
van Strien, T., 150
van Tubergen, F., 140
van Veen, R., 151
van Vliet-Ostaptchouk, J. V., 118
van Zutven, K., 155
Vander Veur, S. S., 598
Vander Wal, J. S., 176, 177
Vandevijvere, S., 663
Vanhoutvin, S. A., 85
VanItallie, T. B., 659
Vanninen, E., 631
Van-Wormer, J., 470
Vanwormer, J. J., 339

Vargas Souto, C. A., 212
Vartanian, L. R., 94, 161, 578
Vasselli, J. R., 29
Vatten, L. J., 13
Vázquez- Sequeiros, E., 539
Vedul-Kjelsas, E., 552
Veierød, M. B., 314
Veith, R. C., 50
Velluzzi, F., 157
Venditti, E. M., 326
Venn, A., 257
Ventelou, B., 159
Venti, C. A., 175
Ventura, A. K., 596
Verbeken, S., 629
Vercellone, A. C., 177
Verhoef, S., 216, 217
Verhoeff, A. P., 140
Verlaan, T., 542
Vermeer, W. M., 100, 598
Vernonroberts, J., 571
Verweij, L. M., 114
Vest, A. R., 382
Vetter, C., 129
Vetter, M. L., 32, 159
Vgontzas, A. N., 130, 131
Victorzon, M., 570
Videhult, P., 652
Viegener, B. J., 404
Vieira, A. R., 14
Villareal, D. T., 224, 226, 228, 230, 231, 232, 397, 401, 461
Vinai, P., 157, 176
Vincent, H. K., 159
Vincent, K. R., 159
Viner, R. M., 640
Vingeliene, S., 14
Vinknes, K. J., 314
Vinter, C. A., 618
Virtanen, K. A., 54, 55
Visscher, T. L. S., 233
Visser, M., 236
Vito, D., 630
Vitousek, K. M., 172, 555
Vogelzangs, N., 157
Vogt, R. A., 269, 441, 460, 568
Vohl, M., 256
Vojta, D., 615
Voks, S., 171
Volger, S., 284, 286, 293, 456, 586
Volkow, N., 177
Volkow, N. D., 177
Volpp, K. G., 341, 522, 525, 526, 528
Volpp, K. G. M., 292, 522
von Kries, R., 596
von Ranson, K. M., 178
Vora, J., 27
Voss-Andreae, A., 144

Vosselman, M. J., 82
Vreugdenburg, L., 211

W

Wabitsch, M., 67
Wada, R., 666
Wadden, S. Z., 259, 283
Wadden, T. A., 6, 16, 32, 153, 154, 155, 157, 161, 171, 213, 214, 215, 230, 249, 253, 254, 256, 259, 260, 263, 264, 265, 267, 269, 270, 271, 283, 284, 286, 287, 288, 289, 291, 292, 293, 294, 295, 298, 299, 300, 301, 304, 311, 324, 336, 337, 338, 339, 340, 343, 344, 355, 357, 367, 393, 441, 444, 453, 454, 456, 457, 458, 459, 460, 461, 466, 482, 511, 561, 567, 568, 569, 577, 578, 581, 587, 605, 623, 636, 640
Wagner, B., 265
Wagner, D. D., 171
Wagner, J. A., 155
Wagner, M. K., 630
Wagstaff, A., 139
Wahid, A., 261
Wainstein, J., 126
Wakefield, D. B., 662
Wakil, S. J., 56
Waldecker, M., 85
Walder, K., 55
Wall, D. E., 93
Wall, M., 152
Wall, M. M., 80, 124
Waller, J., 159, 579
Walley, A. J., 255
Walpole, B., 513
Walsh, B. T., 260
Walter, J., 77
Walters, W. A., 76, 78, 79, 82
Wandel, M., 143
Wang, G. J., 177, 461
Wang, J., 155, 339, 500
Wang, L., 26, 112, 322
Wang, N. Y., 291
Wang, S., 14, 15
Wang, S. M., 610, 612
Wang, S. S., 578
Wang, Y., 11, 70, 185, 607, 609, 610, 612, 616, 618
Wang, Y. C., 18, 19, 432
Wang, Z., 46
Wannamethee, S. G., 195
Wanner, M., 115
Wansink, B., 259, 260, 336
Warburton, D., 106

Ward, C. H., 157, 223
Ward, D. S., 344, 473
Ward, K. J., 640
Wardle, J., 64, 65, 99, 100, 139, 151, 152, 159, 161, 579, 580, 584, 596, 599, 600, 625
Ware, J. E., 158, 217, 223, 224
Ware, J. E., Jr., 262
Wareham, N. J., 50, 143
Warkentin, L. M., 158, 208, 263
Warner, K. E., 666, 667
Warren, C. S., 157
Warren, R., 645
Warrington, N. M., 597
Warschkow, R., 653
Washburn, R. A., 323, 324
Watanabe, M., 125
Waterland, R. A., 595
Waterlander, W. E., 141, 142
Watt, P., 65, 596
Watts, A. W., 152
Waugh, N., 361
Webb, R. M., 442
Webb, V., 336, 393
Webb, V. L., 32, 288, 291, 292, 294, 605
Webber, E. M., 579, 581
Webber, K. H., 511
Webber, L. S., 617
Weber, M. B., 189, 191
Wedel, H., 286
Wee, C., 271
Wee, C. C., 186
Wei, J. Y., 26
Wei, W., 552
Weineland, S., 518, 519
Weinsier, R. L., 441
Weinstein, L. S., 69
Weinstock, R. S., 263, 457, 461
Weintraub, W. H., 645
Weiss, A., 124
Weiss, J. J., 213
Welbourn, R., 571
Welch, C. C., 30
Welk, G. J., 108
Wellman, R. D., 330
Welsh, E. M., 339, 470
Wen, F., 607
Wen, L. M., 115
Wentworth, J. M., 197, 198, 381
Wescott, R. F., 664
West, C. P., 454
West, D. S., 290, 293, 330, 336, 343, 404, 405, 444, 445, 448, 492, 493, 496, 499, 500, 502, 503, 510, 511, 512
Westerterp, K., 217
Westerterp, K. R., 45, 48, 50, 108, 109, 114

Westerterp-Plantenga, M., 217
West-Smith, L., 270
Wetter, T. C., 130
Weyer, C., 52, 54, 81, 441
Wheeler, E., 65, 68
Whelton, P. K., 192, 343, 443, 444
Whisenhunt, B. L., 260
Whitaker, K. L., 151
Whitaker, L. A., 567, 568
Whitaker, R. C., 255, 256, 594, 595
White, A., 79
White, B., 640
White, M. A., 161, 171, 260, 511, 553, 555, 556, 557, 558, 560, 561
Whitehead, M., 137
Whitehead, R. G., 596
Whitehouse, M. J., 357
Whiting, D. M., 544
Whitlock, E. P., 289, 350, 454, 623, 624
Whiton, K., 123
Whittemore, R., 455
Whitt-Glover, M. C., 442, 443
Widom, C. S., 265
Wieland, L. S., 467
Wiig, K., 141
Wijmenga, C., 118
Wilding, J. P., 32, 349
Wilfley, D. E., 172, 178, 437, 553, 554, 568, 579, 605, 622, 623, 624, 625, 628, 632, 641
Wilkinson, J. M., 582
Wilkinson, M. L., 417
Wilks, D. C., 600
Willesen, M. G., 29
Willett, W., 4
Willett, W. C., 3, 9, 10, 11, 111, 313, 317, 330, 598, 605
Williams, D. H., 417
Williams, D. K., 502
Williams, D. L., 27
Williams, G. R., 158, 159, 569
Williams, G. T., 217
Williams, J. B. W., 263
Williams, L. B., 495, 499
Williams, L. K., 159
Williams, N. N., 284, 302, 531, 538
Williams, P. T., 118
Williams, R. A., 97
Williams, R. G., 580
Williams, S. B., 623
Williamson, D. A., 171, 208, 209, 213, 223, 224, 226, 227, 228, 235, 260, 498
Williamson, D. F., 185, 186, 187, 191, 194, 195, 209, 224, 293, 322, 486, 504

Williams-Russo, P., 522
Wilmore, J. H., 111
Wilson, C., 339
Wilson, C. J., 210
Wilson, D. K., 616
Wilson, F. L., 175
Wilson, G. T., 171, 172, 178, 236, 511, 553, 554, 555, 556, 557, 558, 560
Wilson, J. R., 81
Wilson, K. G., 514
Wilson, R., 114, 616
Wilson, S. R., 457
Wilson, T. D., 630
Winett, R. A., 399, 472
Wing, A. L., 261
Wing, R., 261, 630
Wing, R. R., 81, 95, 99, 191, 193, 249, 250, 262, 268, 269, 287, 294, 323, 324, 325, 326, 327, 338, 339, 340, 341, 342, 343, 399, 401, 443, 472, 481, 485, 501, 516, 517, 524, 525, 623, 632
Wing, S., 144
Wingo, B., 444, 445
Winkens, L. H., 150
Winston, G., 442
Winters, C., 324, 325, 327, 340
Wintfeld, N., 432
Wirth, M. D., 131
Wishart, J., 83
Wisniewski, L., 628
Withers, R. T., 115
Withrow, D., 3
Witteman, J. C., 9
Wittert, G. A., 212
Wojtanowski, A. C., 336, 605
Wolever, R. Q., 330
Wolf, A. M., 659
Wolfe, B., 650
Wolfe, B. M., 653
Wolfson, J. A., 100, 598
Wolk, A., 13
Womble, L. G., 171
Won, G. Y., 448
Wonderlich, J., 271
Wonderlich, S. A., 554
Wong, W. W., 580
Wood, A. J. J., 81
Wood, C. L., 318
Woods, G., 461
Woods, M., 258
Woods, S. C., 26, 30, 31, 67
Woodward, E. R., 367
Woodward, M., 188
Wookey, P. J., 31
Woolery, A., 330
Worley, A., 610

Worthley, S., 212
Wray, L. A., 232
Wright, J. A., 255, 594
Wright, K. P., 129
Wright, R. U., 430
Wroblewski, K., 132
Wrotniak, B. H., 628
Wu, G. D., 77, 78, 79
Wu, Y., 124, 616
Wyatt, H. R., 258, 330
Wygand, J. W., 330
Wylie-Rosett, J., 212

X

Xia, J., 46, 54
Xian, Y., 417
Xiao, L., 156, 157, 457
Xiao, Q., 124
Xu, H., 115
Xu, J., 7, 8, 9, 78, 79
Xu, Q., 156
Xu, S., 27, 260
Xu, X., 140
Xu, Z., 76, 78

Y

Yaffe, K., 233
Yamamoto, H., 25
Yamashita, H., 85
Yancey, A. K., 208, 224, 442
Yancey, D. Z., 403
Yancy, W. S., Jr., 226
Yanek, L. R., 495, 499, 502
Yang, C. C., 160
Yang, J., 28, 417, 431, 627
Yang, X., 55
Yang, Y. T., 429
Yang, Z., 432
Yank, V., 457
Yankura, D. J., 217, 224, 226
Yanovski, J. A., 301, 546, 570
Yanovski, S. Z., 260, 301, 546
Yao, S., 543
Yarnall, K. S., 418
Yatsunenko, T., 78, 79, 80, 81
Yavuz, Y., 536
Yeh, H. C., 291
Yeh, M. C., 610
Yenumula, P. R., 379
Yeo, G. S., 66, 70
Yiaslas, T., 476
Yin, B., 45
Yong, L. C., 9
Yoon, J., 140
Yoon, S. S., 8

Yoong, S. L., 132
York, D. A., 50
Yoshida, A., 82
Youn, B. B., 358
Young, J. B., 50, 382
Young, K. M., 623, 624, 627
Young, L. R., 93
Young, R. C., 25
Younossi, Z. M., 15
Yu, J. H., 129
Yu, Y. H., 56
Yu-Poth, S., 313, 314

Z

Zachariae, R., 561
Zachrisson, H. D., 552
Zachwieja, J. J., 51
Zaffanello, M., 600
Zalesin, K. C., 8
Zandberg, L. J., 554
Zee, P. C., 127, 130
Zeelenberg, M., 523
Zeisel, S. H., 418
Zeitler, P., 644
Zeller, M. H., 653
Zellweger, H., 645
Zelter, L., 330
Zemel, B. S., 595
Zenk, S. N., 140
Zerrweck, C., 539
Zhai, L., 124
Zhang, C. Y., 54
Zhang, D., 124
Zhang, N., 432
Zhang, P., 229
Zhang, P. L., 51
Zhang, Q., 233
Zhang, S., 417, 431
Zhang, X., 124, 188
Zhang, Y., 53, 56, 543
Zhao, G., 156, 157, 314
Zhao, P., 144
Zhao, Z., 140
Zheng, Y., 339
Zhou, H., 502
Zhu, J., 65
Zhu, S., 158
Ziauddeen, H., 178
Zickhur, K., 473
Ziegler, O., 653
Zimmerman, M., 156
Zimmet, P., 379
Zinkel, S. R., 601
Zinman, B., 284
Zinn, A. R., 70
Zitman, F. G., 151
Zohoori, M., 233
Zoico, E., 236
Zonderman, A. B., 433
Zou, Z., 124
Zunker, C., 212
Zurlo, F., 43, 46, 48, 50, 51
Zvenyach, T., 418
Zwahlen, M., 11

Subject Index

Note. *f* or *t* following a page number indicates a figure or a table.

Abdominoplasty, 569–570
Acceptance, 514–515, 587
Acceptance and commitment therapy (ACT), 343, 508, 513–519, 517t–518t
Acromegaly, 246, 247t
Activity, physical. *See* Physical activity
Activity thermogenesis, 44f, 46, 47–48. *See also* Physical activity
Addiction model, 177–179
Adherence to treatment, 301, 329, 653–654
Adipex, 351t
Adipose-derived hormones, 32
Adiposity
 carbohydrate-insulin model and, 52
 diabetes and, 10–11
 energy balance and, 43
 gut microbiome and, 82, 86
 medical evaluation and, 243
 overview, 4
 stress and, 151–152
 weight stigmatization and, 161
Adjustable gastric banding (AGB), 368f, 376t, 647–654. *See also* Surgical interventions
Adolescents. *See also* Bariatric surgery for adolescents; Prevention of obesity in youth
 advertising targeting youth and, 662–663, 664f, 667
 bariatric surgery and, 644, 645–647, 646f, 647t
 diabetes and, 651
 motivational interviewing (MI) and, 513
 prevention of obesity in youth and, 616–618, 617f
 self-esteem and, 579
 sleep timing and, 129–130
Adrenocorticotropic hormone (ACTH), 66, 67–68
Adults, treatment of obesity in. *See* Treatment of obesity in adults
Advertising targeting youth, 662–663, 664f, 667
Affordable Care Act (ACA). *See also* Insurance coverage
 commercial-based interventions and, 488
 overview, 19, 425, 428–429, 453–454
 private insurance market and, 430–431
 treatment of obesity in adults and, 304
Affordable Care Organizations (ACOs), 431
African American populations, 437, 439t, 443–445, 446–447. *See also* Minority populations
Age factors
 behavioral assessment and, 255
 body dissatisfaction and, 152
 influence of fitness and physical activity and, 233, 235
 intensive lifestyle interventions (ILIs) and, 228–229, 230–231, 231f, 232–236, 234f
 self-esteem and, 579
Alcohol use and abuse, 43, 271. *See also* Substance abuse/dependency
Alternate-day fasting diets, 311–312. *See also* Dietary treatment; Fasting
American Board of Obesity Medicine (ABOM), 420–422, 421t, 422f, 454
Amylin, 31, 85
Anxiety
 behavioral assessment and, 263
 obesity and, 155, 286
 overview, 150–151, 153–154
 treatment and, 157, 162, 286
 weight stigmatization and, 160
Appetite
 behavioral assessment and, 260
 effects of weight loss on, 215–216, 215f, 216f
 physical activity and, 118–119
 sleep and, 125
 suppression of, 118–119
 weight regain and, 432–433

699

Apps, 45–46, 292
Asian American population, 439t, 445. *See also* Minority populations
Aspiration therapy, 531–532, 533f, 543. *See also* Nonsurgical interventional therapies; Weight loss devices
AspireAssist system, 531, 534f–535f, 550t–551t
Assessment. *See also* Behavioral assessment; Medical evaluations
  adolescents and surgical interventions and, 648–649
  body image and, 567
  depression and, 150
  measuring energy expenditure, 43–46, 44f
  obesity medicine field of health care and, 413–416, 414t
  pharmacotherapies and, 349–350
  physical activity and, 107–109, 108t, 119
  surgical interventions and, 372, 373t
  treatment of obesity in adults and, 284, 285f
  treatment-seeking individuals and, 157
Asthma risks, 3, 15, 383–384, 384f
Atkins type of diet, 315–316, 458
Attractiveness, 565–566, 578. *See also* Body image
Autonomy, 508, 508f
Awareness, public, 660–662, 661f

B

Back pain, 383–384
Bacteroidetes, 82, 83–84, 85
Bardet-Biedl syndrome (BBS), 69–70
Bariatric surgery. *See also* Bariatric surgery for adolescents; Gastric bypass surgery; Obesity medicine field of health care; Surgical interventions
  behavioral assessment and, 270–272
  body contouring following, 387
  choice of, 386–387
  classification of, 367–370, 369t
  cognitive functioning and, 211–212
  compared to physical activity, 325
  complications, 375, 375t
  costs of obesity and, 431
  eating disorders and, 213, 561
  history of, 644–645
  indications and contraindications of, 371, 371t
  leptin and, 53–54
  long-term impact of weight loss and, 197–202, 198t–201t
  mental health and, 157
  NAFLD and NASH and, 15
  obesity medicine field of health care and, 415, 419
  outcomes of, 379–384, 380t, 384f
  overview, 367, 368f, 386, 387–388, 644
  physical activity and, 331
  prevention of comorbidities with, 384–386
  surgery emergencies, 375–379, 376t, 377t
  treatment of obesity in adults and, 285f
  when BMI is equal to or more than 40 kg/m2, 302–303
Bariatric surgery for adolescents. *See also* Adolescents; Bariatric surgery; Surgical interventions
  history of, 644–645
  multidisciplinary team (MDT) and, 647
  outcomes of, 650–652, 650t, 651f
  overview, 645–647, 646f, 647t, 653–654
  patient selection and, 645–646, 646f
  perioperative management, 649
  postoperative follow-up and, 649–650
  preoperative workup, 648–649
  risks and concerns, 652–653
  surgical procedures, 647–648
Barriers to obesity care, 417–419. *See also* Treatment
Basal (resting) metabolic rate (BMR). *See also* Resting metabolic rate (RMR)
  energy balance equations and, 41–42
  energy expenditure and, 57
  measuring energy expenditure, 44f
  overview, 6, 41, 46–47
  weight gain and, 48–52
Beck Depression Inventory–II (BDI-II), 209–210, 223, 253–254, 272
Behavioral assessment. *See also* Assessment
  bariatric surgery patients and, 270–272
  biological factors and, 255–258, 256f, 257f
  environmental factors and, 258–262
  interview and, 254–255
  overview, 253–254, 272
  psychosocial factors, 262–266, 264t, 265f
  sample letters summarizing, 278–280
  surgical interventions and, 459
  temporal factors, 266–268
  treatment and, 268–270
Behavioral economics, 522–529, 523t, 524t, 526f, 527f
Behavioral factors, 53, 441–442, 441f
Behavioral mechanisms, 343–344
Behavioral treatment. *See also* Behavioral weight loss (BWL) treatment; Family-based behavioral weight loss treatment (FBT); Lifestyle interventions; Treatment
  behavior chain, 337, 337f
  behavioral modification, 626t
  behavioral skills and, 339–341
  childhood obesity and, 629–631
  extended-care maintenance programs and, 403–407, 405t
  family-based behavioral weight loss treatment (FBT) and, 627
  format of, 338, 338t
  future directions, 343–344
  initial phase of, 394–403, 395t–397t
  long-term efficacy of, 341–343, 342t
  overview, 289t, 336, 344–345, 393–394, 407, 466
  pharmacotherapies and, 350f, 362–363
  primary care and, 454, 461
  theoretical foundation, 336–338, 337f
Behavioral weight loss (BWL) treatment. *See also* Behavioral treatment
  acceptance and commitment therapy (ACT), 513–519, 517t–518t
  binge-eating disorder (BED) and, 172–173, 173t, 553, 555

Subject Index

eating disorders, 552, 557
motivational interviewing (MI), 508–513, 509f, 510t, 513t
overview, 508, 519
Behaviors, eating, 161, 162, 162f, 177–178, 599–600
Beige (Brite) adipose tissue, 55–56, 82
BELVIQ, 351t, 352f, 353–354
BEST Treatment, 253–254, 255, 270
Beverages, 317–318, 319, 664. *See also* Sugar consumption
Bias, 16, 17t, 487, 581
Biliopancreatic diversion (BPD), 368, 368f, 369, 369t, 370–371, 376t, 387. *See also* Surgical interventions
Biliopancreatic diversion (BPD) with duodenal switch, 368f, 369, 369t, 370–371, 376t, 387. *See also* Surgical interventions
Binge eating. *See also* Binge-eating disorder (BED); Overeating
 addiction model of eating disorders, 178
 effects of weight loss on symptoms associated with eating disorders and, 213, 214f
 family-based behavioral weight loss treatment (FBT) and, 625
 overview, 153, 154, 170, 170t
 self-esteem and, 579
 surgical interventions and, 561
 treatment and, 162
 weight stigmatization and, 162f
Binge-eating disorder (BED). *See also* Binge eating; Eating disorders
 bariatric surgery patients and, 271
 behavioral assessment and, 260–261
 behavioral weight loss (BWL) programs for, 555
 change and, 557, 558t–559t, 560f
 effects of weight loss on symptoms associated with, 213, 214f
 health professionals and, 585
 mental health and, 157–158
 overview, 153, 169–170, 170t, 178–179, 552
 pharmacotherapies and, 555–557

psychological treatments for, 553–555
self-esteem and, 579
surgical interventions and, 561
treatment and, 178
treatment-seeking individuals and, 157
weight stigmatization and, 161
Biological factors. *See also* Genetic factors
 addiction model of eating disorders, 177–178
 appetite and satiety and, 118
 bariatric surgery patients and, 270
 behavioral assessment and, 255–258, 256f, 257f
 binge-eating disorder (BED) and, 171
 minority populations and, 440–441, 441f
 overview, 64–65
 physical activity and, 105–106
 primary care and, 461–462
 sample letters summarizing presurgical assessments, 278–280
Bleeding, 376, 378
Blood glucose, 30–31, 86, 110–111, 110f, 249. *See also* Glucose tolerance
Blood pressure, 8–9, 86, 161, 188, 247. *See also* Hypertension
Body Areas Satisfaction Scale, 214–215
Body contouring, 387, 569–571, 654
Body dissatisfaction. *See also* Body image; Self-esteem
 etiology of, 567–569
 obesity and, 155
 overview, 152–154, 572
 treatment and, 162
Body fat percentages, 249, 318
Body fat stores, 42–43
Body image. *See also* Body dissatisfaction; Self-esteem
 adolescents and surgical interventions and, 650, 651f
 assessment of, 567
 effects of weight loss on, 214–215
 family-based behavioral weight loss treatment (FBT) and, 628
 overview, 565–567, 572
 treatment goals and, 268
 variables that affect, 579–580
Body Image Quality of Life Inventory, 567

Body mass index (BMI)
 adolescents and surgical interventions and, 650, 651f
 barriers to obesity care, 418–419
 behavioral assessment and, 261, 262–263
 behavioral treatment and, 341
 binge-eating disorder (BED) and, 170–171
 biological factors and, 255
 body dissatisfaction and, 152
 brown adipose tissue (BAT) mass and, 55
 childhood obesity and, 601
 depression and, 149–150
 diabetes and, 10
 genetic factors and, 64, 64–65
 intensive lifestyle interventions (ILIs) and, 232–233, 234f
 medical evaluation and, 243–244, 244f, 247
 mortality and, 6, 7f
 night eating syndrome (NES) and, 175
 obesity medicine field of health care and, 415
 overview, 3, 4, 5f, 39f
 pharmacotherapies and, 349–350
 physical activity and, 322
 sedentary time and, 111
 self-esteem and, 577–578, 581
 sleep and, 124–125, 131
 sociocultural factors and, 139, 140
 sugar consumption and, 317–318
 surgical interventions and, 379–380, 388
 treatment of obesity in adults and, 284, 285f, 288
 weight stigmatization and, 160
Body Shape Questionnaire, 213, 567
Body weight, 6, 29, 93–94, 96–97, 96f
Brain-derived neurotrophic factor (BDNF) disruption, 70
Brain-to-gut mechanisms, 24–26. *See also* Gut hormones
Breastfeeding, 595–596
Brown adipose tissue (BAT) mass, 47, 54, 55–56, 82
Built environments, 142. *See also* Environmental factors
Bulimia nervosa. *See also* Eating disorders
 bariatric surgery patients and, 271
 interpersonal therapy (IPT) and, 554

Bulimia nervosa *(cont.)*
  prevalence of, 174–175
  treatment and, 178
  weight loss devices and, 302
Bupropion, 362. *See also*
  Naltrexone SR/bupropion SR
Bypass liners, 531–532, 532*t*,
  533*f*, 534*f*–535*f*, 542–543,
  542*f*. *See also* Nonsurgical
  interventional therapies;
  Weight loss devices

C

Caloric intake, 127–129, 128*f*,
  258–259, 402. *See also*
  Dietary intake; Food intake
Calorie absorption, 368
Calorie reduction
  behavioral treatment and, 339
  effects of on mood, 208–209
  effects of weight loss on appetite,
    cravings and preference and,
    215
  effects of weight loss on mood
    and, 210–211
  effects of weight loss on
    symptoms associated with
    eating disorders and, 213
  obesity medicine field of health
    care and, 415
Calorimetry, 43–44, 45
Cancer risks
  commercial-based interventions
    and, 486
  medical evaluation and, 247
  overview, 3, 11–13, 12*t*, 14*t*
  surgical interventions and, 197,
    385
Carbohydrate oxidization,
  109–110, 110*f*
Carbohydrate-insulin model,
  51–52
Carbohydrates
  dietary treatment and, 319
  energy balance and, 40–41,
    40*f*, 42
  glycemic qualities of, 316–317
  sleep and, 126
Cardiac functioning, 188, 372,
  373*t*, 374*t*
Cardiovascular disease (CVD)
  adolescents and surgical
    interventions and, 651–652
  lifestyle intervention and,
    191–193, 192*t*
  maintenance of weight loss and,
    294

medical evaluation and, 244
obesity medicine field of health
  care and, 416
overview, 3, 6
physical activity and, 261, 331*t*
surgical interventions and, 197,
  382, 384*f*
treatment of obesity in adults
  and, 284, 286, 287, 293–294
Weight Watchers and, 481
Center-based physical activity,
  326–327, 332. *See also*
  Physical activity
Central nervous system (CNS), 24,
  25–26, 30
Child care settings, 607–608
Child Food and Beverage
  Advertising Initiative
  (CFBAI), 662–663
Childhood obesity. *See also*
  Obesity; Prevention of obesity
  in youth
  adjuncts to behavioral
    interventions for, 629–631
  into adulthood, 593–594
  advertising targeting youth and,
    662–663, 664*f*, 667
  eating phenotypes and, 599–600
  energy expenditure and,
    600–601
  family-based behavioral weight
    loss treatment (FBT) and,
    623–629, 624*t*, 626*t*
  motivational interviewing (MI)
    and, 513
  obesogenic food environment
    and, 597–599, 598*f*
  overview, 129–130, 593, 601,
    608–616, 608*f*, 609*t*, 611*f*,
    614*f*, 615*f*, 622, 623
  pharmacotherapies and, 636–642
  prevalence of, 593–594
  prevention in preschool-age
    children, 606–608
  risk factors and, 594–597, 597*f*
  self-esteem and, 579
  treatment and, 631–632
  treatment of obesity in adults
    and, 623
Childhood Trauma Questionnaire
  (CTQ and CTQ-SF), 266
Choice. *See also* Preferences
  energy density and, 97–98
  food prices and, 142
  obesogenic environment
    management and, 100–101,
    101*f*
  portion size and, 94
  self-esteem and, 582

sleep and, 126
variety and, 99–100
Cholesterol, 249, 381–382, 489
Cocaine-amphetamine-related
  transcript (CART), 84
Cognitive dissonance, 508
Cognitive factors, 138*f*, 208,
  211–212, 218, 343–344
Cognitive restructuring, 341
Cognitive-behavioral therapy
  (CBT). *See also* Treatment
  addiction model of eating
    disorders, 178
  binge-eating disorder (BED) and,
    171–173, 173*t*, 553–554, 555
  body image dissatisfaction and,
    571–572
  eating disorders, 261, 552
  family-based behavioral weight
    loss treatment (FBT) and, 628
  maintenance of weight loss and,
    400, 407
  mood disorders and, 263
  night eating syndrome (NES)
    and, 177
  treatment goals and, 268
  treatment of obesity in adults
    and, 285*f*
Cold-induced thermogenesis (CIT),
  47, 55
Collaboration, 508, 508*f*
Commercial-based lifestyle
  interventions. *See also*
  Lifestyle interventions;
  individual programs
  cancer survivors and, 486
  comparisons among, 486
  insurance coverage for, 488
  overview, 480, 486–489, 487*t*
  primary care and, 458
  role of the clinician with, 488
  treatment of obesity in adults
    and, 292–293
Community-based lifestyle
  interventions. *See also*
  Lifestyle interventions;
  individual programs
  Diabetes Prevention Program
    (DPP) Lifestyle Balance
    intervention, 492–493
  family-based behavioral weight
    loss treatment (FBT) and, 629
  lifestyle intervention and,
    493–498, 494*t*–496*t*
  minority populations and, 448
  overview, 492, 505
  prevention of obesity in youth
    and, 613–616, 614*f*, 615*f*,
    618–619

program elements, 498–505, 499t
treatment of obesity in adults and, 292–293
Comorbidities
  adolescents and surgical interventions and, 645–646, 646f, 648–649, 650–652
  binge-eating disorder (BED) and, 170–171
  costs of obesity and, 432
  gut microbiome and, 86
  medical evaluation and, 243–244
  night eating syndrome (NES), 175–176
  overview, 453
  pharmacotherapies and, 349–350, 350f, 359–362, 359t, 361t
  primary care and, 461
  quality of life and, 158
  surgical interventions and, 303, 368, 371, 371t, 375, 380–384
  treatment of obesity in adults and, 284, 285f, 302
Consequences of obesity. *See also* Health status
  behavioral treatment and, 337
  economic costs, 16, 18–19, 18f
  overview, 6–16, 7f, 8f, 10f, 12t, 14f, 19
  social consequences, 16, 17t
Continuing medical education (CME), 419–422, 421t, 422f
Continuous positive airway pressure (CPAP) treatment, 130
Contraceptives, 248t. *See also* Pharmacotherapies
CONTRAVE, 351t, 352f, 357
Coronary artery disease (CAD), 8
Coronary heart disease (CHD), 7–8, 8f, 247
Cosmetic surgery, 387, 569–571
Costs of obesity. *See also* Health care costs; Insurance coverage
  future challenges regarding, 431–434
  historical perspective on, 426–427
  overview, 185–186, 425–426, 431
  personal responsibility and, 433–434
Counseling, 417, 454–457
Cravings, 177–178, 215–216, 215f, 216f

Creatinine alanine aminotransferase (ALT), 249
Crime, 138–139, 140
Cultural factors, 138, 140, 447–448
Cushing syndrome, 246, 247t

D

Decision making, 515, 582
Deep brain stimulation. *See* Electrical stimulation
Degenerative joint disease, 284, 383–384, 384f
Delay discounting (DD), 630–631
Depression
  bariatric surgery patients and, 271
  behavioral assessment and, 263–264, 264t, 265f
  effects of weight loss on mood and, 209–210
  obesity and, 154–155, 154t
  overview, 149–150, 153–154
  pharmacotherapies and, 361–362, 362t
  quality of life and, 158–159
  sleep and, 131
  surgical interventions and, 383–384, 384f
  treatment and, 157, 161–162, 285f, 286
  weight stigmatization and, 160
Deprivation, 138, 139
Desire, sexual, 212–213
Developmental factors, 594, 645. *See also* Adolescents; Age factors; Childhood obesity
Devices for weight loss. *See* Nonsurgical interventional therapies; Weight loss devices
Diabetes
  adolescents and surgical interventions and, 645, 648, 650–651, 654
  behavioral assessment and, 262–263
  cardiovascular disease mortality and, 191, 193
  commercial-based interventions and, 489
  costs of obesity and, 433
  gastric inhibitory polypeptide (GIP) and, 27
  health-related quality of life (HQOL) and, 208
  intensive lifestyle interventions (ILIs) and, 232

  leptin and, 32, 53
  lifestyle intervention and, 188–191, 189t
  medical evaluation and, 244, 246–247, 249
  overview, 9–11, 10f
  pharmacotherapies and, 301, 349–350, 359–361, 359t
  physical activity and, 261
  primary care and, 455–457
  quality of life and, 158–159
  sexual functioning and, 212
  surgical interventions and, 197, 303, 368, 369, 371, 371t, 380–381, 384–385, 384f, 388
  treatment and, 268, 284, 286
  Weight Watchers and, 481
Diabetes Prevention Program (DPP)
  behavioral treatment and, 341–342, 342t
  commercial- and community-based approaches to lifestyle interventions, 293
  extended-care maintenance programs and, 404
  minority populations and, 445–446, 446f, 448–449
  pharmacotherapies and, 360
  primary care and, 455–457
  treatment of obesity in adults and, 290–291
Diabetes Prevention Program (DPP) Lifestyle Balance intervention, 492–493, 497–505, 499t
Diabetes support and education (DSE)
  intensive lifestyle interventions (ILIs) and, 224, 227f, 230f
  maintenance of weight loss and, 294, 295, 295f
Diagnosis
  addiction model of eating disorders, 177
  binge-eating disorder (BED) and, 169–170
  current practice and provision of care and, 417
  eating disorders, 260–261, 552–553
  night eating syndrome (NES), 174–175, 174f
Diagnostic and Statistical Manual of Mental Disorders (DSM), 169–170
Diagnostic and Statistical Manual of Mental Disorders (DSM-5), 177, 260, 263, 264t, 552–553

Diagnostic and Statistical Manual of Mental Disorders (DSM-IV), 171, 176–177
Dialectical behavior therapy (DBT), 172–173, 173t, 552, 554–555. *See also* Treatment
Diet factors, 52, 83–84, 98, 210, 259, 578. *See also* Variety in diet
Dietary intake. *See also* Energy intake; Food intake
  assessment of, 39–40
  community-based lifestyle interventions and, 498
  energy density and, 95–98, 96f
  environmental factors and, 258–260
  glycemic qualities of carbohydrates and, 316–317
  gut microbiome and, 82
  overview, 6, 93
  reduction in, 309
  restriction of, 64, 186–188, 187f, 188, 323–324
  treatment of obesity in adults and, 298–299
  when BMI is less than 30 kg/m2, 289t
Dietary treatment. *See also* Treatment
  adolescents and surgical interventions and, 649
  behavioral treatment and, 341
  childhood obesity and, 629–630
  clinical outcomes, 310
  dietary energy deficit and, 309–310
  family-based behavioral weight loss treatment (FBT) and, 625, 626t
  fiber and whole grains and, 318
  limitations of trials on, 312–313
  macronutrient distributions and, 313–316, 314f, 315f
  maintenance of weight loss and, 318–319, 318f, 401, 402–403
  obesity medicine field of health care and, 415
  options for, 310–312, 311f
  overview, 309, 319
  personalized diets, 312
  pharmacotherapies and, 350f
  sugar consumption and, 317–318
Diet-induced thermogenesis (DIT), 47, 55
Direct calorimetry, 43–44, 45
Disability
  due to obesity, 159
  influence of fitness and physical activity and, 233, 235
  intensive lifestyle interventions (ILIs) and, 235–236
  lifestyle intervention and, 193–194
Disability-adjusted life years (DALYs), 3, 15–16, 19
Discrepancy, 509–510, 510t
Discrimination. *See also* Stigma
  costs of obesity and, 431–432
  overview, 16, 17t, 19, 161
  self-esteem and, 578
Disease model of obesity, 426–427, 433–434, 453–454
Dissatisfaction with body. *See* Body dissatisfaction
Doctors. *See* Health providers
Doubly labeled water (DLW) method, 44–45
Dual-energy X-ray absorptiometry (DXA), 112, 249
Duodenal mucosal resurfacing, 545. *See also* Nonsurgical interventional therapies
Duodenal–jejunal bypass (DJB), 369, 369f, 369t, 542–543, 542f. *See also* Nonsurgical interventional therapies; Surgical interventions
Dyslipidemia, 15, 349–350, 384f, 645–646

E

Eating behaviors, 161, 162, 162f, 177–178, 599–600
Eating Disorder Examination (EDE), 213, 567
Eating Disorder Examination Questionnaire (EDE-Q), 260
Eating disorders. *See also* Binge-eating disorder (BED); Night eating syndrome (NES)
  behavioral assessment and, 260–261
  effects of weight loss on symptoms associated with, 213, 214f
  future directions, 561
  mental health and, 157–158
  obesity and, 169, 552–553
  overview, 169, 178–179, 552
  pharmacotherapies and, 555–557
  surgical interventions and, 561
  weight loss devices and, 302
Eating Inventory (EI), 215
Eating phenotypes, 599–600
Ecological models, 80–81, 661, 661f
Economic environment factors, 441f, 443t
Economic factors, 16, 18–19, 18f, 137, 140–142. *See also* Costs of obesity; Health care costs
Edmonton Obesity Staging System, 245, 245t
Education, 139, 508f
Educational settings
  improving the school environment, 663–665
  prevention of obesity in youth and, 607–608, 609–613, 609t, 611f
  school meals, 665
  weight bias and, 17t
Electrical stimulation, 531–532, 532t, 533f. *See also* Nonsurgical interventional therapies; Weight loss devices
Email-delivered lifestyle interventions, 471–473. *See also* Internet-delivered lifestyle interventions; Remotely delivered lifestyle interventions
Empathy, 508–510, 510t
Employer wellness programs, 430–431
Employment status, 3, 17t, 19, 159, 431–432
Energy balance. *See also* Energy expenditure; Energy intake; Energy stores
  adult gut microbiota and, 81–83
  appetite and satiety and, 118
  behavior related to, 138f
  dynamic energy balance equation, 41–42
  family-based behavioral weight loss treatment (FBT) and, 625
  glucagon-like peptide-1 (GLP-1) and, 26–27
  gut microbiome and, 76–77
  insulin and, 30
  overview, 24, 38–40, 39f, 40f, 57
  peptide YY (PYY) and, 28
  physical activity and, 113–114, 116–118
  short-chain fatty acids (SCFAs) and, 85
  sleep and, 125–129, 126f, 127f, 128f, 131
  static energy balance equation, 41
  substrate balance, 42–43
  weight maintenance and, 40–41
Energy density, 95–98, 96f, 101–102

Energy expenditure. *See also*
    Energy balance; Physical
    activity
  childhood obesity and, 600–601
  energy balance equations and,
    40–42
  family-based behavioral weight
    loss treatment (FBT) and,
    625, 626t
  maintenance of weight loss and,
    56–57, 57f, 401–402
  measuring, 43–46, 44f
  metabolic adaptation and, 52
  molecular mechanisms of,
    53–57, 57f
  overview, 39f, 40f, 57–58, 105,
    119
  preventing weight gain and,
    109–111, 110f
  transportation modes and,
    114–119
  treatment and, 53–57, 57f
  weight gain and, 48–52
  weight loss and, 316
  yoga and, 329
Energy harvest, 83–84
Energy intake. *See also* Dietary
    intake; Energy balance
  childhood obesity and, 599–600
  dietary energy deficit and, 310
  dietary treatment and, 309
  energy balance equations and,
    40–42
  energy density and, 95–98, 96f
  family-based behavioral weight
    loss treatment (FBT) and,
    625, 626t
  overview, 38–40, 39f, 40f, 93
  portion size and, 93–95
  sleep and, 126–129, 127f, 128f
  variety and, 99
Energy stores, 25–26, 40–42, 40f.
    See also Energy balance
Environmental factors. *See also*
    Obesogenic environment
  bariatric surgery patients and,
    270–271
  behavioral assessment and,
    258–262
  behavioral treatment and, 340
  childhood obesity and, 597–599,
    598f
  economic costs, 140–142
  energy density and, 98
  family-based behavioral weight
    loss treatment (FBT) and, 626t
  genetic factors and, 65
  health professionals and, 587
  minority populations and, 441f,
    442, 443t

overview, 137–138, 138f,
    144–145, 186, 262, 659–660
  pharmacotherapies and, 299
  physical environment factors,
    142–144
  public policy and, 660–666,
    661f, 664f
  sample letters summarizing pre-
    surgical assessments, 278–280
  weight gain and, 52
Environmental research framework
    for weight gain prevention
    (EnRG), 138, 138f
Epilepsy, 361–362, 362t
Episodic future thinking (EFT),
    630–631
Erectile functioning, 212–213
Ethnicity. *See also* Minority
    populations
  body dissatisfaction and, 152
  mental health and, 156
  as an obesity treatment variable,
    440–442, 441f, 443f
  overview, 437
  prevalence of obesity and, 4
  self-esteem and, 579–580
  sociocultural factors and, 138, 140
  treatment of obesity in adults
    and, 285f
Evocation, 508, 508f
Evolutionary processes, 38,
    105–106, 440–441
Excess postexercise oxygen
    consumption (EPOC),
    115–116, 119
Executive functioning, 211, 629
Exercise. *See* Physical activity
Experiences of Weight Bias
    questionnaire, 262
Extended-care maintenance
    programs, 403–407, 405t
Extrauterine environment, 80–81

F

Factorial method, 45
Faith-based programs, 446–447,
    501–502
Family factors, 246, 255–256, 580,
    595
Family involvement, 626t, 627–628
Family-based behavioral weight
    loss treatment (FBT). *See
    also* Behavioral treatment;
    Childhood obesity
  components of, 625–629, 626t
  food reinforcement and, 630
  overview, 623–624, 624t,
    631–632

Family-individual-school-based
    (FIS) intervention, 612–613
Fasting, 210–211, 351t. *See also*
    Dietary treatment
Fasting insulin and glucose, 249
Fat, 40–41, 40f, 42–43, 319
Fat mass (FM), 48, 49–50, 51, 53
Fat oxidation, 51, 313
Fat-free mass (FFM)
  leptin and, 53
  overview, 41, 46–47, 48
  weight gain and, 49–50
Feedback, 340–341, 472–473,
    500
Female Sexual Function Index-6
    (FSFI-6), 212
Fiber, 312–313, 318
Financial factors. *See also* Health
    care costs; Insurance coverage
  commercial-based interventions
    and, 488
  community-based lifestyle
    interventions and, 493
  food prices, 142
  future challenges regarding,
    431–434
  historical perspective on,
    426–427
  overview, 425–426, 434
  personal responsibility and,
    433–434
  private insurance market,
    429–431
  public sector coverage, 427–429
  treatment of obesity in adults
    and, 304
Firmicutes, 82, 83–84, 85
Fitness, 233, 235
Follow-up care, 372–375, 373t,
    374t
Food addiction. *See* Addiction
    model
Food advertising, 662–663, 664f,
    667
Food environment, 137–138. *See
    also* Environmental factors
Food insecurity, 599, 667
Food intake, 26–27, 29, 258–260.
    See also Dietary intake
Food preference. *See* Preferences
Food reinforcement, 629–630
Free fatty acids (FFA), 110–111,
    110f
Functional analysis, 337, 337f

G

Gaining of weight. *See* Weight gain
Gallstones, 13–14, 377t

Gamma-aminobutyric acid (GABA), 29, 83
Gastric bypass surgery, 212–213. *See also* Bariatric surgery; Surgical interventions
Gastric inhibitory polypeptide (GIP), 27, 85
Gastric plication (GP), 368, 368f, 369t, 376t, 387. *See also* Surgical interventions
Gastric stimulation. *See* Electrical stimulation
Gastroesophageal reflux disease (GERD), 372, 383, 384f
Gastrointestinal (GI) factors, 24, 24–30, 378. *See also* Brain-to-gut mechanisms; Gut hormones
Gender
  body dissatisfaction and, 152
  depression and, 154–155, 154t
  disability due to obesity and, 159
  effects of weight loss on mood and, 210–211
  intensive lifestyle interventions (ILIs) and, 228–229
  mental health and, 156
  minority populations and, 447–448
  prevalence of obesity and, 4
  sedentary time and, 111
  self-esteem and, 579
  sleep duration and, 124–125
  stress and, 151–152
  treatment and, 161
Generalized anxiety disorder (GAD), 286. *See also* Anxiety
Generalized Anxiety Disorder-7 (GAD-7), 263
Genetic factors. *See also* Genetic syndromes associated with obesity
  appetite and satiety and, 118
  behavioral assessment and, 255–257, 256f, 257f
  childhood obesity and, 596–597, 597f
  common genetic variants, 65–66
  dietary treatment and, 312, 312t
  gut microbiome and, 80–81
  leptin and, 53
  medical evaluation and, 246, 249
  minority populations and, 440–441
  overview, 6, 38, 64–65, 70–71
  severe obesity and, 66
  sugar consumption and, 317
  weight gain and, 52

Genetic syndromes associated with obesity, 66–68, 69–70, 70–71. *See also* Genetic factors
Genomewide association studies (GWASs), 65–66, 70–71, 596–597, 597f
Gestational diabetes, 250–251. *See also* Diabetes
Ghrelin, 28–30, 125
Glucagon-like peptide-1 (GLP-1), 26–27, 360–361
Glucose, 30–31, 86, 110–111, 110f, 249. *See also* Glucose tolerance
Glucose tolerance, 27, 188–191, 189t, 645–646. *See also* Glucose
Glycemic index
  dietary treatment and, 312–313, 316–317
  fiber and whole grains and, 318
  low-glycemic-index diet, 52
  macronutrient distributions and, 313
  maintenance of weight loss and, 319, 402–403
Glycemic load, 210, 316–317
Goal setting, 339, 586, 626t, 627. *See also* Treatment goals
Group interventions
  childhood obesity and, 631
  community-based lifestyle interventions and, 493
  dietary treatment and, 318–319
  extended-care maintenance programs and, 403–407, 405t
  overview, 466
  primary care and, 456–457
  size of groups, 394, 398
  when BMI is less than 30 kg/m2, 289–290
Group Lifestyle Balance Program, 503–504
Growth hormone secretagogue receptor (GHS-R), 29. *See also* Ghrelin
Gut hormones, 24, 25–32. *See also* Brain-to-gut mechanisms; Hormonal factors
Gut microbiome. *See also* Microbiota
  changes in, 82–83
  energy balance and, 81–83
  human studies, 80–81
  mechanisms, 83–85
  overview, 75, 78t–79t, 85–86
  rodent studies, 76–77
  surgical interventions and, 368

H

Hamilton Anxiety Rating Scale (HAM-A), 263
Health care costs. *See also* Costs of obesity; Financial factors; Insurance coverage
  future challenges regarding, 431–434
  historical perspective on, 426–427
  overview, 3, 18, 18f, 425–426, 434
  personal responsibility and, 433–434
  private insurance market and, 429–431
  public sector coverage, 427–429
Health care settings, 17t. *See also* Obesity medicine field of health care; Primary care practice
Health maintenance organizations (HMOs), 430
Health Management Resources (HMR), 458, 482f, 483t, 484–485, 489
Health providers
  advice to, 585–587, 586t
  self-esteem and, 580–582, 585–587, 586t
  specialists, 419–422, 421t, 422f
  training of, 419–422, 421t, 422f
  weight stigmatization and, 162f, 163
Health status. *See also* Consequences of obesity; *individual health conditions*
  adolescents and surgical interventions and, 654
  behavioral assessment and, 257
  health professionals and, 585
  medical evaluation and, 246–247, 247t
  minority populations and, 438–440, 439t, 440f, 441, 443–448, 446f
  overview, 6–16, 7f, 8f, 10f, 12t, 14f, 453
  postoperative complications and, 375–379, 376t, 377t
  self-esteem and, 581–582
  short-term and intermediate effects of weight loss and, 186–188, 187f
  treatment of obesity in adults and, 284–286, 285f

Health-related quality of life
(HRQoL)
  degree of obesity and, 232–233,
    234f
  effects of intensive lifestyle
    interventions on, 224–232,
    225t–226t, 227f, 229f, 230f,
    231f
  intensive lifestyle interventions
    (ILIs) and, 223–224, 235–237
  overview, 3, 16, 19, 158–159
  weight cycling and, 217
  weight loss and, 208, 218
Heart disease. See Coronary heart
    disease (CHD)
Hepatic steatosis, 249
Heritability, 64–65, 255–257,
    256f, 257f. See also Genetic
    factors
High-density lipoprotein
    cholesterol (HDL), 249, 285f,
    381–382, 489
Higher-protein diets, 314–315,
    315f, 319
Hispanic/Latino American
    populations, 437, 439t,
    440f, 445. See also Minority
    populations
History taking in assessment. See
    also Assessment
  behavioral assessment and,
    255–257, 256f, 257f, 264–266
  medical evaluation and,
    245–247, 245f, 246t, 247t
Home environments. See also
    Environmental factors; Family
    factors
  behavioral treatment and, 340,
    399
  family-based behavioral weight
    loss treatment (FBT) and,
    626t, 627–628
  overview, 142–143
Homeostatic model assessment
    levels of insulin resistance
    (HOMA-IR), 249
Homework, 338, 343
Hormonal factors, 6, 30–32, 118,
    125. See also Gut hormones
Hunger
  childhood obesity and,
    599–600
  effects of weight loss on,
    215–216, 215f, 216f
  public policy and, 667
  sleep and, 125
Hypercholesterolemia, 286, 384f
Hypercortisolism, 247, 248
Hyperinsulinemia, 246, 247t

Hyperlipidemia
  medical evaluation and, 244,
    246–247
  pharmacotherapies and, 301
  surgical interventions and,
    381–382
  treatment goals and, 268
  treatment of obesity in adults
    and, 284, 286
Hypertension. See also Blood
    pressure
  adolescents and surgical
    interventions and, 645–646
  binge-eating disorder (BED)
    and, 171
  lifestyle intervention and, 191
  medical evaluation and, 244,
    246–247
  obesity medicine field of health
    care and, 416
  overview, 8–9
  pharmacotherapies and,
    300–301, 349–350
  risk of, 3
  short-term and intermediate
    effects of weight loss and, 188
  surgical interventions and, 382,
    384f
  treatment and, 268, 284, 286
Hyperuricemia, 249
Hypothyroidism, 246, 247, 247t,
    248

I

Impact of Weight on Quality of
    Life Lite (IWQoL), 158, 217,
    262–263
Impulsivity, 125–126, 630–631
Income inequality, 138, 139
Income levels. See also Lifelong
    earnings
  disability due to obesity and,
    159
  overview, 16, 17t, 19, 140–141
  prevalence of obesity and, 4
Indirect calorimetry, 44, 44f, 45
Indirect effects, 344
Individual interventions, 289–290,
    493
Indoor environment of shops,
    143. See also Environmental
    factors
Infancy, 595–597, 597f
Infection, 377t
Infertility risks, 3, 15, 383–384
Inflammation, 15, 84–85, 86
Insomnia, 130–131

Insulin and insulin resistance
  adolescents and surgical
    interventions and, 645–646
  beta-3-adrenergic receptors and,
    54
  cholecystokinin (CCK) and, 26
  glucagon-like peptide-1 (GLP-1)
    and, 26–27
  insulin sensitivity and, 27, 313
  medical evaluation and, 246,
    247, 247t, 248, 249
  overview, 15, 30–31
  pharmacotherapies and, 359
  short-chain fatty acids (SCFAs)
    and, 85
Insurance coverage. See also Costs
    of obesity; Financial factors;
    Health care costs
  commercial-based interventions
    and, 488
  future challenges regarding,
    431–434
  historical perspective on,
    426–427
  overview, 425–426, 434,
    453–454
  personal responsibility and,
    433–434
  private insurance market,
    429–431
  public sector coverage, 427–429
  treatment of obesity in adults
    and, 304
Intensity of physical activity. See
    Physical activity
Intensive behavior therapy (IBT),
    293–294
Intensive lifestyle interventions
    (ILIs). See also Lifestyle
    interventions
  effects of on HRQoL and
    physical functioning,
    224–232, 225t–226t, 227f,
    229f, 230f, 231f
  future directions, 232–236, 234f
  maintenance of weight loss and,
    294–297, 295f, 296f, 297f
  overview, 223–224, 236–237
  when BMI is equal to or more
    than 30 kg/m2, 297–302, 300f
  when BMI is less than 30 kg/m2,
    288–291, 289t
Intentional weight loss. See Weight
    loss
Interagency Working Group
    (IWG), 662–663
Intermittent fasting diets, 311–312.
    See also Dietary treatment;
    Fasting

Internet-delivered lifestyle interventions. *See also* Remotely delivered lifestyle interventions
  extended-care maintenance programs and, 406–407
  maintenance of weight loss and, 407
  overview, 292, 399, 471–473
Interpersonal psychotherapy, 268
Interpersonal relationships, 17*t*
Interpersonal therapy (IPT), 172, 173*t*, 552, 553, 554, 555, 582. *See also* Treatment
Interventions. *See also* Treatment; *individual interventions*
  effectiveness of, 432–433
  energy density and, 97–98
  enhancing physical activity with, 326–328, 327*f*, 328*f*
  long-term impact of weight loss and, 188–202, 189*t*, 192*t*, 196*t*, 198*t*–201*t*
  medical and surgical interventions, 195–202, 196*t*, 198*t*–201*t*
  obesogenic environment management and, 100–101, 101*f*
  overview, 186
  portion size and, 94–95
  psychological functioning and, 161–163, 162*f*
  selecting the best option for, 459, 460*f*
  sleep and, 131–132
  weight loss and, 202
Intragastric botulinum toxin injections, 545. *See also* Nonsurgical interventional therapies
Intragastric silicone balloons. *See* Nonsurgical interventional therapies; Space-occupying devices; Weight loss devices

J

Jejunoileal bypass (JIB), 367, 369*t*
Jenny Craig. *See also* Lifestyle interventions
  minority populations and, 448
  overview, 292–293, 482–483, 482*f*, 483*t*, 488–489
  primary care and, 458
Just-in-time adaptive interventions (JITAIs), 477

L

Labeling, 100–101, 101*f*, 666–667
Laboratory evaluation, 249, 249*t*. *See also* Assessment; Medical evaluations
Laparoscopic adjustable gastric banding (LAGB), 302–303, 368, 369, 369*t*, 370, 376*t*, 386. *See also* Surgical interventions
Laparoscopic gastric plication (LGP), 369*t*, 370, 376*t*, 387. *See also* Surgical interventions
Laparoscopic sleeve gastrectomy (LSG), 369*t*, 370, 376*t*, 386
Late-night eating, 126–129, 128*f*
Lay-led community-based lifestyle intervention, 503–505. *See also* Community-based lifestyle interventions; Lifestyle interventions
Leptin
  cholecystokinin (CCK) and, 26
  energy expenditure variability and, 53–54
  genetic syndromes associated with obesity, 66–67
  leptin resistance, 51–52
  leptin resistance and, 32
  leptin signaling, 84
  medical evaluation and, 246
  overview, 32
  sleep and, 125
  weight gain and, 51–52
Leptin receptor deficiency, 67
Leptin replacement therapy, 53–54
Life events, 245–246, 245*f*, 267
Lifelong earnings, 3, 16, 17*t*. *See also* Income levels
Lifestyle interventions. *See also* Behavioral treatment; Community-based lifestyle interventions; Intensive lifestyle interventions (ILIs); Interventions; Physical activity; Treatment
  adapting for community settings, 493–498, 494*t*–496*t*
  behavioral assessment and, 261
  childhood obesity and, 637, 641
  combining with medications, 299–300, 300*f*, 641
  commercial- and community-based approaches to, 292–293
  long-term impact of weight loss and, 188–195, 189*t*, 192*t*
  minority populations and, 445–448, 446*f*
  obesity medicine field of health care and, 415
  overview, 16, 17*t*, 132, 202, 223–224
  primary care and, 462
  remote delivery of, 291–292, 291*f*
  structured lifestyle interventions, 288–291, 289*t*
  treatment of obesity in adults and, 285*f*
  when BMI is less than 30 kg/m2, 288–291, 289*t*
Lipid homeostasis, 86
Lipid metabolism, 249
Lipid oxidization, 109–110, 110*f*
Lipolysacchardie (LPS), 84–85
Liposuction, 569–570
Liraglutide, 351*t*, 352*f*, 354–355, 638–639
Lisdexamfetamine dimesylate (LDX), 555–556. *See also* Pharmacotherapies
Look AHEAD study
  behavioral treatment and, 341–342, 342*t*, 343
  commercial-based interventions and, 488
  extended-care maintenance programs and, 404
  intensive lifestyle interventions (ILIs) and, 224–232, 225*t*–226*t*, 227*f*, 229*f*, 230*f*
  maintenance of weight loss and, 294–297, 295*f*, 296*f*, 297*f*, 400, 407
  minority populations and, 444–445, 448
  overview, 193–195, 209, 217
  physical activity and, 324
  surgical interventions and, 303
  treatment of obesity in adults and, 286, 290
Loop gastric bypass. *See* Roux-en-Y gastric bypass (RYGB)
Loose skin, 570, 654. *See also* Body contouring
Lorcaserin DEA, 351*t*, 352*f*, 353–354, 638
Loss of control eating, 213, 625. *See also* Binge eating
Loss of weight. *See* Weight loss
Low-calorie, portion-controlled diets, 298–299, 402, 443–444
Low-carbohydrate diets, 312, 313–315, 319
Low-density lipoprotein (LDL)
  commercial-based interventions and, 489
  medical evaluation and, 249

surgical interventions and, 381–382
treatment of obesity in adults and, 285f
Low-energy diets (LEDs), 311, 319. *See also* Dietary treatment
Low-fat diets, 52, 312, 313, 314–315
Low-glycemic-index diet, 52. *See also* Glycemic index
Lymphedema, 383–384

M

Macro-level environmental factors, 144. *See also* Environmental factors
Macronutrient intake. *See also* Carbohydrates; Fat; Protein
dietary treatment and, 312–313
disability due to obesity and, 313–316, 314f
distribution of macronutrients, 315f, 403
effects of weight loss on appetite, cravings and preference and, 215–216
energy balance and, 40–41, 40f
maintenance of weight loss and, 403
oxidation, 40–41, 40f, 42–43
sleep and, 126
substrate balance and, 42–43
Magnet compression bypass anastomosis, 532t, 533f, 544, 544f. *See also* Nonsurgical interventional therapies
Maintenance of weight loss. *See also* Weight loss; Weight management
behavioral treatment and, 340–341, 344, 393–394, 407
community-based lifestyle interventions and, 497
diet principles for, 319
dietary treatment and, 318–319, 318f
extended-care maintenance programs and, 403–407, 405t
gut microbiome and, 85
lifestyle intervention and, 294–297, 295f, 296f, 297f
maintenance training, 400–401
overview, 40–41, 56–57, 57f, 58
pharmacotherapies and, 300–301
primary care and, 461, 462
Maintenance-tailored treatment (MTT), 404, 406

Major depressive disorder, 150, 263–264, 264t. *See also* Depression
Marketing, 662–663, 664f, 667
MATCH (Motivating Adolescents with Technology to Choose Health) interventions, 611
Meal replacements, 294–295, 458, 501
Meal skipping, 258
Meal timing, 126–129, 127f, 128f
Media, 17t, 662–663, 664f
Medicaid, 19, 425, 428
Medical evaluations. *See also* Assessment
advertising targeting youth and, 667
history taking and, 245–247, 245f, 246t, 247t
laboratory evaluation, 249, 249t
overview, 243–245, 244f, 245f, 251
physical activity and, 331, 331t
physical examinations, 247–249, 248t, 249t
surgical interventions and, 372, 373t, 459
treatment planning and, 249–251, 250f
Medical interventions, 195–202, 196t, 198t–201t. *See also* Interventions
Medical Outcome Study 36-Item Short-Form Health Survey (SF-36), 223–224, 225t–226t, 227f, 262–263
Medical Outcomes Study 36-Item Short-Form Health Survey (SF-36), 158
Medicare program, 427–428
Medicare Shared Savings Program (MSSP), 431
Medication-induced weight gain, 247, 248t, 257, 359. *See also* Weight gain
Medications. *See* Pharmacotherapies
Medifast, 458, 482f, 483t, 485–486, 489
Mediterranean diet, 315–316, 316t
Melanocortin-4 receptor (MC4R), 66, 67–68, 246
Mental Component Summary (MCS) subscale of the SF-36, 224, 227f
Mental health. *See also individual mental health diagnoses*
adolescents and surgical interventions and, 648–649
bariatric surgery patients and, 271

behavioral assessment and, 263–264, 264t
binge-eating disorder (BED) and, 171
clinical practice and, 161–163, 162f
obesity and, 154–155, 154t
pharmacotherapies and, 361–362, 362t
risk factors and, 155–158
self-esteem and, 581–582
treatment planning and, 251
weight stigmatization and, 160, 162f
Meso-level environmental factors, 143–144. *See also* Environmental factors
Metabolic adaptation, 49–50, 52–54
Metabolic diseases
gastric inhibitory polypeptide (GIP) and, 27
leptin and, 53
pharmacotherapies and, 362
physical activity and, 331t
quality of life and, 158–159
surgical interventions and, 380–383, 384f
Metabolic equivalents (METs), 329
Metabolic flexibility, 119
Metabolic rate, 39, 48–52, 600–601
Metabolic surgery. *See also* Bariatric surgery; Surgical interventions
choice of, 386–387
classification of, 367–370, 369t
indications and contraindications of, 371, 371t
overview, 387–388
surgery emergencies, 375–379, 376t, 377t
Metabolic thermogenesis. *See* Thermogenesis
Metformin, 359–360, 640–641
Microbiome, gut. *See* Gut microbiome
Microbiota. *See also* Gut microbiome
energy balance and, 81–83
human studies, 80–81
overview, 75–76, 78t–79t, 85–86
rodent studies, 76–77
Micro-level environmental factors, 142–143. *See also* Environmental factors
Migraines, 361–362, 362t, 383–384, 384f

Mindfulness, 330, 515
Mini-gastric bypass. *See* Roux-en-Y gastric bypass (RYGB)
Minnesota Leisure Time Physical Activity Questionnaire, 261
Minority populations. *See also* Ethnicity; Race
  as an obesity treatment variable, 440–442, 441f, 443f
  overview, 437, 438–440, 439t, 440f, 448–449
  self-esteem and, 578
  treatment and, 443–448, 446f
Mobile phones. *See* Smart devices; Telephone-delivered interventions
Moderate- to vigorous-intensity physical activity (MVPA). *See also* Physical activity
  childhood obesity and, 600
  family-based behavioral weight loss treatment (FBT) and, 625
  long-term weight loss and, 324–326
  maintenance of weight loss and, 401–402
  overview, 322–323, 331
  prevention of obesity in youth and, 610–611
  yoga and, 329, 332
Molecular mechanisms, 53–57, 57f
Mood, 208–211
Mood disorders, 157, 171, 263–264, 264t, 265f
Moral character, 576–577
Morbidity
  effects of weight loss on, 188–202, 189t, 192t, 196t, 198t–201t
  maintenance of weight loss and, 294
  overview, 7–9, 8f, 19
  surgical interventions and, 375
  treatment of obesity in adults and, 286
Mortality
  effects of weight loss on, 188–202, 189t, 192t, 196t, 198t–201t
  lifestyle intervention and, 194–195
  maintenance of weight loss and, 294
  overview, 3, 6, 7f, 19
  as a postoperative complication, 379
  short-term and intermediate effects of weight loss and, 186–188, 187f

surgical interventions and, 197, 375, 385–386
  treatment of obesity in adults and, 286
Motivation, 161, 399–400, 404
Motivational interviewing (MI), 508–513, 509f, 510t, 513t, 519
Multidimensional Body-Self Relationship Questionnaire (MBSRQ), 567
Multidisciplinary team (MDT), 644, 647
Multifactorial Assessment of Eating Disorder Syndrome (MAEDS), 209
Multiphase optimization strategy (MOST), 476–477

N

Naltrexone SR/bupropion SR, 351t, 352f, 357, 640, 642. *See also* Pharmacotherapies
Narcolepsy, 130–131
Neighborhood environments, 143–144. *See also* Environmental factors
Neurobiology, 118, 171, 177–178
Neuropeptides
  genetic syndromes associated with obesity and, 66–67
  growth hormone secretagogue receptor (GHS-R) and, 29
  gut microbiome and, 84
  overview, 24–25
  satiation signals and, 25–30
Neuropsychiatric disorders, 361–362, 362t
Night Eating Questionnaire (NEQ), 260
Night eating syndrome (NES), 169, 173–179, 174f, 260–261. *See also* Eating disorders
Nonalcoholic fatty liver disease (NAFLD), 15, 382–383, 384f
Nonalcoholic steatohepatitis (NASH), 15, 382–383
Nonexercise activity thermogenesis (NEAT), 47–48, 50, 52
Nonsurgical interventional therapies. *See also* Weight loss devices
  aspiration therapy, 543
  duodenal mucosal resurfacing, 545
  electrical stimulation, 543–544
  intragastric botulinum toxin injections, 545

magnet compression bypass anastomosis, 544, 544f
  outcomes of, 550t–551t
  overview, 531–532, 532t, 533f, 534f–535f, 545–546
  restrictive procedures, 540–542
  space-occupying devices, 536–540, 537f, 539f
  treatment of obesity in adults and, 301–302
Nutrisystem, 457, 458, 482f, 483t, 484, 489
Nutrition therapy, 285f. *See also* Dietary treatment
Nutritional supplementation, 653–654

O

Obesity. *See also* Childhood obesity; Obesity risks; Treatment of obesity in adults
  body mass index (BMI) and, 4, 5f
  discussions regarding, 286–287
  eating disorders and, 552–553
  historical perspective on, 426–427
  influence of fitness and physical activity and, 233, 235
  medical evaluation and, 243
  mortality and, 6, 7f
  obesity epidemic, 3, 177
  overview, 3, 4, 19, 178–179, 185–186
  self-esteem and, 577–578
  sleep and, 131
Obesity medicine field of health care. *See also* Surgical interventions
  barriers to obesity care, 417–419
  current practice and provision of care, 416–417
  overview, 413, 419–422, 421t, 422, 422f
  recommendations and guidelines for, 413–416, 414t
  specialists and, 419–422, 421t, 422f
Obesity risks. *See also* Obesity; Risk factors
  depression and, 150
  energy expenditure and, 114
  mental health and, 155–158
  sleep disorders and, 130–131
  sleep duration and, 124–125
  sleep timing and, 129–130
  transportation modes and, 114–119

The Obesity Society (TOS), 420
Obesity staging systems, 244–245, 245t. *See also* Medical evaluations
Obesogenic environment. *See also* Environmental factors
　childhood obesity and, 597–599, 598f
　managing, 100–101, 101f
　overview, 39f, 137–138
　sociocultural factors and, 138–140
Obstructive sleep apnea (OSA). *See also* Sleep
　adolescents and surgical interventions and, 645–646
　behavioral assessment and, 262–263
　medical evaluation and, 247
　risk for obesity and, 130–131
　surgical interventions and, 372, 383, 384f
　treatment of obesity in adults and, 284
Oby-Cap, 351t
Online chats, 471. *See also* Internet-delivered lifestyle interventions; Remotely delivered lifestyle interventions
Operant conditioning principles, 337
OPTIFAST, 458, 482f, 483t, 485, 489
Orexigenic agouti-related peptide (AgRP), 83, 84
Orexin deficiency, 131
Orlistat
　childhood obesity and, 637–638, 641–642
　overview, 350–353, 351t, 352f, 353f, 637
Osteoarthritis risks, 3, 14, 247
Overeaters Anonymous, 178
Overeating, 93–95, 100–102, 101f. *See also* Binge eating
Overweight classification
　body mass index (BMI) and, 5f
　mortality and, 6, 7f
　overview, 3, 4, 19
Oxidative stress, 161

P

Pacific Islander American population, 439t, 445. *See also* Minority populations
Packaging, 100–101, 101f

Paffenbarger Physical Activity Questionnaire, 261
Pain, 171, 262–263, 571
Palatability of foods, 93–94, 97–98, 99
Parasympathetic nervous system (PNS), 81
Parental involvement, 626t, 627–628. *See also* Family factors
Pathoenvironmental factors, 38, 39f. *See also* Environmental factors
Patient Health Questionnaire-9 (PHQ-9), 263
Pedometers, 45–46. *See also* Step counting
Percutaneous endoscopic gastrostomy (PEG) tube. *See* Weight loss devices
Perioperative management
　adolescents and surgical interventions and, 649
　mortality and, 379
　obesity medicine field of health care and, 419
　overview, 372–375, 373t, 374t
Perry Preschool Program, 608
Personal responsibility, 433–434, 660, 666–667
Pharmacotherapies
　behavioral assessment and, 257
　binge-eating disorder (BED) and, 173, 173t, 553
　childhood obesity and, 636–642
　combining with psychological treatments for BED, 556–557
　comorbidities and, 359–362, 359t, 361t
　costs of obesity and, 431
　dietary treatment and, 313
　eating disorders, 555–557
　energy harvest and, 83–84
　FDA-approved drugs for short-term use, 357–359
　financial factors and, 429
　gastric inhibitory polypeptide (GIP) and, 27
　genetic factors and, 64
　glucagon-like peptide-1 (GLP-1) and, 27
　liraglutide, 351t, 352f, 354–355
　long-term impact of weight loss and, 195–197, 196t
　lorcaserin DEA, 351t, 352f, 353–354
　medical evaluation and, 247, 248t
　mood disorders and, 263
　naltrexone SR/bupropion SR, 351t, 352f, 357

　night eating syndrome (NES) and, 176
　obesity medicine field of health care and, 415–416, 419
　orlistat, 350–353, 351t, 353f
　overview, 349–350, 350f, 351t, 362–363
　peptide YY (PYY) and, 28
　phentermine, 358–359
　phentermine/topiramate ER DEA, 351t, 352f, 355–356, 358
　primary care and, 460–462
　treatment of obesity in adults and, 285f, 299–301, 300f
Phendimetrazine DEA, 351t
Phenotypes, eating, 599–600
Phentermine, 358–359. *See also* Pharmacotherapies
Phentermine DEA, 351t. *See also* Pharmacotherapies
Phentermine/topiramate ER DEA. *See also* Pharmacotherapies
　childhood obesity and, 639–640, 642
　overview, 351t, 352f, 355–356, 358
Physical activity. *See also* Activity thermogenesis; Energy expenditure; Lifestyle interventions; Moderate- to vigorous-intensity physical activity (MVPA)
　appetite and satiety and, 118–119
　behavioral assessment and, 261
　behavioral treatment and, 339, 341, 344
　childhood obesity and, 600
　clinical applications of, 331–332, 331t
　community-based lifestyle interventions and, 498, 500–501
　compared to bariatric surgery, 325
　considerations for, 329–331
　energy balance and, 57, 116–118
　excess postexercise oxygen consumption (EPOC) and, 115–116
　family-based behavioral weight loss treatment (FBT) and, 625
　genetic factors and, 64
　health professionals and, 587
　influence on obesity and functioning, 233, 235
　intensity of, 106–107, 106t, 401–402

Physical activity (cont.)
  interventions to enhance, 326–328, 327f, 328f
  maintenance of weight loss and, 401–402
  medical evaluation and, 246, 246t
  metrics and energetics, 105–111, 106t, 108t, 110f
  monitoring, 328, 328f
  overview, 6, 105, 119, 322–323, 332
  pharmacotherapies and, 350f
  prevention of obesity in youth and, 618–619
  risk of weight gain and obesity and, 111–114, 112f, 113f
  short bouts of, 327, 327f
  short-term and intermediate effects of weight loss and, 186–188, 187f
  sleep and, 127–129, 128f
  transportation modes and, 114–119
  treatment of obesity in adults and, 285f, 287
  weight loss and, 323–326, 325f
  weight stigmatization and, 161, 162f
  when BMI is less than 30 kg/m2, 289t
Physical Component Summary (PCS) subscale of the SF-36, 224, 227f
Physical environment factors, 137, 142–144, 441f, 443t. See also Environmental factors
Physical examinations, 245f, 247–249, 248t, 249t. See also Medical evaluations
Physical functioning
  degree of obesity and, 232–233, 234f
  effects of intensive lifestyle interventions on, 224–232, 225t–226t, 227f, 229f, 230f, 231f
  influence of fitness and physical activity and, 233, 235
  intensive lifestyle interventions (ILIs) and, 223–224
  treatment goals and, 268
Pittsburgh Sleep Quality Index (PSQI), 216
Plasma blood glucose, 30–31. See also Glucose
Plasma free fatty acids, 110–111, 110f
Plasma ghrelin, 29–30. See also Ghrelin

Plastic surgery, 387, 569–571
Polycystic ovarian syndrome, 246, 247t, 383–384, 384f
Portion size
  behavioral assessment and, 259
  childhood obesity and, 598
  overview, 93–95, 101–102
  portion-controlled diets, 298–299
  sleep and, 125–126
Positive reinforcement, 338, 340–341, 393–394
Poverty, 4, 598–599
Prader–Willi syndrome (PWS), 69
Pre-diabetes, 456–457, 481. See also Diabetes
Preferences, 97–98, 215–216, 215f, 216f. See also Choice
Pregnancy, 250–251
Preschool-age children, 606–608. See also Childhood obesity
Presurgical behavioral assessment, 270–271, 278–280. See also Assessment; Behavioral assessment; Surgical interventions
Prevalence
  binge-eating disorder (BED) and, 170
  body image dissatisfaction and, 567–569
  childhood obesity, 593–594
  minority populations and, 438–440, 439t, 440f
  night eating syndrome (NES), 174–175
  overview, 3, 4, 19, 38, 185–186
Prevention interventions. See also Prevention of obesity in youth
  behavioral treatment and, 344
  diabetes and, 190–191
  effectiveness of, 433
  overview, 162
  physical activity and, 109–111, 110f, 113–114
  preschool-age children, 606–607
  primary care and, 456–457
  public policy and, 202
  surgical interventions as, 384–386
  treatment of obesity in adults and, 287
Prevention of obesity in youth. See also Adolescents; Childhood obesity; Prevention interventions
  community-based lifestyle interventions and, 613–616, 614f, 615f
  overview, 605, 606f, 618–619, 622

prevention in adolescents, 616–618, 617f
  prevention in childhood (6-12 years), 608–616, 609t, 611f, 614f, 615f
  prevention in preschool-age children, 606–608
Primary care practice. See also Health care settings; Obesity medicine field of health care
  barriers to obesity care, 417–419
  behavioral assessment and, 254–255
  behavioral treatment and, 454–458, 455t
  behavioral weight loss (BWL) programs and, 511
  commercial- and community-based approaches to lifestyle interventions and, 458
  current practice and provision of care and, 416–417
  lifestyle intervention and, 293–294
  medical and surgical interventions, 458–459, 460f
  overview, 453–454, 460–462
  self-esteem and, 580–582
Problem Areas in Diabetes (PAID) questionnaire, 210
Problem eating, 260–261. See also Eating disorders
Problem solving, 341, 404, 474
Problem-solving therapy (PST), 404
Profile of Mood States (POMS), 209, 210
Project EAT, 152, 153
Proopiomelanocortin (POMC) neurons, 29, 66, 67–68, 83, 84, 246
Protein
  dietary treatment and, 319
  energy balance and, 40–41, 40f, 42
  macronutrient distributions and, 313
  metabolic adaptation and, 52
Pseudotumor cerebri, 383–384, 384f, 645
Psychological evaluation, 648–649. See also Assessment
Psychological functioning, 17t, 162f, 208–211, 330, 581–582
Psychosocial factors
  bariatric surgery patients and, 271
  behavioral assessment and, 262–266, 264t, 265f

Subject Index

binge-eating disorder (BED) and, 157
consequences of obesity and, 154
minority populations and, 441–442, 441f
overview, 149–154, 163, 208
sample letters summarizing presurgical assessments, 278–280
stress and, 151–152
weight loss and, 208–211, 218
Psychotherapy, 177. *See also* Treatment
Public awareness, 660–662, 661f
Public health, 419, 594, 622
Public policy
addressing the toxic environment and, 660–666, 661f, 664f
costs of obesity and, 426
future directions, 666–668
overview, 186, 202, 659–660

Q

Qsymia, 351t, 352f, 355–356, 358
Quality of life. *See also* Health-related quality of life (HRQoL); Weight-related quality of life
adolescents and surgical interventions and, 645–646
behavioral assessment and, 262–263
body contouring surgery and, 571
impact of obesity on, 158–159
lifestyle intervention and, 193–194
sexual functioning and, 158, 212–213
treatment goals and, 269
weight loss and, 218
Quality-adjusted life-years (QALYs), 158
Questionnaire on Eating and Weight Patterns-Revised (QEWP-R), 260
Questionnaires, 45, 107–108, 258–259. *See also* Assessment

R

Race. *See also* Minority populations
body dissatisfaction and, 152
mental health and, 156

as an obesity treatment variable, 440–442, 441f, 443t
overview, 6, 437
prevalence of obesity and, 4
sleep duration and, 125
Regional diets, 315–316
Reinforcement, positive. *See* Positive reinforcement
Reinforcement pathology, 629–631
Relapse prevention, 404. *See also* Maintenance of weight loss; Prevention interventions
Relationships, 17t, 582
Remotely delivered lifestyle interventions. *See also* Lifestyle interventions
evolution of, 466–467, 467f
extended-care maintenance programs and, 406–407
maintenance of weight loss and, 407
overview, 398–399, 466, 467, 468t–469t, 476–477
treatment of obesity in adults and, 291–292, 291f
types of, 470–476
Resilience, 583–584
Resistance, 32, 508, 509–510, 510t
Resistance exercise, 329, 332. *See also* Physical activity
Respiratory exchange ratio (RER), 109–110, 110f
Respiratory quotient (RQ), 51, 52–53
Responsibility, personal, 433–434, 660, 666–667
Resting energy expenditure (REE), 52, 310, 440–441, 601
Resting metabolic rate (RMR), 41–42. *See also* Basal (resting) metabolic rate (BMR)
Restrictive procedures, 531–532, 532t, 533f, 534f–535f, 540–542. *See also* Nonsurgical interventional therapies; Weight loss devices
Rewards, 344–345, 626t, 627
Ripple effects, 344
Risk factors, 162, 171, 594–597, 597f. *See also* Obesity risks
Rodent studies, 76–77, 85
Roux-en-Y gastric bypass (RYGB). *See also* Surgical interventions
adolescents and, 645, 647–654
complications, 376t
overview, 302–303, 368, 368f, 369, 369t, 370, 387
perioperative management, 372
prevention of comorbidities with, 385–386

S

Safety, 138, 140, 652
Satiety
brain-to-gut mechanisms and, 25
childhood obesity and, 599–600
dietary treatment and, 319
energy density and, 97–98
family-based behavioral weight loss treatment (FBT) and, 625
fiber and whole grains and, 318
macronutrient distributions and, 313
overview, 118–119
physical activity and, 118–119
prebiotics and, 83
satiation signals and, 25–30
surgical interventions and, 368
variety and, 99
Saxenda, 351t, 352f, 354–355
School environment. *See* Educational settings
School-based interventions, 607–608, 609–613, 609t, 611f, 618–619
SCOPE (Specialist Certification in Obesity Professional Education) certification program, 420
Screening
adolescents and surgical interventions and, 648–649
current practice and provision of care, 416–417
obesity medicine field of health care and, 415
pharmacotherapies and, 349–350
treatment and, 162, 285f
Sedentary lifestyle
behavioral assessment and, 261
childhood obesity and, 600
family-based behavioral weight loss treatment (FBT) and, 625
overview, 111
physical activity and, 330–331, 332
risk of weight gain and obesity and, 111–114, 112f, 113f
weight gain and, 52
Self-directed physical activity, 326–327, 332. *See also* Physical activity
Self-efficacy, 337–338, 344, 509–510, 510t
Self-esteem. *See also* Body dissatisfaction; Body image
consequences of, 582
family-based behavioral weight loss treatment (FBT) and, 628

Self-esteem *(cont.)*
 health professional's contribution to, 580–582, 585–587, 586t
 overview, 576–577
 relationship of obesity with, 577–578
 treatment and, 583–585
 variables that affect, 579–580
 weight management and, 582–583
 weight stigmatization and, 161
Self-monitoring
 behavioral treatment and, 339–340, 343
 binge-eating disorder (BED) and, 172
 community-based lifestyle interventions and, 500
 family-based behavioral weight loss treatment (FBT) and, 626t, 627
 remotely delivered lifestyle interventions and, 473–474
Self-regulation, 330, 625
Self-report questionnaires, 45, 107–108, 258–259. *See also* Assessment
Senior centers, 503–504
Severe obesity, 66, 156–157. *See also* Obesity
Sexual functioning, 158, 212–213. *See also* Quality of life
Sexual identity, 152, 210–211, 228. *See also* Gender
Short-chain fatty acids (SCFAs), 83, 85
Single-minded 1 (SIM1) deficiency, 70
Skin tags, 247
Sleep. *See also* Obstructive sleep apnea (OSA)
 behavioral assessment and, 262–263
 duration of, 123–129, 123t, 126f, 127f, 128f
 effects of weight loss on, 216–217
 energy balance and, 125–129, 126f, 127f, 128f
 obesity and, 131
 overview, 123, 132
 sleep disorders, 130–131, 176
 timing of, 129–130
 treatment of obesity in adults and, 284
 weight loss interventions and, 131–132
Sleep-related eating disorder (SRED), 176

Sleeve gastrectomy (SG). *See also* Surgical interventions
 adolescents and, 645, 647–654
 complications, 376t
 overview, 368f, 369, 369t, 386
Small-bowel obstruction, 378–379
Smart devices, 45–46, 292, 473–475. *See also* Remotely delivered lifestyle interventions; Telephone-delivered interventions
Social capital, 138, 139–140
Social cognitive theory, 337–338
Social cohesion, 138, 139–140
Social consequences of obesity, 16, 17t, 19, 262. *See also* Consequences of obesity
Social contributors to obesity, 138–140
Social jetlag, 129
Social media, 475–476
Social networks, 138, 139–140, 626t, 628–629
Social responsibility, 666–667
Social support, 138, 139–140
Social–ecological model, 80–81, 661, 661f
Societal-level economic factors, 141–142. *See also* Economic factors
Sociocultural cultural adaptation strategy, 447
Sociocultural factors
 family-based behavioral weight loss treatment (FBT) and, 625, 626t, 628–629
 minority populations and, 441–442, 441f, 443t
 overview, 137, 138–140
Socioeconomic status (SES)
 childhood obesity and, 598–599
 disability due to obesity and, 159
 mental health and, 156
 minority populations and, 438
 obesogenic environment management and, 100–101, 101f
 overview, 140–141
 prevalence of obesity and, 4
 sociocultural factors and, 138, 139
 transportation modes and, 115
Space-occupying devices. *See also* Nonsurgical interventional therapies; Weight loss devices
 outcomes of, 550t–551t
 overview, 531–532, 532t, 533f, 534f–535f, 536–540, 537f, 539f, 545–546

Space-occupying intragastric silicone balloons. *See* Weight loss devices
Specialists in obesity medicine, 419–422, 421t, 422f. *See also* Health providers
Spontaneous physical activity (SPA), 44f, 50, 52
Src homology 2B adapter protein 1 (SH2B1) deficiency, 68–69
Staging systems, 244–245, 245t. *See also* Medical evaluations
Starvation, 310–311, 314
Step counting, 45–46, 108–109, 327–328. *See also* Physical activity
Stereotypes, 159–160, 581, 585. *See also* Weight stigmatization
Stigma. *See also* Discrimination; Weight stigmatization
 behavioral assessment and, 262–263
 costs of obesity and, 431–432
 depression and, 150
 overview, 16, 17t, 19, 149
 self-esteem and, 576–577
 weight bias and, 17t
Stimulus control, 340, 626t, 627
Stress
 overview, 151–152, 153–154
 treatment and, 161–162, 162
 weight loss and, 267
 weight stigmatization and, 160
Stress urinary incontinence, 383–384, 384f
Substance abuse/dependency, 155, 160, 264–265, 371, 371t
Substance use disorders, 171, 271
Sugar consumption, 317–318, 319, 661, 664, 667
Sugar-sweetened beverages (SSBs), 317–318, 319, 664. *See also* Sugar consumption
Suicidal ideation, 263, 271
Supervised physical activity sessions, 500–501. *See also* Physical activity
Surgical interventions. *See also* Bariatric surgery; Bariatric surgery for adolescents; Gastric bypass surgery; Interventions
 body image dissatisfaction and, 569–571
 financial factors and, 426
 long-term impact of weight loss and, 195–202, 196t, 198t–201t
 overview, 202, 367, 368f, 370–371, 386, 387–388

perioperative management, 372–375, 373t, 374t
primary care and, 458–459, 460–462, 460f
public sector coverage and, 427
sample letters summarizing presurgical assessments, 278–280
sexual functioning and, 212–213
Sympathetic nervous system (SNS), 49, 50–51, 81

T

Taxation, 665–666, 667
Technology, 45–46, 108–109, 112, 328, 328f. *See also* Remotely delivered lifestyle interventions
Telephone-delivered interventions. *See also* Remotely delivered lifestyle interventions; Smart devices
  extended-care maintenance programs and, 406
  maintenance of weight loss and, 407
  overview, 291–292, 291f, 398–399, 470–471
Temporal factors
  bariatric surgery patients and, 271–272
  behavioral assessment and, 266–268
  behavioral treatment and, 344
  sample letters summarizing presurgical assessments, 278–280
Text-based interventions, 473–475. *See also* Remotely delivered lifestyle interventions
Thermic effect of food (TEF), 44f, 46, 47, 57
Thermogenesis, 53, 55, 57, 314, 432–433
Third-party reimbursement for treatment, 425, 434. *See also* Financial factors; Health care costs; Insurance coverage
Thyroid hormones, 81, 249
Thyromegaly, 247, 248
Topiramate, 362, 556. *See also* Pharmacotherapies
TOPS (Take Off Pounds Sensibly), 448, 458
Total daily energy expenditure (TDEE), 45, 46, 47, 48, 50. *See also* Energy balance

Total energy expenditure (TEE), 52, 601
Training, 419–422, 421t, 422f
Transportation modes, 114–119, 141, 144
Treatment. *See also* Behavioral treatment; Dietary treatment; Obesity medicine field of health care; Treatment goals; Treatment of obesity in adults
  addiction model of eating disorders, 178
  barriers to obesity care, 417–419
  binge-eating disorder (BED) and, 171–173, 173t, 553–555
  combining pharmacotherapies with psychological treatments for BED, 556–557
  contraindications to, 250–251
  current practice and provision of care, 416–417
  effectiveness of, 432–433
  energy expenditure and, 53–57, 57f, 58
  glucagon-like peptide-1 (GLP-1) and, 27
  gut microbiome and, 85–86
  gut-to-brain mechanisms and, 32
  identifying goals for, 268–269
  medical evaluation and, 249–251, 250f
  minority populations and, 441–442, 441f
  mood disorders and, 263
  night eating syndrome (NES) and, 176–177
  psychological functioning and, 161–163, 162f
  selecting the best option for, 269–270
  self-esteem and, 580, 583–585
  weight loss maintenance and, 56–57, 57f
  weight stigmatization and, 162f
Treatment goals. *See also* Goal setting; Treatment
  behavioral assessment and, 268–269
  behavioral treatment and, 338
  community-based lifestyle interventions and, 498
  current practice and provision of care and, 417
  health professionals and, 586
  obesity medicine field of health care and, 415
  remotely delivered lifestyle interventions and, 473–474

Treatment of obesity in adults. *See also* Treatment
  barriers to obesity care, 417–419
  behavioral weight loss (BWL) programs for, 511, 512t
  current practice and provision of care and, 416–417
  future directions, 304
  options for when BMI is less than 30 kg/m2, 288–297, 289t, 291f, 295f, 296f, 297f
  overview, 283–284
  selecting the best option for, 284–287, 285f
  when BMI is equal to or more than 30 kg/m2, 297–302, 300f
  when BMI is equal to or more than 40 kg/m2, 302–303
Treatment planning, 249–251, 250f, 287. *See also* Treatment; Treatment goals
Treatment-seeking individuals, 157
Triglycerides, 249, 381
Twin studies, 80–81, 596–597, 597f
Type 2 diabetes. *See* Diabetes

V

Variety in diet, 99–100, 101–102, 402. *See also* Diet factors
Vertical banded gastroplasty (VBG), 368, 369t
Vertical sleeve gastrectomy (VSG), 302–303. *See also* Surgical interventions
Very-low-calorie diet (VLCDs), 298–299, 443–444
Very-low-carbohydrate diet, 52
Very-low-energy diets (VLEDs), 310–312, 311f, 314, 319. *See also* Dietary treatment

W

Waist circumference (WC), 8, 11, 285f, 381
Waist-to-hip ratio (WHR), 10–11
Wearable monitors, 108–109, 112, 328, 328f. *See also* Technology
Weight, 4, 82, 587. *See also* Body weight
Weight and Lifestyle Inventory (WALI)
  behavioral assessment and, 253–254, 256, 272
  eating disorders, 260